# SCIENTIFIC FOUNDATIONS
## OF
## ANAESTHESIA

# Scientific Foundations of Anaesthesia

Edited by

## CYRIL SCURR
M.V.O., F.F.A. R.C.S.

*Consultant Anaesthetist, Westminster Hospital, London*

*and*

## STANLEY FELDMAN
B.Sc., F.F.A. R.C.S.

*Consultant Anaesthetist, Westminster Hospital, London*

LONDON

WILLIAM HEINEMANN MEDICAL BOOKS LTD

*First published* 1970
*Second Edition* 1974

ISBN 0 433 31861 9

*Printed in Great Britain at the Pitman Press, Bath*

. . . the relations of etherization to medical science or physiology . . . is a tempting field of research . . . which cannot be without its influence on the progress of our knowledge of disease.

J. Snow, London, 1847

## PREFACE TO THE FIRST EDITION

John Snow's prophecy that research in anaesthesia would influence our understanding of medicine and disease, has been amply fulfilled. This book is largely concerned with this increase in our knowledge and our expanding appreciation of the physiological processes that maintain life and which may be affected by disease.

No attempt has been made to teach the practical, technical aspects of anaesthesia. Our objective has been to complete a volume which covers the scientific foundations upon which are based the clinical practice of anaesthesia, resuscitation and the care of acutely ill patients in intensive care units. We have tried, not merely to illustrate 'what happens', but also to explain 'why' and 'how'. In order to do this it is necessary to have some knowledge of physics, mathematics and measurement techniques. We have therefore included chapters on the relevant aspects of these subjects.

Although it was originally intended to present the text as short and simple chapters, it soon became evident that these objectives were frequently incompatible with our main aim. In many instances this approach was bound to lead to a superficial, unscientific presentation. We have therefore encouraged authors to present a more detailed coverage of some of the less well appreciated aspects of the subject.

It has been our intention that each chapter should be complete in itself and to this end limited repetition has been unavoidable. Authors have been requested to give a list key of references or further reading that might be of value to anaesthetists, in addition to the usual bibliography. In this way we have tried to present a series of up-to-date chapters reviewing the salient features of the scientific foundations of anaesthesia.

We are most grateful to our many contributors for their co-operation, to members of Magill Department of Anaesthetics of Westminster Hospital for their help with the preparation of proofs and to Mr. Owen Evans of Heinemann Medical Books Ltd., for his advice and assistance.

*July*, 1970                                                                                           C.F.S.
                                                                                                              S.A.F.

# PREFACE TO THE SECOND EDITION

That our first edition was well received has convinced us of the need for a book such as this, based upon a scientific approach to anaesthesia. It will be recalled that our objective was to compile a volume which covered the scientific principles upon which are based the clinical practice of anaesthesia, resuscitation and the care of acutely ill patients in intensive care units. Accordingly we have made no attempt to cover the practical technical aspects of anaesthesia, nor to detail the basis and methods of regional analgesia.

In attempting merely to provide such a foundation for clinical practice, it is clear that this book is not intended to replace full standard texts on physics, pharmacology and the like, but rather to provide an introduction for the clinician to those scientific aspects upon which his practice should be based. We hope too to assist him in the understanding of the ever-increasing volume of investigative work reported in the journals, but again would disclaim any intention of providing a reference book for research workers.

We welcome this opportunity of bringing up to date all the original sections, and to add 10 new chapters covering previous omissions and areas of developing interest.

We are grateful once again to all our contributors for their co-operation and patience in facing delays—not of our making, but of our times. Our warm thanks are due to members of the Magill Department of Anaesthetics of Westminster Hospital, and to Mr. Owen R. Evans and Mr. Richard Emery of William Heinemann Medical Books Ltd. for their advice and assistance.

*February 1974*

C.F.S.
S.A.F.

# CONTENTS

CONTENTS

*SECTION II*

**PHYSIOLOGICAL BASIS OF THE SCIENCE OF ANAESTHESIA**

B. Respiration

*SECTION II*

**PHYSIOLOGICAL BASIS OF THE SCIENCE OF ANAESTHESIA**

C. Neuro-endocrine Systems

*SECTION II*

**PHYSIOLOGICAL BASIS OF THE SCIENCE OF ANAESTHESIA**

D. Metabolic Processes

## SECTION II

### PHYSIOLOGICAL BASIS OF THE SCIENCE OF ANAESTHESIA

E. Body Fluids

## SECTION III

### PHARMACOLOGICAL BASIS OF THE SCIENCE OF ANAESTHESIA

## SECTION IV

### ANAESTHETIC APPARATUS

## SECTION V

### APPENDIX

# LIST OF CONTRIBUTORS

D. BENAZON, M.D., M.R.C.P., F.F.A.R.C.S.
Consultant Anaesthetist, Royal Victoria Hospital, Bournemouth and Poole General Hospital, Dorset.

J. P. BLACKBURN, M.A., M.B., B.Chir., F.F.A.R.C.S., D.I.C.
Consultant in Clinical Measurement, Westminster Hospital, London.

D. M. BURLEY, M.B., B.S., L.R.C.P., M.R.C.S.
Head of Medical Services Department, CIBA Laboratories Ltd., Horsham, Sussex; Clinical Assistant, Rheumatism Unit, Westminster Hospital, London.

I. R. CAMERON, M.A., D.M., M.R.C.P.
Senior Lecturer in Medicine, St. Thomas' Hospital Medical School, London.

J. H. CHAMBERLAIN, M.B., B.S., M.R.C.P.
Consultant Clinical Physiologist, Guy's Hospital, London.

P. CLIFFE, M. B., B. S., B.Sc., Ph.D., F.Inst.P.
Director, Department of Clinical Measurement, Westminster, London.

ELLIS N. COHEN, M.D.
Professor of Anesthesia, Stanford University, California.

C. M. CONWAY, M.B., B.S., F.F.A.R.C.S., D.A.
Consultant Anaesthetist, Westminster Hospital; Honorary Senior Lecturer, Research Department of Anaesthetics, Royal College of Surgeons of England, London.

EDMOND, I. EGER, II, M.D.
Professor of Anesthesiology, University of California Medical Centre, San Francisco, California.

H. BARRIE FAIRLEY, M.B., B.S., F.F.A.R.C.S.
Professor, Department of Anesthesia, University of California, San Francisco; Chief of Anesthesia, Veterans Administration Hospital, San Francisco, California.

S. FARQUHARSON, M.B., B.S., F.F.A.R.C.S.
Consultant, Anaesthetist, Norfolk and Norwich Hospitals.

S. A. FELDMAN, B.Sc., M.B., B.S., F.F.A.R.C.S., D.A.
Consultant Anaesthetist, Westminster Hospital, London.

P. R. FLEMING, M.D., F.R.C.P.
Senior Lecturer in Medicine, Westminster Medical School; Consultant Physician, Westminster Hospital, London.

W. J. GLOVER, M.B., B.Ch., B.A.O., F.F.A.R.C.S.
Consultant Anaesthetist, The Hospital for Sick Children, London.

A. MURRAY HARPER, M.D.
Reader in Surgical Physiology, Wellcome Surgical Research Institute, University of Glasgow; St. Mungo Department of Surgery, Glasgow Royal Infirmary.

D. W. HILL, M.Sc., Ph.D., F.Inst.P., F.I.E.E.
Reader in Medical Physics, Royal College of Surgeons of England, London.

P. J. HORSEY, M.B., B.S., F.F.A.R.C.S.
Consultant Anaesthetist, Southampton Group of Hospitals.

D. C. O. JAMES, M.D., B.S., B.Pharm., M.R.C.Path.
Consultant Pathologist (Blood Transfusion and Transplantation Immunology), Westminster Hospital, London.

R. R. JOHNSTON, M.D.
Assistant Professor, Anesthesiology and Pharmacology, University of California, San Francisco.

JORDAN KATZ, M.D., A.B.A., F.A.C.A.
Professor Anesthesia, University of Wisconsin.

J. J. KENDIG, Ph.D.
Department of Anesthesia, Stanford Medical Centre, California.

A. F. LANT, B.Sc., M.B., Ch.B., Ph.D., M.R.C.P.
Consultant Physician, Westminster Hospital; Senior Lecturer in Therapeutics, Westminster Medical School, London.

J. M. LEIGH, M.B., B.S., F.F.A.R.C.S., D.A.
Consultant Westminster Hospital, Senior Lecturer, Magill Department of Anaesthetics, Westminster Medical School, London.

A. R. LORIMER, M.B., Ch.B., F.R.C.P. (Glas.), M.R.C.P. (Lond. and Edin.)
Consultant Cardiologist, Honorary Lecturer in Medical Cardiology and Medicine, Royal Infirmary, Glasgow.

LAVINIA W. LOUGHRIDGE, M.B., B.Ch., F.R.C.P.
Lecturer in Medicine, Westminster Medical School, London.

J. N. LUNN, M.B., B.S., F.F.A.R.C.S., D.A.
Department Anaesthetics, Welsh National School of Medicine, Cardiff, Wales.

D. GORDON MCDOWALL, M.D., F.F.A.R.C.S.
Professor of Anesthesia, University of Leeds; Honorary Consultant Anaesthetist, Leeds General Infirmary, Leeds.

VINCENT MARKS, M.A., D.M., F.R.C.P. (Edin.), M.R.C.P. (Lond.), F.R.C.Path.
Professor of Clinical Biochemistry, University of Surrey, Guildford.

R. A. MILLAR, M.D., M.Sc., Ph.D., F.F.A.R.C.S.
Professor of Anaesthesia, University of Glasgow.

R. D. MILLER, M.D.
Associate Professor of Anesthesiology and Pharmacology, University of California, San Francisco, California.

J. P. PAYNE, M.B., Ch.B., F.F.A.R.C.S., D.A.
British Oxygen Professor of Anaesthetics, Royal College of Surgeons of England; Consultant Anaesthetist, St. Peter's Group of Hospitals; Consultant in Anaesthetics, Royal Air Force.

C. PRYS-ROBERTS, M.A., M.B., B.S., Ph.D., F.F.A.R.C.S., D.A.
First Assistant, Nuffield Department of Anaesthetics, University of Oxford; Consultant Anaesthetist, United Oxford Hospitals; Fellow of Worcester College, Oxford.

JOHN S. ROBINSON, M.D., F.F.A.R.C.S., D.A.
Professor of Anaesthetics, University of Birmingham.

E. A. SCHWARTZ, M.D.
Department of Physiology, University of California, Los Angeles, California.

S. J. G. SEMPLE, M.D., F.R.C.P.
Professor of Medicine, Middlesex Hospital, London.

I. A. SEWELL, T.D., M.B., B.S., Ph.D., F.R.C.S.
Consultant General Surgeon, Ashton, Hyde & Glossop Hospitals. Visiting Manchester Royal Infirmary.

B. JACQUALINE STORDY, B.Sc. (Lond.)
Lecturer in Nutrition, Department of Biochemistry, University of Surrey, Guildford.

D. A. P. STRICKLAND, B.Sc.
Deputy Director, Department of Clinical Measurement, Westminster Hospital, London.

M. K. SYKES, M.A., M.B., B.Chir., F.F.A.R.C.S.
Professor of Anaesthetics, Royal Postgraduate Medical School; Consultant Anaesthetist, Hammersmith Hospital, London.

G. TAYLOR, F.F.A.R.C.S.
Assistant Professor Department of Anaesthesia, Stanford University Medical Center, Stanford, California.

D. L. THOMAS, B.Sc., Ph.D., M.Inst.P., C.Eng., M.I.E.E.
Department of Clinical Physics and Bio-Engineering, Western Regional Hospital Board, Glasgow.

J. A. THORNTON, M.D., F.F.A.R.C.S., D.A.
Professor of Anaesthetics, University of Sheffield.

J. THURSTON, M.B., B.S., M.R.C.P.
Westminster Hospital, London.

J. R. TRUDELL, Ph.D.
Department Anesthesia, Stanford Medical Center, California.

M. F. TYRRELL, M.B., B.S., F.F.A.R.C.S., D.A.
Consultant Anaesthetist, Westminster Hospital, London.

J. B. WEST, M.D., Ph.D.
Professor of Medicine and Bioengineering, University of California at San Diego Medical School. Late, Reader in Medicine, Royal Postgraduate Medical School and Consultant Respiratory Physiologist. Hammersmith Hospital, London.

*SECTION 1*

# PHYSICAL BASIS OF THE SCIENCE OF ANAESTHESIA

# CHAPTER 1

# PHYSICAL PRINCIPLES PART I

## D. STRICKLAND

### Introduction

In this chapter basic mechanical quantities are defined and discussed. It is helpful when considering physical science, to look for some underlying pattern. It is natural to think in terms of linear relationships between cause and effect, and this aspect will be stressed.

The historical order of the subject will not be adhered to, since revision is often made more efficient by taking as a starting-point some fact or concept which is now well-established. For example, when dealing with the equations of state of gases, the Kinetic theory definition of temperature is taken as basic, and mercury and other thermometers are regarded as imperfect measuring instruments. Reference to chapter 6 can then be made for detailed explanations of temperature as a problem of measurement.

In accordance with current practice the SI system of units (Système Internationale d'Unités) will be used in this chapter, but reference will be made to other units which are still in common use.

### Fundamental Quantities

Mechanical science has developed in terms of certain fundamental quantities, including *mass*, *length* and *time*, which are regarded as analogous to the fundamental axioms of mathematics. It is not easy to produce satisfactory definitions of these quantities, since it is in the nature of definitions that they should refer new concepts back to ones which are already understood. Statements such as 'mass is the measure of the quantity of matter in body', or 'time is the measure of separation of events' lack the precision of other definitions, e.g. 'velocity is the rate of change of displacement with time' for precisely this reason.

It is profitable, however, to extend the discussion of mass by considering how we are aware of it. We do not assess mass by counting atoms and estimating the 'quantity of matter' in one atom. Our immediate awareness of mass is due to the inertial opposition we sense when we shake an object. Again, the fact that we evolved on the surface of a planet makes us aware that the more massive a body is (in the sense of offering inertial opposition to shaking), the more strongly it is pulled towards the centre of the planet. This has sometimes led to confusion between mass and *weight*, a confusion reinforced by the unfortunate use of the same or similar units to measure two quite different quantities.

Whether mass is assessed by inertial opposition to change of motion or by the local earth-surface convenient technique of weighing, it becomes clear that mass is a scalar quantity. By a scalar quantity, we mean one which is fully described by a number and a unit. If one walks two miles the distance covered is described entirely by the number '2' and the unit 'mile'. In contrast a *vector* quantity requires a statement of *direction*. For example, when navigating a ship it is important to know the direction as well as the magnitude of the ship's motion, since 2 miles south is not equivalent to 2 miles north in a crowded shipping lane. To return to mass, two bodies which are separately assessed to have the same mass as the standard kilogram will, when together, produce twice the observed effects (of opposition to motional change, or of weight on the earth's surface) as each separately. Unlike mass, weight is a *vector* quantity requiring, in addition to number and unit, the specification of direction.

Unit lengths, such as the metre, were also primarily defined by reference to some standard separation, such as that between two marks on a specially constructed and preserved object. Greater precision and greater trust in constancy is achieved (at the expense of less direct apprehension) by taking the wavelength of some specific light emanation as standard. Similarly, although the second was originally defined in terms of astronomical observations on the motion of our slightly wobbling and slowing-down planet, it is now compared to the periods of oscillation of identifiable atomic events.

### Displacement, Speed, Velocity and Acceleration

The speed of a moving object is the time-rate at which it covers distance along its path, and this exemplifies a human tendency to define new quantities as the rates of change of more familiar ones. Experience shows that there are differences in both result and technique between running in circles and running straight lines. The distinction hinges on the extension of the scalar concept of distance (which is applicable to paths straight or crooked) to the vector concept of *displacement*. Displacement is distance measured in a specified direction, and a circular tour leaves no resultant displacement despite the distance covered. When direction is associated with speed, we use the specially committed term *velocity* (time-rate of change of displacement) to describe the derived vector quantity. The need for this distinction will become clear when we consider how vector quantities combine, by the well-known triangle of vectors.

When we are moving we are aware of velocity by observations on other objects which we recede from or approach, or whose apparent spatial disposition changes by parallax. Our awareness of *acceleration* (time-rate of change of velocity) is much more direct, due to the jolts and shakings our bodies experience when their velocities *change*. A car-driver may sense an acceleration of less than 1 metre per second in each second (1 m s$^{-2}$), while being completely unaware of his velocity of (say) 30 thousand metres per second towards Jupiter. Another aspect of acceleration that justifies its formal incorporation into our descriptive terminology is that to achieve acceleration on a flat sur-face, an unaided human being must exert some thrust. This is particularly clear when skating, because a velocity, once achieved, requires negligible effort to maintain.

### Force

The abundance of lay terms relating to the activity of pushing, thrusting, lifting and hauling inert objects testifies to its relevance to our way of describing the physical world. The word *force* has been selected for formal definition, and should (in scientific discussion) be precisely used. What a force does depends on where it is applied. For example, it may

1. Compress a resilient object—effecting a *displace-ment*.

2. Keep a body moving on a frictional surface—main-taining *a velocity*.

3. Change the velocity of a body—effecting an *acceleration*.

Any reproducible and measurable effect could have been taken as the basis of definition, and as an interim measure we will consider the acceleration phenomenon. The most obvious definition of unit force is that, freely applied, it gives unit mass unit acceleration in the direction of application. Consequently, the obvious metric unit is the kilo-gramme (kg) times the metre per second per second. The urge to abbreviate and to celebrate have contracted the obvious (1 kg m s$^{-2}$) to the *newton* (N). It must be ad-mitted that we all forget the meaning of such compressed unit-names from time to time, and it is a useful discipline to associate the name with both the quantity defined and with its true meaning. Thus one newton (of force) gives one kg (of mass) an acceleration of 1 m s$^{-2}$. Similarly the CGS unit, the dyne gives 1 g mass an acceleration of 1 cm s$^{-2}$. Conversion factors become obvious in terms of true meanings. Thus, since 1 N gives 1000 g an acceler-ation of 100 cm s$^{-2}$, it is obviously 100 000 times as large as the dyne. A newton is the order of force necessary to support a large cup of coffee.

### Gravitational Units

In the past, complications have been introduced due to parochialism, not only with national units such as the FPS system, but also with the local terrestrial-surface gravita-tional units. Due to the universal attraction between bodies, our local large body (the Earth) forces us continu-ously towards its centre, countered by the resilience of objects that we deform by standing on them. In Fig. 1, a body $E$ in England is being pulled towards a body $P$ in Peru. By symmetry, there will be some comparable body $J$ somewhere around Java exerting an equal force at $E$

which will in consequence be effected as if by the two strings of a catapult. The resultant force passes through the Earth's centre, and the same will be true for all such pairs—in fact this defines the gravitational centre of the Earth. The total force on $E$ depends on its mass ($m$, say), and removing any support under $E$ exposes it to an un-opposed force $W$, or

$$W = km$$

where $k$ depends on the mass of the Earth and on its radius. This force $W$ is the *weight* of the body, at the surface of the Earth. Since force is mass multiplied by acceleration, the factor of proportionality $k$ is the accelera-tion measured when objects fall at the Earth's surface.

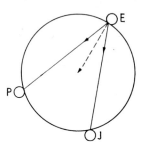

FIG. 1

Usually this is denoted by $g$, the (local) gravitational acceleration of 9·81 m s$^{-2}$ (to three significant figures). Hence the formula

$$W = mg$$

is a special example of the more general law

$$F = ma$$

### Other Aspects of Force

Complex systems, such as air flowing in the lungs, involve forces which fulfil different functions according to where they occur. Friction, such as in viscous drag, de-mands an applied force to maintain even an unchanging velocity, while elastic recoil of tissue and the compression of gases demand forces to maintain displacements. These requirements are in addition to the demands of accelera-tion when the velocities of gases and tissues are changed. In the simplest cases, and in approximations to real situa-tions, there are *linear* laws similar to Newton's $F = ma$. The simplest frictional law is

$$F = rv$$

where $v$ is the velocity and $r$ gives a measure of resistance (frictional force required, per unit velocity maintained), just as $m$ measures inertia as inertial force required per unit acceleration achieved.

For resilient systems the simplest (linear) law is

$$F = sx$$

where $x$ is the displacement caused by force $F$. Here the factor of proportionality, $s$, is the force of compression needed per unit displacement caused, and it assesses the stiffness of the system. Where interest centres on pressure rather than force and on volume rather than linear displacement, analogous relationships can be proposed and their validity investigated. Such analogous relationships illustrate the tendency to look for linear relationships and to define new quantities as ratios of previously defined ones. Lung compliance is an example of this.

### The Triangle of Vectors

If a body is displaced (Fig. 2) from A to B, and then to C it is obvious that the result is the same as if it had gone direct from A to C. We are distinguishing between *distance* (path ABC is obviously greater than path AC) and the vector *displacement*. Having left A and arrived at C by

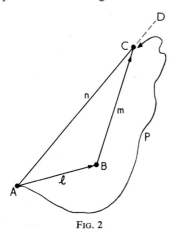

FIG. 2

any path, such as P, the net displacement is still $n$ units of length in the direction A-to-C. The vector displacements A-to-B and B-to-C add according to the triangle rule to give A-to-C. This addition can be regarded as calculation by means of a map.

Mapping is used by navigators to obtain resultant velocities, since velocity is rate of change displacement. For example, suppose that the body moves with velocity $l/t$ in the direction A-to-B, and that simultaneously it is given a velocity $m/t$ parallel to BC. In time $t$ it will arrive at C and the effect will be the same as a single velocity $n/t$ along direction A-to-C. Consequently the same 'map', with a scale interpreted in terms of velocity, can be used to add velocities. Similarly, accelerations, being rates of change of velocities can be mapped and added, while forces, being proportional to accelerations yield to the same technique. The parallelogram of forces (or any vectors) is merely an alternative construction (Fig. 3)

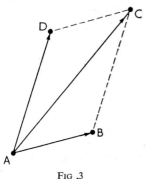

FIG. 3

in which the vector arrows (AB, AD) are for convenience located at the same starting-point on the map, and the resultant is represented in magnitude and direction by the diagonal AC from the same starting-point.

### Resolution of Vectors

In Fig. 4, $J$ represents a joint and interest is focussed on the thrust $F_1$, towards it. This is called the component

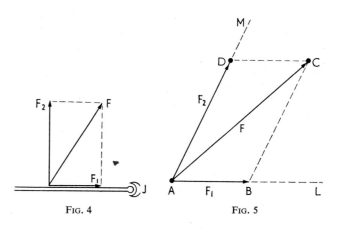

FIG. 4                    FIG. 5

of the total force $F$ in the direction shown, and $F_1$ is one of the pair of forces $F_1$, $F_2$ such that if they were applied simultaneously the effect would be indistinguishable from the single force $F$. The inverse process to combining vectors to obtain their resultant is called *resolving* them into components. In Fig. 5 we wish to know the forces which, acting along two directions AL, AM would produce the same effect as $F$. The parallelogram constructed with a diagonal proportional to $F$ and with sides parallel to AL, AM yields components $F_1$, $F_2$ whose magnitudes can be measured (or calculated by trigonometry) from this map, or 'vector diagram'.

Often the selected directions are perpendicular to one another for the excellent reason that a force along AY (Fig. 6) has no influence on motion along AX, so that

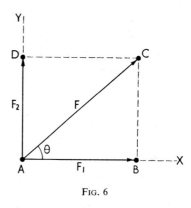

FIG. 6

the resulting perpendicular motions can be analysed separately. For this special case, $F_1$ and $F_2$ can easily be calculated, since

$$AB/AC = \cos \theta$$

$$\text{and} \quad BC/AC = \sin \theta$$

Consequently the formulae

$$F_1 = F \cos \theta$$

$$\text{and} \quad F_2 = F \sin \theta$$

for such situations are frequently used and regarded as obvious.

### Work and Energy

To define the *work* done by a system, and its *energy* (capacity for doing work) requires some refinement of the intuitive and often vague lay concepts from which the terms were borrowed. Energy is manifested in many forms, such as mechanical, electrical, thermal, chemical, nuclear and electromagnetic. In addition, there are lay terms such as 'fatigue' to confuse the issue since one can certainly become 'fatigued' leaning against a wall. When it was realized that energy is conserved when converted from one form to another, it became clear that a definition in terms of mechanical events would serve as a basis.

Other units, such as the calorie, can be related to mechanical units by experimental determination.

In Fig. 7 a force is applied to a body and moves it a distance $x$ from $A$ to $B$. Intuitively one feels that more

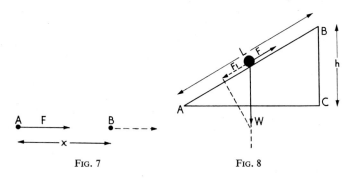

FIG. 7            FIG. 8

work is done if the necessary force $F$ is greater, and that more is done the larger $x$ becomes. Accordingly, the work done is defined as

$$\text{Work} = Fx.$$

The unit of work is therefore the work done when unit force moves its point of application unit distance *in its own direction*. The specification of direction is necessary, as is clear in Fig. 8. Here a body is being pulled up a well-lubricated ramp. Ramps, like gears and levers, are constructed so that a given amount of work can be performed by application of a restricted force, albeit acting over a greater distance. If the body had been raised directly through height $h$, the work done would have been the large force ($W$) multiplied by the small distance ($h$). With the ramp, it is the relatively small force $F$ which is needed to overcome the component $F_1$ of $W$ in the direction shown. The work done is this smaller force multiplied by the correspondingly greater distance $L$ in the direction of that force. Since $h$ is the same fraction ($\sin \theta$) of $L$ as $F$ is of $W$, the work done is the same, with or without the ramp, for

$$Wh = FL$$

It is important to distinguish between useful work done by a machine or a human and the non-productive work done maintaining muscle tone when the human applies force to an unmoving object. Such work involves chemical activity and is difficult to measure, but of course this is no reason why it should not be expressed in mechanical units.

The MKS(SI) unit of work is the newton (of force) multiplied by the metre, and is abbreviated to the joule (J). The CGS unit is the *erg* of work, being that done by a dyne of force moving its point of application through 1 cm in its own direction. Since the newton is 100 000 dynes and the metre is 100 cm,

$$1 \text{ J} = 10^7 \text{ erg}$$

The joule is a convenient unit for measuring the work done by human beings performing simple every-day activities such as raising moderately large drinks from table to lip. Work is as obviously scalar in nature as is volume of liquid.

### Energy. Potential and Kinetic Energy

Since the energy of a system is its capacity for doing work, the same units are involved. Energy units include the calorie which was experimentally determined and is now defined as 4·1868 joules, but the current trend is to express all energies in terms of joules.

When dealing with mechanical energy it is usual, as a matter of convenience, to distinguish between kinetic energy (k.e.) and potential energy (p.e.). If, relative to some point regarded as fixed, a body initially at rest is given a velocity, work has to be done since force must be applied over a distance in order to accelerate the body. This work is in effect stored as kinetic energy, and may in principle be recovered by arranging that the body passes on its energy to whatever stops it. Apart from interchange between mass and energy in nuclear events, energy is simply conserved during interchanges.

The kinetic energy of a body of mass $m$ moving with velocity $v$ with respect to the fixed point (reference frame) is given by

$$\text{k.e.} = \tfrac{1}{2}mv^2$$

This formula, with one factor squared, has many counterparts in energy calculations, and it is instructive to consider it in more detail. It is reasonable that the energy is proportional to the mass, since doubling the mass would, for a given history of acceleration leading up to the velocity $v$, require double the force over the same path. To appreciate the $v^2$ term, imagine a man pushing a car from rest. Suppose that he exerts a constant force, and that by the time $v$ is 1 m s$^{-1}$ he has travelled 10 m. Since the average velocity is 0·5 m s$^{-1}$ this part of the operation would take 20 seconds. If he continues until $v$ becomes 2 m s$^{-1}$, since the force, and hence the acceleration, is constant he will have pushed for 40 seconds. The overall average velocity being 1 m s$^{-1}$, the total distance would be 40 m. He therefore applies the force over *four times* the distance required to reach 1 m s$^{-1}$ in order to produce *double* this velocity. Consequently four times as much energy is expended.

These results are summarized in Fig. 9. Notice that the $v^2$ term is justified by the need to quadruple the distance while doubling the velocity. The factor $\frac{1}{2}$ in the formula can be explained by investigating the detail. The work done by force $F$ acting over distance $x$ is

$$\text{Work} = Fx$$

If the time taken is $t$, the acceleration is $v/t$, so

$$\text{Work} = m(v/t)x$$

Since the average velocity is $\frac{1}{2}v$, the distance $x$ is

$$x = (\tfrac{1}{2}v)t$$

and substitution yields

$$\text{Work} = \tfrac{1}{2}mv^2$$

A further point to note is that, in terms of velocity, this formula is non-linear in contrast with the linear relationships we are pre-disposed to seek. This is solely a consequence of our decision to relate the k.e. to the velocity,

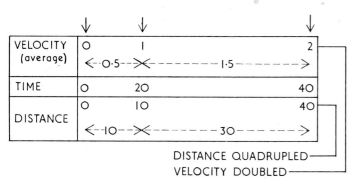

FIG. 9

rather than to the path-length $x$, to which the k.e. is linearly related. This decision is a rational one however, since the k.e. is a function of the velocity no matter how this velocity was achieved. We have chosen the application of a constant force in order to derive the result simply. The same result can be obtained with a varying force by application of the calculus.

It will be seen later that the equation of the state of a perfect gas ($P = RT/V$) involves a non-linear relationship between the parameters $P$ and $V$ by which we elect to describe the state of the gas, although this is based on a linear relationship between mean molecular kinetic energy and the absolute temperature of the sample.

**Potential Energy**

The energy possessed by a mechanical system by virtue of its present geometrical configuration (as opposed to its state of motion) is exemplified by springs which are distorted against the tendency for their molecules to retain their original layout, and by bodies poised under the influence of a gravity. When a body is raised against gravity, work must be done; the body and the Earth somewhat resembling a spring that is being stretched. To raise a mass $m$ through a height $h$ where the gravitational acceleration is $g$ (that is, the weight is $mg$) demands $mgh$ units of work to be done, or

$$\text{p.e.} = mgh$$

Here the energy is linearly related to the height, and height is the obvious parameter to measure.

The simplest spring requires a force $F$ to stretch it a distance $x$ given by

$$F = sx$$

At the beginning of stretching ($x = 0$) the force is zero, so the average is $\frac{1}{2}F$. This gives the result

$$\text{p.e.} = \tfrac{1}{2}Fx$$
$$= \tfrac{1}{2}sx^2$$

which is analogous to the k.e. formula.

**Momentum**

When a body is about to collide with another and give up all its energy, for example, in the form of heat, the parameter that best describes the moving body is its k.e. ($\frac{1}{2}mv^2$). In contrast, in a perfectly *elastic* collision there is no wasted energy, and the best parameter to describe the oncoming body in those circumstances is known as its momentum, $mv$. A vivid distinction between

$$\text{k.e.} = \tfrac{1}{2}mv^2$$

$$\text{and Momentum} = mv$$

is provided by the invention of the elastic-recoil jewellers' window, which returns bricks to would-be robbers. Whereas a conventional window shatters with production of heat and sound and the rupture of the bonds between particles of glass, and leaves a motionless brick in the wreckage, the more sophisticated window reverses the sense of the velocity of the brick. During this operation the brick exerts a force on the window (and vice versa) just as in the case of a gas molecule rebounding from wall of the container. This force is equal to the *rate of change of momentum*, since,

$$F = ma$$

where $a$ = rate of change of $v$,

so $F$ = rate of change of $mv$.

This relationship is in fact a more general definition of force than the interim one given earlier, since it covers cases in which the mass is changing as well as the velocity, as for example when a rocket consumes its fuel.

When dealing with the kinetic theory of gases, use will be made of momentum. If one is concerned with heat exchange, kinetic energy is the relevant parameter, but when considering pressure it is the reversal of momentum that is important. Like velocity, momentum is a vector quantity, and corresponding to the conservation of energy in a closed system there is a law of conservation of momentum in elastic collisions. This law states that, measured in any direction, the algebraic sum of the products of mass and velocity of elastically colliding bodies is unchanged by the collision. At first sight a mathematically inclined criminal might be surprised to see his brick returned with its momentum reversed, but precise measurement would reveal that the jeweller's shop and the Earth had gained momentum in the opposite direction immediately after the impact. The associated velocity change would be exceedingly small because the mass in the case of the Earth is so large. However, astronauts and people in punts do well to avoid throwing massive objects.

## Moments

Figure 10 illustrates a force applied to a lever, causing it to rotate about $P$. It is a common experience that the effectiveness of such of force in imparting twist depends both on the magnitude of the force and on the distance $p$ perpendicular to the line of action. The measure of twist-effectiveness is called the *moment* or *torque* and is defined as the product.

$$\text{Moment} = F \cdot p$$

Although this has the same dimensions as work (both involving force multiplied by distance) it is an important distinction that $p$ is a purely geometrical factor and is measured at right-angles to the line of action. If the lever moves, work will be done, but this will be the product of

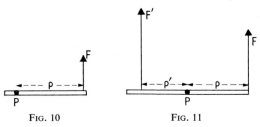

FIG. 10       FIG. 11

$F$ and the distance moved by $F$ *along* its line of action. To maintain this distinction the terms newton and metre are not combined into the joule, and the MKS unit of torque is the newton-metre (N m). Another important distinction between work and torque is that the former is a scalar while the latter requires specification of sense of rotation.

The two most common classes of problem involving moment concern equilibrium (prevention of rotation) and rotary motion as such. Figure 11 shows an equilibrium situation. The clockwise moment due to the larger force $F'$ applied less effectively (smaller $p'$) equals the counter-clockwise product of the smaller force $F$ and the larger $p$, or

$$F'p' = Fp$$

Similarly in Fig. 12 $F'$ is necessarily larger than $F$. Figure 13 illustrates the price paid for the convenience of

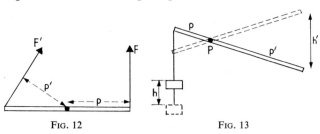

FIG. 12       FIG. 13

exerting a smaller force, since arranging that $p'$ is greater than $p$ requires the user to push for a greater distance *along* the line of action when the lever is used. Geometrically, $h'$ is greater than $h$ by the same factor as $p'$ is greater than $p$. As in the case of the ramp, the work done is exactly the same whether the lever is used or not. Levers and gears (continuous levers) are examples of transformer-like devices in which one factor (force for example) is in effect traded for another (displacement) to satisfy a requirement of matching a load to a source of energy which has limitations set to the manner in which it can supply energy. An interesting example is the lever formed by the fore-arm which trades the large force available by small displacement muscles for the relatively small force but large displacement requirements of the moving hand in human actions such as throwing.

## Rotation of Bodies

The application of a single force can produce a torque, but will tend to cause linear (i.e. translational) as well as rotational motion, as can be seen when one tries to spin a top with one finger. The application of two equal and opposite forces (as when using finger and thumb) produces rotation only, and since this technique has the effect of producing twist without wear on bearings it merits the special name *couple*. The moment (torque) of a couple is simply the sum of the moments due to two forces.

The structure of laws and formulae that describe translational motion is exactly mirrored in the field of rotary motion. Just as force can change linear momentum and impart kinetic energy of translation, so a torque can give angular momentum and establish rotational kinetic energy. Figure 14 shows a small body constrained to move in a circular path. In general this body might be a particle within a solid object, but to establish some new ideas we

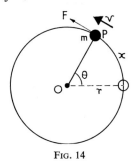

FIG. 14

will consider it separately and imagine that it is provided with a force $F$ that continuously adjusts its line of action so as to be always perpendicular to OP. The torque applied is

$$\tau = F \cdot r$$

and we enquire how much work is done in moving round the arc $x$. The result

$$\text{Work} = Fx$$

is true but unrealistic, since in an extended body each particle has its own value of $x$, the particles nearer O travelling smaller distances $x$ than those further out. However, we feel intuitively that more work is done if we have to apply larger torque, so substituting $\tau/r$ in place of $F$ we see that

$$\text{Work} = \frac{\tau x}{r}$$

In radian measure, the angle $\theta$ is *defined* as the ratio of the arc $x$ to the radius $r$, so

$$\text{Work} = \tau\theta$$

Notice that the angle $\theta$ is common to all particles of a rotating extended body, so $\theta$ is a sensible parameter to involve in calculations. The self-evident result, that the work done is proportional to the torque applied and to the angle turned shows an excellent reason for the existence of radian measure, since the formula is exactly analogous to the translational formula.

$$\text{Work} = Fx$$

This enables us to express kinetic energy more realistically as

$$\text{k.e.} = \tfrac{1}{2}(mr^2)\omega^2$$

By using the special symbol $I$ for the term in parenthesis we obtain two analogous formulae:—

$$\text{k.e.} = \tfrac{1}{2}mv^2 \text{ (Translational)}$$

$$\text{k.e.} = \tfrac{1}{2}I\omega^2 \text{ (Rotational)}$$

In all results for rotary motion the measure of inertia (analogous to mass in the translational case) is $I$, *the moment of inertia*.

In Fig. 14, $I = mr^2$, while for an extended body $I$ is the sum of all the contributions $mr^2$ for all the particles. For storing energy of rotation, the effectiveness of a mass depends on the square of its distance from the axis. This is appreciated by ballet dancers entering a pirouette

TABLE 1

| SOME **TRANSLATORY** QUANTITIES | THEIR **ROTATORY** EQUIVALENTS |
|---|---|
| MASS _ _ _ _ _ _ _ _ _ _ _ m | MOMENT OF INERTIA _ _ _ _ _ $I \; (= \Sigma\, mr^2)$ |
| DISTANCE _ _ _ _ _ _ _ _ x | ANGLE_ _ _ _ _ _ _ _ _ _ $\theta$ |
| VELOCITY_ _ _ _ _ _ _ _ _ v $(=\dot{x})$ | ANGULAR VELOCITY_ _ _ _ $\omega \;(=\dot{\theta})$ |
| ACCELERATION_ _ _ _ _ _ a $(=\dot{v})$ | ANGULAR ACCELERATION _ $\dot{\omega}$ |
| FORCE _ _ _ _ _ _ _ _ _ F | TORQUE _ _ _ _ _ _ _ _ _ $\tau$ |
| LINEAR MOMENTUM_ _ _ mv | ANGULAR MOMENTUM_ _ _ $I\omega$ |
| KINETIC ENERGY_ _ _ _ _ _ $\tfrac{1}{2}mv^2$ | KINETIC ENERGY_ _ _ _ _ _ _ $\tfrac{1}{2}I\omega^2$ |
| ACCELERATION LAW_ _ _ $F = ma$ | ACCELERATION LAW_ _ _ _ _ $\tau = I\dot{\omega}$ |
| LINEAR SPRING_ _ _ _ _ _ $F = Sx$ | ROTATING SPRING_ _ _ _ _ _ $\tau = k\theta$ |
| ENERGY IN SPRING_ _ _ _ $\tfrac{1}{2}Sx^2$ | ENERGY IN SPRING_ _ _ _ _ _ $\tfrac{1}{2}k\theta^2$ |

Had $\theta$ been expressed in degrees the formula would have been

$$\text{Work} = \frac{2\pi}{360}\,\tau\theta$$

which is less obviously analogous.

### Angular Velocity and Moment of Inertia

When the particle in Fig. 14 has been set into motion, the kinetic energy is $\tfrac{1}{2}mv^2$, but $v$ is just as unrealistic a parameter as $x$. However all particles in a rotating body share the same rate of sweeping out angle round the axis, and this *angular velocity* is usually denoted by $\omega$. Suppose that having reached a steady state the period of rotation is $T$ seconds, then

$$\omega = \frac{2\pi}{T} \text{ radians per second}$$

Now in $T$ seconds the particle covers a path $2\pi r$, so

$$v = \frac{2\pi r}{T}$$

Comparing these results shows that

$$v = r\omega$$

with arms outstretched and known in detail by designers of recording galvanometers. The modern long thin galvanometer is intended to have low moment of inertia, in contrast with the fly-wheel which has as much of its mass as possible concentrated at its rim.

Table 1 gives some of the analogous quantities and relationships for translational and rotational motion.

### Centrifugal and Centripetal Force

If a body, such as the mass in Fig. 15, is swinging round on the end of a string, even if its speed is constant, the other aspect of velocity, that is *direction*, is changing continuously. A vector diagram mapping the velocities at two

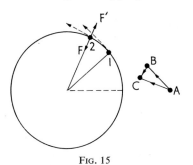

FIG. 15

instants close together shows AB representing the velocity at point 1 and CA that at point 2. The difference between these velocities maps as BC, and it is seen that for small time interval this difference is directed towards the centre of curvature of the path. Now an acceleration consistently directed at right-angles to the path requires a force to maintain it. This force ($F$) is the *centripetal force* provided by the restraining string. The *centrifugal force* ($F'$) exerted on the string is merely an example of Newton's action and reaction law. It can be shown that

$$F = \frac{mv^2}{r}$$

where $v$ is the magnitude of the velocity (speed) and $r$ is the radius of the orbit. The appearance of $v^2$ is due to the fact that doubling $v$ not only doubles the velocity being altered, but halves the time taken to alter it. Similarly, halving $r$ halves the time scale of the motion, which therefore demands greater acceleration.

## Power

The lay term *powerful*, which is applied to people or devices capable of doing considerable work in a short time, is the basis for the formal definition of the power developed by a system as the rate at which it does work. The unit is the joule of work per second, and is abbreviated to the *watt* ($1\ W = 1\ J\ s^{-1}$). The watt is not the exclusive property of the subject of electricity, and it is perfectly valid to speak of the power developed by the muscles of the heart in terms of watts. Other units, such as the horse-power, can be expressed in terms of the watt.

## Pressure

When a surface is bombarded by molecules and the momentum of the molecules (normal to the surface) is reversed, the surface experiences a force. The effectiveness of this force, as far as production of local strain is concerned, depends on the area over which it is distributed. The force per unit area is called the pressure, and may be measured in newtons (N) per square metre; $1\ N\ m^{-2}$ is equivalent to $10^5$ dynes distributed over $10^4$ square centimetres, so

$$1\ N\ m^{-2} = 10\ dyne\ cm^{-2}$$

In our natural environment, we are bombarded by molecules of air of a particular density (about $1\ kg\ m^{-3}$) and of a particular order of temperature (and hence of kinetic energy). The resulting 'atmosphere pressure' is clearly important to us, and measurement shows this to be of the order of $10^5\ N\ m^{-2}$ ($10^6\ dyne\ cm^{-2}$). The reason why the air around us is compressed to the extent that it causes this order of pressure is that the air at the earth's surface is supporting the weight of air stacked vertically above, and, like a pile of cushions, the lower layers are compressed more than the upper ones.

A column of liquid is similarly compressed, but liquids being far less compressible than gases, the variation of density up the column is very small. This suggests a convenient method of producing known pressures at will, and by balancing such pressures against unknown pressures

provides us with a method (the liquid column manometer) of measuring the latter. Since a column of liquid of height $h$, cross-sectional area $A$ and density $\rho$ has a mass $\rho h A$, its weight (a force) at the surface of the earth is $\rho h A g$. Consequently the pressure exerted at the base is $\rho h A g / A$, or

$$P = \rho g \,.\, h$$

For a chosen liquid (e.g. mercury) and chosen planet (e.g. Earth), $\rho$ and $g$ are known, so the pressure produced is proportional to the height of the column. The simplicity and convenience of this technique led to the short-hand reference to the height of a liquid column as a measure of pressure, and the unit '1 mmHg' of course means the pressure caused by a column of mercury 1 mm high at the Earth's surface.

### Classes of Problem Involving Pressure Measurement

When considering the flow of fluids through vessels (blood in arteries or air in air-ways) we are concerned with the *differences* in pressure between two ends of a vessel. If the pressures at both ends are increased by (say) 50 mmHg, the pressure difference is unaltered. In such problems the actual baseline from which pressure is referred is irrelevant. There is an important distinction between problems involving pressure differences and those involving absolute measure of pressure. For example, when considering the solution of gases in a liquid or the compression of gases in a cylinder, the important measure is the actual force per unit area—that is the result of actual bombardment to which the sample is subjected. To clarify this distinction, consider a mercury manometer (Fig. 16)

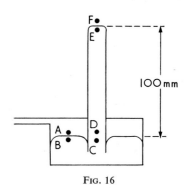

FIG. 16

being used to measure a pressure in a liquid (communicating at A), the measurement taking place on the Earth's surface, with the end (F) open to the atmosphere. Suppose that molecules at A bombard those at B, the pressure to be measured being $P$. Once equilibrium has been reached, mercury no longer moves, so molecules at C are known to be subjected to the same pressure environment (that is bombardment giving rise to the same rate of momentum reversal over unit area) as those at B. The measurement problem has therefore been transferred to assessing the pressure at C. Now this pressure results from the act of supporting the column of mercury (D to E) plus the effect of the bombardment of molecules at E by air molecules at F. For example, suppose the mercury column to be 100 mm high, and the effect of air molecules bombarding E to be the same as would have been caused by an extra column of mercury 760 mm high with no atmosphere above it (atmosphere pressure = 760 mmHg at the time of the measurement). From the point of view of molecules at C (and hence at B and therefore at A), the pressure would be 860 mmHg. If there were oxygen molecules at A and the far end of the tube connected to the manometer were sealed, then this would be the relevant pressure as far as the resulting compression of the oxygen is concerned. This becomes doubly clear if we express the pressure in fundamental terms—i.e. in N m$^{-2}$. We obviously should not ignore the fact that our measuring instrument does not cease at the top (E) of the tube, when describing the number of newtons per square metre to which the oxygen is subjected.

In contrast, suppose that this manometer were measuring an arterial pressure via a catheter or needle, and that another was being used for venous pressure measurement, with a column showing 4 mm. If our interest lay in the difference between arterial and venous pressure it would be correct (but unusual) to quote the arterial pressure as 860 mmHg and the venous pressure as 764 mmHg. By convention we take the baseline value (atmospheric pressure) as understood, and give the results as 100 mmHg and 4 mmHg respectively. It is interesting (and revealing of the state of our understanding) to consider the length of the arterial pressure manometer column in quite different circumstances. Suppose the patient to be in a hyperbaric enclosure in which the density of his local atmosphere had been artificially increased, and that a state of equilibrium had been established. It is unusual to think in terms of the density of the local atmosphere (although the object of the exercise is in fact to present tissues with more oxygen molecules bombarding unit area than is normal outside), and we will enquire what pressure in *excess of* atmosphere was necessary to create this situation. It is important to know what is meant when reference is made to the pressure inside a hyperbaric enclosure, since 2 atmospheres in excess of the outside pressure is not the same thing as 2 atmospheres total. Suppose that, unambiguously, the pressure inside was 1000 mmHg above that outside. If the open end of the manometer lay inside the enclosure, the column would still be 100 mm high. The absolute measure of pressure at A would be 100 mmHg due to the action of the heart, plus the 1760 mmHg due to the local atmosphere with which the patient's tissues are in equilibrium. However, the top of the column would be subjected to the same 1760 mmHg giving 1860 mmHg at A and 1760 mmHg at E, which accounts for the support of a 100 mm column. If the open end of the manometer had been outside, the column would have needed to be 1100 mm high since the air at F would have only contributed 760 mmHg pressure. This agrees with the fact that the patient's arterial pressure would be 100 mmHg above the pressure in the enclosure, or 1100 mm Hg above outside atmospheric pressure. To appreciate fully the meaning of pressure measurements taken this way it is instructive to observe that were it not for the opening to the atmosphere at F the column would need to be 1100

+ 760, or 1860 mm high to back-off the pressure existing in the environment of the patient's artery, and that this figure in turn reflects the fact that we are using mercury on the earth's surface. On the Moon, where weights are one-sixth of Earth-surface values, and where there is no atmosphere the column would be 6 × 1860, or 11 160 mm high. The corresponding length for venous pressure measurement would be 6 × (4 + 1760), or 10 584 mm. An arterial pressure quoted as 11 160 mmHg absolute and a venous pressure of 10 584 mmHg absolute lacks the ring of familiarity, but as far as the patient's haemodynamic status is concerned this represents a pressure difference of 576 mmHg (Moon gravity), or 96 mmHg (Earth gravity).

Although few anaesthetists are likely to be involved with patients in hyperbaric enclosures on the Moon, it is important to appreciate the following facts:

1. That the mercury pressure scale arose from the convenience of observing a length when measuring a pressure.

2. That, no matter what units are used, fluid dynamics calculations are concerned with pressure differences, so that baselines or reference levels are often tacitly omitted.

3. That as far as the environment of molecules at a particular site is concerned, the essential question is how many molecules are concentrated there and how much momentum is involved during collisions over a given area. Since we rarely know (or measure) the density of molecules or their momenta, we relate our observations to the quantity we can measure, that is pressure. For problems of compression the important measure is absolute pressure.

### Other Pressure Symbols and Units

Where there is serious possibility of ambiguity the word 'absolute' may be added to denote pressures referred to true zero (that is, compared with no molecular collisions), and the word 'gauge' is added to denote pressures measured above atmospheric. Accordingly the abbreviations 'a' and 'g' are met, as in Nm$^{-2}$a or lbf in$^{-2}$ g. The abbreviation p.s.i. for pounds-weight per square inch is becoming less often met. In cases where the unit is still used, the modern terminology is 'pounds-force' (lbf) per square inch.

The *pascal* (Pa) is the official SI name for the newton per square metre (Nm$^{-2}$). However, throughout this chapter it is desirable to retain the concept 'force per unit area' clearly, and the fuller form Nm$^{-2}$ is retained.

### Pressure Related to Work

Figure 17 illustrates a syringe being used to eject fluid at a pressure $P$ (absolute), so the force being exerted on the plunger is given by

$$F = P \cdot A$$

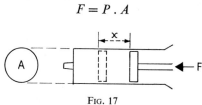

Fig. 17

If the plunger moves some distance ($x$), work will be done, given by

$$\text{Work} = Fx$$
$$= PA \cdot x$$

Now $Ax$ is the volume ejected ($V$, say), so

$$\text{Work} = PV$$

We see from this that we can define pressure either as force per unit area or as work per unit volume. This is made doubly clear by writing

$$\text{Pressure} = \frac{\text{FORCE} \cdot \text{DISTANCE}}{\text{AREA} \cdot \text{DISTANCE}}$$

since cancelling 'DISTANCE' gives the usual definition, while not cancelling it gives the alternative definition.

It is clear that by a 'strong' pump we mean one capable of exerting a large pressure. Similarly, a 'strong' pump is capable of doing a considerable amount of work with each unit volume it ejects. It is as legitimate to measure pressure in joules (of work done) per m³ (of fluid ejected) as by newtons (of force exerted) per m² (of area involved). The simplicity of physicists' calculations of work done by pumps is disguised in medicine by the use of special units. The use of mmHg for pressure spoils the simplicity of

$$\text{Work} = PV$$

More generally, if the pressure changes during the ejection, the work is found by summing the products of pressure and increments of volume ejected, or

$$\text{Work} = \int P \, dV$$

## Temperature

Our main concern with temperature here will be its relevance to the kinetic theory of gases. It is known that heating a body raises the average kinetic energy of its molecules. However, temperature is primarily a lay concept (as a human perception of 'hotness'), and like force and energy awaited formal definition. Unfortunately, the invention of imperfect thermometers preceded the development of kinetic theory. Suppose that scientists had instead developed an instrument for measuring mean molecular kinetic energy. Over the range of human perception a good correlation would have been noted between lay 'temperature' and measured kinetic energy. It would have

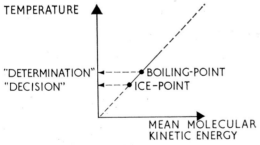

Fig. 18

seemed obvious to *define* temperature as proportional to mean molecular kinetic energy, and to extend the definition

beyond the human range, as in Fig. 18. Four important consequences would have been:

1. The existence of an absolute zero of temperature would have caused no comment.
2. The relationship Temperature = Constant . Mean Molecular K.E. would have been regarded as a mere definition (not a natural law).
3. A decision would have been awaited to set the temperature scale—i.e. to choose the factor of proportionality.
4. There being no thermometers, as we know them, there would have been no preconceived opinion on setting the scale.

To set the scale, suppose that the melting of ice had been chosen as a reproducible phenomenon. Some reasonable number, such as 1000, might have been selected for the point marked 'DECISION' on the figure. This choice would have given reasonable steps in temperature for most medical, domestic and meteorological purposes, and certainly the suggestion of 273 would have been regarded as eccentric. After the scale had been set, the determination of other temperatures (such as that of boiling water) would have been purely a matter of experiment (*see* 'DETERMINATION' on the figure).

The invention of the mercury-in-glass thermometer, for which the convenient end-points (melting-point of ice and boiling-point of water) would have already been decided, would have been seen as making available a cheap instrument. The imperfections of its scale would have been noted as an example of imperfect linearity, rather as some ECG recorders are known to be non-linear. The gas thermometers would have been greeted as instruments of better linearity and precision, and all subsequent experimentation based on thermometers would have been regarded as limited in precision by the imperfections of the measuring instruments.

In contrast, we have inherited a system of temperature scales based on the behaviour of actual thermometers, and the historical order of the subject introduces complications analogous to the assumption that the first recorded ECG traces were definitive and that voltage is only associated with the ECG in some rather esoteric way.

While one may be tolerant of the arbitrary choice of 0 and 100 for the end-points for the centigrade scaling, the choice of 32 and 212 seems in retrospect as unfortunate as measuring the stature of horses in 'hands' and being uncertain whether to start at hoof or fetlock.

From the point of view of anaesthetists, temperature *differences* between actual and normal, and between one site and another, are equally well measured in any agreed scale. Departures from linearity with respect to the kinetic (absolute) scale are rarely important, so that (for example) the definition of the calorie in terms of raising the temperature of a gram of water by 1°C, is perfectly adequate. When dealing with the kinetic theory of gases, however, the absolute scale is involved, and all quantities (such as the gas constant) that are related to it have been determined with the scale as it now stands, with ice melting at approximately 273 degrees.

## Pressure, Volume and Temperature of Gases

In a sample of gas at a known temperature, the molecules are continually interchanging momentum by collisions, and consequently have a spread or spectrum of kinetic energies distributed about an average which is specific for that temperature. In Fig. 19 we imagine that a molecule has been removed from the sample at an instant when its kinetic energy was equal to the average, and transferred to a small box. When a molecule rebounds from the surface of a container, occasions will arise when its reception will have been more vigorous than at others, since the agitation of the molecules of the container is also subject to a spread. On average, the fact that the container is in temperature equilibrium with the gas enables us to simplify the situation in Fig. 19 by assuming that the molecule rebounds without loss or gain of kinetic energy. Our intention is to regard this molecule as undergoing average experiences and to confine our attention to results that would be unchanged if all the molecules in a sample underwent these experiences.

At each impact, the component of the momentum of the molecule perpendicular to the face is exactly reversed

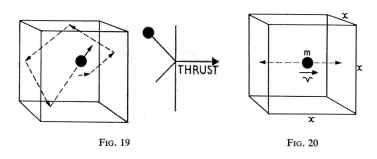

FIG. 19                    FIG. 20

in this simplified model, and the trajectory for one of the collisions is shown in side elevation to the right of the figure. If the container were sufficiently small, the collisions would be frequent enough for each face to experience a pressure due to continual reversals of momentum. Just as we discuss temperature (rather than kinetic energy) because we possess thermometers, so we introduce pressure into our description of the gas because it is measurable and has been correlated with factors of interest to us, both in physics and in medicine. Clearly the molecule rebounds from six faces, and it is necessary to take into account the angles of impact at each face to calculate pressure. Suppose that the molecule had been trapped when it happened to be travelling perpendicular to one face (Fig. 20). Rebounding between two of the six faces, it will exert pressure on one-third of the six. When allowance has been made for the angle of impact and for the longer times between impacts for the six-face rebound (Fig. 19), it is found that the pressure experienced in the two-faced situation is three times as great as when all six faces are involved. In Fig. 20, if $t$ is the time between impacts on one face

$$t = 2x/v$$

Since the momentum is reversed on impact, the force (rate of change of momentum) is

$$F = 2(mv)/t$$
$$= mv^2/x$$

Since the area of the face is $x^2$, the pressure is

$$P = F/x^2$$
$$= mv^2/x^3$$

When allowance is made for this pressure being three times as large as when all faces are affected, the result becomes

$$P = \tfrac{1}{3} mv^2/x^3$$

or, denoting the volume ($x^3$) by $V$,

$$PV = \tfrac{1}{3}mv^2.$$

Notice that this result is proportional to the kinetic energy of the molecule.

If the rest of the molecules are introduced into the box, and the total number in the sample is $N_s$, the result becomes

$$PV = \tfrac{1}{3}(N_s . m)v^2$$

where $v^2$ is called the 'mean value of the squares of the velocities'. Notice in passing that this is not the same as saying that $v$ is the mean velocity. For comparison if we had three square pieces of paper with sides 1, 2 and 3 cm, the mean area would be one-third of 14 cm$^2$. This would correspond to a square of 2·16 cm side, not 2 cm.

Having shown that the product $PV$ is proportional to the number of molecules and their mean kinetic energy, we introduce temperature by reference to the absolute (kinetic theory) scale. For a given *sample* of a given gas (that is given $N_s$ and $m$) this is usually done by noting that $PV$ is proportional to the kinetic energy and hence to the temperature and writing.

$$PV = R_sT$$

where the factor of proportionality $R_s$ is called the *gas constant for that sample*.

The contribution per molecule is expressed by the gas constant per molecule, which is known as Boltzmann's constant ($k$), so

$$PV = N_skT$$

Comparing this with

$$PV = \tfrac{1}{3}N_smv^2$$

gives another interpretation of Boltzmann's constant, since

$$kT = \tfrac{1}{3}mv^2$$

shows that $k$ is two-thirds of the kinetic energy change per molecule corresponding to 1 degree change of absolute temperature.

It is a matter of individual preference which of the many formulations of the ideal gas law (equation of state) is

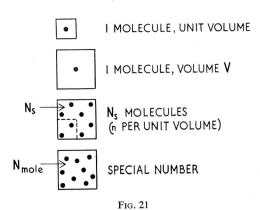

FIG. 21

regarded as basic. One scheme is illustrated in Fig. 21. If we imagine the contribution of *one* (average experience) *molecule* to the pressure in a *unit volume* to be

$$P_1 = kT$$

we need remember that only the temperature of the sample can effect what this molecule does in the unit volume box. Increasing the volume will reduce the rate of collisions and increase the area involved, and the smaller pressure is

$$P = \frac{kT}{V}$$

Increasing the number of molecules to $N_s$ (any number) gives

$$P = \frac{N_s kT}{V}$$

which is sometimes encountered as

$$P = nkT$$

$n$ being the number of molecules per unit volume. Taking some special number of molecules, such as the number in a 1 mole sample (discussed more fully later) gives

$$P = \frac{N_{mole} kT}{V}$$

The product $N_{mole}k$ is the gas constant for a mole sample ($R_m$), so for a mole

$$P = \frac{R_m T}{V}$$

This last formulation has the advantage that $R_m$ is a tabulated quantity.

### Types of Problem Involving the Gas Law

The choice of formula depends on the problem concerned, and it is convenient to divide the problems into two classes. When the gas or gases are in fixed quantities and where we are concerned only with their redistribution, the simplest formula is usually

$$PV = N_s kT$$

It is not necessary to know the actual number or the value of $k$, since these factors cancel in calculations. For example, suppose that a sample of $N_1$ molecules in a volume $V_1$ at pressure $P_1$ and temperature $T_1$ are mixed with another sample of $N_2$ molecules originally at $P_2$ and $T_2$ in a volume $V_2$, so that they occupy the total volume $(V_1 + V_2)$. If the temperature equilibrates to $T_3$, the pressure $P_3$ is given by

$$P_3(V_1 + V_2) = (N_1 + N_2)kT_3$$

But
$$P_1 V_1 = N_1 kT_1$$

and
$$P_2 V_2 = N_2 kT_2$$

Substituting for the quantities $N_1k$ and $N_2k$ gives

$$P_3(V_1 + V_2) = T_3 \left( \frac{P_1 V_1}{T_1} + \frac{P_2 V_2}{T_2} \right)$$

The advantage of working in terms of numbers of molecules is that molecules do not vanish in physical processes such as mixing, diffusion and entering into solution. Their numbers must therefore be accounted for at all stages in the calculations.

When the problem is to establish the *PVT* relationships for a specific sample (such as a given mass) we must, in effect, become 'aware' of the numbers of molecules involved. It would be absurd, however, to calculate the number of molecules and look up the value of Boltzmann's constant, and it is more usual to resort to the form

$$PV = RT$$

Traditionally the standard 'package' of molecules is the mole, so the evaluation of the gas constant $R$ for a given mass involves expressing that mass in terms of molecular 'weight'. This process has the advantage that one is aware of the extent to which one is approximating when taking approximate values for this calculation.

### The Laws of Boyle and Charles (and Gay-Lussac)

In experiments with gases Boyle discovered that at constant temperature a sample of given mass displayed an approximately inverse relationship between pressure and volume, or

$$PV = \text{constant (given mass and given temperature)}.$$

Later work by Charles and by Gay-Lussac showed experimentally that several common gases, when allowed to expand under constant pressure as the temperature was raised, expanded approximately equally for equal temperature increments. In terms of temperature $t°C$, this relationship is approximately

$$\frac{V}{273 + t} = \text{constant (given mass and pressure)}$$

which, in terms of absolute temperature $T$ reduces to

$$V = \text{constant} . T$$

These experimentally determined laws are clearly accounted for by the theoretical relationship

$$PV = RT$$

by restricting the variables $PV$ and $T$ to vary in pairs.

## Avogadro's Hypothesis

For a perfect gas (that is a theoretical material exactly obeying the simple gas law $PV = N_s kT$), Avogadro's hypothesis states that, at a given temperature and pressure the number of molecules per unit volume would be independent of the gas concerned. It is instructive to express this another way. If we confine ourselves to pressure, temperature and volume measurements alone (which we often do, since these are measurable quantities with which we become familiar), there can be no way of knowing which gas is in a container. To illustrate this with simple numbers, imagine that one side of the container of Fig. 19 is free to move, and that, under the impression that a molecule of mass $m$ is trapped, we are holding this side in position. Now suppose that the original sample had contained a trace of heavier gas (for example one having molecules of mass $4m$), and that by chance one of these had been selected on the basis of possessing the average kinetic energy. Now we were expecting a molecule of mass $m$ and velocity $v$, whose kinetic energy would be

$$\text{k.e.} = \tfrac{1}{2}mv^2$$

It is easy to see that a molecule of mass $4m$ having this kinetic energy would have velocity $\tfrac{1}{2}v$, since substituting $4m$ and $\tfrac{1}{2}v$ in the expression for kinetic energy gives

$$\text{k.e.} = \tfrac{1}{2}(4m)(\tfrac{1}{2}v)^2$$
$$= \tfrac{1}{2}mv^2$$

Having half the expected velocity, this molecule takes *twice* as long between impacts, but we find its momentum to be *twice* the expected value $mv$, since

$$\text{Momentum} = \text{Mass . Velocity}$$
$$= (4m)(\tfrac{1}{2}v)$$
$$= 2\,mv$$

Now the force on the wall equals the rate of change of momentum, and since both the momentum and the time lapse between impacts are doubled, the force is exactly the same as the expected molecule would have produced.

We have illustrated this with simple ratios which can be easily visualized, but the result

$$PV = \tfrac{1}{3}mv^2 N_s$$

shows that, for $\tfrac{1}{2}mv^2$ constant the result is independent of $m$ because of compensating adjustment of $v$.

In summary, we see that pressure measurements cannot distinguish between the 'expected' gas and the interloper, which agrees with Avogadro's hypothesis. For a specified volume (1 cm³) at standard temperature (0°C) and pressure (1 atmosphere) the number of molecules is of the order of $2 \cdot 69 \times 10^{19}$, which is Loschmidt's number. Another aspect of this is that a mole sample, which contains rather more than 22 000 times as many molecules will, at standard temperature and pressure, occupy a volume of the order of 22 litres.

## The Mole. Avogadro's Constant

Physical chemistry evolved in a manner which resulted in our inheriting a somewhat arbitrary, though useful, standard 'packet' of matter, the *mole*. In retrospect, it is obvious that atoms combine chemically in integer proportions. For work on a macroscopic scale any sufficiently large number (say $10^{20}$) could be regarded as a convenient packet, both from the point of view of measurability and because (unlike, say, a dozen) such a huge number can accommodate the integer proportions involved in even highly complex molecules.

Again, traditionally, we think of the mass of a given type of atom in terms of (as a ratio of) the mass of some standard particle, as is evident by the use of such terms as 'atomic (and molecular) weight', although it is perhaps unfortunate that the word 'weight' slipped into the terminology at this point. In the past there has been discussion on which particle should be used as reference. Had the universe been tidier in the sense that the masses of all atoms had been exact multiples of the mass of the hydrogen atom, there would have been no discussion. However, even if isotopes having different masses for the same element did not exist, the fact remains that atoms are not multiples of hydrogen atoms, and there are arguments to be made in favour of different reference masses. Essentially the best choice would result in as many of the ratios as possible being near to whole numbers, so that, for approximate work, we effect a 'data reduction' by remembering these numbers for elements of importance to our work. It is also desirable that the reference particle should be unambiguous and not to depend on some local terrestial accident such as the proportion of different isotopes in a 'naturally occurring' sample of some element. Currently references are still found to the chemical scale based on a reference mass of one-sixteenth of that of the average atom in a sample of naturally occurring oxygen, and the physical scale based on one-sixteenth of the mass of isotope oxygen–16. More recent references are becoming unified to the scale in which a value of exactly 12 is assigned to the isotope carbon–12.

Recognizing that the small differences between these scales are relevant for more accurate work, we can simplify the picture by regarding the mole as a sample consisting of a standard number of molecules so selected that we can state the mass of the sample (in grams) to whatever precision we compute the molecular weight. This number is approximately $6 \times 10^{23}$, and is known as Avogadro's constant. The *order* of this number is consequent on the original decision to take the gram as the basic unit of mass, and its *precise value* depends on the atomic weight scale concerned, as well as on the precision of the current best estimate, of course.

Clearly, the importance of the mole is due to its reference to a specified number of molecules. Quantities such as the gas constant per mole and specific heats per mole are listed and may be regarded as constants for a numerically specified sample. Boltzmann's constant is similarly a constant for a specified sample, in this case a sample of one molecule. As such, it is convenient for theoretical work concerning individual molecules and as a parameter in the statistical analysis of macroscopic groups.

### Partial Pressure (Dalton's Law)

Since pressure measurements cannot distinguish between different molecules in a mixed sample, the contribution to total pressure made by a given constituent is in proportion to the number of molecules of that constituent  If all others were removed, then provided that the only influence between constituents had been the random momentary collisions, the remaining molecules would continue with the same average kinetic energy. They would therefore maintain their same contribution (now the only one) to the pressure. The original total pressure must therefore have been the sum of the pressures each constituent produces alone, and these contributions depend only on the number of molecules present, for a given temperature. The simplest form of the gas law, $PV = N_s kT$ illustrates this. If there are two gases, for which we use the suffices 1 and 2, and there are $N_1$ molecules of gas 1 and $N_2$ of gas 2, then

$$PV = (N_1 + N_2)kT$$

because there is no way of distinguishing between molecules as far as $PV$ and $T$ measurements are concerned. Taken in isolation the partial pressures would be given by

$$P_1 V = N_1 kT$$
$$P_2 V = N_2 kT$$

The factors $V$ and $kT$, being common, cancel to give

$$\frac{P_1}{N_1} = \frac{P_2}{N_2} = \frac{P}{N_1 + N_2}$$

This states that the partial pressures and the total pressure are in the same ratios as the separate and combined numbers of molecules. Although we do not normally think in terms of numbers of molecules we usually either know the masses (and the molecular 'weights') of the constituents, or their original separate volumes at given pressure and temperature, or we know their relative abundance in a given mixture. It will be noted that any statement concerning partial pressures in a mixture of gases is merely another way of making a statement of their relative *numerical* abundance, provided that their interactions involve only mutual interchange of kinetic energy in collisions.

### The Gas Law for Real Gases

In Fig. 22 molecule $A$ is approaching the wall of a container. The simple kinetic theory of gases assumes that, apart from momentum interchange on collision, there is no interaction between molecules. In a real gas there are forces of attraction between molecules, so that when $A$ reaches the wall it is doing so against the small force $F$ tending to pull it back into the body of the gas. As a result the pressure actually *measured* will be less than *predicted* by the simplified theory. Van der Waals allowed for this error by replacing $P$ by

$$P + \frac{a}{V^2}$$

where $a$ is a constant for the sample. It will be noted that (for a given number of molecules) the larger the volume the smaller this correction becomes.

Another assumption is that the molecules are of negligible size, so that a molecule such as $D$ colliding with another $E$ can be regarded as indistinguishable from a

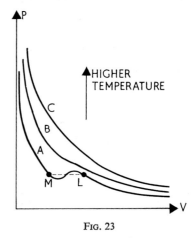

Fig. 22

single molecule $G$ covering the whole distance to the wall. Clearly, when we considered the time taken between collisions with the walls, we should have allowed for the fact that molecules have finite size, and that the distance travelled by molecules $D$ and $E$ is less than it would have been had they been infinitesimally small. This principle is well-known to drivers of shunting engines. Since we measure volume of the container and pressure at its walls, both factors must be corrected, and Van der Waals' equation of state is of the form

$$\left(P + \frac{a}{V^2}\right)\left(V - b\right) = RT$$

where $b$ corrects for the volume error. Although these corrections are small for gases at room temperature, they become important as the liquid phase is approached. In

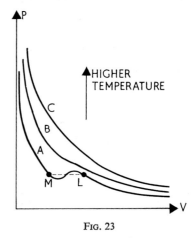

Fig. 23

particular, plotting $P$ versus $V$ for low temperatures gives a curve such as A in Fig. 23, which shows (in contrast to the approximately inverse relationship of curve C) a region over which pressure would be constrained to decrease as the volume decreases. In fact the broken line from L to M is traversed, as part of the sample passes into the liquid phase, and the remainder continues to obey the equation of state. Van der Waal's equation (and other similar empirical equations) also indicates the existence of a critical temperature (for curve B) above which the liquid phase is not entered. For curve B the unstable section just does not occur.

There are several versions of the equation of state for real gases. Some are similar to Van der Waals' equation in that the meaning of the correction terms are argued, and some (such as the 'virial' equations) are basically power-series approximations.

The distinction between gases and vapours, which is related to the critical isothermal curve (B), is taken up later in this chapter.

## Specific Heats of Gases

The definition of specific heat of a solid or liquid as the energy required to raise the temperature of unit mass by one degree presents little conceptual difficulty. When energy is absorbed it is shared among the molecules, and we can expect to account fully for the energy supplied. Some will be manifested by an increase of kinetic energy of motion of the molecules, and some may cause increase in rotational or vibrational energy in molecules more complex than those of the ideal gas.

Suppose that a sample of matter is totally enclosed in a container, so that as the sample expands it must push back the restraining walls of the container. Some of the energy supplied is expended in deforming the container, so less energy is available to be taken up by the sample. Consequently, even when allowance has been made for raising the temperature of the container, more energy is needed to raise the temperature of the sample than would have been required had the expansion not occurred. Now it is important to take into account external constraints. Depending on the circumstances, heating a gas sample may involve anything between the two extremes of complete freedom to expand and complete restraint. It is obviously unsatisfactory to have an infinite number of answers to the question 'what is the specific heat of this gas?', so we define two specific heats corresponding to the two extreme cases.

The specific heat at constant pressure ($c_P$) is the energy required to raise the temperature of unit mass of gas by one degree, expansion being permitted under conditions of constant pressure. This energy is therefore shared between the 'internal' process of raising the energy of the gas molecules and the process of forcing back whatever surfaces are maintaining the constant pressure environment. For unit mass and unit temperature rise we may express this as

$$c_P = \text{Energy gained by gas molecules} + P\Delta V$$

where $\Delta V$ = increase of volume

and $P$ = maintained pressure (constant).

The specific heat at constant volume ($c_v$) is the energy required to produce unit temperature rise in unit mass when the volume is not allowed to increase. Here the container is not pushed back, so

$$c_v = \text{Energy gained by gas molecules}$$

Since the temperature rise and the number of molecules are the same for both cases, the internal energy (that taken up by the gas) is the same, so we have

$$c_p = c_v + P\Delta V$$

This accords with our understanding that whatever energy is demanded by the process of expansion against constraint is not available for the gas molecules. It remains only to assess this energy deficit. For a perfect gas, a unit mass will have the equation of state

$$PV = R_1 T$$

where $R_1$ is the gas constant for the unit mass concerned. If the pressure remains at $P$ and the temperature is raised to $T + 1$ the volume will be given by

$$P(V + \Delta V) = R_1(T + 1)$$

so $$P\Delta V = R_1$$

Consequently, the two specific heats are related by

$$c_p = c_v + R_1$$

A practice often met is to use upper-case letter $C$ for the specific heats of a mole sample and lower-case for any true unit mass (such of 1 gram). Using this convention

$$C_p - C_v = R_m \text{ (1 mole)}$$

$$c_p - c_v = R_1 \text{ (any unit of mass)}$$

As always, the advantage of the mole formulation is that $R_m$ is a known constant for any (perfect) gas, and the requirement is that in actual problems all samples specified by mass must be expressed in terms of moles for the gas in question. Note that the specific heats have been defined so far in terms of energy in *mechanical* units. If they are given in terms of thermal units the formulae require correction. For example, if $C_p$ and $C_v$ are expressed in calories per unit mass per unit temperature rise, multiplying by the number of joules per calorie (Joule's equivalent) puts them on the mechanical unit basis. It is, of course, a historical accident that thermal energy was originally measured in terms of raising an arbitrary unit mass of an arbitrarily chosen substance from a starting temperature defined on the Centigrade scale by one degree of that scale. Reasonable as this decision was at the time, one looks forward to a situation where all units are unified and all tabulated parameters for materials are expressed in terms of those units.

## Specific Heat Ratio, $\gamma$

For the perfect monatomic gas, all the energy taken up by the gas (sometimes called 'internal' energy) appears as kinetic energy of translation. If we compare the two formulations of the equation of state for a given sample,

$$PV = \tfrac{1}{3}N_s m v^2$$

$$PV = R_s T$$

we see that the internal energy is

$$N_s(\tfrac{1}{2}mv^2) = \tfrac{3}{2}R_s T$$

The specific heat at constant volume is the energy supplied

to raise the temperature from $T$ to $T+1$, so for a 1 mole sample

$$C_v = \tfrac{3}{2}R_m$$

Combining this with the result

$$C_p = C_v + R_m$$

gives

$$C_p = \tfrac{5}{2}R_m$$

Thus the ratio of $C_p$ to $C_v$ is given by

$$\gamma = \tfrac{5}{3}$$

This value agrees reasonably with measured values for monatomic gases such as helium, but for diatomic gases the value is nearer to 1·4, which leads us to a further distinction between real gases and the perfect gas. It has been supposed that energy interchanges between molecules is restricted to the distribution of kinetic energy, with three degrees of freedom corresponding to purely translatory motion. When vibrational and rotational energy are taken into account we see that only some of the energy taken up when gas is heated at constant volume appears as kinetic energy in the equation of state. This invalidates the result

$$C_v = \tfrac{3}{2}R_m$$

which is seen to be a low estimate. Attempts to relate values of $\gamma$ to models of real gases met with little success until the limitations of classical mechanics stimulated the development of quantum-mechanics. However, it is clear that disparities between the behaviour of real gases and the predictions for perfect gases, both in relation to heat transfer and to the equation of state can be anticipated in terms of the simplifying assumptions we have made.

### Adiabatic and Isothermal Changes

In general, changes of pressure or volume or both are accompanied by both energy transfer and temperature change. It is convenient to consider one factor being fixed. For example, an isothermal change may be approximated by compressing a gas sufficiently slowly to permit the temperature to remain in equilibrium with the surroundings. Under these circumstances the energy supplied by the source of compression is lost to the surroundings. For a perfect gas the equation predicts that the result of decreasing the volume will be an increase of pressure (due to more frequent bombardment of the walls), and for a real gas one of the empirical equations of state can be used to determine the pressure-volume relationships. For an adiabatic change (approximated by sudden volume changes), the energy supplied (in the case of compression) is contained within the sample, and is manifested by a temperature change. Since all three parameters ($PV$ and $T$) are changing, the problem is to find how any pair ($P$ and $V$ for example) vary during the change, since knowing this enables us to find the third by using the equation of state. For example, suppose that a sample of perfect gas initially occupies a volume $V$ at pressure $P$ and temperature $T$, and is allowed to expand suddenly to occupy a larger volume $LV$ ($L > 1$). Because the gas does work against the restraining container or surroundings, its temperature

will be lower. Suppose that the pressure falls to $P_a$ during the adiabatic expansion, and that the new volume is held constant while the gas absorbs energy from the surroundings, and that when the temperature is back to $T$ the pressure has risen to $P_i$ (corresponding to an isothermal change). For a perfect gas, we know that

$$P_i(LV) = PV$$

or

$$P_i = \frac{P}{L}$$

We expect to find that $P_a$ is less than this, and in fact the result is

$$P_a = \frac{P}{L^\gamma}$$

where $\gamma$ (the ratio of specific heats) is greater than unity. This result is established as an exercise in the use of differential calculus in text-books on heat, and is usually expressed as

$$PV^\gamma = \text{constant}$$

for adiabatic changes. It is important to note that this is not in conflict with the statement that $PV$ is constant if the temperature does not change.

### Surface Tension

Cohesive forces between molecules of a liquid may be sufficiently noticeable at surfaces as to give the impression of a 'skin' under tension. Just as pressure is defined as force per unit area perpendicular to a surface within a volume, so by analogy the force per unit length perpendicular to a line within a surface describes surface tension effects. In Fig. 24, we imagine a surface being maintained across a line $AB$ by distributed forces. Those shown may be thought of as preventing the surface on the side $C$ from breaking away. If $AB = l$, the surface tension is defined as

$$\sigma = \frac{F}{l} \ \text{Nm}^{-1}$$

Just as pressure can be thought of in terms of energy change per unit change of volume (joules per m³) as an alternative to force per unit area (newtons per m²), so surface tension may be related to energy per unit area (joules per m²) instead of as newtons per metre.

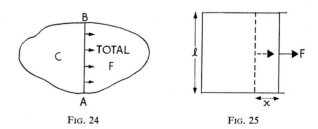

FIG. 24                FIG. 25

If a surface (Fig. 25) is stretched to cover a larger area, the energy required is $Fx$, or $\sigma lx$. Hence

$$\sigma = \frac{\text{Energy change } (Fx)}{\text{Area change } (lx)}$$

This reasoning is extended when surface tension is treated thermodynamically, since on changing its area a surface requires energy changes, just as does a gas when changing its volume. Thus when a surface suddenly enlarges without energy from outside (that is, adiabatically) the temperature drops as the surface energy can increase only at the expense of the internal energy of the liquid.

There are a number of formulae relating surface tension to specific problems. For example, the pressure inside a bubble of gas within a liquid must be such as to maintain its structural integrity. If we imagine the bubble to be halved and fitted with a disk-shaped cap, the thrust on the cap (pressure multiplied by area, or $P\pi r^2$) must exactly equal the total thrust originally maintained by surface tension acting round the periphery.

Consequently

$$P\pi r^2 = \sigma 2\pi r$$

or

$$P = \frac{2\sigma}{r}$$

To this result must be added any hydrostatic pressure due to the bubble being beneath the surface of the liquid.

## Solubility of Gases in Liquids

There is no simple way of anticipating how soluble a given gas will be in a liquid, although in general the more easily liquefied gases tend to be the more soluble. With increase of temperature—and thus of molecular agitation—the general tendency is for a liquid to reject gas molecules, but this is not absolutely invariable, especially where chemical reactions become involved.

The influence of pressure is expressed by *Henry's law*, which states that for most gases, provided that the pressures are not too high nor the temperatures too low, and provided chemical reactions are not involved:

the mass of a gas dissolved by a given volume of solvent, at a given constant temperature, is proportional to the partial pressure of the gas in equilibrium with the solution.

It is useful to envisage this law as stating that the number of gas molecules dissolved into unit volume of the liquid is proportional to the partial pressure. The factor of proportionality is a function of the gas, the liquid, and the temperature.

## Bunsen and Ostwald Solubility Coefficients

These two frequently met measures of solubility are defined here in such a way that the features they share are stressed by identical wording, while differences are indicated by use of italics:

For a given gas dissolved in a given liquid at a stated temperature:

1. The *Bunsen* solubility coefficient ($\alpha$) is the amount dissolved in unit volume of the liquid in equilibrium with the gas at a partial pressure of *one atmosphere*, the amount being expressed as the volume the gas would occupy when at a temperature of 0°C and at a pressure equal to *one atmosphere* (i.e. at standard temperature and pressure, dry—s.t.p.d.).

2. The *Ostwald* solubility coefficient ($\lambda$) is the amount dissolved in unit volume of the liquid in equilibrium with the gas at the partial pressure of the *experiment*, the amount being expressed as the volume the gas would occupy when at the *temperature of the experiment* and at a pressure equal to the *actual partial pressure*.

Examination of these definitions reveals that although they refer to different pressures, within each definition *itself* the same pressure is specified for the act of dissolving and for the assessment of the gas volume. If the gas obeys Henry's law, an increase (for example) of partial pressure will increase the number of gas molecules going into solution, but if it also obeys Boyle's law, the same increase in the pressure to which the volume is referred will compress the gas correspondingly. As a result, for such gases the essential difference between the two coefficients concerns the temperature only, the Bunsen coefficient referring the gas to standard temperature and the Ostwald coefficient leaving it at the actual temperature of the act of solution. For gases which also obey the law of Charles the relationship is:

$$\lambda = \alpha \left(1 + \frac{t}{273}\right)$$

where $t$ is the Centigrade temperature of the solution.

Other facts worth noting are as follows:

(i) The use of s.t.p.d. in the Bunsen coefficient is equivalent, for an ideal gas, to specifying a standard number of molecules per unit volume of gas. Consequently dividing $\alpha$ by 22·4 gives the solubility expressed in moles per litre for 1 atmosphere partial pressure.

(ii) It is advantageous to regard the use of 'atmosphere' in the Bunsen coefficient as merely a form of unit pressure. Naturally, when the gas is dissolved in the presence of water vapour the partial pressure of the gas will be less than the total pressure (as it will if *any* other gas is present), but this does not affect the fact that the definition of the Bunsen coefficient gives the amount dissolved *per 760 mmHg of partial pressure* of the gas concerned. The eventual replacement of all units such as the atmosphere and the mmHg by SI units will do much to remove confusion in such matters.

(iii) Both the Bunsen and the Ostwald coefficients are functions of the actual temperature at which solution takes place. This is because of the nature of matter, and is in no way related to the fact that one of the definitions chooses to assess the volume of dissolved gas at the same temperature, while the other refers the volume to a standard temperature. The Ostwald coefficient takes the stand-point that it may be convenient to assess the volume at the temperature at which the action takes place, while the Bunsen coefficient works in terms of quantity of matter rather than the volume it occupies, but both refer to an act of dissolving which took place at a stated temperature.

## Solubility Units—An Example

Since there are several systems of units in current literature, the following example is given. Taking a value of the Bunsen coefficient for $CO_2$ in plasma as

$$\alpha = 0{\cdot}51 \text{ ml/ml atm}$$

this is seen to be the same as

$$\alpha = 0{\cdot}51 \text{ l/l atm}$$

Expressed in terms of 'volumes percent', this gives

$$\alpha = 51 \text{ ml/100 ml atm}$$

and dividing this by 760 yields

$$\alpha = 0{\cdot}067 \text{ ml/100 ml mmHg}$$

Going back to the 0·51 l/l atm, dividing this by 22·4 gives

$$\alpha = 0{\cdot}023 \text{ mol/l atm}$$
$$= 23 \text{ mmol/l atm}$$
$$= 0{\cdot}030 \text{ mmol/l mmHg}$$

## A Note on Concentration and Related Units

As SI units are more widely introduced a few problems of detail, more apparent than real, will emerge. One concerns the retention of the litre as a volume unit and such derived units as the mole per litre. The twelfth Conférence Générale des Poids et Mesures rescinded the earlier definition of the litre (1·000 028 cubic decimetres) and the word is now again to be employed as a special name for exactly 1 $dm^3$.

Where a particular quantity, such as a concentration, is very well-known in terms of moles per litre (mol l$^{-1}$) there seems little point yet in restating it in moles per cubic metre (mol m$^{-3}$). Although mol dm$^{-3}$ will no doubt appear more often in future, especially for very precise work, medical users may with reason be likely to prefer mol l$^{-1}$. However, when discussing the basic *principles* of a topic such as diffusion, in which volumes, distances and areas all enter into consideration, a certain awkwardness is encountered. This is because if the litre (dm$^3$) is taken as volume, we must either work in relatively unfamiliar length and area (dm and dm$^2$) or tolerate the re-appearance of annoying powers of 10 in equations—a retrograde step. Accordingly, when deriving symbolic *relationships* (such as the diffusion equation) it is better to think in terms of the basic metric units of length, area and volume. Once the necessary results have been achieved it is perfectly reasonable for the particular user to express results in terms of units such as mmol l$^{-1}$ with which he is familiar, and which are quoted in current texts and tables.

## Diffusion of Gases—Some Preliminaries

*Diffusion* is the process whereby a substance spreads through the space available to it, by random molecular motion (as opposed to bulk movement such as is caused by convection). Important situations involving diffusion as a concept include

    1. Redistribution within a simple enclosure, in response to spatial differences of concentration.

    2. Diffusion across membranes or porous barriers, in response to concentration differences between compartments so separated.

*Diffusion-flux* is the name given to the rate of passage (with respect to *time*) of material across unit cross-sectional area perpendicular to the direction of diffusion. For this discussion the symbol $J$ will be used, and the SI unit is the mole-per-second per square metre (mol s$^{-1}$ m$^{-2}$). It is almost invariably better to work in terms of *quantity of material* (in moles), and to convert to volumes if necessary later.

*Concentration* ($c$) is likewise expressed as quantity of the material (gas etc.) per unit volume of space, and will be quoted here in moles per cubic metre (mol m$^{-3}$).

*Concentration gradient* ($dc/dx$) expresses the rate of change of concentration with distance. Here '$x$' is taken as distance measured in the direction in which diffusion is being considered to take place. Since diffusion proceeds from higher to lower concentration regions, the gradient is negative (i.e. 'downwards') in the direction of diffusion. We will express the gradient in terms of moles-per-cubic-metre per metre, or mol m$^{-4}$. In this context 'gradient' is being used in its strict sense—i.e. rate of change with respect to distance.

Five aspects of diffusion will now be considered:

    1. The Fick diffusion equation, and Diffusion Coefficient.
    2. Krogh's diffusion constants.
    3. Diffusion capacity of the lung.
    4. Graham's law.
    5. The more general diffusion equation.

## The Fick Diffusion Equation

This expresses the fact that the rate of diffusion of material across unit area (the diffusion-flux) is greatest where the concentration changes most rapidly with respect to distance, or briefly:

*diffusion-flux is proportional to concentration gradient*

Expressed symbolically this becomes:

$$J = -D\frac{dc}{dx} \text{ mol s}^{-1} \text{ m}^{-2}$$

The negative sign merely formalizes the observation made above, that $dc/dx$ is negative in the direction of diffusion. The factor of proportionality, $D$, is called the *coefficient of diffusion*. It is seen here to mean the diffusion flux caused by unit concentration gradient. The SI unit of $D$ is as follows:

$$\frac{\text{mol s}^{-1} \text{ m}^{-2}}{\text{mol m}^{-4}} \quad \text{or} \quad \text{m}^2 \text{ s}^{-1}$$

Spoken aloud as 'square metres per second' this is an excellent example of a unit which, although impeccably correct, is the result of cancelling out meaningful terms. It also reveals that provided we are consistent in choosing the same measure of quantity in diffusion-flux and concentration gradient (both involving moles, or both involving volumes specified appropriately) the result is independent of this choice. In most current literature, values of $D$ are given in $cm^2\ s^{-1}$ or $cm^2\ min^{-1}$. For example, $CO_2$ diffusing in air has $D$ of the order of $0.14\ cm^2\ s^{-1}$, or $1.4 \times 10^{-5}\ m^2\ s^{-1}$. In water $D$ for $CO_2$ is of the order $15 \times 10^{-4}\ cm^2\ min^{-1}$, or say $0.25 \times 10^{-4}\ cm^2\ s^{-1}$.

## Krogh's Diffusion Constants

For a given gas diffusing through a given liquid, Krogh's diffusion constant ($K$) links the general diffusion coefficient ($D$) with the Bunsen solubility coefficient ($\alpha$). In comparison with

$$J = -D\frac{dc}{dx}$$

we have

$$J = -K\frac{dP}{dx}$$

That is, *Krogh's diffusion constant is the diffusion-flux per unit pressure-gradient.*

To visualize this, consider a region of high partial pressure ($P_1$) and high concentration ($C_1$) separated from a region where they are low ($P_2$ and $C_2$) by distance $x$. From the definition of the Bunsen coefficient, if the concentrations are specified as *volume* of gas (referred to s.t.p.d.) per unit volume of liquid,

$$(C_1 - C_2) = \alpha(P_1 - P_2)$$

where the pressures are expressed in atmospheres for convenience here.

Hence the concentration gradient (numerically, ignoring the sign) is

$$\frac{C_1 - C_2}{x} = \alpha\left(\frac{P_1 - P_2}{x}\right)$$

Generalizing this—that is taking small changes of distance

$$\frac{dc}{dx} = \alpha\frac{dP}{dx}$$

So

$$K = \alpha D$$

At the present the literature does not give tables in SI units, and it may be helpful to interpret values by taking an example. The order of $K$ for $CO_2$ is $7.5 \times 10^{-4}\ cm^2\ min^{-1}\ atm^{-1}$. This actually means that a flux of $7.5 \times 10^{-4}$ ml of gas (referred to s.t.p.d.) crosses each square centimetre in a minute, given a pressure gradient of one atmosphere per centimetre. Now $D$ is given as of the order of $15 \times 10^{-4}\ cm^2\ min^{-1}$, and $\alpha$ as $0.5$ ml/ml atm, so the product $D\alpha$ is $7.5 \times 10^{-4}\ cm^2\ min^{-1}\ atm^{-1}$.

## Diffusion Capacity of the Lung

A cautionary observation on the use of the word 'gradient' is desirable here. Even in everyday English the word has the connotation of a ratio—the ratio of height climbed to distance travelled. Similarly in general scientific use, ratios are almost invariably implied, and we meet potential gradient (volts per metre), temperature gradient (kelvins per metre) as well as velocity gradient (as in viscosity). In this section, concentration gradient and pressure gradient have been used in their strict scientific sense. However, in medicine there are occasions when the word is used somewhat more loosely—it being assumed that the context is clear to workers in the particular field. One such example is met is the common definition of *diffusion capacity of the lung* as:

$$\frac{\text{net rate of gas transfer (ml min}^{-1})}{\text{partial pressure 'gradient' (mmHg)}}$$

The denominator is, of course, a pressure *difference*. Naturally a pressure gradient does exist across the alveolar membrane, but this concerns the diffusion coefficient of the membrane per se.

It will be observed that diffusion capacity is a measure of a flow-type 'effect' per unit driving 'cause'. There are other scientific quantities of this nature, the best known of which is the electrical *conductance* of a *specimen* of conducting material. This is given by

$$\text{conductance} = \frac{\text{current flow (amperes)}}{\text{potential }\textit{difference}\text{ (volts)}}$$

and is the reciprocal of resistance. It should also be noted that the electrical quantity

$$\frac{\text{current density (amperes per square metre)}}{\text{potential }\textit{gradient}\text{ (volts per metre)}}$$

also exists, and is called the *conductivity* of a *material*. This is analogous to diffusion coefficient.

## Graham's Law of Gaseous Diffusion

This states that the rates at which different gases diffuse is *inversely proportional to the square-roots of their molecular masses*, other factors being kept constant. This is easily understood by imagining two different gases in identical environments. Being at the same temperature, their mean molecular kinetic energies will be the same. As a result, the product of molecular mass and the square of the velocity will be the same for 'average' molecules in both gases. Hence, in general, the velocities of the molecules will be inversely proportional to the square-roots of their masses and it is molecular velocity which is primarily involved in diffusion processes.

## The More General Diffusion Equation

The simplest diffusion processes involve dynamic equilibrium, or steady-state conditions. In these, although concentrations vary with distance, continuous withdrawal of molecules (at 'sinks') and replacement (at 'sources') accounts for concentrations not altering with respect to *time*. More generally, concentration may be a function of both position and time. This can happen in quite simple situations, such as when a bolus of material diffuses into the available space. It also happens during the 'transient' phases leading up to or following periods of dynamic equilibrium.

The more general situation can be visualized in the following way. If a small cube of space is imagined with the diffusing gas flowing into one face and out of the other, then if the flux ($J$, in mol s$^{-1}$ m$^{-2}$) is larger over the 'down-stream' face (further in the $x$-direction) than over the opposite face, this would result in a net loss within the cube. In other words, a region of falling concentration is characterized by a (spatial) rise of flux. In fact, if the rate of change of flux with respect to distance is written as $\partial J/\partial x$ and if the small cube has sides of height $h$, the increase of flux at the downstream face compared with the upstream face will be the flux gradient $\partial J/\partial x$ multiplied by $h$. The net rate of loss of gas (bearing in mind that the faces have areas $h^2$) will therefore be

$$\frac{\partial J}{\partial x} \cdot h^3$$

Dividing this by the volume of the small cube gives the rate of fall of concentration, so

$$\frac{\partial c}{\partial t} = -\frac{\partial J}{\partial x}$$

Readers who are unfamiliar with these symbols may find it helps to consider the units. Expressing concentration as mol m$^{-3}$, its rate of change with respect to time will be in mol m$^{-3}$ s$^{-1}$. Corresponding to this, if flux $J$ is expressed in mol s$^{-1}$ m$^{-2}$, its spatial rate of change is in mol s$^{-1}$ m$^{-3}$ also.

Fick diffusion equation, now using partial differential notation to be more general, gives

$$J = -D\frac{\partial c}{\partial x}$$

Taking the rate of change with respect to $x$,

$$\frac{\partial J}{\partial x} = -D\frac{\partial}{\partial x}\left(\frac{\partial c}{\partial x}\right)$$

or

$$\frac{\partial c}{\partial t} = D\frac{\partial^2 c}{\partial x^2}$$

This is known as the diffusion equation for one dimension (i.e. diffusion occurs in the $x$-direction only) It is met as the basis for models of diffusion processes across relatively flat membranes. More complicated versions exist for two- and three-dimensional problems, but the complications are those of mathematical formulation rather than concept.

It is interesting to see how a simple interpretation can be put on what might, to some readers, seem a formidable mathematical equation. For example, suppose that the concentration falls *linearly* with $x$, so that $\partial c/\partial x$ is *constant*. Then the spatial rate of change of $\partial c/\partial x$, or $\partial^2 c/\partial x^2$, will be zero. The diffusion equation shows therefore that the time-rate of change of concentration is zero. This simply means that the region is one steady-state, with diffusion giving rise to gas flow with no net build-up or decay at that point. In contrast, if the concentration gradient ($\partial c/\partial x$) *itself* changes along the stream, the region must be one where the concentration is growing or decaying.

## Vapours, Evaporation and Saturation Vapour Pressure

Reference has already been made, under the heading of the Gas Laws for real gases, to the *critical temperature* of a substance. This is the temperature above which the substance cannot be liquefied by compression. Although the terms 'gas' and 'vapour' are sometimes used as if interchangeable, strictly speaking a substance is a gas when at a temperature above its critical value. Thus although oxygen is a gas at room temperatures, water does not become a true gas until above 400°C, and iron becomes one within the Sun's atmosphere.

Now it is possible for molecules to leave the surface of a liquid (evaporation) or a solid (sublimation) at temperatures below the critical value. The mechanism is that of random movement, whereby the more energetic molecules are able to break away from the attraction of those molecules they leave behind. Molecules so penetrating beyond the interface constitute what is called a *vapour*—that is, gaseous phase at a temperature below the critical value.

Vapours are encountered in two forms: *saturated* and *unsaturated*. A saturated vapour is one which exists in equilibrium with its own liquid, so that as many molecules are in the act of leaving the liquid surface as are returning to it, both processes being random. In such a situation a pressure is exerted by the vapour which is unique for that substance at that temperature. Thus any attempt to compress the vapour results in molecules returning to the liquid phase so that the same number per unit volume remain in the vapour phase. The pressure measured under these circumstances is called the *Saturation Vapour Pressure* (SVP).

In contrast, in a container having too little of a substance in vapour form for there to be a 'reservoir' of liquid, the vapour is said to be unsaturated and behaves as a gas. In particular, compression at fixed temperature is accompanied by rise of pressure, until the SVP is reached, after which condensation results in the maintenance of this steady pressure.

Another contrast between a saturated vapour and a gas concerns variation of pressure with temperature. For a given mass of gas in a fixed volume, the increase of pressure with temperature is approximately linear. For a saturated vapour, rise of temperature shifts the whole spectrum of energies of the liquid molecules upwards. This results not only in a greater chance of any given molecule having sufficient energy to cross the interface, but increases the number possessing the necessary minimum energy to do so. Figure 26 illustrates the progressively steepening graphs of SVP versus temperature. The upper curve is for a more volatile substance (like ether), and the lower one for a less volatile one (like water). Based on the theoretical work of Clapeyron and Clausius there are empirical equations for these curves for various substances. However these are not particularly easy to manipulate algebraically, but can be simply handled by computers. Tables and graphs of SVP versus temperature are in more general use at the present time.

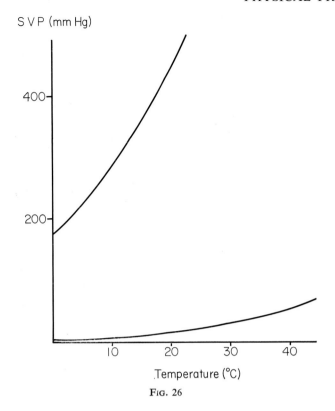

S V P (mm Hg)

Temperature (°C)

FIG. 26

pressure has 'failed' to suppress the establishment of a small local saturated vapour region. It is for this reason that 'Boiling Point' of a liquid is not a uniquely determined temperature, but decreases with reduction of externally maintained pressure. When the pressure maintained at the liquid surface is one atmosphere, the temperature at which boiling occurs is strictly called 'normal boiling point'. In the special case of a liquid boiling against an external pressure due only to its own vapour, saturation is reached for whatever temperature is maintained. It is for this reason that variation of SVP with temperature also gives the variation of boiling point with external pressure. Boiling is merely one situation (with more obvious activity taking place) in which molecules escape across the interface. One well-known aspect of boiling is the need to pressurize cooking-vessels at high altitude in order to reach the necessary temperatures for culinary purposes without losing all the water. An extension of this is the steam sterilizer in which this process is pursued to temperatures above 100°C by pressurizing beyond one atmosphere.

The *latent heat of vaporization* of a substance is the heat energy necessary to convert unit mass from the liquid to the vapour phase at constant temperature. It is usually specified under external pressure conditions of one atmosphere, and so at the normal boiling point of the liquid. The latent heat required is larger if the temperature at which vaporization is accomplished is reduced.

## Mixtures of Gases and Vapours

In practice vapours are often produced in association with gases, such as air. An important example concerns saturated water vapour with air. The contribution to the total pressure made by the saturated vapour is unaffected by the presence of the other gases and (for example) is known to be 47 mmHg for water vapour at 37°C. Thus if a container has saturated water vapour at this temperature, as well as other gases, and if the total pressure is 760 mmHg, only 713 mmHg has to be accounted for by the gases. According to Dalton's Law of Partial pressures the individual contributions due to the various gases (e.g. oxygen, nitrogen, $CO_2$) are in proportion to their relative abundances in that specimen.

## Cooling due to Evaporation

When the more energetic molecules break away from a liquid surface during the process of forming a vapour, this leaves the less energetic ones behind and so lowers the temperature of the bulk of liquid remaining. If the molecules that break free are removed from the vicinity, they cease to belong to the liquid sample. This therefore cools until any further heat loss by this mechanism just balances heat replacement from other sources, such as conduction from warmer bodies in contact with the remaining liquid.

## Boiling and Latent Heat of Vaporization

*Boiling* is the process of conversion from the liquid to the vapour phase, in which bubbles of the vapour form before it escapes from the surface. This means that there is a vapour pressure set up which just equals the external pressure, and the bubble formation can be thought of as if the external

## Humidity

When discussing the water-vapour content of a gas, the term *Absolute Humidity* is used to describe the mass of water contained in unit volume of the gas. For a given temperature, there is a maximum mass of water that can be contained in unit volume of gas, for which the number of molecules of water just account for the known SVP for water at that temperature. For example, the SVP of water at body temperature (37°C) is known to be 47 mmHg, corresponding to an actual content of approximately 50 grams per cubic metre. The term *Relative Humidity* is used to describe the ratio

$$\frac{\text{Actual (absolute) Humidity}}{\text{Maximum possible humidity at that temperature}} \times 100\%$$

Since the partial pressure due to water vapour is proportional to the number of molecules in unit volume, relative humidity is (as a good approximation) the same as the ratio of the actual vapour pressure to the SVP at that temperature. For example, a sample of air at 20°C (at which SVP is 18 mmHg) having a water vapour pressure of 7·2 mmHg has a relative humidity of

$$\frac{7\cdot2}{18} \times 100\% \quad \text{or} \quad 40\%$$

If this specimen were raised to 37°C without water vapour being added, then to a good approximation the relative humidity would fall to

$$\frac{7\cdot2}{47} \times 100\% \quad \text{or} \quad 15\cdot3\%$$

Even if the original specimen had been fully saturated at the lower temperature (i.e. holding $2\frac{1}{2}$ times as much water) at the higher temperature the relative humidity would have only been about 38%.

The converse of this effect is seen when air is cooled and its relative humidity rises. For a sample air having a given water content the temperature to which it can fall before condensation takes place is called the *Dew Point*. This is therefore the temperature at which the actual vapour pressure becomes equal to the SVP. Figure 27 illustrates an example for which the vapour pressure is 18 mmHg, the dew point thus being 20°C.

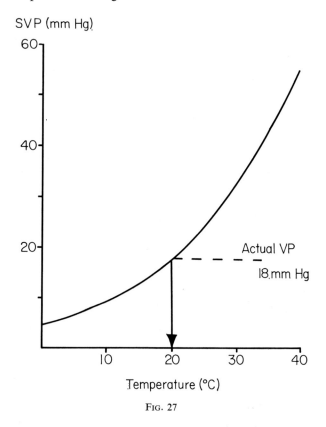

FIG. 27

### Viscosity

On an ideal motorway all vehicles would remain in lane, and for each lane there would be a speed exactly maintained by vehicles in that lane. This situation would be spoiled by vehicles drifting laterally, because (even discounting catastrophes) a mutual 'drag' effect would increase the resistance to flow of traffic. In a similar way, in fluid flow where velocity differentials occur laterally to the direction of flow (compare with adjacent traffic lanes), random lateral movements of particles inject 'out of lane' miscreants, resulting in friction between layers. In passing, it is appropriate that this effect is known as an example of 'transport' phenomena—those in which an effect is transported across a medium by motion of the particles.

Because of adhesion between fluid and the walls of tubes and other channels, it is common to find velocities varying from zero at walls towards maxima away from them. For a channel of a given size and shape there is, for any given fluid,

an upper limit of flow up to which 'lane discipline' is sufficiently well maintained, and motion proceeds as if in layers, constituting *lamina* (streamline) flow. Beyond such limits the flow is *turbulent*, and the lateral motions become macroscopic, producing eddies and swirling paths.

### Newton's Law of Viscous Flow

For lamina flow the viscous drag between two adjacent layers having contact area $A$ is a force $F$ which increases in proportion to $A$. If the symbol $v$ denotes the velocity within a given layer, we are concerned with the lateral velocity gradient, or the rate at which $v$ changes per unit distance across the layers. Denoting distance measured laterally by $s$ (side-ways), the velocity gradient is written as $dv/ds$. To a good approximation $F$ is found to be proportional to this, so

$$F = \eta A \frac{dv}{ds}$$

where $\eta$ is a constant of proportionality for a given fluid. Often known in brief as the *viscosity*, its full name is the *coefficient of dynamic viscosity*. Examination of the defining equation shows that the meaning of $\eta$ is the force per unit area tangential to the motion, per unit lateral velocity gradient.

Another way of expressing Newton's law of viscous flow is

$$\frac{F}{A} = \eta \frac{dv}{ds}$$

which is seen to be an example of the extremely common form

$$\text{Effect} = \text{Constant} \times \text{Cause}$$

The cause, which we have called lateral velocity gradient is often referred to as the *shear rate*. The effect, which is the tangential force per unit contact area, is called the *shear stress*.

### Units of Dynamic Viscosity

In SI units the shear rate is measured in metres per second (axially) per metre (laterally), or $\text{m s}^{-1}\text{ m}^{-1}$. Expressed as $\text{s}^{-1}$ ('per second') this is correct, but scarcely informative. However it follows that the unit of dynamic viscosity is the newton of force divided by the square metre and then divided by 'per second', which reduces to newton seconds per square metre ($\text{N s m}^{-2}$). The corresponding CGS unit is the dyne second per square centimetre ($\text{dyn s cm}^{-2}$), better known as the poise (P) after Poiseuille. Since the dyne is one-hundred-thousandth of a newton and the square centimetre is one-ten-thousandth of a square metre,

$$1 \text{ P} = 0\cdot1 \text{ N s m}^{-2}$$

### Kinematic Viscosity

In many circumstances the density of a fluid must be considered, as well as its viscosity. Examples include flow involving gravitational 'pressure heads' and flow in which accelerations take place. In both cases density enters into the problem since both weight and inertial opposition to acceleration are mass-dependent. In the mathematics of such studies it is found convenient to normalize equations encountered, by dividing throughout by the density and so reducing all relationships to a standard density basis.

*The coefficient of kinematic viscosity* is simply the ratio of the dynamic viscosity to the density of the fluid, or

$$\nu = \frac{\eta}{\rho}$$

The act of dividing N s m$^{-2}$ by kg m$^{-3}$ eventually yields the SI unit as the m$^2$ s$^{-1}$. The CGS unit is called the stokes (St).

Another important application of this ratio concerns turbulent flow. It is not surprising to find that increase of dynamic viscosity tends to reduce turbulence by damping out any disturbances in the flow pattern. The opposite effect is found when the density is increased. This is because any swirling disturbances that are set up tend to persist more when more dense material is involved, for the denser the material is, the more it is able to retain energy within eddies.

### Reynold's Number (Re)

For a fluid flowing in a channel an empirical relationship is found to link the average velocity ($\bar{V}$) above which flow becomes turbulent, with the kinematic viscosity and with the dimensions of the channel. In particular, for a cylindrical tube of diameter $D$ the *dimensionless* number

$$Re = \frac{D\bar{V}}{\nu}$$

is found to have to be in excess of 2000 for turbulence to occur. In this context 'average' velocity means the average across the tube, not the time-average. To interpret this, imagine turbulence just about to occur. An increase of velocity will obviously promote turbulence, and we have already argued that, as far as irregular motion is concerned it is the ratio known as kinematic viscosity which is important. An increase in $D$ is able to promote turbulence simply by removing lateral constraints. However it is very important to examine this from another point of view, since in medicine problems arise in which it is not so much that a given average velocity is involved, but that a given flow has to be considered within vessels of varying diameters.

Re-casting Reynold's number in terms of volume flow ($\dot{Q}$) and also in terms of the data most likely to be well-known gives:

$$Re = \frac{4\rho\dot{Q}}{\pi D\eta}$$

This states that, for a *given flow rate*, turbulence is most likely to occur for dense fluids of low dynamic viscosity in narrow tubes. Naturally this does not contradict the implication suggested by the first formulation of *Re*, that for a given average *velocity* turbulence is more likely if the diameter is large. An example makes this clear: with a *given volumetric flow*, halving the diameter reduces the cross-section area of the vessel four-fold. This quadruples the average velocity, so whereas the $D$ in the numerator of $D\bar{V}/\nu$ is halved, this is more than offset by quadrupling the $\bar{V}$. This is an example of the need for care when interpreting

a formula: it is essential that the correct conditions are imposed when judging the effects of various terms.

### Non-newtonian Fluids

Gases and simple liquids are often quoted as being 'newtonian' fluids. This means that for them Newton's law of viscous flow holds. This in turn implies that their dynamic viscosities ($\eta$) are not affected by the motion itself, and can be taken as constants. *Non-newtonian* fluids do not obey this law because, for them, $\eta$ alters as the shear rate alters. Although blood is a non-newtonian fluid, for much work it is treated as sufficiently near newtonian to simplify models of blood flow, for which there are more than enough complications anyway.

### Poiseuille's Equation

For lamina flow of a newtonian fluid along a cylindrical tube of radius R, the Poiseuille equation gives the *volume flow* as:

$$\dot{Q} = \frac{\pi}{8} \cdot \frac{P}{L} \cdot \frac{R^4}{\eta}$$

Here $P$ is the pressure drop along a length $L$ of tube, so the term $P/L$ means the *axial pressure gradient*. Setting aside the purely numerical term $\pi/8$, the volume flow depends:

1. Directly on the pressure gradient, which may reasonably be thought of as the *cause*.
2. Inversely on the viscosity. This is reasonable, since for a given geometry and velocities, increase of viscosity means increased drag.
3. On the fourth power of the radius.

This third factor ($R^4$) is very significant, as can be seen by imagining a tube to be replaced by one of half the radius. This would result in considerable increase of opposition to flow, since $R^4$ would be reduced sixteen-fold. This will be elaborated later.

### Velocity Profile

Fluid velocity varies from zero at walls towards maxima away from them. It is found experimentally, and can be confirmed mathematically, that although velocity is greatest down the centre of a tube, it varies most rapidly

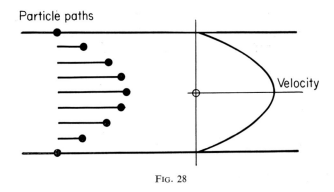

Particle paths

Velocity

FIG. 28

near the walls. A graph of velocity at various positions, versus distance from the axis of a cylindrical tube is shown in Fig. 28, superimposed on a diagram showing representative particle paths over unit time. For lamina flow of a newtonian fluid driven by a *steady* pressure gradient, this shape is found to be a *parabola*. From our point of view it is important that the velocity falls off most rapidly as the wall is approached. However, although the actual velocities are greatest near the centre, the edges are not to be neglected in assessment of total flow, since the low velocities are offset by the relatively larger circumferences than near the central core. Analysis shows that the average velocity is exactly half the maximum, in the parabolic profile case. In this context 'average' velocity $\bar{V}$ means that velocity which, had it applied all across the tube, would have given the same flow as actually occurs. In fact it is found that:

$$\text{Maximum velocity} = \frac{P}{4L\eta} \cdot R^2$$

$$\text{Average velocity} = \frac{P}{8L\eta} \cdot R^2$$

It follows that

$$\dot{Q} = \bar{V} \cdot \pi R^2$$
$$= \frac{\pi P R^4}{8L\eta}$$

Although Poiseuille's equation is a useful qualitative guide, more complicated velocity profiles are met with alternating flows. These are due to acceleration and deceleration effects which, being different between the different velocity layers, break up the simple pattern with overshoot and under-shoot effects. With *turbulent* flows the relatively large-scale lateral movements tend to even out the flow profile. The flatter profiles resulting are reminiscent of toothpaste coming from a tube. The higher opposition to flow associated with turbulent flow is related to the very steep velocity profiles, or high shear rates, near the vessel walls.

### Qualitative Appreciation of Poiseuille's Equation

Returning to Poiseuille's equation, it is instructive to explore the dependence on the fourth power of the radius, by taking a simple example. Consider the consequences of choosing a *smaller* tube (say by halving $R$), while increasing the pressure to maintain the same volume flow. The steps in the argument are:

1. Halving the radius reduces the cross-section area to a quarter, and so enforces a *four-fold* increase in all velocities if the same flow is maintained.
2. Because of the smaller radius, the lateral changes of these velocities are cramped into half the space. Consequently the velocity gradients are increased *eight-fold*.
3. Considering the moving mass of fluid as a whole, there is only a quarter of the area over which the applied pressure can develop the thrust required to move the fluid past the vessel wall. At first sight this would seem to worsen the situation a further four times, requiring a 32-fold increase of pressure.

4. However, because the actual surface area of wall in contact with the fluid is halved (halving the radius halves the circumference), the necessary increase of pressure is not 32-fold but is *16-fold* as predicted by the equation.

This is of considerable importance, not only in the flow of fluids in vessels but also in the recording of remote pressures, such as blood-pressures monitored along catheters. This matter is elaborated in the chapter on Transducers for the Measurement of Pressure.

### Resistance of a Tube

For a given length of circular tube passing steadily flowing newtonian fluid without turbulence, Poiseuille's equation can be written as:

$$\frac{\text{Pressure}}{\text{Flow}} = \frac{8L\eta}{\pi R^4}$$

$$= \text{Constant}$$

By analogy with Ohm's law for the relationship between potential difference and current (electric flow), as is discussed in the next chapter, it is convenient to think of this constant as the resistance of the given tube to flow of the stated fluid.

Where turbulence is set up, either due to generally increased flow or to localized eddies at discontinuities, the resistance ceases to be constant. As with the description of other non-linear effects, various algebraic relationships are met for particular fluids over different flow ranges for a variety of tubes, orifices etc. These are essentially no more than the result of fitting power-series and other algebraic equations to empirical data. One of the simplest is for fully turbulent gas flow through a pipe, for which the resistance is itself roughly proportional to flow. This may be met as:

$$\text{Pressure} = \text{Constant} \times \text{Flow}^2$$

or as

$$\text{Flow} \propto \sqrt{\text{Pressure}}$$

All such empirical approximations are to be regarded as being restricted to known and established situations, and not taken as universal.

### Summary

It has been the object of this chapter to encourage the anaesthetist revising basic science to translate formulae into words. It is strongly recommended that this exercise is carried out initially with texts with which he is already familiar, and which will at some time have provided him with the structure of the subject.

As an example of clarity of text and as a valuable keystone for further study, *Physical Chemistry*, by Gucker and Seifert (English Universities Press Ltd.) is particularly recommended.

# CHAPTER 2

# PHYSICAL PRINCIPLES PART II: Electrical Quantities

## D. STRICKLAND

This chapter has two objectives. The first is to extend the list of physical quantities dealt with in the previous chapter by introducing some of the more useful electrical and magnetic quantities and their associated units. As concepts related to this aspect of science are discussed, important relationships will be detected between electrical quantities, which are analogous to relationships between the more familiar mechanical ones. For example, it is much easier to understand inductive reactance when the underlying concept is recognized as strictly analogous to the opposition experienced when shaking a medicine-ball.

The second objective is to discuss topics, such as linearity, distortion and equivalent circuits, which are of particular use in the understanding of electrical circuits. Electrical and communications engineers have enjoyed a considerable advantage in the past, because their subjects lend themselves to greatly simplifying concepts which allow very rapid assessment of the essentials of apparently complex devices and systems. Because of the strong analogous relationships between the various branches of science, these concepts, theorems and problem-solving stratagems are not restricted to electrical circuits but are of considerable general interest.

## Electric Charge

The earliest observations on the effects of electricity involved the production of what was called 'static electricity' by friction, as when two materials (such as glass and silk) are rubbed together. It was found that two pieces of glass so treated then repelled one another, as did two pieces of silk. In contrast, it was found that a piece of the glass and a piece of the silk attracted one another. It was therefore conceived that these materials had been 'charged' by something which existed in two distinct forms. These ideas were expressed by saying that 'like charges (of electricity) repel one another' and 'unlike charges attract one another.' It only remained to observe that when two bodies oppositely charged come together they could become inert, to justify calling the two forms *positive* and *negative*, implying that they neutralize one anothers' effects. As to which should be called positive—the decision was essentially as arbitrary as the decision of the British to drive on the left. The subsequently discovered *electron* was found to fall into the 'negative' category, while the atomic nuclei were found to be 'positive.'

The quantity of electricity associated with a body is called the *electric charge*. Various units have been defined, but we are here concerned with the coulomb (C). It is advantageous as an interim measure to regard electric charge as basic, and for the moment we will picture the coulomb in terms of the electric charge associated with some measurable amount of ionized material. In fact, an early definition took it as the charge associated with the electrolytic deposition of 0·001118 grams of silver from silver nitrate solution.

## Electric Current

When sources of *moving* electric charge were developed, by analogy with the current of a flowing fluid (litres per minute, or more appropriately cubic metres per second) *electric current* was defined as the rate of passage of electric charge. On this basis we would expect current to be measured in *coulombs per second* ($Cs^{-1}$). The urges to abbreviate and to celebrate tend to obscure the obvious by calling this unit the ampere (1 A = 1 $Cs^{-1}$).

Using the familiar symbols, $Q$ for charge and $I$ for current, we see that a steady current of $I$ amperes (coulombs per second) flowing for $t$ seconds involves the passage of $Q$ coulombs, given by

$$Q = It$$

For various reasons, it has been decided to take the ampere as the SI defined unit, and to regard the coulomb as the charge deposited when one ampere flows for one second.

## Electromotive Force (EMF)

All sources of electric current (cells, generators, etc.) are capable of creating at their terminals (*see* A, B in Fig. 1) excess positive and excess negative charge: that is, they cause separation of charges in otherwise neutral material. When a conducting device (such as a lamp, shown symbolically in the figure) is connected between the terminals, it is the attraction between opposite charges which causes the flow of current. In describing the 'strength' of a pump we have already seen that an important interpretation of pressure is work done per unit quantity of fluid driven by the pump. By analogy the 'strength' (electromotive force) of an electrical generator is the work done when it drives unit quantity of electric charge round an external circuit. For example if in driving 1 coulomb the source does 240 joules of work, we say that the EMF is 240 joules per coulomb. The joule per coulomb is abbreviated to the volt (1 V = 1 $JC^{-1}$), but it is worth thinking in terms of what it means. Thus a 6 volt battery of cells will do 6 joules of work with every coulomb passed, just as a 6 newton per square metre pressure source does 6 joules of work for each cubic metre of fluid pumped.

## 'Conventional' Current Flow

Although both positive and negative charge carriers (ions) can exist in electrolytes and ionized gases, in metals only the loosely bound outer electrons are free to move. Consequently, the flow of electricity may involve the passage of different charges moving in opposite directions in

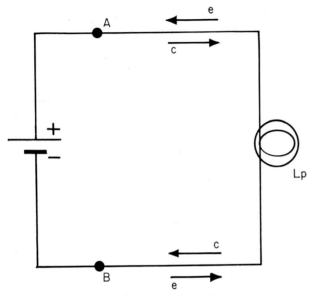

FIG. 1. Note conventional symbol for a cell and for a lamp. Electron flow is indicated by arrows e, conventional current by arrows c.

some situations, while in the system of Fig. 2 charges of one sign only (electrons) flow away from the electron-repelling electrode B towards the positive electrode A. Before the discovery of electrons it was decided *quite arbitrarily* (but of course consistently) to label electrodes positive and negative, and it was postulated that the (unseen) electric current flowed from the one called positive to the one called negative. For many applications it is irrelevant which way the

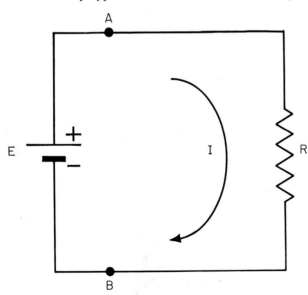

FIG. 2. The zig-zag symbol represents any circuit element offering resistance to current. *I* indicates conventional sense of current.

actual charge carriers flow, and it is very common to encounter a diagram such as Fig. 2 in which *R* represents some circuit element or device in which it is of academic interest whether negative or positive ions or both are involved.

## Resistance to Flow of Electricity

When electrons or ions move through a material under the action of an electric 'field' (region of attraction one way and repulsion the other for a given charged particle), collisions occur. This has two important consequences:

    1. The material becomes heated as energy is imparted to the molecules affected.
    2. These collisions constitute resistance to the flow of current.

Such resistance is analogous to the resistance of an airway to the extent that it imposes a restriction on the current that can be forced through by a given EMF. In his famous experiments Ohm quantified the concept of resistance and we would say that a resistance of *R* units restricts the current from a source of EMF *E* volts to *I* amperes, where

$$I = \frac{E}{R}$$

The unit of *R* is thus the volt per ampere, which is abbreviated to the Ohm. ($1 \; \Omega = 1 \; VA^{-1}$).

## Potential Differences

In an anaesthetic circuit pressure differences exist between various points due to the resistances to flow caused by tubing, bends, joints, etc. Similarly no electrical circuit consists of a single resistance, since there is always at least the 'internal' resistance of the source, due to material imperfections. Consequently electrical circuits consist of at least two parts, such as *r* and *R* in Fig. 3, which

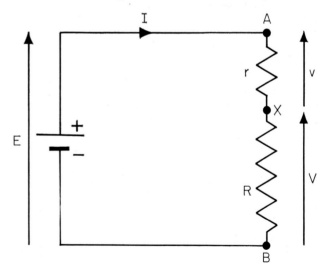

FIG. 3. The addition of potential differences *v* and *V* to equal the applied EMF *E*, following from the scalar nature of energy.

has two elements in series. For example, *R* might represent an obvious 'load,' such as a lamp and *r* might represent the internal resistance of the source.

For every coulomb of charge passing between A and B, the work done is $E$ joules, because the EMF is $E$ joules per coulomb. Some of this is dissipated as heat in $R$ and the rest within $r$. The number of joules per coulomb dissipated between X and B is called the potential difference ($V$ volts), or the potential of X relative to B. This compares directly with the pressure difference between two points in a fluid flow system. Ohm showed that this potential difference is

$$V = I R$$

and we similarly find that for AX

$$v = Ir$$

Now energy is not only conserved, but is scalar, so the total energy delivered by the source for each coulomb passed, must equal the sum of the energies dissipated in the circuit. For this reason we find that potential differences in series are simply additive, or

$$E = V + v$$

It therefore follows that

$$E = I(R + r)$$

In words, this means that resistances in series are additive.

The analogy between electrical and fluid resistances is important. A resistive circuit element is one which dissipates energy when flow takes place, and it is this energy dissipated, for unit charge passed, that we call potential difference in the electrical case. In fluid systems this corresponds to pressure difference, given by energy dissipated per unit volume passed.

**Power Related to Electric Current**

By definition of the volt (joule per coulomb), if $Q$ coulombs pass between terminals $X$ and $B$ across which a potential difference of $V$ volts exists, $VQ$ joules of work is done. If it takes $t$ seconds to do this, the power (rate of doing work) is

$$W = VQ/t \text{ joules per second}$$

or $\qquad W = VI \text{ watts}$

It is mainly due to the non-coherent units of pressure and flow encountered in medicine that this simple relationship is better known than its fluid flow counterpart:

$$\text{Power} = \text{Pressure difference} \times \text{Flow}$$

For example a flow of 6 litres per minute ($10^{-4}$ cubic metres per second) occurring with a pressure difference of 12 kNm$^{-2}$ (90 mmHg) requires the pump to develop a power of

$$W = 12\,000 \times 10^{-4}$$
$$= 1\cdot2 \text{ watts}$$

**Electrical Components other than Resistance**

In mechanical systems we encounter four common classes of component:

1. *Dissipative components* such as frictional resistance.
2. *Potential energy storage components* such as springs.

3. *Kinetic energy storage component* such as flywheels, and

4. Components which *transform*, or adjust the level of mechanical thrusts and motions, such as levers and gears.

Similarly in electrical circuits we meet

1. *Resistive* elements which dissipate energy.
2. *Capacitors* which store energy electrostatically.
3. *Inductors* which store energy electromagnetically, and
4. *Transformers* which adjust levels of voltage and current.

The concepts underlying these are important, not only for the understanding of electrical apparatus, but also for appreciating the problems of electrical safety and reduction of electrical interference (*see also* the chapter on the Measurement and Recording of Biological Electrical Potentials).

**Capacitance**

In Fig. 4 $X$ and $Y$ represent two conducting bodies separated from one another by an insulating (or dielectric) gap, and connected to a source of EMF. Because like charges repel one another, some of the excess electrons at terminal B avail themselves of the opportunity to spread out on Y, *temporarily* constituting a current in YB. Although these electrons are unable to cross the gap, actually their arrival repels some electrons from $X$, and these electrons are attracted to the positive terminal A anyway. Consequently a transient current flows, conventionally along AX and YB, completing the circuit. This leaves the pair XY in a 'charged' state, manifested in two ways:

1. A potential difference $V$ is associated with the separated charges: this rises to equal the EMF $E$, at which point the process stops.
2. An 'electric field'—a region in which attraction in a specific direction is experienced by any charged body— is set up in the gap.

If, during the transient flow, $Q$ coulombs of negative charge arrive at Y and leave X (as shown by the excess positive charge $+Q$ remaining), it is found that the charge $Q$ is proportional to the potential difference $V$, or

$$Q = CV$$

The factor of proportionality $C$ is constant for a given pair of conducting bodies XY. It is the charge in coulombs established per volt of potential difference set up. This is reminiscent of compliance, defined as volume taken up per unit change of pressure difference set up, and $C$ is known as the Capacitance of the system. The unit is essentially the coulomb (of charge stored) per volt (of potential difference necessarily set up), and is abbreviated to the farad, so

$$1 \text{ F} = 1 \text{ coulomb per volt}$$

**Aspects of Capacitance**

Although some applications of capacitance involve the energy storage aspect, it is more important that during transient conditions and in cases where sources of EMF are alternating, the action across the insulated gap discussed above can give rise to current flow *without* direct connection. This is deliberately used in electrical circuits involving capacitors (devices made to exhibit known capacitance). Such devices have capacitances in the range of picofarads (1 pF = $10^{-12}$ F) to thousands of microfarads.

3. The induction of EMFs, as in electrical generators and transformers.

The magnetic effects near permanent magnets, due to electron movements at molecular level can be thought of similar as to those produced near conductors by the gross movement of electrons. It is the second and third categories

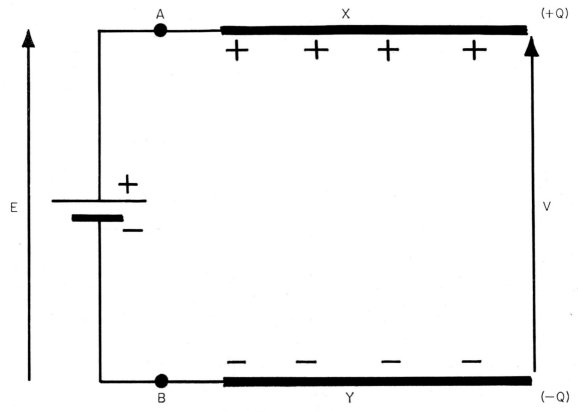

Fig. 4. Charging a capacitor.

However, capacitance can exist between any two separate conducting bodies, such as a patient and an electrical cable, or an anaesthetist and his patient. (This matter is discussed in the chapter on Biological Electrical Potentials.) Three factors determine the capacitance between two bodies. Capacitance increases if the area of the bodies is increased, since this gives more opportunity for the charges to spread. Similarly, decreasing the distance between the bodies intensifies the field and permits more electrons to arrive at one and repel electrons from the other. Finally the introduction of an insulating material, in place of a vacuum or air, can increase capacitance by a factor depending on the material used.

## Some Aspects of Magnetism

Magnetic fields are regions in which certain types of phenomena are observed, including:

1. The attraction and repulsion of magnets and magnetizable pieces of metal.
2. Interaction with current-carrying conductors, as in meters and motors.

of phenomena which are relevant here and to assist in the visualization of these, some aspects of 'magnetic flux' will be recapitulated. Although in the historical development of the subject, magnetic flux came relatively late, our present purposes are better served by taking over this concept as a starting point.

## Magnetic Flux

The phenomena of electromagnetism are visualized—a first step towards explanation—by imagining lines indicating the presence of these phenomena, as illustrated in Fig. 5. Here, within and around both a permanent magnet and a conductor (in the form of turns of wire) carrying current, the closed loops drawn are representative of lines of magnetic flux. In passing, the reason for coiling the conductor is simply to arrange more of it to lie close to the region where the effects are desired to be produced. The term 'flux' suggests that, in the absence of human sensory awareness, early workers supposed that some form of influence (possibly even a substance) actually flowed around magnetic circuits. These lines are drawn so as to be most

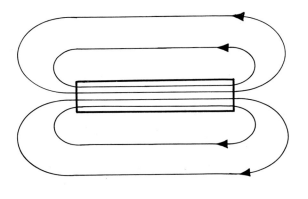 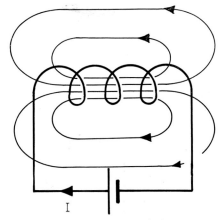

FIG. 5. Magnetic flux due to a bar magnet and due to a current-carrying coil. As far as observed effects are concerned, the source is irrelevant.

densely packed where the observed effects are most pronounced. In addition, at any point the direction associated with these lines coincides with the direction in which a north-seeking pole would be attracted. Of course, these convenient lines are simply an aid to visualization just as are lines of longitude, contour lines and isobars.

### Electromagnetic Induction

Figure 6 represents a conductor AB, either as a single 'turn' or more generally a number ($N$) of turns, lying within a region of magnetic flux. It is found that an EMF can be induced within the conductor if its relationship to the flux is made to vary either by

1. moving the conductor or the magnetic circuit producing the flux, relative to one another, so that a different amount of flux threads (or 'links' with) the conductor, or

2. altering the amount of flux, without moving the conductor or the flux source. The easiest way of doing this is to *produce* the flux by passing current through some other conductor and simply varying this 'magnetizing' current.

Thus if $\phi$ webers of flux link with $N$ turns, and $\phi$ is changing, then the resulting EMF is $N$ multiplied by $d\phi/dt$, in volts. Notice that the observed phenomenon is the appearance of an EMF, and we imagine changing flux linkage to visualize this process, rather as a meteorologist feeling a strong wind might picture this in terms of a region of high isobar density having moved across the weather map.

### Flux Density

Since the packing density of lines of flux is imagined as representing the local concentration of observed effects, we formalize this by defining *flux density* (usual symbol $B$) as the number of flux lines passing through unit cross-sectional area—i.e. per unit area normal to their direction. The unit of flux density is therefore the weber per square metre, abbreviated to the *tesla*:

$$1 \text{ T} = 1 \text{ Wb m}^{-2}$$

### The Motor Effect and the Moving Coil Meter

Figure 7 illustrates a section of a conductor carrying a current $I$ amperes, and lying perpendicular to magnetic flux

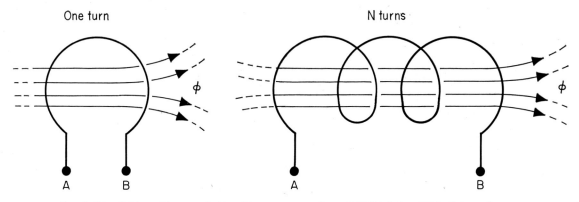

One turn        N turns

FIG. 6. Flux linking with a conductor with one or more 'turns.' EMF is induced if the linkage *changes*.

Whatever the mechanism, it is found that *the more rapid the change, the larger is the EMF.*

Induction of an EMF in this way enables us to quantify magnetic flux. The unit is the weber (Wb), and it is defined so that flux linkage changing at the *rate* of 1 weber *per second* (in one turn) causes an EMF of 1 volt to appear.

of density $B$ teslas. If the length XY is $L$ metres it is found that a force $F$ newtons acts as shown, mutually perpendicular to the flux and to the conductor. $F$ is larger for stronger flux density, for greater current and for greater length of conductor, i.e.

$$F = BIL \text{ newtons}$$

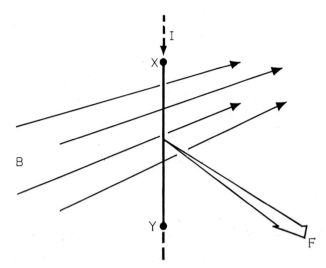

FIG. 7. Force on a conductor carrying a current within a region of magnetic flux—the Motor Effect.

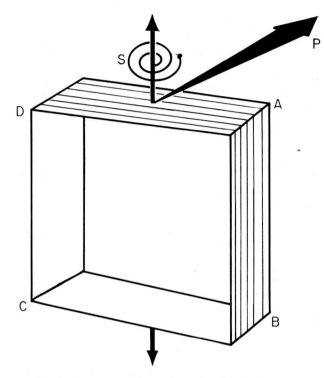

FIG. 9. Arrangement of restoring spring $S$ and pointer $P$. Several turns are wound on a frame A B C D.

Recording devices based on the moving coil meter movement rely on this effect. If the rectangular coil ABCD in Fig. 8 is arranged always to lie in the same plane as the magnetic flux as shown, then a current $I$ *to be measured* causes a force $BIL$ to pull the side AB out of the plane of the diagram, and an equal force to push CD into that plane. The coil will be twisted by a torque given by $WBIL$ newton

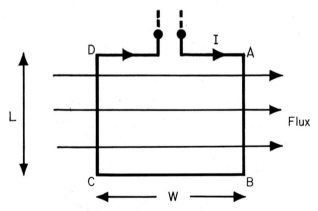

FIG. 8. The rectangular coil—basis of moving-coil meters.

metres, and measurement of this torque permits $I$ to be measured. To do this the coil (which usually has many turns—say $N$) is pivoted and allowed to twist against a restoring spring for which the opposing torque is proportional to the angle of rotation $\theta$. Hence the rotation ceases when

$$NBWL \cdot I = S\theta$$

$S$ being the stiffness coefficient of the spring. Fig. 9 illustrates the arrangement, showing the rectangular pivoted frame on which the turns are wound, the restoring spring $S$ and a pointer $P$ fixed to the frame. To ensure that, even as it rotates, the coil always lies coplanar with the flux and that B is constant, curved pole pieces $NS$ (shown in Fig. 10) are used, with a fixed soft iron cylinder $C$ to concentrate the flux and make it radial as required. The coil is mounted

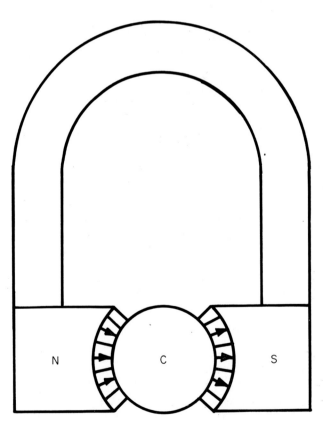

FIG. 10. Obtaining a radial uniform magnetic flux.

coaxially with C and its sides swing within the gaps *NC* and *CS*.

### Electromagnetic Induction and the Generation of Electricity

If a coil is rotated in a magnetic field the effect is the reverse of the motor effect, and an EMF is generated. One of the simplest examples is when a rectangular coil rotates in a uniform (as opposed to radial) field. Here the flux linkage alternates from maximum when the plane of the coil is at right-angles to the flux, through zero when they are coplanar and to maximum in the reverse direction after 180 degrees rotation. This gives rise to a sinusoidally varying EMF (*see* chapter on Mathematics), such as is encountered with the alternating current (a.c.) mains electricity supply. The advantages of a.c. supplies include:

1. Ease of transmission, and
2. Greater flexibility from the point of view of the user.

These both depend on the fact that 'transformers' can increase or decrease the size of an alternating EMF as required. For transmission of power it is easier to work at

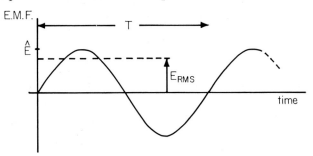

FIG. 11. The sinusoidal waveform, showing period (*T*), peak amplitude (*Ê*) and RMS measure.

very high voltages (with correspondingly low currents in the cables), the voltage being brought down to safer values before handing over to the consumer. Within apparatus the 240 volt public supply may be stepped up for some purposes and down for others.

Certain 'geometrical' aspects of the sinusoidally alternating waveform are of importance. In Fig. 11 the time *T* for a complete cycle of alternation is called the period, or periodic time. The number of cycles per second is known as the frequency (*f*) and

$$f = 1/T$$

Until recently the unit of frequency was called the cycle per second (c/s) but it is now called the hertz (Hz). Thus if *T* is 20 milliseconds, *f* is 50 Hz.

The peak amplitude reached is shown as *Ê*, but it is usual to specify sinusoidal EMFs by the steady value which would produce the same heating effect. Since a high value of *E* causes a proportionally high value of current *I* in a load, the power delivered, being given by *EI* depends on the *square* of *E*. As a result the effective equivalent steady value is often called the RMS (square root of the mean of the squares) value, $E_{RMS}$. This value gives more prominence to the higher excursions of *E* than the intermediate values and may be shown to be

$$E_{RMS} = \hat{E}/\sqrt{2}$$

It is this value which is actually quoted, so the 240 volt a.c. mains actually alternates with a peak value of $240\sqrt{2}$, or 340 volts.

### Mutual- and Self-induction

In Fig. 12 current $I_1$ from an alternating supply (represented by the circuit symbol shown) causes magnetic flux which also alternates. An EMF $E_2$ is consequently induced in a conductor such as *S* linked by changing flux due to the current $I_1$. The magnitude of the EMF induced in the 'secondary' circuit *S* is found to be proportional at all times to the rate of change of flux linkage, and hence of the

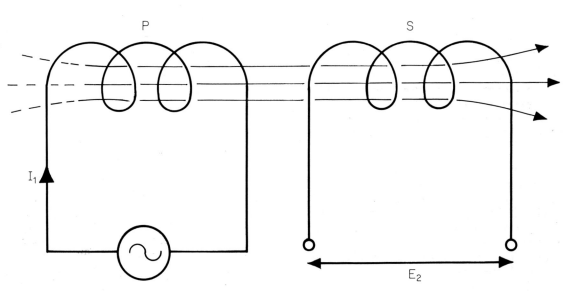

FIG. 12. Mutual induction: when the current ($I_1$) in *P* changes, the resulting changing flux induces an EMF ($E_2$) in *S*.

current in the 'primary' circuit causing this flux. Symbolically

$$|E_2| \propto \frac{dI_1}{dt}$$

$$= M\frac{dI_1}{dt}$$

The factor of proportionality $M$, which gives the secondary EMF caused by unit rate of change of primary current is called the coefficient of mutual inductance. Its unit is the henry (H), which is short for the volt per ampere-per-second.

Mutual inductance is deliberately created in devices known as transformers, but is also important in explaining some forms of electrical interference, as will be seen in the chapter on 'The Measurement and Recording of Biological Potentials.'

In transformers the use of very tight coupling, by winding $P$ (primary) and $S$ (secondary) on top of one another, often on cores of ferromagnetic materials which encourage the establishment of flux, makes it possible efficiently to create an alternating EMF in the secondary circuit, the energy being transferred by magnetic linkage with the primary circuit. If the secondary winding has more turns than the primary, the induced EMF can be larger than the supply EMF, and vice versa if the secondary has fewer turns. This enables, for example, the mains supply to be transformed up in EMF for some requirements, and down for others.

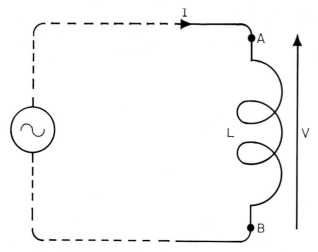

FIG. 13. Self-induction: here the alternating flux is caused by the a.c. $I$. (The broken lines are to suggest that the circuit causing the current is not under discussion.)

*Self-inductance*, as the name suggests, concerns EMF induced in a circuit due to a changing current flowing in the circuit itself, in contrast to current in an adjacent circuit. In Fig. 13 an electrical source causes changing current $I$ to flow in a circuit represented by the coil AB. The consequent changing flux links the circuit itself, and an EMF is induced between the terminals AB just as truly as if the flux had been caused by some other source. In this case the number of volts induced by unit rate of change of current is called the (coefficient of) self-inductance, or simply the

inductance, of the circuit. The common symbol is $L$, and the unit is the henry, as for mutual inductance.

**Electrical and Mechanical Analogues**

In the simplest law of sliding friction the force ($F$) of opposition experienced is approximately proportional to the velocity of the moving surface ($v$), or

$$F = rv$$

corresponding to Ohm's Law for electrical resistance

$$V = RI$$

The simplest spring opposes a movement (displacement, $x$) by a force

$$F = Sx$$

where $S$ expresses the stiffness. If this is re-written as

$$x = CF$$

where $C$ is the reciprocal of $S$, a measure of compliance. This is seen to be analogous to the capacitance law

$$Q = CV$$

This analogy also is consistent with that for resistance, because if charge $Q$ is taken as analogous to displacement $x$, this agrees with current $I$ (rate of change of charge) being analogous to velocity $v$ (rate of change of displacement).

Inductance is found to be analogous to mass, because if we denote by $V$ the potential difference induced between the terminals of a circuit exhibiting inductance $L$ henries, measured in the sense of *opposing* a rate of change of current $dI/dt$, we find

$$V = L\, dI/dt$$

This is precisely analogous to the result

$$F = ma$$

for a mass $m$ being accelerated, since

$$a = dv/dt$$

These analogous quantities are listed, together with consequent extensions in Table 1. They enable us to relate

TABLE 1

| Mechanical Concept, etc. | | Electrical Analogue | |
|---|---|---|---|
| Displacement | $x$ | Charge | $Q$ |
| Velocity | $v = dx/dt$ | Current | $I = dQ/dt$ |
| Force | $F$ | Potential difference | |
| | | p.d. | $V$ |
| Friction resistance | | Electrical resistance | |
| law | $F = rv$ | law | $V = RI$ |
| Compliance law | $F = x/C$ | Capacitance law | $V = Q/C$ |
| Inertia law | $F = mdv/dt$ | Inductance law | $V = LdI/dt$ |
| ork definition Work | $= Fx$ | P.D. definition   Work | $= VQ$ |
| Power law      Power | $= Fv$ | Electrical power Power | $= VI$ |
| Kinetic energy   K.E. | $= \frac{1}{2}mv^2$ | Energy in inductance | |
| | | Energy | $= \frac{1}{2}LI^2$ |
| Potential Energy  P.E. | $= \frac{1}{2}CF^2$ | Energy in capacitance | |
| | | Energy | $= \frac{1}{2}CV^2$ |

the less familiar concepts of electrical circuits to events such as accelerations, displacements, thrusts and so on which we experience with our own bodies and the many simple mechanical devices encountered every day. In this table, the compliance $C$ refers to $1/S$ for a simple spring. This is itself analogous to volume compliance, as met by anaesthetists. Also, to preserve the obvious similarity between p.e. and energy in a capacitance, the former is expressed as $\frac{1}{2}CF^2$, but substitution yields the more familiar $\frac{1}{2}Sx^2$.

### Impedance and Phase Concepts

If a finger is rubbed to and fro along a table, with a sinusoidal motion (fastest in the centre, slowing towards the extremes), the frictional resistance force is felt to be maximal when the velocity is maximal, and zero when the velocity is zero. In the same way, the potential difference across a resistor is found to be 'in phase with' the current through it.

In contrast, if a heavy object is shaken from side to side, the inertial opposition forces are felt to be greatest at the instants when the velocity is zero (at the lateral extremes of the shaking), and zero when the velocity is maximum (in the middle of the shake). This is expressed by saying that the force is a quarter of a cycle out of phase with the velocity, or that they are 'in quadrature.' Figure 14 illustrates the analogous phenomenon for the inductor. Since $V$ depends on the rate of change of $I$ it is maximal when $I$ changes most rapidly—on coming through zero.

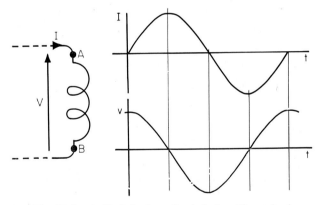

FIG. 14. Inertia-like behaviour of an inductor. $V$ is maximal when $I$ is changing most rapidly, and zero when $I$ passes through its peak.

Not only are $V$ and $I$ in quadrature, but it is found that, for a given current amplitude the peak value of $V$ is larger the more rapidly $I$ changes—that is, the higher the frequency. The ratio of the peak value of $V$ to that of $I$ is (to distinguish the phenomenon from resistance) called the *reactance* of the inductor ($X$). $X$ is obviously greater for larger inductance ($L$), since the larger $L$ is for a given peak current, the more it opposes the changing current. In fact it is found that

$$X = 2\pi fL \text{ ohms}$$

Notice that this opposition to a.c. is in no way due to resistance. Even a copper conductor an inch thick will oppose and set a limit to a *changing* current.

Capacitance also exhibits quadrature phase relationship between current and potential difference, the only distinction being that, because it takes time for a capacitor to establish a p.d. when a current flows, the p.d. lags a quarter of a cycle behind the current. With the inductor the 'inertia-like' opposition to changing current results in the latter lagging behind the potential difference. It is also found that the reactance (size of $V$ divided by size of $I$) varies with frequency, but since a higher frequency provides less time for the capacitor to charge before the current reverses, it is found that the reactance *falls* as frequency increases. Also, since a large capacitance means one that can take on a relatively large charge before the opposing p.d. becomes appreciable, it is not surprising to find that the reactance falls with larger capacitance. It is found that, for a capacitor

$$X = \frac{1}{2\pi fC} \text{ ohms}$$

The appearance of $2\pi$ in the formulae for reactances of inductors and capacitors is a simple consequence of the geometry of the sinusoid. Whether measured graphically or deduced by using the differential calculus, it is found that the steepest rate of rise, had it been maintained, would have caused peak amplitude to be reached in the fraction $1/2\pi$ of a cycle.

As in mechanical systems, the two electrical energy storing devices ($L$ and $C$) behave differently from one another as frequency is changed, one increasing its opposition to a.c., the other lowering it. In general circuits may have mixtures of components, resistive and reactive, and the opposition to a.c. is not simply proportional or inversely proportional to frequency as with pure reactances, but varies in a more complicated way. For mixed circuits the term Impedance is used to suggest opposition. Thus

$$\text{Impedance } (Z) = \frac{\text{size of p.d. across circuit}}{\text{size of current through it}}$$

$R$ (resistance) and $X$ (reactance) are thus special cases of $Z$ (impedance), $R$ being used for purely dissipative components, and $X$ for purely energy-storing ones.

It is important to appreciate, even if only in quite general terms, that for circuits in general, impedances and the phase relationships between current and potential difference can vary with frequency. Reference will be made to this in discussions of applications of electrical circuitry and devices.

### Resonance

By pressing down gradually on the roof of a car, the opposition developed by the springs when given time to act can be easily felt. In contrast, to become aware of the inertia of the car it is necessary to press down sharply, because inertial opposition depends on acceleration instead of displacement. By pressing up and down at the frequency at which the car shakes 'naturally,' the inertial opposition and the stiffness opposition can be made to cancel one another. For example, the moment when the springs are most compressed and pushing upwards most strongly is the moment when the mass is undergoing greatest deceleration.

Similarly, half a cycle later the springs are pulling down most forcibly at the instant when the tendency to overshoot requires to be controlled by downwards acceleration. With the inertial and compressional forces fighting one another, the man rocking the car at the correct rate merely has to overcome the third physical component, the frictional resistance. It should be noticed that, as in other analogous oscillatory systems, a mass and spring continuously interchange energy between two forms—kinetic and potential here.

*Resonance* is the general term for phenomena in which two mechanisms that oppose changes of condition nullify each other's effects at some special frequency, so permitting much greater oscillatory changes than either would alone. When such a system oscillates freely after some initial impulse, the resonance is said to be natural, or free. Forced resonance merely refers to the response of such a system to a maintained sinusoidal excitation.

### The Series Resonant Circuit

Figure 15 shows a circuit having the three electrical components R, L and C in series with one another. The source of EMF is to be regarded as being fixed in magnitude (E volts) but adjustable in frequency. Here the inductor and

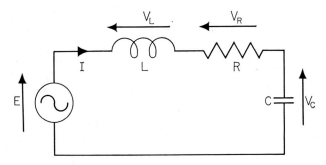

FIG. 15. Series resonant circuit.

the capacitor are the two energy-storing devices, the forms of energy being magnetic and electric respectively. To understand how this circuit is analogous to the mass-spring-friction system, the following facts are required:

1. The reactance of the inductor is given by

$$X_L = 2\pi f L \text{ ohms}$$

2. That of the capacitor is

$$X_C = \frac{1}{2\pi f C} \text{ ohms}$$

3. The p.d. across the inductor ($V_L$) leads the current by a quarter of a cycle, while that across the capacitor ($V_C$) lags the current by the same amount.

4. Consequently $V_L$ and $V_C$ are exactly in *anti-phase* (i.e. half a cycle out of phase) with one another.

5. At the one frequency ($f_0$ say) at which $X_L$ equals $X_C$, the p.d.s. $V_L$ and $V_C$ not only oppose one another, but, being equal in size, they cancel out exactly.

6. At this frequency only R exerts any effective opposition, so the current I is maximal at $f_0$.

The resonant frequency is easily deduced, since

$$2\pi f_0 L = \frac{1}{2\pi f_0 C}$$

or

$$f_0 = \frac{1}{2\pi \sqrt{LC}} \text{ Hz}$$

Notice that larger inductance (analogous to greater mass) and larger capacitance (analogous to *less* stiff springs) both cause reduction in resonant frequency. In the chapter on Transducers for the Measurement of Pressure the analogous result is quoted for catheter-manometer systems, and the same ideas apply to spring-controlled meter movements, acoustical resonant cavities and many other systems.

The behaviour of the series resonant circuit illustrates other important ideas when considered over a range of frequencies above and below resonance.

### 'Resonance Curves'

Figure 16 shows how the impedance of the series circuit can be visualized as it varies with frequency. Since the reactance of the inductor ($X_L$) is proportional to frequency ($f$) the graph of $X_L$ versus $f$ is the straight line shown. The reactance of the capacitor ($X_C$) is inversely proportional to

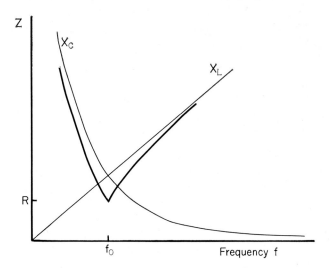

FIG. 16. Variation of impedance Z with frequency for series resonant circuit. $X_L$ and $X_C$ curves show how the reactances vary separately.

frequency as shown by the curve labelled $X_C$. We have already noted that at the resonant frequency the impedance ($Z$) is at its lowest value, being due to R alone, thus giving the minimum point on the graph of Z versus $f$. For frequencies so high that $X_C$ and R are trivial compared with the rising $X_L$, the impedance approximates to $X_L$ as shown. At frequencies well below resonance $X_C$ becomes dominant, so the impedance tends more closely to $X_C$.

Figure 17 shows the current as maximal, for a given magnitude of source EMF, when Z is minimal. The magnitude of I being given by the magnitude of E divided by that of Z, varies from zero at the extremes of zero and infinite frequency, with maximum value E/R at $f_0$.

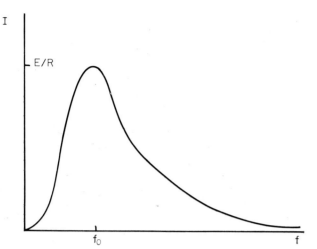

Fig. 17. 'Resonance curve,' showing variation of current for series resonant circuit with EMF of fixed size but variable frequency.

## Parallel Resonant Circuits

When an inductor and capacitor are in parallel, as in Fig. 18, the circuit formed behaves in the opposite way to the series resonant circuit. Since the current $I_L$ lags the p.d. while $I_C$ leads the p.d., it is now the *currents* which tend to cancel, so the total current ($I$) required from a source connected between AB tends to become smaller as resonance is reached. In practice the unavoidable resistances in the circuit (typified by a series resistance $R$ associated with the inductor) prevent $I_L$ from being exactly in antiphase with $I_C$, so the total ($I$) reaches a *minimum* (rather than zero) at resonance. The impedance is thus high (but not infinite) at resonance.

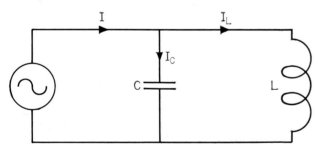

Fig. 18. Ideal parallel resonant circuit. In practice there are resistive losses, often represented by a resistance in series with $L$.

## Sharpness of Resonance

Common experience suggests that resonant systems with relatively low losses and relatively large energy storage are more 'sharply tuned'—that is, vary more abruptly in response just away from the resonant frequency—than more noisey systems. Examples include under-damped catheter-manometer combinations, high quality crystal bowls and electrical resonant circuits intended to pick out signals at some specific frequency. A very simple example is the series resonant circuit already discussed. If the resistance is increased from $R$ to some higher value the consequent reduction of the resonant current is less important in itself than is the flatter resonance curve, suggesting less pronounced variation as the resonant frequency is passed through.

This concept forms the basis of *tuning*—the process by which a signal of a desired frequency is selected from a background of others. This was first used in radio receivers, but is important in electro-medical equipment such as carrier-amplifiers, ultrasonic generators and telemetery systems, and all electronic devices containing oscillators.

## Stray and Unseen Components

Mechanical devices have unavoidable limitations, due to the requirements of physical materials and structures. Examples include the irreducible mass of a moving pointer, the springiness of a connecting-rod and the friction in a bearing. Electrical devices have similar limitations, of which the most obvious is the self-resistance every component has because it is made of real matter. Less obviously, because every circuit passing a current is linked by its own magnetic flux, each component has some self-inductance. Even though such inductance may be very small compared with that of a purpose designed inductor, its effect may become important at high enough frequencies.

At frequencies encountered in most electro-medical work, capacitance is more significant. Between any two parts of any device, when potential differences occur, capacitance effects are produced. When a.c. is involved, such *self-capacitances* give rise to current flow across gaps, just as real as are met with manufactured capacitors. Particularly important examples of such effects are the *stray* capacitance between pairs of leads, the capacitance between parts of the wiring of apparatus, and the capacitances involving patients, electrical apparatus and anaesthetists discussed in the chapter on recording biological electrical signals.

## The Importance of Parallel (Shunt) Impedances

Many of the phenomena associated with electronic devices cannot be adequately understood without knowledge of how components behave in parallel with one

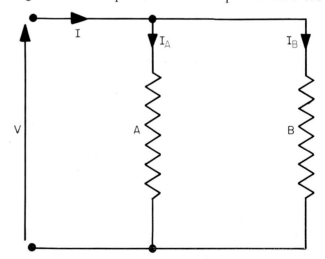

Fig. 19. Resistances in parallel. Since each current is proportional to $V$, they are simply additive.

another, as are the resistances $A$ and $B$ in Fig. 19. Just as two roads in parallel act as by-passes to one another and oppose the flow of traffic less than either alone, so the combined resistance ($R$, say) of this circuit will be less than either *A* or *B*. Since the total current *I* is the sum of the two currents shown,

$$I = I_A + I_B$$

Now the two resistances share the same potential difference *V*, so

$$I = \frac{V}{A} + \frac{V}{B}$$

A single equivalent resistance *R* taking the same total current, given the same p.d. would require that

$$I = \frac{V}{R}$$

so

$$\frac{1}{R} = \frac{1}{A} + \frac{1}{B}$$

In words, *the reciprocals of parallel resistances are additive*. Obviously the reciprocal of *R* is larger than either reciprocal, being the sum of the two, so *R* is smaller than either *A* or *B*, as anticipated. The result is sufficiently important to have available in the following more convenient form:

$$R = \frac{AB}{A + B}$$

The ideas introduced above can be extended to cover parallel reactances, and (most generally) impedances. A particularly important situation, in which one of two parallel components is capacitive, is shown in Fig. 20. This

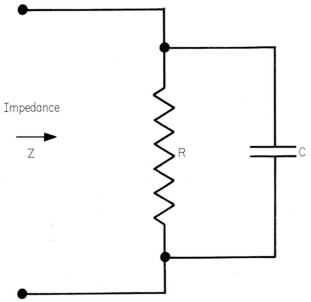

FIG. 20. Resistance and reactance in parallel. The effect of the capacitor, compared with that of the resistor, depends on frequency.

covers cases where *C* is stray, as well as where *C* is deliberately introduced. Such a deliberately introduced capacitor is often called a *decoupling* capacitor, intended to divert unwanted alternating currents from some circuit, represented here by *R*. It is instructive to see how the action of such a circuit can be argued without recourse to mathematics:

1. For currents at frequencies high enough for the reactance ($1/2\pi fC$) to be small compared with *R*, most of the current flows through *C*. *R* may be thought of as being short-circuited, in effect, by the low reactance of *C*. Clearly the impedance will fall towards zero as the frequency is raised indefinitely.

2. At frequencies low enough for the reactance of *C* to become very large compared with *R*, in particular as d.c. is approached, little current flows through *C*, which becomes less and less important. The impedance therefore tends towards *R* as the frequency is decreased.

3. Notice that at both extremes *it is the smaller impedance that dominates a parallel combination*, by accepting the major part of the current. This is the opposite effect to that met with series components, where the larger one dominates by imposing the main restriction on the current, and by taking the major share of the available p.d. across its terminals. To the motorist it is self-evident that with a high impedance road in series with a wide one, the minor road dominates the situation. With a by-pass it is the better road that dominates, provided of course that traffic divides according to the ease of the roads, and not by some mass act of malevolent stupidity on the part of the other motorists.

### Equivalent Circuits

Knowledge of the operation of individual electrical components is only one aspect of understanding circuits, and the same observation applies to the study of mechanical, hydrodynamic and other analogous systems such as are met in acoustics and in the many models of physiological systems currently being investigated. There are certain extremely powerful analytical tools available to the electrical and electronic engineers, and these are being more and more widely used in other analogous fields. A simple example is the concept of there being, for a given complex circuit, one or more simpler circuits which are to stated extents and under defined circumstances equivalent to the actual circuit. A very simple example of this is often taken as so obvious that it is often not formally stated: the assumption that circuit elements can be regarded as 'lumped' between two terminals each. Reflecting on the fact that all components have self-resistance and inductance 'distributed' throughout their structures, and capacitance distributed over their parts, reveals that the simple series and parallel components shown on diagrams are simplifications. In fact, at higher frequencies than those for which a given lumped equivalent circuit can be regarded as a good enough approximation, either more elaborate equivalent circuits have to be postulated, or full acceptance has to be made of the distributed nature of components. This is not only true in electronics, but extends to such topics as cardiovascular and respiratory models. However, at any state in an investigation it may become possible to imagine some simplified model which is equivalent to a complex system to some acceptable degree.

Two of the most profoundly important concepts used routinely by engineers are linked together and will be discussed next. Although they have mathematical aspects which are important to the engineer, the underlying ideas are common-sense ones, and are as important to the non-mathematically orientated reader as to the engineer who uses the associated mathematics intelligently rather than by rote.

### Linear Components and Devices

A linear device is one which produces some measurable effect which is simply proportional to some measurable quantity regarded as the cause. Simple examples that have been met include mass, for which acceleration is proportional to applied force, resistance for which current is proportional to p.d. and capacitance with p.d. proportional to charge stored. Similarly, provided they do not employ ferro-magnetic cores so permeated by flux that they have become saturated, transformers yield secondary EMF's proportional to the rates of change of their primary currents. Sometimes devices are accepted as being only approximately linear in their behaviour, often over some restricted range. An example is lung-compliance. If pressure change is regarded as cause and volume uptake as effect, the extent to which it is useful to regard the relationship between these as linear is well-known to respiratory physiologists.

The really important aspect of linear devices is expressed as the *Principle of Superposition*. This states that the response of a linear device to the sum of simultaneous and different stimuli is the same as the sum of the responses to the stimuli taken one at a time. For example, no matter how complicated an electrical circuit is, provided it is made up of linear components, its response to a complex signal made up of a mixture of d.c. and alternating currents of different frequencies can be understood by taking the signal components one at a time, finding how the circuit responds to each and then adding together these responses to get the total response. For example, to understand how a stethoscope modifies the characteristics of a heart sound, or how an amplifier affects a signal to be recorded or how a bed of rock transmits an earthquake wave, the same processes are involved:

1. Determine if the system concerned is linear.
2. If so, find how it treats any given signal component in isolation.
3. Sum the individual responses to individual components of the signal.

When a system or device is *non-linear*, either it must be treated as a complex of linear approximations, or its response to specific stimuli must be argued in detail for those stimuli. Sometimes this process is simple—a ratchet screwdriver is non-linear in its response to alternating twists of the user's wrist, but its action can be understood by thinking about the nature of a typical 'input' twist and the precise nature of the device. However, with really complicated non-linear systems the behaviour of each part may depend on the current state of its response and detailed prediction of behaviour may become a matter for computer-assisted analysis. A very obvious example of a non-linear system concerns the flow of fluid along a tube for which the elastic properties depend on the extent to which it is stretched. Clearly the flow response to some small pressure

component will be different if this is superimposed on a small standing (mean) pressure than it will if the mean pressure is so large as to stretch the tube to near its limit.

### Thévenin's Equivalent Circuit Concept

The objective here is to investigate a way of thinking about complicated circuits that reduces them (conceptually, as well as mathematically) to the trivially simple circuit of Fig. 22. The concept is contained in a theorem of the same name, and it applies to electrical circuits, acoustic, mechanical, hydrodynamic and other analogous assemblages, and indeed to all systems existing or yet to be evolved, provided that they consist of components which are linear in the sense described above. Stated for electrical circuits:

*Any assemblage of linear components, no matter how complex, can be replaced as far as its effect at two terminals AB are concerned, at any stated signal frequency, by a single source of EMF in series with a single impedance connected to AB.*

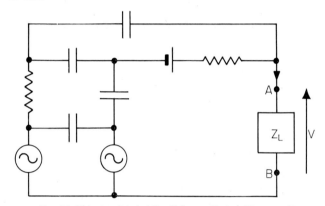

FIG. 21. This circuit is (arbitrarily) complicated. However, it is possible to think simply about it when the concern is with what happens at some external 'load' $Z_L$.

For engineers the theorem also tells how the EMF and the impedance can be calculated, but it is more important here to discuss the ideas further. Figure 21 shows an arbitrarily selected circuit with more than one source and several linear components. They are linear in that for each of them any change in the magnitude of the current through it would produce a proportional change in p.d. across it. The sources are also assumed to have linear internal impedances, simply included with the other components. The box marked $Z_L$ (denoting 'load' in this context) takes a current ($I$) when connected across AB. It is almost trite to say that there could be an infinite number of possible circuits which, if connected across AB would send the same current through $Z_L$. It is even true that there are, given a free hand in choosing the EMF and impedance, an infinite number as simple as that in Fig. 22. Obviously if some circuit did not quite do this, adjustment of its EMF the nature and size of the impedance, or both could always be made on an *ad hoc* basis until the result was just right. However, Thévenin was being more subtle. His object was not merely to derive an equivalent circuit delivering the correct current into some particular load, but to choose $E$ and $Z$ so that the equivalence holds *no matter what value of $Z_L$ happens to be connected*. This restricts the choice, but increases the usefulness of the exercise, for we wish to be able to think of any linear circuit as replaced by an easily visualized equivalent that holds no matter what circuit is attached to follow it. The uniqueness of the equivalent can easily be appreciated by the following argument. To hold for the extreme case where $Z_L$ is an open-circuit, $E$ must be equal to whatever p.d. appears across AB when $Z_L$ is

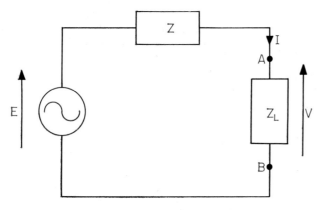

FIG. 22. Thévenin's equivalent and simple circuit. $E$ and $Z$ are chosen so that $Z_L$ is treated as it was by the complex original circuit.

removed. This fixes $E$. At the other extreme, with $Z_L$ a short-circuit the equivalent circuit gives a current of $E/Z$. Since this must equal the short-circuit current delivered by the original circuit, this in turn fixes $Z$. The full statement of the theorem shows that:

1. $E$ must be made equal to the open-circuit p.d. that would appear across the terminals, and
2. $Z$ must equal the impedance which would be measured looking back into AB with all internal EMF's 'switched off,' but with their internal impedances remaining. It is a relatively easy matter, for those interested, to show that this impedance is the same as gives the short-circuit current when divided into $E$.

Although to the engineer this theorem is important for answering specific problems, the really important idea is that of *legitimately* regarding some complex device as if it had been much simpler. It is perfectly reasonable to ask, in connection with a new blood-pressure transducer, or a new physiological signal amplifier, 'What is the equivalent source circuit that represents this device at its output terminals?' An engineer will be able to calculate these from knowledge of the contents, but all users can enquire about and subsequently think in terms of the Thévenin equivalent circuit.

### Input and Output Impedances

Much human activity consists of connecting devices together, so that the output of one device provides the input to the next. Thévenin has shown that, for linear devices a circuit can be simplified in the imagination, as far as the current delivered to the following circuit is concerned. Thévenin's equivalent series impedance ($Z$) is sometimes known as the *source impedance* and sometimes as the *output impedance* of the circuit, as seen by a circuit connected

across AB. The *input impedance* of a circuit is the impedance which, connected across the previous circuit, demands the same current as does the actual circuit at its input terminals.

With this in mind, it is easy to see that the trivial-looking circuit in Fig. 22 is really quite important. If $Z_L$ is the input impedance of a device or circuit, and if $E$ and $Z$ are the Thévenin EMF and output impedance of the previous circuit, then these three quantities ($E$, $Z$ and $Z_L$) are all that is required for determining the signal passed on to the second device from the first. This is quite general, and so it is worth examining and interpreting the result for $V$, the p.d. passed on in this otherwise apparently unimportant-looking circuit. For this exercise $Z$ and $Z_L$ will be treated as resistances. Similar considerations apply in more general cases of impedances, with differences which become more important as the subject is dealt with in greater detail.

Ohm's law, applied to $Z_L$ gives

$$V = IZ_L$$

while, applied to the whole circuit it gives

$$I = \frac{E}{Z + Z_L}$$

Consequently

$$V = \frac{EZ_L}{Z + Z_L}$$

If this result is (merely typographically) rearranged to look as follows:

$$V = \left(\frac{Z_L}{Z + Z_L}\right) . E$$

its interpretation at once becomes clear, especially when expressed in words:

The output terminal p.d. ($V$) is the same fraction of the total EMF as the 'load' resistance ($Z_L$) is of the total resistance.

To illustrate the simplicity of this, if an electromanometer transducer with an output impedance of 1 kΩ is connected to an amplifier with an input resistance of 100 kΩ, the fraction of the source EMF passed on will be 100/101. In contrast, if an electrode with a resistance of 50 kΩ were connected to the same amplifier, only the fraction $\frac{2}{3}$ would go on to be amplified.

### Attenuators and Potential Dividers

An *attenuator* is a circuit for reducing a signal, usually by splitting an applied p.d. into fractions and rejecting what is not required. The simplest form consists of two resistors such as $A$ and $B$ in Fig. 23(a). The output voltage is given by the fraction $B/(A + B)$ of the input. More complicated circuits are made when special additional properties are wanted, in particular when it is vital to present constant resistance to both the previous and the following circuits even when attenuation is altered.

The term *potential divider* is applied to the simple circuit. Potential dividers may be fixed, stepped variable or continuously variable. Stepped variable attenuators (Fig. 23(b)) enable overall amplification in such equipment as ECG recorders and cathode-ray oscilloscopes to be altered in calibrated steps, by switching different resistors in as needed. Continuous variable potential dividers are typified by the volume controls on radio receivers, and by the 'preset' screwdriver adjustments found on many equipments. These latter are no different in principle from the others; they are simply adjusted infrequently.

that is connected, the resistance between them decreases. Used as a rheostat this would compensate for an increase in the resistance of the circuit with which it was in series.

### Wheatstone's Bridge as Two Potential Dividers

The following circuit was invented to solve a particular problem—that of finding an unknown resistance in terms of known ones. The same circuit configuration appears in

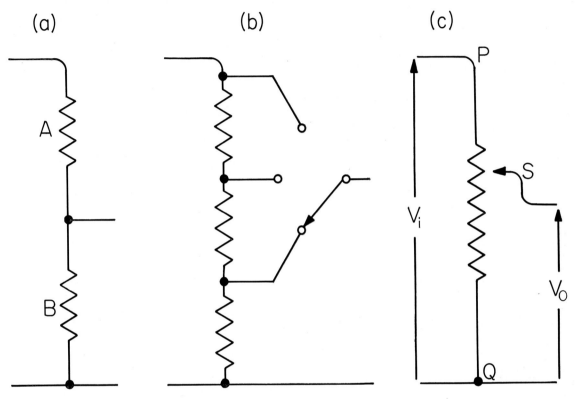

FIG. 23. (a) Fixed; (b) Switched and (c) continuously variable potential dividers.

The simplest form of continuously variable potential divider uses a resistor manufactured with a sliding contact that can ride from one end to the other. The circuit symbol is shown in Fig. 23(c), where an adjustable fraction of the applied p.d. is being selected. If the resistance between $S$ and $Q$ is $x$ ohms and the total between $P$ and $Q$ is $r$ ohms, the fraction

$$\frac{V_0}{V_i} = \frac{x}{r}$$

is variable between 0 and 1 as $x$ is varied from 0 to $r$ by sliding $S$ from the end $Q$ towards $P$. The term *potentiometer* has become associated with such potential dividers because an early method of measuring a potential difference involved comparing it with a tapped fraction of a known EMF. Another word still encountered is *rheostat*. This relates to one particular use of a variable resistance inserted in series with a circuit whose resistance alters, in order to keep the current constant by compensating for resistance changes. A potential divider such as that shown can be used as a simple variable resistance by connecting between $S$ and $Q$ (or $S$ and $P$). As the slider is moved towards the other end

many applications, and since it illustrates several ideas it is worth treating as an example.

In Fig. 24 two potential dividers are energized by the same source of EMF. The potential difference ($V$) between the terminals A B is to be regarded as an output to a following circuit: in the original use this was a sensitive meter for establishing a null condition ($V = 0$). For convenience, the conductor marked $X$ is taken as a reference for potentials, just as sea-level can be taken as a reference for heights. Denoting the potential of $A$ with respect to $X$ by $V_{AX}$ (and similarly for $V_{BX}$), it follows that

$$V = V_{AX} - V_{BX}$$

This is precisely analogous to saying that the difference between the heights of two camps $A$ and $B$ on Everest equals the height of $A$ above sea-level minus that of $B$, also referred to sea-level.

Now each of $V_{AX}$ and $V_{BX}$ can be written as a fraction of $E$, so

$$V = \left(\frac{Q}{P + Q}\right) \cdot E - \left(\frac{R}{R + S}\right) \cdot E$$

Two aspects of this result are important. When $Q$ is the same fraction of $P + Q$ as $R$ is of $R + S$ the bridge is said to be *balanced*, and $V$ is zero. This is often expressed as follows:

$$\frac{Q}{P + Q} = \frac{R}{R + S}$$

so
$$QR + QS = PR + QR$$
or
$$QS = PR$$

This enables (say) $R$ to be found in terms of the other three. The second important aspect is that alterations in one or more of the 'arms' of the bridge, provided that the changes are small in relation to the starting values of the resistances,

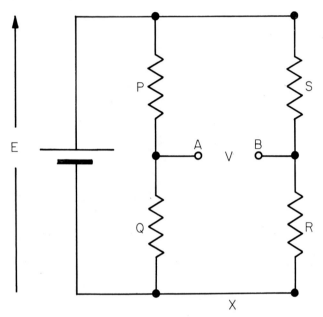

FIG. 24. The Wheatstone Bridge circuit. To assess $V$, AX is regarded as the output terminals of one potential divider and BX those of another.

give rise to an output $V$ that is reasonably linearly related to the resistance changes. This principle is used in very many circuits and devices. Examples will be found in this book, in the chapters on temperature measurement, on transducers for the measurement of pressure and on the analysis of gases and vapours.

### The Concept of Filtering

In the chapter on Mathematics and Shapes the importance of Fourier's Theorem is stressed. To summarize, Fourier's theorem states that any repetitive waveform can be analysed into component sinusoids, the lowest frequency-component (the fundamental) repeating at the same rate as the signal, and the others being whole multiples (harmonics) of this. The complete theorem goes on to show how the amplitudes and relative phases of the various components of a given waveform can be calculated.

More advanced versions of this theorem establish that any waveform, even if non-repetitive, can be considered in terms of sinusoidal components, although not harmonically related unless the waveform is repetitive. Children 'listening

to the sea' in shells are actually selecting from random background noise those frequency-components to which the shell-ear cavities are broadly tuned.

Circuits involving reactive components, such as the simple resistor by-passed by a capacitor, the resonant circuits discussed earlier, and even ostensibly resistive circuits at frequencies at which stray capacitances and inductances are noticeable, affect the various frequency-components of complex signals to different extents. When such variations of the signal passed on are unwanted, they are regarded as *amplitude/frequency* distortion. This is normally accompanied with variations of relative phases of different components, as between input and output, known as *phase/frequency distortion*.

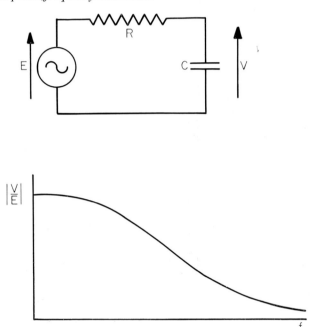

FIG. 25. Illustrating low-pass filtering. The ratio of the output $V$ to the input $E$ decreases as the reactance of the capacitor falls.

*Filters* are circuits in which the transmission of signals in some bands of frequency and rejection of others is deliberate. The principles and processes are the same as for distortion—only the intention is different. Filters vary in complexity, being more so the more stringent the conditions placed on

(a) the sharpness required—i.e. the rapidity of transition between frequencies passed and those attenuated,

(b) constancy of output within pass-bands,

(c) constancy of impedance presented to the circuits to which they are attached, with variation of frequency.

Discussion of such circuits is inappropriate here, but the description of the behaviour of two simple circuits having crude filter characteristics is justified by the useful ideas that emerge and by the frequency with which these circuits occur in electronic devices.

### Single CR Low and High Pass Circuits

In Fig. 25, $R$ is either an actual resistor or the Thévenin equivalent source resistance for a more complicated circuit.

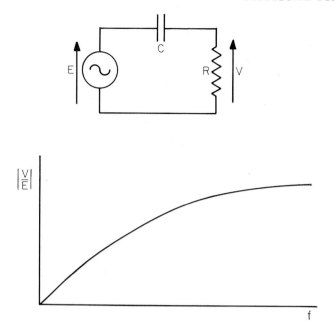

FIG. 26. Illustrating high pass filtering. Here the output is greater when less voltage is dropped across C.

At low frequencies C tends towards an open-circuit, making the current through R and thus the fraction of E lost across R negligible. The ratio of the size of V to that of E is plotted, the graph being called the *amplitude/frequency response curve* of the circuit.

Figure 26 is an example of an a.c. *coupling circuit* often met in electronic circuits, and particularly noticeable in ECG amplifiers. It is a crude high-pass filter, being obviously the converse of the previous circuit. Here it is the p.d. across R which is passed on and that across C discarded. Strictly speaking it rejects 'very low' frequencies (such as polarization effects from skin electrodes), where 'low' means frequencies for which $1/2\pi fC$ is large compared with R. It is often loosely stated to 'block d.c.,' although examination of the response curve shows that d.c. is merely the ultimate low frequency.

**Exponential Waveforms**

In the chapter on Mathematics and Shapes, exponential decay is dealt with as an important phenomenon in many diverse branches of science. In electronic circuits the simple CR combination just discussed is the most common circuit exhibiting exponential effects, when energized with d.c. If a direct voltage E (Fig. 27) is suddenly switched across a capacitor and resistor at a time when the capacitor is discharged ($V_C = 0$), all of E is momentarily developed across R. As the capacitor charges, the rise of $V_C$ makes $V_R$ fall (since their sum must always equal E). By Ohm's law the current falls proportionately from the initial $E/R$ towards zero. Since smaller current means less rapid establishment of charge Q, the p.d. across the capacitor *rises less rapidly the more the process continues*. The fall of I illustrates

C may be an actual capacitor, or some stray capacitance as discussed earlier. The circuit acts as a frequency-dependent potential divider. At frequencies high enough to make the reactance of C small compared with R, the p.d. across the capacitor becomes a very small fraction of E. As the frequency is decreased C begins to dominate the circuit and the p.d. across R becomes trivial. Briefly, at high frequencies C tends towards a short-circuit, and V tends towards zero.

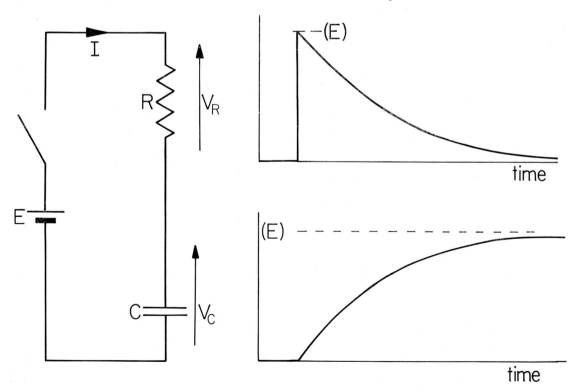

FIG. 27. Exponential waveforms for a circuit illustrating the phenomena described in the chapter on Mathematics and Shapes.

precisely what an exponential decay is—one for which the rate of change decreases as the quantity falls. The time-constant is the time taken for the fall to reach 36·8% (i.e. $1/e$) of the starting value, as discussed more fully in the mathematics chapter. For the $CR$ circuit it can be shown to be given by

$$\text{Time constant} = CR$$

the result being in seconds when the capacitance is in farads

and the resistance is in ohms. Obviously a larger capacitance takes more charge and a larger resistance reduces the charging current. A time constant of a few seconds is often encountered with the input circuits of ECG recorders, and the exponential decay curve can be seen in the recovery from a step calibration signal.

Similar exponential decay of current is met when a charged capacitor is discharged through a resistor. The effect is analogous to the gradual closing of a door with a spring and a hydraulic damper.

## CHAPTER 3

# TRANSDUCERS FOR THE MEASUREMENT OF PRESSURE

## P. CLIFFE

Electronic instrumentation is frequently used to detect changes of electrical potential produced by the flow of electric currents within the body. The electrocardiograph and electroencephalograph are familiar examples of such instruments which produce their recordings from electrodes directly attached to the patient. However, the use of electronic methods is clearly not confined to the measurement of electrical quantities alone but may be applied to measure the magnitude of almost any physical property. Temperature, light intensity, displacement, xelocity acceleration, force, pressure, flow, sound intensity are but a few examples. By means of suitable devices each of these physical quantities may be converted into electrical signals which vary proportionately with the physical quantity under investigation. By suitable processing such as amplification, the information may be displayed by producing a proportional deflection on a cathode ray oscilloscope or pen recorder.

Devices which convert one type of physical quantity into another are called transducers. For example, a thermocouple converts thermal into electrical energy and is a thermo-electric transducer, while a mechanoelectric transducer produces an electrical signal from a mechanical change. Some transducers are named directly in this way so that a photoelectric cell which converts light energy to electrical energy is a photoelectric or opticoelectric transducer. A pen recorder is thus an example of an electro-mechanical transducer. While the cathode ray oscillograph may be regarded as an electro-optical transducer and a pH meter as a chemico-electric transducer, some form of energy conversion occurs in most electro-medical instruments. It is therefore more usual to retain the specific name of the instrument and to confine the use of the term transducer to mechano-electric and electro-mechanical transducers.

Most sensing devices used in clinical medicine are of the type which convert some mechanical quantity into an

electric signal, and they may be termed input transducers in that they feed information about a patient into the processing devices of the associated instrument. There are many advantages resulting from the use of transducer systems and many of the measurements commonly made in medicine would not be possible without them. Thus:

1. The *sensitivity* may be very great or may be readily varied. For example, a mechano-electric transducer can measure a displacement as small as $10^{-6}$ centimetres.

2. A transducer may be applied to relatively *inaccessible sites*, e.g. intracardiac or intravascular sites.

3. The transducer can be made capable of a *high frequency response*.

4. *Loading* of the system under investigation may be negligible. Photo-electric cells may be adapted to measure movements of objects to which no mechanical connection is made at all. For example, eye movements have been measured by directing light onto the cornea and following the movement of the reflected beam by means of a photo-electric cell.

5. The selection of suitable transducers for different physical quantities allows these to *be presented simultaneously* and compared. Blood pressure, pulse rate, body temperature, respiratory volume and flow are but a few examples.

6. The electrical signals generated by a transducer may be processed and *derived results* may also be presented with the original information. For example, a pneumotachograph is an instrument for sensing a respiratory flow and if the electrical flow signal is integrated the tidal volume results. Far more complex processing than this can be effected by computers and nowadays transducers can be directly connected to them.

In the present section the use of transducers will be illustrated by considering the methods available for the measurement of blood pressure.

## MEASUREMENT OF BLOOD PRESSURE

### Indirect Methods

The sphymomanometer is the commonest device for measuring systolic and diastolic pressures. A stethoscope allows the systolic pressure to be identified when the intra-arterial pressure just exceeds the cuff pressure, while diastole is identified by the changing character of the Korotkoff sounds.

The Oscillotonometer, widely used in anaesthesia, uses a second cuff to replace the stethoscope of the sphygmomanometer. Both cuffs are connected to a cylindrical airtight box, the top of which contains a pressure scale and pointer, as in Fig. 1.

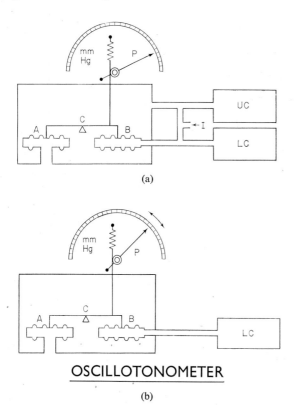

OSCILLOTONOMETER

(b)

FIG. 1(a) and (b). Oscillotonometer principle.

The instrument case contains two pressure sensitive capsules A and B. Of these, A is relatively stiff and its inside surface is open to atmosphere. B is more sensitive and is compressed much more readily than A for a given applied pressure. The capsules are cross connected by a lever system pivoted at C. The lever actuates the pointer P via a mechanical link.

In using the instrument:

1. Inflate both cuffs and oscillometer case via the inlet. Blow up above systolic pressure.
Capsule A is compressed and the pointer P is displaced to indicate the pressure in the system. Capsule B is unaffected because its internal and external pressures are equal. *See* Fig. 1(a).

2. Release the pressure in the system by small incre-

ments and after each fall of pressure operate a lever to detect whether systolic point has been reached.

Operation of the lever produces the condition shown in Fig. 1(b) in which only the lower cuff is connected to the sensitive capsule, but the box is still pressurized. Blood passing under the upper cuff causes pressure pulsations in the lower cuff which are transmitted by the sensitive capsule B to the pointer. Systole is detected by a sudden increase in amplitude of the oscillations.

3. When the systolic point is detected the lever is released and this returns the system to Fig. 1(a). The sensitive capsule is not actuated and the displacement of the stiff capsule A deflects the pointer to show the systolic pressure.

The diastolic pressure is detected in a similar manner, except that it is the level at which the oscillations of the needle suddenly *decrease* in amplitude.

In newer forms of oscillometer the pressure can be released slowly and continously and the oscillations can be observed without the interruption of operating the 'change-over' lever. This is effected by connecting the cuffs by means of a fine capillary tube, which offers sufficient resistance to pulsatile air flow but allows the steady level to be slowly changed in both cuffs. Again, when systole and diastole are detected the lever is released to read the true pressure in the upper cuff.

### Crystal Detectors

Various instruments have appeared in which a piezo-electric crystal has been used as a detector. This is a device which produces an EMF across opposite faces when compressed. The materials may be prepared as discs or plates, and if placed over the brachial artery or a digital artery will produce a pulsatile waveform which can be amplified and displayed by a meter of oscilloscope.

Other instruments have used microphones to pick up the Korotkoff sounds. These devices suffer from interference from external noise, and from difficulties of locating and maintaining position at the arterial site. If the ECG is recorded simultaneously the microphone can be activated only when the Korotkoff sounds occur, so that interference not associated with cardiac activity is eliminated.

A recent suggestion has been made of placing a flat piezo-electric plate in a small pocket in the inside wall of the rubber bag of the sphygmomanometer cuff. It is claimed that the disadvantages of other crystal systems are eliminated.

Another detector, applied to a finger, consists of a small lamp and photocell placed on the finger pulp. The intensity of light reaching the photocell varies with capillary blood flow. These may be used in conjunction with a sphygmomanometer cuff and give some indication of systolic level. This arrangement has proved useful in children undergoing anaesthesia.

### Direct Methods

#### Electromanometry

An electromanometer is a transducer which when attached to an intravascular catheter produces an electrical signal proportional to blood pressure. It can be made to follow the rapid pulsatile changes which occur and hence the waveforms of arterial and venous pressures may be transcribed by suitable recorders.

Before dealing with the details of electromanometers themselves, it is instructive to consider some of the principles which apply to the sensing and measurement of quantities which vary with time. Fig. 2 shows a selection of familar waveforms together with others encountered in the apparatus of clinical measurement. As indicated they

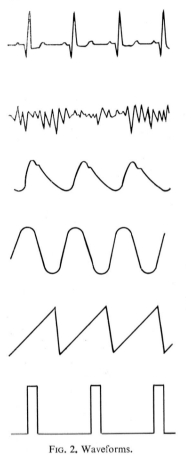

FIG. 2. Waveforms.

are an ECG waveform, an EEG waveform, an arterial pressure waveform, the variation with time of the voltage of the alternating current mains, the voltage time variation on the time base on a monitor oscilloscope which moves the spot from side to side on the screen and a pulse from an electronic stimulator.

If each of these waveforms and the millions being handled each day had to be considered individually and in detail the task would be impossible. However, it was shown by Fourier at the beginning of the 19th century that no matter how complex a waveform is, it can be analysed as the sum of a number of simple waveforms. These simple waveforms are called sinusoids or simple harmonic waveforms. They have the same shape as the a.c. mains voltage shown in the diagram. Suppose we wish to build up the waveform of the stimulator. It is possible to start with a smooth sinusoid having the same repetition rate as the pulse and an amplitude which can be calculated.

This sinusoid is called the first harmonic or fundamental of the stimulator waveform. To this is added a second sinusoid of twice the repetition rate that is the second harmonic. It must also have the correct amplitude and be displaced in time correctly relative to the first harmonic, that is the phase difference between the first and second harmonics must be correctly chosen. To these is now added a third harmonic with three times the repetition rate of the first and again with the correct amplitude and phase. This process is continued and for the stimulator waveform twenty or thirty sinusoids may be required. When all the corresponding ordinates are added the waveform of the stimulator will be closely approximated. If the repetition rate for the stimulator is one per second then the frequency of the thirtieth harmonic will be 30 cycles per second.

For clinical purposes the waveform of an arterial pressure may be interpreted adequately without recourse to Fourier analysis, however, the understanding and assessment of a blood pressure transducer suitable for arterial pressure cannot be satisfactorily achieved without this approach. The sharper the waveform under examination the more harmonics will be required to represent it. Thus for example, far fewer harmonics would be necessary for the arterial pressure waveform than for the time base or the stimulator. However, if the blood pressure transducer is faithfully to reproduce the waveform it must be capable of responding to the highest frequency contained in the harmonic series by which the arterial waveform is represented. The frequency response of a transducer is thus an important quantity for it determines whether the device will be able to follow adequately the most rapidly moving parts in a particular waveform. These ideas are well known to 'hifi' enthusiasts who appreciate for example that if the higher harmonics of the violin are to be faithfully reproduced the apparatus must be capable of

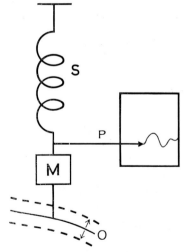

FIG. 3. Analog of a recording system.

following these high frequencies up to some 15–20 thousand cycles per second although of course this is far in excess of the fundamental frequency of the note being played.

In order to see how adequate frequency requirements

may be achieved it is necessary to consider the principles underlying the operation of mechanical transducers. The simple recording system shown in Fig. 3 serves to illustrate.

Suppose that $O$ is a moving object such as the chest wall and that its displacement time pattern is to be recorded on the drum via a pointer $P$. $M$ is a mass suspended from a spring $S$. Why may this simple mass/spring arrangement be regarded as an analog of a recording system? Any mechanical recording device inevitably has mass because it is made of metal, wire, etc. This is represented by $M$.

The spring is the essential measuring element. Thus as the chest wall moves, it exerts forces on the simple recorder and these are balanced by the spring at each displacement, which is then recorded.

A simple recorder such as this would clearly suffer from a number of disadvantages. Firstly, if the mass were large and the spring not particularly stiff then the mass/spring system would only be capable of relatively slow movement and may not be able to follow the changes in displacement of the object at $O$. Secondly, the mass/spring system might unduly load the object and prevent its free movement. The frequency response of the recorder could clearly be increased by reducing the mass as far as possible and making the spring relatively stiff. In fact it is

the instrument. It will later be seen that the frequency of the mass/spring system should be nearly twice that of the highest harmonic in the waveform being recorded. Secondly, the system must be correctly damped. Damping may be defined as the dissipation of energy within an oscillating system and the rate of dissipation of this energy must be correctly chosen by proper adjustment of the resistance of the viscous medium.

Consider how these principles may be applied to an electromanometer. Fig. 4 shows that the electromanometer consists essentially of a flexible diaphragm mounted in a chamber and connected usually via a catheter to the source of pressure to be measured. The system is filled with saline. Fluctuations of pressure cause displacements of the diaphragm which are sensed electrically. Just as for the simple recorder the behaviour of this system is controlled by three essential physical properties.

1. The 'mass' or fluid inertia of liquid which oscillates in the catheter. The equivalent mass now however turns out to be rather different from that in the simple recorder. The reason is that inertia is that property which opposes change in motion of a mass. As liquid oscillates within the catheter manometer system it moves

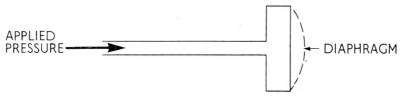

FIG. 4. Electromanometer principle

possible to show that the frequency of oscillation of the mass and spring on their own is $F = \dfrac{1}{2\pi}\sqrt{\dfrac{S}{M}}$. This result incorporates the idea that the stiffer the spring and the lighter the mass the higher will be the natural frequency of oscillation of the system. In practice it is necessary to arrange that this frequency is considerably in excess of that of the movement of the object $O$. Even so, a simple recorder of this type would suffer from another serious disadvantage. As the object $O$ moves, unless the mass and spring system were restrained in some way, there is nothing to stop it breaking into its own free oscillation and this would introduce artefacts into the tracing in the form of higher frequency ripples super-imposed on the displacement tracing of $O$. Suppose that the mass were surrounded by a viscous oil. If the oil were correctly chosen it would be possible to damp out these free oscillations by dissipating their energy as heat in the oil. The resistance offered by the oil ensures that the recorder follows smoothly the movements of the object $O$. These principles apply to many mechanical transducers including electromanometers, pen recorders and galvanometers. For correct operation two requirements have to be met. Firstly the value of the mass and spring elements must be so adjusted to give an adequate frequency response for

with a relatively high velocity in the narrow catheter as compared with the more or less negligible movement in the wide chamber. Thus the fluid inertia is most effective in the catheter. It is possible to show that the fluid inertia is proportional to $\dfrac{\rho L}{A}$

where $\rho$ = the density of the liquid in the system

$L$ = the length of the catheter

and $A$ = the area of cross section of the catheter.

This shows the mass factor increases as the catheter diameter is reduced and just as in the simple recorder, if the mass factor increases, the frequency response of the system will be reduced.

2. The stiffness of the diaphragm.

This corresponds with the stiffness of the spring in the simple recorder and the frequency response of the transducer increases with diaphragm stiffness.

3. The viscous resistance of the catheter to movement of liquid along it. This factor provides the damping in the system and controls free oscillation of the liquid within it.

Fortunately, for the correct operation of an electromanometer in practice, it is not necessary to make a separate assessment of these three factors. The alternative approach is to investigate the behaviour of the transducer when subjected to rapid changes in pressure. It is then possible to decide whether the catheter/transducer system is able to respond adequately to the higher harmonics in the pulsatile pressure waveform. Two methods are available and they are complementary.

1. Step response method. This involves applying a sudden pressure change or step to the catheter and transducer which, of course, are liquid filled as for the measurement of an actual intra-vascular pressure. A simple device for doing this is shown in Fig. 5. The tip of

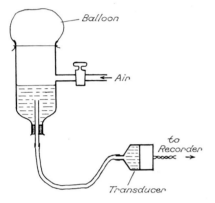

FIG. 5. Step response test for an electromanometer.

the catheter is fitted into a small vessel which can be pressurized and which is terminated by a balloon. By introducing air through the side arm the balloon is blown

For a given diaphragm if the catheter is relatively wide and short damping is likely to be low, the step of pressure is not accurately reproduced but the system overshoots and then oscillates as shown in Fig. 6(a). For clarity this diagram is drawn for a rising pressure step, but the principle is the same. If the diameter of the catheter is now greatly reduced the system cannot follow the rapid pressure change but slowly falls to the final pressure value as shown in 6(b). The reason for this result is that as the diameter of the catheter is decreased the viscous resistance to the movement of liquid within it increases and it can no longer follow a rapid change. In addition the fluid inertia increases with decreasing catheter size and this again limits the frequency response of the system. By adjusting the size of the catheter between these limits a value can be reached for which the pressure just returns to the steady value without oscillating as in Fig. 6(d). Damping is then said to be critical. However, even this condition is not the optimal arrangement and if a small overshoot is permitted such as in Fig. 6(c) this is found to be the best compromise in terms of the time taken to return to the steady value. Fig. 6 indicates that it is possible to quantitate damping and it can be shown that a damping factor $D$ may be defined where $D = R/2\sqrt{MS}$. ($R$ = viscous resistance) Referring to the simple recorder, this is clearly reasonable, for the greater the viscous resistance the greater will be the rate of energy dissipation and damping. Furthermore the larger the mass and the stiffer the spring the greater is the energy stored in the mass/spring system and further oscillations will be necessary to dissipate its energy of oscillation,

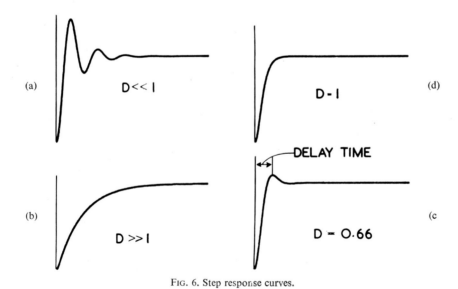

FIG. 6. Step response curves.

up so that the pressure within the system may be say 50 mm. Hg. The balloon is then suddenly burst and the resulting tracing observed on the recorder used with the pressure transducer. There are several possible results depending on the relationship of the catheter length and diameter to the stiffness of the transducer diaphragm.

i.e. the damping will be less. $D$ expressed in this way has a convenient range of values. Thus for critical damping when the system just does not oscillate $D$ is equal to 1. If $D$ is very much less than 1 as in Fig. 6(a) we get the oscillatory condition. The optimum condition is when $D$ is equal to 66 per cent of critical damping as shown in 6(c). Again it is unnecessary to assess $R$ $M$ and $S$ separately in order to determine damping because it turns out that the overshoot is directly related to $D$ and when $D = 66$ per cent of critical the overshoot is 6 per cent of the initial applied pressure. This condition represents the best compromise that can be obtained

2. The frequency response method. The extent to which the transducer will respond to rapidly changing pressures may be investigated directly. An arrangement for doing this is shown in Fig. 7. By means of a reciprocating piston an approximately sinusoidal pressure variation may be applied having a constant pressure

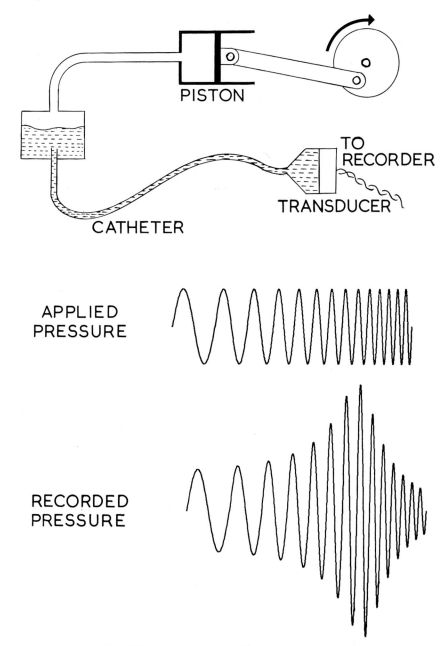

FIG. 7. Frequency response test for an electromanometer

with a transducer limited by resistance and inertia and in this way the catheter can be matched to the transducer.

It should be emphasized that it is insufficient to go to the maker and buy a particular blood pressure transducer and then attach any catheter to it and expect it to produce undistorted arterial traces. The catheter is an integral part of the transducer system and has to be matched to if it is to perform satisfactorily.

amplitude. Ideally, as the frequency is increased the pressure amplitude should remain constant. In practice this is not the case and if the damping is less than the optimal value it is found that within a particular frequency range the amplitude increases considerably. This range is around the natural frequency of the transducer catheter system. This situation compares with Fig. 6(a) and in an actual pressure tracing, free vibrations of the measuring system distort an arterial waveform. The extent to which the peak amplitude is affected depends on the damping. When the catheter is adjusted for optimal damping as in Fig. 6(c) the amplitude of the sinusoidal applied pressure remains constant within ±2 per cent up to two-thirds of the natural frequency of the catheter transducer system. In practice it is usually considered that the higher harmonics of an arterial waveform lie in the region of about twenty cycles per second. Under these circumstances a catheter transducer having a natural or resonant frequency of thirty cycles per second would be sufficient for the purpose. By then applying sufficient damping, either by the correct choice of catheter or by introducing a constriction into the catheter line, the damping can be made optimal and the frequency response up to twenty cycles a second will be uniform.

### Phase Relationships in Electromanometers

When an impulse is applied to the tip of a catheter a delay will occur before this impulse reaches the diaphragm. This delay is due to the inertia of the liquid within the catheter and yielding of the catheter wall. It has been seen that a complex pressure waveform can be built up

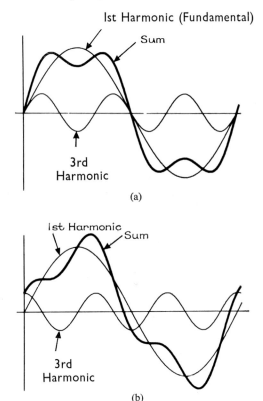

FIG. 8. Phase distortion.

of harmonics and if these harmonics are delayed by different amounts during their passage along the catheter then the waveform will be distorted. This is illustrated in Fig. 8(a) and 8(b). This shows a first harmonic (the fundamental) together with its third harmonic. At the initial instant of time shown these are in phase. If corresponding

ordinates are added together the resultant is shown by the thick line. Referring now to Fig. 8(b), it will be seen that at the initial time instant the phase of the third harmonic has been reversed. Clearly the resultant waveform is changed in shape. Similarly in an arterial waveform if the various harmonics are displaced, one relative to another, due to passage along the catheter the arterial waveform will be distorted. The extent to which this relative displacement occurs depends on the damping within the system and distortion results from this course if the damping is either above or below the optimal value. At the optimal value, that is 66 per cent of critical damping, it may be shown that while all the harmonics in the complex pressure waveform are delayed due to inertia, they are all delayed by an equal time interval and therefore the waveform as a whole is unchanged.

In most cases the delay time for a given catheter can usually be neglected. However it may be measured by the apparatus of Fig. 5. A second transducer similar to that under test is connected directly to the pressure chamber. The response of this transducer to a sudden impulse is compared with that to which the catheter is attached, by viewing on a cathode ray oscilloscope. The time separation of the two responses is due to the delay time of the catheter and this may become important where an accurate time assessment is required of different events within the cardiac cycle.

In the preceding discussion it has always been assumed that the catheter manometer system is liquid filled. The presence of small air bubbles has a profound effect on the damping and is a common cause of over-damped traces in practice. The velocity of movement of the liquid within the catheter is greatly increased due to the compression of the air bubble. The adjustment of an electromanometer system may be summarized as follows.

1. The diameter and length of the catheter must be correctly selected to ensure optimal damping. This condition results if the system responds to a pressure step by a 6 per cent overshoot.

2. If the catheter diameter is reduced a stiffer diaphragm must be employed. This allows the velocity of liquid movement in the catheter to be minimized for a given pressure change.

Diaphragm stiffness is stated by the manufacturer as a 'volume displacement'. It is usually expressed by the number of cubic millimeters yield per 100 mm. Hg. applied pressure. Typical values range from 0·1–0·01 cu.mm. per 100 mm. Hg. The lower values would be suitable for arterial measurements with catheters of the order of 0·5 mm. internal diameter and up to about 100 cm. in length. The other values are suitable for venous pressures where a more restricted frequency range is sufficient.

Other requirements of electromanometers which are inherent in their design include:

1. Adequate sensitivity.
2. Stability of the transducer, amplifier and recorder. This is clearly necessary in order to avoid baseline drift.
3. Linear response of the system.
4. Low hysteresis associated with diaphragm yield.

5. Ease of handling particularly in relation to the elimination of bubbles and the ability to sterilize the transducer.

### Sensing of Diaphragm Movement

Two types of blood pressure transducer are commonly in use and available commercially. They differ in the way in which the diaphragm movement is sensed. The strain gauge instrument utilizes a change in electrical resistance while the electromagnetic transducer employs a change in electrical inductance for this purpose.

### Strain Gauge Transducer

If a wire is stretched its electrical resistance increases. This change in resistance is not accounted for in terms of the decrease in area and increase in length but it depends on the atomic structure of the metal. Fig. 9 shows how

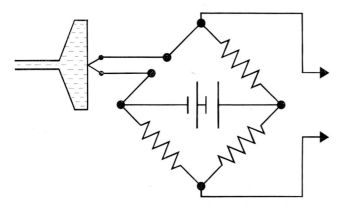

FIG. 9. Diaphragm movement sensed by a strain gauge in a bridge circuit.

this property is used to measure the displacement of the diaphragm in the strain gauge transducer. A wire in tension is attached to the diaphragm and forms one half of a Wheatstone bridge. As the diaphragm moves the tension in the wire alters, that is its strain changes, and a proportional potential difference is produced.

Examples of this type of transducer are made by the Statham Company. Some details are as follows:

| Type | P 23 D | P 23 G |
|---|---|---|
| Pressure Range | 0–75 cm. Hg. | 0–75 cm. Hg. |
| Excitation | 10 volts AC or DC | 10 volts AC or DC |
| Bridge Resistance | 300 ohms | 350 ohms |
| Output Voltage | 50 microvolts/mm. Hg. at 10 volts excitation | 20 microvolts/mm. Hg. at 10 volts |
| Volume Displacement | 0·04 cu. mm./100 mm. Hg. | 0·01 cu. mm./100 mm. Hg. |

The very low volume displacement of the P 23 G allows its use for recording via very narrow tubes, e.g. frequency responses of 30 cycles per second may be obtained with a metre of nylon tube of 0·4 mm. internal diameter.

| Type | SP 37 (miniature) |
|---|---|
| Pressure Range | 0–300 mm. Hg. |
| Excitation | Basically 3 volts DC or AC (but adaptable) |
| Bridge Resistance | 200 |
| Output Voltage | 50 uV/V/cm. Hg. |
| Volume Displacement | 4 × 10⁻⁴ cu. mm./mm. Hg. for transducer 8 × 10⁻⁴ cu. mm./mm. Hg. for dome. |

| Type | Statham P 23 BB (for Venous pressure) |
|---|---|
| Pressure Range | ±50 mm. Hg. |
| Sensitivity | 3·6 mv/cm. Hg. at 12 volts excitation |
| Excitation | 12 volts RMS or DC Max. |
| Volume Displacement | 3·1 cu. mm./100 mm. Hg. |
| Frequency Response | Approx. 7 c/s through 50 cm. catheter, 1 mm. diameter, 1 mm. bore. |

### Silicon Strain Gauge

Instead of using a wire strain gauge, the transducing element may consist of a signal crystal silicon diaphragm, into which is fused a fully active four arm bridge using recent techniques associated with integrated and microminiature circuits. The transducer has high sensitivity, and is in fact about ten times more sensitive than conventional transducers. Because the crystal diaphragm is stiff the volume displacement is low.

Good temperature stability is claimed by the manufacturers for these transducers. Comparative measurements have, however, shown the semi-conductor gauge to have greater thermal drift than its equivalent wire strain gauge or electromagnetic manometer. Typical characteristics.

| Type | SE 4–81 |
|---|---|
| Pressure Range | 0–±300 mm. Hg. |
| Sensitivity | Approx. 25 mv/100 mm. Hg. at 10 V excitation |
| Input and output impedance | 1000 ohms |
| Max. excitation voltage | 10 volts RMS or DC |
| Volume displacement | 0·01 cu. mm./100 mm. Hg. |

### Operation of Bridge Systems

The Wheatstone bridge of Fig. 10 has been redrawn as two potential dividers $AB$ and $CD$. Suppose the supply is a direct voltage as indicated in Fig. 10 and suppose that $P$ is positive with respect to $Z$ by $E$ volts. In the simplest case in which all arms $A$, $B$, $C$, $D$ are equal, the potential divider $AB$ causes $X$ to be $\frac{1}{2}E$ volts above $Z$ which may be taken as the reference point. Similarly, $Y$ will be $\frac{1}{2}E$ volts above $Z$ in potential so $X$ and $Y$ are at the same potential. Using $X$ and $Y$ as output terminals will therefore give zero output (null, or balance condition). Now suppose

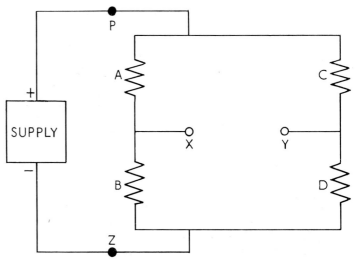

FIG. 10. Principle of operation of bridge system.

that for some reason the resistance of $A$ is increased. More volts will be dropped across $A$ and so the potential of $X$ will fall respect to the reference point $Z$. If $C$ and $D$ had been unaltered the potential of $Y$ would not have changed, so with $XY$ as output terminals an output signal arises with $Y$ positive with respect to $X$. The same result could have been achieved if $D$ had been increased (taking $Y$ nearer to $P$ in potential), or if $C$ or $B$ had been reduced. In fact correctly sensed changes of any one, two, three or all four arms would produce a signal between $X$ and $Y$. The opposite changes (e.g. a reduction of $A$ and/or $D$ and increase of $B$ and/or $C$) would produce an output of the opposite sense, that is $Y$ negative with respect to $X$. This is what would happen in Fig. 10 on passing from a negative to a positive pressure applied to the transducer. Suppose that the bridge were balanced for zero pressure. When a positive pressure is applied the potential of $Y$ with respect to $X$ might be positive. Under these circumstances, if a negative pressure is applied to the bridge, the polarity of the output terminals will be reversed.

### Electromagnetic Transducer

The principle is shown in Fig. 11. A small iron core attached to the diaphragm moves within a coil which forms the two arms of an inductive bridge. This is similar to the resistive bridge but two of the resistive arms are now replaced by inductors. The bridge is supplied by an alternating current with a frequency of several thousand cycles

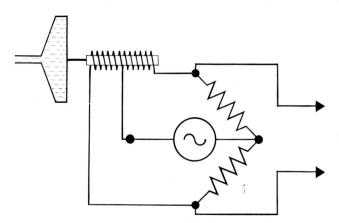

FIG. 11. Principle of inductive pressure transducer.

per second. As the iron moves, the inductance is changed in the two arms and the effect in the bridge is similar to that of changing the value of arm $A$ relative to $B$ in Fig. 10.

When an alternating supply replaces the direct one the same argument applies but now the output signal between $X$ and $Y$ is an alternating one. The amplitude of the output signal depends on the degree of unbalance. Thus for zero pressure when the bridge is balanced the output is zero. On applying a pressure, a sinusoidal voltage output is obtained of which the amplitude varies proportionately to the applied pressure and thus it is the envelope of the output voltage which carries the shape of the arterial waveform. This signal is illustrated in Fig. 12 for an arterial waveform.

In order to recover the pressure waveform as a direct signal which may be applied to a pen recorder or oscilloscope, a circuit is used which eliminates the negative going portion of the bridge output and also filters out the carrier wave to leave simply the pressure waveform. This circuit also achieves one other function and this is related to what happens in the alternating bridge when the pressure passes through zero. It has been seen that the output signal between $Y$ and $X$ is na alternating one. It is found that if the potential of $Y$ with respect to $X$ is in the same phase as that of $P$ to $X$ when a positive pressure is applied to the transducer, then phase reversal between $X$ and $Y$ will occur if a negative pressure is applied so that the bridge is unbalanced in the opposite way. The circuit into which the bridge output is fed recognizes this change of phase when

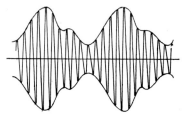

Fig. 12. 'Carrier' output from inductive transducer.

the pressure passes through zero and its output can produce a positive voltage for a positive pressure and a negative voltage when the pressure is reversed. The apparatus used with alternating bridges is usually called a carrier amplifier and the means of recognizing when a zero is passed through is achieved by a circuit known as a phase sensitive detector. These circuits have been described in detail elsewhere. (Cliffe and Strickland, 1964.)

In certain transducers of this type the inductors are arranged on either side of the diaphragm which itself acts like the iron core. In one model the coils which form the inductors and the diaphragm are immersed in oil, and separated by plastic 'buffer' diaphragms from the liquid which connects to the catheter. In this type, pressures may be applied simultaneously at both ends, that is the transducer forms a differential manometer.

An interesting application of a differential pressure

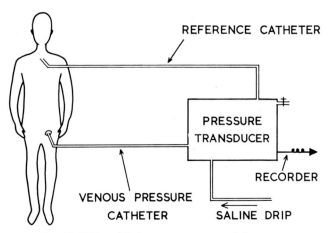

FIG. 13. Differential electromanometer used for venous pressures.

transducer has been described by Blackburn (Blackburn, 1968) for the measurement of central venous pressure. The mean value of central venous pressure may range between 5 and 10 millimetres of mercury. Consequently if a single ended transducer is connected to the patient via a catheter, then any change in the patient's position relative to the transducer will produce variations in indicated pressure, due to changes in hydrostatic pressure between the patient and the transducer. This is likely to occur when an operating table is tilted during surgery or when the patient moves about in the post operative period. To avoid the necessity of continually repositioning the transducer the differential arrangement shown in Fig. 13 may be employed. One side of the transducer is connected via a catheter directly to the vein within which the pressure is required. The other side of the transducer is liquid filled and the tip of an open ended catheter connected to it is positioned at some suitable reference point, for example the sternal angle. The pressure measured by the transducer will then be difference between the measuring and reference points independently of the position of the patient.

Typical data for Inductive Transducers.

Sanborn

| Type | 267 A 267 B | 268 A 268 B |
|---|---|---|
| Range | −100 to +400 mm. Hg. | −40 to +40 mm. Hg. |
| Sensitivity | Quoted as 1 cm. per deflection/1 mm. Hg. | 1 cm. deflection per 0·1 mm. Hg. |
| Volume Displacement | 0·03 cu. mm./100 mm. Hg. | 0·3 cu. mm./100 mm. Hg. |

The Types 267A and 267B have the same characteristics, but 'A' indicates single ended and 'B' indicates differential. Similarly for the 268 series.

### Intravascular Transducers

In recent years miniature strain gauge bridges and electromagnetic transducers have been incorporated into the tip of catheters. A pressure may then be sensed directly intravascularly without the necessity of a liquid connection to an external transducer. They have the advantage of a very high frequency response sufficient in fact to record intra-cardiac sounds. However certain problems arise with respect to thermal drift and recalibration in situ.

### Other Transducers

Other physical principles have been utilized in the production of transducers for medical use. In one, the diaphragm is used as one movable plate of a condenser. Together with the fixed plate it forms an electrical capacitor. The capacitance varies with pressure applied to the diaphragm.

One of the earlier and very reliable manometers was that of Hamilton in which the movement of the diaphragm was measured by reflecting a beam of light off a small mirror attached to it onto a moving photographic plate. The manometer was stable but insensitive and difficult to adjust. This instrument has been modified by arranging the reflected light beam to fall on a double vacuum photo cell, the output of which can be made proportional to the applied pressure. However these transducers are currently less commonly used than the strain gauge and electromagnetic types already described.

In the present chapter attention has been particularly directed to the use of transducers for the measurement of blood pressure. They have also been widely applied to elucidate the physiology of the respiratory. (Fry et al., 1957; McCall et al., 1957; Stott, 1957); alimentary (Jacobson, 1963); urinary (Rose, 1944); systems and have yielded useful information in the practice of obstetrics (Smyth, 1957).

The range of pressures covered is from a fraction of a centimetre of water to several hundred millimetres of mercury but whatever the application the general principles outlined still apply.

### Practical considerations

#### Adjustment of Electromanometers

It has already been seen that in order to reproduce pressure waveforms without distortion it is necessary to arrange that when a sudden pressure change is applied to the catheter manometer system the indicated pressure shall overshoot by about 6 per cent. Under these circumstances damping will be 66 per cent of critical and the required waveform will be recorded with minimal amplitude and phase distortion. With the particular tube or needle attached to the transducer one should ensure that the system is capable of an oscillatory response. The damping should then be adjusted to make the overshoot about 6 per cent. This may be achieved:

1. By arranging a needle valve in the liquid line and adjusting for correct overshoot.
2. By constricting the liquid line by a length of hypodermic needle tubing. In this way definite constrictions may be arranged for particular transducers when used with particular catheters or needles.
3. By adjusting an electrical damping control on the transducer amplifier.

Attention has already been drawn to the importance of ensuring that the liquid filled system is air free.

Pressure recordings during surgery should be capable of running unattended for several hours. The amplifying equipment currently available is sufficient with occasional recalibrations but the hydraulic connections to the transducer may be inadequate.

Fig. 14 shows a system of taps used by the author in conjunction with a Statham strain gauge electromanometer. The catheter can be flushed continuously at a very slow rate controlled by the needle valve N. Tap T2 serves to direct saline into the transducer chamber during filling but is not otherwise used. Tap T1 may be used to connect the transducer to an external pressure for calibrating purposes without interrupting the flow of saline through the catheter. The needle valve D, by introducing a constriction into the line, allows damping to be adjusted. Visual adjustment of damping is usually adequate for surgical monitoring but the control may be preset for a catheter of a given diameter if required. The transducer head may be sterilized with the usual disinfectants and well washed before use.

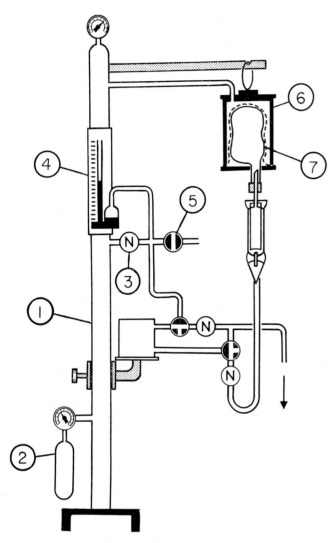

FIG. 15. Calibrating and control system for use with electromanometers.

Transducers of this kind are used in combination with a control unit resembling a transfusion stand and shown in Fig. 15. The central column (1) is pressurized by an oxygen cylinder (2) using an Adams regulator. The column is used (a) to pressurize the plastic bags used for transfusion and (b) to provide a calibrating pressure for the transducer. Should small gas leaks occur in the system, they are automatically compensated. The calibrating pressure is controlled by a needle valve (3) and read on the mercury manometer (4) mounted on a column. Tap (5) serves to restore the calibrating pressure to zero. With this arrangement, the coagulation of blood in catheters and needles is prevented by the slow saline drip which need not be interrupted when the transducers are recalibrated. The plastic transfusion bag is contained in a perspex cylinder (6) which can be pressurized via a plastic sleeve (7), shown dotted in Fig. 15. If the seams of the bag are imperfect, or if the bag empties, oxygen under pressure cannot enter the giving set. The system allows a constant pressure to be applied to the bag as it empties, ensuring a constant drip rate through the transducer catheter. The system may be operated virtually unattended for many hours.

Another more elaborate system designed especially for remote recording is described by Melrose (1968).

A rotating disc tap is employed in which sequential positions serve to connect the source pressure to the transducer, to calibrate and simultaneously flush the catheter, and to check the zero. A motorized version of the system can be operated by a switch from a remotely placed recording room.

## REFERENCES

Blackburn, J. P. (1968), *British Medical Journal*, **4**, 825.
Cliffe, P. and Strickland, D. A P. (1964), *Anaesthesia*, **19**, 1.
Fry, D. L., Hyatt, R. B., McCall, C. B. and Mallos, A. J. (1957), *J. App. Physical*, **10**, 210.
Jacobson, B. (1963), *Med. Elect. Biol. Engng.*, **1**, 165.
McCall, C. B., Hyatt, R. B., Noble, F. W. and Fry, D. L. (1957), *J. App. Physical*, **10**, 215.
Melrose, D. G. (1968). In: *Measurement and Precision in Surgery*. H. J. B. Atkins, Ed. Blackwell, 1968.
Rose, D. K. (1944), *Medical Physics*, Vol 3, p. 295. O. Glasser, Ed. New York: Year Book Publishers.
Smyth, C. N. (1957), *J. Obstet. Gynae. Brit. Emp.*, **64**, 59.

## CHAPTER 4

# METHODS OF MEASURING BLOOD FLOW

### A. M. HARPER, A. R. LORIMER and D. L. THOMAS

The number and variety of techniques available for the measurement of blood flow have increased markedly in recent years. Electronic engineering and radioisotopes have contributed to the proliferation of methods and their modifications which present themselves to a potential rheologist. It will not be possible to deal with all the techniques in this chapter—only those which have an application to the study of organ or tissue blood flow in the patient will be discussed.

Some methods will be dealt with in much more detail than the remainder because they illustrate a general principle from which other methods have evolved.

The following is a general classification of the techniques which will be discussed in this chapter:

GROUP (I): Methods of measuring flow through individual vessels.

(a) Flowmeters—electromagnetic and ultrasonic.
(b) Indicator dilution techniques for segmental venous flow.

GROUP (II): Methods using diffusible indicators.

GROUP (III): Methods for measuring cardiac output and regional blood flow using non-diffusible indicators.

GROUP (IV): Miscellaneous:

(a) Plethysmography.
(b) Thermocouples.

## GROUP 1(a): BLOOD FLOWMETERS— ELECTROMAGNETIC AND ULTRASONIC

The basic quantity measured by these flowmeters is blood velocity. This measurement may be correlated with the actual blood flow, the accuracy of the correlation depending on the type and design of the particular flow probe. The design is a complex problem and herein lies the art of the flow probe designer. The flow probes (transducers) may be divided into two main classes: those for intact vessels, typical of which are the cuff types, so called because they are fitted like a cuff round the vessel, and those for catheterized vessels, for example catheter-tip mounted probes.

### Electromagnetic Blood Flowmeters

The basic principle of the electromagnetic flowmeter is illustrated in Fig. 1. An electric field E is induced which is perpendicular in direction and proportional in magnitude to both the applied magnetic field B and the blood velocity $v$:

$$E = v\mathrm{B} \sin \theta$$

where $\theta$ is the angle between the field (B) and the velocity ($v$).

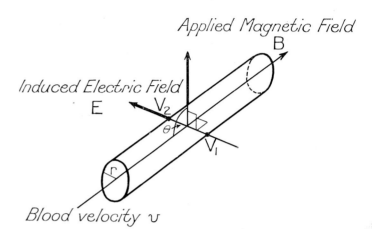

FIG. 1. Basic principle of electromagnetic flowmeter (*see* text).

The magnetic field does not have to be perpendicular to the blood velocity, though it is normally so arranged because then $\sin \theta = 1$ and the largest signal is obtained. Since the induced electric field is measured by means of the potential difference $(\phi_1 - \phi_2)$ between two electrodes mounted on opposite sides of the vessel, we have

$$(\phi_1 - \phi_2)/2r = v\mathrm{B} \sin \theta$$

where $r$ = the radius of the blood vessel.

If we write $F$ for the flow rate and let $\theta$ be a right angle we find that

$$F = \pi r(\phi_1 - \phi_2)/2\mathrm{B}$$

A more sophisticated treatment referred to a particular flow probe would lead to a slightly different numerical factor and would also involve some dependence on the

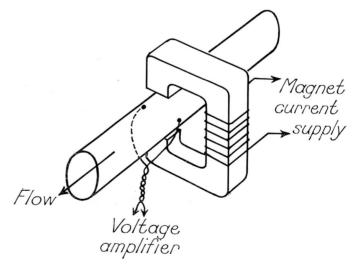

FIG. 2. Type of flow probe suitable for large vessels.

velocity profile, i.e. the graph of velocity plotted against the radial position within the blood vessel. As might be expected, one of the factors by which the merit of a flow probe is assessed is the degree of independence of the flow signal from velocity profile.

Figure 2 is a diagrammatic illustration of the U-type or C-type of electromagnetic flow probe, so called because

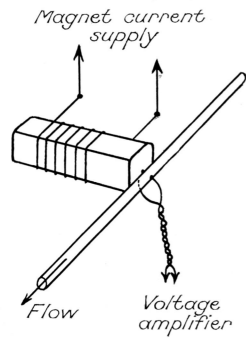

FIG. 3. Type of flow probe suitable for small vessels.

of the shape of the electromagnet. It requires a large amount of clear space around the blood vessel, and, as such, the design is more appropriate to probes for larger vessels. However, a homogeneous magnetic field is readily obtained and this allows for accurate flow measurements. On the other hand the I-type, again descriptive of

shape (Fig. 3), is appropriate for smaller vessels and is less demanding in terms of access. In return for these benefits, some inhomogeneity of the magnetic field and a resulting degree of inaccuracy in flow measurement must be accepted. In the catheter-tip type (Fig. 4) the flow is around rather than through the probe; however, the basic principle remains the same and the catheter must be small enough not to disturb the blood flow significantly. In this method the magnetic field is very inhomogeneous and the measured quantity is blood velocity rather than blood flow rate in the vessel as a whole. This re-emphasizes the point that the electromagnetic method essentially measures blood velocity. Total flow rate is obtained by summing all the values of velocity over the blood vessel cross-section (i.e. integration); it is only with the cuff type probe that this can be made an inherent property of the probe.

The exciting magnetic field is always alternating for the reason that the flow-induced potentials of a steady field could not be distinguished from the larger electro-chemical potentials which are always present. Typically, the frequency of the alternating field is a few hundred cycles a second which gives a sampling rate which is sufficiently high for the fastest varying flows encountered in the vascular system. Sinusoidal or square-wave excitation may be used, special advantages for each system being claimed by its proponents. Square-wave excitation provides a method of sampling the flow signal which is easy to understand and whose translation into electronic circuitry is straightforward. The system using sinusoidal excitation of the magnetic field is more elegant, more sophisticated and more efficient. The last point is an important one, because it means that for an output signal of a given size, sinusoidal excitation requires less current and therefore dissipates less heat and uses a smaller magnet than square-wave excitation. These may be important considerations especially if chronic implantation of the probes is envisaged.

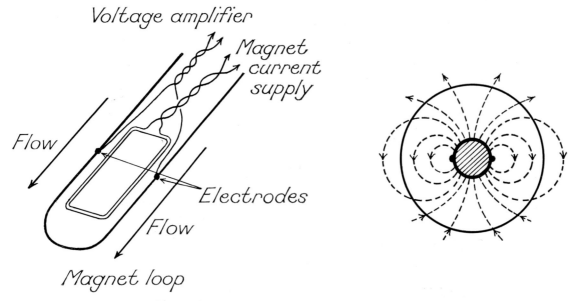

FIG. 4. Diagram of catheter-tip probe and its magnetic field.

However, as mentioned previously, square-wave excitation is easier to understand and Fig. 5 shows the basic block diagram of a square-wave instrument. Figure 6 shows the various wave forms appearing at different stages of the electronic processing. It will be seen that the signal from the flow probe consists of two parts: (a) spikes of large amplitude, called transformer spikes, which result from the cyclical reversal of the electro-magnet current; and (b) the flow signal proper which is of very much smaller amplitude and lies mainly between these spikes. An electronic gate is used so that only the flow-induced signal is passed and not the signal induced at each reversal

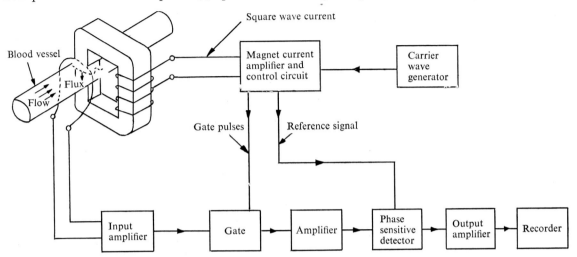

FIG. 5. Basic block diagram of the square-wave electromagnetic flowmeter. (From Hognestad, H. [1966], *Med. Eng. Res.*, **5**, 28)—reproduced by kind permission of the author and publishers.

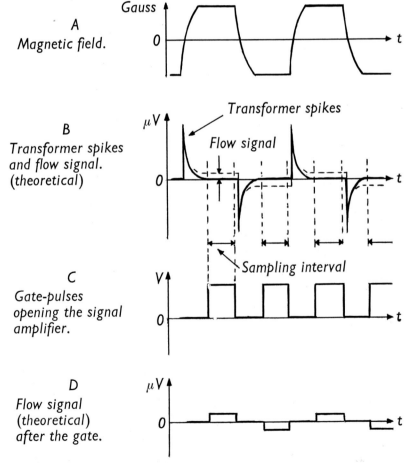

FIG. 6. Theoretical wave forms in the square-wave electro-magnetic flowmeter. (From Hognestad, H. [1966], *Med. Res. Eng.*, **5**, 28)—reproduced by kind permission of the author and publishers.

of the electromagnetic field. After the gate the flow signal contains alternate positive and negative excursions which are in phase with the exciting magnetic field. These are rectified by the phase-sensitive detector to provide a smooth positive signal corresponding to flow in the forward direction or a smooth negative signal corresponding to flow in the reverse direction. An output amplifier and recorder for flow rate and integrator for total flow complete the system.

Much of the literature is pre-occupied with the problem of base line shift, i.e. the presence of an unwanted unpredictable signal which is either constant in time or subject only to slow variations. It is a very real problem which results necessarily from the miniaturization of the flow transducers and the inhomogeneity of biological material. However, the sophistication of modern flowmeters is such as to minimize this source of error.

Some practical remarks on the use of electromagnetic flowmeters are appropriate. Normally these flowmeters are precalibrated in the sense that each flow probe will have a number indicative of its sensitivity to which the amplifier gain is made to correspond by means of a calibrated dial. It is easy to check this calibration if a test flow is run into a graduated cylinder. It is advisable to check all the probes periodically in this manner, and for this purpose it is convenient to use one per cent saline solution instead of blood and apply a correction to take account of the different electrical properties of the two fluids. However, it is even better to calibrate the probe *in vivo* on each occasion that it is used. This is done by placing the probe in position round the vessel, inserting a needle attached to a syringe into the lumen distal to the probe, and clamping the vessel distal to the needle. A measured amount of blood can be withdrawn into the syringe and the calibration factor adjusted accordingly. At the same time one should check that the electronic zero and the zero obtained when the vessel has been clamped do not differ by more than the amount specified for the instrument. Electronic zero refers to the signal output when the magnetic field is switched off. Some instruments provide for reversing the magnetic field, in which case the output signal will reverse in sign but should remain the same size (in this case the average is the zero error). To obtain an occluded zero the flow is stopped by a clamp or other physical means and the magnetic field is left switched on. In using electromagnetic flow probes it has to be realized that the size of the signals being picked up is very small, only of the same order of magnitude as electrophysiological signals recorded from the skin surface: because of this it is essential to ensure that the probe makes good contact. Firstly, the probe must be a snug fit around the vessel in which it is proposed to measure flow; a comprehensive range of probe sizes is therefore essential. Care must be taken to ensure that the flow probe does not loosen as a result of vasoconstriction during the course of an experiment. Secondly, the probe must be sufficiently wet to ensure adequate electrical contact with not only the blood vessel but also the surrounding tissue; it is usually necessary to bathe the site in saline.

## Ultrasonic Blood Flow Detectors

At the present time many of these instruments are qualitative rather than quantitative. This is because they can only measure velocity: to obtain flow rate one must independently measure the blood vessel's cross-section. Despite this limitation, these instruments have considerable use for examining patterns of blood flow not readily accessible to other methods of measurement—for example, foetal and placental blood flow. Another application is for peripheral circulation where the technique allows the superficial vascular system to be quickly surveyed.

Ultrasonic flowmeters utilize the properties of sound waves travelling through a moving fluid. One of the main reasons for using ultrasound rather than ordinary sound is the requirement that the wavelength be small compared with the dimensions of the system being investigated. Typically, the frequencies used are between one and ten megahertz, for example 1·5 megahertz (one and a half million cycles per second) corresponds to a wavelength of one millimetre in tissue.

One way of obtaining the velocity of the moving fluid is to measure the difference in transit time of up-stream

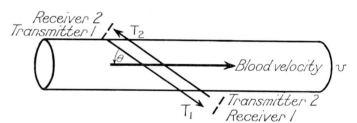

FIG. 7. Basic principle of ultrasonic flowmeter using transit time difference.

and down-stream ultrasonic pulses; this is illustrated in Fig. 7. Transducers, which act as both transmitters and receivers, are placed on either side of the blood vessel so that the line joining them makes a small acute angle $\theta$ with the blood velocity. If the distance between the two transducers is $L$, the blood velocity $v$, and the velocity of ultrasound $c$, then it may be shown that the down-stream and up-stream transit times $T_1$ and $T_2$ respectively are given by

$$T_1 = L/(c + v \cos \theta)$$
$$T_2 = L/(c - v \cos \theta)$$

then approximately (because $v$ is very much smaller than $c$)

$$T_2 - T_1 = (2Lv \cos \theta)/c^2$$

Since $c$ is known and $L$ and $\theta$ are geometrical properties of the transducer assembly, an instrument arranged to measure the time difference $T_2 - T_1$ can be calibrated directly in terms of the blood velocity $v$.

One type of ultrasonic flow detector suited for external use employs the principle of the Doppler frequency shift. A familiar example of this effect is the apparent drop in pitch of a moving sound source as it approaches, passes by and recedes. The effect also occurs when sound from a stationary source is reflected by a moving object. A valid way of describing this is to say that the observer hears an image of the sound source reflected in a moving mirror, and it can be deduced that the line of sight velocity of the image is twice that of the mirror. Figure 8 shows a transmitter-receiver transducer angled to a blood vessel: the receiver detects an image of the transmitter reflected in the 'mirror' of moving blood corpuscles, and the image is moving towards the receiver with the velocity $2v \cos \theta$.

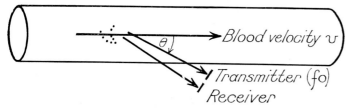

FIG. 8. Basic principle of ultrasonic flowmeter using Doppler frequency shift.

It can be shown that the Doppler effect causes a fractional change in frequency equal to the ratio of the velocity of the moving source to the velocity of the ultrasound.

$$\text{Explicitly } f - f_0 = (2fv \cos \theta)/c$$

(where $f$ = the received frequency and $f_0$ = the transmitted frequency).

The equation is similar to that for transit time difference shown on page 31. A popular way of using the Doppler type of instrument is to present the beat frequency (i.e. the difference or $f - f_0$) directly as an audio output and to rely for interpretation on the ear of a trained observer; in effect this is to use the instrument as an ultrasonic stethoscope. Alternatively, the beat frequency may be used to provide an output giving the blood velocity ($v$) directly. This is the method of choice if one wishes to study pulse waveforms in individual blood vessels.

The equations for transit time difference and Doppler frequency shift give both the direction and magnitude of the velocity. However, although there is no technical barrier to preserving both items of information, instruments can be bought which do not give the direction of the velocity but only preserve its magnitude: this is of importance when considering possible applications.

As with electromagnetic flow probes, certain precautions are necessary with ultrasonic probes to ensure optimum performance. As ultrasound is almost completely reflected at any interface with air, it is therefore necessary to provide an acoustic coupling medium between the transducer and the tissue in which measurements are being made. A variety of substances can be used, for instance olive oil or specially prepared gels.

The attenuation of ultrasound in body tissues has a bearing on the choice of ultrasound frequency. The fact that penetration decreases with frequency conflicts with the need to reduce wavelength in order to obtain better resolution. For each situation a compromise is necessary. It may be useful to carry out investigations at different frequencies but this requires different transducer heads and corresponding switching facilities in the electronic circuitry. Commonly used frequencies lie in the range from one to ten megahertz, the latter being appropriate for transducers which can be placed close to the blood vessel of interest. In contrast, two megahertz may be required for foetal and placental investigations.

## GROUP 1(b): INDICATOR DILUTION TECHNIQUES FOR SEGMENTAL VENOUS FLOW

If an indicator is injected into a vein and the blood sampled 'down-stream' from the site of injection, then the degree of dilution will depend on the blood flow—provided that there has been complete mixing of the indicator in the blood. If the rate at which the indicator has been injected and the degree of dilution which it has undergone after mixing with the blood flowing through the vessel is known, then the flow through the vessel can be determined by simple proportion.

For instance, if an indicator is injected into a vein at 1 ml/min and contains $W$ g of indicator per ml, and the down-stream blood sample contains $\frac{1}{100} \times W$ g of indicator per ml, then the flow is 100 ml/min or $F$ ml/min = $f(C)/(c)$ where $f$ = quantity of indicator injected in ml/min, $C$ = concentration of indicator injected and $c$ = concentration of indicator in blood sample.

The success of the method will depend on:

(1) Complete mixing of the indicator with the blood.

(2) The absence of tributaries entering the vein between the site of injection and the site of sampling.

(3) The absence of indicator in the venous blood 'up-stream' of the injection site—or, alternatively, a knowledge of its concentration.

(4) The smallness of volume of injected indicator flow compared with volume of blood flow.

A suitable technique consists of inserting a double lumen catheter into the vessel under study. The indicator is injected at a constant rate and emerges through fine holes drilled into a stainless steel head of the catheter. This disperses the indicator into fine jets and facilitates mixing. The blood is sampled down-stream through a side hole in the catheter.

The indicator can be a radioactive tracer such as [131]I labelled serum albumin, Evans blue dye or similar substances. Alternatively, cold saline can be used—the degree of dilution of coldness determining the flow. This can be measured by thermistor probes inserted into the vessel itself. For a critical evaluation of thermal dilution techniques the reader is referred to Lowe (1968).

## GROUP II: METHODS USING DIFFUSIBLE INDICATORS

In this group are the methods which depend on using indicators which diffuse rapidly between blood and tissue. Such indicators are oxygen, nitrous oxide, and radioactive isotopes of the inert gases krypton and xenon. They are used to measure the rate of uptake or of clearance of the indicator by the tissues of the organ under study.

### The Fick Principle

The methods described in this group are derived from the Fick principle, first proposed in 1870, which states that in the steady state the quantity of a substance taken up by an organ in unit time was the product of the arterio-venous difference and the blood flow. For example,

$$\text{Blood flow} = \frac{\text{oxygen consumption}}{\text{arterio-venous oxygen content difference}}$$

### Inhalation Techniques—Kety Schmidt Method

Probably the first successful application of a diffusible indicator to the measurement of organ blood flow in man was by Kety and Schmidt who used $N_2O$ to measure cerebral blood flow. It is appropriate to describe their method to illustrate some of the general principles of the methods in this group.

Patients inhale a mixture of 15 per cent $N_2O$ in air over a period of 10 minutes. Blood samples are taken at intervals from an artery and from the main venous drainage of the organ under study (i.e. internal jugular bulb, coronary sinus, etc.). These samples are analysed for $N_2O$ content and the arterial and venous time concentration curves are plotted (Fig. 9).

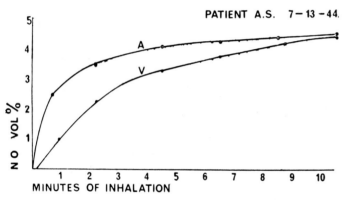

FIG. 9. Arterial and cerebral venous concentrations of $N_2O$ plotted against time of inhalation of $N_2O$. (From Kety, S. S. and Schmidt, C. F. (1945), *Amer. J. Physiol.*, **143**, 53)—reproduced by kind permission of the authors and publishers.

The original Fick equation can be expressed as:

$$F = \frac{Q(t)}{Ca(t) - Cv(t)} \tag{1}$$

where $F$ = flow in unit time, $Q(t)$ = quantity of substance taken up in time unit, $Ca(t)$ = concentration in arterial blood, and $Cv(t)$ = concentration of the venous blood, both at time $t$ in minutes after the start of inhalation.

In integral form

$$F = \frac{\int_0^T Q(t)\, dt}{\int_0^T (Ca - Cv)\, dt}$$

where $T$ = total time of inhalation.

However, one cannot measure the quantity $\int_0^T Q(t)\, dt$ of $N_2O$ taken up by the brain, but quantity = concentration $C \times$ weight $W$. Figure 9 shows that following a ten-minute period of inhalation, the arterial blood, the venous blood and presumably the tissue are approximately in equilibrium for $N_2O$. Therefore the brain concentration will be the same as the final venous concentration $Cv(T)$ measured at the end of 10 minutes inhalation. Therefore the numerator of the Fick equation $\int_0^T Q(t)\, dt$ can be expressed as $Cv(T) \times W$.

As the arterio-venous difference for $N_2O$ is changing throughout the period of inhalation, the denominator of the Fick equation must be expressed as $\int_0^T (Ca - Cv)\, dt$, that is the sum of all the arterio-venous differences over all the little bits of time ($dt$) during the period of inhalation ($t$).

Equation (1) can now be expressed as:

$$F = \frac{Cv(T) \times W\lambda}{\int_0^T (Ca - Cv)\, dt} \tag{2}$$

The constant $\lambda$ is introduced as the ratio of the solubilities of nitrous oxide in brain tissue and blood, i.e. the final venous concentration will only reflect the brain concentration if the gas is equally as soluble in blood as in brain tissue. This is true with nitrous oxide ($\lambda = 1$) but deviates from unity with krypton and xenon.

In equation (2), everything is known except $W$, the weight of the brain. However, dividing both sides of the equation by $W$, the following equation is obtained:

$$F/W = \frac{Cv(T)\lambda}{\int_0^T (Ca - Cv)\, dt} \tag{3}$$

In other words, instead of expressing flow in units per minute through the entire organ, it can be expressed in units per unit weight per minute. Whatever answer obtained for the right hand side of the equation (let it be 5) could be expressed as a flow of 5 g blood per g of brain per minute or 5 Kg of blood per Kg of brain per minute. However, if the partition coefficient ($\lambda$) is calculated as the ratio of the solubilities of 1 g of brain and 1 ml of blood, then the final flow calculation can be expressed as ml blood per g brain per minute or more usually ml/100 g/min.

In summary, the Kety-Schmidt technique requires intermittent samples of arterial and venous blood which are analysed for $N_2O$ content. The numerator of equation (3) is the concentration in the venous blood at the end of the period of inhalation. The denominator is the integrated arterio-venous difference or the area between $A$ and $V$ on Fig. 9. The final result is expressed as flow in ml per unit weight of tissue per minute.

### Limitations of the Kety-Schmidt Method

In the original method $N_2O$ was inhaled for 10 minutes. This was thought long enough for equilibration to be reached between blood and tissue. However, in conditions of slow flow, equilibration may not have been reached in 10 minutes and the blood flow will be over-estimated. This error can be reduced by extending the period of inhalation, by using an indicator of lower solubility (for instance the radioactive isotope $^{85}$Kr) or by extrapolating the arterio-venous difference to infinite time (Lassen and Munck, 1955).

It is also essential for the method that the venous blood samples are truly representative of the venous drainage from the organ under study.

### Modifications of the Kety-Schmidt Method

The following are some of the more widely used modifications of the original method.

(1) The use of a radioactive rare gas isotope like $^{85}$Kr or $^{133}$Xe instead of $N_2O$ as the indicator has the enormous advantage of avoiding the tedious and time-consuming analysis of $N_2O$ in blood. For example, $^{85}$Kr can be delivered to the patient in a concentration of 0·1 mCi per litre of air and the blood samples can easily be analysed for radioactivity using standard techniques (*see* Lassen and Munck, 1955).

(2) Instead of sampling the arterial and venous blood at intervals and calculating the integrated $A - V$ difference, the same effect can be achieved if continuous samples of arterial and venous blood are withdrawn with automatic withdrawal syringes. Subtraction of the concentration of indicator in the venous syringe ($\int Cv \, dt$) from that in the arterial syringe ($\int Ca \, dt$) will give the integrated $A - V$ difference. This has the obvious attraction of saving in the number of analyses which have to be undertaken.

(3) In order to overcome difficulties in measurement of 'low flow' situation where the venous blood and the tissue are not in equilibrium for the indicator at the end of 10 minutes of inhalation, Lassen and Munck (1955) have suggested that the period of inhalation be extended to 15 minutes and that a mathematical correction be introduced to extend the measurement of the $A - V$ difference to infinite time.

(4) The use of the desaturation curve (i.e. taking samples of arterial and venous blood for, say, 15 minutes after an equal or longer period of inhalation) will have the advantage of reducing the need for such exact control of the concentration of indicator delivered to the patient during inhalation.

Lassen and Klee (1965) have discussed the advantages and disadvantages of the modifications to the Kety-Schmidt method. They suggest the subject should inhale $^{85}$Kr in air for at least 15 minutes, and up to 30 minutes when slow flow values were expected. The samples of arterial and venous blood could be taken either during the 15 minute inhalation period, or during the desaturation phase following a 30 minute inhalation.

### Intra-arterial Injection Techniques

The original Kety-Schmidt method gives flow per unit weight through the whole organ under study and requires both arterial and venous cannulation. The intra-arterial injection of the inert diffusible gases $^{85}$Kr and $^{133}$Xe depends on measuring the rate of clearance of the isotope from the organ by means of external detectors. It obviates the need for venous blood samples from the organ under study and permits measurements of flow through fairly small volumes of tissue.

### Theory

Two important physical properties of krypton and xenon make them suitable for this type of study. Firstly, when carried to the cerebral tissue by the arterial blood, entry into and subsequent exit from the tissue will depend solely on diffusion and solubility. Secondly, as the solubility of the gas is so much higher in air than in blood or tissue, a high proportion of it will, on reaching the lungs in the venous blood, be excreted into the alveolar air.

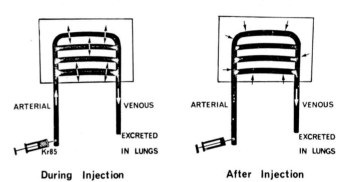

FIG. 10. Basic principle of inert gas clearance method with intra-arterial injection. (Harper, A. M. and Bell, G., 1966, in *Wound Healing*, Ed. Illingworth; Publ. Churchill: London)—reproduced by kind permission of the publishers.

Therefore, there will be no effective arterial recirculation. Accordingly, if an injection of $^{85}$Kr or $^{133}$Xe, dissolved in saline, is made into the internal carotid artery, the isotope will equilibrate rapidly between the blood and brain tissue. When the injection is stopped, the arterial blood (now containing no isotope) will wash the gas out of the brain tissue, and the rate of 'washout' or clearance will depend on the blood flow (Fig. 10). The more rapid the clearance the faster the blood flow and vice versa.

### Methods

#### Beta Counting

As the beta emissions of $^{85}$Kr have a maximum range of only 2·5 mm in tissue, this isotope can be used to measure blood flow through the superficial cortex of an organ such as the brain or kidney. To illustrate—the surface of a kidney is exposed and an end window Geiger-Müller tube placed 1 mm above a selected area on its surface. The G.M. tube is connected to a ratemeter and direct writing recorder. The range of the ratemeter is set at between 100 and 1,000 counts per second maximum deflection and the time constant at 1 second. A catheter with side holes at its tip is inserted into the femoral artery and advanced up the aorta until the side holes lie opposite the ostium of the renal artery. $^{85}$Kr, dissolved in saline, is injected into the catheter. The actual amount of $^{85}$Kr injected is immaterial as long as enough is given to ensure maximum count rate of over 100 cps. When the injection has been given, the clearance curve obtained on the recorder is transposed onto semilogarithmic paper. The $T\frac{1}{2}$ value is calculated for a straight line drawn through the initial part of the clearance curve. The $T\frac{1}{2}$ is the time in minutes taken for radioactivity to fall by half from its initial value, assuming an exponential decay. Flow can then be calculated as ml/g/min from the formula:

$$\text{Flow ml/g/min} = \frac{\lambda \times \log_e 2}{T\frac{1}{2}} \qquad (\textit{Vide infra})$$

### Gamma Counting

After an injection into the artery supplying the organ, the gamma emissions of $^{85}$Kr and $^{133}$Xe can be recorded by means of scintillation crystals mounted externally. The latter isotope is more commonly used. As an illustration, regional blood flow in the brain can be measured as follows. Scintillation crystals (an array can be used) are mounted over various points of the patient's scalp. The crystals are collimated with lead so that each 'looks' at a defined brain volume. The size and overlap of the volumes of the brain seen by adjacent crystals will depend on the size of the crystals and the design of the collimator.

The signals from the scintillation crystals and their associated photomultipliers are fed through pulse height analysers into a multi-channel digital tape-recorder. From the tape-recorder the impulses from each crystal can be fed through a ratemeter to a scaler and chart recorder. The following information will be received:

    (1) From the ratemeter and chart recorder—the shape of the clearance curve.
    (2) From the scaler—the time integral of the radio-activity during the clearance period.

For measurement of regional cerebral blood flow about 2 mCi of $^{133}$Xe dissolved in 2 ml of saline are injected over one or two seconds into a catheter in the internal carotid artery. The clearance is recorded for at least 10 minutes. These measurements are usually done in association with routine cerebral angiography.

### Calculation of Blood Flow

The calculation of the mean blood flow through the volume seen by each crystal can be obtained by using the formula:
Flow in ml per g of brain per minute:

$$\frac{\lambda b \times (H_{\max} - H_{10})}{A_{10}}$$

where $\lambda b$ = tissue:blood partition coefficient for whole brain for $^{85}$Kr (Lassen and Munck, 1955) or $^{133}$Xe (Veall and Mallett 1965)
$H_{\max}$ = maximum height of clearance curve ($H_{10}$ being height at 10 minutes)
$A_{10}$ = area under clearance curve or total integrated counts after 10 minutes.

The mathematical proof of this equation is given by Zierler (1965), and the basic principles are given in Appendix I of this chapter. The use of the 10-minute period is, like the original Kety-Schmidt equation, an approximation, and longer periods may be needed when very low flows are expected. The height of the clearance curve is obtained from the direct writing recorder and the area from the scaler (Fig. 11).

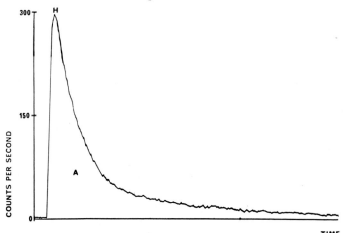

Fig. 11. $^{133}$Xe clearance curve from brain. $H$ = maximum height and $A$ = area under curve. (Harper, A. M., 1969, in *Cerebral Circulation*, Ed. McDowall; Publ, Little, Brown & Co.: Boston)—reproduced by kind permission of the editor and publishers.

Clearance curves can also be treated in another way—namely, by 'exponential stripping'. As two exponential components can usually be extracted from a cerebral clearance curve of $^{85}$Kr or $^{133}$Xe, these components probably reflect flow through grey and white matter. In practice, the clearance curve is replotted on semilogarithmic paper. A straight line drawn through the 'tail' of the curve is subtracted from the primary curve (Fig. 12) and the '$T\frac{1}{2}$' of the resulting exponential

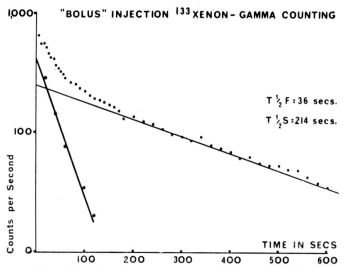

Fig. 12. Semilog. plot of clearance curve showing exponential stripping in fast ($F$) and slow ($S$) components. (Harper, A. M., 1969—in *Cerebral Circulation*, Ed. McDowall; Publ. Little, Brown & Co.: Boston)—reproduced by kind permission of the editor and publishers.

components is calculated. The 'T$\frac{1}{2}$' is the time taken for the radioactivity to decline to half its initial value. Blood flow can be calculated separately for each exponential:

Flow ml/g/min for fast (grey) or slow (white) component:

$$= \frac{\lambda \times \log_e 2}{T\frac{1}{2}}$$

$$= \frac{\lambda \times 0.693}{T\frac{1}{2}}$$

where $\lambda$ = cerebral grey or white matter: blood partition coefficient.

However, the brain is unusual in having a fairly clearly defined bimodal distribution of blood flows. If the technique is applied to an organ such as the kidney, up to four exponential components can be extracted and it is by no means certain what these represent. Under these circumstances it is probably safer to use the $H/A$ formula.

### Applications of Intra-Arterial Injection Method

The technique can be used to measure flow through any organ whose arterial supply can be cannulated exclusively. As well as the brain, it is used to measure renal blood flow and myocardial blood flow. As the latter appears to be a fairly homogeneous tissue with a relatively mono-exponential clearance, flow can be calculated from the T$\frac{1}{2}$ of a semilogarithmic plot of the clearance curve following injection of $^{133}$Xe into the coronary artery (usually in association with coronary angiography).

### Intra-tissue Injection

In the two types of method so far described in this group (i.e. Kety-Schmidt technique and the intra-arterial injection techniques) the tissue has been labelled by isotope carried in the arterial blood. It is also possible to measure the blood flow following direct intra-tissue injection of the indicator.

The clearance of radioactive sodium has been used for some years to measure flow through muscle. However, as sodium is to some extent diffusion limited, it is probably better to use $^{133}$Xe.

The technique applied to the measurement of blood flow through the anterior tibial muscle as described by Lassen *et al.* (1964) is as follows. 0.5 mCi of $^{133}$Xe dissolved in saline is injected into the anterior tibial muscle of the resting patient. The rate of disappearance of the isotope is measured with a scintillation crystal mounted above the site of injection. The detector is coupled to a ratemeter and the clearance curve recorded on a logarithmic potentiometer (the last obviates the necessity for replotting the clearance curve on semilogarithmic paper). The resting clearance rate is measured for 5 minutes and then a cuff is inflated above the knee to greater than systolic blood pressure. During this induced ischaemia the patient is asked to move his foot up and down until pain prevents any further exercise. The cuff is then released and the xenon clearance is followed during the subsequent reactive hyperaemia (Fig. 13).

The flow is calculated by drawing a tangent through the clearance curve and applying a formula similar to that given on page 35.

This technique has proved valuable in assessing the severity of vascular disease of the legs and in assessing the results of surgery. It is simple to use and appears less liable to technical error than plethysmography.

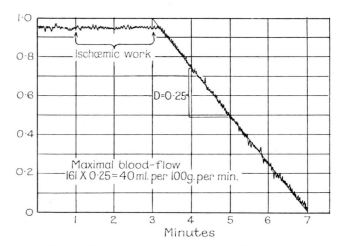

Fig. 13. $^{133}$Xe clearance curve in healthy subject obtained with a logarithmic potentiometer. The graph indicates the period of cuff obstruction of blood-flow in the leg during which muscular work to the point of exhaustion is carried out. Maximal slope, D, after release of cuff pressure is 0.25 of the total amplitude of the logarithmic potentiometer. Maximal M.B.F. is consequently 161 × 0.25 = 40 ml per 100 g per min. Maximal reactive hyperaemia sets in about 0.2 min after cuff release. (Lassen, N. A., Lindbjerg, J., and Munck, O., *Lancet*, 1: 686: 1964)—reproduced by kind permission of the authors and publishers.

However, care must be taken that no gas bubbles are injected or that isotope is not lost into the subcutaneous tissue since either may lead to a falsely slow clearance rate.

### Summary of Methods in Group II

All the methods in Group II involve labelling the tissue with a diffusible indicator (usually $^{133}$Xe or $^{85}$Kr) and measuring the rate of uptake or clearance from the tissue. The tissue can be labelled in three ways:

(a) by inhalation,
(b) by direct intra-arterial injection,
(c) by direct tissue injection.

If (a) then arterial and venous blood samples are required. If (b) or (c), no blood samples are needed but the rate of clearance of the indicator is measured with external detectors.

The choice of labelling technique will depend on the tissue being investigated and often on the associated investigations being undertaken. To give a few examples:

(1) Where metabolic studies are required and venous samples are needed for oxygen and other measurements, then inhalation techniques with cannulation of, say, jugular or renal veins or coronary sinus should be used.

(2) Where regional cerebral blood flow estimations are required and associated cerebral angiography is being carried out, then intra-arterial injection into the carotid artery should be used—similarly for coronary or renal blood flow.

(3) For muscle blood flow studies the direct intra-tissue injection should be used.

The methods described will give blood flow per unit weight of tissue. They all have the great advantage that they will reflect true tissue perfusion (any blood going through $A - V$ shunts will not be reflected in the clearance curves).

## GROUP III: NON-DIFFUSIBLE INDICATOR DILUTION METHODS

Methods using indicator dilution principles are now frequently used for measuring blood flow through organs and for cardiac output determinations. Numerous substances have been used as indicators, mainly dyes and radioisotopes.

In the normal subject any appropriate indicator injected into a systemic vein will pass through the pulmonary circulation and then be distributed throughout the body by the arterial system. There are several important requirements for a suitable indicator. It should not by itself alter circulatory haemodynamics; it must be detectable and measurable at the peripheral sampling site; and it should remain within the circulation during at least its first passage through the body, although subsequent elimination is an advantage.

### Theory

In the first instance, it is easier to consider a simple model. Suppose a tube with a mixing chamber has a steady flow of water at $Q$ ml/sec (Fig. 14).

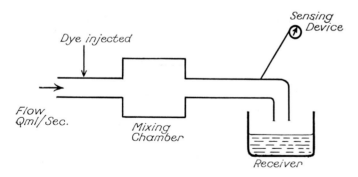

FIG. 14. Basic principles of dye dilution technique (*see* text).

The indicator is injected proximal to the mixing chamber, from which the effluent is collected until all the indicator has passed out of the chamber. Let this time equal $t$ seconds and let $I$ mg be the amount of indicator injected, the mean concentration of indicator in the effluent being $\bar{c}$. The total

flow through the system is $Qt$ ml. Since $I$ mg of indicator was injected, the measured mean concentration can be expressed as:

$$\bar{c} = \frac{I}{Qt} \quad \text{and thus} \quad Q = \frac{I}{\bar{c}t} \text{ ml/sec}$$

Thus a flow such as cardiac output can be expressed as:

$$\text{Cardiac output } (L/\text{min}) = \frac{60\ I}{\bar{c} \times 1,000}$$

In this equation 60 converts seconds to minutes and 1,000 converts millilitres to litres.

The passage of indicator through the tubing distal to the mixing chamber can be detected by a suitable photo-electric device or scintillation crystal (depending on whether a dye or radioisotope is used) and recorded as a time-concentration curve. However, such a model system ignores the problem of recirculation which occurs in many human studies. In man, dye injected into the right side of the circulation is mixed in the right ventricle, passes through the pulmonary circulation and is then distributed by the arterial system before returning to the right side of the heart at a rate that depends on the circulation time. The fall of the time-concentration curve in man never reaches zero before being interrupted by recirculation. Fortunately, the down-slope of such curves is usually exponential and can be replotted on semilogarithmic paper to become a straight line (Fig. 15).

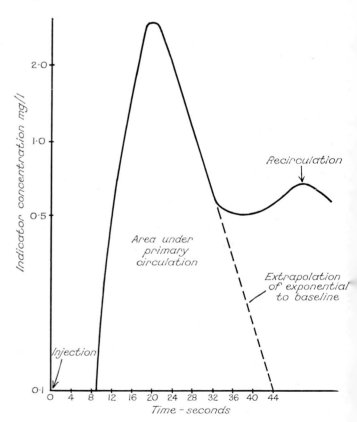

FIG. 15. Semilog. plot of time-concentration curve as used to calculate cardiac output.

Extrapolation of the downslope enables a reasonable estimate to be made of the way in which the time-concentration curve would have behaved in the absence of recirculation. The value of $\bar{c}t$ is the area under the time-concentration curve.

Various methods are available for measuring this area. The simplest is to sum the heights of the curve at one-second intervals, reading the later heights after recirculation from the extrapolated line so that the effect of recirculation can be corrected. Other methods such as planimetry have previously been used.

More recently general purpose analogue computers have been programmed to calculate the area under the exponential. Several small special purpose devices have also been developed specifically for application in measurement of cardiac output and provide a more or less immediate digital display of the result. A small computer for calculating cardiac output from thermal dilution curves is also available. In this situation recirculation does not occur and only simple integration of the thermal dilution curve is required (Cowell and Bray, 1970).

## Indicator Substances

These include both dyes and radioisotopes such as [131]I labelled human serum albumin or [51]Cr labelled red blood cells.

Indocyanine green is now the most frequently used dye. It has a peak spectral absorption at 800 nm (nanometers) at which wavelength the absorption of both oxyhaemoglobin and reduced haemoglobin is identical and changes in their relative amounts in the blood do not affect the detection of the dye. A method currently in use for cardiac output measurement is as follows: A Teflon cannula is inserted percutaneously into a brachial artery and a venous catheter is passed from an opposite arm vein to the junction of the superior vena cava and the right atrium. Ten milligrams of indocyanine green are injected as a bolus from an injection chamber of known volume, followed by a flushing injection of saline. Arterial blood is withdrawn at a constant rate by a pump through a densitometer. A time-concentration curve of the injected dye is obtained on a recorder. Both pen and ultra violet recorders are suitable and it is important to ensure that an adequate height of deflection above the base line is obtained. It is also possible to record directly on to a tape recorder for subsequent data retrieval and analysis. The system is calibrated by the serial sampling of dyes of varying concentrations. It is important to ensure that the dye solution is freshly prepared (less than 6 hours old) and that the patient's own blood is used with the dye samples in the calibrating procedure. After the dye time-concentration graph has been recorded, it is transposed on to semilogarithmic paper which facilitates calculation of the area under the exponential. The area under the primary circulation curve can then be obtained. With this calibration method an equilibrium specimen of blood for dye concentration is not necessary. The amount of dye injected is known and the calibration curve indicates the deflection produced by a given amount of dye. Repeat estimations can be undertaken as required.

## Measurement of Limb and Organ Blood Flow with Non-diffusible Indicators

Dye or radioisotope injection has also been used to measure forearm blood flow. For instance, dye can be injected at a constant rate into the brachial artery and sampled from a vein in the antecubital-fossa. In contrast to plethysmography, such techniques do not interrupt venous outflow from the limb and therefore do not alter the pressure gradient nor cause abnormal accumulation of vaso-active metabolites, either of which might alter the blood flow. The major problem associated with accurate measurement of limb blood flow has been the need to ensure adequate mixing of the indicator with blood. Approaches which have been used to improve mixing include jet injection of indicator and intra-arterial injections of large volumes of up to 34 ml/min. Unfortunately, jet injections have been reported as causing haemolysis. Overbeck and his colleagues (1969) attempted to overcome these difficulties by using a stainless steel needle with holes drilled behind a blocked tip. A specially designed infusion pump is used to deliver 8 ml/min at up to 1,500 mmHg pressure. Using [131]I albumin as an indicator, limb blood flow can be calculated as follows:

$$F = \frac{A}{B - C}$$

where $F$ = limb (forearm and hand) blood flow in ml/min
$A$ = radioactivity infused per minute into the brachial artery
$B$ = radioactivity in venous blood per ml
$C$ = radioactivity in contralateral brachial artery per ml.

Studies using this method have suggested that total forearm and hand blood flow in man may be calculated accurately. The system appears to produce satisfactory mixing and does not cause haemolysis. It is sometimes desirable, but difficult, to study separately changes in blood flow to skin and muscle, and one method is that of simultaneous cannulation of both the deep and superficial veins of the forearm to allow measurement of muscle and skin blood flow.

## Surface Counting of Non-diffusible Isotopes

These methods all employ indicator dilution principles and have been used mainly for measurement of cardiac output with more recent application being in the measurement of renal blood flow and glomerular filtration rate.

The concept of injecting a suitable radioisotope intravenously and then following the passage of radioactivity through the heart by means of an externally placed detector has been attractive to many workers. It is simple for the patient, avoids arterial cannulation and results are quickly available. It has the disadvantage that the number of studies is limited by the radiation administered although the use of newer isotopes with a short half life, such as 99 m technetium, reduces radiation dosage and allows multiple studies. One method of praecordial counting (Lorimer et al., 1968) consists of the intravenous injection of 35–40 mCi of [131]I serum albumin from a calibrated injection chamber. The

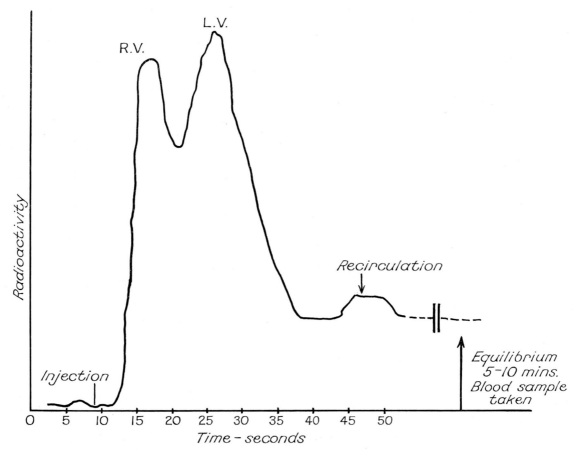

FIG. 16. Time-concentration curve during praecordial counting after injection of [131]I serum albumin. Peaks indicate right and left ventricular activity.

external detector is positioned over the fourth left interspace at the sternal edge and consists of a simple lead collimator containing a $2 \cdot 5 \times 2 \cdot 5$ cm² sodium iodide crystal linked to a ratemeter and pen recorder. Two peaks of radioactivity are recorded after injection (Fig. 16).

The first is due mainly to right ventricular appearance and washout and the second to left ventricular appearance and washout. This washout is exponential and can be replotted in the same way as with indocyanine green to give the area under the primary circulation curve. A venous sample is taken at 10 minutes after injection when mixing is complete for measurement of blood radioactivity and a simultaneous equilibrium value for praecordial radioactivity is obtained. Cardiac output is calculated from:

$$\text{Cardiac output } (L/\text{min}) = \frac{60\,I \times 1{,}000}{A \times \dfrac{C}{d}}$$

where   $I$ = total radioactivity injected
      $A$ = area under curve
      $C$ = radioactivity per ml of a blood sample taken at equilibrium
      $d$ = height of deflection of recorder at equilibrium

Comparison of the results obtained from praecordial counting and other methods suggest that valid results are given by the former and that the reproducibility of the

method is similar to that of Fick or dye dilution methods. The technique is simple and atraumatic, requiring only two venepunctures.

One disadvantage in the use of a radioisotope such as [131]I serum albumin is that the cumulative radioactivity makes this method impractical for an investigation requiring more than three of four measurements of cardiac output. However it is now possible to obtain albumin bound 99 m technetium which hopefully will facilitate repeated measurements.

The recent development of gamma scintillation cameras capable of recording sequential radioisotope images from the praecordium has meant that anatomical features as well as chamber volume and flow measurements can be made with respect to heart, lung and great vessels (Ishii and MacIntyre, 1971; Kriss et al., 1971). Scintiphotographic images produced by gamma emitting radioisotopes can be recorded in rapid sequence as the isotope flows through the circulatory system. The field of view of a gamma camera is large enough to include the heart and major portions of each lung field. 99m technetium as sodium pertechnetate is injected intravenously. Gamma rays striking the crystal are converted to electronic signals and collected by an analyser which can retain and display radioactivity corresponding to the distribution of isotope in the gamma camera field. As the isotope bolus flows through the heart and great vessels the rapidly changing sequence of images can be recorded at short intervals of for example 0·5 seconds or less and then transferred for storage. At the end of the investigation, data can be retrieved, displayed on an oscilloscope and areas of interest selected for analysis (Fig. 17).

By means of an appropriate storage and play back system indicator dilution curves can be recorded from individual vascular compartments such as right atrium, right ventricle and lung fields. Volume and flow measurements have been made by several groups of workers. Although such techniques require expensive equipment for data acquisition, storage and analysis, it seems likely that much information will be gained from these methods in the future.

Ram, Holroyd and Chisholm (1969) have reported a similar method for measuring glomerular filtration rate using the contrast media of intravenous pyelography. They gave a single injection of [131]I labelled diatrizoate with external counting, blood sampling and calculation similar to those used in measurement of renal plasma flow. The disappearance curve of the injected isotope was replotted on semilogarithmic paper and the mono-exponential decay which was observed during the two-hour period after injection was extrapolated to zero time. The authors accept that the method of curve analysis is empirical but believe that satisfactory correlation with endogenous creatinine clearance values are found. This method may

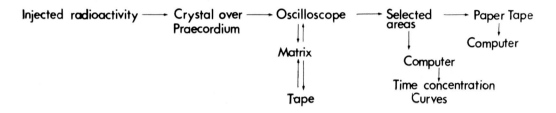

Fig. 17. Diagram of study of circulatory kinetics using a gamma camera system.

## Measurement of Organ Blood Flow by Surface Counting of Radioisotopes

Methods of measuring renal blood flow or glomerular filtration rate usually involve the continuous infusion of para-aminohippurate or inulin, with also perhaps the need for bladder catheterization and accurate timing of urine and blood samples. Ram and his co-workers (1968) have investigated a single injection method using [131]I labelled hippuran for the measurement of renal plasma flow. An external scintillation counter was placed over the sternal end of the second left interspace and the biological decay of 30mCi of injected radioisotope was followed on a pen recorder and replotted on semilogarithmic paper. This usually gave a straight line for the first ten to twenty minutes of the decay curve and could readily be extrapolated to zero time. A blood sample was taken at twenty minutes for measurement of radioactivity.

The renal plasma flow was calculated from:

$$RPF = kv \text{ (ml/min)}$$

where

$$k = \frac{\log_e 2}{T\frac{1}{2}(\text{min})}$$

$v$ = apparent volume distribution hippuran or

$$\frac{\text{activity injected}}{\text{plasma radioactivity per ml}}$$

Overall, the external counting method tended to give consistently higher values than other techniques, possibly due to slow leakage of isotope from blood into tissue spaces.

eventually prove to be clinically useful, although it has not yet been shown to be of definite value when compared with inulin clearances in patients with reduced glomerular filtration rates.

## GROUP IV: MISCELLANEOUS TECHNIQUES

### Plethysmography

Plethysmography describes a physiological measuring technique for determining local blood flow in a digit, limb, or tissue segment by means based on the measurement of a change in volume. The initial applications were simple. The limb under study, usually the hand and forearm, was enclosed in a rigid water-tight chamber filled with fluid and linked to a recorder. Fluctuation in the volume of the limb due to changes in blood flow displaced the incompressible fluid from the chamber. The amount displaced was recorded. Burch (1947) has used a similar device to measure flow in the fingertip, which is sealed in a rigid, air-tight capsule with a proximal inflatable cuff. Sudden inflation of the cuff to a pressure above the venous occlusion pressure, but below the systolic arterial pressure, prevents outflow of blood but arterial inflow continues. The volume of the fingertip increases, displacing fluid from the capsule and activating a sensing device. Environmental temperature and temperature of the water in the plethysmograph are both important factors in altering local blood flow and have to be carefully controlled.

Probably the most frequently used apparatus for measuring limb blood flow by venous occlusion plethysmography is the Whitney strain gauge (Whitney, 1953). This is a relatively thick-walled rubber tube with a very small lumen which is filled with mercury. The electrical resistance of the mercury is balanced in a Wheatstone bridge circuit and an increase in length of the column of mercury results in an increase of electrical resistance which can be recorded. When used in conjunction with venous occlusion the increase in girth of a segment of a limb may be measured and hence the increase in volume due to blood also measured. The strain gauge is small, easily fitted and is comfortable for the patient. One disadvantage is the lack of a suitable means of direct calibration. However, Ardill, Fentem and Williams (1968) attempted a dynamic calibration by infusing 0·9 per cent saline via the brachial artery into a segment of the forearm after the circulation had been arrested by a pneumatic cuff. Two strain gauges were used. In five experiments the inflow recorded by the proximal-gauge was within 10 per cent of the inflow expected from a knowledge of the rate of infusion and the volume of the limb between the two cuffs. Despite the apparent simplicity of the method, there are disadvantages in that the choice of a representative site in the forearm is difficult and the pattern of results obtained from adjacent segments of forearm may vary considerably according to the factor or factors responsible for changing local limb flow.

An inverse relationship is present, the larger the volume the smaller being the impedance. Allwood and Farncombe (1967) have described the use of surface electrodes and a transistorized impedance measuring circuit to record changes in impedance in the forearm and calf during venous occlusion plethysmography. Volume changes were simultaneously measured with a water-filled plethysmograph or a mercury-in-rubber strain gauge. A close inverse relationship was found between variations and electrical impedance. However, correlation was poor in the presence of vasoconstriction, due possibly to redistribution of blood in the segment.

### Qualitative Estimations of Local Blood Flow with Heat

The rate of heat transfer between the outside of a copper disc and the skin over which it is placed can be used to give a quantitative estimation of local blood flow (Hatfield and Troncelliti, 1950). Alternatively, a heated thermocouple in the form of a needle can be inserted into the tissue under study. The principle as enunciated by Betz (1968) is that the temperature of a constantly heated point in a tissue is dependent on the conduction of heat through the tissue, and on the convection

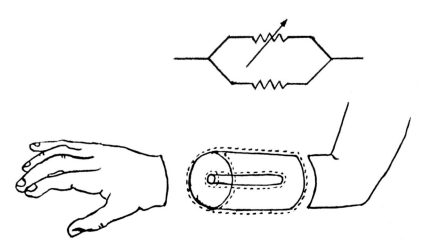

FIG. 18. Electrical impedance plethysmography. Schematic diagram showing change in volume in a limb segment due to accumulation of blood and its electrical analogue of a fixed and variable resistance in parallel. (Allwood, M. J., 1968, in *Blood Flow Through Organs and Tissues*, Ed. Bain and Harper; Publ. Livingstone: Edinburgh)—reproduced by kind permission of the author and publishers.

### Electrical Impedance Plethysmography

The principles of electrical impedance plethysmography depend upon the fact that living tissue such as the human limb segment is an ionic conductor which shows a characteristic impedance to the passage of a high frequency alternating electrical current. The impedance of a particular tissue segment is due to both the impedance of the intervening tissues and the volume of blood contained within the segment. Since the impedance contribution of the tissue remains constant at any given time, changes in the total observed impedance following venous occlusion represent changes in the ratio of blood to tissue (Fig. 18).

of heat by the blood. A probe with two thermocouple junctions is inserted into the tissue. If one junction is heated, the temperature difference between the heated and unheated junction can be recorded continually and the rate of heat clearance derived. From the latter a quantitative estimate of blood flow can be calculated.

### CHOICE OF METHODS

Before undertaking the measurement of blood flow through an organ or tissue, the clinician will ask himself very carefully what it is he wants to measure. This may seem paradoxical but it can be illustrated as follows. The measurement of blood flow to a limb with arterial disease can be assessed with an electromagnetic flowmeter on the artery supplying the limb, with a plethysmograph on a digit, or by injecting $^{133}$Xe into the muscle of the limb. What information can be obtained from each method? The electromagnetic flowmeter will measure the total volume of blood going to the limb but tell nothing about its distribution; the plethysmograph on a digit will give a better indication of skin blood flow and will give an indication as to whether the needs of the extremities are being met; and the xenon clearance will tell whether the tissue perfusion in a selected area of muscle is adequate.

Therefore, the information given by each method is different and the question 'what does one want to measure' is an important one. Just as important is whether or not the method selected will be hazardous or uncomfortable to the patient. For instance, the use of electromagnetic flow probes will obviously be restricted to the operating theatre, and there will be many circumstances where it would not be desirable to puncture an artery to carry out a xenon clearance study.

How frequently or how often the measurement of flow must be repeated may be a factor in deciding the method. Other questions which must be taken into consideration are whether one is interested in actual tissue perfusion or in the total organ flow and whether metabolic studies, such as oxygen uptake, are required.

It is unfortunate that the ease and simplicity of a method of measuring blood flow is often in inverse proportion to the quality and usefulness of the data it produces. None of the techniques is easy. They are all beset with traps, and artefacts abound. However with patience, care and practice, good results will be obtained as long as there is full understanding of exactly what is being measured and that the information taken from the results is that which the method was designed to produce.

## APPENDIX I

### Indicators and Tracers in Steady-State Biological Systems*

A steady-state system is one through which there is a continuous flow of material, and in which the quantity of material in any part of the system, and the rate of flow between any two parts remains constant. Many biological systems behave in ways that closely approximate to this state—the examples of blood flow described in this chapter are all typical.

Under ordinary conditions, there is no way of distinguishing one part of the flow in the system from another; indeed often there is nothing within the system to indicate directly to the observer that there is in fact any such flow. Such a system can be studied only when a tracer, possessing distinctive characteristics recognizable by the observer, constitutes part of the flow.

Consider a steady-state system having a flow $F$, and let a quantity of non-diffusible tracer (e.g. labelled blood)

* This appendix is based on a paper by Orr and Gillespie (1968).

be administered instantaneously at time zero. A fraction $f(t)$ of the tracer is contained in a defined part at time $t$. Since the fates of the tracer and of the material under study are identical, the same fraction $f(t)$, of the quantity $F\delta t$ of the material that entered the system during a time $\delta t$, is in the defined part at a time $t$ after entry. In other words—there will be in the system at any time a fraction $f(t)$ of the material $F\delta t$ that entered the system $t$ seconds earlier. The total amount of the material in the part of the system is therefore the sum of the contributions from all the material that entered the system at all times between $t = 0$ and $t = \infty$ before the defined time. Therefore

$$C = \int_0^\infty f(t)F \, dt = F \int_0^\infty f(t) \, dt = F\theta$$

where $C$ stands for capacity and refers to the total amount of the material, and $\theta$ is the total integral with respect to time of the tracer fraction $f(t)$. $\theta$ is called the Occupancy: it can be shown that $\theta$ is the mean duration of time that the tracer particles remain within the system.

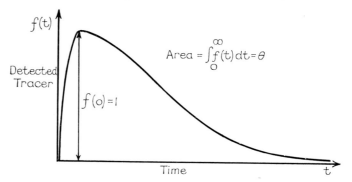

Fig. 19. Tracer-time curve for unit bolus injection (see text).

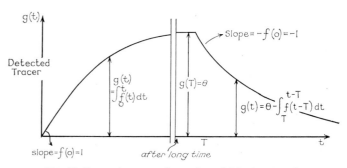

Fig. 20. Tracer-time curve for prolonged injection at unit rate (see text).

Since no particular part of the system was defined, the relation

$$\theta/C = 1/F$$

holds for all parts: this is called the Occupancy Principle. It states that the ratio of occupancy to capacity is the same for all parts of the system and equals the reciprocal of the entry flow into the system. The Occupancy Principle is valid regardless of the time course of administration of tracer and the proof is readily extended to cover this more general case. Also, it is significant that recirculation effects present no special problems.

Use of the Occupancy Principle has the effect of transferring the information available from the tracer directly to the material under study (in this case, blood). Attention is therefore focused on the real biological system instead of being distracted by the ambiguities inherent in the detail of the slope of short regions of the tracer-time curve.

In Figs. 19 and 20 the tracer-time curves for unit bolus injection and continuous injection at unit rate are compared. As already noted, the area under the curve in Fig. 19 is the occupancy notwithstanding the fact that any real bolus injection cannot be instantaneous but requires a finite time interval. However, provided the injection time of the tracer is much shorter than the mean transit time of the tracer within the system (or more strictly the occupancy $\theta$), the maximum height of the curve will be approximately $f(0)$ which is unity. This fact is used to calibrate the amplitude of the tracer time curve in the actual experimental situation: in other words—$\theta$ is given by the ratio of the total area under the curve to the maximum height of the curve (or the initial height in the ideal case of an instantaneous bolus).

In Fig. 20 we have a continuous injection at unit rate starting at $t = 0$ and finishing at $t = T$ a time sufficiently long for the system to have achieved equilibrium with the tracer. It is obvious (or if not, it may be easily proved) that the clearance curve is just the uptake curve turned upside down: it is therefore purely a question of convenience which is chosen for study. Taking the uptake curve it can be seen that it starts rising at zero time with a slope of $f(0)$ which is unity, at time $t$ its value is $\int_0^t f(t)\,dt$ which is called $g(t)$. For the long time $T$, $g(T)$ approaches $\int_0^\infty f(t)\,dt$ which equals $\theta$. Again, in the experimental situation the amplitude of the tracer curve must be calibrated, and here $\theta$ is given by the ratio of final height to initial slope.

The comparison we have just made between bolus and continuous administrations of tracer makes clearer the fact that the information obtained from the tracer time curve does not depend on the time course of administration of tracer, provided that the latter is known. Therefore, one is perfectly free to choose the method of tracer administration purely from a practical viewpoint, for example high specific activity of the tracer and long equilibration times favour bolus injection, whereas converse factors favour continuous injection. This important independence property of the tracer technique was pointed out by Meier and Zierler in 1954.

Using the Occupancy Principle, various relationships mentioned in the course of this chapter may be derived. Mathematical rigour is not claimed. The aim is to show that these are variations on a theme—a theme which embodies a remarkably simple but far-reaching property of steady-state biological systems.

## Cardiac Output

As mentioned above, the occupancy per unit blood volume is the integral of the tracer concentration curve for unit quantity of tracer. To find this, the detector response $x$ must be related to indicator concentration $i$: $Kx = i$, say. The factor $K$ is determined by noting the detector response for a known indicator concentration, for example by waiting until the indicator is completely mixed with the blood stream and then determining $i$ directly by withdrawal of a blood sample. Thus occupancy per unit volume:

$$\theta/C = \left[ \int_0^\infty Kx(t)\,dt \right]/I$$

where $I = $ total amount of tracer.

The cardiac output is the rate of flow which is the reciprocal of this quantity; therefore

$$\text{Cardiac output} = I/\int_0^\infty Kx(t)\,dt$$

In the Occupancy Principle the part of the system that is 'looked' at is arbitrary provided that the whole flow passes through that part. This proviso could be met by a precordial counting technique if the detector 'looked' at the whole heart. It is not met by the dye dilution techniques which give answers whose accuracy depends on how typical blood flow at the sampling site is of the whole flow.

## Kety-Schmidt Equation for Diffusible Tracers

The Occupancy Principle is valid and applicable to both diffusible and non-diffusible tracers: purely for the sake of simplicity the discussion, so far, has been restricted to non-diffusible tracers.

In the context of this chapter the quantity of tracer which has passed from the blood stream into the brain (or other organ) is of interest. For this reason the relevant blood tracer concentration is the arterio-venous difference and the total amount of tracer is that taken up by the brain (which is given by $Cv(T)\lambda W$). Therefore, considering occupancy per unit blood volume (the actual total blood volume is irrelevant in this context),

$$\theta/C = \left[ \int_0^\infty (Ca - Cv)\,dt \right]/Cv(T)\lambda W$$

The reciprocal gives the blood flow for the whole brain, hence blood flow per unit mass of brain

$$F/W = Cv(T)\lambda/\int_0^\infty (Ca - Cv)\,dt$$

## Radioactive Tracer Uptake and Clearance Techniques

In the Kety-Schmidt method, the tracer concentrations are measured in the blood stream; radioactive tracers eliminate this need for blood sampling because they are directly detectable in the tissue of the organ under study. The Occupancy Principle allows the equation of the blood occupancy-capacity ratio (from which is derived the blood flow) with the occupancy-capacity ratio for the organ tissue—the latter being measured. Because the tracers used diffuse through the tissue, whereas the blood does not, it is useful to the understanding of the process to imagine that the radioactive tracer accompanies a continuous steady flow of a stable isotope of the same chemical element. This has no bearing on the real physical situation as will be seen from the fact that the size of this steady flow of stable isotope does not need to be specified and may therefore in the conceptual situation be made infinitely small.

Writing $F'$ for the stable isotope flow per unit mass of tissue we have

$$1/F' = \theta \text{ blood}/C \text{ blood} = \theta \text{ tissue}/C \text{ tissue}$$

But the blood flow $F$ is related to $F'$ by

$$FC \text{ blood} = F'$$

because $C$ blood is simply the measure of the stable isotope concentration in the blood. Therefore the blood flow per unit mass of tissue is

$$F = C \text{ tissue}/C \text{ blood} \times \theta \text{ tissue} = \lambda/\theta \text{ tissue}$$

where $\lambda$ is the ratio of solubilities of the radioactive tracer (or equally its stable isotope) in tissue and blood. The occupancy $\theta$ tissue is obtained from the activity-time curve in the way described for Figs. 19 and 20, i.e. area/height for bolus injection or height/slope for continuous steady injection (either uptake or clearance). Where the activity curve has a simple exponential character both ratios are given by $T\frac{1}{2}/\log_e 2$.

## APPENDIX II

### The Detection of Radioactive Tracers

The majority of radioactive isotopes used as biological tracers emit $\beta$-particles (otherwise called $\beta$-rays). Many isotopes emit $\gamma$-rays as well. When sampling techniques are used, $\beta$-counting is generally the more sensitive method, but when it is desired to measure the amount of radio-activity somewhere within the body, the short range of $\beta$-particles in tissue—seldom more than a few millimetres—is a serious limitation. In these circumstances, it is necessary to count $\gamma$-rays because they possess the same properties as high energy X-rays and penetrate tissue easily. In Fig. 21 the basic differences between $\beta$- and $\gamma$-counting are illustrated.

In general, a Geiger counter is used for detecting high energy $\beta$-particles, plastic or liquid scintillation counters are used for low energy $\beta$-particles, and a sodium iodide scintillation counter for $\gamma$-rays. Although only the sodium iodide counter is an efficient $\gamma$-ray detector, the $\gamma$-ray sensitivity of the others must be taken into account when the $\beta$-particles which are being counted are accompanied by $\gamma$-rays—a commonly occurring situation. The converse problem does not arise because the sodium iodide $\gamma$-ray detector may be easily screened from the short-range $\beta$-particles by a small thickness of aluminium.

A difference between the Geiger counter and the scintillators, in particular sodium iodide, is that the pulse height output from the latter is related to the energy of the ingoing radiation. It is usual to use this property

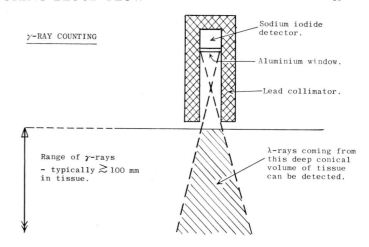

γ-RAY COUNTING

Sodium iodide detector.
Aluminium window.
Lead collimator.

Range of $\gamma$-rays - typically $\gtrsim$ 100 mm in tissue.

λ-rays coming from this deep conical volume of tissue can be detected.

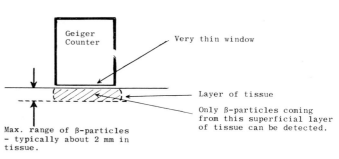

Geiger Counter

Very thin window

Layer of tissue

Only $\beta$-particles coming from this superficial layer of tissue can be detected.

Max. range of $\beta$-particles - typically about 2 mm in tissue.

Fig. 21. Schematic diagrams of Geiger counter and Scintillation counter.

to discriminate against unwanted pulses due to background radiation and noise. This is called 'pulse height analysis's in its simplest form it consists of eliminating all pulse: below the height which characterizes the radiation of interest.

PROPERTIES OF RADIOACTIVE ISOTOPES
COMMONLY USED IN CIRCULATION STUDIES

| Isotope | Radioactive Half-life* | Principal Radiations and their Energies |
|---|---|---|
| $^{51}$Cr | 28 days | Decays by capture of orbital electron (inverse $\beta$ decay) $\gamma$ 0·320 MeV |
| $^{131}$I | 8·1 days | $\beta$- 0·606 MeV (2·2 mm)† $\gamma$ 0·364 MeV |
| $^{85}$Kr | 10 years | $\beta$- 0·67 MeV (2·5 mm)† $\gamma$ 0·514 MeV |
| $^{32}$P | 14 days | $\beta$- 1·71 MeV (8 mm)† No $\gamma$-ray |
| $^{99m}$Tc | 6 hours | No $\beta$-particle $\gamma$ 0·140 MeV |
| $^{133}$Xe | 5·3 days | $\beta$- 0·346 MeV (1·0 mm)† $\gamma$ 0·081 MeV |

* Not to be confused with the physiologically determined halving time $T\frac{1}{2}$ which is much shorter.
† Figures in mm refer to maximum range in tissue.

$^{81m}$K — 13 sec — obtained from Rb.

Because radioactive decay is a statistical process, the detector pulse rate is subject to statistical fluctuations. In the simpler (analogue) type of instrument these fluctuations are smoothed by the ratemeter, the output of which then feeds a chart recorder. This is satisfactory provided it has been possible to optimize ratemeter and recorder settings in a trial run of the experiment; otherwise there may be degradation or loss of experimental information. Furthermore, although the chart record is valuable for showing the shape of the tracer-time curve, some inevitable inaccuracy occurs at the stage when measurements—height, area, etc.—are made from the curve. These difficulties are completely avoided if a digital ratemeter feeding a numerical printer is used. The original signal from the radiation detector is preserved as the number of counts in consecutive small time intervals and integrals are now found directly by accumulating the total number of counts during the integration period. Apart from advantages of greater accuracy, digital instrumentation has special value in multi-channel investigations since the onerous task of simultaneously achieving optimum adjustment of several analogue ratemeters and chart recorders is avoided. In such cases a simplified analogue display is usually retained because of its excellent ability to convey quantitative information visually.

## REFERENCES

Allwood, M. J. (1968), *Blood Flow Through Organs and Tissues*, Ed. Bain and Harper, p. 22. Edinburgh: Livingstone.

Allwood, M. J. and Farncombe, M. (1967), *J. Physiol.* **189**, 33.

Ardill, B. L., Fentem, P. H. and Williams, R. L. (1968), *Blood Flow Through Organs and Tissues*, Ed. Bain and Harper, p. 25. Edinburgh: Livingstone.

Betz, E. (1968), *Blood Flow Through Organs and Tissues*, Ed. Bain and Harper, p. 169. Edinburgh: Livingstone.

Burch, G. A. (1947), *Amer, Heart J.*, **33**, 48.

Cowell, T. K. and Bray, D. G. (1970), *Electron Power*, **16**, 150.

Harper, A. M. (1969), *Cerebral Circulation*, Ed. McDowall, Boston, Little, Brown and Co. (in press).

Harper, A. M. and Bell, G. (1966), *Wound Healing*, Ed. Illingworth, p. 181. London: Churchill.

Hatfield, C. A. and Troncelliti, M. V. (1950), *Surg. Clin. N. Amer.*, **30**, 1585.

Hognestad, H. (1966), *Med. Res. Eng.*, **5**, 28.

Ishii, Y. and MacIntyre, W. J. (1971), *Circulation* **44**, 37.

Kety, S. S. and Schmidt, C. F. (1945), *Amer., J. Physiol.*, **143**, 53.

Kriss, J. P., Enright, L. P., Hayden, W. G., Wexler, L. and Shumway N. E. (1971) *Circulation*, **43**, 792.

Lassen, N. A. and Munck, O. (1955), *Acta physiol. scand.*, **33**, 30.

Lassen, N. A. and Klee, A. (1965), *Circulation Res.*, **16**, 26.

Lassen, N. A., Lindbjerg, J. and Munck, O. (1964), *Lancet* **i**, 686.

Lorimer, A. R., Boyd, G., McCall, D., Mills, R. J. and Moran, F. (1968), *Blood Flow Through Organs and Tissues*, Ed. Bain and Harper, p. 79. Edinburgh: Livingstone.

Lowe, R. D. (1968), *Blood Flow Through Organs and Tissues*, Ed. Bain and Harper, p. 6. Edinburgh: Livingstone.

Meier, P. and Zierler, K. L. (1954), *J. appl. Physiol.*, **6**, 731.

Orr, J. S. and Gillespie, F. C. (1968), *Science*, **162**, 138.

Overbeck, H. W., Daugherty, R. M. Jr. and Haddy, F. J. (1969), *J. clin. Invest.*, **48**, 1944.

Ram, M. D., Evans, K. and Chisholm, G. D. (1968), *Brit. J. Urol.*, **4**, 425.

Ram, M. D., Holroyd, M. and Chisholm, G. D. (1969), *Lancet* **i**, 398.

Veall, N. and Mallett, B. L. (1965), *Phys. med. Biol.*, **10**, 375.

Whitney, R. J. (1953), *J. Physiol.*, **121**, 1.

Zierler, K. L. (1965), *Circulation Res.*, **16**, 309.

*References for further reading:*

(1) *Blood Flow Through Organs and Tissues* (1968), Ed. Bain and Harper. Edinburgh: Livingstone.

(2) *New Findings in Blood Flowmetry* (1968), Ed. Cappelen. Norway: Universitetsforlaget.

(3) *Cerebral Circulation* (1970), Ed. McDowall. Boston: Little, Brown & Co.

*CHAPTER 5*

# THE MEASUREMENT OF GAS FLOW AND VOLUME

### JOHN N. LUNN

This chapter is concerned with some aspects of the measurement of volume flowrate of gas and of discrete volumes of gas. The methods of measurement used at each stage as gases pass from the anaesthetic machine to, and from, the patient will be described in sequence.

### Gas Flow into the Breathing System—Continuous Flow

It is important to distinguish between volume flowrate and velocity because, although the latter is never used in anaesthesia, the two terms are sometimes confused. Volume flowrate is a measure of the volume passing a point in unit time (e.g. litres/second) whereas velocity is a measure of the average *speed* with which a given, small, quantum of gas is travelling (e.g. metres/sec).

In order to clarify this difference consider two tubes with very different cross-sectional areas. When gas is flowing at a given rate along both tubes the volumes delivered per unit time at the end of each tube will be identical. However, the speed of a quantum (which necessarily must be small in relation to the whole volume of the system) is much greater in the smaller tube. When gas is passed through the same tubes at identical velocities then the volume reaching the collection point in unit time will be very different and will be in proportion to the cross-sectional areas of the tubes.

### Flowmeters

These are devices used for measuring, or giving an output proportional to, volume flowrate. Many of the commonly used instruments fall into the latter category and volume flowrate is determined. Previous calibration of the flowmeter is, of course, essential.

There are two types of flowmeters in common use.

### 'Constant-pressure Flowmeters' (Variable Orifice*)

The flowmeters, commonly Rotameters (Fig. 1(a)), found on anaesthetic machines are in this group. The bobbin, with fluted edges to encourage rotation, is supported by the stream of gas flowing through a calibrated tube whose bore is wider at the top than at the bottom. The greater the flow, the higher the bobbin is forced up the tube, but the pressure lost, between the top and bottom of the bobbin, remains constant because its weight is also constant. The increase in diameter is gradual and there is, therefore, a limit to the range of flows which can be measured on any one flowmeter with one taper. However, on some Rotameters dual tapers

---

* The word 'orifice' is used in this connection in a functional and general sense to refer to the pathway or space through which gas flows. The precise definition of orifice—an aperture whose diameter exceeds its length—does not necessarily apply to all aspects of flowmeter function.

are used in order to allow a wider range of flow to be metered, whilst maintaining reasonable accuracy throughout the range. The scale usually starts from 10% of the maximum flowrate.

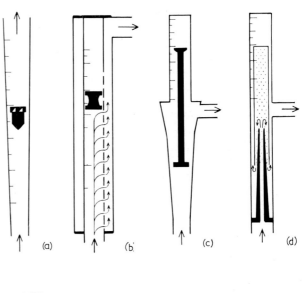

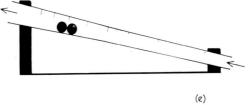

Fig. 1. Diagram of constant-pressure flowmeters (a) Rotameter; (b) Coxeter; (c) Heidbrink; (d) McKesson: (e) Connell.

An alternative, and earlier, version of a constant-pressure flowmeter (Coxeter, Fig. 1(b)) is one in which the escape of gas from the measuring tube is through a series of holes. The tube has parallel sides and, in this case, the bobbin rises up the tube to the point which reveals the appropriate number of holes to allow the gas to escape. This arrangement results in the bobbin being forced up the tube at fixed increments of flow and precludes precise measurement of flow between any two points.

Other flowmeters (Heidbrink; McKesson, Fig. 1(c) and (d)) have been manufactured whose internal dimensions change rapidly. This means that a wide range of flows can be metered by one tube albeit with some loss of precision. In another design (Connell, Fig. 1(e)) the tube is inclined and gas flow is indicated by the position of two ball-bearings. It was originally claimed that the second ball-bearing eliminated oscillation but in modern inclined-flowmeters the single ball-bearing does not oscillate noticeably.

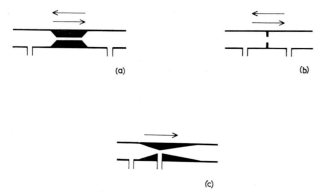

Fig. 2. Diagram of the airflow resistances of constant-orifice flowmeters: (a) Tube; (b) Orifice; (c) Venturi.

### 'Constant-orifice Flowmeters' (Variable Pressure)

In this type there is a progressive increase in pressure drop, with increasing rates of flow, across a restriction in a tube. Pressure gauges (Bourdon) or water manometers (Foregger) are calibrated to indicate flowrate. The restriction is either a long narrow tube (Fig. 2(a)) so that the pressure drop is proportional to flowrate, or an orifice (Fig. 2(b)) in which case the pressure drop is proportional to the square of flowrate. The magnitude of this pressure difference can be shewn to be related to the ratio between the diameters of the tubes and of the constriction (Ower and Pankhurst, 1967). A constant-orifice flowmeter is designed to generate a pressure difference great enough not to require a manometer with very high sensitivity. The relatively slow response of a water manometer is not a disadvantage because continuous flow is usually also steady. The pneumotachograph, normally used to measure rapidly varying flow can be regarded as another form of constant-orifice flowmeter but the differential manometer used with it needs to have a very fast response (see later).

### Other Flowmeters

The water-sight flowmeter is both a variable pressure and a variable orifice device. A tube with a series of holes dips into water. As flow increases both the number of orifices, through which the gas flows, and the pressure in the tube, increase. The number of holes in use indicates the volume flowrate.

So far the only resistance to gas flow which has been discussed is the orifice. There are, however, many different forms of airflow resistance. An orifice may be either a hole in a flat plate or a nozzle with tapering sides. The orifice may be prolonged into a tube or the nozzle and tube may be, as it were, combined in a venturi. Other forms of airflow resistance are mentioned in connection with pneumotachography. Details of design, including the sites and sizes of points for pressure sensing in relation to the airflow resistance, are beyond the scope of this chapter: minimal

standards have been published by the British Standards Institution (1964).

The venturi tube (Fig. 2(c)) can be regarded as a compromise between the tube and orifice type of airflow resistance. The acceleration of gas molecules through the throat of the venturi results in a loss of pressure which is compared with the pressure upstream from the constriction of the venturi tube. In a perfect venturi the downstream pressure is equal to the upstream pressure.

### Accuracy of Rotating Bobbin Flowmeters

In the absence of back pressure, flowmeters on modern anaesthetic machines are stated to have an accuracy of the order of ± 5 per cent of the indicated flow plus ± 0·5 per cent of the maximum flow. This presupposes a high standard of technical maintenance and care. A flowmeter of this type must be mounted exactly in the vertical position. If it is not the bobbin is inevitably tilted in one direction with an increased risk of friction. Dirt in the tube may encourage the bobbin to stick and gas passes by at a flowrate *different* from that indicated. Rotation of a Rotameter bobbin is essential for accurate readings. If such a bobbin is not rotating gas may be flowing but the indicated value is not precise.

Static electric charges are generated when two insulators in contact are separated from one another. The persistence of these charges depends upon the efficiency of the material of the surfaces as insulators. The better insulators hold the charge more than conductors which allow the charge to dissipate quickly. If static charges do accumulate they may be great enough to cause a flowmeter bobbin to stick. The degree of inaccuracy in flowmeter readings is very variable but as a result of the cessation of rotation of the bobbin the concentrations of gas mixtures issuing can be significantly altered without this being obvious from the rotameter readings.

There are a number of possible factors which may predispose to the generation and persistence of static electric charges in modern anaesthetic practice. Anaesthetic gases are very dry; moisture improves conductivity and thus the dissipation of static charges. However, humidification of gases prior to their passage through flowmeters would also increase inaccuracy. Hagelsten and Larsen (1965) suggest that automatic ventilators, which cause intermittent depression of the bobbins of flowmeters, are responsible for the accumulation of static charges. Clutton Brock (1972) did not confirm this but demonstrated that movement or rocking of anaesthetic machines might be a factor. The use of non-conductive material in flowmeter construction and the absence of metal conductors at the top or bottom of the tube are also important factors.

One solution to the problem of static electricity which has been suggested by Clutton Brock (personal communication, 1972) is that manufacturers should return to a modification of Ewing's inclined flowmeter with a steel ball-bearing as the indicator. As the ball does not move constantly there is no static charge generated. A temporary solution is to coat the inside of the tube with stannic oxide; a permanent solution is to use some other conductive material in the manufacture of flowmeters. There is now one commercial version of the Ewing tube available in Britain. In addition Rotameters Ltd., are producing tubes whose internal surface is a conductor and is connected at both ends to earth by a gold-plated band. Finally, ionizing radiations could also be employed to aid the dispersion of static charges.

A further source of error is the presence of leaks between the calibrated tube of the flowmeter and the flowmeter block or through cracks in the calibrated tube.

Flowmeters supplying driving gas to some ventilators, humidifiers and nebulizers may have to function against considerable back-pressure. Back-pressure may not alter the *actual* flowrate of gas but it does alter the indicated flow. Pressure-compensated flowmeters with a controlling needle-valve distal to the calibrated tube should be used in conjunction with these devices if accurate flow metering is desired. The accuracy then depends upon the driving-gas pressure remaining equal to the pressure at which the flowmeters were calibrated.

Serious errors could arise if a flowmeter calibrated for one gas were to be used for another, because of differences in density, and or, viscosity (see later). The extent of the error would depend upon the position of the bobbin in the flowmeter and also upon the shape of the bobbin in relation to the cross-sectional area of the flowmeter. At the lower end of a tapered tube the area through which the gas passes is relatively small compared with the distance which it has to travel in order to pass the bobbin. Providing the flow is not great it will, as it passes the bobbin, be laminar or smooth. (Immediately above the bobbin and, indeed because of it, flow may be turbulent). At the other end of the flowmeter tube the ratio between the length of the passage for the gas and the cross-sectional area of the flowmeter is reversed, and the passage corresponds to an orifice. Flow through this region is therefore turbulent. (*See* General Problems of Flow Measurement—later.)

### Gas Flow within the Breathing System—Intermittent Flow

In intermittent flow the volume flowrate is changing rapidly and therefore a fast-response system is essential if the changes are to be followed faithfully.

**Pneumotachography.** (Synonymous American usage, pneumotachygraphy.)

A pneumotachograph is a fast-response measuring system based on a form of constant-orifice flowmeter. It consists of an airflow resistance, across which a pressure drop occurs, a differential pressure transducer and a means of recording the output. There are a number of designs of airflow resistance which are suitable. Most of these are essentially bundles of small bore tubes with thin walls placed longitudinally in the gas pathway. These provide a linear resistance so that pressure drop varies directly with flowrate. In one design two strips of metal, one with transverse corrugations, are wound together round a central rod (e.g. Fleisch pneumotachograph, Fig. 3). Multiple pressure sensing points are from an annular groove in the wall of the tube. Another design is a single orifice plate which causes a pressure drop proportional to the square of the flowrate. Mesh screens are also used as linear airflow resistances.

The restrictions in flow pathways so far discussed have been designed to produce a substantial drop in pressure. In pneumotachographs, which can be, and often are, inserted into the patient's airway, care is taken to keep the pressure drop as small as possible. This not only helps to maintain laminar flow, but also avoids imposing additional airway resistance upon the patient.

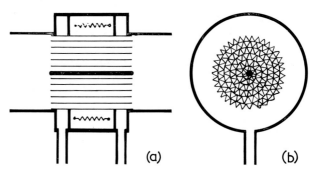

Fig. 3. Diagram of Fleisch pneumotachograph airflow resistance: (a) Longitudinal section; (b) Transverse section through the pressure sensing connection.

As the flow increases the pressure drop also increases, at first proportionally, but later, due to turbulence, non-linearity occurs. The useful range of airflow resistances is therefore limited at low flows, by a small pressure difference and at high flows, by non-linearity. Pneumotachographs have, therefore, to be constructed specifically for the particular range of flows to be measured. The wider the range of flows the greater the departure from exact proportionality and, even within the designated range, each airflow resistance becomes marginally non-linear at the higher flowrates. Any distortion of the resistance by condensate, damage or dirt will, of course, further alter this relationship. The requirement to select an appropriate airflow resistance for all anticipated flowrates is clear.

In this selection it is important to remember that the highest, or peak, rate of flow is much greater than the average flow. In sinusoidal flow, the peak flow is about three times the average flow. In measuring a flowrate which declines exponentially (expiratory flow) the rate is initially at least ten times the average flow.

The airflow resistance in the expired gas pathway is near room temperature and is cooler than the warm moist gas that is passing through it. Condensation occurs unless preventive measures are taken; in one commercial version a small heating coil surrounds the resistance. The increase in pressure drop caused by condensation is particularly troublesome with metal mesh-screens; but the use of plastic has reduced this effect. Wide mesh screens also reduce the effect of condensation particularly when provision is made for drainage of the water. Although commercial airflow resistances are usually calibrated in terms of pressure drop this calibration must be repeated in the conditions of the study.

The pressure difference created by the airflow resistance is usually very small, of the order of 1 to 2 mm $H_2O$, and is sensed by a differential pressure transducer whose electrical output is then amplified and displayed. The manometer needs to be selected carefully. For use when there is a large, sudden, difference in pressure, particularly during most forms of intermittent positive pressure ventilation, it is important that the measuring system is symmetrical on both sides of the airflow resistance, in terms of both capacity and resistance, otherwise the transducer will respond to the initial increase in pressure on the side with the smaller capacity. This will appear as volume but it is clearly due to faulty measurement technique. A similar error occurs when screens which buckle are used as airflow resistances during intermittent positive pressure ventilation.

In order to use a pneumotachograph for the measurement of volume, integration, either by electronic or graphic means, must be performed (*see* chapter on Mathematics and Shapes, Section V). This process is to determine the area under the line representing flow against time and individual inspiratory and expiratory tidal volumes can then be calculated.

### Ionization Pneumotachograph

This pneumotachograph, first described in 1949 (Lovelock), would appear to have solved some of the physical problems of pneumotachography mentioned above. Ionization of gas is achieved from a source of alpha particles—Americium 241; the ions are then collected and the collec-

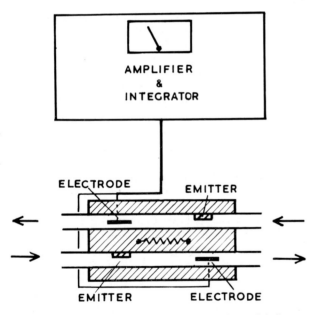

FIG. 4. Diagram of the Ionization Pneumatachograph indicating the principle of its function.

tion current is amplified (Fig. 4). This current is proportional to gas flow, is virtually unaffected by changes of the composition of the gas mixture, temperature, pressure or humidity (Jeretin *et al.*, 1971). By using two detectors bidirectional flow can be recorded.

### Other Flowmeters for use During Intermittent Flow

Flow measuring devices utilizing a *venturi* to cause a measurable pressure difference can be used in reciprocating flow to record volumes in both directions (Ventigrator).

Unfortunately this system generates turbulent flow and the small pressure drop at the lower flow rates gives low sensitivity but the large pressure difference at high flow rates increases sensitivity (Nunn and Ezi Ashi, 1962). In addition changes in the density of the gases affect the pressure drop considerably.

The rate of cooling (inspiration) or warming (expiration) of a *thermistor* has been used in a respiration monitor, particularly for small children (Millar, 1963) but this cannot be made quantitative. However, in the *Respiratory Flowmeter* (Birchover) recently announced, the combination of a venturi and a thermistor appears to be a novel and ingenious solution to the problem of humidity in ventilation measurements. A venturi tube is placed within the expired gas pathway so that ambient air is entrained. This air then cools a thermistor mounted in the entrainment port; the change in temperature is related to the entrained air which, in turn, is related to expiratory gas flow through the venturi.

The speed of transmission of sound between a fixed transmitter and fixed receiver is dependent upon the velocity of air passing between them. This is the basis of an *ultrasonic* flowmeter which is incorporated into a system for lung function testing (Biomedical Engineering, 1969). Preliminary reports from Conway (personal communication, 1972) suggest that this is unaffected by the pressure of the gas flow and less affected than other instruments by the composition of the gas mixture.

### Anemometers

These are devices which are used in meteorology to measure wind speed and also to indicate direction. There are many different designs—for example, the cup, the swinging plate, the Pitot tube and the vane. The cup anemometer is bulky; it has three of four cups mounted so that they are filled sequentially with gas and cause the rotation of an indicator. The swinging plate anemometer is mounted vertically on knife edges and is deflected by the current of gas—the angle of inclination of the plate being proportional to the speed of gas flow. Neither of these two anemometers is known to have been applied in anaesthesia. The vane anemometer (c.f. windmill) has a number of flat plates attached to radial rods. These rods cause a spindle to rotate which carries a pointer to indicate rate of rotation and hence gas speed.

Anemometers are commonly placed in anaesthetic or breathing systems to measure minute-volume in situations where reciprocating flow is occurring although they may only respond to flow from one direction.

### Wright Respirometer

This is a modified vane anemometer; a single plate or vane is mounted on a rotor between jewelled bearings. A stator is necessary to direct the gas onto the vane (Fig. 5). It is cylindrical in shape and has a number of slots cut through it—these have the effect of directing the gas onto the periphery of the vane. The rotation of the vane is transmitted through a system of gears to pointers moving over the dials. This latter mechanism is protected from moisture by a mercury seal which is vulnerable to damage. The vane does not move in response to flow in the reverse direction because there is no stator to deflect the gas. Vanes of this type respond to wind speed or velocity and therefore the volume displayed is dependent upon factors which alter velocity. When the gas passes through the slots in the stator its velocity is changed. The velocity here bears a relationship, though not necessarily a linear one, to the volume which has passed.

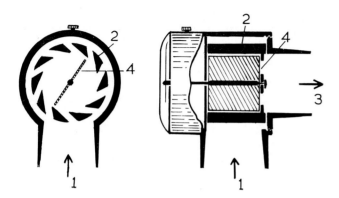

FIG. 5. Diagram of the Wright Respirometer. (1) Gas inlet; (2) Stator with slots; (3) Gas outlet; (4) Vane. (Reproduced with permission of authors and publishers from *Automatic Ventilation of the Lungs*, Mushin, W. W., Rendell-Baker, L., Thompson, P. W. and Mapleson, W. W. (1969), 2nd edition. Oxford: Blackwell Scientific Publications Ltd.

Changes in the composition of gas mixtures, in humidity, in instantaneous rates of gas flow and damage by rough handling (not to say dropping), all impose limitations on the accuracy of this device (Nunn and Ezi Ashi, 1962; Lunn and Hillard, 1970). Nevertheless for clinical purposes its use is justifiably widespread. The Drager volumeter (Fig. 6) responds to flow in two directions and consists of two rotors which interlock. Although this instrument is more accurate and larger than the Respirometer, it is both more expensive and affected by moisture.

### Electronic Anemometers

Graphical recording of ventilation is impossible with either of the two anemometers described. In order to minimize some of the disadvantages mentioned above and to provide this facility recent improvements in design have been made. In an electronic version of the Wright Respirometer detection of the rotation of the vane is achieved by means of a photoelectric cell. The light shining upon the photoelectric cell is intermittently shielded by the vane as it rotates. The output of the cell is processed electronically and either tidal volume or minute-volume can be displayed. The vane has been strengthened by corrugations in order that, it is claimed, flow above 1·5 litres per minute and up to 300 litres per minute can be detected.

Another vane anemometer (Spiroflo, Fig. 7) with a stator which causes the gas to swirl onto the vane mounted in the axis of gas flow uses a different method of detection. In this case the electrical output of a capacitative transducer is altered. The output is proportional to flow rate and tidal or minute-volume can be displayed.

It is claimed for both these electronic anemometers that they are not only less vulnerable to physical damage but also less affected by moisture than the non-electronic versions. Both instruments can be battery-operated and both provide facility for graphical recording; in addition the necessity, during minute-volume determinations, for independent timing is removed.

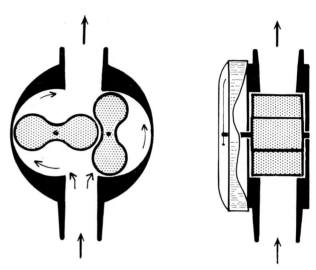

FIG. 6. Diagram of the Drager Volumeter. (Reproduced with permission of authors and publishers from *Automatic Ventilation of The Lungs*, Mushin, W. W., Rendell-Baker, L., Thompson, P. W. and Mapleson, W. W. (1969), 2nd edition. Oxford: Blackwell Scientific Publications Ltd.

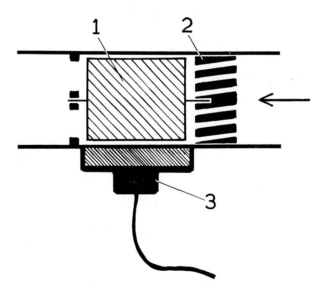

FIG. 7. Diagram of the Spiroflo. (1) Vane; (2) Stator (swirl-plate); (3) Transducer.

### General Problems of Flow Measurement

Some of the sources of inaccuracy have already been considered in relation to specific instruments but there are others which have a more general interest and importance.

The factors determining whether flow of fluids through tubes is laminar or turbulent were defined by Reynolds

(1883). These are the mean velocity ($\bar{u}$), viscosity ($\eta$), density ($l$) and the radius ($r$) of the tube; they are related in the equation, Reynold's Number,

$$Re = \frac{\bar{u}\eta r}{l}$$

When this figure is less than 1,000, flow is laminar, if it is greater than 1,500, flow is turbulent ($R_e$ is dimensionless). It can be calculated (Cooper, 1960) that, for air and oxygen, the critical volume flowrate at which laminarity ceases in a smooth-walled tube, and the transition towards turbulent flow begins, is $28.5 \times r$ litres/minute (where $r$ is the radius of the tube in centimetres). If the diameter of a tube changes (e.g. corrugated rubber tubing) or, if there is a change in direction (e.g. Cobb and Magill suction endotracheal tube connectors) turbulent flow will result and will continue for some distance downstream.

In laminar flow the pressure drop, and therefore the indicated flowrate, is influenced by the viscosity* of the gas. Thus if the viscosities of two gases are similar, and laminar flow occurs, approximately equal flowrates will be recorded for both gases on one instrument calibrated for either. In turbulent flow the effect of density predominates, but because of the square-law relationship between pressure drop and flowrate interchangeability is impossible. This is the factor which adversely affects the performance of flowmeters when used for gases other than the designated gas and also the Ventigrator.

The density of a gas is affected by ambient temperature and pressure; viscosity is affected by the former only. Bobbin flowmeters are calibrated at designated temperatures (usually 15°C or 20°C) and pressures; in precise work corrections are made to allow for these variations. Under hyperbaric conditions the difference between indicated and actual flow through a bobbin flowmeter becomes clinically important because the density of gas is increased (McDowall, 1964). (The actual flow of gas at 2 atm is 71 per cent of that indicated at the same barometric pressure.)

An increase in temperature of 1°C, between 20°C and 40°C, increases the viscosity of a gas by about 0.2 per cent (Grenvik, 1966); this is unlikely to be important clinically but is important in investigations utilizing pneumotachography to measure the difference between inspired and expired volumes (Smith, 1964; Hobbes, 1967).

Some bobbin flowmeters (gap meters) are scaled without reference to a particular gas and calibration charts are available for different gases. Corrections are not usually applied to anemometer measurements.

### Gas Flow in the Breathing System—Volume

Gas volume measurements in association with anaesthetized patients are usually made of expired gas on the assumption that errors due to leaks will probably be smaller. An underestimate of expiration is less hazardous clinically than an underestimate of inspiration.

Measurement of gas volumes can be very precisely achieved by the use of water displacement from calibrated

---

* Viscous forces are those shearing forces within a moving column of air or other fluid. When exerted against the boundaries of a tube it is as if these forces are causing the air to adhere to the walls.

vessels. For obvious reasons this method is not used in anaesthetic practice but it remains of fundamental use. Gas has first to be collected into air-tight containers such as a Douglas bag. The contents can then be passed from the bag through a variety of gas meters or spirometers. Corrections must be applied for atmospheric conditions (water vapour, barometric pressure and temperature) and for losses through the walls of such bags which, in the case of a polyvinylchloride bag (60 cm square; 0.25 mm thick), may amount to 200 ml per hour of a mixture of 80 per cent nitrous oxide in oxygen (Cooper, 1959).

### Spirometers

The general design of these is a double walled cylindrical chamber, containing water in the space between the walls, with a light-weight cylinder bell inverted over it so that the water forms an air-tight seal for the contents of the bell. The weight of the cylinder is balanced by a counter-weight or weights suspended over a pulley system. This pulley system can carry a pen so that a record may be made on a rotating drum.

Systems utilizing mechanical parts are prone to inaccuracy from inertia. Smoothly running pulleys are essential and many ingenious methods are used to overcome this problem. Once moving, the bell may fail to stop at the instant at which gas ceases to enter it, and either an overestimate of volume will be recorded or the bell may oscillate. A significant depression of the water level can occur with high rates of gas inflow which will cause the gas to be exposed to a positive pressure. A further problem is the correct, leak-free, function of all valves in the system.

There are a number of different spirometers each having a special use but, in general, spirometers are of limited value during anaesthesia because of the need to supply fresh anaesthetic gases to the system and to absorb carbon dioxide. However, the traditional bag-in-box system has been adapted by Nunn (1956) so that spirometers can be used satisfactorily in anaesthetic systems during spontaneous ventilation by arranging to remove an equivalent volume to the fresh gas flow from the measuring system by continuous suction.

### Dry Spirometers

These are much more convenient to use than water displacement spirometers but they demand the highest standards of construction. The gas collection vessel is often a wedge-shaped bellows with plastic sides. These bellows must be light enough to allow a rapid response and also to avoid an increase in pressure within the system (back-pressure). The maximum back-pressure should not exceed 1.5 cm $H_2O$ in order to avoid errors in volume determinations (Cotes, 1966).

### Special-purpose Spirometers

Special adaptations of these spirometers exist which incorporate timing devices so that forced expiratory volumes within specified times can be recorded. It is clearly essential that inertia be low and it is suggested that movement of the bellows should commence after 100 ml has entered them (Cotes, 1966). Movement of the pen carriage is triggered by movement of the bellows. One such spirometer is the Vitalograph (Fig. 8) which, in spite of having a high inertia and failing to meet minimal requirements regarding back-pressure (Drew and Hughes, 1969) is widely used. There is another spirometer (McDermott) which meets these specifications (Collins *et al.*, 1964).

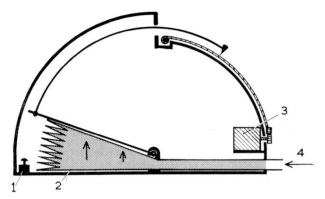

FIG. 8. Diagram of the Vitalograph. (1) Switch released by movement of the bellows; (2) Book bellows; (3) Motor which drives the chart; (4) Gas inlet into the book bellows.

However, it must be freely admitted that precision instruments, which are more costly, may not be justified in clinical work. Assuming that vital capacity is measured with the same instrument as is used for forced expiratory volume in one second (or 0·75 sec) then the clinically useful relationship $FEV_{1sec}$ as percentage of vital capacity will be less seriously in error.

### Peak Flow Measurement

Peak expiratory flow is sometimes measured and a pneumotachograph, suitably calibrated, may be used for this purpose. For convenience in the ward the Wright Peak Flowmeter (Fig. 9) is preferred (Wright and McKerrow, 1959). The vane is forced around on its horizontal axis by

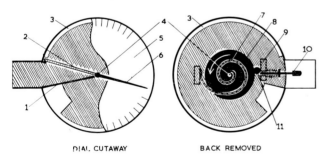

DIAL CUTAWAY          BACK REMOVED

FIG. 9. Diagram of the Wright Peak Flowmeter. (1) Fixed plate to direct gas; (2) Vane; (3) Annular slot; (4) Shaft; (5) Dial; (6) Pointer; (7) Spiral spring; (8) Brake disc; (9) Fixed block; (10) Push button zeroing knob; (11) Floating disc.

the expiratory flow and a gradually increasing pathway is opened up for the expired gas which then escapes to the atmosphere through an annular slot. The vane carries with it the brake disc and its rotation is resisted by the slight tension of a spiral spring. The vane is held at its maximum

reading by the brake disc which becomes jammed against a block by a small floating disc. This floating disc falls into place under the action of gravity when the brake disc ceases to move, and therefore does not function properly unless the meter is held in the correct manner: recent models have a handle designed to encourage the user to do this. The final position of the pointer represents the balance between forces due to the air pressure on the vane and the tension of the spiral spring. After the reading has been made, the brake disc is released by a push button whose action is to dislodge the floating disc so that the vane and the pointer are returned to the zero stop by the spiral spring.

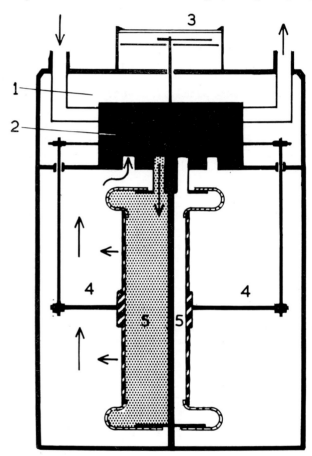

FIG. 10. Diagram of a dry gas meter. (1) Valve section; (2) Valve box; (3) Display: dial and pointer; (4) Measuring sections; (5) Bellows.

### Dry Gas Meters

There are a number of these: the most common in medical use is the Parkinson Cowan meter which has the same basic design as those used throughout Britain in metering domestic gas. The description which follows would apply in general to all of these meters: in detail they vary considerably. There are three sections (*see* Fig. 10); the one at the top contains the valve and display mechanisms; the two identical hermetically sealed sections below each contain bellows. Gas enters the bellows in the sealed section, or into the chamber outside the bellows. As the bellows fill so the gas in the surrounding chamber is forced out of the meter. When the bellows are full, gas enters the outer chamber and compresses the bellows, so that the gas contained is discharged to the exterior. A similar mechanism comes into operation in the other section a quarter of a cycle later.

The movements of the pair of bellows control the opening and closing of the valves across the ports into, and out of, each section. In addition the movement of the bellows is mechanically transmitted so that the pointer moves around the dial.

The arrangement of the valves is such that the pressure drop is kept at a minimum; nevertheless observation of the rotation of the pointer indicates that this is greater in some phases of the operation. In domestic meters the pressure drop is stated not exceed 1·3 cm $H_2O$ at the maximum flowrate of 100 litres/minute. The arrangement also ensures that both bellows are not completely empty at the same moment.

Provided that the cumulative volume over a full cycle is measured, both adult, and neonatal, minute-volume ventilation can be accurately registered but leaks are more likely to cause serious errors at low flows. With suitable precautions and, using a well-maintained meter, an accuracy of ± 1 per cent is claimed (Adams *et al.*, 1967).

## Wet Gas Meters

Although the dry gas meter is capable of much greater accuracy than many clinical meters even higher levels of accuracy are required, and achieved, in other fields. The wet gas meters (*see* Fig. 11), or gas clocks, are a group of

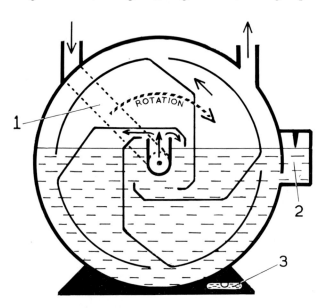

FIG. 11. Wet gas meter. Gas pathway is shown by solid arrows; rotation by broken arrow. (1) Entrance port to hollow spindle; (2) Water level; (3) Spirit level.

instruments whose accuracy may be as good as ± 0·1 per cent. Their limitation is that the maximum flow rate which may be passed is about 8 litres/minute. In order to visualize the mechanics imagine four chambers which rotate about

a central axis. The gas enters through the hollow spindle and passes to each chamber in sequence thus maintaining the rotation of the spindle. As the central inlet to each chamber rotates it passes beneath the water level and thus becomes sealed. The water causes the gas to be displaced peripherally through the outlet of the chamber situated on its circumference. The rotation of the spindle is displayed on a calibrated dial. It is clear that both the filling with water and precise levelling, are critical. In practice the chambers are spirals with different points of entry and exit like a 'multi-start' screw thread. Gas passes axially and causes the tube to rotate as above. This is a precision instrument but it is valuable in an anaesthetic laboratory in the calibration of other apparatus.

## General Problems in Gas Volume Measurement

Cotes (1965) suggests maximum levels of additional resistance which can be tolerated in any apparatus for measuring ventilation. The pressure drop should not exceed 5 cm $H_2O$ at 85 litres/minute if ventilation is between 0 and 10 litres/min and not over 2·5 cm $H_2O$ at 10–30 litres/min. It is customary for this reason to use wide-bore tubing and connections but in the presence of back-pressure or of residual pressure these may contribute a further source of error because of the additional compressible volume and the compliance of the tubing. A volume of 1 litre is compressed to approximately 999 ml by the application of 1 cm $H_2O$ pressure (Cooper, 1959)—so in large volume systems residual pressure should be kept at a minimum when accuracy is important. In a metre of distensible rubber tubing 1–4 ml are 'lost' for each cm $H_2O$ applied pressure (Mushin *et al.*, 1969). A further hazard of additional compliance is that once filled it may discharge through pathways other than the measuring system.

The author is pleased to thank Professor W. W. Mushin and Dr. W. W. Mapleson for many helpful discussions about this subject over several years. The skilful drawing of all the diagrams by Mr. E. K. Hillard is also gratefully acknowledged.

## References

Adams, A. P., Vickers, M. D. A., Munroe, J. P. and Parker, C. W. (1967), "Dry Displacement Gas Meters," *British Journal of Anaesthesia*, **39**, 174.

Biomedical Engineering (1969), "Ultrasonic Flowmeter," **4**, 524.

British Standard 1042:Part 1:1964, "Methods for the Measurement of Fluid Flow in Pipes. Part 1: Orifice, Plates, Nozzles and Venturi Tubes." London: British Standards Institution.

Clutton-Brock, J. (1972), "Static Electricity and Rotameters," *British Journal of Anaesthesia*, **44**, 86.

Collins, M. M., McDermott, M. and McDermott, T. J. (1964), "Bellows Spirometer and Transistor Timer for the Measurement of Forced Expiratory Volume and Vital Capacity," *Journal of Physiology*, **172**, 39P.

Cooper, E. A. (1959), "The Estimation of Minute Volume," *Anaesthesia*, **14**, 373.

Cooper, E. A. (1960), "Suggested Methods of Testing and Standards of Resistance for Respiratory Protective Devices," *Journal of Applied Physiology*, **15**, 1053.

Cotes, J. E. (1966), "Respiratory Function Tests in Pneumoconioses," *International Labour Organization*. Geneva, p. 93.

Cotes, J. E. (1968), *Lung Function*, p. 23. Oxford: Blackwell Scientific Publications. 2nd Edition.

Drew, C. D. M., Hughes, D. T. D. (1969), "Characteristics of the Vitalograph Spirometer," *Thorax*, **24**, 703.

Grenvik, A., Hedstrand, U., Sjögren, H. (1966), "Problems in Pneumotachography," *Acta Anaesthesiologica Scandinavica*, **10**, 147.

Hagelsten, J. O., Larsen, O. S. (1965), "Inaccuracy of Anaesthetic Flowmeters caused by Static Electricity," *British Journal of Anaesthesia*, **37**, 637.

Hobbes, A. F. T. (1967), "A Comparison of Methods of Calibrating the Pneumotachograph." *British Journal of Anaesthesia*, **39**, 899.

Jeretin, S., Martinez, L. R., Tang, I. P. and Ito, Y. (1971), "Pneumotachography by the Ionization Principle," *Anesthesiology*, **35**, 218.

Lovelock, J. E., Wasilewska, E. M. (1949), "An ionization Anemometer," *Journal of Scientific Instruments*, **26**, 367.

Lunn, J. N., Hillard, E. K. (1970), "The Effect of Repairs on the Performance of the Wright Respirometer," *British Journal of Anaesthesia*, **42**, 1127.

McDowall, D. G. (1964), "Anaesthesia in a Pressure Chamber," *Anaesthesia*, **19**, 321.

Millar, R. A., Marshall, B. E. (1963), "A Respiration Monitor for Use during Anaesthesia," *British Journal of Anaesthesia*, **35**, 447.

Mushin, W. W., Rendell-Baker, L., Thompson, P. W. and Mapleson, W. W. (1969), "Automatic Ventilation of the Lungs," p. 43. Oxford: Blackwell Scientific Publications Ltd. 2nd Edition.

Nunn, J. F. (1956), "A New Method of Spirometry Applicable to Routine Anaesthesia," *British Journal of Anaesthesia*, **28**, 440.

Nunn, J. F. and Ezi-Ashi, T. I. (1963), "The Accuracy of the Respirometer and Ventigrator," *British Journal of Anaesthesia*, **34**, 422.

Reynolds, O. (1883), *Philosophical Transactions*, **174**, 935.

Smith, W. D. A. (1964), "The Measurement of Uptake of Nitrous Oxide by Pneumotachography. I. Apparatus, Methods and Accuracy," *British Journal of Anaesthesia*, **36**, 363.

Wright, B. M., McKerrow, C. B. (1959), "Maximum Forced Expiratory Flow Rate as a Measure of Ventilatory Capacity," *British Medical Journal*, **ii**, 1041.

**References for further reading:**

British Standard 1042 (1964), "Methods for the Measurement of Fluid Flow in Pipes. Part I." London: British Standards Institution.

*Methods in Medical Research*, Volume II (1966), "Flow Direction Technics," Ed. D. L. Fry. Chicago, U.S.A.: Year Book Medical Publishers.

Ower, E. and Pankhurst, R. C. (1966), "The Measurement of Air Flow," London: Pergamon Press.

*CHAPTER* 6

# THE MEASUREMENT OF TEMPERATURE

P. CLIFFE

## Physical Meaning of Temperature

The physical definition of temperature can be established by considering the way in which information about it is obtained. In common with the measurement of any other physical quantity, a property of matter is chosen which varies with temperature; e.g. length of a metal, volume of a liquid, pressure or volume of a gas, pressure of a saturated vapour, colour of a substance, electrical resistance of a metal or semi-conductor, or the EMF developed across the junctions of dissimilar metals.

For illustration, consider Fig. 1, in which the length of a metal rod is chosen. The property of length defines the

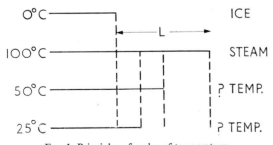

Fig. 1. Principles of scales of temperature.

'scale' of temperature. Now to give the scale quantitative significance, measure the value of the property (length of the rod) at two fixed temperatures, namely, that

of pure melting ice and that of steam, at standard atmospheric pressure. The choice of a graduation system, e.g. 0 and 100 units on the Centigrade graduation, then defines a temperature difference of 100°C. Alternatively, the choice of 32 and 212 units is made for the Fahrenheit graduation system.

For the temperatures at any other point on the 'scale' the assumption is made that increments in temperature are proportional to the corresponding increments in the measured property, i.e. temperature changes are defined in this example as being proportional to the changes in the length of a metal rod which they produce. Hence, the measurement of temperature is reduced to that of measuring the length of the rod. For example, 50°C is the temperature of the rod which has increased by $L/2$, and so on.

Clearly, the choice of another 'scale', such as a gas scale or resistance scale, would again require temperature by definition to vary linearly with the change in volume or pressure of the gas or the electrical resistance. As they are not closely related properties, the different scales would not agree.

In view of this apparently unsatisfactory nature of the definition of temperature, scientists in the last century sought means whereby a temperature scale may be defined independently of any material substance.

One approach involved the study of gas thermometers. For example, it would be possible arbitrarily to define temperature as proportional to changes in pressure in a constant volume hydrogen thermometer of specified design with the pressure of the gas specified at the ice point. However, when gases other than hydrogen are used in such a gas thermometer the measured values of temperature are found to differ slightly. If the pressure of gas at the ice point is indefinitely reduced it can be shown that at this limit all gases behave in the same way and have the properties of an 'ideal' gas. The ideal gas scale of temperature may thus be defined, as for the constant volume hydrogen scale, and by measurement of the properties of actual gases extrapolated to zero pressure, corrections may be made to the constant volume hydrogen scale. This can be done, although within the range of 0–100°C the corrections are only of the order of 0·003°C. The ideal gas scale turns out to be identical with another 'theoretical' scale, called the thermodynamic scale, defined in terms of the efficiency of an ideal heat engine.

The modern definition of temperature is related to the thermodynamic scale, and is essentially based on the accurate definition of fixed points such as the ice and steam points, but extended to cover a wide range of temperature from a fraction of a degree absolute to thousands of degrees centigrade. The present day specifications are laid down in 'The International Practical Temperature Scale of 1968' published by H.M.S.O.

### Application to Thermometers

In medicine, temperature measurements may be required in patients or in apparatus. Where the temperature of patients is required the usual thermometers are:

1. Mercury in glass (the clinical thermometer)
2. Thermocouple
3. Resistance (metal)
4. Thermistor (resistance of semi-conductor).
   In scientific apparatus, the above types are also used, but frequently 'dial' thermometers are employed. These are commonly:
5. Dial thermometers—mercury in steel
   vapour pressure
   bimetallic elements

### 1. Clinical Thermometers

Within the limited accuracy (±0·1°C) required from a clinical thermometer, it remains probably the most satisfactory instrument for routine clinical use. Its disadvantages include:

(a) Breakage
(b) Slow response, due to relatively high thermal capacity
(c) Unsuitability for remote reading
(d) Unsuitability for recording
(e) Difficulty of application to unconscious patients, and
(f) Unsuitability for subcutaneous or intracavity temperatures, e.g. from sites in the oesophagus, nasopharynx, or rectum.

Electrical thermometry overcomes these disadvantages.

Another important use of the mercury thermometer relates to the calibration of electric thermometers. The mercury thermometer may be obtained in a wide variety of ranges and accuracies and these can be checked by the National Physical Laboratory by comparison with a standard. The resulting accuracy of calibration is usually adequate for most medical applications.

### 2. Thermocouples (Fig. 2)

When a circuit made of two dissimilar metals has the two junctions maintained at different temperatures an electromotive force (EMF) is developed. The arrangement of metals is called a 'thermocouple' and the effect is called the Seebeck Effect.

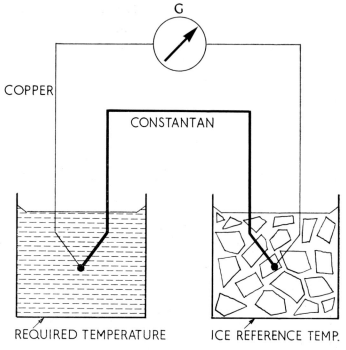

FIG. 2. The principle of the thermocouple.

The relationship between the EMF developed and the temperature difference between the junctions is approximately parabolic in form, and may be represented by

$$E = At + Bt^2$$

Where $E$ is the EMF developed for a temperature difference of $t$°C, while $A$ and $B$ are constants which depend on the metals forming the thermocouples. The effect of the non linear factor $B$ varies with the metal pair. For copper and constantan (an alloy of copper and nickel) the maximum deviation from linearity between 0°C and 100°C is between 2–3°C, although for other combinations it is less. In practice, the metal junctions are made by silver soldering or welding.

In order to measure temperature it is necessary to maintain the temperature of one junction constant when the other can be used to determine the required temperature provided the EMF of the thermocouple is measured. If

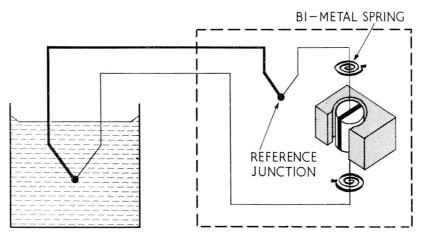

FIG. 3. Mechanical cold junction compensation in thermo-electric thermometer.

the galvanometer, G, has a high resistance compared with the thermocouple so that there is negligible potential difference across the couple, then the potential difference across G is equal to the EMF and the current through G is proportional to the EMF.

This simple arrangement is associated with certain difficulties. From the practical standpoint the use of ice may be inconvenient. Furthermore, if the metal at the galvanometer terminals differs from that which terminates the thermocouple, then further thermojunctions are formed. If they differ in temperature they will produce thermo-EMF's. The law of intermediate metals states that, provided the temperature remains unchanged, any different metal may be placed in one part of the leads joining two thermojunctions, without changing the overall EMF. Clearly this requires no variation in temperature at the galvanometer terminals.

These objections have been overcome in one commercial instrument as shown in Fig. 3.

The 'cold junction' is mounted in a small copper cylinder about 5 mm. long and 5 mm. in diameter. The junction is mounted very close to the terminals of a sensitive reflecting galvanometer of which the upper suspension is connected to a bimetallic spiral spring. Because of their close proxmity within a small metal box, the junction, the bimetallic spring and the terminals, are at approximately the same temperature. This is further ensured by enclosing the instrument in a stout metal case, the conductivity of which encourages a uniform temperature inside.

As room temperature changes, that of the junction changes, and this is just compensated by movement of the bimetal spring, so that the net effect is that of a constant reference temperature. The non-linear relationship between galvonometer deflection and temperature is corrected by the use of a non-linear galvanometer scale. However, for the thermocouples supplied the effect is small and only careful observation would reveal that the scale divisions are not equal.

This instrument is available in 2 models for reading 0–50°C or for 16–46°C ($\pm$0·1°C). The thermojunctions are of nichrome and constantan, which produce an EMF

of 46·5 microvolts per degree centigrade. They are supplied in a large variety of forms: needles of approximately 22 gauge, as applicators for rectal and intra-oesophageal use, as loops for attaching to the skin, etc. By a manually operated switching device up to fifteen junctions may be read sequentially. The advantages of this type of instrument are:

(a) The junctions may be very small and versatile
(b) The thermocouples respond rapidly on account of their low thermal capacity.
(c) The accuracy is adequate

Although a sensitive galvanometer is employed, no special levelling is required. The movement may be clamped so that the instrument can be carried about in a case without special precautions.

### Recording with Thermocouples

Certain problems are encountered in recording from thermocouples, partly because the voltage output per degree centigrade is only about 50 microvolts and partly because the cold junction temperature has to be kept constant. While for laboratory use the cold junction may be maintained in melting ice in a vacuum flask, this procedure is often inconvenient in the operating theatre.

One very satisfactory method of overcoming the difficulty, is to use the principles embodied in Fig. 3. The galvanometer scale can be replaced by a double photo-electric cell. Light reflected from the galvanometer mirror is distributed between the cells as the coil is deflected, and the photocell output is proportional to the angular deflection. Correction circuits can linearize the EMF-temperature relationship and the amplified output is applied to a multipoint chart recorder.

An electrical method of cold junction compensation, Fig. 4, is to arrange the thermojunction in series with a resistance bridge circuit in which only one arm is temperature dependent. Thus the temperature coefficient of resistance of nickel is relatively high, $68 \times 10^{-4}$ per degree centigrade, while constantan is very low, $0·2 \times 10^{-4}$ per degree centigrade. As the ambient temperature varies, the bridge unbalance can be arranged to compensate for

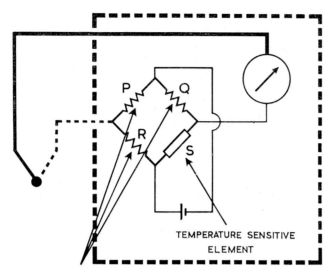

TEMPERATURE STABLE
ELEMENTS

FIG. 4. Electrical cold junction compensation.

the change of thermal EMF which would occur at the cold junction; $P$, $Q$, and $R$ are of constantan, and $S$ is of nickel.

Another approach is to maintain the reference junction at some other constant temperature. A useful device is the small thermostatically controlled oven, employed industrially for controlling the temperature of crystals used as control devices in crystal oscillators. The arrangement is shown in Fig. 5. The oven consists of a thick walled aluminium tube which has a mercury contact thermometer embedded in the wall. The contact thermometer has two

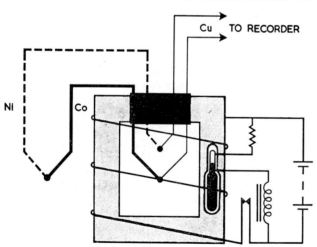

FIG. 5. Constant temperature oven for reference junction.

wires sealed into the stem so that the mercury thread connects them at a prearranged temperature. The cylinder has a heating coil of wire wound in close thermal contact with its surface, but electrically insulated from it.

The relay is arranged so that when the thermometer makes contact, the heating coil switches off. The purpose of the relay is to prevent the relatively large current in the heating coil from passing through the thermometer. The oven is surrounded with insulation and its temperature remains constant within $\pm 0.1°C$.

With this system a multichannel recording arrangement may be produced as shown in Fig. 6. The needle or other type applicators plug into a junction box. From here, a multicore cable continues to a potentiometer recorder via an oven. The wires of the cable are formed from the same material as the appropriate members of the thermojunctions so that no further thermocouples are introduced. The cable leads into the thermostatically controlled oven at 40°C where thermojunctions are formed with copper. The remainder of the connections are in copper and no further 'stray' thermojunctions are introduced. The input to the multichannel potentiometric recorder amplifier is via automatically operated switches and the temperatures

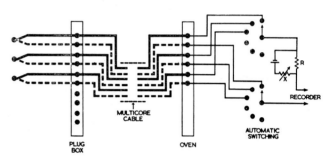

FIG. 6. Multichannel recording with thermocouple.

of applicators are printed sequentially. By introducing a direct 'back off' voltage via $R$ into one of the leads, 'zero' may be set at any required level.

### 3. Platinum Resistance Thermometry

The resistance of a metal varies with temperature according to the relation:

$$R_t = R_0 (1 + at + bt^2)$$

where      $R_t$ = resistance at temperature $t°C$

            $R_0$ = resistance at ice temperature

$a$ and $b$ are constants which have been accurately determined for various metals.

For a 100 ohm coil of platinum, the resistance change near ice temperature is about 0.4 ohm per °C.

Knowing the values of $a$ and $b$, if the resistance of a coil is accurately measured at the ice point, an unknown temperature may be determined from the above relation if $R_t$ is accurately measured. When used in this way a platinum resistance thermometer is capable of much higher accuracy than is usually required medically, e.g. a few thousandths of a °C. The practical arrangement is as in Fig. 7, which shows a modified Wheatstone bridge. The fixed arms $P$, $Q$ and $R$ of the bridge may be wound with constantan, which has a negligible temperature coefficient of resistance and is thus thermostable.

In order that no resistance error is introduced by the connecting leads to the coil, a second pair of 'false' leads is included in the thermometer housing and these are connected into the opposite-fixed arm $Q$. Hence, the resistance of the actual leads is balanced out.

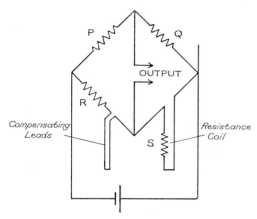

FIG. 7. Bridge circuit for a resistance thermometer.

The current through the coil must be limited to avoid self-heating. For example, for a 100 ohm coil, the power dissipated should be limited to about 0·1 milliwatt, so that the current through the coil should not exceed 1 milliampere. Thus a change of temperature of 1°C would produce a change of bridge output voltage of approximately 400 microvolts, compared with about 40 microvolts per degree centigrade for a thermocouple. Resistance coils may be made sufficiently reproducible as to be readily interchangeable.

For medical use the chief disadvantage has been the physical size of the coil and correspondingly slow response time. While the rectal and oesophageal thermometers have been produced commercially, smaller probes are not readily available.

Although high accuracy of temperature measurement is possible with bridge circuits if the resistance is measured by balancing the bridge, it is often desirable to have a direct reading instrument. This is possible, because as the thermometer coil resistance changes the bridge is unbalanced, and the resulting current may be related to temperature, and read directly from a suitable meter.

Two problems arise with bridge circuits;

(i) The resistance of the detecting element does not vary linearly with temperature. For platinum, between 0° and 100°C the maximum error arising from assuming a linear relationship is approximately 0·4°C.

(ii) If the resistance of one arm of a bridge is changed in equal steps, the corresponding steps of unbalance current in the galvanometer will not be equal, i.e. the relation between resistance change in one arm and unbalance current is non-linear. The problem may be resolved in three ways:

(a) *Non-linear scale*

As for the thermocouple, the resistance thermometer may be calibrated against a standard and a special non linear scale can be prepared for the galvanometer so that actual temperature and observed temperature are made equal.

(b) *Selection of bridge parameter*

Commercial galvanometers are normally supplied with linear scales. If one of these is used for the bridge,

and the temperature range is restricted, e.g. to 20°C within the physiological range, it is possible to limit the non-linear error by the correct choice of bridge resistances. The principle is discussed below in the section on thermistors.

(c) *Electronic Linearization*

By electronic circuits, using diodes, it is possible to correct the slope of any curved characteristic, piece by piece, until it becomes linear within specified limits. This technique can be applied to the outputs of bridge circuits.

### 4. Thermistor Thermometers

The thermistor is a semiconducting element consisting of a heavy metal oxide which has a large negative temperature coefficient of resistance. Oxides of manganese, nickel, cobalt, iron and zinc have been used. Thermistors are produced by compressing such oxides in powder form to beads, rods or discs, and sintering the mixture at high temperature into a solid mass. Electrodes are applied by firing on metal colloids, applied as paints or by fusing the material around wires.

For biological use, minute beads ranging in diameter from 0·006 to 0·1 in. are available, which may be sealed into the tip of hypodermic needles. Fig. 8 shows a photomicrograph of such a bead (STC/U.23) compared with the head of a match. They have a very small thermal capacity and can respond to a change of temperature rapidly–in

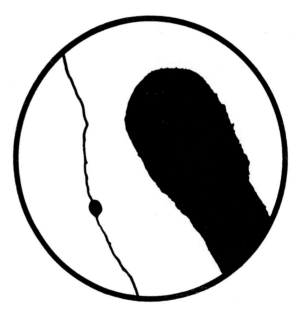

FIG. 8. Thermistor bead compared with a match.

as little as 0·2 seconds. However, they are not as stable as metal resistance elements and most thermistors show an ageing as an increase of resistance with time over a period of months. In addition, they may exhibit hysteresis effects if subjected to rapid large temperature fluctuations and it is sometimes recommended that they be recalibrated if subjected to temperature changes of greater than 10°C

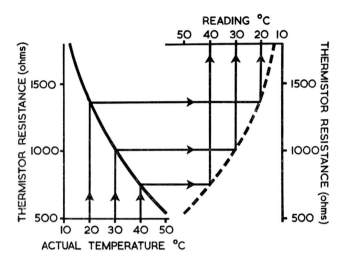

FIG. 9. Principle of linearizing thermistor characteristics when used in bridge circuits.

per minute, or to greater changes than 50–60°C. Furthermore, variations occur from one to another of the same type so that individual calibrations are necessary, although matched pairs are now available.

The variations of resistance of EMF with temperature are non-linear for resistance thermometers and thermocouples, but the deviation from linearity is relatively small. This is not so for the thermistor where the resistance varies exponentially with the reciprocal of the absolute temperature. Compared with the metallic resistor the resistance change is large, e.g. the thermistor approximately halves its resistance for a 20°C increase in temperature. Because of this relatively large sensitivity the thermistor is well suited to the measurement of small temperature changes, such as that within the pulmonary artery during thermal dilution procedures for measuring cardiac output.

Thermistors are used in bridge circuits, but because of their relatively high resistance compared with metal coils, no special requirements are necessary regarding compensating leads. The problems of non-linearity are dealt with as described previously.

The principle of selecting bridge parameters to provide linear but limited ranges of temperature-resistance relations is shown in Fig. 9. The left hand curve (solid line) shows the variation of resistance of the thermistor with increasing temperature. Notice that the resistance decreases as shown when the temperature rises. Furthermore, the out of balance current is not proportional to the change of resistance but follows a curve. This is shown on the right hand side (dotted curve) of Fig. 9, where the temperature reading is, of course, the out of balance current suitably calibrated as a temperature. By arranging that the bridge constants are such that the shape of the right hand curve for the bridge is the same as the left hand curve for the thermistor, the reading will correspond with the actual temperature.

## 5. Dial Thermometers

(a) *Bimetallic* If a flat spiral spring is made up of two differing metal ribbons in contact, then on heating, the spring will tend to wind (or unwind) because of the difference in expansion between the metals. This movement may be transferred to a pointer.

(b) *Pressure Gauge Types.* In the Bourdon gauge, the "spring" consists of a hollow ribbon of metal which unwinds as the pressure inside it is increased and this movement causes a needle to rotate against a scale. Attached to the pressure gauge via a capillary is a steel tube filled with mercury, or a metal tube filled with a volatile liquid in the presence of its saturated vapour. The pressure changes produced by changing the temperature of the active element may be calibrated so that the dial reads in temperature units. The accuracy is about $\pm \frac{1}{4}$°C and the minimum range usually about 30°C.

*CHAPTER 7*

# METHODS FOR THE ANALYSIS OF GASES AND VAPOURS

## D. W. HILL

### Introduction

Various methods used in the analysis of gases are described in this chapter and the underlying principle used in the measurement has been emphasized so that the reader may be able to understand the working of the apparatus and the limitations of the technique. The earliest and simplest methods of gas analysis involved chemical processes but these have been largely superseded by physical or physico—chemical methods which are usually simpler and quicker to perform.

### Volumetric Gas Analysers

### The Haldane Gas Analyser

In the Haldane gas analyser a known volume of the gas mixture to be analysed is presented in turn to a series of absorbents and the diminution in volume is noted in each case. Since each absorbent is specific for a particular component, the percentage by volume of that component is simply given by the ratio of (change in volume/total volume) × 100 per cent.

Figure 1 is a diagrammatic representation of a Haldane apparatus (Haldane, 1920). The gas sample is first drawn into the 10 ml. calibrated burette (A) through the inlet C by raising and lowering the reservoir of mercury (D). For each analysis the mercury level is carefully adjusted to operate with a fixed volume of gas. After manipulating the taps the mercury is raised forcing the gas into the absorption pipette (B). As absorption proceeds, reagent passes from the reservoir (G) into (B). Several different pipettes are normally available to hold the various reagents. Typical absorbents would be 20 per cent NaOH for carbon dioxide and alkaline pyragallol (10 gm. sodium dithonite + 1 gm. anthraquinone + 25 ml. N. KOH) for oxygen. The mercury meniscus at $L_1$ and $L_2$ must always be precisely level when volumes are measured in order to ensure that the pressure inside the burette A is at atmospheric. The water jacket (W) serves to stabilize the burette temperature.

Lloyd (1960) has described a development of Haldane's apparatus which makes for a greater accuracy (0·02 per cent total gas volume). A screw control levels the mercury reservoir. The main assembly is made from a single glass structure without joints to eliminate leakage, and it is completely immersed in a water bath. In volumetric gas analysis no gas must be lost before the initial measurement, at each absorption only the gas under study must be removed and the carbon dioxide analysis is performed before the oxygen absorption. All measurements must be made with the gas in contact with solutions of the same vapour pressure, for example, in Haldane's method all

measurements are taken with the bulk of the gas in contact with acid rinse (a film of N/10 HCl being retained on the surface of the mercury in A.) Nunn (1958) describes in detail the problems involved in estimating gas mixtures

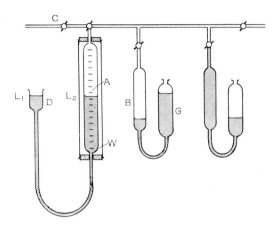

FIG. 1. Schematic diagram of the Haldane volumetric gas analyser.

containing nitrous oxide by Haldane's method. He overcomes these by the use of an all-glass apparatus and saturated sodium hydroxide solution (nitrous oxide being virtually insoluble in sat. NaOH) as the $CO_2$ absorber.

A simplified version of the Haldane apparatus has been devised by Campbell (1960) for use with the re-breathing method, for the estimation of blood $CO_2$ tension, (Howell, 1962). A simple volumetric absorption analyser for $CO_2$ has also been described (Nunn, 1958).

### The Scholander Gas Analyser

The Haldane apparatus needs relatively large volumes of gas. The micro-gas analyser of Scholander (1947) allows the determination of $O_2$, $N_2$ and $CO_2$ in 0·5 ml. sample volumes with an accuracy of 0·015 per cent. The gas sample is introduced by means of a calibrated pipette into a reaction chamber (B) connected to a micrometer burette (H). The chamber terminates in an indicator drop in a capillary tube leading to a compensating chamber (A). Absorbents for the gases concerned are tilted in turn into the reaction chamber without causing any change in the total liquid content of the system. The side-arm (C) holds the $CO_2$ absorber, whilst side-arm (D) holds the oxygen absorber. During gas absorption mercury is fed into the reaction chamber from the micrometer burette so as to keep the position of the drop constant. The percentage

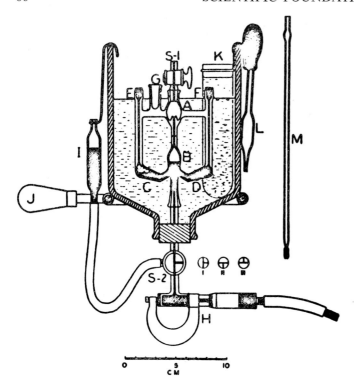

FIG. 2. The Scholander micro-gas analyser. (After Scholander, 1947.)

is an acid-saponin-ferricyanide solution. The saponin haemolyses the cells, the lactic acid liberates $CO_2$ from the carbonates and the carbamino compound, and the potassium ferricyanide which is an oxidizing agent converts haemoglobin and oxyhaemoglobin to methaemoglobin to liberate all the oxygen that was associated with

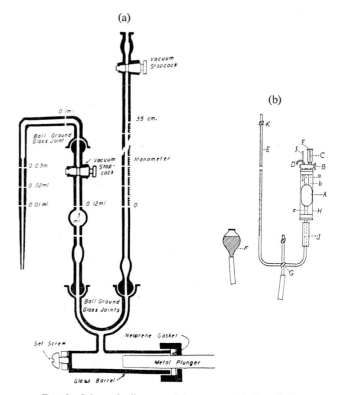

FIG. 3. Schematic diagram of the manometric Van Slyke apparatus, (a) micro version, (b) macro version.

by volume of the gas component can be simply expressed in terms of the ratio of the micrometer readings. In the Scholander apparatus the reagents chosen all have the same vapour pressure.

### Manometric Gas Analysers

#### The Manometric Van Slyke Apparatus

The manometric Van Slyke apparatus gives a greater accuracy and precision than the volumetric version. The manometric system measures the changes in pressure, rather than volume, which take place when specific components of the gas mixture are absorbed. This is done at a constant volume and temperature.

The Van Slyke and Neill apparatus (1924) is illustrated in Figure 3. The burette (A) has a double stopcock B to which is attached a measuring cup (C) and an outlet tube (D). These are used to introduce or remove samples or reagents. The burette is connected to the manometer (E) and to the mercury levelling bulb and reservoir (F). The bulb can be shut-off from the apparatus by means of the stopcock (G). The burette is mounted in a water jacket (H) containing a thermometer (I), and is usually calibrated at 0·5, 2 and 50 c.c. By lowering the mercury level to the 50 c.c. mark a vacuum is produced inside the burette and this extracts free gases from the sample. The extracted gases are compressed to 2 or 0·5 c.c. at each stage and the pressure read from the manometer.

Blood for gas analysis is collected and stored anerobically. In order to liberate both the dissolved and combined gases it is necessary to employ a "releasing agent". This

haemoglobin in the original sample. The releasing solution is first de-gassed by reducing the atmospheric pressure within the apparatus, then the blood is added and the burette agitated. The released gases are then extracted by creating a vacuum. The carbon dioxide is absorbed with sodium hydroxide and the oxygen with sodium hydrosulphite. The flexible joint (J) allows for a "to and fro" motion of the burette assembly during agitation. This motion is accomplished by means of a crank and eccentric drive from an electric motor.

### Physical Methods

Physical methods for the analysis of gas and vapour mixtures are becoming of increasing interest to anaesthetists because of the speed of response, their convenience and the presentation of their results as an electrical output signal. Some instruments are designed to give an output which is proportional to the concentration of one particular component of a mixture, and ideally they should only respond to a physical property which is specific to the component under investigation. In practice this is not always possible and it becomes necessary to consider the effects produced by a mixture of constituents. Other analysers such as gas chromatographs and mass spectrometers are designed to analyse a range of components present in a mixture. From this it becomes evident that ideally the anaesthetist needs to have at his disposal a range of analysers to cover the commonly encountered gases and vapours. The situation is further complicated by the fact that it is usually necessary to provide a range of standard calibration mixtures in order to be able to check the accuracy of each instrument's reading. For routine clinical monitoring a simple oxygen analyser and a halothane analyser may be all that is required. However, for research purposes these will need to be supplemented by a range of infra-red analysers and at least one gas chromatograph.

## Paramagnetic Oxygen Analysers

There is a clinical need for a compact analyser specific for oxygen which could be used for example, to indicate the oxygen concentration in circle anaesthetic systems and in oxygen tents. The development of suitable analysers has been made possible by the paramagnetic property of oxygen molecules. When oxygen molecules are introduced into a non-homogeneous magnetic field they experience a force which is proportional to the oxygen partial pressure, if the temperature is constant. A simple oxygen monitor can be made by using a quartz suspension to mount two small hollow glass spheres shaped like a dumb-bell between the pole pieces of a powerful permanent magnet. The pole pieces are shaped so that the field is markedly non-uniform. The spheres are filled with nitrogen. In the simplest form a stream, of a few milli-litres per minute, of the gas mixture to be analysed, is drawn past the dumb-bell-shaped assembly by means of a sucker bulb. Oxygen molecules, being paramagnetic, experience a force which moves them along the direction of the field gradient so that they tend to displace the dumb-bell. The force on the dumb-bell is proportional to the oxygen partial pressure. The quartz suspension carries a small mirror from which a beam of light is reflected on to a scale calibrated in terms of oxygen concentration or partial pressure. A silica gel drying column is placed in front of the inlet to the chamber of the analyser. Descriptions of the construction and application of direct reading paramagnetic oxygen analysers are given by Pauling, Wood and Sturdevant (1946), Hobson and Kay (1956) and Woolmer (1955).

The suspended dumb-bell comprises two thin-walled glass spheres 4 mm. in diameter sealed to a 6 mm. long glass rod. Mounted above on the fibre suspension is a 2 mm. × 2 mm. glass mirror. The magnetic force acting on the spheres between the pole pieces is proportional to the product of the magnetic field strength, the field gradient and the difference in volume susceptibility between the spheres and the surrounding gas. The force acting on each sphere gives rise to a turning moment which deflects the mirror, Pauling, Wood and Sturdevant (1946) give details of methods of compensating for the effect of ambient temperature changes on the calibration of this type of oxygen analyser.

A greater accuracy can be achieved by the use of a null

balance method, Munday (1958). The deflection of the spot of light in the paramagnetic analyser is opposed and nullified by means of passing a current through a coil attached to the dumb-bell. The ten-turn helical potentiometer which controls the value of the backing-off current is calibrated directly in terms of oxygen concentration. Thus for a range of 0–100 per cent oxygen each potentiometer calibration interval is equivalent to 0·1 per cent $O_2$. A typical accuracy is plus or minus 0·1 per cent $O_2$ over a plus or minus 5°C variation in temperature, with an optimal sampling flow of 100 ml. per minute. The deflection of the instrument is exponential, the 90 per cent response time being less than 8 seconds. Nunn (1964) has checked the performance of this arrangement in detail and finds it to be as accurate as the Lloyd-Haldane chemical analyser for oxygen (Lloyd, 1958).

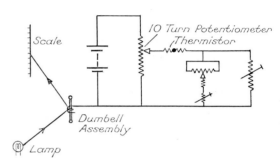

Fig. 4. Schematic diagram of a null-balance paramagnetic oxygen analyser. (Courtesy Servomex Controls Ltd.)

A schematic diagram of the null-balance type DCL101 oxygen analyser by Servomex is shown in Figure 4. The thermistor (temperature sensitive resistor) compensates for the effects of ambient temperature changes upon the analyser's calibration. The calibration is linear with oxygen tension since in the null-balance condition the dumb-bell always operates in the same portion of the magnetic field. With the earlier direct reading analysers the calibrations were individual for each instrument, depending as they did on the magnet's characteristics.

An electric direct reading oxygen analyser type OA150 by Servomex Controls Ltd. is illustrated in Figure 5. The deflection of the dumb-bell reflects light from a mirror on to one or other of a pair of photo-cells. The difference in output signals from the photo-cells is fed to a differential amplifier whose output current supplies the dumb-bell coil. Any deflection of the suspension is thus continuously nulled. The panel meter reads the coil current which is proportional to the oxygen tension. Two scales are provided 0–25 per cent and 0–100 per cent. Ellis and Nunn (1968) have evaluated the OA150 and find that the sensitivity is adequate for clinical purposes (0·25 per cent on the 0–25 per cent range and 1 per cent on the 0–100 per cent range).

One disadvantage of the paramagnetic oxygen analyser lies in the fact that it is not sufficiently fast to be able to follow oxygen changes in a single breath and can only handle relatively low sampling rates. The 99 per cent response time is of the order of 1 minute.

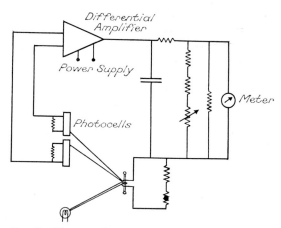

Fig. 5. Direct reading paramagnetic oxygen analyser. (Courtesy Servomex Controls Ltd.)

## Thermal Conductivity Analysers

Changes in the composition of a gas stream may produce significant alterations in the thermal conductivity of the stream. As a result, the temperature of a heated wire filament situated in the stream may rise or fall and this will be accompanied by corresponding electrical resistance changes in the wire which can be detected with a sensitive Wheatstone bridge arrangement. In a typical thermal conductivity cell (Katharometer) four platinum filaments would be used in a constant current circuit (Jessop, 1966). It is arranged that the gas of interest does not flow over two of the filaments. These act as reference arms for the bridge and provide compensation for changes occurring in the ambient temperature. The other two arms are surrounded by the gas stream in which one component is of interest. The active and reference filaments are arranged as shown in Figure 6. The difference in the thermal conductivity of air and carbon dioxide enables the thermal

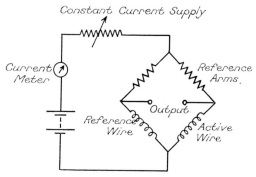

Fig. 6. Katharometer bridge circuit.

conductivity technique to be used for the estimation of $CO_2$ in expired air or oxygen. Variations in the proportions of oxygen and nitrogen in the sample stream will have little effect since they have almost the same thermal conductivity. Changes in water vapour of the stream are eliminated, as far as thermal conductivity changes are concerned, by arranging to saturate the gas fed to both the active and

reference filaments. The four filaments are mounted in a metal block to ensure that ambient temperature changes will affect all filaments equally.

Fundamentally, thermal conductivity analysis is not specific to any one component of a gas mixture, and considerable ingenuity may be required in the choice of the gas mixture passing over the reference filaments to ensure that the active filaments only respond to changes in the concentration of the component of interest (Jessop, 1966). This, together with the fact that the conventional katharometer operating at atmospheric pressure is too slow to follow gas composition changes in individual breaths, means that thermal conductivity analysers are rarely encountered in anaesthesia. Miniature wire katharometers, however play an important part in gas chromatography.

By reducing the pressure of the gas surrounding the filaments to a few millimetres of mercury absolute it is possible to increase the speed of response to a katharometer so that it can follow the $CO_2$ concentration changes in individual breaths. A detailed description of thermal conductivity gas analysers applied to respiratory physiology is that of Visser (1957).

## Infra-red Gas Analysers

The best accuracy using thermal conductivity analysers is with binary or quasi-binary gas mixtures. When it is required to know the composition of a gas stream whose proportions can vary widely, then it may be more convenient to use several infra-red gas analysers plus a paramagnetic oxygen analyser, nitrogen usually being measured by difference. Infra-red gas analysers depend for their operation upon the fact that many gases and vapours can absorb specific wavelengths of infra-red radiation. As long ago as 1863 infra-red absorption was used to measure the $CO_2$ concentration in respiratory gases (Tyndall, 1863). The main absorption bands arise from vibrational energy changes in the sample molecules. Rotational energy changes must also be taken into account, and it is found that each vibrational energy level has a series of rotational levels associated with it. The vibration-rotation band of a diatomic molecule should consist of two branches known as the P-branch and the R-branch. Figures 7 and 8 illustrate the similar situation found with linear triatomic molecules such as $N_2O$ and $CO_2$. In anaesthetic studies the commonly encountered infra-red gas analysers are of the non-dispersive type shown in Figure 9. This is a double-beam-in-space arrangement using a hot wire spiral and mirrors to form a sample beam and a reference beam. The beams are occluded simultaneously twice per revolution of the motor-driven chopping disk to give an interruption frequency which usually lies within the range 6–60 Hz. The chopper disk has four segments, of which the metal has been cut away from two opposite segments, Figure 10. When the opaque pair of segments is not in the way, the two infra-red beams fall one on to each half of a balanced condenser microphone detector (Luft, 1943). This consists of two identical chambers separated by means of a thin flexible metal diaphragm. The chambers are filled to an absolute or partial pressure of a few centimetres of mercury pressure with a sample of the pure gas or vapour to be analysed. Thus the detector of an infra-red $CO_2$ analyser would contain a low pressure of $CO_2$, whilst that of an analyser for di-ethyl ether would contain a low pressure of di-ethyl

windows of the sample cell are made of a substance such as calcium fluoride which will transmit infra-red wavelengths to about 5 micro-metres. The reference beam tube is usually filled with an inert gas such as nitrogen. Assuming that when the gas to be tested is present in the sample cell there will be a significant absorption of infra-

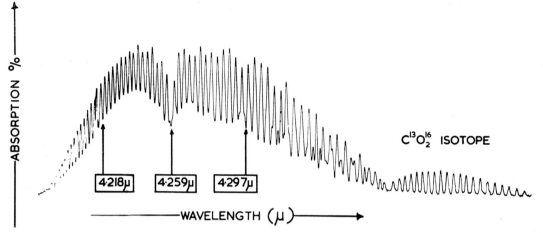

FIG. 8. Absorption spectrum for carbon dioxide.

ether vapour. The advantage of this arrangement is that the detector filling can only absorb those infra-red wavelengths which are covered by the absorption bands of the substance to be analysed. By means of adjustable shutters it is first arranged that the strengths of the two beams falling on the detector are made equal without the presence of

red energy, and the sample beam falling on to the detector will be weaker than the reference beam. The consequent asymmetrical warming of the detector contents will cause the pressure in the reference half of the detector to rise to a higher value than that in the sample half. As a result, the flexible diaphragm is pushed over towards the sample half of the detector. As the chopper disk revolves, so the diaphragm is caused to vibrate at the chopping frequency.

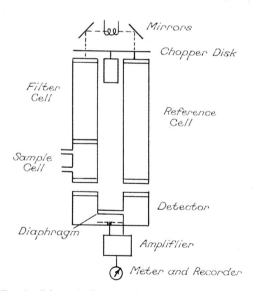

FIG. 9. Schematic diagram of a non-dispersive infra-red gas analyser.

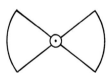

FIG. 10. Design of a chopper disk for a non-dispersive infra-red gas analyser.

The diaphragm is arranged to form one half of a parallel plate capacitor. In some forms of analyser the capacitor is supplied with a constant electrical charge and the resulting voltage changes at the chopping frequency are amplified by means of a three-stage amplifier tuned to the chopping frequency, synchronously rectified and then smoothed and displayed on a panel meter or recorder. The meter or recorder is normally calibrated in terms of per cent concentration or parts per million by volume. In other types of analyser, the capacitor forms one part of the tuning circuit of a radio frequency oscillator used in an amplitude modulation system. Changes in the sample concentration alter the amplitude of the modulated carrier. After demodulation the signal corresponding to concentration is again fed to a meter or recorder. The radio frequency system avoids the 'noise' and insulation problems associated with the use of an electrometer valve encountered in the constant charge system. For laboratory,

any specimen in the sample cell. The beam passing through the sample cell is known as the sample beam, whilst the second beam is called the reference beam. The beams pass down metal tubes whose interior surfaces have been internally honed and gold plated so that they are highly reflective. Multiple reflections ensure that the efficiency of the beam transmission down the tube is high. The as opposed to industrial, use the constant charge system works well and is widely used in a number of medical infra-red gas analysers. The condenser microphone is supplied with a voltage of the order of 100 V d.c. through a high resistor and the voltage variations appearing across the detector are measured with an amplifier having an electrometer valve input stage. A detailed account of a number of different infra-red gas analyser systems is that of Hill and Powell (1968).

Cross-sensitivity effects arise from the overlapping of the absorption bands of the wanted component of the sample with those of unwanted components in the sample mixture (Hill and Powell, 1967). The apparent increase in sensitivity arising from the contributions of other sample components can be reduced, if not eliminated, by means of optical interference filters (Heavens, 1955, Francon, 1963) to select a band which is clear of overlap, or by the use of a gas filter cell placed in each beam and filled with the interfering substance(s). The gas filter cell is usually filled with 100 per cent of the interfering substance. Then any wavelength capable of being absorbed by the interfering substance will be completely absorbed in the filter cell before it can fall on the detector. With infra-red gas analysers for $CO_2$ a cross-sensitivity is often observed for $N_2O$. This arises from the fact that the portion of the $CO_2$ absorption band due to the $C_{13}O_2$ isotope (about 1 per cent abundance) overlaps the neighbouring band of $N_2O$ in the region of 4·3 micro-metres. The use of paired filter cells filled with $N_2O$ will eliminate the interference.

Cormack and Powell (1972) provide a detailed account of the methods they adopted to increase the accuracy of their Luft-type infra-red $CO_2$ analyser from 0·1 to 0·01 per cent $CO_2$. They found that the largest source of drift was due to room temperature changes. Legg and Parkinson (1968) discuss the calibration of $CO_2$ analizers.

### The Gas Discharge Nitrogen Meter

The recording of nitrogen wash-out curves is still an important technique in the evaluation of pulmonary

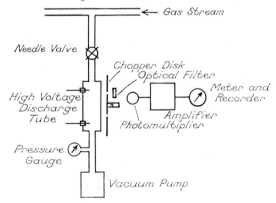

FIG. 11. Schematic diagram of a gas discharge nitrogen meter.

function. For this purpose a fast-response analyser is required which is specific for nitrogen. The gas-discharge nitrogen meter of Lundin and Akesson (1954) is well suited for this application and is often employed for the

preliminary assessment of patients in anaesthetic studies. A rotary oil vacuum pump draws a sample of the patient's expired air into a discharge tube which operates at an absolute pressure of a few torr, Figure 11. A d.c. voltage of about 1,500 V is placed across the electrodes in the tube and excites the familiar purple colour discharge which is characteristic of the presence of nitrogen. This purple light is arranged to be interrupted by means of a rotating segmented chopping disk driven by a synchronous electric motor. After chopping, the light passes through optical filters, in order to select only those bands corresponding to the purple emission, and falls on to a photo-cell. The output from the cell is amplified by means of a tuned amplifier and fed to a fast response recorder. The response time of the analyser is of the order of 20 milli-seconds so that it is well able to measure the nitrogen concentration present in individual breaths.

### The Ultra-violet Halothane Meter

The ultra-violet halothane meter designed by Robinson et al. (1962) is an instrument which is specific for halothane and which is convenient for clinical use where only a limited accuracy is required. It operates upon the principle that halothane absorbs ultra-violet light strongly with maximum absorption in the region of 200 nano-metres. There is no convenient light source at this wave-length but halothane will still absorb significantly at the 234 nano-metre emission of a low pressure mercury lamp. Referring to Figure 12, a 6 watt lamp is suitable, mounted in an envelope made of an ultra-violet transmitting glass. Light from the lamp (L) passes through a cylindrical stainless steel cuvette (C) (2·5 cm. long by 1 cm. i.d.) fitted with quartz windows, and falls upon an ultra-violet sensitive photo-cell $P_1$. A second photo-cell, $P_2$ monitors the intensity of the lamp and acts as a reference. The output voltages developed across the ten-megohm load resistances of the photo-cells are fed one to each side of a

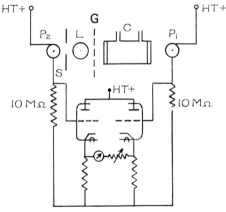

FIG. 12. Schematic diagram of an ultra-violet halothane analyser.

balanced triode cathode follower stage. A panel meter scaled 0–5 per cent v/v halothane and a recorder are connected between the cathodes. The halothane meter is calibrated against an accurate vaporizer or known halothane mixtures in cylinders. A lever arrangement can raise a metal gauze (G) so that it partially occludes the beam on the cuvette side, and a shutter (S) is available to adjust the intensity of the light falling on the reference cell to be equal to that falling on the sample photo-cell. With the lamp off, the zero control of the cathode follower is adjusted to bring the meter to zero. With no halothane present, the shutter is adjusted to zero the meter again. A known halothane concentration is then sucked into the cuvette using a small pump and the gain control adjusted to give the correct meter reading. The gauze is next raised and the halothane removed from the cuvette. The meter reading due to the gauze is noted. This can be used as a check on the correct function of the instrument. The halothane meter is a useful device, but does tend to suffer from a long warm-up time, of the order of an hour. Ultraviolet light decomposes halothane and can produce toxic irritant by-products. If it is necessary to return the effluent from the cuvette back to the gas circuit, then it should be passed through soda lime to remove the impurities.

**The Drager Narkotest**

The Drager Narkotest is an ingenious non-electrical arrangement for the routine measurement of inspired halothane vapour concentrations up to 3 per cent v/v. The mixture of gas and halothane vapour having a low humidity enters the Narkotest via the bottom port. In an open anaesthetic circuit arrangement the gas and vapour stream will have come from the manifold of the anaesthetic machine and thus will be dry. The Narkotest is also well suited for mounting in the inspiratory limb of a closed circuit as shown in Figure 13. By the time expired gas from the patient has travelled back to the Narkotest it will have cooled down to the ambient temperature so that there will be no condensation of water within the Narkotest. The Narkotest is not recommended for use in the expiratory limb of a circle because of the problem of condensing water vapour, but it should be possible to use it in this position if a trap is arranged to collect condensed water.

On entering the Narkotest the gas and vapour stream passes between four strips of silicone rubber. There is no chemical reaction between the halothane vapour and the rubber, but the adsorption of the vapour by the rubber causes the strips to increase in length. The strips are coupled to an axle carrying a pointer by means of a terylene thread. A light lever carrying a pointer at its end is fixed to the axle, the pointer sweeping over a scale calibrated from 0–3 per cent v/v halothane in 0·2 per cent v/v steps. The system is sensitive to temperature and humidity changes and compensation against these effects is provided in the following manner. The upper end of the strips is fixed to a pivoted metal plate, the other end of which is anchored with a nylon thread. The effect of an increasing humidity is to lengthen the rubber strips but at the same time the humidity stretches the nylon thread which takes up the increase in length of the rubber and thus minimizes any motion of the pointer. The lower end of the rubber strips is secured by means of a bimetal strip. As the temperature increases so does the length of the

rubber strips, but this is taken up by the bending down-wards of the bimetal. A more subtle effect arises from the fact that the uptake of halothane vapour by silicone rubber is also temperature dependent, decreasing with increasing temperature. This is compensated by the action of a bimetallic ring which is attached to the pointer pivot. With increasing temperature the action is to increase the effective moment of the counter balance weight for the pointer and thus to reduce the deflection. The set zero knob is a mechanical control which is used to line up the pointer with the zero scale mark. If the Narkotest has

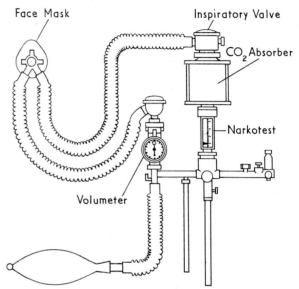

FIG. 13. Use of the Drager Narkotest in a circle anaesthetic system.

been set up at 25°C to read 1 per cent this will become a reading of 1·2 per cent at 33°C. The effect of water vapour on the silicone rubber and nylon thread is different, but after the elapse of five to ten minutes the correct compensation for water vapour will have occurred.

The resistance to gas flow of the chamber containing the rubber strips is low, being 3·6 mm. of water at a flow of 30 litres per minute. The response time of the Narkotest is flow rate dependent. The time to achieve half the final reading is 8 seconds at eight litres per minute and 40 seconds at one litre per minute. At one litre per minute it takes 90 seconds to achieve 90 per cent of the final value. The direction of flow through the Narkotest is of no consequence, and it is sufficient that the instrument be mounted vertically as judged by eye.

The accuracy of the Narkotest is quoted as plus or minus 0·15 per cent v/v over the range 0–3 per cent. In one model tested by the author againt a calibrated re-fractometer at 1 per cent the Narkotest read 1·06 per cent whilst at 3·2 per cent it read 3·25 per cent.

Unfortunately the action of the Narkotest is not specific for halothane. A 70/30 per cent mixture of nitrous oxide and oxygen will produce a reading on the Narkotest equivalent to about 0·25 per cent halothane. Hence if nitrous oxide is to be present, the zero reading of the Narkotest should first be set up on the halothane-free nitrous oxide oxygen mixture which will be used. With regard to sensitivity to carbon dioxide, 10 per cent $CO_2$ in oxygen will give a reading equivalent to 0·1 per cent halothane.

The Narkotest is particularly sensitive to ether, and should not be used in the presence of ether or of cyclopropane. A measured concentration of 2 per cent v/v di-ethyl ether gave the equivalent reading of 1·5 per cent v/v halothane on the Narkotest, 3 per cent ether was equivalent to 2·2 per cent halothane and 4 per cent ether gave full scale (3 per cent halothane). In spite of these limitations the Narkotest fulfils a useful requirement for a simple halothane monitor which can be used in a closed circuit.

## The Rayleigh Refractometer

The measurement of the optical refractive index of a binary gas or vapour mixture provides a stable method for the factory calibration of gas and air machines for obstetrical practice, dental anaesthetic machines and anaesthetic vaporizers. The refractive index of a gas mixture is defined as:

$$\mu = \frac{\text{velocity of light in vacuo}}{\text{velocity of light in the gas}}$$

The velocity of light in the mixture will depend upon the number of molecules present, i.e. on the density and thus upon the temperature and pressure of the gas. The refractive index is usually referred to the standard conditions of 0°C and 760 mm. Hg. by assuming that $(\mu - 1)d$ is constant where "$d$" is the density.

Changes occurring in the refractive index of a mixture can be accurately measured by means of an optical instrument known as a Rayleigh refractometer. The principles of its use are set out by Edmondson (1957), Hanson and Maimon (1959) and Luder (1964). Figure 14a, b (after Edmondson, 1957) illustrate the principle of the instrument.

White light from the filament lamp A is focussed by lens B on to the vertical slit C which is situated at the focus

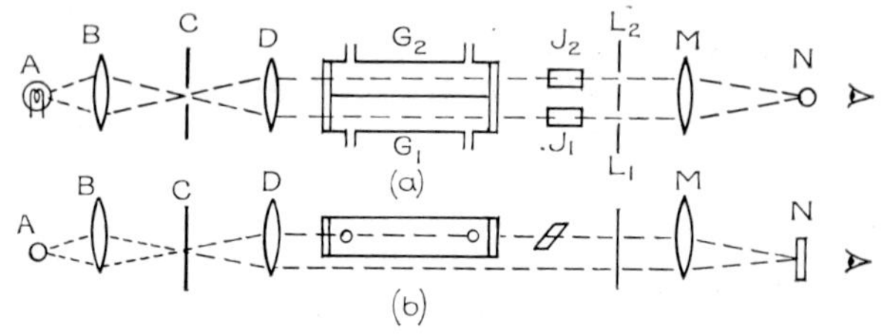

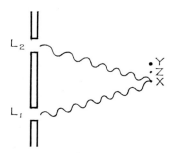

FIG. 14. (a) Plan view, and (b) side elevation of a Rayleigh refractometer.

of lens D. Light emerging from D is now parallel and passes through two similar metal tubes fitted with optical glass windows and inlet and outlet ports. These tubes are made gas tight and do not communicate with each other. One tube $G_1$, the sample cell, contains the gas mixture to be analysed, the other $G_2$, the reference cell, contains a gas of known refractive index. After passing through the

tubes the two beams of light pass through a pair of optically flat glass plates $J_1$ and $J_2$. These plates are mounted at an angle, $J_1$ being fixed, whilst $J_2$ can be slowly rotated so as to alter its angle of slope compared with $J_1$. After leaving the plates the rays pass through the vertical slits $L_1$ and $L_2$ and a lens M which brings them to a focus at N. This is a cylindrical lens eyepiece which magnifies in the horizontal plane only. Two other beams of light from D pass underneath the gas cells $G_1$ and $G_2$ but not through the glass plates $J_1$ and $J_2$. This light is also viewed through N by the observer at O.

If the light was monochromatic (of a single wavelength) the observer O would see a picture as in Figure 15a. The

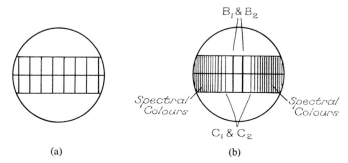

FIG. 15. Fringe pattern as seen in the eyepiece of a Rayleigh refractometer with (a) monochromatic light, (b) white light.

horizontal line across the middle is a shadow due to the bottom wall of the tubes $G_1$ and $G_2$. The upper vertical lines arise from optical interference between the beams of light passing through $G_1$ and $G_2$. The lower vertical lines arise from interference between the beams of light passing beneath $G_1$ and $G_2$. The formation of the fringes is illustrated in Figure 16. The point X is situated in the axis mid-way between the slits and is equidistant from each slit. Light waves passing through each slit are exactly in step and since the distances $L_1X$ and $L_2X$ are equal they will still be in step at X where they will reinforce each other to give a light band. Consider a point Y such

FIG. 16. Formation of the refractometer fringes.

that the distance $L_1Y$ is one light wavelength less than $L_2Y$, then the waves will reinforce again at Y to produce a second bright band. Half-way between X and Y at Z the path length for the two waves will differ by one half a wavelength and at Z the waves will arrive exactly out of step so they will cancel each other out to produce darkness.

Thus there will appear in the eyepiece N a series of alternate vertical dark and light bands of light.

Suppose that the gas in cell $G_1$ is replaced with a gas having a slightly greater refractive index than that in $G_2$. The light waves passing through $G_1$ will now be relatively retarded and the rays arriving at the point A will no longer be exactly in step. Light passing through $L_1$ will however now be in step at some point X with light from $L_2$ which has taken the longer path $L_2X$. The same effect applies to all the interference bands so that the observer sees that the bands or fringes move over to the left. The lower set of bands, below the horizontal line A in Figure 15 are formed from light which has not passed through $G_1$ and $G_2$ and so remains stationary.

With monochromatic light such as that of the green line from a mercury discharge lamp, it is not at all easy to distinguish one fringe from another. It is important to be able to do this in order to count the fringe shift produced when the gas mixture in $G_2$ is changed.

By using a white light source the view seen in the eyepiece is changed to that of Figure 15b. At the centre is a fringe of bright light with two sharply defined black fringes $B_1$, $B_2$ on either side. The next pair of dark fringes $C_1$ and $C_2$ are less well defined, further fringes hardly being visible, The edges of the field of view display the colours of the rainbow. When the composition of the gas in $G_1$ is changed, the central bright fringe and bands $B_1$ and $B_2$ shift to the left whilst the lower fringes remain stationary. On slowly rotating glass plate $J_2$ so that the beam through $G_2$ has to pass through a greater thickness of glass, the light which has passed through the reference cell $G_2$ can be retarded by the same amount as the light passing through the sample cell $G_1$. This has occurred when the fringes pattern in the upper and lower halves of the field of view are again matched up. The angle through which $J_2$ has been turned can be calibrated against the refractive index change or against the percentage of one gas or vapour in the reference gas.

In order to calibrate the refractometer to measure refractive index changes directly, monochromatic light from a mercury or sodium lamp must be used. With only the gas present in $G_1$ and $G_2$ the black fringes of Figure 15a are aligned and the reading of the rotation scale attached to $J_2$ noted. By moving $J_2$ the pattern is shifted by one fringe and the reading again noted. This procedure is repeated for several fringes and a mean dial change (D) found which gives rise to a shift of one fringe. This is equivalent to a refractive index change of $(\Delta\mu)$. Then

$$\Delta\mu = \frac{\lambda}{L} = D$$ where $\lambda$ is the length of the cells $G_1$ and $G_2$

in cm. and $\lambda$ is the wavelength in cm. of the light source.

The source is changed to white light and the upper an lower fringes of Figure 15b aligned. The gas or vapour mixture is introduced into $G_1$ and $J_2$ moved to re-align the fringes. Let the dial reading change be $D_1$ then the refractive index change due to the mixture is $D_1 \times D_2$. If the refractive index of the pure vapour at ambient temperature and pressure is $\mu_1$, and that of the carrier gas is $\mu_2$ then a 100 per cent vapour mixture in $G_1$ would produce a refractive index change of $(\mu_1 - \mu_2)$. By simple proportion the percentage vapour present in the mixture which gave a refractive index change of $D_1 \times D_2$ can be found.

The refractive indices of some gases and vapours of interest at 0°C and 760 mm. Hg. are:

| | |
|---|---|
| Oxygen | 1·000272 |
| Nitrogen | 1·000297 |
| Air | 1·0002918 |
| Nitrous oxide | 1·000515 |
| Carbon dioxide | 1·0004498 |
| Chloroform | 1·001455 |
| Trichloroethylene | 1·001784 |
| Halothane | 1·00151 (white light) |
| Water vapour | 1·000257 |

Rayleigh Refractometers are today widely used by manufacturers of anaesthetic vaporizers and anaesthetic machines to establish the calibration of their products. At least one manufacturer has four in constant use for checking vaporizers. The Test House of the British Standards Institution also uses refractometers to check on the accuracy of trichloroethylene inhalers for midwifery use. Rayleigh Refractometers are about 4 feet long, but portable refractometers which can be held in the hand have been developed for use in mines to measure methane concentrations in air. They can also be used by anaesthetists to check on the accuracy of vaporizers.

Hulands and Nunn (1970) give a useful account of possible applications in anaesthesia for portable refractometers.

## Gas Chromatography

The technique of gas chromatography is of particular interest to anaesthetists since it provides a means of analysing multi-component gas and vapour mixtures, and also a convenient method for the analysis of volatile anaesthetic agents in blood. Gas chromatography has been put to a wide variety of uses, for example, the identification and estimation of barbiturates in urine.

The heart of a gas chromatograph is the chromatographic column. This is a glass or stainless steel tube, typically several feet long, with an outside diameter of $\frac{1}{8}$ in. or $\frac{1}{4}$ in. For work near ambient temperature with gases it is possible to use a nylon tube. For the analysis of organic vapours, the column would be carefully packed with an inert supporting phase such as crushed, sieved firebrick or Celite (a diatomaceous earth) having a typical mesh range of 80–100. This support is coated before packing with 10–30 per cent by weight of a suitable stationary phase. For general purpose use, this might be dinonyl phthalate, but for the analysis of halothane vapour concentrations silicone fluid is the best stationary phase. The column is mounted inside a forced air circulation oven which, for the analysis of anaesthetic vapours, would be thermostated in the region of 70–100°C. The column is perfused with a steady flow of an inert carrier gas such as helium, hydrogen, argon or nitrogen at a flow rate of the order of 20–60 ml. per minute. A sample of the liquid or gas mixture to be investigated is injected on to the front of the column. For gases the sample volume is in the range 1–20 c.c., whilst for liquids it is 1–5 micro-litres. The sample is first vaporized and then swept through the column whose function is to separate the gases in a sample by retarding each in order according to their affinities for the stationary phase. In many cases, this is in the order of their boiling points. Assuming that the resolution provided by the column is adequate, it is necessary to detect the consequent separate emergence of each component from the far end of the column. Several types of detecting device are available, and these will be discussed in detail. At any instant the output voltage from the detector is proportional to the concentration of the component concerned in the gas passing through the detector. The effect of the absorption column is not necessarily the same for all components. As the bolus of a particular component passes through the detector an associated recorder traces out a peak on the chart. The area under the peak is proportional to the amount of the component present. When the peaks are well separated and sharp, it is often sufficient to work with peak heights rather than with peak areas. The gas chromatograph is calibrated by letting it sample standard mixtures, whose concentrations preferably bracket the unknown peaks. The gas chromatograph is not a continuous analyser and needs feeding with discrete samples.

## Sampling Systems for Gas Chromatographs

Gas chromatographs are normally fitted with an injection port which can be heated independently of the column. The port carries a silicone rubber septum which can be easily renewed. Beneath the septum is a glass liner, which again can be taken out, in this case for cleaning. By means of a micro-syringe fitted with a 2 in. long needle, the liquid sample can be injected through the septum almost on to the top of the column which is plugged with a small amount of glass wool. The injection port is fed with the carrier gas stream and is heated, perhaps to 100°C or higher. The liquid sample is rapidly vaporized, any solid residue being trapped on the glass liner.

A sample of a gas or vapour stream can be collected in a gas-tight syringe and injected through the septum. Incidently, the life of the septum is extended by the use of side opening needles having a smooth tip. A greater degree of reproducibility is obtained by using a gas-sampling valve to inject a consistent sample volume (Hill and Hook, 1960; Cundall et al., 1966). The sampling valve can be motor driven when the chromatograph is wanted for repetitive monitoring.

## Detectors

For the analysis of gases such as oxygen, nitrogen, carbon dioxide and nitrous oxide it is necessary to use a thermal conductivity detector or katharometer. In its simplest form, the effluent from the column flows past a small heated metal wire spiral. The spiral loses heat to the walls of the detector by conduction through the carrier gas stream. As a result the wire attains an equilibrium temperature. When a sample component bolus surrounds the wire, the resulting thermal conductivity of the gas may be greater or less than that of the carrier gas alone. As a result, the temperature of the wire, and thus its electrical resistance will alter. A second, identical wire is perfused only with the carrier gas and serves as a reference. The two wires form opposite arms of a Wheatstone bridge circuit which is fed from a constant current supply. The out-of-balance voltage from the bridge is fed, via an attenuator, to a potentiometric recorder. This would normally have a 1 mV. sensitivity, a 1 second balancing time and a chart speed of 1 in. in 3 or 5 minutes. For thermal conductivity detection the carrier gas should be helium or hydrogen since the thermal conductivities of these gases are so much higher than those of the others.

For general purpose working with organic vapours, the *flame ionization detector* is the method of choice. With this arrangement, the effluent from the column is fed into a small flame which is kept burning from an independent mixture of hydrogen and oxygen. The passage of the bolus of organic vapour into the flame causes it to burn more strongly. The flame burns between a pair of electrodes (Butler and Hill, 1962), or inside a concentric cylinder electrode, the needle jet from which the flame issues being the other electrode. A polarizing voltage of about 200 V d.c. is placed across the electrodes and the resulting ionization current amplified by means of an electrometer amplifier and fed to a potentiometric recorder. The flame ionization detector was described by McWilliam and Dewar (1958), and its mode of action has been investigated by Ackman (1968). A suitable electrometer amplifier is that of Gabriel and Morris (1966). The great advantage of the flame ionization detector is that the standing signal in the absence of a peak is small, less than $10^{-9}$ A. This contrasts with the katharometer where the bridge must be kept accurately balanced, the balance being affected both by changes in temperature and flow rate. The flame detector has a linear dynamic range of the order of 1,000 to 1. It does, however, require the use of hydrogen, and it destroys samples passing through it.

For the analysis of halothane, chloroform, trichloroethylene and methoxyflurane in blood, the *electron capture detector* of Lovelock (1963) has some outstanding advantages, since it is particularly sensitive to halogenated compounds. Basically it consists of a small volume ionization chamber containing a tritiated zirconium foil as the cathode. The foil emits free electrons in the form of beta particles of low energy, and activities in the range 20–500 mC. are suitable. When the column elutes a strongly electron capturing compound into the chamber, the ionization current decreases, the chamber being polarized with only 8–10 V d.c. The standing current is arranged to be backed-off, and the polarity of the associated electrometer amplifier is set so that the small diminution in current due to the passage of a gas through the detector is recorded as a positive-going peak on the chart recorder.

## Applications of Gas Chromatography

A katharometer chromatograph having two columns in parallel can be used to analyse the blood gas contents of oxygen, nitrogen, carbon dioxide and nitrous oxide, (Hill, 1966), Figure 17. The molecular sieve column separates oxygen and nitrogen and permanently adsorbs $CO_2$ and $N_2O$. The Porapak column (crossed linked polymer beads) will not resolve oxygen and nitrogen. It lets these through as a combined peak, whilst splitting $CO_2$ and $N_2O$. In earlier work, activated charcoal was used in place of Porapak. A conventional acid-sapponin-fericyanide Van Slyke releasing agent solution is first degassed by passing the carrier gas (helium or hydrogen) vigorously through it for some 3 minutes. The solution is contained in a reaction vial fitted with a rubber septum. By means of

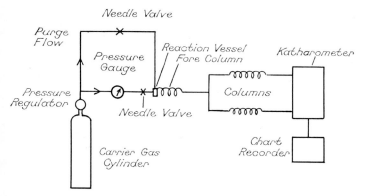

FIG. 17. Parallel column katharometer gas chromatograph arranged for the analysis of blood gas contents.

a three way tap, the vial is next sealed off, and 80–100 micro-litres of blood is added. Whatever the sample volume used, it must be kept the same during the calibration procedure. The vial is well shaken for a further 3 minutes whilst the blood gases are being liberated. The vial is next opened to the carrier gas which sweeps the blood gases on to the column system. The first column, filled only with firebrick, holds back the water from the blood sample and delays the peaks from the molecular sieve column. Subsequent blood samples can be loaded every $3\frac{1}{2}$ minutes. The instrument is calibrated for $CO_2$ by injecting known potassium carbonate solutions. Oxygen and nitrous oxide are calibrated by injecting known volumes of these gases. Nitrogen is often of no particular interest, except that a small nitrogen peak provides a check on the fact there has been no leak in of air. By increasing the sensitivity this arrangement is convenient for the estimation of nitrogen in blood.

For the analysis of ether vapour, halothane vapour and cyclopropane in expired air, a dinonyl phthalate column is very suitable when used with a katharometer. A molecular sieve column can be run in parallel for the estimation of oxygen, Hill (1960). Halothane needs to be extracted from blood, suitable extractants being n-heptane or carbon tetrachloride. A 1:1 dilution is used. The blood is shaken up with the heptane and left overnight at about 2°C in a refrigerator. This gives an average 98 per cent extraction (Butler and Hill, 1968). Cervenko (1968) added ether to the carbon tetrachloride as an internal marker in order to avoid the need to inject a precise volume into the

chromatograph. The blood was then spun for 15 minutes at 2,000 r.p.m., and 5 micro-litres of the plasma containing $CCl_4$ and halothane injected. The average recovery was 95 per cent. This process requires 15 minutes, and samples cannot be loaded on to the flame ionization detector chromatograph at less than 10 minute intervals because of the need to clear the large carbon tetrachloride peak when using an integrator.

Davies (1970) describes a reaction chamber for the analysis of blood-gases by means of a katharometer detector gas chromatograph. Eighty microlitres of blood are required for each analysis, duplicate analyses requiring eight minutes. Calibration for carbon dioxide is performed with potassium carbonate solution, for oxygen by using room air and for nitrous oxide by using cylinder nitrous oxide. Reproducibility studies were carried out by analysing one blood sample ten times: the coefficients of variation for oxygen, carbon dioxide and nitrous oxide were in each case approximately 0·5 per cent. Davies carried out comparisons of oxygen and carbon dioxide contents of whole blood by gas chromatography and the manometric Van Slyke method. For oxygen the correlation coefficient was 0·999 and for carbon dioxide it was 0·995.

The great sensitivity of the electron capture detector to halothane means that the blood can now be diluted 1,000:1 with n-heptane, and the halothane peak will still be greater than the heptane peak. Blood samples can now be loaded at 3 minute intervals. The apparatus is suitable for work in the operating room, since nitrogen is the only gas required. Standards are prepared by weighing halothane in heptane, and these should be made up each day. A 4 foot column filled with Celite impregnated with 35 per cent by weight of silicone fluid type MS550 and run at 40°C is suitable. Jones et al. (1972) describe a neat method for the analysis of methoxyflurane in blood by gas chromatography. The methoxyflurane is extracted from the blood by equilibration with silicone fluid. Because of its non-volatility, injection of the silicone extractant into the gas chromatograph results in a methoxyflurane peak after one minute and this is not accompanied by a solvent peak. The method permits the storage of blood samples for several days prior to chromatography. A linear calibration was found over the range 1–20 mg/100 ml and the coefficient of variation in blood at the 10 mg/100 ml level was ±1·8 per cent.

## Mass Spectrometry

Although they are expensive, mass spectrometers offer the advantage of being able to give a rapid analysis of several components in a gas or vapour sample. For example, it is possible to monitor breath-by-breath changes in the expired oxygen, nitrogen and carbon dioxide concentrations. The interior of the mass spectrometer operates at a low pressure, and a small sample of the gas mixture is drawn into the instrument by a vacuum pump. An incident beam of electrons produces ionization in the sample, and a combination of electric and magnetic fields then separates out the various molecular species in terms of their ratios of electric charge to mass. Each species is collected at a separate electrode and the resulting currents are scanned at intervals and presented on a fast recorder. Mass spectrometers have performed elegantly in lung function studies, Fowler and Hugh-Jones (1957), but conventional models are unable to separate $CO_2$ and $N_2O$. The ionization process gives rise to a 'cracking' pattern of subsidiary peaks due to the break up of the larger molecules. Even with a substance such as ethyl alcohol the resulting pattern needs care in interpretation.

Conventional mass spectrometers have tended to be bulky in construction because of their need to employ a large, powerful magnet. This situation has been radically changed with the development of the quadrupole mass spectrometer. With this arrangement, ions of a specific charge-to-mass ratio are separated by means of a combination of d.c. and radio frequency electric fields. By suitably choosing the field conditions, only ions of a particular ratio pass through the quadrupole head to the collected electrode where the ion current is measured by means of a low-noise

analyse simultaneous changes in the concentration of oxygen, nitrogen, carbon dioxide and water vapour in the breath. By knowing the partial pressure of water vapour, the fractional concentrations of the gases can be directly determined. Scheid *et al.* (1971) describe an automatic control system for use with a mass spectrometer which corrects for the partial pressure of water vapour in the sample by stabilizing the sum of the mass spectrometer signals for all component gases other than water vapour. It also corrects for pressure changes.

An interesting development is the connection of a mass spectrometer to an arterial catheter fitted with a silicone rubber membrane at its tip for the continuous *in vivo* measurement of blood-gas tensions (Wald *et al.*, 1970). In addition to monitoring $O_2$, $N_2$ and $CO_2$ these workers were able to monitor $N_2O$ in blood by monitoring the fragment ion peak (NO) at mass 30 where no other compound normally found in the body produces a response. Both $N_2O$ and $CO_2$ coincide at the normal mass to charge ratio of 44.

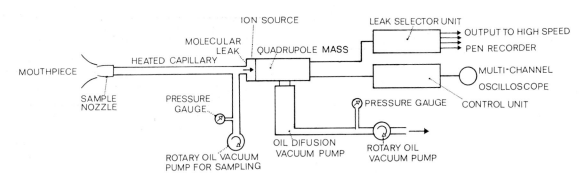

FIG. 18

photomultiplier. Figure 18 shows the schematic arrangement of a quadrupole mass spectrometer for respiratory studies. The head is maintained under a high vacuum by means of an oil diffusion pump baked by a two stage rotary oil pump. A second rotary oil pump is used to suck the sample gas stream into the analyser. The inlet system design is critical for a fast response. Typically, it consists of a 1 metre long stainless steel capillary which is electrically heated by passing a current through it. At a sampling rate of about 25 ml per minute at the inlet, the pressure at the end of the capillary is about 5 torr. Sample gas diffuses through the molecular leak into the high vacuum of the head where the gas molecules are bombarded by electrons from the ion source to form ions. A response time of 100 ms is possible for 0–90 per cent of a square wave input of dry air. The delay, or transit time, of the sample down the capillary is less than 150 ms. Both stainless steel and glass vacuum manifolds have been employed. A typical mass range would be 2–100 with the possibility of observing the whole spectrum and monitoring four selected peaks. A 30 minute start-up time is required with no refrigerant needed for the pumps. Roboz (1968) gives a description of the physical principles of a quadrupole mass spectrometer.

A quadrupole mass spectrometer can be set-up to

### Calibration Techniques for Gas Analysis

Physical methods of gas analysis require to be standardized against mixtures of known composition. If commercially analysed cylinders of the required mixtures are not available, these can be prepared for gas and vapour mixtures by the method of Hill (1960). Cylinders filled to 2,000 p.s.i. can take up to three weeks to mix in the vertical position, so that they should be rolled at first to mix their contents. Gas mixing pumps are invaluable for the preparation of small volumes of gas mixtures for the calibration of analysers or tonometry. Vapour mixtures are best prepared in alloy cylinders under pressure, but alternatively an accurate vaporizer can be employed, Hill (1963). A full account of the preparation of accurate gas and vapour mixtures is that of Hill and Powell (1968). De Grazio (1968) describes the use of a small (500 ml.) glass mixing vessel fitted with a magnetic stirrer for the production of standard gas mixtures for use with a gas chromatograph.

Since the variation of the saturated vapour pressure with temperature is accurately known for many liquids, it is possible to produce a wide range of calibration vapour mixtures by saturating a known flow of carrier gas with the vapour of the liquid concerned held at a known temperature.

This arrangement is described by Nunn *et al.* (1970). With carrier gas volume flows between 100 and 700 ml per minute, dew point determinations confirmed a saturation of better than 99·5 per cent at the water bath temperature.

## REFERENCES

Ackman, R. G. (1968), "The Flame Ionization Detector. Further Comments on Molecular Breakdown and Fundamental Group Responses," *J. Gas Chromatog.*, **6**, 497.

Amman, E. C. B. and Galan, R. D. (1968), "Problems Associated with the Determination of Carbon Dioxide in Infra-red Absorption," *J. appl. Physiol.*, **25**, 333.

Butler, R. A. and Hill, D. W. (1962), "Estimation of Volatile Anaesthetics in Tissues by Gas Chromatography," *Nature*, **189**, 488.

Campbell, E. J. M. (1960), "Simplification of Haldane's Apparatus for Measuring $CO_2$ Concentration in Respired Gases in Clinical Practice," *Brit. med. J.*, **1**, 457.

Cervenko, F. W. (1968), "Halothane in Blood and Tissues," *Proc. Roy. Soc. Med.*, **61**, 528.

Cormack, R. S., and Powell, J. N. (1972). Improving the performance of the infra-red carbon dioxide meter *Brit. J. Anaesth.* **44**, 131.

Cundall, R. B., Hay, K. and Lemeunier, P. W. (1966), "A Gas Sampling Valve for use in Vapour Phase Chromatography," *J. Sci. Instrum.*, **43**, 652.

Davies, D. D. (1970). A method of gas chromatography for quantitative analysis of blood-gases, *Brit. J. Anaesth.*, **42**, 19.

De Grazio, R. P. (1968), "A Gas Mixing and Sampling Flask," *J. Gas Chromatog.*, **6**, 468.

Edmondson, W. (1957), "Gas Analysis by Refractive Index Measurement," *Brit. J. Anaesth.*, **29**, 570.

Ellis, F. R. and Nunn, J. F. (1968), "The Measurement of Gaseous Oxygen Tension Utilising Paramagnetism. An Evaluation of the 'Servomex' OA 150 Analyser," *Brit. J. Anaesth.*, **40**, 569.

Fowler, K. T. and Hugh-Jones, P. (1957), "Mass Spectrometer Applied to Clinical Practice and Research," *Brit. med. J.*, **i**, 1205.

Francon, M. (1963), *Modern Applications of Physical Optics.* New York: Interscience.

Gabriel, W. P. and Morris, R. A. (1966), "A Flame Ionization Meter for Gas Chromatography," *J. Sci. Instrum.*, **43**, 104.

Haldane, J. S. (1920), *Methods of Air Analysis*, 3rd edition. London: Griffin.

Hanson, D. H. and Maimow, I. A. (1959), "Gas Analysis by Optical Interferometry," *Anal. Chem.*, **31**, 77.

Heavens, O. S. (1955), *Optical Properties of Thin Films.* London: Butterworths.

Hill, D. W. (1960), "The Application of Gas Chromatography to Anaesthetic Research." In: *Gas Chromatography*, Ed. R. P. W. Scott, p. 344. London: Butterworths.

Hill, D. W., and Hook, J. R. (1960). Automatic gas-sampling device for gas chromatography, *J. Scient. Instrum.*, **37**, 253.

Hill, D. W. (1961), "Production of Accurate Gas and Vapour Mixtures," *Brit. J. appl. Physiol.*, **12**, 410.

Hill, D. W. (1963), "Halothane Concentrations Obtained with a Drager 'Vapor' Vaporizer," *Brit. J. Anaesth.*, **35**, 285.

Hill, D. W. and Stone, R. N. (1964), "A Versatile Infra-red Gas Analyser using Transistors," *J. Sci. Instrum.*, **41**, 732.

Hill, D. W. and Powell, T. (1967), "Cross-sensitivity Effects in Non-dispersive Infra-red Gas Analysers using Condenser Microphone Detectors," *J. Sci. Instrum.*, **44**, 189.

Hill, D. W. (1966), "Methods of Measuring Oxygen Content of Blood." In: *Oxygen Measurements in Blood and Tissues.* Eds. J. P. Payne and D. W. Hill. London: Churchill.

Hill, D. W. and Powell, T. (1968), *Non-dispersive Infra-red Gas Analysers.* London: Adam Hilger Ltd.

Hobson, A. and Kay, R. H. (1956), "Two Designs for a Paramagnetic Oxygen Meter," *J. Sci. Instrum.*, **32**, 176.

Howells, J. B. L. (1962), "Re-breathing Methods for Measurement of Blood $CO_2$ Tension," *Brit. J. Anaesth.*, **34**, 617.

Jessop, G. (1966), "Katharometers," *J. Sci. Instrum.*, **11**, 177.

Jones, P. L., Moloy, M. J., and Rosen, M. (1972). A technique for the analysis of methoxyflurane in blood gas chromatography, *Brit. J. Anaesth.*, **44**, 124

Legg, B. J. and Parkinson, K. J. (1968), "Calibration and Infra-red Gas Analysers for use with Carbon Dioxide," *J. Sci. Instrum.*, **1**, 1003.

Lloyd, B. B. (1958), "Developments of Haldane's Gas Analysis Apparatus," *J. Physiol. (Lond.)*, **143**, 5.

Lovelock, J. E. (1963), "Electron Absorption Detectors and Technique for use in Quantitative and Qualitative Analysis," *Anal. Chem.*, **35**, 474.

Luder, M. (1964), "Measurement of Halothane Concentrations with the Interferometer," *Der Anaesthetist*, **13**, 360.

Luft, K. F. (1943), "Uber eine neue methode der registrierenden gasanalyse mit hilfe der absorption ultraroter strahlen ohne spektrale zerlegung," *Z. Tech. Phys.*, **24**, 97.

Lundin, G. and Akesson, L. (1954), "A New Nitrogen Meter Model," *Scand. J. Clin. Lab. Invest.*, **6**, 251.

McWilliam, I. C. and Dewar, R. A. (1958), "Flame Ionization Detector for Gas Chromatography." In: *Gas Chromatography*. Ed. D. H. Desty, p. 142. London: Butterworths.

Nunn, J. F. (1958a), "Respiratory Measurements in the Presence of Nitrous Oxide," *Brit. J. Anaesth.*, **30**, 254.

Nunn, J. F. (1958b), "The Drager Carbon Dioxide Analyser," *Brit. J. Anaesth.*, **30**, 264.

Nunn, J. F. (1964), "Evaluation of the Servomex Paramagnetic Analyser," *Brit. J. Anaesth.*, **36**, 666.

Nunn, J. F., Gill, D. and Hulands, G. H. (1970). Apparatus for preparing saturated vapour concentrations of liquid anaesthetic agents, *J. Physics, E.*, **3**, 331.

Pauling, L., Wood, R. E. and Sturdevant, J. H. (1946), "Oxygen Meter," *J. Amer. Chem. Soc.*, **68**, 795.

Robinson, A., Denson, J. S. and Summers, F. W. (1962), "Halothane Analyser," *Anesthesiology*, **23**, 391.

Roboz, J. (1968). Introduction to mass spectrometry instrumentation and techniques, p. 105. New York: Interscience.

Scheid, P., Slama, H., and Piper, J. (1971). Electronic compensation of the effects of water vapour in respiratory mass spectrometry, *J. Appl. Physiol.*, **30**, 258.

Scholander, P. F. (1947), "Analyser for Accurate Estimation of Respiratory Gases in One-half Cubic Centimetre Samples," *J. biol. Chem.*, **167**, 235.

Tyndall, J. (1865), "On Radiation. The Rede Lecture. Tracts," *Royal College of Surgeons of England*, **139A, 4**, 1.

Visser, B. F. (1957), *Clincial Gas Analysis Based on Thermal Conductivity.* Utrecht: Kemink and Zoon.

Woolmer, R. F. (1956), "The Pauling Oxygen Analyser as an Aid to the Anaesthetist," *Brit. J. Anaesth.*, **28**, 315.

# ELECTRODE SYSTEMS FOR THE MEASUREMENT OF BLOOD-GAS TENSIONS CONTENT AND SATURATION

### D. W. HILL

A knowledge of the acid-base balance condition and of the oxygen and carbon dioxide tensions in the arterial blood is important in the management of many patients. The development of suitable electrode systems, which can be used in clinical situations, and require only small sample volumes of blood, has made these measurements possible on a routine basis in many centres. However, care is still required in handling the blood samples and in calibrating the apparatus.

Currently, the trend is for the electrode systems for pH, $P_{O_2}$, and $P_{CO_2}$ measurements to be mounted on a trolley together with their associated amplifiers and cylinders of calibration gases. The outer jackets of the electrodes are perfused with a stream of water at body temperature from a circulating water bath. Provision is made for placing blood samples and calibration buffer solutions in the water bath, and for bubbling calibration gas mixtures through heat exchanger coils placed in the bath. A small-volume tonometer is usually available in order that blood samples can be readily calibrated with known gas mixtures. With some systems an additional attachment may also be provided to give a read-out directly in terms of oxygen saturation. In effect, the trolley becomes a mobile blood-gas laboratory that can be located close to the operating room, or taken to the bedside in an intensive care ward.

A comparison of four commercial blood-gas analysis systems under working conditions is discussed by Miller and Tutt (1967).

### The Concept of pH

An acid has been defined, Bronsted (1923), as a substance having a tendency to lose a hydrogen ion (proton) and a base as one with a tendency to gain a proton. The relationship between an acid and a base may then be expressed in the form

$$\text{Acid} \leftrightharpoons \underset{\text{Proton}}{H^+} + \text{Base}$$

An acid in aqueous solution dissociates into a positively charged hydrogen ion and a negatively charged non-metallic ion, e.g. $HCl \leftrightharpoons H^+ + Cl^-$. In the case of a base, the dissociation is into a positive metallic ion and a negative hydroxyl ion, e.g. $NaOH \leftrightharpoons Na^+ + OH^-$. The strength of an acid should be governed by its tendency to give up protons, so that a strong acid such as HCl will be almost completely dissociated. A normal (molar) solution of HCl contains 36·5 g. of HCl in one litre of water. If the HCl is completely dissociated there would be 35·5 g. of $Cl^-$ ions and 1 g. of $H^+$ ions. Sørensen introduced the concept of pH to express in logarithmic terms the hydrogen ion concentration of a solution. The letter p stands for "Potenz"

or "Power" and $C_H = 10^{-p}$ where $C_H$ is the hydrogen ion concentration. Thus the pH of a 1 molar HCl solution is $0 (10^0 = 1)$ since the hydrogen ion concentration is 1 g./L.

The degree of dissociation of pure water is very small, $H^+$ and $OH^-$ ions being produced in equivalent proportions, so that pure water is neutral. A litre contains $10^{-7}$ g. of $H^+$ ions, giving a pH of 7. A weak acid, such as acetic acid, is less completely dissociated than a strong acid. A litre of a molar solution of acetic acid contains about $10^{-2·4}$ g. of $H^+$ ions, the pH being 2·4.

A base, even when fully dissociated, will produce a smaller concentration of $H^+$ ions so that its pH in solution will be greater than 7.

### The Interpolation Technique for the Measurement of Blood $P_{CO_2}$

Since there is a logarithmic relationship between blood pH and $P_{CO_2}$ a straight line graph will be obtained if pH is plotted on a linear scale against $P_{CO_2}$ on a logarithmic scale.

Given this straight line graph for a certain blood sample, then the $P_{CO_2}$ of the sample can be read if the blood pH is known. This is the basis of the interpolation method of measuring $P_{CO_2}$. In practice, two points are required in order to define the line. The blood is equilibrated in turn with two gas mixtures of known $P_{CO_2}$, and the blood pH measured at each tension. The gas $P_{CO_2}$'s should fall on either side of the blood pH if possible. If the pH of the blood at the two levels of $P_{CO_2}$ is plotted on semi-log paper a straight line will result (Fig. 1). This is the isopleth for the blood sample and by interpolation of the pH of the blood specimen before equilibration, on this line, its $P_{CO_2}$ can be determined. By comparing this isopleth with standard isopleths the base excess can be determined.

In its original form, Astrup (1956), and Astrup and Shroder (1956), blood (or plasma), volumes of 1·5 to 2·0 ml. were required. However, the method lends itself to the use of very small blood volumes, 0·1 ml. This volume of blood is sucked up into a small pH electrode, and its pH determined. The blood is then equilibrated with two gas mixtures of known $P_{CO_2}$ and the pH again determined. Miniature vibrating tonometers enable equilibration to be achieved with small blood volumes (Kelman et al., 1966). Astrup's method also gives the base excess and standard bicarbonate values for the sample.

If plasma is used with the interpolation technique there is a considerable difficulty in separating the plasma without changing the $P_{CO_2}$ (Nunn, 1959). When whole blood is used, a small error arises if the initial sample is desaturated (Astrup, 1959). The accuracy of the method, however, is comparable with that of others and is not affected by the presence of anaesthetic gases.

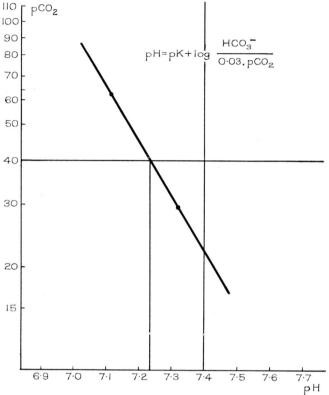

$$pH = pK + \log \frac{HCO_3^-}{0.03 . pCO_2}$$

FIG. 1. Relationship of log $P_{CO_2}$ to pH.

## The Carbon Dioxide Electrode

The design of a practical electrode for the direct measurement of the partial pressure (tension) of carbon dioxide in blood has been described by Severinghaus and Bradley (1958). It is modified from that of Stow, Baer and Randall (1957). The $CO_2$ electrode is basically a pH-sensitive glass electrode arranged to measure the pH of a very thin film of an aqueous sodium bicarbonate solution. The solution is separated from the blood (or gas) sample by a polytetrafluoroethylene (Teflon) membrane. This is permeable to carbon dioxide gas molecules, but not to ions which might affect the pH of the bicarbonate solution.

Figure 2 illustrates the mode of action of the $CO_2$ electrode. The bicarbonate solution is held between the

INTERIOR OF GLASS ELECTRODE

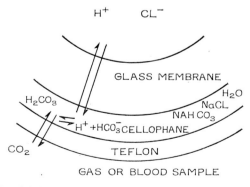

FIG. 2. The mode of action of the carbon dioxide electrode.

dome-ended glass electrode and the Teflon membrane by a matrix consisting of a thin layer of cellophane, glass wool, or sheer nylon stocking. The matrix layer is stretched over the end of the glass electrode and held in place by a rubber band. In one design the Teflon membrane is held in place over the end of a Perspex tube by means of a rubber O-ring. The tube is then inverted and a few ml. of sodium bicarbonate solution added to the rear of the Teflon. The pH glass electrode with its cellophane covering is then gently inserted into the Perspex tube and brought up to the rear of the Teflon, gentle agitation being employed to remove any remaining air bubbles from around the tip of the electrode. In addition to the pH-sensitive glass electrode, a reference calomel electrode is also required and this is mounted in the electrode housing in contact with electrolyte. Teflon is a good insulating material, so that the inside of the $CO_2$ electrode is completely insulated from both the cuvette and the water bath.

When carbon dioxide gas molecules dissolve in the sodium bicarbonate electrolyte layer, the carbon dioxide reacts with the water to form carbonic acid, thus lowering the pH of the solution. The pH change is a linear function of the logarithm of the $CO_2$ tension. This relationship holds, if a glass wool matrix is used, over the range 0·2 per cent to 100 per cent $CO_2$. However, if cellophane is used, the relationship becomes non-linear for $CO_2$ concentrations below about 1·5 per cent. The maximum sensitivity in terms of pH change for a given change in $CO_2$ tension is obtained by using a bicarbonate concentration of about 0·01 moles/litre. The sensitivity is reduced to about one half when pure distilled water is used as the electrolyte. It falls gradually when bicarbonate concentrations greater than 0·01 moles/litre are used since the concentration of carbonate ions now becomes significant. The response time is quicker with the more dilute electrolyte, so that if a loss of sensitivity of the order of 5 per cent can be tolerated, there may be advantages in reducing the strength of the electrolyte to 0·001 moles/litre.

The response time of the $CO_2$ electrode is of the order 0·5 to 3 minutes depending upon the pH change involved, the thickness of the Teflon membrane, and the direction of the pH change, the bicarbonate concentration, and the presence of a catalyst for the hydration reaction of $CO_2$. The speed of response is greater for an increasing $P_{CO_2}$ than it is for a decreasing $P_{CO_2}$. The enzyme carbonic anhydrase (present in red blood cells) can be added to the electrolyte in order to reduce the response time of the electrode. Of the other possible membrane materials, polyethylene is reliable, but in considerably less permeable than Teflon. Rubber and silastic (silicone rubber) membranes tend to become water-logged and slow the response time. Drifts in the electrode calibration may become troublesome with these alternative materials.

The response time of a 1 $\mu$m. thick Teflon membrane alone is quoted by Severinghaus as being about one minute to reach 95 per cent of the final $CO_2$ equilibrium value. The cellophane spacer used beneath the Teflon membrane has been shown to slow the response time of the electrode, particularly at low values of $P_{CO_2}$, and also to cause non-linearity of the calibration curve at the low $CO_2$ partial pressures. The use of a piece of sheer nylon stocking reduces the response time and improves the linearity of the electrode. It is also possible to use powdered glass wool for the spacer layer and this offers the advantage of a rapid response time. The response is considerably faster in an electrode with glass wool than it is in an electrode with no spacer at all. Thus the glass wool is catalysing the reaction of $CO_2$ with water. With a $\frac{3}{8}$-$\mu$m. thick Teflon membrane and glass wool powder it is possible to achieve a 95 per cent response time of 20 seconds. The response time of the catalytic electrode is now set almost entirely by the response time for the membrane itself, one minute in the case of a 1 $\mu$m. thick Teflon membrane.

## Calibration of a $CO_2$ Electrode

Calibration gas mixtures should not be run through the cuvette of the electrode for long periods—this avoids cooling and drying of the electrode. The gas mixtures should not be run at a slow flow rate through a long piece of plastic or rubber tubing, since under these circumstances they may lose $CO_2$ before reaching the cuvette. If an extensive calibration is being carried out, then the cuvette should be periodically flushed through with a dilute detergent-anti-foam mixture in order to keep the membrane moist. Normally the output meter used with the $CO_2$ electrode will be calibrated directly in terms of $P_{CO_2}$ in mm. Hg, a typical range being 15–150 mm. Hg. Two calibration gas mixtures are employed. The first is flushed through the cuvette and the instrument set to read this value. The second mixture is next flushed through and the sensitivity control altered to make the reading correct. The first gas mixture is now replaced in the cuvette and the procedure repeated until both mixtures read correctly on the scale.

If only a sensitive pH meter is available for use with the $CO_2$ electrode, two known gas mixtures should be placed in turn in the cuvette and the pH readings $R_1$ and $R_2$ noted. Let the corresponding $CO_2$ percentages for the mixtures be $\%_1$ and $\%_2$. The sensitivity of the electrode system $S$ is given by $S = (R_1 - R_2)/(\log\%_1 - \log\%_2)$. Suppose that an unknown sample contains $x$ per cent $CO_2$ where $\%_1 > \%_x > \%_2$. Then $\log\%_x = (R_x - R_2)/S + \log\%_2$ or $\log\%_x = \log\%_1 - (R_1 - R_2)/S$. The $P_{CO_2}$ of the sample is then found by multiplying $\%_x$ by (barometric pressure–water vapour pressure at the temperature of the sample). An approximate calibration may be obtained by plotting on semi-log graph paper. $P_{CO_2}$ or $\%CO_2$ is plotted on the logarithmic scale against instrument reading on the linear scale. There should be no difference in reading between equivalent blood and gas samples.

## Handling of Blood Samples for the $CO_2$ Electrode

The cuvette of the electrode should be filled with a gas mixture containing a $P_{CO_2}$ of about the same value as is to be expected from the blood sample. A large difference between the gas and blood $P_{CO_2}$ may introduce inaccuracies. If pure $CO_2$ has been used for checking the sensitivity, the cuvette should be carefully washed out in order to remove any dissolved $CO_2$ from the cuvette walls and membrane. A bubble-free blood sample is taken into a heparinized syringe and immediately capped, agitated, and stored in a water bath kept at the electrode temperature. The cuvette volume of the Severinghaus $CO_2$ electrode is about 0·1 ml. and the minimum blood sample volume needed is about 0·3 ml. After filling the cuvette slowly, an interval of 10 seconds is allowed for residual gas to diffuse from the walls and membrane, and an additional 0·5 ml. of blood is passed through. The lower stopcock of the cuvette is then closed, but the upper one is left open in order to prevent pressure changes occurring in the cuvette. One to two minutes is allowed for equilibrium to be complete before the reading is taken.

Freshly drawn blood at body temperature continues to use oxygen and therefore to produce carbon dioxide. Thus its oxygen tension will fall and its carbon dioxide tension rise (Severinghaus, 1959; Nunn, 1962). The process of metabolism can be retarded by storing the blood samples in iced water in a Dewar flask. Lunn and Mapleson (1963) found that this treatment limited changes in the carbon dioxide tension of whole blood to within 2½ per cent of the initial value for periods of at least two hours and possibly up to four hours. After storing, the cells and plasma must be re-mixed by rolling the syringe between the hands (Severinghaus, 1960; Nunn, 1962).

## Effects of Temperature Changes on the $CO_2$ Electrode

It is necessary that the temperature of the electrode be held constant to within $\pm$ 0·1°C by means of an efficient water bath. This follows since the combined effects of temperature changes upon the sensitivity of the pH electrode and upon the $P_{CO_2}$ of the blood sample amount to a total variation in sensitivity of 8 per cent per °C.

## $P_{CO_2}$ Electrode "Read-out"

Essentially, the requirements for the $CO_2$ electrode amplifier are those of a sensitive pH meter. The entire range of $CO_2$ concentration from 1 per cent to 100 per cent v/v is covered in a pH range of less than 2 pH units. The associated pH meter should be such that it can be read to within 0·001 pH unit. In order to avoid loading the glass electrode, the input resistance of the meter should be at least 1000 meg-ohms. The latest types of instruments for blood-gas analysis are provided with an on-line digital display of the output from the electrode concerned.

## Dynamic Response of the $CO_2$ Electrode

Lunn and Mapleson (1963) discuss the performance of the $CO_2$ electrode in detail. It can be assumed that the chemical reaction within the bicarbonate solution and the response time of the pH measurement system are rapid compared with the over-all response time of the electrode, also that the bicarbonate solution and the gas in the cuvette are each perfectly mixed. That this is true follows from the size of the cuvette and the diffusion coefficient of carbon dioxide in gas and water. The carbon dioxide tension of the bicarbonate solution will then respond to a small change in the carbon dioxide tension of the sample in an exponential fashion with a time constant equal to the product of the capacity of the bicarbonate solution for carbon dioxide and the resistance of the Teflon membrane to the diffusion of carbon dioxide. In practice, Lunn and Mapleson (1963) found that for a gas sample the time constant of the $CO_2$ electrode depended upon the carbon dioxide tension of the bicarbonate solution. Above a $CO_2$ tension of 50 mm. Hg, the time constant was steady at 0·2 minutes. However, for lower tensions the time constant increased rapidly, being approximately 5 minutes for a tension in the bicarbonate solution of 1 mm. Hg. In each case a 0·01 molar bicarbonate solution was used without a catalyst. For a small step change in the $CO_2$ tension of the gas sample a simple exponential response was observed from the electrode.

### The Use of a $CO_2$ Electrode to Estimate the $CO_2$ Content of Whole Blood

Severinghaus (1962) reported that by diluting whole blood in the ratio 20 to 1 with 0·01 molar hydrochloric acid, both the bicarbonate and carbamino $CO_2$ of the blood are converted to free $CO_2$ in solution. This can then be measured with a $CO_2$ electrode. The blood can be diluted anaerobically by means of a 20 ml. syringe, a 1 ml. syringe and a three-way stopcock. The dead-space of the 20 ml. syringe and stopcock are first filled with the hydrochloric acid. The remaining stopcock dead-space is then washed out with blood and exactly 1 ml. of blood put into the 1 ml. syringe. The stopcock is closed and its dead-space washed out with hydrochloric acid from the 20 ml. syringe. The volume of HCl in the syringe is set at 19 ml. and the stopcock turned to connect together the 1 ml. and 20 ml. syringes. The contents of the syringes are mixed by pushing the plungers alternately. The $P_{CO_2}$ of the mixture is measured by means of the $CO_2$ electrode. The system is standardized by means of a solution containing exactly 25 mM./litre of sodium carbonate. The $CO_2$ content of the sample blood is given by multiplying the observed blood $P_{CO_2}$-carbonate solution $P_{CO_2}$ ratio by 25. It is important to make the standard solution from sodium carbonate and not from sodium bicarbonate since the latter contains both carbonate and water. Before weighing out the carbonate it should be heated to 150°C for two hours in order to drive off water.

Linden *et al.* (1965) use 0·1 molar hydrochloric acid, 20 ml. of acid being added to 1 ml. of blood as before. The acid destroys the erythrocytes and releases the carbon dioxide carried in combination in the blood. Using arterial dog blood, Linden *et al.* (1965) obtained a good agreement between $CO_2$ contents determined by the traditional technique of Van Slyke and Neill (1924) and the use of the $P_{CO_2}$ electrode. The average content agreed to within ± 0·32 mM. The average difference was 0·081 mM, the $P_{CO_2}$ electrode system giving the higher result.

Kelman (1967) describes a digital computer program to convert the carbon dioxide tension into whole blood $CO_2$ content at various temperatures and in the presence of metabolic acidosis or alkalosis.

### Cation Electrodes

The availability of membrane materials which are selectively permeable to a particular ionic species has led to the production of electrodes which are responsive to particular ions such as $Na^+$ and $K^+$. Eisenman *et al.* (1957) devised a glass electrode made from a mixture of sodium aluminium and potassium oxides at pH 7·6. The electrode was insensitive to calcium, magnesium, ammonia and lithium ions except when these were present in unusual concentrations. Friedman *et al.* (1959) used a flow-through cuvette sodium electrode to continuously record the concentration of sodium in the femoral arteries of dogs. They were able to detect sodium concentration changes of only a few milli-equivalents per litre produced by the action of pressor and depressor agents.

### Polarographic Electrodes for the Measurement of the Oxygen Tension of Blood

The technique of polarography as used in the oxygen electrode is to produce an electrical current by means of the electrochemical reduction of oxygen. For a constant concentration of oxygen in the solution to be measured, the amount of oxygen reduced, and hence the current produced, will depend on the value of the potential applied to the polarizable electrode. Figure 3 shows a simple

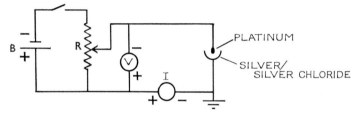

FIG. 3. Basic polarographic system for the measurement o blood oxygen tension.

polarographic system. A potentiometer *VR* allows a proportion of the voltage from a mercury battery *B* to be applied across the polarographic cell consisting of a platinum cathode and a silver/silver chloride anode immersed in the solution whose oxygen tension is to be measured. The cell current (of the order of one microampere) is measured by means of the sensitive galvanometer. A typical calibration curve is given in Figure 4 (Lubbers, 1966). The curve was obtained from four known gas mixtures, and passes through the origin. $CO_2$ had no effect on the current obtained for oxygen. Up to some 400 mV, increasing the polarizing voltage applied across the cell will cause a corresponding increase in the cell current. However, in Figure 4, at 400 to 800 mV there is a plateau region and the current changes little with increasing voltage. Under these conditions each oxygen molecule reaching the surface of the platinum cathode will be almost instantly reduced, the reduction current then being proportional to the amount of oxygen reaching the electrode per unit time. In general, the current is proportional to the oxygen available to the electrode while in the sample, and not necessarily to the oxygen tension of the sample. The main condition that must be observed to ensure that the electrode current is proportional to the oxygen tension of the sample, is that the oxygen should be transported only by diffusion to the cathode. In a homogeneous sample the amount of oxygen transported to the anode by diffusion will depend upon the difference in oxygen tension of the sample and that existing at the anode surface. Since the oxygen tension at the anode surface of a correctly working cell is zero, the cell current will be

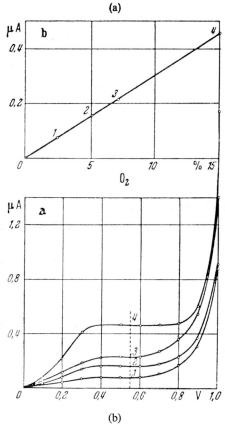

(a)

(b)

FIG. 4 (a), (b). Calibration curve for an oxygen electrode placed in solutions of known oxygen tension. (After Gleichmann and Lubbers, 1960.)

proportional to the oxygen tension of the sample. A constant zone of diffusion is established in front of the anode surface.

The development of a suitable platinum electrode for the measurement of the oxygen tension of blood has taken some sixty years. The main trouble has been in the "poisoning" action on the electrode of blood cells and proteins. Bartels (1951) measured the oxygen tension of whole blood by means of a dropping mercury electrode in which the cathode surface was constantly renewed. However, each blood sample required a separate calibration curve. The platinum electrode is more convenient to use in principle, but requires frequent cleaning in order to remove protein deposits (Inch, 1958). Davies and Brink (1942) showed that bare platinum electrodes could be used for oxygen tension measurements when the platinum surface was protected by an agar or collodion membrane.

### The Clark Electrode

Although the membrane covered electrodes were more stable and more accurate than the bare electrodes, they suffered from the disadvantage that the cell current had to

traverse both the membrane and the sample before reaching the reference electrode. Clark (1960) placed both the platinum cathode and the reference electrode within a membrane so that the membrane would completely insulate the electrode from the sample. The cell was now virtually unaffected by the characteristics of the blood sample other than its oxygen tension. The oxygen consumption of the original Clark-type electrode is by no means negligible, therefore the blood sample used with this electrode must be agitated, otherwise the reading from the electrode will diminish with time owing to the depletion of oxygen by the action of the electrode in the immediate vicinity. Severinghaus and Bradley (1958) used a Clark-type electrode together with a rotating magnet in the sample cuvette to produce stirring. A detailed description of the use of a Clark-type oxygen electrode is given by Bishop (1961). McConn and Robinson (1963) found that with a Clark-type electrode, the ratio of the current obtained for water equilibrated with air to the zero or background current is a constant. A series of calibration curves for the same electrode, Figure 5, had a common point of intersection on the oxygen tension axis. That is to say that zero electrode current was not given by a solution having zero oxygen tension, but occurred at a definite oxygen tension (the intercept) which McConn and Robinson called the electrode constant. From a knowledge of this constant for a particular electrode it is possible to

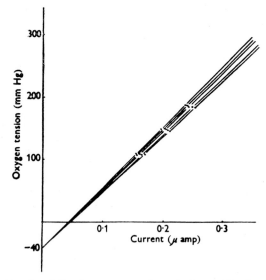

FIG. 5. Calibration curves used to obtain a calibration constant for an oxygen electrode. Curves taken at two-hourly intervals. (After McConn and Robinson, 1963.)

calibrate the electrode rapidly using water equilibrated with air. A blood oxygen tension can then be determined in eight minutes.

The requirements for a fast response and a calibration which is independent of the blood flow are mutually contradictory for membrane-covered blood oxygen tension electrodes. A theoretical evaluation is compared with results from practical electrodes by Schuler and Kreuzer (1967).

Mapleson *et al.* (1970) have shown that the response time of Clark-type electrodes can be variable from day to day, and that on the average the response is considerably slower than had hitherto been suspected. With the electrodes and membranes used by them, 100 per cent response occupied more than 10 minutes and the response was different for different blood tensions. Although the system was fundamentally linear, incomplete response leads to a considerable apparent non-linearity and hysteresis. The incompleteness of response can be corrected mathematically.

## The Use of an Oxygen Electrode to Measure the Oxygen Content of Whole Blood

It is possible to make use of an oxygen tension polarographic electrode to measure the oxygen content of a sample of whole blood in a similar fashion to the $P_{CO_2}$ electrode. The method is given in detail by Linden *et al.* (1965). 0.5 ml. of blood is diluted with 20 ml. of a solution of saponin and potassium ferricyanide, using the two syringe technique employed in the measurement of carbon dioxide content with a $P_{CO_2}$ electrode. The solution consists of 6 g. of potassium ferricyanide and 3 g. of saponin per litre of distilled water, it is made freshly each day and stored in a 500 ml. bottle partially immersed in a water bath at $38° \pm 1°C$. Adding the solution to the blood sample produces haemolysis and the release of oxygen from combination with the haemoglobin. The oxygen remains in a physically dissolved state in the solution and its tension is then measured with the polarographic electrode.

Once the oxygen is in physical solution the tension and concentration are linked by the Bunsen solubility coefficient $\alpha$. This is defined as ml. $O_2$ at NTP/ml. solution at a partial pressure of 760 mm. Hg. If $V$ ml. of saponin-ferricyanide solution be used and the oxygen tension of this solution be $P_s$ mm. Hg then the oxygen content of this volume is $\alpha . V(P_s/760) . (311/273)$ ml. The oxygen content provided by the $v$ ml. of blood is obtained by difference, i.e. in $v$ ml. of blood there are

$$\alpha(311/273)(P_m/760)(V + v)(P_s/760)/(v).$$

In 100 ml. of blood there will be

$$(100/v) . \alpha . (311/273)(1/760) . [P_m - P_s . V/(V + v)]$$

ml./100 ml. Since $\alpha$, $V$ and $v$ are constants, the oxygen content $CO_2 = K[P_m - P_s . V/(V + v)]$ ml./100 ml., where $K$ is a constant. The factor $v/(V + v)$ represents the dilution of the oxygen dissolved in the saponin-ferricyanide solution occurring as the result of the addition of $v$ ml. of blood. Linden found this to have a value of 0.975 by filling the two syringes and three-way tap with water and weighing.

Linden *et al.* determined the value of the constant $K$ by analysing nine samples of dog blood of varying oxygen content with the manometric technique of Van Slyke and Neill (1924), and also taking readings on each blood with the oxygen electrode arrangement.

Linden *et al.* determined the value of the constant K by analysing nine samples of dog blood of varying oxygen contents with the manometric technique of Van Slyke and Neill (1924), and also taking readings on each blood with the oxygen electrode arrangement.

Solymar *et al.* (1971) have described a neat stainless steel cell for the routine determination of blood oxygen content using a polarographic oxygen electrode.

## Polarographic Electrodes for the Measurement of Tissue Oxygen Tensions

A need exists for a relatively simple method for the determination of tissue oxygen tensions both in experimental animals and man. This need was particularly apparent to radio-biologists concerned with the effect of oxygen in increasing the sensitivity of tumours to ionizing radiation. By means of a local extracorporeal circulation it is possible to drop the oxygen tension of the surrounding well-perfused tissue whilst leaving the poorly perfused tumour at a relatively higher oxygen tension. For this type of work, a simple polarographic electrode consisting of a gold or platinum wire 0.004 in. in diameter covered in epoxy resin except for the tip and mounted inside a hypodermic needle may be used (Montgomery and Horwitz, 1950; Montgomery, 1957; Johansen and Krog, 1959). The reference electrode can consist of a chlorided silver plate covered with ECG electrode paste and strapped on to an arm or leg. Each electrode pair is polarized at 600 mV and the polarographic current recorded with a simple battery powered electrometer on the lines of that described by Cater, Phillips and Silver (1956). These electrodes are calibrated by placing them in a physiological saline solution equilibrated with air at the start and finish of the experiment. The electrode is used in the tissue without any protective membrane so that poisoning by protein will occur. However, a change in calibration of up to 10 per cent is normally acceptable over a period of an hour or two. Cater, Phillips and Silver describe a bare noble metal electrode, and Cater and Silver (1961) describe an ultra-micro-needle electrode in which the cathode surface area is of the order of 1–5 square microns. Electrodes of this size retain the rapid response of the larger electrodes, but do not appear to suffer from many of the disadvantages, i.e. they can be made insensitive to stirring, they consume extremely small amounts of oxygen, and they cause little mechanical damage to tissues on insertion. They are still affected by the electrophoretic deposition of protein and are easily damaged, Silver (1966) describes a micro-Clark type of electrode based upon a 25–50 micron platinum wire electropolished down to a one micron tip and fused into a thin glass insulation. The cathode is covered with a thin membrane of the histological mountant DPX and used with a silver reference electrode mounted in the same assembly as the cathode.

Walker *et al.* (1968) describe a membrane-covered flush-type oxygen electrode developed for the measurement of the tissue $P_{O_2}$ of human foetal scalp.

### Fuel Cells

Weil *et al.* (1967) report the use of a modified solid oxide fuel cell to analyse the oxygen concentration of gases. The cell response is linear from 1·0 per cent to 99·6 per cent v/v oxygen. Continuous or single breath analysis is possible since the cell's time constant is only 0·2 second. A comparison between the modified Westinghouse type 203C cell and a Scholander apparatus gave a mean difference between the two methods of 0·008 per cent v/v with a standard deviation of 0·015 per cent v/v.

### Catheter-tip Oxygen Electrodes

Parker *et al.* (1971) describe a useful catheter-tip oxygen tension transducer using a silver-lead galvanic cell. A diamel-coated wire of 180 $\mu$m diameter is positioned and sealed within a lead cylinder with epoxy resin (Araldite resin AY105 with hardener HT972). The silver-lead assembly is sealed into the end of an etched polytetrafluoroethylene tube of 0·8 mm outside diameter. Contact to the lead cylinder is made by cold welding an insulated copper wire to the back of the lead cylinder. Both the silver and the copper wire are connected to a miniature autoclavable plug. The assembly is dipped into a saturated solution of $K_2CO_3$ and $KHCO_3$ and allowed to dry and then fitted into a cap of polytetrafluoroethylene having a wall thickness of about 25 $\mu$m. This is sealed onto the polytetrafluoroethylene catheter containing the wires using silicone rubber adhesive, the contact surfaces having previously been etched. It is also possible to use a polyvinyl chloride membrane which is easier to produce. At this stage the cell is inactive. It is activated when required by holding the tip in steam for two minutes to form a thin film of electrolyte on the inside of the membrane. To sterilize the device it is autoclaved at 134°C for three minutes. This provides both activation and sterilization. After activation, the cell consists of a silver cathode and a lead anode in contact with a thin film of saturated $K_2CO_3$ and $KHCO_3$. Oxygen is reduced at the cathode according to the equation $O_2 + 2H_2O + 4e^{-2} \rightarrow 4(OH^-)$. At the anode lead is converted to lead hydroxide according to the equation $2Pb + 4(OH^-) \rightarrow 2Pb(OH)_2 + 4e^-$. The electrons released flow through the external load resistor (2·2 k$\Omega$) of the cell, the current flowing being proportional to the rate of reduction of oxygen at the silver surface. A typical sensitivity would be about 1 nano-ampere per mm Hg $pO_2$. Parker *et al.* (1971) describe a suitable operational amplifier circuit for displaying the cell current on a potentiometric pen recorder.

### Catheter type

A demand exists for an oxygen polarographic electrode whose dimensions are sufficiently small that the electrode can be mounted at the tip of a catheter for *in vivo* work. The use of a Clark-type of electrode is necessary in order to obtain a calibration which is stable over extended periods. Beneken, Kolmer and Kreuzer (1968) describe a catheter-tip electrode which has an outer diameter of only 2 mm. The central platinum cathode 300 microns in diameter is insulated by a plastic (polyvinyl chloride) or glass tube. The outer silver anode supports a Teflon membrane 3 or 6 microns in thickness which is held in place by a silver ring. The electrolyte is a phosphate buffer solution of pH approximately 9. The length of the electrode assembly is 10 mm. The current output of the electrode is about 4 micro-amps for a 300 micron diameter cathode in 100 per cent oxygen at 37°C. The calibration curve is said to be linear up to 100 per cent oxygen with a constant environmental temperature, and it passes through the origin. The calibration varies from electrode to electrode, but for an individual electrode it remains within 2 per cent over 34 days. When used in the gas phase its reading is not influenced by the presence of $CO_2$, ether, trichloroethylene, halothane or $N_2O$. The electrode is polarized with 800 mV.

The particularly interesting property of the electrode, apart from its small size, is its fast speed of response, 0·20–0·25 seconds for a 95 per cent deflection with a change in concentration between 0–100 per cent in both directions. This is two to three times longer than that obtained with a mass spectrometer. With the electrode it is also possible to detect cardiogenic oscillations present on the alveolar portions of the oxygen tension tracing. It has been ascertained that these oscillations are in fact due to $Po_2$ changes and not due to a mechanical effect of pressure or flow on the electrode.

This electrode arrangement can also be used for the continuous recording *in vivo* of blood oxygen tension (Kreuzer *et al.*, 1960). When used in gas streams rapid diffusion ensures that there is no flow dependency for linear gas velocities from 0–312 cm. per second. However, with liquids the calibration is flow dependent, above flow velocities of 8–10 cm./sec. the $Po_2$ reading becomes constant. Kreuzer *et al.* report that static pressures in the range 0–120 cm. $H_2O$ did not affect the output of the electrode, but that rapid pulsatile pressures did.

An even faster speed of response for an oxygen electrode is claimed by Friesen and McIlroy (1970). Using a 3 micrometre thick polytetrafluoroethylene membrane they achieved an 80 milli-seconds response time and this could be further reduced to 40 milli-seconds by manually stretching the membrane to just below its breaking point. The speed of response was now adequate for alveolar sampling during heavy exercise.

### Oximeters

Oximeters are instruments designed to measure the percentage oxygen saturation of haemoglobin in whole blood. They operate upon the principle that in the red region of the spectrum at about 650 nanometres there is a large difference between the optical absorption coefficients of oxygenated and reduced haemoglobin, whilst in the near infra-red region at about 800 nanometres there exists an isobestic point, i.e. the absorption coefficients are equal. In an oximeter, filters are used to select wavebands centred on 650 and 800 nm from the output of a source of light which is usually an incandescent lamp. If the oximeter is of the transmission type, the filtered light is shown through a narrow cuvette containing the blood sample and falls on to a pair of semi-conductor photocells, one for each filter. It can be shown (Reichert, 1966) that the ratio of the optical densities of the blood at the red and infra-red wavelengths is linearly related to the percentage oxygen saturation. The lamp supply is well stabilized and the ratio of the output signals from the red and infra-red photocells can be obtained with a divider circuit or a ratio recorder. Care must be taken to ensure that the blood is kept moving during the measurement to prevent sedimentation of the cells occurring which would affect the reading obtained.

When an oximeter is to be used with an extracorporeal circulation, then a wide bore cuvette is required in order to provide a low resistance to the flow of blood. The diameter will be too large for sufficient transmitted light to be received by the photocells and so use is made of light reflected backwards from the blood. Rodrigo (1953) has shown that a plot of the logarithm of the reciprocal of the reflected red light against the percentage oxygen saturation yields a straight line. In a two wavelength instrument, the ratio of the reflected red and infra-red intensities is linearly related to the oxygen saturation.

Oximeters require to be calibrated and this can be carried out against blood samples prepared in a tonometer and having known oxygen saturations. The blood is first fully oxygenated and the haemoglobin capacity for oxygen measured with a Van Slyke apparatus or a gas chromatograph. The blood is then tonometered with gas mixtures of known oxygen tensions and the oxygen content for the haemoglobin determined for each mixture. The percentage saturation is then given by the ration (content/capacity) × 100 per cent.

With conventional transmission and reflection oximeters, the blood sample must be fed into the oximeter. An interesting development which allows continuous recording of oxygen saturation *in vivo* is the fibre optic reflection oximeter. The oximeter is coupled to the patient by means of a flexible fibre optic cardiac catheter. Typically, this would contain approximately 200 fibres each about one metre long inside a radio opaque polytetrafluoroethylene sleeving having an outside diameter corresponding to a No. 7 French gauge (2·33 mm). About 25 cm from the proximal end, the fibres are divided at random into two halves and brought out as separate bundles.

Polyani and Hehir (1960) have described the construction of a fibre optic oximeter. A projection lamp fed from a stabilized supply shines a beam of white light through a series of optical interference filters located around the periphery of a disk rotated by a synchronous electric motor. Alternate filters of the total of six are centred at 650 and 800 nanometres. An image of the projection lamp filament is focussed onto the end of one side branch of the fibre optic catheter. Thus alternate pulses of red and infra-red light are fed down the catheter. After reflection from blood at the tip, the pulses are fed back down the second fibre bundle to a photomultiplier situated in the oximeter. Gating circuits are employed to separate out the signals due to the red and infra-red wavelengths. These signals are fed into a ratio circuit and its output displayed on a pen recorder. Under these conditions the ratio of the reflected light intensities in the red and infra-red is linearly related to the percentage oxygen saturation. At present, the slope of the calibration line appears to vary from catheter to catheter. The catheters must be handled with care, as the breakage of individual fibres leads to cross-talk between the fibre bundles and degrades the signal-to-noise ratio of the instrument. The response time of the circuitry is set at about 100 ms which is fast enough to allow individual cardiac pulsations to be followed. Enson *et al.* (1962) have discussed the performance of a fibre optic oximeter.

Ramirez *et al.* (1969) and Lindstrom (1970) have shown that it is possible to mount a reflecting diaphragm at the tip of the fibre optic catheter and obtain an arterial blood pressure transducer with a frequency response sufficiently wide that it can also be used to record heart sounds. With a 1 mm diameter diaphragm approximately 12 mm thick, the pressure range −50 to 300 mmHg is obtainable with a frequency response from d.c. to 1,500 Hz. Prototypes are now being produced in which both oxygen saturation, heart sounds and blood pressure can be recorded from a single fibre optic catheter.

## REFERENCES

### $CO_2$ electrode references

Bartels, H. and Reinhardt, W. (1960), "Einfache methode zur Sauerstoffdruckmessung im Blut," *Pflügers Arch.*, **271**, 105.

Cambino, S. R. (1961), "Collection of Capillary Blood for Simultaneous Determinations of Arterial pH, $CO_2$ Content, $P_{CO_2}$ and Oxygen Saturation," *Am. J. clin. Path.*, **35**, 175.

Fatt, I. (1964), "Rapid-responding Carbon Dioxide and Oxygen Electrodes," *J. appl. Physiol.*, **19**, 550.

Gleichmann, U. (1960), "Fortlaufende messung des Kohlensauredruckers im artetiellen Blut," *Pflügers Arch.*, **272**, 57.

Gleichmann, U. and Lubbers, D. W. (1960), "Die messung des Kohlensaurdruckers in Gasen und Flussigkeiten mit der $P_{CO_2}$ Elektrode uniter besonderer Berucksichtigung der Gleichzeitigen Messung von $P_{O_2}$, $P_{CO_2}$ und pH im Blut," *Pflügers Arch.*, **271**, 456.

Hertz, C. H. and Siesjö, B. (1959), "A Rapid and Sensitive Electrode for Continuous Measurement of $P_{CO_2}$ in Liquids and Tissues," *Acta Physiol. Scand.*, **47**, 115.

Kelman, G. R. (1967), "Digital Computer Procedure for the Conversion of $P_{CO_2}$ into Blood $CO_2$ Content," *Resp. Physiol.*, **3**, 111.

Lunn, J. N. and Mapleson, W. W. (1963), "The Severinghaus $P_{CO_2}$ Electrode: A Theoretical and Experimental Assessment," *Brit. J. Anaesth.*, **35**, 666.

Nunn, J. F. (1962), "Measurement of Blood Oxygen Tension: Handling of Samples," *Brit. J. Anaesth.*, **34**, 621.

Robinson, J. S. (1962), "pH and $P_{CO_2}$ Measurements in Blood," *Brit. J. Anaesth.*, **34**, 611.

Severinghaus, J. W. and Bradley, A. F. (1958), "Electrodes for Blood $P_{O_2}$ and $P_{CO_2}$ Determination," *J. appl. Physiol.*, **13**, 515.

Severinghaus, J. W. (1959), "Recent Developments in Blood $O_2$ and $CO_2$ Electrodes," in *pH and Blood Gas Electrodes*, ed. Woolmer, R. F. London: Churchill.

Severinghaus, J. W. (1960), "Methods of Measurement of Blood and Carbon Dioxide during Anesthesia," *Anesthesiology*, **21**, 717.

Severinghaus, J. W. (1962), "Electrodes for Blood and Gas $P_{CO_2}$ and Blood pH," *Acta anaesth. Scand.*, Suppl. 11, 207.

Snell, F. (1960), "Electrometric Measurements of $CO_2$ and Bicarbonate Ion," *J. appl. Physiol.*, **15**, 729.

Stow, R. W., Baer, R. F. and Randall, B. F. (1957), "Rapid Measurement of the Tension of Carbon Dioxide," *Arch. Phys. Med. Rehabil.*, **38**, 646.

### Cation electrode references

Eisermann, G., Rudin, D. O. and Casby, J. U. (1957), "Glass Electrode for Measuring Sodium Ion," *Science*, **126**, 831.

Friedman, S. M., Jamieson, J. D., Hinks, J. A. M. and Friedman, C. L. (1959), "Drug-induced Changes in Blood Pressure and in Blood Sodium as Measured by a Glass Electrode," *Amer. J. Physiol.*, **196**, 1049.

## Tonometer references

Adams, A. P. and Morgan-Hughes, J. O. (1967), "Determination of the Blood-gas Factor of the Oxygen Electrode using a New Tonometer," *Brit. J. Anaesth.*, **39**, 107.

Fahri, L. E. (1965), "Continuous Duty Tonometer System," *J. appl. Physiol.*, **20**, 1098.

Kelman, G. R., Coleman, A. J. and Nunn, J. F. (1966), "A Microtonometer used with a Capillary Glass pH Electrode," *J. appl. Physiol.*, **21**, 1103.

Laue, D. (1951), "Eine neues tonometer zur raschen aquilibrierung von blut mit verschieden gastrucken," *Pflügers Arch. Ges. Physiol.*, **254**, 142.

Thornton, J. A. and Nunn, J. F. (1960), "Accuracy of Determination of $P_{CO_2}$ by the Indirect Method," *Guy's Hosp. Rep.*, **18**, 203.

## Oxygen electrode references

Adams, A. P. and Morgan-Hughes, J. O. (1967), "Determination of the Blood-gas Factor of the Oxygen Electrode using a New Tonometer," *Brit. J. Anaesth.*, **39**, 107.

Bartels, H. (1951), "Potentiometrische bestimmung des sauerstoffdruckes im vollblut mid der quecksilbertropfelektrude," *Pflügers Arch. Ges. Physiol.*, **254**, 107B

Beneken Kolmer, H. H. and Kreuzer, P. (1968), "Continuous Polarographic Recording of Oxygen Pressure in Respiratory Air," *Resp. Physiol.*, **4**, 109.

Bishop, J. M. (1960), "Measurement of Blood Oxygen Tension," *Proc. Roy. Soc. Med.*, **53**, 177.

Bradley, A. F., Stupfel, M. and Severinghaus, J. W. (1956), "Effect of Temperature on $P_{CO_2}$ and $P_{O_2}$ of Blood *in vitro*," *J. appl. Physiol.*, **9**, 201.

Cater, D. B., Phillips, A. F. and Silver, I. A. (1956), "Apparatus and Techniques for the Measurement of Oxidation-reduction Potentials, pH and Oxygen Tension *in vivo*," *Proc. Roy. Soc. B.*, **146**, 289.

Cater, D. B. and Silver, I. A. (1961), "Electrodes and Microelectrodes used in Biology," in *Reference Electrodes*, ed. Ives, D. J. C. and Janz, J. C. New York: Academic Press.

Clark, L. C. (1956), "Monitor and Control of Blood and Tissue Oxygen Tensions," *Trans. Amer. Soc. Art. Int. Org.*, **2**, 41.

Davies, P. W. and Brink, F. Jr., (1942), "Micro-electrodes for measuring local oxygen tensions in animal tissues," *Rev. Scient. Instrum.*, **13**, 524.

Fatt, I. (1964), "Rapid Responding Carbon Dioxide and Oxygen Electrodes," *J. appl. Physiol.*, **19**, 550.

Friesen, W. O. and McIlroy, M. B. (1970), "Rapidly Responding Oxygen Electrode for Respiratory Gas Sampling," *J. Appl. Physiol.*, **29**, 258–259.

Gleichmann, U. and Lubbers, D. W. (1960), "Die Messung des Sauerstoff-Druckes in Gasen und Flussigkeiten mit der Pt-Elektrode unter besonderer Beruchsichtigung der Messung im Blut," *Pflügers Arch. Ges. Physiol.*, **281**, 32.

Hedley-White, J. and Laver, M. B. (1964), "Solubility in Blood and Temperature Correction Factors for $P_{O_2}$," *J. appl. Physiol.*, **19**, 901.

Hedley-White, J., Radford, E. P. and Laver, M. B. (1965), "Nomogram for Temperature Correction or Electrode Calibration during $P_{O_2}$ Measurement," *J. appl. Physiol.*, **20**, 785.

Inch, W. R., (1958), "Problems associated with the use of the exposed platinum electrode for measuring oxygen tensions in vivo," *Can. J. Biochem Physiol.*, **36**, 1009.

Johanson, K. and Krog, J. (1959), "Polarographic Determination of Intravascular Oxygen Tensions *in vivo*," *Acta Physiol. Scand.*, **46**, 228.

Kelman, G. R., Coleman, A. J., and Nunn, J. F. (1966), "Evaluation of a microtonometer used with a capillary glass pH electrode," *J. Appl. Physiol.*, **21**, 1103.

Laver, M. B. and Seifen, A. (1965), "Measurement of Blood Oxygen Tension in Anaesthesia," *Anesthesiology*, **26**, 73.

Linden, R. J., Ledsome, J. R. and Norman, J. (1965), "Simple Methods for the Determination of the Concentrations of Carbon Dioxide and Oxygen in Blood," *Brit. J. Anaesth.*, **37**, 77.

Mapleson, W. W., Horton, J. N., Ng, W. S. and Imrie, D. D. (1970), "The Response Pattern of polarographic Oxygen Electrodes and its Influence on Linearity and Hysteresis," *Med. and Biol. Engng.*, **8**, 585–592.

McConn, R. and Robinson, J. S. (1963), "Notes on the Oxygen Electrode," *Brit. J. Anaesth.*, **35**, 679.

Miller, J. N., and Tutt, P. (1967), "A comparison of four blood gas analysis systems in working conditions," *Bio-Med. Engng*, **2**, 456.

Morgan, F., Kettel L. J. and Cugell, D. W. (1966), "Measurement of Blood $P_{O_2}$ with the Microcathode Electrode," *J. appl. Physiol.*, **21**, 725.

Montgomery, H. and Horwitz, O. (1950), "Oxygen Tension of Tissues by the Polarographic Method," *J. clin. Invest.*, **29**, 120.

Montgomery, H. (1957), "Oxygen Tension of Peripheral Tissue," *Am. J. Med.*, **23**, 697.

Nunn, J. F. (1962), "Measurement of Blood Oxygen Tension; Handling of Samples," *Brit. J. Anaesth.*, **34**, 621.

Nunn, J. F., Bergman, N. A., Bunatyan, A. and Coleman, A. J. (1965), "Temperature Coefficients for $P_{CO_2}$ and $P_{O_2}$ of Blood *in vitro*," *J. appl. Physiol.*, **20**, 23.

Parker, D., Key, A. and Davies, R. (1971), "A Disposable Catheter-tip Transducer for Continuous Measurement of Blood Oxygen Tension *in vivo*," *Bio-Med. Engng.*, **6**, 313–317.

Polgar, G. and Forster, R. E. (1960), "Measurement of Oxygen Tension in Unstirred Blood with a Platinum Electrode," *J. appl. Physiol.*, **15**, 706.

Rhodes, P. G. and Moser, K. M. (1966), "Sources of Error in Oxygen tension Measurement," *J. appl. Physiol.*, **21**, 729.

Schuler, R. and Kreuzer, F. (1967), "Rapid Polarographic *in vivo* Oxygen Catheter Electrodes," *Resp. Physiol.*, **3**, 90.

Solymar, M., Rucklidge, M. A. and Prys-Roberts, C. (1971), "A Modified Approach to the Polarographic Measurement of Blood $O_2$ Content," *J. Appl. Physiol.*, **30**, 272–275.

Van Slyke, D. D. and Neill, J. M. (1924), "The Determination of Gases in Blood and Other Solutions by Vacuum Extraction and Manometric Measurement," *J. biol. Chem.*, **61**, 523.

Walker, A., Phillips, L., Powe, L. and Wood, C. (1968), "A New Instrument for the Measurement of Tissue $P_{O_2}$ of Human Fetal Scalp," *Amer. J. Obstet. Gynec.*, **100**, 63.

Weil, J. V., Sodal, I. E. and Speck, R. P. (1967), "A Modified Fuel Cell for the Analysis of Oxygen Concentration of Gases," *J. appl. Physiol.*, **23**, 419.

## Oximeter references

Enson, Y., Briscoe, W. A., Polyani, M. L. and Cournand, A. (1962), "*In vivo* Studies with an Intravascular and Intracardiac Reflection Oximeter," *J. appl. Physiol.*, **17**, 552.

Lindstrom, L. H. (1970), "Miniaturized Pressure Transducer Intended for Intravascular Use," *I.E.E.E. Trans. Bio.-Med. Engng.*, BME **17**, 207.

Polyani, M. L. and Hehir, R. M. (1960), "New Reflection Oximeter," *Rev. Sci. Instrum.*, **31**, 401.

Ramirez, A., Hood, W. B., Jr. and Polyani, M. L. (1969), "Registration of Intravascular Pressure and Sound by a Fibre Optic Catheter," *J. Appl. Physiol.*, **26**, 679.

Reichert, W. J. (1966), "The Theory and Construction of Oximeters," in *Oxygen Measurements in Blood and Tissues*, p. 81. Eds. J. P. Payne and D. W. Hill. London: Churchill.

Rodrigo, F. A. (1953), "Determination of Oxygenation of Blood *in vitro* by Using Reflected Light," *Am. Heart J.*, **45**, 809.

## Interpolation technique references

Astrup, P. (1956), "A Simple Electrometric Technique for the Determination of $CO_2$ Tension in Blood and Plasma, Total Content of $CO_2$ in Plasma and Bicarbonate in 'Separated' Plasma at a Fixed $CO_2$ tension (40 mm. Hg)," *Scand. J. Clin. Lab. Invest.*, **8**, 33.

Astrup, P. and Schroder, S. (1956), "Apparatus for the Anaerobic Determination of the pH of Blood at 38°C," *Scand. J. Clin. Lab. Invest.*, **8**, 30.

Astrup, P. (1959), "Ultra-micro-method for Determining pH, $P_{CO_2}$ and Standard Bicarbonate in Capillary Blood," in *Symposium on pH and Blood Gas Measurement*, p. 81, ed. Woolmer, R. F. London: Churchill.

Astrup, P., Anderson, O. S., Jorgensen, K. and Engel, K. (1960), "The Acid-base Metabolism: a New Approach," *Lancet*, **i**, 1035.

Nunn, J. F. (1959), "The Accuracy of the Measurement of Blood $P_{CO_2}$ by the Interpolation Technique," in *Symposium on pH and Blood Gas Measurement*, p. 60, ed. Woolmer, R. F. London: Churchill.

Nunn, J. F. (1960), "Measurement of Blood Carbon Dioxide Tension," *Proc. Roy. Soc. Med.*, **53**, 180.

Sorensen, S. P. L. (1909), "Etudes enzymatiques, Part 2. Sur la mesure et L'importance de la concentration des ions hydrogenes dans leurs reactions enzymatiques," *Compt. Rend. Trav. Lab. Carlsberg*, **8**, 1.

*CHAPTER* 9

# THE DETERMINATION OF pH

## M. K. SYKES

In 1923 Brønsted defined an acid as a molecule capable of donating a hydrogen ion, and a base as a molecule capable of accepting a hydrogen ion. The "strength" of an acid or base may be related to the abundance of hydrogen or hydroxyl ions. This in turn depends on the concentration of the substance present in the aqueous solution and on the degree of dissociation. In practice the concentration of $H^+$ ions varies from 1 g./litre for a molar solution of the strongest acids, to $10^{-14}$ g./litre for the strongest alkalis. To cover this wide range of concentrations Sørensen (1909) proposed that a logarithmic scale should be used so that $pH = -\log_{10}(H^+)$ where $(H^+) = $ the concentration of $H^+$ ions.

Water is unique in that it has equal proportions of $H^+$ and $OH^-$ ions; the concentration of $H^+$ ions is therefore $10^{-7}$ g./litre and the pH is 7·0. Since a base, even when it is fully dissociated, contains a smaller concentration of $H^+$ ions than water, its pH must be greater than 7. The converse applies to acids. The relationship of the concentration of $H^+$ ions to pH is shown more clearly in Table 1. It will be noted that a change in pH from 7·4 to 7·2 represents a greater change in hydrogen ion concentration than a change from pH 7·6 to 7·4.

### TABLE 1

THE RELATION OF pH TO HYDROGEN ION CONCENTRATION

| pH Scale | nanoequiv/l. | |
|---|---|---|
| 7·0 | 100 | |
| 7·2 | 63 | |
| 7·4 | 40 | i.e. ten-fold change in concentration for 1 pH unit. |
| 7·6 | 25 | |
| 7·8 | 16 | |
| 8·0 | 10 | |

## Methods of Measurement

Although most of the hydrogen ions in the body are within the cells it is not possible to make a direct measurement of intracellular pH. Measurements are therefore usually confined to extracellular fluids and blood. There are three methods in common use.

### Indirect Measurement

In biological fluids pH can be calculated from $P_{CO_2}$ and plasma bicarbonate by utilizing some form of the Henderson-Hasselbalch equation:

$$pH = pK' + \log \frac{(HCO_3^-)}{0·03 \times P_{CO_2}}$$

It has now become apparent that a constant value of pK' of 6·10 can no longer be accepted since pK' varies with temperature, $P_{CO_2}$ and the non-respiratory component of acid-base balance (Severinghaus, Stupfel and Bradley, 1956; Siggaard-Andersen, 1962). Although the estimate of pH obtained by this method is satisfactory for most clinical purposes (Ludbrook, 1959) it is not adequate for accurate work.

### Colorimetric Methods

The use of coloured indicator dyes for measurement of pH was widespread before electrometric measurements were simplified but it is now less commonly used. For a rapid but very inaccurate estimation ($\pm 1$ pH unit) a "universal" indicator may be used. This consists of a mixture of indicators which cover a wide pH range (*e.g.* BDH Universal indicator pH 4·0 — 11·0). A few drops of the indicator are added to the liquid under test and the colour compared with a chart which relates the colour to the pH. Greater accuracy ($\pm 0·4$ units) can be obtained by using this type of indicator in the form of test papers. More accurate measurements ($\pm 0·3$ pH units) can be obtained by using a simple comparator. This consists of a small stand backed by an illuminated ground glass screen. The solution under test is mixed with the appropriate concentration of indicator in a tube and the colour is then compared with the colour of the indicator in a number of other tubes containing buffers of known pH. Further precision can be achieved by the use of instruments which measure the absorption of white (polychromatic) light. Such instruments are known as absorptiometers and commonly utilize a photo-electric cell to measure the intensity of the transmitted light. Measured amounts of indicator are added to the test solution and to a series of buffer solutions and the light transmission is then compared. Still greater accuracy is obtained by using a spectrophotometer which utilizes monochromatic light either in the visible or ultra-violet spectrum. The accuracy of techniques utilizing this type of instrument approaches that of electrometric measurement but the cost and technical complexity are also comparable. Methods utilizing light absorption are difficult to apply to turbid solutions and many indicators undergo specific reactions with proteins. For these reasons indicator techniques are now rarely used for clinical estimations of the pH of plasma.

## Electrometric Methods

Most measurements of pH are now made by means of pH-sensitive electrodes. The hydrogen electrode has always been the standard by which other methods are judged for, of all electrodes, its response to hydrogen ions is the most clearly understood. However, the technical difficulties associated with its use have precluded its employment in the clinical field. The quinhydrone electrode is simpler technically but lacks versatility. The glass electrode is extremely versatile, does not affect the

solution to be measured and can be used with oxidizing or reducing solutions and with colloidal suspensions. It can be adapted for micro-measurements, and can be used for measurements in flow systems or even *in vivo*. It is therefore the electrode of choice for clinical work.

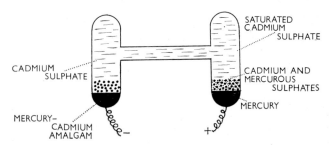

FIG. 2. The standard Weston cell.

## Measurement of pH with the Glass Electrode

When a metal is placed in a solution of one of its salts there is a tendency for the metal ions to go into solution thus leaving the metal with an excess negative charge. If two different metals and their salts are separated by a porous partition, as in the Daniel cell (Fig. 1) an electromotive force (EMF) is produced because there is a greater tendency for the zinc ions to go into solution than for copper ions to do so. The EMF of the whole cell may be regarded as the difference between the separate EMF's produced by the two half-cells.

The EMF of a cell depends not only on the nature of the solution but also on its concentration. By maintaining a constant concentration it is possible to maintain a constant EMF. This is accomplished in both half-cells of the Weston standard cell (EMF 1·018 volts at 20°C). When a current flows, cadmium ions enter the solution from the cadmium amalgam (negative terminal) and mercurous ions leave the solution to form mercury at the positive terminal. However, the concentration of the solutions in the cell is accurately maintained since the solutions remain saturated with both sulphates (Fig. 2).

In the measurement of pH two half-cells are used (Figs. 3 and 4). One, the reference electrode, resembles half of the Weston cell but uses mercury and a saturated solution of mercurous chloride ($Hg_2Cl_2$) or calomel. This is connected to the solution under test by a salt bridge of saturated potassium chloride solution, the actual junction being

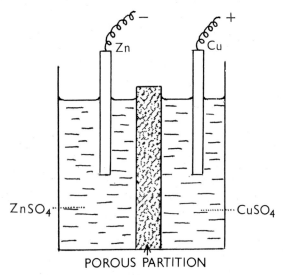

FIG. 1. The Daniel cell.

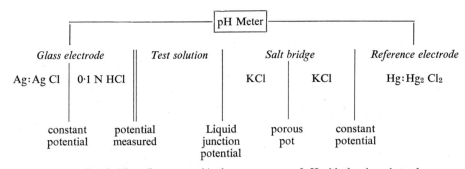

FIG. 3. The cell system used in the measurement of pH with the glass electrode.

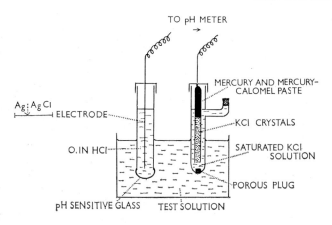

FIG. 4. The glass-calomel electrode system.

formed at a porous plug or at the end of a capillary tube. The EMF produced by this cell remains constant as long as the temperature is kept constant.

The other half-cell is the glass electrode. This consists of a glass tube with a bulb of pH-sensitive glass sealed onto the end. The bulb contains an electrolyte, usually N/10 HCl, into which a silver wire dips to effect an electrical connection. Again, the combination of a metal and its salt ensures a stable potential within the cell. The outside of the pH-sensitive glass makes direct contact with the test solution, the potential developed between the glass and test solution depending on the concentration of hydrogen ions in the solution. It is the variation in this potential which indicates the difference in pH between buffer and test solution.

In addition to the three potentials already mentioned there is a fourth, the liquid junction potential, which is generated at the junction between the test solution and salt bridge. This kind of potential is always developed at the interface between two solutions of different compositions or strengths because of differences in ionic transport across the boundary layer. The magnitude of this potential depends on a number of factors, but in any individual electrode system the commonest cause of variation in the liquid junction potential is a variation in the geometry of the junction itself. For this reason electrode manufacturers take great care to design a liquid junction which can be accurately reproduced each time a measurement is made.

If a reproducible liquid junction potential can be achieved it becomes apparent that the only variable EMF in the system is that generated at the surface of the glass electrode. The total EMF of the system should therefore be governed solely by the temperature and the pH of the test solution. By applying thermodynamic principles it can be shown that the EMF of the cell should be approximately 61·5 mV. per pH unit change at 37°C. Unfortunately this theoretical relationship does not apply in practice. There are three reasons for this. Firstly, the thermodynamic *activity* of a solution is not accurately related to the *concentration* of ions except in infinite dilution. This is because attractions arise between migrating anions and cations. Secondly, the exact magnitude of the liquid junction potential is not known. The liquid junction potential can be minimized by using concentrated solutions of potassium chloride (Semple, 1961), and it is possible to design electrode systems which do not rely on a liquid junction, but even so the accuracy of pH measurement can be no better than the accuracy of the convention used to estimate the activity of the chloride ion at the reference electrode. This limits the accuracy of "true" pH determination to ±0·02 units at the best (Semple, 1967). The third source of innaccuracy is the variability in the response of the glass electrode. The "asymmetry potential" (the potential developed across the glass due to the difference in hydrogen ion concentration on the two sides) decreases with time and after 6–12 months the electrode ceases to function effectively. In addition, the electrode is easily poisoned by protein deposition or other contaminants and may not be linear over all parts of the pH scale.

For these reasons it is necessary to refer the pH measurement to a conventional scale of pH which is, in turn, defined in terms of a number of buffer solutions. The pH electrode is therefore standardized against two known buffers so that the proportionality factor (mV. per pH unit change) can be determined and all measurements are then compared with a known buffer so that the actual value of pH can be determined with reference to an agreed standard.

### Buffers

Buffer solutions are solutions composed of a weak acid and its salt with a strong base, or a weak base and its salt with a strong acid. These dissociate to produce a constant concentration of hydrogen ions at any given temperature and show little variation in pH on the addition of small quantities of a strong acid or base. Unfortunately a number of different pH scales exist and one of the oldest, that of Sørenson, differs by 0·04 pH units from some of the scales used to-day. The choice of scales is now limited to the British Standard Scale (BS) or that of the National Bureau of Standards (NBS) in the U.S.A. Whilst the NBS scale is based on the theoretically derived value of pH, the BS scale ignores this completely and defines the standard on the basis of a phthalate buffer; furthermore, none of the BS buffers are near the pH of blood. For these reasons most workers now prefer the NBS scale (Report of *ad hoc* Committee on Methodology, 1966). However, as was pointed out previously, such a theoretical scale is based on certain assumptions and even if these are correct there is still the unknown potential at the liquid junction. Not only is this junction variable in the individual cell, but it also varies with the design of the electrode and with the composition of the test solution (Siggaard Anderson, 1961). It may therefore differ with buffer and blood (Kater, Leonard and Matsuyama, 1968). For these reasons measured blood pH probably does not bear a fixed relation to the hydrogen ion concentration of the sample.

In clinical practice two buffers are usually used to set up the electrode system. The primary standard for blood pH measurements is a mixture of $KH_2PO_4$ (0·0087 molal) and $Na_2HPO_4$ (0·0304 molal). This has a pH of 7·386 at 37°C. A second buffer is used to adjust the gain of the pH meter. A mixture of the same salts in 0·025 molal concentrations is usually used, the pH of this being 6·840 at 37°C (Bates 1962).

**Measurement of Potential**

The EMF developed by a glass electrode assembly is approximately 61·5 mV./pH unit at 37°C, but the internal resistance of the cell is high. Consequently, if the potential

one of the voltmeters described above as a null detector in a bridge circuit. An exactly equal and opposite voltage is applied to balance the EMF produced by the glass electrode system; the voltage required is then calibrated against the EMF of a standard cell.

As mentioned previously, the EMF of a glass electrode system varies somewhat from day-to-day. The fact is ignored in some commercial pH meters which assume a constant mV/pH unit ratio. The reading can be corrected by noting the pH difference between known buffers and then applying an appropriate correction factor. This

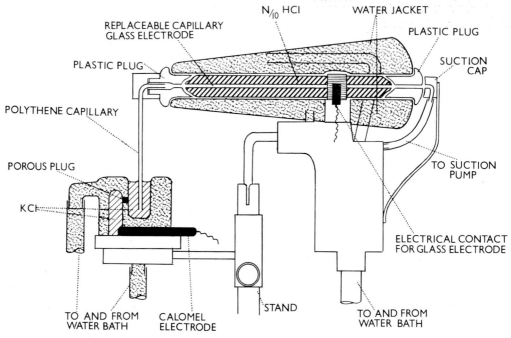

REPLACEABLE CAPILLARY GLASS ELECTRODE

N/10 HCl

WATER JACKET

PLASTIC PLUG

PLASTIC PLUG

SUCTION CAP

POLYTHENE CAPILLARY

POROUS PLUG

KCl

TO SUCTION PUMP

ELECTRICAL CONTACT FOR GLASS ELECTRODE

TO AND FROM WATER BATH

CALOMEL ELECTRODE

STAND

TO AND FROM WATER BATH

FIG. 5. The Radiometer micro-electrode system.

across the cell is measured when a current is flowing the reading obtained will be lower than the true EMF. It is, therefore, essential to measure the potential difference when little or no current is flowing. This can be be achieved in one of two ways. In the first method the small voltage generated by the electrode system is amplified and displayed on a meter. Since the internal resistance of the electrode system is of the order of 100 megohms the input impedance of the meter should be at least 10,000 megohms. (If the input impedance of the meter is less than this it will act as a shunt across the cell and the voltage measured will be a fixed proportion of the true voltage). In addition, the amplifier must be linear and extremely stable. These requirements can be met in various ways, e.g. by the use of an electrometer valve, a vibrating condenser electrometer or by a chopper amplifier. The electrometer valve was used in earlier pH meters but the more recent pH meters employ one of the other two methods. In both cases the aim is to convert the DC voltage to AC which can then be easily amplified. After amplification the output is rectified back to DC and displayed on a meter. The second method of measuring the potential without drawing current from the cell is to use

process is facilitated by reading the output directly in millivolts. Modern accurate pH meters have a buffer adjustment control, which enables the user to align the buffer reading on the scale with the pH of a known buffer, and a span control which enables the user to adjust the sensitivity of the instrument so that it matches the difference in pH between two known buffers. The latter adjustment corrects for variations in electrode output.

### Electrode Systems

A number of electrode systems are available for the measurement of pH under anaerobic conditions. The capillary micro-electrode re-introduced by Sanz (1957) revolutionized measurements on small samples and led to the development of the ultra-micro method described by Siggard Andersen, Engel, Jørgensen and Astrup (1960).

Since the equipment developed by the latter authors is widely distributed it's use will be described to illustrate the details of the measurement of pH.

**Technique of Measurement**

The whole system can be mounted on a trolley or can stand on a bench (Fig. 5). The calomel reference electrode is mounted on a small stand and is maintained at 37°C by water circulated from a central water bath. This should be left on continuously since the calomel electrode adjusts extremely slowly to changes in temperature. The calomel half-cell is connected to the solution under test by a saturated solution of KCl. This solution is divided into two portions which are connected by a porous plug. The solution surrounding the calomel electrode needs occasional replenishment via a side arm. The solution contained in the cup becomes rapidly contaminated by the solution under test and needs frequent replacement. Evaporation of the solution in the cup may be prevented by a cork when not in use.

The glass electrode consists of a removable glass cylinder which contains a capillary of pH sensitive glass down the centre. The pH sensitive glass is surrounded by N/10 HCl. A silver/silver chloride wire lies in the HCl and is connected to a metal contact on the outside of the glass electrode. This connects it with the electrical lead to the pH meter. The glass electrode is fixed inside the glass water-jacket by two plastic plugs. Through one of these passes a polyethylene capillary tube, the outer end of which can be dipped into the sample or into the KCl bridge in the cup of the calomel electrode. The other end of the glass capillary can be connected to a suction pump by pressing the suction cap over the end of the plastic plug. This enables samples of buffer or blood to be drawn into the capillary and subsequently disposed of. A pin on the handle of the glass electrode assembly is fitted into a slot on the stand when a measurement is made. This action depresses a switch which activates the pH meter and ensures mechanical stability whilst the measurement is being made.

Before making a measurement, the temperature of the water bath is checked. The gain of the instrument is then adjusted so that the meter scale matches the span between the two known buffers*. On some Radiometer pH meters this procedure can be facilitated by utilizing the electrical zero of the meter. For this reason the manufacturer's instructions should be closely followed.

When the gain has been correctly adjusted, the 7·386 buffer is once again sucked into the electrode. The buffer adjustment is now used to align the needle with this point on the scale and all blood readings are referred to this buffer standard, the buffer being inserted before and after each blood reading to check that no drift has occurred. Re-standardization of the span control is rarely needed more than once or twice a day but the buffer adjustment may have to be manipulated frequently to re-align the scale with the buffer value.

Certain aspects of technique are important. First, the temperature of the electrode must be controlled accurately at $37 \pm 0.1°C$. To ensure this degree of accuracy it is essential to maintain an adequate flow of water round the system. The pump, water bath and thermostat should be checked frequently and all tubing should be of plastic and of minimal length and maximum bore. The outside of the electrodes and leads should be kept scrupulously clean

and dry and the KCl in the cup of the reference electrode should be changed frequently. The glass electrode should be flushed thoroughly with saline or buffer after blood samples have been taken into the capillary (water may precipitate globulins) and the electrode should always be left filled with buffer or saline. If the electrode response becomes sluggish the capillary should be cleaned of protein film by filling with 1% pepsin in N/10 HCl for 15–30 minutes; it should then be thoroughly flushed with saline or buffer. Flushing with hydrogen peroxide may also help. Blood on the porous plug in the reference electrode can usually be removed with a small test tube brush, but brushing with a small quantity of hydrogen peroxide may be required if the plug is heavily contaminated. Care should be taken to ensure that no hydrogen peroxide diffuses into the calomel cell since it may cause irreparable damage.

When making any measurement it is essential to introduce the buffer or blood into the capillary in two stages to ensure that complete ionic equilibrium is obtained. The capillary is filled completely with the solution (taking care that no air bubbles are present) and the solution left in contact with the electrode for 10–15 seconds. A second aliquot of sample is then aspirated into the electrode and the reading made when the position of the needle on the dial becomes steady. Drift or a sluggish response is an indication for cleaning the electrode as described above.

**Sources of Error in pH Measurement**

Errors in pH measurement occur frequently despite the apparent simplicity of the technique. Anyone who wishes to convince himself of this fact should attempt to duplicate all blood pH measurements on two electrode systems. Even with meticulous care agreement to within 0·005 of a pH unit will be the exception rather than the rule! Indeed, the author has on a number of occasions noted errors of up to 0·3 pH units when the same blood sample has been measured on two electrode systems which were set up on the same pair of buffers and which gave almost identical readings on a third buffer. The only way to guard against such errors is to check the electrode system at least once a day. This can be accomplished either by comparing a pH reading of a *blood* sample with that determined on another electrode system, or by the use of a stabilized serum preparation (G. W. Burton —*see* Adams, Morgan-Hughes and Sykes, 1967 and 1968). Ox serum is usually used and 1 per cent sodium azide is added as a preservative. The serum should be preserved at $-25°C$: it then remains stable for several years. However, if stored at room temperature it seems to remain stable for up to 12 weeks. The buffer line of the ox serum is first determined on two electrode systems by equilibrating samples with 4 and 8 per cent $CO_2$ in $O_2$ in the microtonometer and measuring the pH. These results are plotted on a pH/log $P_{CO_2}$ nomogram. The buffer line of this preparation is then checked daily on the electrode system, deviations of the buffer line from the original value indicating malfunction of the electrode system.

For a further discussion of sources of error the reader is referred to the papers quoted above.

* The precision buffers manufactured by Radiometer Ltd., are most useful for this purpose and may be obtained from V. and A. Howe & Co. Ltd., 46 Pembridge Road, London, W.11. A similar range of buffers is manufactured by British Drug Houses Ltd., Poole, Dorset.

## Temperature Corrections

If the blood is sampled at one temperature, stored anaerobically and read in an electrode system maintained at another temperature it is necessary to apply a correction factor to the observed reading, there being a rise in pH as the temperature of the blood falls or vice versa. The reason for the change in pH is that the degree of ionization of the protein elements of blood is reduced as temperature falls. This releases more cation ($Na^+$ and $K^+$) for the carriage of $CO_2$ as $HCO_3^-$ and the bicarbonate content of the plasma increases. $P_{CO_2}$ therefore falls and pH rises (Brewin *et al.*, 1955).

The factor commonly used to correct pH for temperature changes is that of Rosenthal (1948), namely pH rises 0·0147 of a pH unit for each °C fall in temperature. Recently it has been shown that this factor is affected by the respiratory and, to a lesser extent, the non-respiratory state of the blood (Burton, 1965). However, the significance of a pH measurement at low body temperatures is not clear and most units utilizing induced hypothermia assess the non-respiratory component at 37°C and only adjust the $P_{O_2}$ and $P_{CO_2}$ values to body temperature.

## Blood Sampling and Storage

Blood samples may be venous, capillary or arterial. Venous samples taken from the antecubital vein are completely unreliable as the pH is influenced by the degree of stasis introduced by the tourniquet, the activity of the muscles, and the proportions of skin and muscle blood flow being obtained. Brooks and Wynn (1959) have shown that "arterialized" venous blood obtained from the back of the hand without constriction and under certain specified conditions may provide a useful estimate in some cases. Astrup has proposed that capillary blood should be used. In the warm vasodilated ear of a patient at rest this may yield a reasonable comparison with arterial blood, but in babies and under certain conditions (Cooper and Smith, 1961) the relation to arterial blood pH is very variable.

Arterial blood is therefore used whenever possible. Almost any palpable artery may be used, the sample being obtained by direct puncture by needle or indwelling catheter inserted under direct vision or by the Seldinger (1953) technique. Catheters may be left in the radial or brachial arteries for 24 to 48 hours but the femoral artery should be treated with more circumspection.

If the blood sample is to be obtained by direct puncture it is best to use a glass syringe, the plunger of which has been lubricated with silicone oil before autoclaving. The dead space of the syringe and needle is filled with heparin (1,000 units/ml.) and the needle is inserted at an angle of 60° to the artery. When the artery is pierced the blood will flow into the syringe in a pulsatile manner and it should be allowed to flow into the syringe at its own rate. Plastic syringes may also be used for direct puncture but it is usually easier to insert the needle into the artery first and then to attach the syringe when a free flow of blood has been obtained. The barrel of the syringe should be well lubricated with heparin by taking about 1 ml. of heparin into the syringe, holding the syringe with its nozzle uppermost and then working the plunger up and down a few times. The syringe is then tapped to allow the air bubbles to rise to the surface of the heparin and any bubbles and excess heparin are expelled before attaching the syringe to the needle in the artery. A slight force must be applied to the plunger to overcome the friction present in plastic syringes but care must be taken not to apply excessive pressure for this may cause the syringe to leak or may even cause dissolved gas to come out of solution, so altering the pH.

After sampling, firm pressure must be applied to the artery. The required duration and extent of pressure cannot be predicted but should be related to the size of needle used and to such other factors as the arterial pressure, use of anticoagulants, etc. For direct puncture an occlusive pressure of 2–3 minutes duration followed by more gentle pressure for a further 2–3 minutes is usually adequate. However, the artery must always be observed for a further 5–10 minutes and it is a wise precaution always to apply a pressure dressing. Many of the complications of arterial puncture are attributable to haematoma formation: this should never occur.

The syringe should be capped with a plastic or metal cap and then rotated between the palms to mix the sample. Mixing should be repeated before the pH is measured and the measurement should be completed as soon as possible after sampling. If immediate analysis is impossible the syringe should be stored in ice and water. Under these conditions the pH falls approximately 0·004 pH units per hour.

## The Value of pH Measurements

Measurements of the pH of blood reflect changes in the extra-cellular compartment of the body but this may bear little relation to changes in the intracellular compartment. Changes within the cells cannot be measured directly and little is known about the significance of intracellular changes in pH. However it is also important to realize that changes in the blood may not parallel changes in other body fluids. For example an acute non-respiratory acidosis will cause a fall in blood pH but a rise in CSF pH.

From the Henderson-Haselbalch equation (p. 107) it may be seen that pH depends on the ratio between the quantities of base and acid present. Using the bicarbonate system as an example the ratio of $HCO_3^-$ to $CO_2$ is normally 20:1. Any increase in bicarbonate or decrease in $CO_2$ will therefore cause an alkalemia and any reduction in bicarbonate or increase in $CO_2$ will cause an acidaemia (Report of *ad hoc* Committee on Acid-base Terminology, 1966). It is obvious therefore that the significance of acid-base changes cannot be decided on the basis of a measurement of pH alone. However, if one of the other two variables (i.e. $HCO_3^-$ or $P_{CO_2}$) is measured then the full acid-base picture can be derived from the Henderson-Hasselbalch equation or from one of the nomograms based on it.

Changes in either the respiratory or non-respiratory components of acid-base balance are usually compensated by an alteration in the other component so that the pH is returned towards 7·4, but the rate at which this compensation occurs varies. For example a change in the non-respiratory component usually induces a rapid but opposing change in the respiratory component so that pH is quickly returned towards normal levels. On the other hand the non-respiratory response to a respiratory change takes a matter of hours or days to develop: marked changes of pH may therefore result from acute changes of $P_{CO_2}$. In both situations the direction of the primary change is indicated by the direction of change in pH, for compensation is seldom complete. It is, however, unwise to base clinical judgements on such an assumption for two reasons. Firstly, there may be some complicating factor which causes an alteration in one of the components independently of the primary change. For example a patient with respiratory failure may also have been treated with diuretics for heart failure. The pH, instead of being on the acid side of normal (indicating a primary respiratory disturbance) might then be above 7·4. This would wrongly suggest a primary non-respiratory alkalosis with compensating respiratory acidosis. The second reason for treating this assumption with caution is that there may be an alteration in the respiratory state due to the disturbance caused by blood sampling. For example a patient in chronic respiratory failure with a high $P_{CO_2}$ and compensatory increase in bicarbonate may develop a pH above 7·4 due to transient over-breathing at the moment of sampling. All pH values must therefore be considered in relation to the patient's history and present state. If this is done then pH may provide much useful clinical information. As an example one can consider again the patient with chronic obstructive airways disease who develops acute respiratory failure due to an infection. The $P_{CO_2}$ will rise and cause a marked fall in pH. The bicarbonate will then rise gradually over the next one to two days until the pH is restored towards normal. If the patient has a high $P_{CO_2}$ and a low pH on admission it suggests that the bicarbonate level is normal and that the patient is suffering from acute respiratory failure. If however the pH on admission is not low when the $P_{CO_2}$ is high it suggests that the $CO_2$ retention has existed for some time and that the patient has a compensating non-respiratory alkalosis. The difference between these two situations may well affect the plan of treatment.

### Conclusions

In conclusion, it should be remembered that a pH measurement is only as accurate as the worker and the apparatus. Accurate pH measuring equipment seldom costs less than £600 and a competent worker usually considerably more. One has only to compare pH determinations made by a number of different workers on the same system or by the same workers on different systems, to realize how wide can be the variation in results. However, if care is taken, reproducible results can be obtained and the measurement of blood pH can then provide an invaluable guide to the acid-base status of the patient.

### REFERENCES

Adams, A. P., Morgan-Hughes, J. O. and Sykes, M. K. (1967), "pH and Blood-gas Analysis: Methods of Measurement and Sources of Error Using Electrode Systems," Part 1, *Anaesthesia*, **22**, 575.

Adams, A. P., Morgan-Hughes, J. O. and Sykes, M. K. (1968), "pH and Blood-gas Analysis: Methods of Measurement and Sources of Error Using Electrode Systems," Part 2, *Anaesthesia*, **23**, 47.

Bates, R. G. (1962), "Revised Standard Values for pH Measurements from 0 to 95°C," *J. Res. Nat. Bur. Std. A.*, **66A**, 179.

Brewin, E. G., Gould, R. P., Nashat, F. S. and Neil, E. (1955), "An Investigation of Problems of Acid-base Equilibrium in Hypothermia," *Guy's Hosp. Rep.*, **104**, 177.

Brønsted, J. N. (1923), "Einige Bemerkungen uber den Begriff der Säuren und Basen," *Rev. trav. chim. Pays-Bas*, **42**, 718.

Brooks, D. and Wynn, V. (1959), "Use of Venous Blood for pH and Carbon-dioxide Studies. Especially in Respiratory Failure and During Anaesthesia, *Lancet*, **1**, 227.

Burton, G. W. (1965), "Effects of the Acid-base State Upon the Temperature Coefficient of pH of Blood," *Brit. J. Anaesth.*, **37**, 89.

Cooper, E. A. and Smith, H. (1961), "Indirect Estimation of Arterial $P_{CO_2}$," *Anaesthesia*, **16**, 445.

Kater, J. A. R., Leonard, J. E. and Matsuyama, G. (1968), "Junction Potential Variations in Blood pH Measurements," *Ann. N. Y. Acad. Sci.*, **148**, 54.

Ludbrook, J. (1959), "Estimation of $P_{CO_2}$ by Means of the Henderson-Hasselbalch Equation": p. 34 in *A Symposium on pH and Blood Gas Measurement*, Ed. by R. F. Woolmer. London: Churchill.

Report of the *ad hoc* Committee on Acid-base Terminology: Current Concepts of Acid-base Measurement (1966), *Ann. N. Y. Acad. Sci.*, **133**, 251.

Report of *ad hoc* Committee on Methodology: Current Concepts of Acid-base Measurement (1966), *Ann. N. Y. Acad. Sci.*, **133**, 259.

Rosenthal, T. B. (1948), "The Effect of Temperature on the pH of Blood and Plasma in Vitro," *J. biol. Chem.*, **173**, 25.

Sanz, M. C. (1957), "Ultramicro Methods and Standardization of Equipment," *Clin. Chem.*, **3**, 406.

Seldinger, S. I. (1953), "Catheter Replacement of the Needle in Percutaneous Arteriography," *Acta radiol.*, (Stockh), **39**, 368.

Semple, S. J. G. (1961), "Observed pH Differences of Blood and Plasma with Different Bridge Solutions," *J. Appl. Physiol.*, **16**, 576.

Semple, S. G. C. (1967), "Problems in Measurement and Interpretation of Blood Acid-base State," *Bio-med. Engng.*, **2**, 500.

Severinghaus, J. W., Stupfel, M. and Bradley, A. F. (1956), "Variations of Serum Carbonic Acid pK' with pH and Temperature," *J. appl. Physiol.*, **9**, 197.

Siggaard Andersen, O., Engel, K., Jørgensen, K. and Astrup, P. (1960), "A Micro Method for Determination of pH, Carbon Dioxide Tension, Base Excess and Standard Bicarbonate in Capillary Blood," *Scand. J. Clin. Lab. Invest.*, **12**, 172.

Siggaard Andersen, O. (1961), "Factors Affecting the Liquid-junction Potential in Electrometric Blood pH Measurement," *Scand. J. Clin. Lab. Invest.*, **13**, 205.

Siggaard Andersen, O. (1962), "The First Dissociation Exponent of Carbonic Acid as a Function of pH," *Scand. J. Clin. Lab. Invest.*, **14**, 587.

Sørensen, S. P. L. (1909), "Etudes Enzymatiques. Part 2 Sur la mésure et l'importance de la concentration des ions hydrogènes dans leurs reactions enzymatiques," *Compt. rend. trav. lab. Carlsberg*, **8**, 1.

### OTHER SUGGESTED READING

Bates, R. G. (1964), *Determination of pH. Theory and Practice.* New York: John Wiley.

Davenport, H. W. (1969), *The ABC of Acid-base Chemistry.* 5th Edition. Chicago: University of Chicago Press.

Mattock, G. (1961), *pH Measurement and Titration.* New York: The Macmillan Co.

Nunn, J. F. (1962), "Nomenclature and Presentation of Hydrogen Ion Regulation Data," in *Modern Trends in Anaesthesia*, 2: Aspects of Hydrogen Ion Regulation and Biochemistry in Anaesthesia. Edited by F. T. Evans and T. C. Gray. London: Butterworths.

Siggaard-Andersen, O. (1967), "Therapeutic Aspects of Acid-base Disorders," in *Modern Trends in Anaesthesia*, 3: Aspects of Metabolism and Pulmonary Ventilation. Edited by F. T. Evans and T. C. Gray. London: Butterworths.

*SECTION II*

# PHYSIOLOGICAL BASIS OF THE SCIENCE OF ANAESTHESIA

## A.  Cardiovascular System

# CHAPTER 1

# CARDIAC PERFORMANCE

JULIAN M. LEIGH

## Introduction

The heart pump is of such complexity that it defies an exact mechanical or electrical description. Recent literature on cardiac performance is however extensive. Terminology to describe various aspects of myocardial function has correspondingly increased to such an extent that the clinician may find it difficult to discourse with the research worker. It should be evident, for example, that when the clinician discusses the 'forcefulness of the apex beat' and 'the jugular venous pressure' as measured in the neck, he is discussing indices of cardiac performance of the same type as the research worker with his 'force-velocity-length' relations, etc. An understanding of the scientific principles allows this gap to be bridged. Additionally, much of the terminology is confusing even for those actively engaged in the study of this subject. The same term has sometimes been used by different authorities for different features of myocardial function. The most abused of these is 'contractile state'. Accordingly, this term will not be employed at all in what follows.

In principle the haemodynamic function of the normal heart is to receive the venous return volume and to pump the *same volume* back into the circulation. The venous return volume thus controls the cardiac output. Since the former is dictated by the demands of the peripheral organs or tissues, it is apparent that the cardiac output is regulated by tissue demands for nutrients. This chapter deals with the unique mechanisms which enable the heart, and in particular ventricular muscle, to function as a highly efficient demand pump capable of achieving outputs of 3–25 litres per minute in health. Even under conditions of disease the cardiac output may be maintained—at least at rest—by the ventricular compensating mechanisms:— elevation of left ventricular end-diastolic pressure, ventricular hypertrophy, and increased sympathetic nervous system activity.

## Regulation of Cardiac Output

Cardiac output is a simple function of,

Pulse rate × stroke volume

While the pulse rate is normally an extrinsic reflex phenomenon, the stroke volume is essentially a function of the effectiveness of the heart pump, as it responds to the venous return volume. It is determined by:–

I *The preload*—ventricular end-diastolic fibre length or volume, or pressure.

II *Inotropy (myocardial contractility)*.

III *The afterload*—aortic or pulmonary impedance.

## I Ventricular Preload

Myocardial performance, in particular the force of myocardial contraction, is profoundly influenced by the initial fibre length. This is stated in the *Frank-Starling relation*, i.e., the greater the initial fibre length, the more forcibly does the ventricle contract. For any given level of inotropy, myocardial force is dependent upon ventricular end-diastolic volume. This, in turn, is dependent upon several factors but more importantly on venous return, or more correctly upon the *tendency for venous return*. The factors which may be considered to modify the venous return are:

(a) *Blood volume:* Ventricular end-diastolic volume is influenced by total blood volume. The most extreme impairment is seen in haemorrhagic 'shock' in which both stroke volume and cardiac output become reduced. Even with a normal blood volume the distribution of blood may influence venous return and ventricular filling.

(b) *Posture:* The upright posture tends to reduce intrathoracic and end-diastolic filling pressure and to reduce cardiac output due to blood pooling in extra-thoracic areas. This is important during general anaesthesia where head-up tilts of 10–25 degrees are often employed, for example, during induced hypotension.

(c) *Intrathoracic pressure:* This is usually negative during spontaneous ventilation. It constitutes the *thoracic pump* which promotes cardiac filling and increases end-diastolic volume. During intermittent positive pressure ventilation, a higher mean intrathoracic pressure is maintained and thus venous return is reduced and with it end-diastolic volume. This will tend to reduce cardiac output.

(d) *Intrapericardial pressure:* Pericardial effusion, for example, interferes with ventricular distensibility and limits end-diastolic volume.

(e) *Venous tone:* Veno-constriction augments cardiac filling and occurs in the early stages of acute blood loss, in exercise and in response to sympathomimetic amines and cardiac glycosides. However many drugs, including ganglionic blocking agents and alpha adrenergic blockers decrease venous tone and will reduce cardiac filling.

(f) *Muscle pump:* Contracting skeletal muscle together with unidirectional venous valves promote venous return. This effect is largely obtunded during anaesthesia.

(g) *Atrial contribution:* Normally atrial contraction contributes 20–30 per cent of ventricular filling. This is not important at rest in the normal subject but during exercise, tachycardia, and in patients with ventricular hypertrophy or with heart disease in general, it is a very important factor in maintaining cardiac output.

## II Inotropy (Myocardial Contractility)

There is undeniable difficulty over the definition of this abstract *quality* due to the fact that, as yet, no primary or derived *quantity* can be used alone to describe it. Myocardial contractility has been taken to include force of contraction, cardiac output and ventricular stroke work, the rate of rise of ventricular pressure ($dp/dt$) and the ventricular function curve and its slope, etc. It has been suggested that the mechanics of myocardial contraction are best considered in terms of the 'force-velocity' relationship so that for any given preload, afterload and heart rate, myocardial contractility may be defined by the slope of the force-velocity curve. Recently further derived indices have been advocated as better indications of myocardial contractility (*vide infra*).

The factors which affect myocardial contractility are much more easy to appreciate and are as follows:–

(a) *The sympathetic nervous system:* This is the single most important determinant of myocardial contractility. An increase in activity of this system leads to an increase in contractility. Circulating catecholamines will have a similar effect.

(b) *Positive inotropic agents:* These drugs include sympathomimetic agents, particularly those with prominent beta effects, the glycosides, calcium and theophylline. All these agents improve the force of myocardial contraction at a given end-diastolic volume.

(c) *Negative inotropic agents:* These include quinidine, local anaesthetic agents such as lignocaine and procaine, and the barbiturates. Many general anaesthetic agents, and in particular halothane, also depress myocardial contractility.

(d) *Physiological depressants:* Hypoxia, hypercapnia and acidosis depress myocardial contractility.

(e) *Ventricular integrity:* Should an area of myocardium become necrotic or non-functional due to coronary artery disease or cardiomyopathy, ventricular performance at any given level of end-distolic volume would be reduced. Although the remaining myocardium may function normally, the presence of the abnormal portion may lead to ventricular asynergy with a deleterious effect on stroke output (Herman *et al.*, 1969).

## III Ventricular Afterload

The volume of blood ejected by the ventricle is a function of the shortening of ventricular fibres during systole. For any given level of diastolic fibre length, in a given inotropic state, this is dependent upon the afterload imposed on the ventricles by the aortic or pulmonary impedance since this pressure dictates both the opening and closing pressures of the respective valves and therefore limits stroke volume. If the afterload is very high then stroke volume must be low. If it is very low, the ventricular emptying must be complete. The normal function lies in between and afterload is dependent upon mean arterial pressure.

The foregoing is an introduction to the factors determining cardiac performance. The characteristics of the *Frank-Starling* and *inotropic* mechanisms may be best examined in terms of the differences which they exhibit in the force-velocity-length interrelationships.

Before discussing these in detail let us first discuss the mechanics of myocardial contraction.

### Mechanics of Myocardial Contraction

There are two phases:

(i) *The isometric contraction phase*, during which force is developed in the muscle (like taking up slack) but in which no shortening occurs.

(ii) The *ventricular ejection phase*, when shortening does occur and in which external work is performed without a further increase in force. These two phases are illustrated in Fig. 1 which shows simultaneous

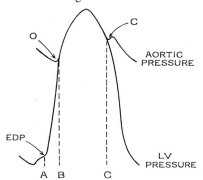

FIG. 1. Simultaneous left ventricular and aortic pressure waveforms. EDP = end-diastolic pressure; O = opening of aortic valve; C = closure of aortic valve; AB = isometric contraction phase; BC = ventricular ejection phase.

recording of intraventricular and aortic pressure. At *A* the isometric contraction phase begins and there is a rapid rise of pressure in the ventricle but with no ejection. At *B*, the semilunar valves open and ejection begins accompanied by a rise of pressure in the aorta. At *C*, the valves close marking the end of ejection and pressure at both sites decreases to the diastolic level. Obviously, cardiac performance must be thought of as a function of time. Determination of cardiac output in the arbitrary time-base of one minute, or even of its division by the pulse rate to derive stroke volume may not convey physiological information which is critical enough for the analysis of cardiac performance. This is because the cardiac output can vary independently of changes in the state of the myocardium. A more useful approach involves separate examination, with respect to time, of events occurring during the isometric contraction phase rather than those during the ventricular ejection phase.

There are certain problems inherent in the evaluation of these events in the intact subject and we must first turn to a simple model, i.e. the isolated papillary muscle in which myocardial fibres are in a parallel formation. Fig. 2a shows the classical arrangement for studying such a muscle. The muscle (*M*) with its stimulating electrodes (*E*) is connected to a tension transducer (*TT*) and to a lever (*L*) on a fulcrum (*F*). A small preload weight (*P*) is attached to the other end of the lever; this stretches the muscle to a given length. A stop (*S*), Fig.

2b, is then put in place so that the muscle cannot stretch any further. A large afterload weight (*A*) is then attached to the other end of the lever, further stretching cannot occur because of the stop. When the muscle is then stimulated via the electrodes it will contract against the

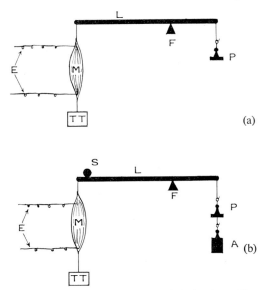

FIG. 2. Arrangement for study of isolated papillary muscle preparation.

total load. The events which occur are shown in Fig. 3 which shows shortening against time and tension against time. *AB* represents the isometric contraction phase in which tension develops but in which there is no shortening. At *B* the tension has developed such that the force

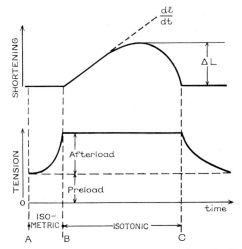

FIG. 3. Shortening-time and tension-time plots of a single papillary muscle contraction.

equals the afterload. Once the afterload is matched, isotonic shortening occurs and the load is lifted. By repeating the experiment with different afterloads a series of such graphs can be obtained, Fig. 4. The characteristic initial velocities of shortening ($dl/dt$) can also be obtained for each afterload. If the several initial velocities of shortening are replotted as a function of load (force), Fig. 5, the force-velocity relation of the

given papillary muscle under its specific conditions of inotropy and specific pre-load can be drawn. This is an inverse relationship, i.e., the velocity of muscle shortening decreases as the total load which it carries

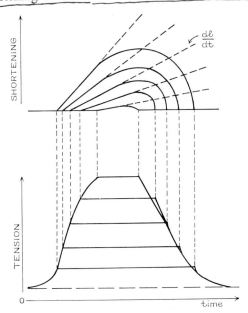

FIG. 4. Shortening-time and tension-time plots of papillary muscle contractions at different afterloads. The initial velocities of shortening $dl/dt$ are shown.

increases. If the curve is now extrapolated to zero afterload, the velocity of shortening is maximal ($V_{max}$). Conversely, when the load is increased until there is no external shortening but only force is generated, the maximum isometric tension ($P_0$) is obtained.

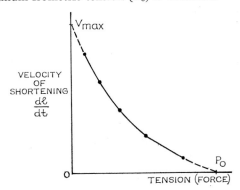

FIG. 5. Force-velocity curve showing extrapolation to $V_{max}$ and $P_0$.

Also inherent in the force-velocity relation is other mechanical information, i.e., external work and power. Both work and power are zero when the load is zero or when the load is greater than $P_0$, i.e., when there is no change in length. Thus both work and power are *dependent on the load* and work and power cannot be used in themselves as indices of changes in myocardial contractility unless the load itself is unaltered.

Work = force × distance (or length)
Power = Force × velocity

The inter-relationship between force, velocity and length can be represented in a three-dimensional diagram, Fig. 6, where force is plotted on the $x$ axis, velocity on the $y$ axis and length on the $z$ axis. Power is represented on the force-velocity plane and work on the force-length plane.

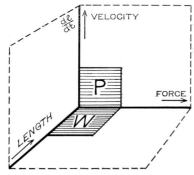

FIG. 6. The three-dimensional relationship between force, velocity and length and their mechanical derivatives work and power.

## Force-Velocity Diagram

The two fundamental processes by which myocardial performance may be altered can be represented on the force-velocity diagram. That is:—

(i) a change of initial muscle length by alteration of preload.

(ii) a change of inotropic state (myocardial contractility).

In the first case there is an increase in isometric tension which is common to all muscles, i.e., an increase in initial fibre length produces an increase in the force of contraction (which correlates in the intact heart with the Frank-Starling phenomenon). In terms of the force-velocity relationship this means that, in a force velocity curve $P_0$ (the maximum isometric tension) goes to the right without a change in the maximum velocity of shortening, $V_{max}$. (Fig. 7).

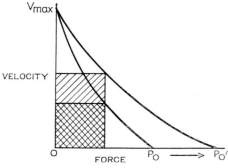

FIG. 7. Force-velocity diagram showing the Frank-Starling effect. $P_0$ shifts to the right with an increase in initial fibre length. Note that there is an increase in ventricular power at a given load denoted by the increase in the shaded area. But note also that this effect decreases at low levels of load.

On the other hand, when there is an inotropic intervention, there is an increase in $V_{max}$ as well as in $P_0$ (Fig. 8). Thus it can be seen that $V_{max}$ is unique for a given inotropic state and it *alone* provides an indication of changes in that state of the myocardium.

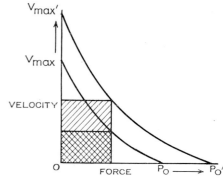

FIG. 8. Force-velocity diagram showing the effect of a positive inotropic intervention. The whole curve is shifted to the right. Note that there is an increase in ventricular power at a given load—denoted by the increase in the shaded area. But note also that this effect is maintained at low levels of load.

## Velocity-Length Diagram

When muscle shortening occurs from different initial lengths with a constant load, this is demonstrable on the velocity-length diagram. For a given inotropic state the instantaneous velocity of shortening is essentially independent of the length from which the muscle began shortening, although it is still a function of instantaneous

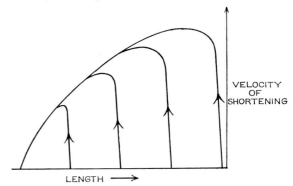

FIG. 9. Velocity-length diagram from different initial fibre lengths but at a constant state of contractility.

muscle length and all the velocities of shortening join to form a common pathway, Fig. 9. If contractility is improved by an inotropic intervention, the velocity-length relation is shifted upwards to a new common pathway, Fig. 10.

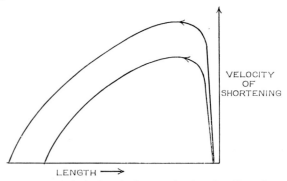

FIG. 10. Velocity-length diagram showing the effect of a positive inotropic intervention at constant initial fibre length.

## Force-Velocity-Length Relations in the Intact Heart

These three parameters now become, pressure, ventricular ejection rate (flow) and stroke volume and can still be represented on a three dimensional diagram with work and power now being *pressure × volume* and *pressure × ejection rate* respectively* and still being represented on the same surfaces. However, the circumstances of rigorously controlled experimentation which can be applied to the papillary muscle preparation, no longer apply. Length cannot be fixed at will, nor can preload or afterload. In fact, there is no isotonic phase as afterload changes throughout ejection. This time interval is therefore referred to as *the ventricular ejection phase.*

A single ejecting ventricular beat can be represented by a complex line on a three-dimensional diagram, Fig. 11. AB represents that part of isometric contraction during

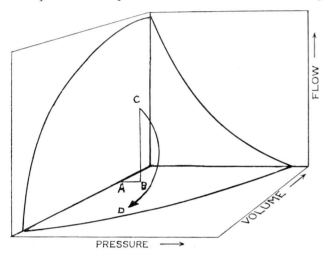

Fig. 11. Three dimensional pressure–volume–flow course of a single ejecting ventricular beat. AC = isometric contraction. CD = ventricular ejection.

which there is a rise in pressure without either a change in flow or volume. BC represents the instant in which the aortic valve opens and in which ejection rate becomes maximal with virtually no change in volume at constant pressure. C represents the end of isometric contraction. From here onwards the developed pressure produces work against the afterload. This is manifest (segment CD) by ejection of the stroke volume at decreasing rate while the pressure first rises and then falls. (See also Fig. 1.)

Preload is represented in the intact heart by end-diastolic ventricular pressure (end-diastolic volume), and the afterload by mean aortic or pulmonary arterial pressures. The inotropic state is now, however, much more difficult to express.

```
*            Work = force × distance = dyn cm
or,          Work = pressure × volume = dyn cm⁻² × cm³
                  = dyn cm
       1 dyn cm = 1 erg = 10⁻⁷ joule
             Power = force × velocity = dyn cm sec⁻¹
or,          Power = pressure × ventricular ejection rate
                  = dyn cm⁻² × cm³ sec⁻¹ = dyn cm sec⁻¹
   1 dyn cm sec⁻¹ = 10⁻⁷ watt
```

The entire situation of myocardial contractility may be described in a three dimensional diagram, Fig. 12, by a surface, the slope of which follows a force velocity relationship and the orientation of which, with respect to intraventricular pressure, ventricular ejection rate and stroke volume represents a given state of contractility.

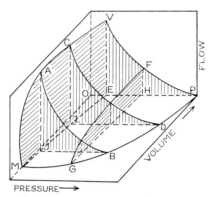

Fig. 12. Three dimensional figure of a contractility surface VPM. The MV edge of the surface represents the maximal flow–volume relation. It is not attached along its full length to the flow–volume plane because it follows the end-diastolic pressure line ME. Three force–velocity 'supports' of the surface VPE, CDI, and ABJ are shown. The lines VP, CD, and AB represent isovolume lines. PM is the maximal pressure–volume attachment of the surface. FGH is an isotonic 'support' of the surface.

An elevation of the surface would generally indicate increased ventricular function and a depression of the surface would indicate decreased ventricular function.

In order to perform controlled experiments on the intact heart, resort has to be made to the experimental animal 'heart-lung preparation' in which preload and afterload can be controlled.

Alternatively, experiments can be carried out with a Walton and Brodie strain gauge arch with which ventricular fibre length can be fixed, i.e., measurements are carried out of $P_0$ (maximal isometric tension) under chosen conditions. This instrument can of course be applied to the heart *in situ* during surgery.

## Assessment of Ventricular Contractility in the Intact Subject

How much of what has been learned from examination of the isolated papillary muscle can be applied to the assessment of ventricular contractility in the intact subject? It is evident that misleading information may be obtained by considering events during the ejection phase of ventricular activity, as these are accompanied by changes in load during the material time (i.e. ejection is not isotonic). What is required is a graphical representation of the *instantaneous rate of change of myocardial fibre length*. This is impossible, but it is possible to obtain a graphical representation of the <u>instantaneous rate of change of intraventricular pressure</u>, i.e., the first derivative of the intraventricular pressure or $dp/dt$. Fig. 13 shows an intraventricular pressure trace with its first derivative $dp/dt$.

When isovolumetric contraction begins $dp/dt$ rises slowly and then rapidly to reach a maximum or $dp/dt$ max.

This value usually occurs at the instant of opening of the aortic valves, i.e., at the peak isovolumetric pressure. A similar negative peak occurs during isovolumetric relaxation.

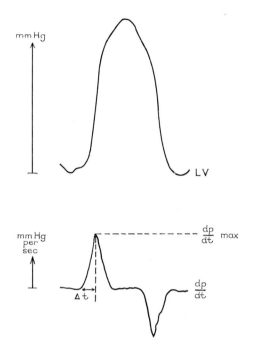

FIG. 13. Simultaneous recording of left-ventricular pressure and its first derivative d$p$/d$t$. $\Delta t$ is the time taken to reach d$p$/d$t$ max.

When there is an improvement in the myocardial contractility, d$p$/d$t$ max. is increased and vice versa. However, d$p$/d$t$ max. is also sensitive to haemodynamic parameters and if these are also changing, d$p$/d$t$ max. does not solely represent myocardial contractility.

### Haemodynamic Factors Affecting d$p$/d$t$ max.

(a) If there is an increase in ventricular preload, i.e., a rise in end-diastolic pressure, the rate of rise of ventricular pressure in the isovolumetric phase is increased.

(b) If the afterload, i.e., mean arterial pressure is increased, there is again a rise of d$p$/d$t$ max.

(c) There is also an increase of d$p$/d$t$ max. associated with tachycardia.

Thus d$p$/d$t$ max. cannot be used alone to assess changes in contractility unless the pulse rate, preload and afterload are kept constant.

Various attempts have been made to correct d$p$/d$t$ max. by using a haemodynamic parameter which when related to it cancels the effect of the change. In this respect, parameters derived from the isovolumetric phase of contraction are again much more useful than those derived from the ejection phase. Various indices have been derived, for example—comparison of the change in d$p$/d$t$ max. with the time taken to reach d$p$/d$t$ max., i.e., the distance $\Delta t$ in Fig. 13; also the isometric time tension index, d$p$/d$t$ max/IIT, where IIT is the integrated isometric systolic tension (a constant fraction of the mean systolic

tension during the isometric contraction phase). d$p$/d$t$ max. may also be compared for this purpose with left ventricular end-diastolic pressure, the peak developed isovolumetric pressure, or the instantaneous developed pressure at the time of d$p$/d$t$ max. This latter index—d$p$/d$t$ max.IP appears to be by far the best of these indices (Prys-Roberts et al., 1972).

The above assessments all involve the use of invasive and potentially hazardous techniques of investigation.

### Non-Invasive Correlates of Ventricular Contractility

One of the most promising developments in recent times is the possibility of obtaining good correlation between data obtained from the body surface and myocardial contractility. Additionally, the advent of small computers raises the possibility of real-time, beat by beat, assessment of contractility.

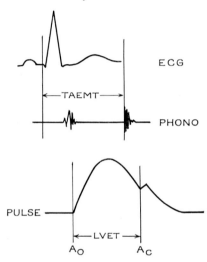

FIG. 14. Simultaneous records of ECG, phonocardiogram and arterial pulse wave-form. The total active electromechanical time (TAEMT) is from the onset of the Q wave of the ECG to the first deflection of the second heart sound, i.e., the $Q - S_2$ interval. Ao and Ac represent opening and closure of the aortic valve and the time–interval between them is the left ventricular ejection time (LVET). TAEMT − LVET = PEP (the preejection period).

The necessary data are obtained from the following simultaneous recordings:–

1. ECG
2. phonocardiogram
3. pulse wave-form, e.g. from a force transducer over a carotid artery.

The next requirement of this method involves the determination of the systolic time intervals, i.e., the pre-ejection phase (PEP) and the left ventricular ejection time (LVET) which together constitute the total active electromechanical time (TAEMT).

The ECG and the phonocardiogram are essentially transmitted without delay so they can be referred to one another on the same scale (Fig. 14). Therefore as $S_2$ signifies closure of the aortic valve then $Q-S_2$ is the TAEMT of the ventricle in that cardiac cycle.

Although the pulse wave-form is offset, opening and closing of the aortic valves ($Ao - Ac$) is constant wherever the pulse-wave is obtained, i.e., $Ao - Ac = $ LVET, and $QS_2 - $ LVET $= $ PEP.

While Weissler and his colleagues (1969) have demonstrated some correlation between PEP/LVET ratio and changes in cardiac performance, Reitan and his colleagues (1972) have demonstrated better correlation between changes in contractility and the index $1/PEP^2$.

On line computation of PEP may be readily performed with a small analogue computer (Blackburn *et al.*, 1972a). Investigations of this parameter have shown that when carbon dioxide was administered to both dogs and man, $1/PEP^2$ appeared to give a reliable indication of the changes in contractility associated with the subsequent catecholamine release, or the direct depressant effects produced by carbon dioxide or propranolol administration (Blackburn *et al.*, 1972b). However, with great changes in preload and afterload such as those occurring during Valsalva manoeuvres, this parameter cannot differentiate between contractility and the Frank-Starling mechanism (Blackburn *et al.*, 1973).

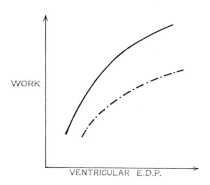

Fig. 15. Ventricular function curves. The dotted curve demonstrates depressed pump-effectiveness i.e., less work is performed at a given venticular end-diastolic pressure. The interpretation of these curves has to be guarded since they may represent the net results of simultaneous changes in heart rate, afterload and contractility. Note that time, the most important relation in terms of myocardial function, is not a feature of this method of display. Nevertheless, this is an extremely useful approach. The type of change shown is seen to a greater or lesser degree with most volatile anaesthetic agents.

## Quantities Derived from the Ventricular Ejection Phase

Many quantities may be derived during the ventricular ejection phase though they are influenced by preload and afterload. In the experimental situation data obtained

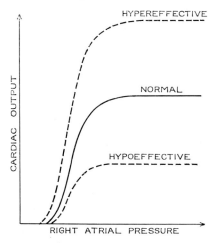

Fig. 16. Cardiac function curves (after Guyton) represent another way of looking at the pump-effectiveness of the heart. In this case the response is to changes in right atrial pressure. The upper displaced curve (hypereffective) represents increased pump-effectiveness from any cause e.g. autonomic stimulation, athletic training, hypertension with cardiac hypertrophy. The lower trace (hypoeffective) represents diminished pump-effectiveness from any cause, e.g. myocardial infarction, sympathetic blockade, drug depression, cardiomyopathy and congenital or acquired valvular disease.

from a Starling heart lung preparation are more meaningful because the preload and afterload can be controlled at will.

$$\text{The stroke volume is obviously} = \frac{\text{cardiac output}}{\text{heart rate}}$$

$$\text{The mean stroke ejection rate is} = \frac{\text{stroke volume}}{\text{LVET}}$$

Work and power can be derived as mentioned earlier and these can be related to the ventricular end-diastolic pressure (preload). Ventricular function curves (Fig. 15) which are plots of ventricular stroke work against ventricular end-diastolic pressure, at a given level of afterload,

TABLE 1

ANALAGOUS COMPARISONS OF SOME OF THE PARAMETERS CONCERNED IN CARDIAC PERFORMANCE

|  | *Papillary Muscle* | *Intact Heart* | *Intact Subject* | *Clinical* |
|---|---|---|---|---|
| Preload | Preload (fibre-length) | Vent. E.D.P. mean atrial p. | Vent. E.D.P. mean atrial p. | Jugular venous pressure |
| Afterload | Afterload | Mean aortic (or pulmonary artery pressure) | Mean aortic (or pulmonary artery pressure) | |
| Vel. of shortening | $\dfrac{dl}{dt}$ | $\dfrac{dv}{dt}$ | $\dfrac{dp}{dt}$ | |
| Net shortening | $\Delta l$ | Stroke Vol. | Stroke Vol. | Character of apex beat |
| Vent. work | Force × distance | Press. × vol. | Press. × Vol. | |
| Vent. power | Force × $\dfrac{dl}{dt}$ | Press. × $\dfrac{dv}{dt}$ | Press. × $\dfrac{dv}{dt}$ | |

can be useful in studying the changes in inotropic state produced by pharmacological agents including anaesthetics.

The cardiac function curve, popularized by Guyton, relates preload, as right atrial pressure (central venous pressure) to cardiac output (Fig. 16). These plots show a series of isolines, each representing a given state of pump-effectiveness.

Table 1 summarises the analogous comparisons of some of the various parameters in the isolated muscle, the intact heart and the intact subject.

It is appropriate to append to this discussion the following comments by J. R. Blinks (1967). 'It would be a great step forward if investigators abandoned the habit of thinking of myocardial contractility as something to be assessed in terms of some particular index, and regarded their measurements only as ways of getting an idea of the changes occurring in the fundamental relationship between force, velocity, length and time. That is the heart of the matter. The various measurements that can be made all provide glimpses of that relationship. Some provide better glimpses than others and the window that provides the best view in one situation may not be best for the next. Certainly, the better picture can be pieced together from several different glimpses than from one alone'.

## REFERENCES

Blackburn, J. P., Conway, C. M., Leigh, J. M., Lindop, M. J., Reitan, J. A. and Robbins, R. (1972a), "An Analogue Device for Measuring the Pre-Ejection Period (PEP)," *Cardiovasc. Res.*, **6**, 444.

Blackburn, J. P., Conway, C. M., Leigh, J. M., Lindop, M. J. and Reitan, J. A. (1972b), "Pa$_{CO_2}$ and the Pre-ejection Period: The Pa$_{CO_2}$/Inotropy Response Curve," *Anesthesiology*, **37**, 268.

Blackburn, J. P., Conway, C. M., Davies, R. M., Enderby, G. E. H., Edridge, A. W., Leigh, J. M., Lindop, M. J., Phillips, G. D. and Strickland, D. A. P. (1973), "Valsalva Responses and Systolic Time Intervals During Anaesthesia and Induced Hypotension," *Brit. J. Anaesth.* (in press).

Blinks, J. R. (1967), "Editorial," *Anesthesiology*, **28**, 800.

Herman, M. V. and Gorlin, R. (1969), "Implications of Left Ventricular Asynergy," *Amer. J. Cardiol.*, **23**, 538.

Noble, M. I. M., Trenchard, D. and Guz, A. (1966), "Left Ventricular Ejection in Conscious Dogs," *Circulat. Research*, **19**, 139.

Prys-Roberts, C., Gersh, B. J., Baker, A. B. and Reuben, S. R. (1972), "The Effects of Halothane on the Interactions between Myocardial Contractility, Aortic Impedance, and Left Ventricular Performance. I: Theoretical Considerations and Results," *Brit. J. Anaesth.*, **44**, 634.

Reitan, J. A., Smith, N. T., Borison, S. and Kadis, L. (1972), "The Cardiac Pre-ejection Period: A Correlate of Peak Ascending Aortic Blood Flow Acceleration," *Anesthesiology*, **36**, 76.

Weissler, A. M., Harris, W. S. and Schoenfeld, C. D. (1969), "Bedside Technics for the Evaluation of Ventricular Function in Man," *Am. J. Cardiol.*, **23**, 577.

*The following are recommended for further reading and reference material:—*

Eisele, J. H., Trenchard, D., Stubbs, J. and Guz, A. (1969), "The Immediate Cardiac Depression by Anaesthetics in Conscious Dogs," *Brit. J. Anaesth.*, **41**, 86.

Guyton, A. C. (1968), "Regulation of Cardiac Output," *Anesthesiology*, **29**, 314.

Linden, R. J. (1968), "The Heart-ventricular Function," *Anaesthesia*, **23**, 566.

Shimosato, S. and Etsten, B. E. (1971), "The Effects of Anesthetic Drugs on the Heart: A Critical Review of Myocardial Contractility and its Relationship to Hemodynamics," pp. 17–72 in *Clinical Anaesthesia: A Decade of Clinical of Progress*. L. Fabian Ed. Oxford: Blackwell.

Siegel, J. H. (1969), "The Myocardial Contractile State and its Role in the Response to Anesthesia and Surgery," *Anesthesiology*, **30**, 519.

*Symposium on Ventricular Function:* "Clinical Applications Based on New Understandings of Pathophysiology." D. T. Mason and B. L. Segal, Eds. (1969), *Am. J. Cardiol.*, **23**, 485–583.

*CHAPTER 2*

# THE METABOLIC REGULATION OF CIRCULATORY TRANSPORT

## C. PRYS-ROBERTS

The prime function of the cardiovascular system is the transport of the substrates and metabolites of cellular respiration. The regulatory mechanisms of the system are organized to maintain adequate blood flow through the tissue capillaries for this purpose. In normal healthy man, the cardiovascular system is characterized by its ability to adapt rapidly to alterations in tissue metabolism, and to maintain preferential blood flow to those tissues or organs whose need is greatest in relation to function. The co-ordination of cardiac and peripheral vascular activity necessary for such adaptation depends on the complex interplay of local factors and the adjustments of vascular tone induced by the autonomic nervous system. This chapter deals with those aspects of cardiovascular performance and regulation which are disturbed by the induction, maintenance and recovery from anaesthesia. Emphasis will be laid on the role of tissue oxygen demand in the regulation of the circulation and, in particular the failure of oxygen supply in relation to this demand consequent on depressed cardiovascular function.

## Circulatory Regulation

### Local regulation of tissue blood flow

Local circulatory control mechanisms may be visualized as providing optimal exchange function between the blood and the interstitial fluid, their effects being achieved by adaptation of regional blood supply, and by alteration of the distribution of capillary blood flow. Primarily, these local mechanisms promote increased flow to those tissues where metabolism is increased, but may also exert a protective influence against the effects on the tissues of undesirable circulatory changes. They may be a stabilizing influence in maintaining constant flow in the face of variations of perfusion pressure (metabolic autoregulation). The latter is of special importance in relation to cerebral blood flow (*see* Chapter 4). Of the numerous factors which appear to be involved in such local control, the influence of mechanical stretch (transmural pressure changes) and alterations of chemical environment on myogenic activity appear to predominate. The former is outside the scope of this discussion, but is well covered in the review by Mellander and Johansson (1968).

Functional hyperaemia in a tissue is intimately related to local chemical factors, of which oxygen lack and accumulation of metabolites are most important. Specific vasodilator metabolites play some part in blood flow regulation in certain organs; for instance, adenosine nucleotides in relation to coronary blood flow (Berne, 1964) and bradykinins in sweat and salivary glands (Hilton and Lewis, 1956). However, the absence of a universally distributed 'vasodilator transmitter' emphasizes the role of oxygen

lack as the predominant agency mediating vasodilator activity. That oxygen lack alone can produce depression of myogenic activity in blood vessels has been shown by Guyton *et al.* (1964), Ross *et al.* (1964) and by Skinner and Powell (1967). The latter authors emphasized the additive effects of raised plasma potassium levels in association with oxygen lack in causing dilation of the pre-capillary resistance vessels, thus reinforcing the hypothesis of Dawes (1941) and Kjellmer (1965a). Increased carbon dioxide tensions, and the metabolites of anaerobic glycolysis also exert vasodilator activity on the pre-capillary resistance vessels, but their influence is quantitatively much weaker than that of oxygen lack (Kjellmer, 1965b). Alterations of carbon-dioxide tensions are particularly active in the control of the cerebral and splanchnic segments of the circulation.

### Neurogenic Circulatory Regulation

The efferent nerve impulses in the sympathetic and parasympathetic systems, which mediate cardiac and peripheral vascular control, arise from bilateral neuronal systems extending from the cerebral cortex to the spinal cord (Peiss, 1964). Efferent activity in these neuronal systems is modulated by afferent information reaching the cerebral cortex and the vasomotor centres of the hypothalamus and medulla from somatic and visceral sensory nerve endings. The influence of somatic sensory information from exteroceptors (pain, temperature) and proprioceptors (muscle spindles), and from special sense organs (auditory, visual and olfactory stimuli) is largely mediated through alterations in the 'arousal' of the cortex and higher cerebral centres. Vasoactive reflexes mediated through medullary and mid-brain centres arise from intravascular sensory mechanoreceptors (baroreceptors) and chemoreceptors and their afferent nerves (Heymans and Neil, 1958; Folkow, Heymans and Neil, 1965). They are primarily concerned with the fine adjustments of vascular tone necessary to maintain optimal resistance to blood flow throughout the whole cardiovascular system. These adjustments are generated from 'pressor' and 'depressor' zones located respectively in the lateral (facilitatory) and medial (inhibitory) descending reticular formations (Wang, 1964). Pressor activity causes neurogenic vasoconstriction of both arterial and venous segments, cardioacceleration, and augmented myocardial contractility, whereas activation of the depressor zones results in cardiac slowing, but not vascular dilatation. Peripheral vascular dilatation is generally mediated by inhibition of 'pressor' activity, the major exception being resistance vessels in muscles which are actively dilated by cholinergic sympathetic fibres (Uvnäs, 1960; Wang, 1964).

## Integration of Neurogenic and Local Control Mechanisms

Local regulation of blood flow may be regarded as serving the interests of each individual organ or tissue, whereas the neurogenic reflex mechanisms subserve the interests of the animal as a whole. The circulatory adjustments which arise from the cortico-hypothalamic areas invoke immediate enhancement of cardiac rate and contractile force, constriction of most vascular beds, but active dilatation of the resistance vessels in skeletal muscle. Such vasodilatation is augmented locally by the production of heat and metabolites which suppress the neurogenic constrictor influence on some pre-capillary sphincters. Such combined mechanisms are admirably suited to accompany sudden, widespread muscular activity, and apply to the onset of muscular exercise as much as to the general 'alarm' reactions involved in fight and flight (Abrahams, Hilton and Zbrozyna, 1960).

In general, neurogenic control of pre-capillary resistance vessels is relatively ineffective if the vessels are exposed to the dilator actions of oxygen lack, carbon dioxide excess and metabolites (Kjellmer, 1965b), whereas the post-capillary resistance and capacitance vessels are predominantly sensitive to neurogenic control, particularly at low levels of sympathetic activity (Mellander, 1960; Folkow, Heymans and Neil, 1965). The competitive influence of neurogenic constrictor and local chemical dilator mechanisms may be exemplified by the responses to haemorrhage (Mellander and Johansson, 1968). Early in the course of haemorrhage, all consecutive vascular sections are constricted, and in particular, muscle blood flow which may fall to an extent that causes the accumulation of anaerobic metabolites. As the accumulation continues, the dilator effect of these metabolites predominates over the neurogenic control of the pre-capillary and sphincter resistance sections. Since the post-capillary resistance sections are relatively unaffected by metabolites and oxygen lack, and remain constricted, transcapillary pressure increases from within and fluid is lost from the plasma into the interstitial fluid space (Lundgren, Lundvall and Mellander, 1964). The beneficial effects attributed to alpha-adrenergic blocking therapy in haemorrhagic shock (Nickerson, 1963) may be explained on the basis of a reversal or reduction of this loss by inhibiting vasoconstriction in the post-capillary sections.

## Circulatory Transport in Relation to Metabolism

When cellular activity is increased in a large mass of tissue it induces functional hyperaemia. The resulting changes in general haemodynamics are likely to be profound. Cardiovascular adaptation to increased metabolism has been extensively reviewed by Grande and Taylor (1965) and they have given prominence to the relationship between cardiac ouput (and its determinants, heart rate and stroke volume) and work-load and oxygen uptake. The significance of this relationship may not appear to be connected with anaesthesia, but a consideration of the consequences of cardiovascular depression or excitation by anaesthetic agents or techniques cannot be complete without reference to it.

## Cardiac Output and Oxygen Consumption

The output of the heart should not be considered purely as a 'driving force' of blood flowing to the tissues, but more as the sum of all the autoregulated flows through each tissue or organ in the body, the performance of the heart as a pump being influenced as much by its load (the vascular impedance) as by agencies acting on the myocardium. In this respect, the primary variations related to metabolic demand are those of changes in the calibre of peripheral arterioles, and these are reflected back as changes in left ventricular load. Changes in ventricular performance are secondary to regulatory mechanisms discussed earlier.

It is well established that cardiac output is closely related to the total body oxygen consumption, both at rest and during exercise. It is also worth emphasizing that the body oxygen stores are meagre, and thus tissue oxygen consumption must equal the pulmonary uptake of oxygen except for transient periods in which an oxygen 'debt' may be built up. Resting or 'basal' conditions are both difficult to define and achieve in man, and within any well-defined segment of the population, a wide range of values of cardiac output and oxygen uptake have been described. It is recognized that resting cardiac output is related to the subject's age (Brandfonbrener, Landowne and Shock, 1955) and lean body mass (Schröder et al., 1966) to a much greater degree than to surface area, and that the relation to weight$^{0.66}$ permits a better correlation between different species, both large and small (Guyton, 1963). Based on this relation (Fig. 1), we might expect the standard actuarial male (45 years old and weighing about 70 kg) to have a cardiac output of 5·6 litres/minute (cardiac index of 3·4 litres/minute/m²), both values being marginally higher than those predicted by Guyton (1963).

A similar relation holds for oxygen consumption (uptake), and from the predictions of Boothby, Berkson and Dunn (1936); it can be calculated from the Fick relation that such a hypothetical individual would have an arterio-venous oxygen-content difference ($Ca_{O_2}-C\bar{v}_{O_2}$) of about 4·15 ml/100 ml. This value agrees well with the mean value of 4·25 ml/100 ml derived from 17 sources in the literature (Prys-Roberts, 1968a). It is clear that the inter-relation of cardiac output, oxygen uptake and $Ca_{O_2}-C\bar{v}_{O_2}$ are tightly constrained in the resting state throughout life (Fig. 2). A number of factors may cause a deviation from this normal state, of which varying degrees of exercise constitute the most common events in everyday life. A number of studies have been carried out to determine the relation between cardiac output and oxygen uptake in normal, young and old, trained and untrained subjects of different sizes and occupation. The range of the exercise response is also shown in Fig. 2, from which it will be apparent that as oxygen uptake increases with work load, the reduced availability of oxygen consequent on the progressive failure of the heart to maintain its output to meet the demand, is reflected in the increased capillary extraction of oxygen and increased $Ca_{O_2}-C\bar{v}_{O_2}$. The exercise capability is limited by the extent of the extraction which can occur, and is particularly limited by the haemoglobin concentration and thus the oxygen capacity.

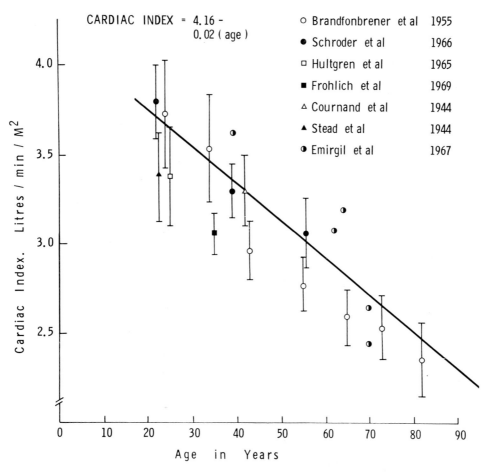

FIG. 1. Relation between cardiac index (litres/minute/m²) and age.
Based on data from:
○ Brandfonbrener, Landowne and Shock (1955).
● Schröder, Dissmann, Kauder and Schüren (1966).
▲ Stead, Warren, Merrill and Brannon (1944).
△ Cournand, Riley, Breed, Baldwin and Richards (1944).
◑ Emirgil, Sobol, Campodonico, Herbert and Mechkati (1967).
■ Frohlich, Tarazi and Dustan (1969).

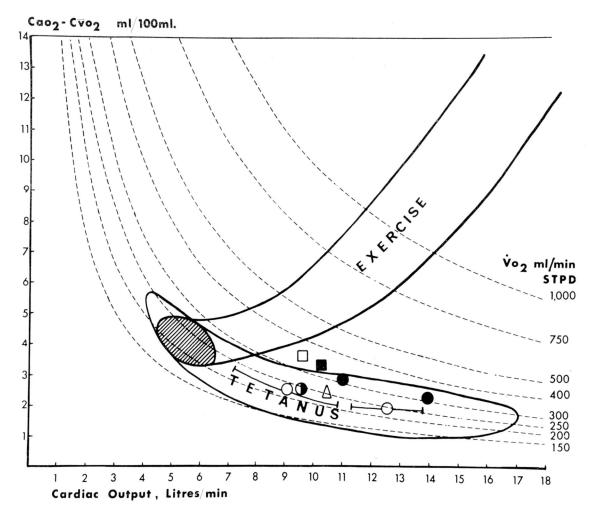

FIG. 2. Relation between cardiac output and arteriovenous $O_2$ content difference ($Ca_{O_2} - C\bar{v}_{O_2}$) at various values of oxygen uptake ($V_{O_2}$). The hatched area, representing the range of normal values in resting man, and the band representing the relationship to exercise in normal man, are derived from the data of numerous authors (tabulated in Prys-Roberts, 1968a). A number of disease states in which cardiac output is excessive in relation to metabolic demand is typified by the relation in patients with tetanus (data from Corbett, Kerr, Prys-Roberts, Smith and Spalding, 1969). Other symbols denote the relation in:

*Chronic Anaemia.*

—○—⊣  Brannon, Merrill, Warren and Stead (1944). Left hand symbol represents patients with Hb concentration 5–9 gm/100 ml, right hand symbol Hb < 5 gm/100 ml.

● Roy, Bhatia, Mathur and Virmani (1963). Right hand symbol: Hb = 4·5 gm/100 ml, Left hand symbol: Hb = 3 gm/100 ml.

○ Wade and Bishop (1962).

△ Leight, Snider, Clifford and Hellems (1954): data from patients with sickle cell anaemia.

*Hyperthyroidism.*

□ Theilen, Wilson and Tutunji (1963).

■ Wade and Bishop (1962).

Reduction of oxygen capacity in the form of chronic anaemia is associated with markedly increased cardiac output, but although $Ca_{O_2}-C\bar{v}_{O_2}$ is reduced at rest (Fig. 2), the availability of oxygen ($Ca_{O_2}$ × Cardiac Output) to the tissues may be compromised despite the marked increase in cardiac output which occurs. Reduction of haemoglobin concentration to less than 5 gm/100 ml may cause a 100 per cent increase of cardiac output at rest in both iron-deficiency anaemia (Brannon, Merrill, Warren and Stead, 1944; Roy, Bhatia, Mathur and Virmani, 1963) and sickle cell anaemia (Leight, Snider, Clifford and Hellems, 1954). Hypermetabolic states such as hyperthyroidism are also associated with increased cardia coutput and low $Ca_{O_2}-C\bar{v}_{O_2}$ at rest (Fig. 2), but recent evidence suggests that the hyperdynamic circulatory state is caused by increased sympathetic nervous activity (Mazzaferri and Skillman, 1969). A similar situation may occur in certain patients with severe tetanus, who also show other signs of sympathetic overactivity (Corbett, Kerr, Prys-Roberts, Smith and Spalding, 1969). Functional hyperaemia induced by experimental focal limb sepsis, and by septic shock, may cause a 50 per cent increase of cardiac output, but only 12 per cent increase in total body oxygen uptake (Hermreck and Thal, 1969).

## Anaesthesia

Total body oxygen uptake is reduced by general anaesthesia, though estimates of degree vary widely according to the method of measurement, age and size of the subject and the nature and depth of anaesthesia. Oxygen uptake falls by between 15 and 25 per cent of the predicted basal value following induction of anaesthesia, and remains at this level throughout anaesthesia (Severinghaus and Cullen, 1958; Nunn and Matthews, 1959; Theye and Tuohy, 1964; Prys-Roberts et al., 1968; Marshall et al., 1969; Cullen et al., 1969). Increasing the inspired concentration of halothane from 0·8 per cent to 2·5 per cent caused a 17 per cent decrease of oxygen uptake (Theye and Sessler, 1967). Allocating the distribution of the overall reduction of oxygen consumption is difficult since estimates differ widely, depending on whether studies were performed in vitro or in vivo. Fink and his colleagues (1969) have observed that rat heteroploid cells in vitro reduce their oxygen consumption by nearly 50 per cent in response to a number of anaesthetic agents, whereas Matteo and his colleagues (1969) found a great variation in the response of brain, heart and liver slices to different anaesthetic agents. In vivo estimates of cerebral oxygen uptake by a number of authors show a decrease of between 15 and 49 per cent (Theye and Michenfelder, 1969), whereas myocardial oxygen uptake may only be reduced about 5 per cent under halothane anaesthesia (Theye, 1967).

Most anaesthetic agents, administered under controlled conditions, with constant artificial ventilation, cause a reduction of cardiac output, but the changes seen during spontaneous ventilation are dependent on at least one other variable, of which the carbon-dioxide tension of the arterial blood is of importance. The arterio-venous $O_2$-content difference may not vary outside the normal range (3·5–5.0 ml/100 ml), because the reduction of cardiac out-

put is usually commensurate with that of oxygen uptake during spontaneous ventilation or artificial ventilation (Fig. 3) in which arterial $P_{CO_2}$ is maintained within the normal range (Prys-Roberts et al., 1968). During hypercapnia, however, a hyperdynamic circulatory state is maintained as a result of the increased sympathetic activity, although this response may be markedly modified by certain anaesthetic agents. The cardiac output change in response to hypercapnia is attenuated by general anaesthetic agents as compared to that of conscious man, the effects being least marked during anaesthesia with 15–20 per cent cyclopropane (Cullen, Eger and Gregory, 1969), whereas the response during nitrous oxide-relaxant technique lies between that of 'light' cyclopropane anaesthesia and that of halothane (1 per cent inspired) which markedly attenuates the response (Prys-Roberts et al., 1968). During hypercapnia, the reduced $Ca_{O_2}-C\bar{v}_{O_2}$ compared with that during eucapnia, reflects the disproportionately raised cardiac output in relation to the unaltered oxygen uptake, both during artificial and spontaneous ventilation (Fig. 3). Many of the cardiovascular changes observed during halothane anaesthesia with spontaneous ventilation, such as unaltered or raised cardiac output, reduced systemic vascular resistance and skin vasodilatation (Johnstone, 1956; Wyant et al., 1958; Payne, Gardiner and Verner, 1959) should more correctly be attributed to the varying degree of hypercapnia which inevitably ensues (Larson et al., 1969). The sympathetic stimulatory effects of hypercapnia counteract, to some degree, the myocardial depressant effects of halothane and many other agents, and undoubtedly contribute to the maintenance of adequate cardiovascular function during halothane anaesthesia with spontaneous ventilation.

Hypocapnia induced by passive alveolar hyperventilation during anaesthesia has the opposite effects to those of hypercapnia, although here again, the effects are modified by the anaesthetic agents and techniques used, and especially the age and physical state of the patient. During anaesthesia with either the nitrous oxide-relaxant technique or with halothane, cardiac output is significantly reduced during hypocapnia, although arterial pressure does not fall to a commensurate degree (Prys-Roberts et al., 1967; Prys-Roberts et al., 1968); whereas the effect is minimal in the conscious subject and during anaesthesia with 20 per cent cyclopropane, but marked during anaesthesia with 25–30 per cent cyclopropane (Cullen, Eger and Gregory, 1969). The reduction of cardiac output during hypocapnia is not due to depressed myocardial function (Ng et al., 1967), nor to reduced sympathetic nervous activity (Moster et al., 1969). Under the influence of a local reduction of $P_{CO_2}$, the resistance vessels constrict in most vascular compartments, thus there is an increase in systemic vascular resistance (Prys-Roberts et al., 1967, 1968). If cardiac output is maintained against a raised resistance, then arterial pressure must rise, and baroreflex activity increases in the afferent limb, and inhibits central sympathetic drive. Since the resistance vessels remain constricted due to the local effects of low $CO_2$, inhibition of peripheral vascular sympathetic tone has little effect, and the main inhibitory response is directed through the cardiac

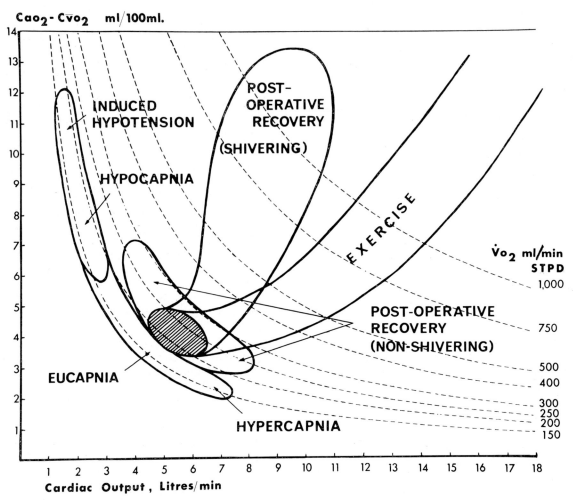

FIG. 3. Relation between cardiac output, oxygen uptake ($\dot{V}o_2$) and $Cao_2 - C\bar{v}o_2$ during various aspects of anaesthesia. The normal range (hatched area) and the band representing the relation during exercise are as in Fig. 2. The relation during anaesthesia with 1 per cent halothane in oxygen is shown by the left hand enclosure (data from Prys-Roberts, Kelman, Greenbaum, Kain and Bay, 1968). The enclosure covers the relation during spontaneous ventilation (eucapnia) and artificial ventilation over a $Pa_{CO_2}$ range from 16–26 mmHg (hypocapnia), through 36–48 mmHg (eucpania) to 52–84 mmHg (hypercapnia). The induced hypotension enclosure merges with that for hypocapnia, the data are from Prys-Roberts, Lloyd, Kerr and Patterson (in preparation). The post-operative recovery enclosures show the responses of non-shivering and shivering patients described by Bay, Nunn and Prys-Roberts (1968). The circulatory response during shivering lies well to the left of the normal response to increased metabolic demand during exercise, from which we imply that cardiac function is depressed not only at rest but also in a stress situation.

sympathetic nerves. Reduction of stroke volume occurs, not specifically because of the reduced adrenergic augmentation of contractility, but because the ejection of blood from the ventricle cannot be maintained against a raised resistance unless myocardial contractile force is augmented by adrenergic activation or an increase in the left ventricle end-diastolic pressure causes an increased force of contraction by the Frank-Starling mechanism. The heart rate does not change significantly during hypocapnia, which is in keeping with the findings of Bristow *et al.* (1969) that the baroreflex control of heart rate is markedly attenuated by anaesthesia. Due to the shift in the oxygen dissociation curve the actual availability of oxygen may be reduced during hypocapnia caused by passive hyperventilation despite the enhanced uptake of oxygen by the blood. This is reflected in the increased $Ca_{O_2}$–$C\bar{v}_{O_2}$ (Fig. 3). There is no reason to believe that the increased oxygen extraction during hypocapnia is in any way harmful, unless the fall in cardiac output is so great, as it may be in the elderly, that it may jeopardize the perfusion of vital organs.

### Deliberate Hypotension

Although this subject is dealt with in detail in a later chapter (Chapter 6), the effect of deliberate hypotension on the relation between cardiac output and oxygen uptake deserves mention at this point. No causal relationship has been established between the fortuitous reduction of cardiac output to a degree which is commensurate with the fall of oxygen uptake during light anaesthesia, but it is axiomatic that if cardiac output is disproportionately reduced in relation to oxygen uptake, then increased extraction of oxygen at the tissue capillaries must occur, with the consequent desaturation of mixed venous blood. The use of high concentrations of halothane (1–4 per cent inspired) together with intermittent positive pressure ventilation (IPPV) is very successful in producing arterial hypotension, but does so at the cost of reducing cardiac output by myocardial depression without significant change in vascular resistance (Prys-Roberts, Lloyd, Kerr and Patterson, in preparation). Under these conditions, the desaturation of mixed venous and jugular venous blood may be severe (Fig. 3). The lowest values indicate that despite the use of high inspired oxygen concentrations, the supply of oxygen is barely adequate for the needs of the body. When arterial hypotension is induced with ganglion blocking-agents (e.g. trimetaphan or hexamethonium), cardiac output will be better maintained, and the values of $Ca_{O_2}$–$C\bar{v}_{O_2}$ tend to remain within the normal range. The addition of low concentrations of halothane (0·5 per cent to 1 per cent) to the inspired gas mixture in ganglion-blocked patients impairs the oxygen transport much less than that caused by hypotension induced with halothane alone.

### Recovery from Anaesthesia

During emergence from anaesthesia, total body-oxygen uptake returns rapidly to levels which are not significantly different from the predicted basal values for individual patients (Bay, Nunn and Prys-Roberts, 1968). Two pat-terns of ventilatory and circulatory response can be elicited during this recovery period, the first characterized by an increase in both ventilation and cardiac output in response to the moderate increase in metabolic rate. Blood gas tensions and $Ca_{O_2}$–$C\bar{v}_{O_2}$ remain within normal limits under these conditions. The second pattern is characterized by a failure of either ventilation or cardiac output, or both, to increase in response to the metabolic demand, thus $Ca_{O_2}$–$C\bar{v}_{O_2}$ remains high and mild arterial hypoxaemia may occur without significant atelectasis or marked ventilation/perfusion abnormalities (Prys-Roberts, 1968b). The second response is especially likely to occur in elderly patients (Renck, 1969) but does not occur in patients receiving antihypertensive drugs (Prys-Roberts, Meloche and Foëx, 1971). Although heart rate may increase to pre-anaesthetic levels, stroke volume lags behind, and since right ventricular end-diastolic pressures are not unduly low, and are occasionally raised, it may be assumed that the decreased stroke volumes reflect decreased myocardial contractility. This hypodynamic response is unlikely to jeopardize the patient's safety during this period, since with normal levels of oxygen uptake the reserve of oxygen extraction available is more than enough to compensate for the decreased oxygen availability (cardiac output × arterial $O_2$ content).

Post-operative shivering may increase oxygen uptake to levels found during exercise. This may occur after almost any technique or combination of agents for general anaesthesia, and is not specifically related to alterations of body temperature during and after anaesthesia (Prys-Roberts, 1968b). Overt shivering, rigidity and clonic movements occur frequently following anaesthesia, and there is a general impression which is not supported by reliable data that its incidence is higher after the use of halothane. Shivering causes a marked increase in total oxygen uptake at an early stage of emergence, usually between 15 and 30 minutes after withdrawal of anaesthesia, and metabolism may be increased to between 300 and 600 per cent of the predicted basal level (Bay, Nunn and Prys-Roberts, 1968). A paradoxical cardiovascular response to this demand usually develops, since although cardiac output may be increased to more than double the basal level, the overall blood flow is inadequate to maintain oxygen transport. This hypodynamic response is shown in Fig. 3, and may be prolonged in the older patient. It is likely that the attenuated cardiac response to increased oxygen demand is to some extent due to residual depression of myocardial contractility. This would seem to be inevitable with most anaesthetic agents, but is recognized as being particularly marked after anaesthesia with halothane or methoxyflurane. Full recovery of myocardial contractility in the intact animal may take as long as one hour from the time of withdrawal of 1 per cent halothane anaesthesia, even when rapid pulmonary elimination of the agent is encouraged by maintaining passive hyperventilation (Prys-Roberts, Gersh, Baker and Reuben, 1972). In elderly patients, the author has found evidence of decreased contractility, assessed by measuring the pre-ejection period, and of decreased cardiac output up to 3 hours after withdrawal of anaesthesia.

It has already been stressed that a hypodynamic circulatory state presents no serious danger to the patient who recovers consciousness without shivering, since the compensatory mechanisms for increased oxygen extraction seem to be adequate. When shivering occurs, however, the hypodynamic circulatory response presents a potentially severe hazard to the patient, since the limits of capillary oxygen extraction are rapidly reached, and the dangers of arterial hypoxaemia may go unrecognized because of the marked skin vasoconstriction which occurs during post-operative shivering (Prys-Roberts, 1968b).

in combination, of reduced cardiac output, low haemoglobin concentration, arterial hypoxaemia, and breathing 100 per cent oxygen; these are shown in Table 1.

From the calculations shown in this table, it will be clear that moderate degrees of hypoxaemia do not seriously jeopardize the oxygen availability, nor does their treatment with 100 per cent oxygen breathing make a startling improvement. On the other hand, the combination of preoperative blood loss and a hypodynamic circulation reduces the $O_2$ availability to almost one-half the normal value; the combination of shivering and moderate

TABLE 1

RELATIONSHIPS BETWEEN OXYGEN REQUIREMENTS, OXYGEN AVAILABILITY AND CIRCULATORY TRANSPORT UNDER A VARIETY OF CLINICALLY COMPATIBLE CONDITIONS DURING RECOVERY FROM ANAESTHESIA. THE COMPARISONS ARE MADE AGAINST THE PREDICTED NORMAL VALUES FOR A 45 YEAR OLD, 70kg MAN BREATHING AIR AND 100 PER CENT OXYGEN.

(NS: non-shivering)

| | Insp. gas | Cardiac output l/min | $O_2$ Uptake ml/min | $Ca_{O_2} - C\bar{v}_{O_2}$ ml/100 ml | Hb gm % | $Pa_{O_2}$ mmHg | $Ca_{O_2}$ ml/100 ml | $Sa_{O_2}$ % | Available $O_2$ ml/min | $O_2$ uptake as % of available $O_2$ % |
|---|---|---|---|---|---|---|---|---|---|---|
| Normal | Air | 5·4 | 250 | 4·6 | 14·4 | 90 | 19·4 | 97 | 1,050 | 23·8 |
| Normal | 100% $O_2$ | 5·0 | 250 | 5·0 | 14·4 | 600 | 21·8 | 100 | 1,090 | 22·9 |
| Post-operative (NS) hypoxaemic | Air | 5·4 | 250 | 4·6 | 14·4 | 60 | 18·2 | 91 | 982 | 25·5 |
| Post-operative (NS) hypodynamic | Air | 3·5 | 250 | 7·1 | 14·4 | 90 | 19·4 | 97 | 679 | 36·8 |
| | 100% $O_2$ | 3·5 | 250 | 7·1 | 14·4 | 600 | 21·8 | 100 | 763 | 32·7 |
| Post-operative (NS) Anaemic and hypodynamic | Air | 3·5 | 250 | 7·1 | 11·0 | 90 | 14·8 | 97 | 519 | 48·2 |
| | 100% $O_2$ | 3·5 | 250 | 7·1 | 11·0 | 600 | 17·1 | 100 | 598 | 41·8 |
| Post-operative Shivering Hypodynamic | Air | 10·0 | 1000 | 10·0 | 14·4 | 90 | 19·4 | 97 | 1,940 | 51·5 |
| | 100% $O_2$ | 10·0 | 1000 | 10·0 | 14·4 | 600 | 21·8 | 100 | 2,180 | 46·0 |
| Hypodynamic and hypoxaemic | Air | 10·0 | 1000 | 10·0 | 14·4 | 60 | 18·2 | 91 | 1,820 | 55·0 |

It is perhaps worth placing in its proper perspective, the relative importance of reduced cardiac output (in relation to demand), and arterial oxygen tension measurements in the post-operative period. Much attention has been paid to $Pa_{O_2}$ values of between 50 and 60 mmHg as representing a serious threat to the patient's safety, and yet in terms of available oxygen to the tissues, such a reduction of $Pa_{O_2}$ represents a reduction of oxygen saturation (assuming a normal value of 97 per cent) of not more than 12 per cent. If no change of cardiac output occurred, such a reduction would result in a 12 per cent reduction in the available oxygen; whereas if the patient is maintained on 100 per cent oxygen during the post-operative period, and has a 30 per cent reduction of cardiac output, the available oxygen will also be reduced by 30 per cent. A number of possible variations on this theme have been calculated in order to show the effects, both singly and

hypoxaemia in a patient with a hypodynamic circulatory response to the increased $O_2$ uptake during shivering, reduces the oxygen availability to less than 50 per cent of the normal value. None of these disturbances could have been recognized by routine post-operative observation of the patient, since cyanosis would be unlikely to be obvious under ordinary lighting conditions, and the hypodynamic response could not be interpreted from measurements of blood pressure and heart rate. It is also worth noting that the administration of 100 per cent oxygen, although a step in the right direction, makes an insignificant improvement.

The best single index of inadequate circulatory response under any given circumstances is the measurement of the arterio-venous $O_2$ content difference ($Ca_{O_2} - C\bar{v}_{O_2}$). True mixed venous blood should be sampled only from the right ventricle, or pulmonary artery; but for clinical assessment of the patient, samples from the right atrium or *superior vena cava* are quite satisfactory since the difference in $O_2$ content between blood samples drawn from these sites and those from the pulmonary artery will not be more than 1 ml/100 ml.

## ACKNOWLEDGEMENT

The author wishes to thank the Department of Medical Illustration, Radcliffe Infirmary, Oxford, for preparing the diagrams in this chapter.

## REFERENCES

Abrahams, V. C., Hilton, S. M. and Zbrozyna, A. (1960), "Active Muscle Vasodilatation produced by Stimulation of the Brain Stem: its Significance in the Defence Reaction," *J. Physiol. (Lond.)*, **154**, 491.

Bay, J., Nunn, J. F. and Prys-Roberts, C. (1968), "Factors Influencing Arterial $Po_2$ during Recovery from Anaesthesia," *Brit. J. Anaesth.*, **40**, 398.

Berne, R. M. (1964), "Metabolic Regulation of Blood Flow," *Circulation Res.*, **15**, Supp. I, 261.

Boothby, W. M., Berkson, J. and Dunn, H. L. (1936), "Studies of the Energy of Metabolism of Normal Individuals: A Standard for Basal Metabolism with a Nomogram for Clinical Application," *Amer., J. Physiol.*, **116**, 468.

Brandfonbrener, M., Landowne, M. and Shock, N. W. (1955), "Changes in Cardiac Output with Age," *Circulation*, **12**, 557.

Brannon, E. S., Merrill, A. J., Warren, J. V. and Stead, E. A., Jr. (1944), "The Cardiac Output in Patients with Chronic Anemia as Measured by the Technique of Right Atrial Catheterization," *J. clin. Invest.*, **24**, 332.

Bristow, J. D., Prys-Roberts, C., Fisher, A., Pickering, T. G. and Sleight, P. (1969), "Effects of Anesthesia on Baroreflex Control of Heart Rate in Man," *Anesthesiology*, **31**, 422.

Corbett, J. L., Kerr, J. H., Prys-Roberts, C., Smith, A. C. and Spalding, J. M. K. (1969), "Cardiovascular Disturbances in Severe Tetanus due to Overactivity of the Sympathetic Nervous System," *Anaesthesia*, **24**, 198.

Cournand, A., Riley, R. L., Breed, E. S., Baldwin, E. de F. and Richards, D. W., Jr. (1944), "Measurement of Cardiac Output in Man using the Technique of Catheterization of the Right Auricle or Ventricle," *J. clin. Invest.*, **24**, 106.

Cullen, D. J., Eger, E. I., II., and Gregory, G. A. (1969), "The Cardiovascular Effects of Carbon Dioxide in Man, Conscious and during Cyclopropane Anesthesia," *Anesthesiology*, **31**, 407.

Dawes, G. S. (1941), "The Vasodilator Action of Potassium," *J. Physiol. (Lond.)*, **99**, 224.

Emirgil, C., Sobol, B. J., Campodonico, S., Herbert, W. H. and Mechkati, R, (1967), "Pulmonary Circulation in the Aged," *J. appl. Physiol.*, **23**, 631.

Fink, B. R., Kenny, G. E. and Simpson, W. E. (1969), "Depression of Oxygen Uptake in Cell Culture by Volatile, Barbiturate and Local Anesthetics," *Anesthesiology*, **30**, 150.

Folkow, B., Heymans, C. and Neil, E. (1965), "Integrated Aspects of Cardiovascular Regulation," in *Handbook of Physiology. Circulation*, Sect. 2, Vol. 3, Chapter 49, pp. 1787–1823. Washington, D.C.: Amer. Physiol. Soc.

Frohlich, E. D., Tarazi, R. C. and Dustan, H. P. (1969), "Re-examination of the Hemodynamics of Hypertension," *Amer. J. med. Sci.*, **257**, 9.

Grande, F. and Taylor, H. L. (1965), "Adaptive Changes in the Heart, Vessels, and Patterns of Control under Chronically High Loads," in: *Handbook of Physiology. Circulation*, Sec. 2, Vol 3, Chapter 74, pp. 2615–2677. Washington, D.C.: Amer. Physiol. Soc.

Guyton, A. C. (1963), *Circulatory Physiology: Cardiac output and its regulation*, London: Saunders.

Guyton, A. C., Ross, J. M., Carrier, O. Jr., and Walker, J. R.

(1964), "Evidence for Tissue Oxygen Demand as the Major Factor causing Autoregulation," *Circulation Res.*, **15**, Suppl. 1, 60.

Hermreck, A. S. and Thal, A. P. (1969), "Mechanisms for the High Circulatory Requirements in Sepsis and Septic Shock," *Ann. Surg.*, **170**, 677.

Heymans, C. and Neil, E. (1958), "*Reflexogenic Areas of the Cardiovascular System*," London: Churchill.

Hilton, S. M. and Lewis, G. P. (1956), "The Relationship between Glandular Activity, Bradykinin Formation and Functional Vasodilatation in the Submandibular Salivary Gland," *J. Physiol. (Lond.)*, **134**, 471.

Johnstone, M. (1956), "The Human Cardiovascular Response to Fluothane Anaesthesia," *Brit. J. Anaesth.*, **28**, 392.

Kjellmer, I. (1965a), "On the Competition between Metabolic Vasodilatation and Neurogenic Vasoconstriction in Skeletal Muscle," *Acta physiol. scand.*, **63**, 450.

Kjellmer, I. (1965b), "Studies on exercise hyperaemia," *Acta physiol. scand.*, **64**, Suppl. 224, 1.

Larson, C. P., Jr., Eger, E. I., II., Muallem, M., Buechel, D. R., Munson, E. S. and Eisele, J. H. (1969), "The Effects of Diethyl Ether and Methoxyflurane on Ventilation: II. A comparative study in man," *Anesthesiology*, **30**, 174.

Leight, L., Snider, T. H., Clifford, G. O. and Hellems, H. K. (1954), "Hemodynamic Studies in Sickle Cell Anaemia," *Circulation*, **10**, 653.

Lundgren, O., Lundvall, J. and Mellander, S. (1964), "Range of Sympathetic Discharge and Reflex Adjustments in Skeletal Muscle during Haemorrhagic Hypotension," *Acta physiol. scand.*, **62**, 380.

Marshall, B. E., Cohen, P. J., Klingenmaier, C. H. and Aukberg, S. (1969), "Pulmonary Venous Admixture before, during and after Halothane: Oxygen Anesthesia in Man," *J. appl. Physiol.*, **27**, 653.

Matteo, R. S., Hoech, G. P., Jr. and Hoskin, F. C. G. (1969), "The Effects of Cyclopropane and Diethyl Ether on Tissue Oxygen Consumption and Anaerobic Glycolysis of Brain *in vitro*," *Anesthesiology*, **30**, 156.

Mazzaferri, E. L. and Skillman, T. G. (1969), "Thyroid Storm," *Arch. intern. Med.*, **124**, 684.

Mellander, S. (1960), "Comparative Studies on the Adrenergic Neuro-hormonal Control of Resistance and Capacitance Vessels of the Cat," *Acta physiol. scand.*, Suppl. 176.

Mellander, S. and Johansson, B. (1968), "Control of Resistance, Exchange, and Capacitance Functions in the Peripheral Circulation," *Pharamacol Rev.*, **20**, 117.

Moster, W. G., Reier, G. E., Gardier, R. W. and Hamelberg, W. (1969), "Cardiac Output and Postganglionic Sympathetic Activity during Acute Respiratory Alkalosis," *Anesthesiology*, **31**, 28.

Ng, M. L., Levy, M. N. and Zieske, H. A. (1967), "Effects of Changes in pH and of Carbon Dioxide Tension on Left Ventricular Performance," *Amer. J. Physiol.*, **213**, 115.

Nickerson, M. (1963), "Sympathetic Blockade in the Therapy of Shock," *Amer., J. Cardiol.*, **12**, 619.

Nunn, J. F. and Matthews, R. L. (1959), "Gaseous Exchange during Halothane Anaesthesia: the Steady Respiratory State," *Brit. J. Anaesth.*, **31**, 330.

Payne, J. P., Gardiner, D. and Verner, I. R. (1959), "Cardiac Output during Halothane Anaesthesia," *Brit. J. Anaesth.*, **31**, 87.

Peiss, C. N. (1964), "Supramedullary Cardiovascular Regulation," in: *Effects of Anesthetics on the Circulation*, Eds. Price, H. L. and Cohen, P. J. Springfield: C. C. Thomas.

Prys-Roberts, C. (1968a), "Some Physiological Effects of Artificial Ventilation during Anaesthesia," Ph.D. Thesis, University of Leeds.

Prys-Roberts, C. (1968b), "Post-anesthetic Shivering," in: *Common and uncommon problems in anesthesiology*, Ed. Jenkins, M. T. Clinical Anesthesia Series 3/1968. Philadelphia: F. A. Davis.

Prys-Roberts, C., Meloche, R. and Foëx, P. (1971), "Studies of anaesthesia in relation to hypertension. 1. Cardiovascular responses of treated and untreated patients," *Brit. J. Anaesth.*, **43**, 122.

Prys-Roberts, C., Gersh, B. J., Baker, A. B. and Reuben, S. R. (1972), "The effects of halothane on the interactions between myocardial contractility, aortic impedance and left ventricular performance. 1. Theoretical considerations and results." *Brit. J. Anaesth.*, **44**, July issue in the press.

Prys-Roberts, C., Kelman, G. R., Greenbaum, R. and Robinson, R. H. (1967), "Circulatory Influences of Artificial Ventilation during Nitrous Oxide Anaesthesia in Man. II. Results: The relative influence of mean intrathoracic pressure and arterial carbon dioxide tension," *Brit. J. Anaesth.*, **39**, 533.

Prys-Roberts, C., Kelman, G. R., Greenbaum, R., Kain, M. L. and Bay, J. (1968), "Hemodynamics and Alveolar-arterial $Po_2$ Differences at Varying $Pa_{CO_2}$ in Anesthetized Man." *J. appl. Physiol.*, **25**, 80.

Renck, H. (1969), "The Elderly Patient after Anaesthesia and Surgery," *Acta anaesth. scand.*, Suppl. 34.

Ross, J., Jr., Kaiser, G. A. and Klocke, F. J. (1964), "Observations on the Role of Diminished Oxygen Tension in the Functional Hyperaemia of Skeletal Muscle," *Circulation Res.*, **15**, 473.

Roy, S. B., Bhatia, M. L., Mathur, V. S. and Virmani, S. (1963), "Hemodynamic Effect of Chronic Severe Anemia," *Circulation*, **28**, 346.

Schröder, R., Dissmann, W., Kauder, H. G. and Schüren, K. P. (1966), "Altersabhängigkeit und Körperbezugsmasse des Herzzeitvolumens mit einem Beitrag zur Methodik der Farbstoffverdünnungskurven," *Klin. Wschr.*, **44**, 753.

Severinghaus, J. W. and Cullen, S. C. (1958), "Depression of Myocardium and Body Oxygen Consumption with Fluothane," *Anesthesiology*, **19**, 165.

Skinner, N. S., Jr. and Powell, W. J., Jr. (1967), "Action of Oxygen and Potassium on Vascular Resistance of Dog Skeletal Muscle," *Amer. J. Physiol.*, **212**, 533.

Stead, E. A., Jr., Warren, J. V., Merrill, A. J. and Brannon, E. S. (1944), "The Cardiac Output in Male Subjects as Measured by the Technique of Right Atrial Catheterization: Normal values with observations on the effect of anxiety and tilting," *J. clin. Invest.*, **24**, 326.

Theilen, E. O., Wilson, W. R. and Tutunji, F. J. (1963), "The Acute Hemodynamic Effects of Alpha-methyldopa in Thyrotoxic Patients and Normal Subjects," *Metabolism*, **12**, 625.

Theye, R. A. (1967), "Myocardial and Total Oxygen Consumption with Halothane," *Anesthesiology*, **28**, 1042.

Theye, R. A. and Michenfelder, J. D. (1968), "The Effect of Halothane on Canine Cerebral Metabolism," *Anesthesiology*, **29**, 1113.

Theye, R. A. and Sessler, A. D. (1967), "Effect of Halothane Anesthesia on Rate of Canine Oxygen Consumption," *Anesthesiology*, **28**, 661.

Theye, R. A. and Tuohy, G. F. (1964), "Oxygen Uptake during Light Halothane Anesthesia in Man," *Anesthesiology*, **25**, 627.

Uvnäs, B. (1960), "Central Cardiovascular Control," in: *Handbook of Physiology. Neurophysiology*, Sect. 1, Vol 2, Chapter 44, pp. 1131–1162. Washington, D.C.: Amer. Physiol. Soc.

Wade, O. L. and Bishop, J. M. (1962), *Cardiac Output and Regional Blood Flow*, Oxford: Blackwell.

Wang, S. C. (1964), "Bulbar Regulatory Mechanisms," in: *Effects of Anesthetics on the Circulation*, Eds. Price, H. L. and Cohen, P. J. Springfield: C. C. Thomas.

Wyant, G. M., Merriman, J. E., Kilduff, C. J. and Thomas, E. T. (1958), "The Cardiovascular Effects of Halothane," *Canad. Anaesth. Soc. J.*, **5**, 384.

CHAPTER 3

# THE PULMONARY CIRCULATION

JULIAN M. LEIGH

## Introduction

Volatile anaesthetic agents gain access to the circulating blood through the media of the respiratory gases, the alveoli and the pulmonary capillary blood flow. The anaesthestist relies upon this, sometimes for induction but mostly for the maintenance of anaesthesia in the modern 'anaesthetic sequence'. At the same time he fulfils his responsibilities to the patient by ensuring gaseous homeostasis via the same route. For these reasons the pulmonary circulation is an important area for his interest.

The existence of the pulmonary circulation was an essential feature of William Harvey's postulations on the unidirectional circulation of the blood (1628). In 1669 Richard Lower in 'Tractatus de Corde' described how venous blood became arterialized in traversing the lungs and that the absorption of a vital chemical from the air was involved. In 1868 Adolph Fick at a meeting of the Physical-medical association of Wurzburg theorized on the determination of stroke volume, based upon the exchange of the respiratory gases and their arterio-venous content difference. The figure which he arrived at was 77 cc per beat and thus a cardiac output or pulmonary blood flow of 4·9 litres per minute.

## General Features of the Pulmonary Circulation

The pulmonary circulation is unique among the regional circulations in that it is in series rather than in parallel. The right ventricular output passes through one capillary bed but the left ventricular output becomes subdivided to pass through several capillary networks which are in parallel with each other. It is also unique in that it has its own heart pump, the right ventricle.

The pulmonary vessels can be seen on a plain chest film and are responsible for most of the markings in the lung fields. Under conditions of a very high pulmonary blood flow these markings are more pronounced. The opposite, i.e., a paucity of markings, is seen where there is a low pulmonary blood flow.

The pulmonary circuit is a low resistance and therefore a low pressure system in contrast to the systemic circulation, which has a resistance about ten times as high. The systemic circuit has a higher systolic pressure than the pulmonary circuit, that is 120 mmHg compared to 20 mmHg systolic. The mean capillary pressure in the systemic circulation is about 20 mmHg whereas in the pulmonary circulation it is about 10 mmHg and is pulsatile. The systemic circulation contains twice as much blood as the pulmonary. The pulmonary capillary blood volume is about 60–100 cc and the capillary transit time varies from about 1 sec down to about 0·4 seconds depending upon cardiac output.

The cardiac output subserves the demands of the systemic organs and is regulated by the venous return volume and the Starling mechanism. Since the pulmonary circuit is in series, the flow through it is modified at the same time. As an average size adult the cardiac output in health can vary from about 3 litres per minute during sleep to 25 litres or more per minute during exercise, the pulmonary circuit must cope with these flows firstly without disturbing its function and secondly without overloading its heart pump. The resistance in the system is kept down under conditions of high flow due to its high compliance. The latter results from the distensibility of the large vessels, by dilatation of already opened capillaries and by recruitment of hitherto unopened capillaries.

The function of the pulmonary circulation is the exchange of respiratory gases according to their tension gradient with the alveolar gas. In this way something like 360 litres of oxygen are exchanged for 288 litres of carbon dioxide in a single day. The pulmonary capillaries and their accompanying 350,000,000 alveoli provide a gas exchange surface of some 70 square metres, that is about 40 times the body surface area. The capillary blood volume is spread out on this area as if in a sheet about 4 microns thick.

It is important that intracapillary blood pressure does not exceed the osmotic pressure of the plasma proteins lest transudation of plasma and pulmonary oedema ensue. The mean capillary blood pressure in the pumonary circuit is of the order of 10 mmHg and is much lower than the plasma colloid osmotic pressure of about 25 mmHg. This large gradient between intrapulmonary capillary pressure and the osmotic pressure is highly important in keeping the lung dry for proper function.

The demonstration of arterio-venous anastomoses within the lungs has been achieved by a variety of workers but not always confirmed by others. (Liebow 1962, Tobin, 1966). It would be surprising if they did not exist since a–v anastomoses are an important feature of other circulations. Their possible role in the lung could be to by-pass a high flow load away from the capillaries, i.e., to relieve what would otherwise be an excessive pressure load on them.

The low resistance characteristics of the pulmonary circuit are reflected in the structure of its different elements. The right ventricle is one third the thickness of the left ventricle, reflecting its lower work load. The main pulmonary arteries are elastic conducting vessels only about twice as thick as the venae cavae and one third the thickness of the aorta. The muscular pulmonary arteries range from 1,000–100 microns in diameter and are characterized by circularly orientated smooth muscle between two elastic laminae. In the systemic arteries muscularization occurs at a much larger diameter. Pulmonary arterioles are vessels of less than 100 microns diameter, the walls consist of a single elastic lamina and an endothelial lining.

There is no muscular media except at the origin from the parent artery. The pulmonary capillaries are about 4 microns in diameter. The walls or septa between alveoli consist of capillary endothelium and alveolar epithelium.

### Vasomotor Control in the Pulmonary Circulation

Experimental stimulation and pharmacologic challenges are capable of demonstrating vasomotor reactions in the pulmonary circuit. The presence of pulmonary vasomotor nerves is undisputed but their importance under physiological conditions is difficult to assess. This is especially so since all the distributional characteristics of the pulmonary bed are present in the denervated lung of the adrenalectomized animal and also in the completely isolated but perfused lung. The particular features of interest are: *the autoregulation of flow at alveolar level by oxygen tension and the passive hydrostatic effects of gravity on pulmonary blood flow.*

### The effect of oxygen

In 1946 Von Euler and Liljestrand demonstrated that alveolar hypoxia caused a rise in pulmonary artery pressure in the cat. This response to hypoxia is enhanced by extra-cellular acidosis and by hypercapnia. The characteristic response of muscular pulmonary arteries to alveolar hypoxia is thus to *constrict*. This is important at the local level since the mechanism will divert perfusion to better ventilated alveoli without a rise in main pulmonary artery pressure. However, when alveolar hypoxia is generalized and continuous as it is in the permanent inhabitants of the high altitude situation these, whether animals or man, suffer a state of chronic pulmonary hypertension with hypertrophy of the muscular pulmonary arteries and the right ventricle. A state which is amenable to reversal by oxygen therapy or return to low altitude. The arterial constriction associated with alveolar hypoxia raises two questions. Firstly, as the arteries are proximal to the capillaries, how can they 'sense' the change in oxygen tension? And secondly, how is it that hypoxia which is a dilator of systemic arteries causes constriction of pulmonary arteries?

Firstly, it is apparent from the thin walls of the small arteries and veins that they could participate in gas exchange. That alveolar gas does indeed penetrate into quite large arteries has been demonstrated in the most elegant manner by Sobol and his colleagues (1963) Fig. 1.

If a breath of hydrogen is taken, it gets into the blood stream and travels round the circulation producing an acute change in potential as it passes. This can be sensed by a platinum tipped hydrogen sensitive electrode. In this particular experiment a double lumen catheter with a hydrogen electrode at its tip and another one 4 cm proximally was passed through the right heart to a wedged position in the pulmonary artery. The hydrogen electrode at the tip is giving the output 'PC' and the one 4 cm proximally the output PA, confirmed by the pressure tracings in the top right hand corner of the figure. A third hydrogen electrode was placed in the brachial artery-BA. The time lines are one second apart. At the arrow a breath of hydrogen was taken. Not only did the inhaled hydrogen appear at the wedged position within 2 seconds but it also appeared virtually at the same time,

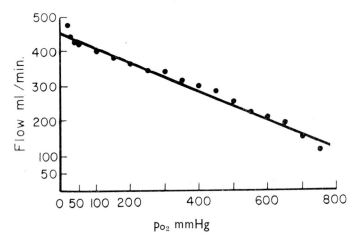

Fig. 2. From Assali *et al.* (1963). The negative correlation between the flow permitted by the isolated lamb ductus arteriosus (ordinate) and the oxygen tension of the perfusate (abscissa).

at the pulmonary artery electrode. The fact that BA electrode does not register a change in potential for a further 5 seconds shows that there is not sufficient time for the hydrogen to have recirculated. The findings demonstrate that the gas has rapidly penetrated pulmonary arteries of 1·5–3·0 mm in diameter. Since such arteries do contain smooth muscle this is strong evidence that they are directly accessible to alveolar gas and could therefore influence the distribution of blood according to the composition of that gas.

Having demonstrated that the alveolar gases can get

into vessels which can influence distribution it is necessary to consider the problem of the arterial muscle which constricts in the face of hypoxia.

Lundholm and Mohme-Lundholm (1963) believe that the contractile process of systemic vascular smooth muscle depends upon the continuing production of high energy compounds. Evidence points to a direct relationship between oxygen availability and the contractile strength of systemic vascular smooth muscle. This is very well demonstrated by the ductus arteriosus in which tonic contraction in the face of an increased oxygen tension is an essential feature of the transition from foetal to neonatal existence. Figure 2 is from the work of Assali and his colleagues (1963) and shows the flow permitted by the isolated ductus when the oxygen tension of the perfusate was varied over the range shown. Measurements *in vivo* on the foetal lamb when ventilated with different mixtures have also demonstrated this effect (Born *et al.*, 1956).

By contrast hypoxia has the opposite effect on the pulmonary artery (Fig. 3). The tracing is from a cat anaesthetized and ventilated with a double lumen tube in place. The lungs were denervated and the total pulmonary blood flow was controlled. The lower trace shows the flow in the left pulmonary artery obtained by an electromagnetic flow meter and the upper trace shows ventilation pressure. When the ventilation of the left lung was discontinued (Fig. 3A and 3B), the left pulmonary artery flow fell as a result of hypoxic vasoconstriction. In Fig. 3B the ventilation of the lung was recommenced at the arrow. Some hyperinflations were given to achieve re-expansion and the flow rate immediately rose.

When Lloyd (1967) investigated the contractile properties of isolated strips of pulmonary artery, he found that the responses to changes in oxygen tension were the reverse of those *in vivo*. This showed that the muscle

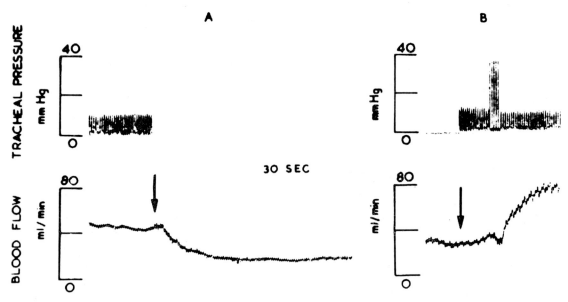

Fig. 3. (from Barer, 1966). Tracings from a cat anaesthetized with a double lumen tube in place. Upper trace airway pressure. Lower trace left pulmonary artery flow. In A, at the arrow, ventilation of the left lung ceased and pulmonary blood flow fell away as a result of hypoxic vaso-constriction. In B, at the arrow, ventilation of the left lung was recommenced. Some hyperinflations were given to achieve re-expansion and the flow rate immediately rose.

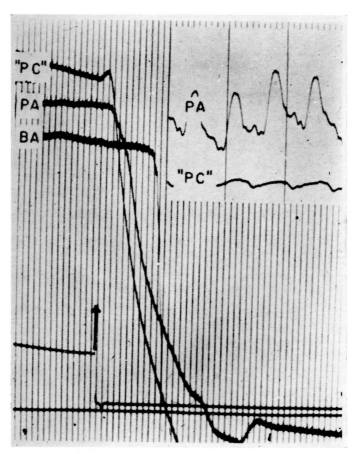

FIG. 1. From Sobol *et al.* (1963). A double lumen catheter was wedged in the pulmonary artery. The pressure tracings (inset) confirm that the tip was wedged 'PC' and the second lumen, 4 cm proximally, was in the pulmonary artery PA. Each lumen was also equipped with a platinum tipped hydrogen sensitive electrode. The potential measured at these is shown in the main part of the Fig, 'PC' and PA respectively. A third hydrogen electrode was placed in the brachial artery-BA. The time lines are one second apart. At the arrow a breath of hydrogen was taken in. A sudden change in potential at both the 'PC' and PA electrode occurred virtually simultaneously two seconds later while the change in potential at the BA electrode did not occur for a further five seconds. The findings demonstrate that the gas has rapidly penetrated pulmonary arteries of 1·5–3·0 mm diameter.

TABLE 1

Recent findings on pharmacological factors affecting hypoxic pulmonary vasoconstriction. Barer (1966) using the cat, favours the alpha agonist whereas Hauge (1968) and Hauge and Melmon (1968) using the rat, favour histamine as the mediator.

| Possible Mediator | Antagonist | Effect on Hypoxic Pressor Response | |
|---|---|---|---|
| | | Barer (1966) | Hauge et al. (1968) |
| Noradrenaline | Dibenamine | Reversed | — |
| | Phenoxybenzamine | Reversed | None |
| | Phentolamine | — | Sl. Attenuation |
| | Guanethidine | Attenuated | None |
| | Reserpine | Attenuated | None |
| Histamine | Mepyramine | Sl. Attenuation | — |
| | Diphenhydramine | — | Reversed |
| | Chlorpheniramine | — | Reversed |
| | Pyrilamine | — | Reversed |
| | Tripelennamine | — | Reversed |
| | Promethazine | — | Reversed |
| Serotonin (5 HT) | LSD | None | — |
| | Methysergide | — | None |
| ATP | 2, 4 xylenol | — | None |
| Bradykinin | Sodium Salicylate | — | None |

itself responds like any other vascular smooth muscle. The pressor response to alveolar hypoxia therefore involves an activating mechanism present in the lung which over-rides the tendency for the muscle itself to relax consequent upon oxygen deprivation. The available evidence points to this being a humoral response.

The search for a chemical mediator consists of two basic steps. Firstly, the postulation and demonstration that a given substance is a pulmonary vasoconstrictor and secondly, that treatment with a substance which is a blocking agent of the first will attenuate or abolish the pressor response to hypoxia. One difficulty with this kind of work is that the blocker may not be specific and since the doses used are difficult to select, different workers are not entirely in agreement with each other. However, it seems that histamine and noradrenaline may be involved. Table 1 abstracts the findings of two of the workers in this field. On the left is the postulated constrictor, next the blocking agent and in the two right hand columns the effect of the blocking agent on the hypoxic pressor response, according to Barer (1966) and Hauge (1968) and Hauge and Melmon (1968). The former favours the alpha agonist (noradrenaline) whereas the latter workers favour histamine as the mediator. Further experiments by the latter workers appear to be confirmatory, since after the exhibition of semi-carbazide which is a specific antihistaminase, the hypoxic pressor response was potentiated.

## Pulmonary Oxygen Toxicity

The pathogenesis of this condition is still poorly understood. Conscious normal men get symptoms of airway irritation after about 12 hours of 100 per cent oxygen at 1 ATA. In conscious dogs consolidation of lung tissue and death occur within approximately 30–80 hours. The rate of development and degree of lung damage are proportional to the inhaled oxygen tension and the duration of exposure. The picture is one of damage to the alveolar-capillary membrane similar to that seen with toxic pneumonitis with oedema, haemorrhage and cellular infiltration.

## The Effect of Gravity

Because the pulmonary circulation is a low pressure system, the pulmonary blood flow is subject to hydrostatic effects due to gravity. These effects may be illustrated by a four zone model (Hughes et al., 1968). For full discussion of the effects of gravity on pulmonary blood flow.

## Ventilation/Perfusion Relationships

Of special importance to proper lung function is the relationship or matching between ventilation ($V$) and perfusion ($Q$). Figure 4 is a model which explains the matching of ventilation and perfusion. This model permits there being two conditions of the alveoli, i.e., open (the two on the right) and closed (the one on the left), and two kinds of capillary similarly open and closed. There are thus three kinds of relationship established. On the left there is perfusion without ventilation causing a right to left shunt of venous blood and on the right is the reciprocal situation, i.e., ventilation without perfusion, resulting in alveolar dead space. Only in the centre is the situation ideal, i.e., an open capillary in contact with an open alveolus, so that gaseous equilibrium can occur. The vertical hatching in the bronchial tree represents the anatomical dead space ventilation. The latter plus the cross-hatched area is the total physiological dead space.

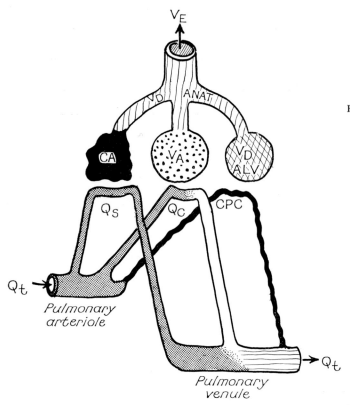

FIG. 4. Model to explain the possible relationships (matching) between ventilation and perfusion. The model states that matching can be explained 'as if' there were two kinds of alveoli and two kinds of pulmonary capillary, i.e., open and closed. There are thus three possibilities; perfusion without ventilation, on the left; ventilation without perfusion, on the right; the ideal situation is shown in the centre. CA = closed alveolus. CPC = closed pulmonary capillary. $Q_t$ = cardiac output. $Q_s$ = shunted blood flow. $Q_c$ = ideal pulmonary capillary blood flow. ($Q_t = Q_s + Q_c$). $V_E$ = ventilatory volume measured during expiration. $V_D$ ALV = alveolar dead space ventilation. $V_D$ ANAT = obligatorily 'wasted' anatomical dead space ventilation. ($V_D$ ALV + $V_D$ ANAT = physiological dead space ventilation) $V_A$ = ideal alveolar ventilation. ($V_E = V_A + V_D$ ANAT + $V_D$ ALV.)

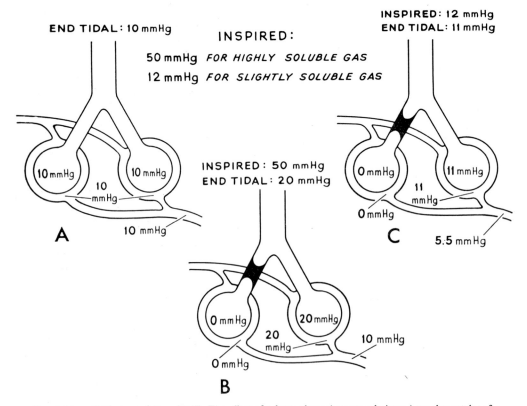

FIG. 5. From Saidman and Eger (1967). The effect of a large shunt (venous admixture) on the uptake of anaesthetic agents (for full description see text).

B. Highly soluble gas.
C. Slightly soluble gas.

The venous admixture effect of the shunt past the closed alveolus is represented by the change in shading in the right hand side of the venule. This model is a useful one because the volumes represented by all these shaded areas can be quantitated if suitable measurements are taken. (*See appendix to this chapter.*) However, it must be remembered that there are 350,000,000 alveoli and therefore there are possibly 350,000,000 variants of the inter-relationships.

partial pressure, and therefore the effect on the effluent pulmonary venous blood is that the partial pressure in this two unit model is the average of the two, i.e., 10 mmHg, which is no different from that in the ideal arrangement in Fig. 5A. On the other hand, the end-tidal tension is 20 mmHg, i.e., double.

Figure 5C shows the effect of a shunt on the slightly soluble gas. The arrangement is as previously, i.e., with the left hand airway blocked off and the alveolar ventilation

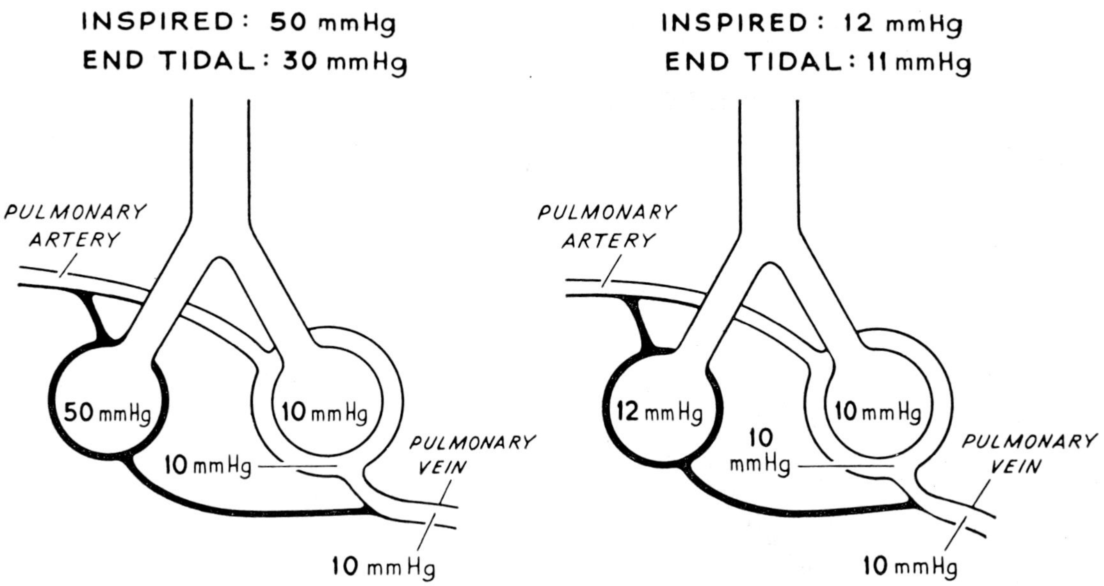

INSPIRED: 50 mmHg
END TIDAL: 30 mmHg

PULMONARY ARTERY

50 mmHg    10 mmHg

PULMONARY VEIN

10 mmHg

10 mmHg

INSPIRED: 12 mmHg
END TIDAL: 11 mmHg

PULMONARY ARTERY

12 mmHg    10 mmHg

10 mmHg

PULMONARY VEIN

10 mmHg

FIG. 6. From Saidman and Eger (1967). The effect of a large dead space on the uptake of anaesthetic agents (for full description *see* text).

### The Effect of Alterations in V/Q on the Uptake of Anaesthetic Agents

The effect of alterations in shunt and dead space on the uptake of anaesthetics have been elaborated by Saidman and Eger (1967) utilizing a simple V/Q model. In Fig. 5A, the ventilation and perfusion are ideally matched. Inhalation of a highly soluble gas and a slightly soluble gas is being considered. In order to achieve an alveolar partial pressure of 10 mmHg a very much higher inspired tension of the highly soluble gas, i.e., 50 mmHg has to be given than the insoluble gas, i.e., 12 mmHg. Because there is no V/Q abnormality, the effluent pulmonary venous blood has a partial pressure equal to that in the alveoli, and the end-tidal tension (mixed alveolar tension), which in this model is the average tension in the two alveoli is also equal to that in the alveoli and in the pulmonary venous blood.

Figure 5B shows the effect of a shunt on the highly soluble agent. The shunt is shown in this case as the result of the blockage of the alveolus on the left. Alveolar ventilation is assumed to be the same and therefore the alveolus on the right becomes doubly ventilated, which effectively doubles the partial pressure of the highly soluble agent. The partial pressure in the effluent blood from this alveolus is thus 20 mmHg. However, the shunted blood from the non-ventilated alveolus has a zero

doubled to the right hand unit. This has a very small effect on the alveolar partial pressure of the insoluble agent because the inspired to end-tidal gradient was very small in the first place. There is only a rise of 1 mmHg in this partial pressure, which is also reflected in the end-tidal partial pressure; however, the effect in the blood phase is much more significant. The partial pressure in the blood from the ventilated alveolus becomes halved, as it was with the soluble agent, but the effluent pulmonary venous blood partial pressure is very much lower than in the ideal situation, i.e., 5·5, as opposed to 10 mmHg. Thus a shunt has a greater effect on an insoluble agent. In practice induction with a soluble anaesthetic agent would not be faster than with an insoluble one, a rather more normal anaesthetic time course would ensue with a soluble than with an insoluble anaesthetic and the inspired concentration would have to be raised less with the soluble agent to achieve a normal rate of induction.

Figure 6 shows the effect when alveoli are ventilated but not perfused, i.e., there is an increase in dead space. The same two agents are being considered. The alveolus on the left has no perfusion so in neither case is the effluent pulmonary venous blood partial pressure affected—both are 10 mmHg. However, the non-perfused alveoli undergo no exchange with the blood and thus the anaesthetic agent partial pressure in them is in equilibrium with the inspired. The end-tidal partial pressure in the two unit model is the average of the two alveolar partial pressures and is very much higher in the case of the highly soluble agent (on the left) than in the ideal situation shown earlier, i.e., 30 mmHg instead of 10 mmHg. The effect on the insoluble agent (on the right) is minimal. This would mean that with a souble agent the patient would not be as deeply anaesthetized as the end-tidal partial pressure would suggest, if indeed it was measured.

The choice of the two unit model of course greatly exaggerates these effects. While they are of theoretical interest they are probably seldom of major clinical significance.

### The Effects of V/Q Abnormalities on Oxygen and Carbon Dioxide Homeostasis

(a) *Shunting:* The result of pulmonary shunting is that the pulmonary venous effluent blood has a lower arterial oxygen content than that of the end-pulmonary capillary blood. The ratio of shunt flow to cardiac output, the $Qs/Qt$ ratio, can be derived from an application of the Fick principle. An indirect estimate of the shunt flow may also be obtained from the alveolar to arterial oxygen tension gradient ($A - a_{O_2}$ gradient), i.e., the gradient between the oxygen tension in the ideal capillary or ideal alveolus and that in the pulmonary venous blood. The relationship between $A - a$ oxygen gradient and the oxygen content difference, which is of course the clinically important quantity, is non-linear because of the shape of the oxygen dissociation curve, thus when considering alveolar to arterial oxygen tension gradients at least one of the figures must be quantitated.

Hypoxaemia in association with anaesthesia has been reviewed by Payne (1967). An increase in alveolar to arterial oxygen tension gradient under conditions of a constant inspired oxygen tension has been shown to occur after premedication and after the induction of anaesthesia itself, especially when IPPV is employed, with prolongation into the post operative period if surgery is lengthy. The effect is increased with age as there is a negative correlation between age and arterial oxygen tension. Earlier workers in this field showed that $A - a_{O_2}$ gradient became progressively larger as anaesthesia continued, however this has not been confirmed recently (Panday and Nunn, 1968; Lumley *et al.*, 1969).

The increase in $A - a_{O_2}$ gradient is not associated with alveolar hypoventilation as the arterial $P_{CO_2}$ is not raised. Although it was first considered to be associated with atelectasis this has not been demonstrated by X-ray studies; also since the lesion is amenable to oxygen administration, frank atelectasis is an unlikely explanation.

There remain two possible explanations:

*Firstly:* if there is a fall in cardiac output at a constant oxygen consumption, it is obvious that as output falls mixed venous oxygen content falls and therefore the venous admixture effect of a constant shunt will be a greater depression of arterial oxygen tension at a given alveolar oxygen tension. This has been demonstrated in a theoretical study by Kelman and his colleagues (1967). However it is possible that shunt values do not remain constant during changes in cardiac output. Sykes and his co-workers (1970) have shown that in the high output state produced by over-transfusion in dogs there is an increase in $Qs/Qt$ ratio. At the other end of the scale, work carried out by the author and M. F. Tyrrell, in which dogs had their cardiac outputs lowered, showed that $Qs/Qt$ ratio decreases with cardiac output, an effect which tends to offset the effect of progressive venous desaturation until very low levels are reached (Fig. 7). Each line represents the regression line for an individual dog, $Qs/Qt$ ratio is on the ordinate. In the GBA group the blood pressure and cardiac output were lowered with pentolinium tartrate, and the decrease in shunt ratio as blood pressure fell is shown. In the HALO group, blood pressure and cardiac output were lowered with halothane and $Qs/Qt$ ratio also decreased. In the HAEM group the effect of haemorrhage and a fall in cardiac output on $Qs/Qt$ is shown; once more there is a decrease. The control group is plotted against time and there was very little change in $Qs/Qt$ ratio.

The *second* and probable cause is maldistribution of ventilation and perfusion. In this respect there could be two possible mechanisms for the increase in shunting:—

(i) Decreased aeration due to the effect of small airways closure during expiration.

(ii) An increase in shunting through non-aerated areas resulting from a disorder of the hypoxic pressor response.

Evidence has accumulated to substantiate (i) above particularly after abdominal surgery (Spence and Alexander, 1972; Alexander *et al.*, 1972). The arguments are as follows: FRC is reduced after surgery and more so after upper abdominal surgery; the net increase in transpulmonary pressure as a result of the causal process brings the airways closing point (CP) closer to the end-tidal position (ETP). Alexander and his colleagues (1972) have reported significant negative correlation between the index (ETP−CP) and the $A-a_{O_2}$ gradient. Davis and Spence (1972) have shown that the situation is worse in the elderly and that these also obtain least benefit from an increase in inspired oxygen concentration. These facts further substantiate the above explanation since it is well known that closing volume becomes closer to end-tidal volume with increasing age.

There is also evidence that the second hypothetical mechanism, i.e. a disorder of the hypoxic pulmonary pressor response, may also contribute to the hypoxaemia. Sykes and his colleagues (1973) have demonstrated the abolition of this response in the isolated perfused cat lung during the administration of 1–1·5% halothane, 0·5–0·75% trichlorethylene, 2–4% ether and 74% nitrous oxide. While these findings cannot necessarily be extrapolated to the human situation, they provide presumptive evidence of a contributory role of clinical anaesthetics, at least in early post-operative hypoxaemia.

Instances of gross shunting associated with anaesthesia are seen, for example with the use of an endobronchial blocker, although hypoxic vasoconstriction would tend to offset this. The worst form is seen in the chemical pneumonitis associated with acid aspiration, where shunting through areas of oedematous non-ventilated lung occurs, and these can be seen on a plain chest X-ray.

(b) *Dead Space:* Changes in dead space during anaesthesia are associated with changes in cardiac output and the consequent passive changes in capillary perfusion. These may be particularly seen during haemorrhage and can be achieved by measurement of the arterial to end-tidal carbon dioxide gradient. Figure 9 is from a clinical study by the author and P. W. R. Smethurst. The record was made during a facio-maxillary procedure on a male patient aged 45. Hypotension was induced by means of a trimetaphan infusion, during controlled ventilation with

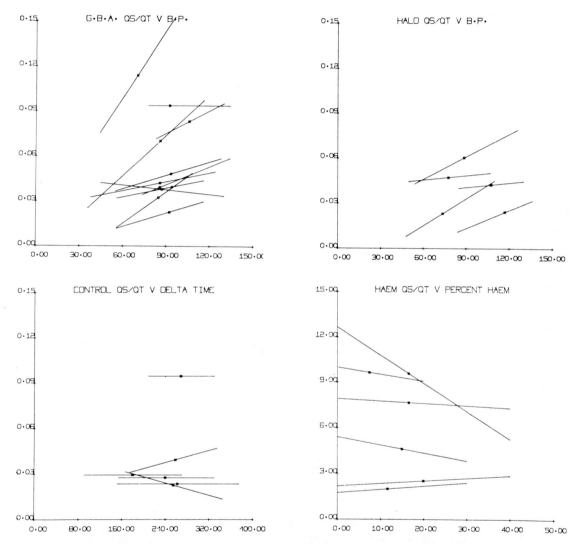

FIG. 7. Regression of $Q_s/Q_t$—shunt ratio—(ordinate) in anaesthetized ventilated dogs. G.B.A.—blood pressure and cardiac output lowered with pentolinium tartrate (abscissa—mean arterial blood pressure mmHg). HALO—blood pressure and cardiac output lowered with halothane (abscissa—mean arterial blood pressure mmHg). HAEM—blood pressure and cardiac output lowered by haemorrhage (abscissa—percentage of estimated blood volume removed). CONTROL—anaesthesia unvaried (abscissa—time in minutes). This work demonstrates that $Q_s/Q_t$ decreases when blood pressure and cardiac output are lowered by pentolinium tartrate, halothane and haemorrhage when compared with the effect of the passage of time alone.

induced hypotension. Figure 8 shows the changes in dead space ratio (VD/VE) in the experiments mentioned earlier. The values are on the ordinate and are of total functional dead space, i.e., including anatomical and apparatus dead space which are of course unchanged in each animal. It can be seen that the dead space ratio increased in association with the fall in blood pressure and cardiac output produced by ganglion blockade, by halothane and by haemorrhage in contrast with the control group.

Assessment of the changes in alveolar dead space alone

nitrous oxide/oxygen and trichlorethylene. The upper tracing is of blood pressure from 0–200 mmHg and the lower is end-tidal carbon dioxide concentration from 0–10 per cent. The changes in blood pressure are quite clearly seen to be accompanied by parallel changes in end-tidal carbon dioxide concentration. The arterial to end-tidal gradients at the two times of sampling were 9·0 and 5·4 mmHg respectively, giving alveolar dead space ratios of 24 per cent during the hypotension and 13·5 per cent at the higher blood pressure.

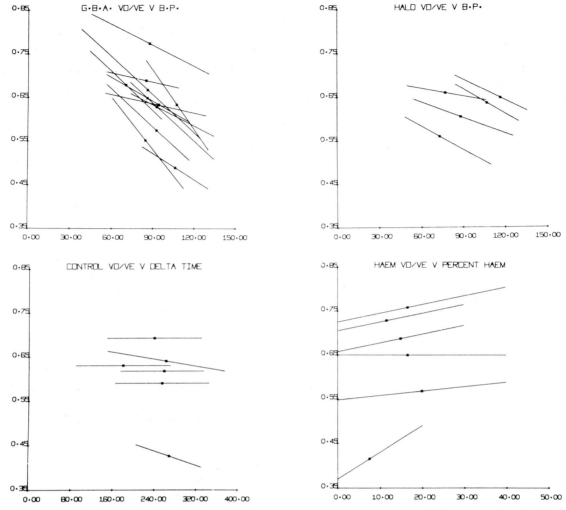

Fig. 8. Regression of VD/VE—physiological dead space ratio—(ordinate) in the same groups of dogs as are shown in Fig. 7. The values on the ordinate are of *total functional* physiological dead space, i.e., including apparatus dead space which was of course unchanged in each individual animal. This work demonstrates that VD/VE increase when blood pressure and cardiac output are lowered by pentolinium tartrate, halothane and haemorrhage when compared with the effects of the passage of time alone.

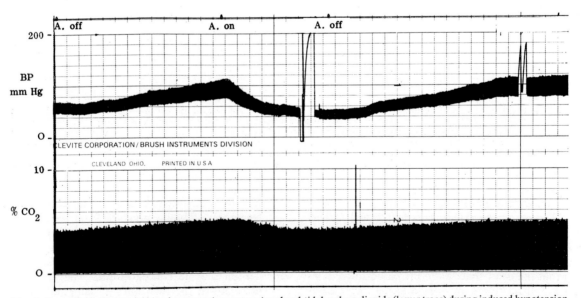

Fig. 9. Record of intra-arterial blood pressure (upper trace) and end-tidal carbon-dioxide (lower trace) during induced hypotension by trimetaphan (arfonad) in a male patient aged 45 during controlled ventilation with nitrous oxide/oxygen and trichlorethylene. 'A off' and 'A on' denote stopping and starting the arfonad infusion. The two interruptions in the arterial tracing represent times when arterial blood was sampled. The time scale is one minute per division. Blood pressure changes are clearly paralleled by changes in the end-tidal carbon dioxide concentration. The $a$-ETpP$_{CO_2}$ gradients at times of sampling were 9·0 and 5·4 mmHg respectively; the ratios of VD ALV/VE were 24 per cent during the hypotension and 13·5 per cent at the higher blood pressure.

## The Effects of Drugs on the Pulmonary Circulation

Finally, it is appropriate to ask whether individual para-anaesthetic drugs or anaesthetic agents themselves exert any specific and significant effects on the pulmonary circulation of intact animals or man. There is little work on this because firstly, before any phenomenon can be demonstrated to have an active vasomotor effect on the pulmonary circulation it must be proved to act independently of changes in the systemic circulation and of changes in respiration. Ideally flow and respiratory tract pressure should be constant when drugs are assessed. Having achieved this, if possible, measurements of changes in vascular tone require that the pressure drop across the pulmonary circuit be measured. Pulmonary arterial pressure is of course easy to obtain by catheterization, i.e., persuading the catheter to traverse the tricuspid and pulmonary valves. This is a relatively easy as the catheter travels with the blood stream. However, the distal part of the circuit cannot be approached with such ease. Left heart catheterization is carried out against the blood stream and it is virtually impossible to persuade the tip of a catheter through the mitral valve. There are several manoeuvres for obtaining access to the left atrium—sometimes it can be entered through a patent formen ovale from the right atrium; alternatively the atrial septum can be deliberately breached by a trans-septal puncture from the right atrium; when it is absolutely necessary more heroic procedures can be adopted; for example, puncture at the sternal notch and successive puncture of aorta, pulmonary artery and then left atrium; percutaneous puncture of the left ventricle and then a transmitral approach; an endobronchial approach; or finally a percutaneous approach from the rear. Of course, none of these can be justified, for the purposes of research in the human subject. Recourse is usually made to a wedged pulmonary artery catheter. It is considered that as no flow past the wedged catheter can occur, the static column of blood ahead of the catheter is in continuity with the left atrium and therefore accurately reflects the left atrial pressure. However, this technique is very liable to artefacts and some workers prefer to use the left ventricular end-diastolic pressure.

Since the pressure gradient across the pulmonary circuit is very small, any errors in measurement will grossly affect the calculated derived resistance. High fidelity measurements and careful technique are thus required. Since both the controlled conditions required and the measurements indicated are virtually impossible to achieve, especially during clinical anaesthesia itself, it is not surprising that information is lacking in this field. It is probable that under clinical conditions any effect on the pulmonary circulation is overridden by the systemic effects.

There are however, two studies, one by Goldberg and his colleagues (1968) on intact, unsedated dogs in whom monitoring apparatus had been implanted previously and the other by Price and his colleagues (1969) on twelve healthy male volunteers. The former study demonstrated that thiamylal, a thiobarbitrate somewhat similar to thiopentone, caused an increase in pulmonary vascular resistance and the latter that cyclopropane raised pulmonary vascular resistance.

## Summary

As the pulmonary circuit is in series, the flow through it is governed by events in the systemic circulation. Its function is gaseous exchange and the low resistance in the circuit is subservient to this function. Regional flow is affected by the passive hydrostatic effects due to gravity, and by the active, probably humorally mediated, effects of the intra-alveoar oxygen tension, although excessive oxygen is toxic to the alveolar capillary membrane.

When perfusion is wasted there is a shunt effect which can be evaluated by the alveolar to arterial oxygen tension gradient, and when perfusion is reduced there is a dead space effect which can be evaluated by the arterial to end-tidal carbon dioxide gradient. As far as the state of anaesthesia is concerned, there is a partially explained increase in alveolar to arterial $O_2$ gradient in association with that state. Changes in dead space are associated with the low cardiac output state of induced hypotension. Specific effects of individual agents on the pulmonary circulation are difficult to measure and probably masked under clinical conditions by systemic events.

## APPENDIX

### SOLUTION OF THE VENTILATION/PERFUSION MODEL

**Ventilation**

Solution of the ventilation compartments of the model usually consists of deriving the ratio of each subdivision to expired tidal volume ($V_E$).

Referring to Fig. 4,

$$V_{D \mid ALV} + V_{D\ ANAT} = V_{D\ PHYS}$$
$$\text{and } V_{D\ PHYS} + V_A = V_E$$

The full interrelationship between these quantities may be expressed with reference to the gas R line in an $O_2/CO_2$ diagram (Fig. 10).

In this diagram AI is the gas R line and,

$$A\bar{E} \propto V_{D\ PHYS}$$
$$A\acute{E} \propto V_{D\ ALV}$$
$$\acute{E}\bar{E} \propto V_{D\ ANAT}$$
$$\bar{E}I \propto V_A$$
$$\text{and, } AI \propto V_E$$

As can be seen, the co-ordinates of these defined points make up a series of similar triangles. Since, in similar triangles, the ratios of any pair of similar sides are equal, derivation of the various equations is easy (Leigh and Tyrrell, 1968). Thus:

$$\frac{V_D}{V_E} = \frac{A\bar{E}}{AI} = \frac{Pa_{CO_2} - P\bar{E}_{CO_2}}{Pa_{CO_2}} \quad \text{(Bohr equation)}$$

$$\frac{V_{D\ ALV}}{V_E} = \frac{A\acute{E}}{AI} = \frac{Pa_{CO_2} - P\acute{E}_{CO_2}}{Pa_{CO_2}}$$

$$\frac{V_{D\ ANAT}}{V_E} = \frac{\acute{E}\bar{E}}{AI} = \frac{P\acute{E}_{CO_2} - P\bar{E}_{CO_2}}{Pa_{CO_2}}$$

$$\frac{V_A}{V_E} = \frac{\bar{E}I}{AI} = \frac{P\bar{E}_{CO_2}}{Pa_{CO_2}}$$

The following measurements are required:—

$Pa_{CO_2}$, using a direct-reading electrode or interpolation from pH.

$P\bar{E}_{CO_2}$, measured on expired gas (collected classically through a one-way valve into a Douglas bag) with a direct reading electrode, Haldane apparatus or infa-red $CO_2$ analyser.

$P\acute{E}_{CO_2}$, measured during tidal expiration using the write-out from an infa-red $CO_2$ analyser for accuracy,

To convert percentage $CO_2$ to tension multiply by (barometric pressure − 47)/100.

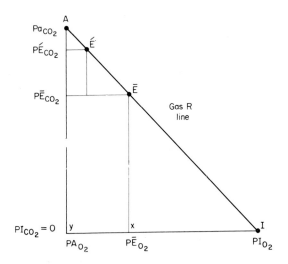

FIG. 10. Geometric interrelationship of the respiratory gases in the $O_2/CO_2$ diagram (Abscissa = $P_{O_2}$, ordinate = $P_{CO_2}$).

A = ideal alveolar gas. $\acute{E}$ = end-tidal gas. $\bar{E}$ = mixed expired gas. I = inspired gas. $Pa_{CO_2} = PA_{CO_2}$. AI is the gas R line. For further explanations see text.

Finally if $V_E$ is measured, then the ventilation model can be fully quantitated.

### Ideal Alveolar Oxygen Tension

The ideal alveolar oxygen tension ($PA_{O_2}$) is the key figure in the ventilation/perfusion model as it is assumed to exist both in the $V_A$ compartment and the $Q_c$ compartment. The equation for its calculation may be easily obtained from Fig. 10.

$$\frac{Iy}{Ix} = \frac{AI}{\bar{E}I}$$

$$\therefore \quad \frac{P_{I_{O_2}} - PA_{O_2}}{P_{I_{O_2}} - P\bar{E}_{O_2}} = \frac{Pa_{CO_2}}{P\bar{E}_{CO_2}}$$

$$\therefore \quad PA_{O_2} = P_{I_{O_2}} - Pa_{CO_2}\left(\frac{P_{I_{O_2}} - P\bar{E}_{O_2}}{P\bar{E}_{CO_2}}\right) - \text{Nunn Equation}$$

In addition to the measurements mentioned above the following are required: $P_{I_{O_2}}$ and $P\bar{E}_{O_2}$; these can be measured directly by polarographic electrode, or by Haldane apparatus or paramagnetic oxygen analyser. Both the latter give $O_2\%$ which requires conversion to tension.

### Perfusion

Quantitating the perfusion part of the model involves solution of the *shunt equation*, which may be derived as follows:

Referring to Fig. 4,    $Qt = Qc + Qs$,

and, since    $Qc = Qt − Qs$

$\therefore$    $Qt = (Qt − Qs) + Qs$

The oxygen flow through these compartments is:—

$$Qt.Ca_{O_2} = (Qt − Qs)\, C\acute{c}_{O_2} + Qs.C\bar{v}_{O_2}$$

(*where C = content; $\acute{c}$ = end-pulmonary capillary; $\bar{v}$ = mixed venous*)

$\therefore$    $Qt.Ca_{O_2} = Qt.C\acute{c}_{O_2} − Qs.C\acute{c}_{O_2} + Qs.C\bar{v}_{O_2}$

$\therefore$    $Qt\,(Ca_{O_2} − C\acute{c}_{O_2}) = Qs\,(C\bar{v}_{O_2} − C\acute{c}_{O_2})$

$$\therefore \quad \frac{Qs}{Qt} = \frac{Ca_{O_2} − C\acute{c}_{O_2}}{C\bar{v}_{O_2} − C\acute{c}_{O_2}}$$

which may be rewritten:—

$$\frac{Qs}{Qt} = \frac{C\acute{c}_{O_2} − Ca_{O_2}}{C\acute{c}_{O_2} − C\bar{v}_{O_2}}$$

$Ca_{O_2}$ is measured on arterial blood; $C\bar{v}_{O_2}$ is strictly only measurable on blood obtained from the pulmonary artery. These content measurements in cc $O_2$/100 cc blood can be made by chemical and volumetric methods (e.g. on a Van Slyke's apparatus), by gas chromatography, by derivation from saturation measurements (oximetry) or from $P_{O_2}$ (polarography). Both the latter have to be converted to content assuming a normal saturation curve.

End-pulmonary capillary blood cannot, of course, be sampled but the basic assumption of the model is that this blood is in equilibrium with ideal alveolar gas. The ideal alveolar oxygen tension ($PA_{O_2}$) is therefore calculated from the Nunn equation—*vide supra*—and thence $C\acute{c}_{O_2}$ assuming a normal saturation curve. Finally, the $Qs/Qt$ ratio can be obtained and the normal value is less than 0·04 (4%). If the cardiac output is also measured, $Qs$ can be fully quantitated.

*The animal work carried out by the author and Dr. M. F. Tyrrell was supported by a grant from the Medical Research Council.*

### REFERENCES

Alexander, J. I., Horton, P. W., Millar, W. T., Parikh, R. K. and Spence, A. A. (1972), "The effect of Upper Abdominal Surgery on the Relationship of Airway Closing Point to End Tidal Position," *Clin. Sci.*, **43**, 137.

Assali, N. S., Morris, J. A., Smith, R. W. and Manson, W. A. (1963), "Studies on Ductus Arteriosus Circulation," *Circ. Res.*, **13**, 478.

Barer, Gwenda (1966), "Reactivity of Vessels of Collapsed and Ventilated Lungs to Drugs and Hypoxia," *Circ. Res.*, **18**, 366.

Born, G. V. R., Dawes, G. S., Mott, J. C. and Remick, B. R. (1956), "The Constriction of the Ductus Arteriosus caused by Oxygen and by Asphyxia in Newborn Lambs," *J. Physiol.*, **132**, 304.

Davis, A. G. and Spence, A. A. (1972), "Postoperative Hypoxemia and Age," *Anesthesiology*, **37**, 663.

Fick, A. (1870), "Uber die Messung des Blutquantums in den Herzventrikeln," *Sitsungsb. der phys-med Ges. zu Wurzburg*, **XIV**, XVI.

Goldberg, S. J., Linde, L. M., Gaal, P. G., Momma, K., Takahashi, M. and Sarna, G. (1968), "Effects of Barbiturates on Pulmonary and Systemic Haemodynamics," *Cariovasc. Res.*, **2**, 136.

Harvey, W. (1628), *Exercitatio de Motu Cordis et Sanguinis*, Trans. K. J. Franklin (1957), Springfield, Illinois: Thomas.

Hauge, A. (1968), "Role of Histamine in Hypoxic Pulmonary Hypertension in the Rat: I. Blockade or potentiation of endogenous amines, kinins and ATP," *Circ. Res.*, **22**, 371.

Hauge, A. and Melmon, K. L. (1968), "Role of Histamine in Hypoxic Pulmonary Hypertension in the Rat: II. Depletion of histamine, serotonin and catecholamines," *Circ. Res.*, **22**, 385.

Hughes, J. M. B., Glazier, J. B., Maloney, J. E. and West, J. B. (1968), "Effect of Lung Volume on the Distribution of Pulmonary Blood Flow in Man," *Resp. Physiol.*, **4**, 58.

Kelman, G. R., Nunn, J. F., Prys-Roberts, C. and Greenbaum, R. (1967), "The Influence of Cardiac Output on Arterial Oxygenation: a Theoretical Study," *Brit. J. Anaesth.* **39**, 450.

Leigh, J. M. and Tyrrell, M. F. Unpublished observations.

Leigh, J. M. and Smethurst, P. W. R. Unpublished observations.

Liebow, A. A. (1962), "Recent Advances in Pulmonary Anatomy," in *Pulmonary Structure and Function*, p. 2. London: J. and A. Churchill.

Lloyd, T. C. (1967), "Influence of $P_{O_2}$ and pH on Resting and Active Tensions of Pulmonary Arterial Strips," *J. appl. Physiol.*, **22**, 1101.

Lower, R. (1669), *Tractatus De Corde*. Trans. K. J. Franklin in R. T. Gunther's *Early Science in Oxford* (1932), Vol. IX. Oxford: Oxford University Press.

Lundholm, L. and Mohme-Lundholm, E. (1963), "Dissociation of Contraction and Stimulation of Lactic Acid Production in Experiments on Smooth Muscle under Anaerobic Conditions," *Acta physiol. scand.*, **57**, 111.

Lumley, Jean, Morgan, M. and Sykes, M. K. (1969), "Changes in Arterial Oxygenation and Physiological Dead Space under Anaesthesia," *Brit. J. Anaesth.*, **41**, 279.

Panday, J. and Nunn, J. F. (1968), "Failure to Demonstrate Progressive Falls of Arterial $P_{O_2}$ during Anaesthesia," *Anaesthesia*, **23**, 38.

Payne, J. P. (1967), "Recent Studies in Oxygenation and Oxygen Therapy and their Clinical Significance," in *Modern Trends in Anaesthesia: 3, Aspects of Metabolism and Pulmonary Ventilation*, p. 132. London: Butterworths.

Price, H. L., Cooperman, L. H., Warden, J. C., Morris, J. J. and Smith, T. C. (1969), "Pulmonary Haemodynamics during General Anaesthesia in Man," *Anaesthesiology*, **30**, 629.

Saidman, L. J. and Eger, E. I. (1967), "The Influence of Ventilation/Perfusion Abnormalities upon the Uptake of Inhalation Anaesthetics," in *Clinical Anaesthesia. Lung Disease*. p. 79. Oxford: Blackwell.

Sobol, B. J., Bottex, G., Emirgil, C. and Gissen, H. (1963), "Gaseous Diffusion from Alveoli to Pulmonary Vessels of Considerable Size," *Circ. Res.*, **13**, 71.

Spence, A. A. and Alexander, J. I. (1972), "Mechanisms of Postoperative Hypoxaemia," *Proc. Roy. Soc. Med.*, **65**, 12.

Sykes, M. K., Adams, A. P., Finlay, W. E. I., Wightman, A. E. and Munroe, J. P. (1970), "The Cardiorespiratory Effects of Haemorrhage and Overtransfusion in Dogs," *Brit. J. Anaesth.*, **42**, 573.

Sykes, M. K., Davies, D. M., Chakrabarti, M. K. and Loh, L. (1973), "The Effect of Inhalational Anesthetic Agents on the Pulmonary Vasculature of the Isolated Perfused Cat Lung," *Brit. J. Anaesth.*, in press (abstract).

Tobin, C. E. (1966), "Arteriovenous Shunts in the Peripheral Pulmonary Circulation in the Human Lung," *Thorax*, **21**, 197.

Von Euler, U. S. and Liljestrand, G. (1946), "Observations of the Pulmonary Artery Blood Pressure in the Cat," *Acta physiol. scand.*, **12**, 301.

*CHAPTER* 4

# FLUID DYNAMICS OF THE CEREBRAL CIRCULATION

## D. GORDON McDOWALL

The cerebral circulation is unique in that all its adjustments and variations must take place within an almost completely closed space. The concept of Monro (1783) and Kellie (1824) is, of course, a completely valid one but it has led to many misconceptions. For example, physiologists believed for many years that the circulation within the closed skull has to behave entirely passively and be influenced only by changes in blood pressure (Hill, 1896). Today most of the misconceptions concern the relationship between intracranial pressure and atmospheric pressure. The following discussion will commence with an account of the normal physiology of intracranial pressures (Section I) and intracranial volumes (Section II) and conclude with a discussion of the alterations in intracranial pressures and volumes produced by disease (Section III).

## 1. INTRACRANIAL PRESSURES

### Arterial Pressure

The pressure in the main vessels to the brain (2 internal carotids and 2 vertebrals) is virtually the same as in the brachial artery under normal conditions. However, both carotid and vertebral arteries can actively constrict so that a considerable pressure gradient between aorta and circle of Willis can occur. Spasm of these vessels is well known to radiologists, and experimental work with isolated segments of carotid artery has demonstrated that a considerable range of active constriction is possessed by this vessel (Mchedlishvili, 1969). In the quoted study it was shown that serotonin was a potent vaso-constrictor of the carotid artery. Similar changes in vertebro-basilar resistance have been demonstrated by Soderberg and Weckman (1959).

The circle of Willis is a very important feature of intracranial fluid dynamics in that is acts to equalize pressure between the different arterial inputs. Thus, if one of the inputs is obstructed, blood from the other arteries moves round the arterial circle to supply all the efferent vessels.

From the circle of Willis the blood is distributed to the fore brain either via surface pial arteries or through perforating branches. There is a further drop in pressure in these small arteries which also have the ability to vary their calibre by active muscular constriction. Many adrenergic nerve fibres are present on the surface of these vessels and it is likely that they can produce active changes in arterial diameter (Falck, Nielsen and Owman, 1968). Shulman (1965) has measured the pressure in the small pial arteries of the brain of the dog and has reported it to equal $63 \pm 26$ mm Hg at a mean aortic pressure of $137 \pm 19$ mm Hg, while in the cat Kanzow and Dieckhoff (1969) obtained a comparable result, i.e. pressure was 60 per cent of aortic. Symon (1967) however, has found the pressure in these small arteries to be between 80 and 90 per cent of central arterial pressure in dogs and monkeys. There is, therefore, a drop of between 10 and 50 per cent in arterial blood pressure before the cerebral arterioles are reached. It is probable that spasm of these medium sized cerebral arteries can considerably increase the pressure drop proximal to the arterioles.

It remains true, however, that the major resistance to flow and the most active point of flow control is the cerebral arteriole. The calibre of these vessels is controlled by the smooth muscle in their walls but the mechanisms whereby smooth muscle tone is controlled are still the subject of disagreement. Space will not allow a discussion of blood flow control mechanisms here but the interested reader is referred to recent accounts by Betz (1970), Harper (1970), Millar (1970) and McDowall (1971).

### Venous Pressure

Up until the point of the arteriolar resistance all pressures have been considered in relation to atmospheric pressure but, of course, atmospheric pressure is of only indirect importance within the closed skull. As Abercrombie put it in 1828 'the brain is closely shut up from atmospheric pressure and all influences from without, *except what is communicated through the blood vessels which enter it*'. The true reference pressure for intravascular pressures within the skull is the intracranial pressure which can most easily be measured in the cerebrospinal fluid. This pressure is 100–150 mm $H_2O$ or 7–10 mm Hg throughout the cerebrospinal fluid space in the horizontal position. The source of this intracranial pressure will be considered later. In the context of our present discussion on venous pressure it is clear that the pressure in the thin-walled capillaries and veins (which in the brain have virtually no muscular coat) cannot be below the general intracranial pressure otherwise they would collapse. In fact, because there is still some downstream resistance to be overcome, the pressure in these thin walled veins has to be above the CSF pressure and has been measured in the dog to be approximately 130 mm $H_2O$ in excess of CSF pressure (Shulman, 1965). It should be noted in passing that the brain is one of the few sites where pulsatile venous flow is normal; the pulsations being transmitted to the veins by the CSF.

From the thin walled cerebral veins, the blood enters the various dural sinuses. Within these sinuses the blood is partially protected from the general intracranial pressure because of the relatively rigid dural walls. In some species indeed certain of the sinuses run in channels in bone. Along the length of the sinuses the venous pressure falls from the point of entry, i.e., the mouth of the cerebral veins to the point of exit, i.e., the jugular bulb where the pressure is close to atmospheric. For instance, in the dog the venous pressure in the anterior part of the superior sagittal sinus is $90 \pm 31$ mm $H_2O$, while at the torcula it has fallen to $46 \pm 24$ mm $H_2O$ (Shulman, Yarnell, and Ransohoff, 1964).

The pressure in the jugular bulb is close to atmospheric because the jugular vein is exposed to atmospheric pressure in the loose tissues of the neck. It is for this reason that the pressures within the skull cannot be considered to be totally independent of atmospheric pressure (or more strictly the tissue pressure of the neck) though as Abercrombie said, the relationship is still via the blood vessels which enter the brain. Atmospheric pressure sets the pressure in the jugular bulb which in turn sets all the pressures upstream of it, each point in the cerebral circulation after the arterioles, having a pressure equal to atmospheric plus the pressure required to overcome the resistance of the vascular segment between that point and the jugular bulb.

### Cerebro-spinal Fluid Pressure

Why should the intracranial pressure be 100–150 mm $H_2O$ above atmospheric pressure? The reason is concerned with the formation and reabsorption of CSF. CSF is formed mainly in the choroid plexuses which secrete CSF against the resistance of the reabsorptive channels. It is reabsorbed at the arachnoid villi into the venous sinuses, mainly the superior sagittal sinus. These villi consist of coiled microtubules (Welch and Friedman, 1960) and therefore reabsorption of CSF is a mechanical process requiring a pressure gradient to force CSF through the microtubules and into the venous blood. The CSF pressure, therefore, has to be equal to the pressure in the venous sinuses at the site of the arachnoid villi plus the pressure required to overcome the flow resistance of the microtubules. In the study of Shulman (1965) undertaken in the dog, the pressure difference available to force CSF across the arachnoid villi was approximately 50–60 mm $H_2O$. It is the pressure required to overcome the resistance of the arachnoid villi and the resistance between the arachnoid villi and the jugular bulb which sets the intracranial pressure. The source of the intracranial pressure is the secretory pressure of the choroid plexuses.

## VARIATIONS IN INTRACRANIAL PRESSURE WITH PULSE AND RESPIRATION

The intracranial pressure oscillates with the arterial pulse. This pulsation arises in part from the pulsatile changes in cross-sectional area of the cerebral arteries and arterioles and in part from the pulsatile volume changes in the choroid plexuses (Bering, 1955). Fig. 1 is a record of CSF pressure in one lateral ventricle of a patient during surgery for a cerebral tumour. The pulsations of pressure with the arterial pulse can be clearly seen. Fig. 2 shows similar pulsations in a patient breathing spontaneously; in this case the measurements were made in the lumbar space.

Bering (1955) maintains that these pulsations arise in the lateral ventricles where the bulk of the choroid plexus system is, and that they therefore have their greatest amplitude in the lateral ventricles. His measurements showed these oscillations to be progressively damped during transmission caudally in the CSF axis, e.g. pulsations in the lumbar theca were only 40 per cent of those in the lateral ventricle in Bering's study. If this is so then during systole the pressure must be higher in the lateral ventricles than in more caudal areas of the CSF space while during diastole the converse will be true. There will also be a time lag in the transmission of the CSF pressure wave from the site of origin in the choroid plexuses to the lumbar space and the combined effects of the phasic pressure differences and the time lag will be to propel and mix CSF around the cerebrospinal axis.

This view of the origin of the arterial pulsations of the CSF has not been universally accepted for two reasons. Firstly, inspection of the brain shows marked pulsations apparently largely originating in the major arteries at the base of the brain, while little pulsatile movement can be discerned in the choroid plexuses. Secondly the experiments of Dunbar, Guthrie and Karpell (1966) demonstrate that, at least in the lumbar space, the arterial pulsations are derived from the local arterial supply to the cord. It should be noted, however, that there is still a time lag between intracranial arterial pulsation and lumbar CSF pulsation (of 1/25–2/25 second) because the arterial pressure wave reaches the brain before it reaches the lumbar spinal cord. Therefore, the mechanism proposed by Dunbar et al to explain CSF arterial pulsations would still provide a force tending to propel and mix cerebrospinal fluid. The pulsations of the brain arising from the pulsatile volume changes of the cerebral arteries probably also act to produce movement of cerebral interstitial fluid, thus preventing local accumulation of excessive concentrations of metabolites. This is one of the reasons for favouring pulsatile flow during extracorporeal perfusion.

CSF pressure also varies with respiration as can be seen in Fig. 1, although the direction of the changes in this figure is opposite to the normal since the patient was being ventilated by intermittent positive pressure. Fig. 2 is a record of lumbar CSF pressure obtained in a patient breathing spontaneously. It shows, as reported by Weed and McKibben in 1919, that CSF pressure falls during inspiration and rises during expiration, these changes probably following changes in intrathoracic venous pressure.

The large variations in intrathoracic venous pressure produced by coughing, abdominal compression, etc., also produce changes in cerebrospinal fluid pressure (Bethune, Currie, and Watson, 1968). In these situations the rise in intrathoracic pressure is transmitted via the jugular and vertebral veins to the intracranial veins. These latter dilate when their intraluminal pressure increases, since they are devoid of a muscular coat. In this way intracranial blood volume rises and so CSF pressure is increased. This rise in CSF pressure has, of course, the satisfactory effect of lessening the change in transmural pressure produced by a sudden elevation of venous pressure thus lessening the likelihood of tissue oedema formation or venous or capillary rupture.

These are the changes which occur with brief alterations in venous pressure but when a more prolonged elevation in cerebral venous pressure occurs, as, for instance, during pressure on the neck by poor positioning on the operating table, the CSF pressure first rises but then falls towards its normal value (Bedford, 1935). The secondary fall is due to increased reabsorption of CSF and to movement of CSF from the cranial space to the spinal theca.

## EFFECT OF POSTURE ON INTRACRANIAL PRESSURE

It is on this topic that most of the confusion about intracranial fluid dynamics arises. One of the first difficulties that complicates any simple hydrostatic explanation is that the pressure in the jugular bulb need not change between the supine and the erect position, because the jugular veins are subject to atmospheric pressure in the neck. Since the jugular bulb pressure does not change, the hydrostatic pressure difference between the head and the right atrium cannot exert an effect on intracranial pressure. The pressure in the dural sinuses will, however, fall by the hydrostatic pressure difference between the sinus and the jugular bulb in the erect position. In the case of the superior sagittal sinus this would involve a reduction in venous pressure of about 100 mm $H_2O$ between supine and erect positions which, allowing for a 50 mm $H_2O$ pressure gradient to overcome flow resistance, would give a pressure in the superior sagittal sinus of —50 mm $H_2O$. Given that a gradient of 50–60 mm $H_2O$ is required to drive CSF across the arachnoid villi, this would make the CSF pressure at the vertex just about atmospheric.

There is another factor, however, which must be taken into account and that is the hydrostatic pressure of the CSF fluid volume between the head and the lumbar thecal sac. The CSF might be expected to fall into the lumbar thecal space on moving from supine to erect, thus lowering intracranial pressures. This does indeed occur but only to a limited extent and that for two reasons: (1) the spinal theca has rather a low compliance; and (2) more importantly, the skull is almost a rigid box. As Davson (1960) has pointed out, if a glass tube, closed at the top and filled with fluid, is held perpendicularly, with the open end at the foot, fluid does not run out of the tube because the pressure at the foot of the tube is no greater than atmospheric. Since, therefore, the pressure at the foot of such a tube is not increased the lumbar theca should not be distended and no CSF should flow out of the intracranial space. This is, however, not quite the situation in man assuming the erect position because the intracranial dura is not as rigid as is a closed glass tube and so its sags and allows some increase in lumbar CSF pressure and some movement of CSF from intracranial space to spinal theca. Furthermore, dilatation of intracranial cerebral veins will act to increase the apparent distensibility of the intracranial contents. Thus, in the lateral position lumbar CSF pressure is normally in the range 100–150 mm $H_2O$, but in the sitting position it rises to 350–400 mm $H_2O$. However, if the full hydrostatic pressure difference were to be added to the lumbar CSF pressure this should rise to 700 mm $H_2O$ in the sitting position. Since lumbar CSF pressure rises somewhat on moving from supine to erect, intracranial pressure must fall in this change of position,

but it will quickly rise again since the reduced intracranial pressure will slow the rate of reabsorption of CSF at the arachnoid villi. CSF will therefore accumulate and the pressure will increase until a sufficient CSF-venous pressure gradient has been regained.

Bethune *et al.* (1968) have measured the intracranial pressure in patients with closed skull and they state: 'elevating the head reduces the pressure though even when standing it would not appear to fall below atmospheric pressure'. It must be emphasised that these remarks apply to the CSF pressure and not to the pressure in the venous sinuses which can certainly be subatmospheric.

## INTERACTIONS BETWEEN ARTERIAL, VENOUS AND CSF PRESSURES

### (a) Arterial and CSF Pressures

If the arterial pressure falls quickly, CSF pressure falls with it because a sudden fall in arterial pressure reduces cerebral blood flow and cerebral blood volume before autoregulation has time to become effective. If, however, time is allowed for autoregulation to become effective, then CSF pressure returns to normal as cerebral blood flow regains its previous level. Thus CSF pressure is not affected by the level of blood pressure unless the blood pressure falls below the lower limit of autoregulation. The same applies to systemic hypertension.

In the opposite sense, changes in CSF pressures are said not to affect blood pressure unless the CSF pressure is elevated to near arterial level when cerebral blood flow is reduced sufficiently to produce medullary ischemia (Wright, 1938). When this occurs, blood pressure rises in the well known Cushing response (Cushing, 1901).

### (b) Venous and CSF Pressure

As we have already seen, any rise in cerebral venous pressure is in the short term mirrored by a change in CSF pressure. Such changes occur with coughing, jugular compression, etc., and also when cerebral blood flow increases. An increase in cerebral blood flow raises cerebral venous pressure by at least three mechanisms: (1) arteriolar vasodilatation allowing the transmission of a greater part of the arterial blood pressure to the venous side; (2) increased cerebral blood volume leading to increased cerebrospinal fluid pressure with secondarily elevated cerebral venous pressure; and (3) increased blood flow through the rather rigid dural sinuses causing a rise in pressure in these sinuses which backfires into the surface cerebral veins. Therefore, in any circumstance in which cerebral blood flow is increased both cerebral venous and CSF pressure rise in parallel in the short term, e.g. halothane administration (McDowall, Barker and Jennett, 1966), although with time the CSF pressure returns to its control value through a compensatory fall in CSF volume.

If CSF pressure is acutely raised e.g. experimentally by injecting fluid into the CSF space, then it is usually said that cerebral venous pressure changes only slightly. This, however, is only true of pressures within the dural sinuses which, because of their relatively rigid walls, are largely

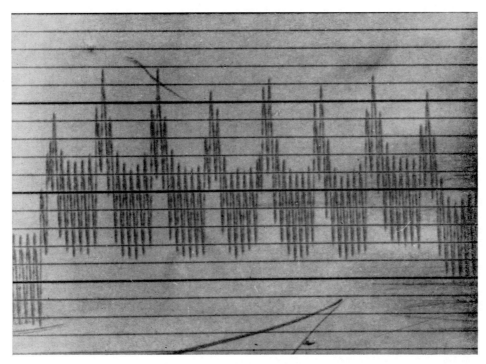

Fig. 1. This trace is a record of C.S.F. pressure measured in the lateral ventricle of an anaesthetized patient. Pulsations in C.S.F. pressure in time with the arterial pulse and with the respiration can be seen, these latter being the inverse of the normal since this patient was being ventilated by IPPV. (Reproduced from International Anesthesiology Clinics, "The Cerebral Circulation." Ed. McDowall, D. G., by kind permission of Little, Brown & Co., Boston.)

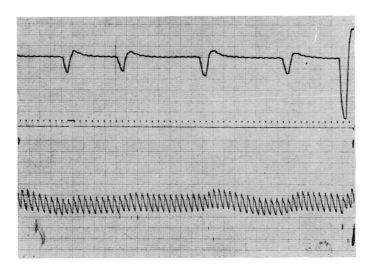

Fig. 2. Record of lumbar C.S.F. pressure in a patient breathing spontaneously. The upper trace is a record of pressure changes in a tambour stretched around the patient's chest. This record has no quantitative significance but serves to time the phases of respiration; downward deflections representing inspiration and upward ones expiration. The lower trace is of lumbar C.S.F. pressure and shows pulsations in phase with both the arterial pulse and respiration. C.S.F. pressure falls during inspiration and rises during expiration. It falls again during the expiratory pause which is prolonged in this patient who was bradypnoeic following Droperidol-Fentanyl. The large inspiratory deflection at the extreme right represents a deep inspiration in response to command. The C.S.F. pressure scale is 25 mm $H_2O$/large square and the time trace is in seconds.

immune from acute intracranial pressure changes. The maintenance of normal dural venous pressure in situations of elevated CSF pressure, allows CSF reabsorption at the arachnoid villi to increase, thus producing a compensatory mechanism. The subarachnoid cerebral veins are, unlike the dural sinuses, not protected from the effects of raised intracranial pressure and therefore their pressure must rise unless the veins are to collapse. It is clear, therefore, that as long as blood continues to flow through the brain the pressure in the subarachnoid veins must always be in excess of the general intracranial pressure. Therefore, when the CSF pressure rises, the pressure in the cerebral veins increases but the arterioles relax so that total cerebrovascular resistance remains constant (Shulman and Verdier, 1967). This compensation continues until the cerebral arterioles are fully dilated which occurs at an intracranial pressure of 30 mm Hg (450 mm $H_2O$).

This increased subarachnoid venous pressure with near normal dural venous pressure must mean that there is an increased pressure gradient at the points of entry of the subarachnoid veins into the dural sinuses. The source of this increased pressure gradient is the 'nipping' of the entry cuffs of the veins into the sinuses by the elevated CSF pressure (Wright, 1938).

## II. INTRACRANIAL VOLUMES

The total volume contained within the skull is about 1500 mls, of which the brain occupies about 90 per cent. The remaining space is filled with blood (about 5 per cent) and cerebrospinal fluid.

The size of the interstitial fluid volume space of the brain has been hotly contested for several years now since discrepancies were apparent between the space as measured by electron microscopy (almost zero) and that measured by tracer dilution. There now appears again to be a degree of agreement that the space is approximately 10–15 per cent of total wet weight of brain.

The total cerebrospinal fluid volume is approximately 120–140 mls. This volume of CSF can, however, alter in response to various physiological and pathological changes and in most cases the changes in CSF volume are opposite or compensatory to initial changes in cerebral blood volume. Thus, in hypocapnia cerebral blood volume falls and cerebrospinal fluid volume increases and the same sequence of changes is seen in hypothermia (Rosomoff, 1961 and 1963). It is for this reason that during hypocapnia CSF pressure, after an initial drop, returns to the control value. In addition to compensation by increased or reduced reabsorption of CSF, quicker compensation for changes in the volume of intracranial contents can be produced by shifting CSF from the intracranial compartment to the spinal compartment, the extra space in the spinal compartment being provided by compression of subarachnoid and epidural veins. This mechanism can be seen most dramatically when an intracranial balloon is inflated in an experimental animal, for the CSF pressure rise which occurs lasts only a few minutes. The pressure then returns to a level which is only slightly above the initial value. Fig. 3 is from the work of Fitch, McDowall,

Ellis, Paterson and Hain (1970) and shows the rapid adjustment of intracranial pressure seen in this experimental situation.

Cerebrospinal fluid volume is maintained fairly constant by the balance achieved between formation and reabsorption. CSF is produced at a rate of about 0·4 ml/min in man (Rubin et al., 1966); rather more than half of this is formed by the choroid plexuses, and the rest comes from the interstitial fluid of the brain (Davson and Bradbury, 1965; Bering, 1965). In steady state conditions,

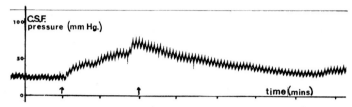

FIG. 3. The record shows the changes in intracranial pressure induced by the injection of 1 ml of fluid into an intracranial extradural balloon in the dog. The fluid was injected over two minutes between the arrows and the intracranial pressure rose by approximately 50 mm Hg. However, within 4 minutes the intracranial pressure had returned to within 10 mm Hg of its initial value. This compensation must have been achieved by moving about 1 ml of blood and C.S.F. out of the skull during this period.

the volume absorbed is obviously the same as the volume formed but when conditions change e.g. if cerebral blood flow falls due to hypocapnia, then the reduced CSF pressure slows the rate of CSF reabsorption through the microtubules of the arachnoid villi until CSF volume has increased sufficiently to produce a normal CSF pressure. Once this normal CSF pressure is achieved, absorption once again balances formation. Changes in CSF volume over the normal range of CSF pressure seem to be produced by variations in the rate of reabsorption since CSF production rate is not affected (Rubin et al., 1966; Cutler et al., 1968).

## III. ALTERATIONS IN INTRACRANIAL PRESSURES AND VOLUMES PRODUCED BY DISEASE

### (a) Occlusion of the Internal Carotid Artery in the Neck

As is well known, the internal carotid arteries are commonly involved in atheromatous obliteration of their lumen. It has been clearly established that obstruction of a carotid artery does not reduce carotid flow until the cross sectional area is reduced to less than 5 sq mm (i.e. an 80–90 per cent reduction) (Brice, Dowsett and Lowe, 1964). Even when carotid obliteration becomes complete, the changes in cerebral blood flow may be remarkably slight. Thus, in a study of cerebral arterial pressures in the monkey, Symon (1967), demonstrated that complete occlusion of one internal carotid artery caused a reduction of only 14 per cent in the pressure in the ipsilateral middle cerebral artery. Occlusion of the contralateral carotid artery had virtually the same effect, thus demonstrating the pressure equalizing function of the circle of Willis.

Bilateral carotid occlusion caused a fall of 50 per cent in middle cerebral artery pressure since the monkey, like man, receives the greater part of it's cerebral blood flow via the carotids. Furthermore, the margin of safety is very wide since cerebral blood flow has to be reduced to 15 per cent of normal before cerebral necrosis occurs (Zulch and Behrend, 1961).

Despite the above experimental evidence, cerebral infarction not infrequently occurs in man after unilateral carotid obliteration. This is due to individual variability in the efficiency of the circle of Willis, which is frequently the site of abnormalities (Riggs and Rupp, 1963). It may also occur if a patient with a complete carotid obstruction is suddenly rendered hypotensive, because at low blood pressure a marginally adequate anastomotic flow may become inadequate (Adams, 1967). It must be remembered that many of these patients are normally hypertensive so that an apparently 'normal' blood pressure during anaesthesia, for example, may be inadequate to maintain cerebral perfusion. The other danger which arises from acute hypotension in a patient with a partial carotid stenosis is that the slowing of blood flow may initiate thrombus formation at the site of the stenosis.

Necrosis following internal carotid occlusion (or stenosis plus hypotension) occurs in two patterns: (1) in the territory of one of the main intracerebral arteries; or (2) in a 'water shed area'. The arterial territory usually involved is the middle cerebral artery because it is furthest from collateral supply from the other internal carotid and from the basilar supply. The size of the infarct can vary widely depending upon the functional efficiency of the circle of Willis in any particular patient, and upon the collateral circulation supplied on the cortical surface by cortical branches of anterior and posterior cerebral arteries.

Necrosis in association with internal carotid stenosis may also occur in a 'water shed' pattern, e.g. in the boundary zone between the zones of supply of the anterior and middle cerebral arteries. The precipitating cause of such an infarct is usually an episode of systemic hypotension acting on a cerebral circulation compromised by stenosis of a major neck vessel, though symmetrical water shed infarcts can occur in the absence of major vessel pathology if hypotension is severe or prolonged (Adams, 1967).

### (b) Occlusion of Intracranial Arteries

Similar considerations apply as with neck vessels except that the territory involved is limited to the distribution territory of the occluded vessel. Complete occlusion will usually produce some area of necrosis but the extent of this will depend on the site of the occlusion within the artery, the rapidity of occlusion, and on the efficiency of the anastomoses with cortical branches of neighbouring vessels.

An interesting situation sometimes arises in cases of partial obstruction of an intracranial artery in which hypocapnia may actually cause an increase in blood flow in the affected territory. This occurs when the degree of vessel stenosis is such that the distal intraluminal pressure is below the autoregulatory range. The arterioles of the involved artery are then maximally vasodilated and little affected by changes in $Pa_{CO_2}$. If hypocapnia is now induced the arterioles in the surrounding normal territories constrict so that the arterial pressure in the circle of Willis rises and blood flow to the partially obstructed region is improved. This bizarre situation has been termed intracerebral steal, but, since the impoverished area benefits by the new distribution of flow resources, Lassen's term 'Robin Hood Syndrome' is more apt as well as being more dramatic (Lassen and Palvolgyi, 1968). Certainly Soloway et al. (1968) have demonstrated that hyperventilation reduces the area of cerebral infarction which occurs in the dog after applying an occlusive clip to the middle cerebral artery.

### Intracranial Tumours

As an intracranial tumour increases in size, space must be made for it within the skull. Initially the required room is found by the displacement of blood and CSF from the skull. Thus, the cerebral venous blood volume is reduced and CSF is moved out of the skull and into the spinal dural sac. At first, therefore, growth of the tumour proceeds without producing large increases in intracranial pressure since the total volume of the intracranial contents is not altered. It should be noted that this adjustment is made at the expense of those compensating mechanisms which normally provide the buffer against acute changes in cerebral blood volume produced, for example, by coughing or straining.

As the tumour continues to grow these compensatory reductions in the volumes of the fluid compartments are fully taken up. Any further small expansion of the tumour now produces a large rise in pressure because of the compressed state of the intracranial contents. One might anticipate that when the intracranial pressure begins to rise CSF volume would be further reduced by increased reabsorption of CSF through the arachnoid villi. Unfortunately, however, the relative immunity enjoyed by the sagittal sinus pressure to acute changes in CSF pressure does not seem to apply to more sustained pressure changes perhaps because chronically elevated pressures are more effective in compressing the sinus dural walls. Shulman et al. (1964), for example, have shown that in chronically hydrocephalic dogs the pressure in the superior sagittal sinus was elevated to virtually the same degree as the general intracranial pressure. This means that the compensation which might have been afforded by an increased CSF—dural venous pressure gradient is lost.

Fig. 4 is a diagramatic representation of the relationship between the growth of an intracranial tumour and the change in intracranial pressure. It is self-evident that in the intracranial situation there must eventually be a precipitous terminal rise in intracranial pressure but the more interesting phase is the period of nearly complete compensation for the tumour growth. How long this phase lasts depends on the rate of tumour growth and its siting in relation to the CSF pathways. The dependence on rate of growth is partly related to the possibility that the extent of compensation possible is greater when a tumour grows slowly. At its simplest this latter point can readily be demonstrated in animal experiments for in the dog 3–4 ml of fluid given into an intracranial balloon over two or three minutes may kill the animal while 8–12 ml are required if infusion is given over six hours.

As has already been pointed out, the stage of slow pressure increase is achieved by the exhaustion of normal

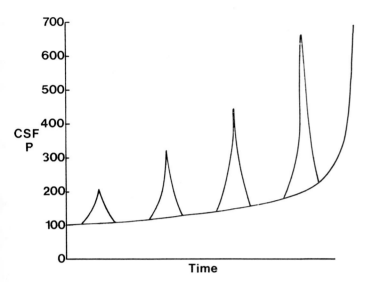

FIG. 4. The continuous line is a diagramatic representation of the changes in intracranial pressure which occur as a tumour grows within the skull. It will be seen that there is a stage of nearly complete compensation for the tumour growth during which little change in pressure occurs. This is followed by a decompensated stage in which intracranial pressure increases rapidly with only a small further increase in tumour volume. Since the earlier stage of compensation is achieved by infringing on the reserves which are normally available to cope with acute changes in intracranial blood volume, any sudden change in this latter volume will produce an abnormally great intracranial pressure increase. The peaks shown on the diagram represent the effects of administering Halothane at various stages during the progression of tumour growth. Halothane, by increasing cerebral blood flow and intracranial blood volume produces a progressively greater increase in intracranial pressure as intracranial compression develops. It is important to note that these large pressure increases due to Halothane and other volatile anaesthetics occur on top of base line intracranial pressure which need not be greatly elevated. The heights of the peaks in this diagram have been obtained from the work of Jennett, Barker, Fitch and McDowall (1969).

compensatory mechanisms so that the intracranial pressure becomes very sensitive to changes in cerebral blood volume. This instability of intracranial pressure in this phase is evidenced by the appearance of 'plateau waves' in these patients (Lundberg, 1960). These plateaux are large increases in CSF pressure on top of an only moderate elevated base line pressure. They last for 5–20 minutes and are thought to be triggered by small changes in intracranial blood volume which in normal subjects would be readily accommodated. A further evidence of the delicately balanced intracranial situation in these patients is seen if a volatile anaesthetic agent is administered. The intracranial pressure change which results from the anaesthe-

tically induced increase in intracranial blood volume is markedly greater than in 'normal' patients (Fitch and McDowall, 1970A). This is diagramatically illustrated in Fig. 4 which shows an increasing effect of halothane administration on intracranial pressure as cerebral compression progresses. It is important to note that large CSF pressure increases can be produced by volatile anaesthetic drugs even when the 'base line' CSF pressure is not greatly elevated, and that these changes can occur in the absence of respiratory depression or hypoxia, though of course they are greatly accentuated in the presence of these latter factors.

An intracranial tumour growing in one compartment of the brain, produces brain distortion and this, rather than the generalized intracranial pressure increase is responsible for many of the clinical signs. It may also produce pressure gradients within the brain if its growth in one compartment leads to a pressure change which is not transmitted throughout the intracranial contents. Failure of pressure equalization is usually the result of tentorial herniation with supratentorial lesions and herniation of the cerebellum into the foramen magnum with posterior fossa lesions (Langfitt, et al., 1964). One of the possible dangers of administering a volatile anaesthetic to a patient with an intracranial tumour is that the intracranial pressure change may be greater in the compartment with the tumour than elsewhere and this pressure gradient may lead to herniation (Fitch and McDowall, 1970B).

Alterations in cerebral blood flow are produced by intracranial tumours. Firstly, as is well known, cerebral blood flow begins to fail when the intracranial pressure rises above about 400–500 mm $H_2O$ or 30 mm Hg (Kety, Shenkin and Schmidt, 1948). During plateau waves intracranial pressure frequently exceeds this value and cerebral blood flow is consequently reduced during these periods (Cronqvist and Lundberg, 1968).

In addition, however, cerebral blood flow is affected by the presence of an intracranial tumour even when intracranial pressure is not greatly elevated. Thus, in the case of a supratentorial tumour there is a global reduction in cerebral blood flow throughout the involved hemisphere for reasons which are not yet clear. There are also small areas of increased cerebral perfusion in and around the tumour which are thought to be due to local tissue acidosis produced by tissue compression. Furthermore, there are alterations in the mechanisms of cerebro-vascular control so that vessels in the region of the tumour may respond paradoxically to changes in $Pa_{CO_2}$ and/or they may fail to autoregulate to acute blood pressure changes. Finally, brain distortion by tumour growth can mechanically angulate individual cerebral vessels, usually the posterior cerebral arteries, to produce local derangements in cerebral perfusion. The picture is thus a complicated one and the interested reader is referred for a full account to the recent review by Miller (1970).

## ACKNOWLEDGEMENTS

The author was greatly helped in the preparation of this review by discussions with Mr. A. E. Wall, Mr.

R. M. Gibson and Mr. J. Currie, Consultant Neurosurgeons at Leeds General Infirmary. The measurements shown in Fig. 1 and 2 were made in collaboration with Dr. W. Fitch, M.R.C. Research Assistant, University of Leeds.

## REFERENCES

Abercrombie, J. (1828). *Pathological and Practical Researches on Diseases of the Brain.* Edinburgh.

Adams, J. H. (1967), "Patterns of Cerebral Infarction," *Scot. med. J.*, **12**, 339.

Bedford, T. H. B. (1935), "The Effect of Increased Intracranial Venous Pressior on the Pressure of the Cerebrospinal Fluid," *Brain*, **58**, 427.

Bering, E. A. (1955), "Choroid Plexus and Arterial Pulsation of Cerebrospinal Fluid," *Arch. Neurol. Psychiat.*, **73**, 165.

Bering, E. A. (1965), "The Cerebrospinal Fluid Circulation." In: *Cerebrospinal Fluid and the Regulation of Ventilation.* (C. McC. Brooks, F. F. Kao and B. B. Lloyd, Eds.), p. 385. Oxford: Blackwell.

Bethune, D. W., Currie, J. C. M. and Watson, B. M. (1968), "Physiological Pressure Variations within the Cerebrospinal Fluid Pathways in Man," *J. Physiol.*, **196**, 136P.

Betz, E. (1970), "Influence of c.s.f. pH on the Regulation of the Cerebral Circulation." In: *The Cerebral Circulation*, (D. G. McDowall Ed.), p. 525. International Anesthesiology Clinics Series. Boston: Little, Brown & Co.

Brice, J. G., Dowsett, D. J. and Lowe, R. D. (1964), "Haemodynamic Effect of Carotid Artery Stenosis," *Brit. med. J.*, **2**, 1363.

Cronqvist, S. and Lundberg, N. (1968), "Regional Cerebral Blood Flow in Intracranial Tumours with special reference to Cases with Intracranial Hypertension," *Scand. J. Lab. and Clin. Invest.*, Suppl. 102.

Cushing, H. (1901), "Concerning a Definite Regulatory Mechanism of the Vasomotor Centre which Controls Blood Pressure during Cerebral Compression," *Bull. Johns Hopk. Hosp.*, **12**, 29.

Cutler, R. W. P., Page, L., Galicich, J. and Watters, G. V. (1968), "Formation and Absorption of Cerebrospinal Fluid in Man," *Brain*, **91**, 707.

Davson, H. (1960), "Intracranial and Intraocular Fluids." In: *American Handbook of Physiology*, Section I, Vol. III, p. 1761. Washington: American Physiological Society.

Davson, H. and Bradbury, M. (1965), "Formation and Drainage of the Cerebrospinal Fluid. Basic concepts." In: *Cerebrospinal Fluid and the Regulation of Ventilation.* (C. McC. Brooks, F. F. Kao and B. B. Lloyd, Eds.), p. 385. Oxford: Blackwell.

Dunbar, H. S., Guthrie, T. C. and Karpell, B. (1966), "A Study of Cerebrospinal Fluid Pulse Wave," *Arch. Neurol.*, **14**, 624.

Falck, B., Nielsen, K. C. and Owman, Ch. (1968), "Adrenergic Innervation of the Pial Circulation", *Scand. J. Lab. and Clin. Invest.*, Suppl. 102.

Fitch, W. and McDowall, D. G. (1970A), "Hazards of Anaesthesia in Patients with Intracranial Tumours." In: *The Cerebral Circulation.* (D. G. McDowall, Ed.). International Anesthesiology Clinics Series. Boston: Little, Brown & Co.

Fitch, W. and McDowall, D. G. (1970B), "Further Studies of the Effects of Anaesthetic Danger on Intercranial Pressure," *Proc. Roy. Soc. Med.* In press.

Fitch, W., McDowall, D. G., Ellis, F. R. Paterson, G. M., and Hain, W. R. (1970). "Effect of Elevated Atracranial Pressure on Cardiac Output and Other Circulatory Parameters," *Brit. J. Anaesth.*, **42**, 90.

Harper, A. M. (1970), "General Physiology of Cerebral Circulation." In: *The Cerebral Circulation.* (D. G. McDowall, Ed.), p. 473. International Anesthesiology Clinics Series. Boston: Little Brown & Co.

Hill, L. (1896). *The Physiology and Pathology of the Cerebral Circulation.* London: Churchill.

Jennett, W. B., Barker, J., Fitch, W. and McDowall, D. G. (1969), "Effect of Anaesthesia on Intracranial Pressure in Patients with Space-occupying Lesions," *Lancet*, **1**, 61.

Kanzow, E. and Dieckhoff, D. (1969), "On the Location of the Vascular Resistance in the Cerebral Circulation," *Proc. Int. CBF Symposium, Mainz.* In press.

Kellie, G. (1824), "On Death from Cold and Congestion of the Brain," *Trans. med. chir. Soc., Edinburgh*, **1**, 84.

Kety, S. S., Shenkin, H. A. and Schmidt, C. F. (1948), "Effects of Increased Intracranial Pressure on Cerebral Circulatory Functions in Man," *J. clin. Invest..* **27**, 493.

Langfitt, T. W., Weinstein, J. D., Kassell, N. F. and Simeone, F. A (1964), "Transmission of Increased Intracranial Pressure, 1. Within the Craniospinal Axis," *J. Neurosurg.*, **21**, 989.

Lassen, N. A. and Palvolgyi, R. (1968), "Cerebral Steal during Hypercapnia and the Inverse Reaction during Hypocapnia Observed by the 133 Xenon Technique in Man," *Scand. J. Lab. and Clin. Invest.*, Suppl. 102.

Lundberg, N. (1960), "Continuous Recording and Control of Ventricular Pressure in Neurosurgical Practice," *Acta psychiat. Scand.*, **36**, Suppl. 149, p. 1.

McDowall, D. G., Barker, J. and Jennett, W. B. (1966), "Cerebrospinal Fluid Pressure Measurement during Anaesthesia," *Anaesthesia*, **21**, 189.

McDowall, D. G. (1971), "The Cerebral Circulation." In: *General Anaesthesia*, Vol. I, p. 272. (T. C. Gray and J. F. Nunn, Eds.). London: Butterworths.

Mchedlishvili, G. I. (1969), "The Spasm of the Internal Carotid Artery," *Proc. Int. CBF Symposium, Mainz.* In press.

Millar, R. A. (1970), "Neurogenic Control of the Cerebral Circulation. In: *The Cerebral Circulation.* (D. G. McDowall, Ed.), p. 539. International Anesthesiology Clinics Series. Boston: Little, Brown & Co.

Miller, J. D. (1970), "The Effect of Space occupying Lesions on Cerebral Circulation." In: *The Cerebral Circulation.* (D. G. McDowall, Ed.). International Anesthesiology Clinics Series. Boston: Little, Brown & Co.

Monro, A. (1783). *Observations on the Structure and Functions of the Nervous System.* Edinburgh: Creed and Johnston.

Riggs, H. E. and Rupp, C. (1963), "Variation in form of circle of Willis," *Arch. Neurol.*, **8**, 8.

Rosomoff, H. L. (1961), "Effect of Hypothermia and Hypertonic Urea on Distribution of Intracranial Content," *J. Neurosurg.*, **18**, 753.

Rosomoff, H. L. (1963), "Distribution of Intracranial Contents with Controlled Hyperventilation: Implications for Neuroanesthesia," *Anesthesiology*, **24**, 640.

Rubin, R. C., Henderson, E. S., Ommaya, A. K., Walker, M. D. and Rall, D. P. (1966), "The Production of Cerebrospinal Fluid in Man and its Modification by Acetazolamide," *J. Neurosurg.*, **25**, 430.

Shulman, K. (1965), "Small Artery and Vein Pressures in the Subarchnoid Space of the Dog," *J. Surg. Res.*, **5**, 56.

Shulman, K., Yarnell, P. and Ransohoff, J. (1964), "Dural Sinus Pressure," *Arch. Neurol.*, **10**, 575.

Shulman, K. and Verdier, G. R. (1967), "Cerebral Vascular Resistance Changes in Response to Cerebrospinal Fluid Pressure," *Amer. J. Physiol.*, **213**, 1084.

Soderberg, U. and Weckman, N. (1959), "Changes in Cerebral Blood Supply caused by changes in the Pressure Drop along Arteries to the Brain in the Cat," *Experientia*, **15**, 346.

Soloway, M., Nadel, W., Albin, M. S. and White, R. J. (1968), "The Effect of Hyperventilation on Subsequent Cerebral Infarction," *Anesthesiology*, **29**, 975.

Symon, L. (1967), "A Comparative Study of Middle Cerebral Pressure in Dogs and Macaques," *J. Physiol.*, **191**, 449.

Weed, L. H. and McKibben, P. S. (1919), "Pressure Changes in the Cerebrospinal Fluid following Intravenous Injection of Solutions of Various Concentrations," *Amer. J. Physiol.*, **48**, 512.

Welch, K. and Friedman, V. (1960), "The Cerebrospinal Fluid Valves," *Brain*, **83**, 454.

Wright, R. D. (1938), "Experimental Observations on Increased Intracranial Pressure," *Aust. New Z. J. Surg.*, **7**, 215.

Zulch, K. J. and Behrend, R. C. H. (1961), "The Pathogenesis and Topography of Anoxia, Hypoxia and Ischemia of the Brain in Man." Page 144 in: *Cerebral Anoxia and the Electroencephalogram.* (H. Gastant and J. S. Meyer, Eds.). Illinois: Thomas.

CHAPTER 5

# PLACENTAL CIRCULATION

## GORDON TAYLOR

The placenta has been defined as an apposition or fusion of the foetal membranes to the uterine mucosa for physiological exchange. In particular the apposition of foetal and maternal circulations facilitates respiration, excretion and nutrition of the foetus. The anatomy and the regulation of both placental circulations are of the utmost importance when considering the physiology of pregnancy. The current concepts of the placental circulation are summarized in succeeding sections. A more detailed account may be found elsewhere (Martin 1965).

### Development of Placental Circulations

After ovum implantation the trophoblast encounters and erodes maternal endometrial capillaries. Maternal blood is released and percolates through the labyrinth of clefts produced by the trophoblastic syncytium (Hamilton and Boyd, 1960). Expansion of the trophoblast brings about invasion and erosion of endometrial veins. A sluggish maternal circulation from capillaries to veins is thus produced.

In the second week the ovum is covered in villi which contain mesoderm and vascular primordia. Embryonic blood vessels undergo proliferation and by the third week have produced an anastomosing network of channels within the villi. Vessels developing on the inner surface of the chorion and in the body stalk provide the connection between the vascular network in the villi and the embryonic heart. The trophoblast grows rapidly in the first 12 weeks, and the multiple branching villi now fill what can be recognized as the intervillous space.

The maternal circulation also develops rapidly. In the fifth week the trophoblast invades the endometrial arteries, and arterial inflow into the intervillous space is established. As the foetus grows so the placental site enlarges and more maternal vessels open into the intervillous space. By the end of the third month the placenta is in a mature form with its complement of 100–200 foetal cotyledons.

### The Uteroplacental Circulation

The uteroplacental circulation is maternal in origin and consists of the intervillous space and the arteries and veins supplying this space. The customary terminology of radial and spiral arteries as branches of the uterine artery appears to have no functional significance in the pregnant uterus. Instead these branches should be referred to as uteroplacental arteries or coiled arteries (Harris and Ramsey, 1966b). The reason for the change is that both radial and spiral arteries may open directly into the intervillous space.

In the mature placenta about 60–100 arterial openings may be found in the base of the placenta (Boyd and Hamilton, 1967). However, there appears to be a decrease in the number of arterial openings as gestation progresses. This may reflect the dual action of the trophoblast in breaching the main trunk of some arteries in several places, and occluding branches of others. The uteroplacental veins form a network around the arteries and have thin walls. The veins lack valves and are subject to external compression. Villi may be seen in these veins, but do not appear to produce occlusion although they may function as physiological ball valves.

Angiography to demonstrate the uteroplacental circulation in monkeys was pioneered by Borell, and he has used a similar method to illustrate the uteroplacental circulation in the human (Borell et al., 1965). These studies have shown a striking similarity between the monkey and human uteroplacental circulation.

By radiographic and other studies (Harris and Ramsey, 1966a) the uteroplacental arteries may be seen to discharge their contents in fountain-like spurts into the intervillous space. Blood leaving these arteries has a pressure of between 60–70 mm. of mercury. Freese (1968) suggests that a single uteroplacental artery lies beneath the central space of each cotyledon. This area is devoid of villi with consequent minimal loss of pressure and velocity of the entering maternal blood. Due to this umbrella shape of the central space, the maternal blood moves laterally and enters spaces between the villi. Pressure and velocity is gradually lost due to increasing resistance by the villi. After bathing the villi the blood returns to the pelvic veins via the uteroplacental veins.

Further support for this concept of the maternal placental circulation is provided by direct pressure measurement within the intervillous space and pelvic veins. When the uterus is in the relaxed state the intervillous space has a pressure range of 6–10 mm. of mercury. The pelvic venous pressure is slightly lower.

### Factors Affecting Uteroplacental Circulation

The total uterine blood flow is partitioned between the placenta and the myometrium. Current techniques do not allow separation of the two fractions. Obviously blood perfusing the myometrium will not participate in maternal-foetal exchange. In the pregnant uterus at term the myometrial flow must be a significant fraction of the total uterine flow, as the uterus increases some 20 times in weight during pregnancy. Total uterine blood flow is believed to be of the order of 600–800 ml./min. which represents about 10 per cent of the cardiac output at term.

It is a well known clinical observation that excessive uterine contraction is often associated with evidence of foetal asphyxia. Radioangiography illustrates that for every increase in the interuterine pressure there is a diminution of blood entering through the uteroplacental arteries. Intrauterine pressure of 36 mm. of mercury will abolish all arterial flow in monkeys (Harris and Ramsey, 1966b). In the human, pressures of about 50 mm. of mercury markedly reduce the arterial inflow (Borell *et al.*, 1965). Exit of blood through uteroplacental veins is suspended during contractions. At this time because of obstruction to outflow of blood, the intervillous space pressure will increase. All these factors have a bearing on the welfare of the foetus during a contraction.

In hypotensive conditions caused by hypovolaemia or sympathetic blockade, uterine blood flow may be reduced and evidence of foetal asphyxia may be apparent. Hypotension is often corrected when the blood volume is restored. Adverse changes in the foetus may be accentuated when a vasopressor drug such as methoxamine is used. This drug is known to decrease the uterine blood flow in animals (Eng *et al.*, 1971). Ephedrine, however, appears not to affect uterine blood flow to the same extent as methoxamine (Schnider *et al.*, 1968).

The evidence that hypertension is associated with a fall in uterine perfusion is indirect. Radio-active sodium injected into the myometrium or the intervillous space is believed to reflect uterine blood flow. In pregnancies complicated by hypertension and pre-eclampsia, the disappearance time of the sodium was found to be considerably prolonged. Towards the end of the normal pregnancy sclerotic changes appear in the walls of the uteroplacental arteries. These changes are accentuated in a pregnancy associated with hypertensive states and may be of a magnitude to obliterate the vascular lumen.

### Foetal Circulation

Within the umbilical cord there are three vessels; one vein and two arteries. The umbilical vein conveys oxygenated blood from the placenta to the foetal inferior vena cava. The umbilical arteries take origin from the internal iliac arteries in the foetus and return blood to the placenta.

Each primary villus receives at its origin an arterial and a venous branch of the umbilical vascular system. As the foetal cotyledon ramifies into minor villi, so the vessels divide and an extensive capillary network develops. Arterio-venous shunts to eliminate portions of the capillary network have not been demonstrated. The blood flow in the umbilical circuit is controlled by the interaction of foetal artery pressure and umbilical vascular resistance.

Extensive physiological studies of the umbilical circulation have been carried out in foetal lambs. The umbilical arteries receive about 57 per cent of the combined output of the two ventricles. Umbilical flow increases as the foetus matures and reaches a rate of 300 ml./minute at term. As the placental vascular bed is the major resistance within the umbilical circulation, Dawes (1962) has suggested that the increase in umbilical flow during certain periods of the pregnancy could be largely accounted for by the decrease in vascular resistance. Towards the end of pregnancy the increase in umbilical flow was almost entirely due to the rising foetal blood pressure.

### Regulation of Foetal Circulation

Reduction of maternal oxygen tension or a decrease in uterine blood flow can induce hypoxaemia in the foetal lamb. To compensate to some extent for this there is a greater rate of blood flow caused by an increase in foetal heart rate and a rise in foetal blood pressure. The oxygen extraction from the maternal blood is therefore more complete. This compensatory mechanism would appear to be mediated by the foetal autonomic nervous system. There are limits to this compensation and when severe anoxia occurs there is an increase in umbilical vascular resistance, probably due to release of foetal catecholamines. The heart rate may increase but as anoxia supervenes it falls precipitously. Umbilical flow then falls accentuating the foetal hypoxia. A similar series of events can be observed with the human foetus.

Panigel (1962) has shown that the umbilical and cotyledonary vessels will constrict when the oxygen tension is increased and dilate when the carbon dioxide tension is raised. Umbilical vasoconstriction can also be produced by catecholamines, histamine, posterior pituitary extract, ergot alkaloids and serotonin. Nitrites and papaveretum will cause vasodilatation. These effects are due to direct action upon the vessel wall as neural structures cannot be demonstrated in the umbilical cord. Physical stimuli such as manipulation or tension will produce marked constriction of umbilical vessels particularly the arteries. This is of some importance when one considers that entanglement of the cord around the neck or one of the limbs occurs in 30 per cent of all deliveries.

### Placental Circulation and Placental Exchange

So far the maternal and foetal circulations in the placenta have been discussed independently. The most important aspect of these circulations lies in the exchange of substances between them. This exchange will be affected by the course of foetal and maternal blood streams and the flow rates. The most efficient arrangement would be a countercurrent flow pattern which exists in sheep and rabbits. Here the circulations are arranged in parallel to one another, blood flowing in opposite directions. In the primate placenta a countercurrent flow pattern is not seen. Foetal blood makes a complete circuit through the artery to capillary and on to vein. During its course the foetal blood is exposed to maternal blood which is arterial at the inflow orifices and venous at the outflow orifices and of intermediate composition elsewhere in the intervillous space.

There is considerable evidence for this pattern of placental circulation in man. Blood samples from the intervillous space for $P_{O_2}$ and $P_{CO_2}$ and pH give values which are towards the maternal venous level. Therefore instead of a diffusion gradient there is a spectrum of gradients throughout the placenta. Some radiographic studies in humans indicate that the uteroplacental arteries may be shut off from time to time during relaxation of the uterus. The role of this phenomenon in regulation of uterine blood flow is unknown, but it does have implications for placental exchange. The problem may be analogous to ventilation-perfusion ratios in the lung.

The evaluation of the data relating to the transfer of respiratory gases across the placenta is extremely difficult. Normal obstetric practice is open to many variables and several reports available are based on the investigation of few cases. With these limitations certain salient facts emerge from the many papers on this subject.

The total uterine blood flow is about 600–800 ml./minute when the pregnancy is at term. The principle points relating to the transfer of respiratory gases across oxygen dissociation curve for foetal haemoglobin lies to the left of the curve for the adult.

A number of factors may influence the transfer of respiratory gases across the placenta. The most obvious of these is the disruption of the placental site as a result of premature separation or haemorrhage. Somewhat more insidious is toxaemia of pregnancy which is primarily a disease of the mother. Placental insufficiency forms part of the pathology of this disease, probably due to a diminution of maternal blood flow through narrowed utero-placental arteries. A similar form of placental insufficiency

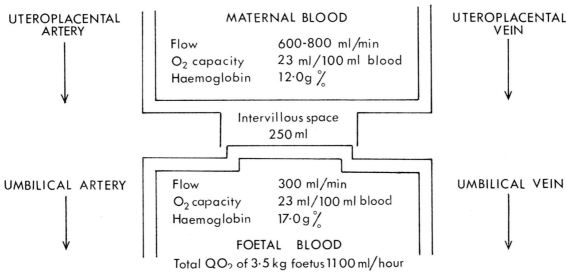

FIG. 1. Circulatory and respiratory parameters in the placenta (after Crawford 1965 Obstetric Anaesthesia).

the placenta are summarized in Figure 1. The arterio-venous difference across the uteroplacental vessels is about 4·7 ml. oxygen per 100 ml. of blood, indicating therefore that uterine and placental oxygen consumption is 2,100 ml./hour. It is believed that the average size placenta uses oxygen at the rate of 90 ml./hour. Neonatal studies indicate that a 3·5 kg. infant requires 1,300–1,400 ml. oxygen per hour. In utero without having the need of work, of respiration or temperature maintenance, the oxygen requirement is probably much less, about 1,100 ml./hour. This leaves about 900 ml./hour of oxygen which is available for uterine tissue which is in excess of that calculated from previous studies. From the above calculations it can be seen that the uterus and the placenta appear to consume about half the oxygen available within the utero-placental circulation. It is possible that a shunt mechanism in the uterus occurs during maternal oxygen deprivation which will allow preferential arterial blood supply to the placental site.

The oxygen tension of uteroplacental vessels has been found to be 95 mm./Hg. in the artery and 33 mm./Hg. in the veins. This compares with an oxygen tension of 28 mm./Hg. in the umbilical vein and 17 mm./Hg. in the umbilical artery. Foetal oxygen carriage is affected by two other factors, namely that foetal oxygen carrying capacity is about 23 ml./100 ml. blood, and secondly the

may be seen in association with essential hypertension and chronic glomerulonephritis of the mother. Other diseases such as maternal diabetes mellitus and rhesus incompatibility which are associated with oedema of the placenta may cause an increase in the time taken for diffusion of respiratory gases, particularly oxygen.

It would appear that maternal age and gestational duration are important in the efficient transfer of respiratory gases across the placenta. Evidence is available which suggests the perinatal mortality rises with increasing maternal age. In a normal pregnancy the placenta permits satisfactory transfer of respiratory gases, but, beyond the fortieth week there would appear to be increasing perinatal mortality related to the length of postmaturity. This perinatal mortality may be caused by a diminution of oxygen supply rather than the retention of carbon dioxide and fixed acids.

Maternal hypoxia from any cause and severe maternal hypotension will produce a pronounced fall in the oxygen saturation in foetal blood. Coincidentally with this there will be an increase in carbon dioxide and the level of fixed acids. Maternal hypercarbia can lead to foetal acidosis but the foetus excretes fixed acids with comparative ease. However a prolonged labour with associated severe maternal metabolic acidosis will decrease the ability of the foetal blood to accept oxygen.

Labour can interfere with the transfer of respiratory gases due to almost complete isolation of the contracting uterus from maternal arterialized blood, particularly during the second stage. The adverse effects may be compounded when the contractions are long or the interval between them is short. In addition the mother may further aggravate the situation should she hold her breath and push between contractions. A period of uterine quiescence is essential to allow the foetal circulation to rectify the lowered oxygen tension and the accumulation of carbon dioxide.

Placental transfer of respiratory gases may also be compromised by interference with umbilical blood flow. This is often due to the many types of cord entanglement and compression that have been described. Foetal asphyxia from either maternal or foetal causes has been detected in the past by a variation from the range of normality in the foetal heart rate, and by the appearance of meconium in the draining liquor. For many years it has been accepted that the only really reliable sign has been persistent foetal bradycardia. Foetal tachycardia and meconium stained liquor are thought to be only incidental signs in certain cases of diagnosed foetal asphyxia. In recent years Beard *et al.* (1967) have made a valuable contribution in popularizing the work of Saling using sampling of foetal capillary blood from the scalp through the partially dilated cervix.

Blood is collected into heparinized capillary tubing and the micro-Astrup technique used to determine the pH and base deficit together with the $P_{CO_2}$. Direct measurement of the $P_{CO_2}$ has confirmed the accuracy of this technique.

Provided blood uncontaminated with liquor can be obtained, accurate assessment of the foetal acid-base balance may be deduced and a decision made with regard to delivery of the foetus. This decision may be made with confidence in spite of the continued presence of one or more of the traditional signs of foetal asphyxia.

### The Placental Transfer of Anaesthetic Drugs

For all practical purposes the placental barrier closely resembles the blood brain barrier and therefore factors affecting drug transfer will be similar. From this point of view the transfer of substances of a molecular weight greater than 600 is determined primarily by the lipid solubility of the drug. An example of a drug with high lipid solubility is bupivacaine. Next in order of importance is the dissociation constant. Succinylcholine is highly ionized and therefore crosses the placenta with difficulty. The third factor may be the presence of a high concentration of a drug in the maternal circulation which will facilitate transference due to the large gradient across the placental membrane. Fourthly, the placenta contains a number of enzymes such as amine oxidase which breaks down catechol amines and impedes transfer into the foetal circulation. Finally the rate of transference of drugs may be influenced by pathological changes in the placenta. This has little bearing in the clinical situation as there would be coincident diminished oxygen supply to the foetus.

Transference of drugs across the placental membrane as described above assumes that both foetal and maternal circulations are maintained at a satisfactory level. On occasions, maternal hypotension may ensue, and therefore interfere with the rate of drug transfer. The immature brain of the foetus and the young neonate has been found to be markedly deficient in myelin. Drugs of poor lipid solubility may in fact affect the neural tissue of such brains much more easily than the adult brain. An example of this is the effect of morphine upon the newborn rat which is found to be very sensitive compared with the adult rat. Enzyme systems in the neonate are known to be poorly developed and therefore some drugs, e.g. those of the barbiturate group are not readily metabolized by the neonate.

When a drug is given intravenously it is carried round the body in bolus formation for one or two circulations. The drug presents itself at the placental site in a highly concentrated form. Variants of this can be produced by increasing the rapidity of the injection and giving higher concentrations of drugs. Intra-muscular injection never produces the concentrated bolus formation, but rather a steady trickle into the maternal circulation. Many volatile anaesthetic agents may act in a similar way to an intravenous injection. High concentrations of vapours required for the induction of anaesthesia are taken into the lungs and the maternal circulation. Transfer of volatile anaesthetics will occur readily to the foetal circulation if the maternal blood levels are high.

In obstetrics the dangers of administering concentrated drugs intravenously may be largely offset if the drugs are injected during the early part of a uterine contraction. This is obvious from a discussion earlier in this chapter as it has been shown that the uterus may be almost isolated from the maternal circulation during a contraction.

All the gases and vapours at present in use in anaesthetic practice cross the placenta with ease. However, the concentrations of these agents in cord blood are always lower when compared with maternal blood, but there is distinct evidence that, because of the free passage of these agents across the placenta, neonatal depression may result following administration to the mother.

Agents such as thiopentone and pethidine and certain of the phenothiazine derivatives also cross the placenta easily. Neontal depression can occur as a result of administration of these drugs, but with pethidine and other narcotics this can be largely offset by using one of the narcotic antagonists. The muscle relaxants do not cross the placenta freely. Of those in use at present, gallamine has been isolated in cord blood, therefore it would appear that the use of this drug should be discouraged in obstetric anaesthesia.

Regional analgesic techniques are part of the routine obstetric practice in the United States and in many centres in the United Kingdom. Lignocaine and bupivacaine are commonly used. Both drugs are highly lipid soluble and can be detected in cord blood, using suitable analysing techniques. When correct clinical dosage is used, neonatal depression is not seen. Recent investigations have shown the cord concentration of bupivacaine is very low and somewhere in the region of 20–40 per cent of the maternal level.

## Summary

The arrangement of the adjacent maternal and foetal circulations in the placenta provides the foetus with the physiological requirements for life for forty weeks while in the uterus. During that time oxygen and nutrient substances are taken in by the foetus while carbon dioxide and other waste products are removed. Interference with either of the circulations within the placenta or as a result of outside influences will affect the foetus in a harmful fashion. It is therefore of importance that neither circulation should be allowed to be impaired. Most commonly used anaesthetic drugs are highly lipid soluble, and therefore cross the placenta with ease. Care should be taken to keep the levels of these drugs to a minimum if neonatal depression is not to occur.

### REFERENCES

Beard, R. W., Morris, E. D. and Clayton, S. G. (1967), "pH of Foetal Capillary Blood as an Indicator of the Condition of the Foetus," *J. Obstet. Gynaec., Brit. Cwlth.*, **74**, 812.

Borrell, U., Fernstrom, I., Ohlson, L. and Wiqvist, N. (1965), "Influence of Uterine Contractions on the Uteroplacental Blood Flow at Term," *Amer. J. Obst. Gynec.*, **93**, 44.

Boyd, J. D. and Hamilton, W. J. (1967), "Development and Structure of the Human Placenta from the End of the Third Month of Gestation," *J. Obstet Gynaec., Brit. Cwlth.*, **74**, 161.

Crawford, J. S. (1965), "The Principles and Practice of Obstetric Anaesthesia", 2nd Ed., p. 48. Oxford: Blackwell.

Dawes, G. S. (1962), "The Umbilical Circulation," *Amer. J. Obstet. and Gynec.*, **84**, 1634.

Eng, M., Berges, P. U., Ueland, K., Bonica, J. J. and Parer, J. T. (1971), "The Effects of Methoxamine and Ephedrine in Normotensive Pregnant Primates", Anesthesiology, **35**, 354.

Freese, U. E. (1968), "The Uteroplacental Vascular Relationship in the Human," *Amer. J. Obstet. Gynec.*, **101**, 8.

Hamilton, W. J. and Boyd, J. D. (1960), "Development of the Human Placenta in the First Three Months of Gestation," *J. Anat.*, **94**, 297.

Harris, J. W. S., Ramsey, E. M. (1966a), "The Morphology of Human Uteroplacental Vasculature," *Caernegie Inst. Wash. Pub.* 625 *Contrib. Embryol.*, **38**, 45.

Harris, J. W. S. and Ramsey, E. M. (1966b), "Comparison of Uteroplacental Vasculature and Circulation in Monkey and Man," *Carnegie Inst. Wash. Pub.* 625 *Contrib. Embryol.*, **38**, 61.

Martin, Chester B. (1965), "Placental and Fetal Physiology," *Anesthesiology*, **26**, 447.

Panigel, M. (1962), "Placental Perfusion Experiments," *Amer. J. Obst. Gynec.*, **84**, 1664.

Shnider, S. M., De Lorimier, A. A., Holl, J. W., Chapler, F. K. and Morishima, H. O. (1968), "Vasopressors in Obstetrics", *Amer. J. Obst. Gynec.*, **102**, 911.

*CHAPTER 6*

# HYPOTENSION

### MALCOLM F. TYRRELL

### Systemic Arterial Pressure

In the healthy young adult systemic arterial pressure is 120 mm. Hg. systolic and 80 mm. Hg. diastolic. The arterial pressure may be measured directly at many sites using intra-arterial cannulae and pressure transducing devices, but more usually it is measured indirectly at the brachial artery using auscultatory or oscillometric methods. The values of systemic arterial pressures are lower in infants and higher in the elderly, where systolic pressures in excess of 200 mm. Hg. may be anticipated (Fig. 1). During normal sleep systolic pressure commonly falls to 80 to 100 mm. Hg. and such levels are often encountered during anaesthesia. With such wide normal variation it is impossible to define hypotension precisely and it is better to relate hypotension to a pre-existing control level than to set arbitrary pressure levels.

### Mean Arterial Pressure

This is the average arterial pressure throughout the cardiac cycle. Due to the shape of the arterial pressure wave form the mean arterial pressure is nearer the diastolic than the systolic pressure. Fig. 2 illustrates the mean

pressure; here the area of the curve above the mean pressure line must equal the sum of the two shaded areas

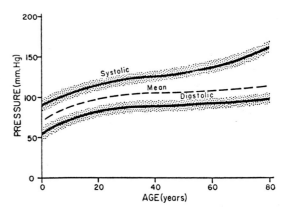

FIG. 1. Changes in systolic, diastolic and mean arterial pressures with age. Shaded areas show normal range. From, *Textbook of Medical Physiology* by Guyton (1966). 3rd Ed. Saunders: Philadelphia.

below. Mean pressure may be obtained mechanically, by introducing a high resistance to flow between the cannula and transducer, or electronically. An approximation to mean arterial pressure may be given by the expression:

$$\frac{\text{Systolic Press.} + 2 \text{ Diastolic Press.}}{3}$$

In the young adult, mean arterial pressure is 90–100 mm. Hg. and shows a positive correlation with age (Fig. 1).

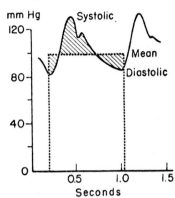

FIG. 2. Mean Arterial Pressure. The area of the curve above the rectangle equals the sum of the two areas below. From, *Physiology and Biophysics of the Circulation* by Burton (1965). Year Book Medical Publishers, Chicago.

Arterial pressure is normally maintained at a higher level than is required to provide adequate tissue blood flow; this allows for instantaneous increases in regional blood flow by local vasodilation. Mean arterial pressure represents the effective pressure head driving blood through the circulation and it is upon the relationship between pressure and resistance that tissue blood flow and perfusion depends.

### Flow, Pressure and Resistance Relationships

The relationships between flow, pressure and resistance may be expressed by three forms of a separate equation, analogous to the relationships governing electrical current, potential difference and resistance (Ohm's Law).

(1) $\Delta P = FR$      $(V = IR)$

(2) $F = \dfrac{\Delta P}{R}$    $\left(I = \dfrac{V}{R}\right)$

(3) $R = \dfrac{\Delta P}{F}$    $\left(R = \dfrac{V}{I}\right)$

where $P$ = Pressure (more accurately pressure difference)
      $F$ = Flow
      $R$ = Resistance

In terms of the circulation as a whole:–

Pressure    = Mean systemic arterial pressure
Flow        = Cardiac output
Resistance = Total peripheral resistance

The overall tissue blood flow and the adequacy of the circulation is dependent upon whether flow meets tissue demands. This depends upon the relation $\dfrac{\Delta P}{R}$ which is of more importance than a simple statement of pressure alone.

## FACTORS AFFECTING PRESSURE AND RESISTANCE

There are three independent mechanisms by which arterial pressure is regulated and all of these involve alterations in peripheral vascular tone.

These mechanisms are:

(1) Regulation by the autonomic nervous system
(2) Regulation by the kidneys
(3) Regulation by the endocrine system

Fifty per cent of the resistance to blood flow resides in the arterioles, the calibre of which are controlled by nervous and humoral mechanisms; the resistance in an individual arteriole may vary hundreds fold. In this property rests the unique position of the arteriole in the regulation of peripheral resistance and arterial pressure and in the overall distribution of cardiac output.

Regulation of arterial pressure by the autonomic system is largely reflex and concerned with acute changes, such as those occurring during exercise and changes in posture. More importantly in the present context, the autonomic system is active during the pressure changes associated with the reduced flow following such conditions as haemorrhage and myocardial infarction. The mechanisms concerned with arterial hypotension are:

(*a*) **Pressoreflexes.** Pressor receptors are found in the carotid sinus and in the walls of the aorta and other large arteries including the pulmonary artery. A fall in arterial pressure diminishes excitation of these receptors and reduces the afferent input to the vasomotor centre. There follows a general increase in sympathetic activity associated with raised catecholamine levels resulting in arteriolar constriction and increased myocardial contractility and heart rate. In haemorrhage, venous constriction also occurs, so tending to maintain arterial pressure.

(*b*) **Ischaemic responses.** Very low arterial pressures are associated with hypoxia of the vasomotor centre, and this results in increased sympathetic activity.

Regulation of the blood pressure by the endocrine and renin-angiotensin system is concerned with chronic changes and is referred to elsewhere.

## FACTORS AFFECTING FLOW

Flow (or cardiac output) may be derived as

Cardiac output = Stroke volume × Heart rate

This statement does not necessarily mean that if the heart rate increases then the cardiac output will increase; this will depend upon whether at the same time stroke volume is increased, maintained or decreased.

**Stroke volume.** As the left ventricle may be incompletely filled during diastole and incompletely emptied during systole, it will be seen that stroke volume is dependent upon the difference between diastolic and systolic volumes.

Diastolic volume is determined by the effective ventricular filling pressure and the distensibility of the ventricular walls, which itself varies with the phase of the cardiac cycle and rate of distension.

Effective ventricular filling pressure is the pressure

difference inside and outside the ventricle at the end of the diastolic period. Extracardiac pressure is measured in the pericardial or pleural space and is influenced by respiration and by pathology of the pericardium and lungs. Haemorrhage into the pericardium will increase extracardiac pressure and restrict ventricular filling, thus producing a reduction in stroke volume.

The pressure inside the ventricle is related to central venous pressure, which itself reflects the relation between total blood volume and vascular capacity. Circulating volume may be reduced by whole blood loss, by plasma and by saline loss. Central venous pressure will be decreased in such cases. The capacity of the venous system is very variable and small losses of blood may be compensated by constriction of venous reservoirs.

Systolic volume of the heart is determined by myocardial contractility. Ventricular ejection demands work output and adequate coronary blood flow. In coronary artery insufficiency contractility is reduced, and with it stroke volume and cardiac output. Central venous pressure will be elevated. The degree of ventricular contraction is determined by sympathetic discharge and by pacemaker activity.

**Heart rate.** This is dependent upon inherent pacemaker activity and influenced by autonomic balance. Fainting attacks result from acute hypotension following bradycardia and peripheral vasodilation, an inappropriate reflex response. Stimulation of visceral efferent fibres may also produce such autonomic inbalance.

## SHOCK

The literature on shock and hypotension is bedevilled by semantics and definitions. From the clinical standpoint the term is used to describe a patient with acute systemic arterial hypotension accompanied by pallor, weakness, sweating and a rapid, thready pulse. Much of this symptomatology is associated with sympathetic overactivity.

Guyton (1966) defines shock as 'An abnormal state of the circulation in which cardiac output is reduced enough that the tissues of the body are damaged for lack of adequate tissue blood flow'. This is a useful definition in that it emphasizes that flow is of overall importance and that shock and hypotension are not necessarily synonymous. Severe shock may exist in the presence of a normal systemic pressure and conversely adequate perfusion may be present despite profound hypotension. Decreased cardiac output, increased total peripheral resistance and a decreased effective circulating volume initiate and both directly and indirectly sustain the shock state.

Since shock results from an inadequate cardiac output, then any factor reducing cardiac output may cause shock. The reduced cardiac output may be caused in two ways:

(A) Reduced Venous Return.

This may result from diminished circulating volume, decreased vasomotor tone or a greatly increased peripheral vascular resistance. Such mechanisms play a part in the following:

(1) Haemorrhagic shock
(2) Endotoxic shock

(3) Anaphylactic shock
(4) Mechanical obstruction to venous return
(B) Reduced Pumping Ability of the Heart.

(1) Cardiogenic shock

### Haemorrhagic Shock

Haemorrhagic shock has received the greatest attention in clinical and laboratory research, although many of the phenomena associated with haemorrhagic shock are common to all forms.

Circulating volume may be reduced by whole blood loss, or by plasma or electrolyte loss. Reduced circulating volume results in a decrease in venous return with a subsequent fall in cardiac output. Should cardiac output and with it tissue blood flow fall to a critical level then shock will result. Up to 10 per cent of the blood volume may be removed with minimal effects, but a greater loss results in a reduced cardiac output. Systemic arterial pressure is maintained until 20 per cent of blood volume is removed and then declines. Sympathetic overactivity maintains arterial pressure by increased peripheral vasoconstriction rather than cardiac output and this mechanism protects the vulnerable cerebral and coronary circulations.

The descriptive terms used in shock, such as non-progressive or compensated, progressive and irreversible shock are really laboratory definitions. Shock in experimental animals is studied by controlled arterial haemorrhage into a reservoir set at an appropriate level above the heart. The animal bleeds into the reservoir until a desired degree of hypotension is achieved, usually 30–40 mm. Hg. This level is held for varying time intervals and by adjustment of the reservoir the animal may be retransfused. Depending upon the level of hypotension and its duration, there are two possible outcomes:

(1) Reinfusion may be followed by recovery with a normal arterial pressure and this may be termed non-progressive or compensated shock.
(2) If the level of hypotension or its duration exceeds a critical level, then arterial pressure falls progressively despite retransfusion or additional transfusion. This is termed irreversible shock. It is a matter of conjecture whether this condition has its counterpart in clinical practice.

Much controversy surrounds the aetiology of irreversible shock. The most reasonable assumption is that tissue hypoxia is responsible, but of what tissues and by what mechanism remains obscure. There have been many theories:

(1) For many years it was held that the liver elaborated a vasodilator material that was causative. This has since been identified as ferritin, which is without effect on the circulation.
(2) Following almost total suppression of the splanchnic blood flow in shock, bacteraemia and endotoxin released from Gram negative organisms in the bowel have been implicated in the production of irreversible shock (Fine, 1954). Further, reduced blood flow to certain organs,

particularly the liver, reduces the ability of the reticulo-endothelial system to perform essential detoxication. However, there is conflicting evidence for the protection given by antibiotics in this situation, and for the protection obtained in bacteria-free animals.

Much of this experimental work has been performed on dogs, where cessation of splanchnic blood flow is almost complete under profound sympathetic activity. In man this is probably not the case, and evidence suggests that the renal circulation suffers greatest stagnation in human shock.

(3) Recently the role of oxygen debt has been implicated in initiating the irreversible stage of shock. Crowell and Smith (1964) measuring oxygen consumption in bled dogs have demonstrated that shock becomes irreversible in the dog when the oxygen deficit reaches 150 ml. $O_2$/Kgm. irrespective of the rate at which the deficit accumulated. It has also been shown that animals receiving hyperbaric oxygen withstand greater circulatory trauma than animals breathing atmospheric air. However, dogs have a higher metabolic rate and acquire an oxygen debt at a much faster rate than man.

A further observation by Broder and Weil (1964) showed that in shock, when serum excess lactate exceeds 4 m-mole/L then survival is rare. This suggests that there is a level of cellular damage beyond which recovery is unlikely.

(4) Wiggers and Werle (1942) first pointed out that progressive myocardial failure was a significant factor in haemorrhagic shock. More recently Crowell and Guyton (1961) have demonstrated progressive left ventricular failure in hypovolaemic hypotension despite retransfusion, and other workers have shown left ventricular failure and decreased myocardial contractility in haemorrhagic, endotoxic and cardiogenic shock. Myocardial cells are inadequately perfused during shock, despite coronary artery autoregulation, and myocardial contractility suffers from the metabolic acidosis accompanying shock and from the products of cell injury.

(5) Microcirculatory stagnation with subsequent alterations in blood rheology and coagulation properties have led many workers to suggest these changes are basic in perpetuating shock. Hardaway (1963) has suggested that increasing blood viscosity together with the acidosis, toxins and other factors accompanying shock result in blood hypercoagulability and microthrombus formation in the capillaries. This would intensify the stagnant anoxia of shock.

## Microcirculation in shock

The microcirculation appears to be a final common path in all shock states. Factors governing total cardiac output have been discussed, but the share each individual circuit receives of the cardiac output is dependent upon the resistance that circuit offers to blood flow. This resistance resides in three sites:

(1) The arteriole
(2) Precapillary sphincter
(3) Postcapillary sphincter

The sphincters perform a further function. By their activity relative to each other they govern the hydrostatic pressure within the capillary itself; hence they govern the direction of net flow across the capillary wall between the plasma and the extracellular fluid.

The sphincters are influenced both by sympathetic activity and by local metabolites, pH and hypoxia. For the same catecholamine concentrations, precapillary sphincter constriction is greater than the post-capillary. In this way capillary presure is reduced and this facilitates the inflow of fluid into the intravascular space with augmentation of blood volume. This response is of value in early shock where circulating volume is maintained although the haematocrit is reduced.

Metabolites, acidosis and hypoxia relax the precapillary more than the postcapillary sphincter. Mellander and Lewis (1963) have shown that in the late stages of haemorrhagic shock the resistance of the postcapillary sphincter exceeds that of the precapillary, the direction of fluid flow is reversed and interstitial oedema occurs. This may explain the change in fluid shift seen in irreversible shock, and the capillary pooling and stagnation seen particularly in the splanchnic beds of the experimental animals. It also explains the observation that arterial pressure cannot be maintained in irreversible shock despite retransfusion and overtransfusion.

## Endotoxic Shock

Gram negative organisms are commonly implicated in the production of endotoxic shock, but it is probable that one third of cases in man are due to Gram positive organisms. Endotoxin stimulates the sympathetic system to produce arteriolar and venular constriction. This progresses to give the characteristic picture of capillary stagnation, in the dog seen as engorgement of the bowel, liver and kidneys. Sequestration of blood in these areas results in hypovolaemia, reduced venous return and central venous pressure and hence reduced arterial pressure.

## Anaphylactic shock

This denotes the rapid, severe reaction following the injection of an antigen to which the subject is sensitized. In man this results in intense bronchospasm and often systemic arterial hypotension. Shock resulting from antigen-antibody reactions usually follows drug administration or the injection of venom by insects. The antigen-antibody reaction leads to histamine release and this is responsible for generalized vasodilation, reduced venous return and cardiac output and subsequently arterial hypotension. Emergency treatment consists of adrenaline, given intravenously if necessary. Ventilation and oxygenation must be maintained.

## Cardiogenic Shock

The initial event in cardiogenic shock is reduced myocardial contractility leading to reduced cardiac output and arterial hypotension. Hypotension may reduce coronary blood flow and in this way a vicious cycle is instituted. The commonest cause of cardiogenic shock is coronary insufficiency leading to myocardial ischaemia or infarction. Other causes include acute myocarditis, extremes of heart rate, cardiac tamponade and the terminal phase of chronic myocardial failure. Unlike other forms of shock, failure of the heart as a pump results in a raised central venous pressure due to the inability to pump into the circulation the blood that is in the venous reservoir.

## RATIONALE OF TREATMENT IN SHOCK

Treatment in shock should aim at increasing effective blood flow through the microcirculation. Recently the pathogenesis of shock has been much more clearly elucidated following experimental work and the creation of 'shock teams' in the clinical situation. The aim is to base treatment upon the haemodynamic diagnosis since most cases of shock show a mixed picture and do not fall tidily into categories such as 'haemorrhagic', 'endotoxic' or 'cardiogenic'. The measurements upon which diagnosis is made are cardiac output, systemic arterial and central venous pressures, blood gas and acid-base status and estimates of excess lactate production (MacLean, 1966).

**Intravenous fluids.** In haemorrhagic shock blood volume must be restored as soon as possible. Whole blood should be used, but recently the use of Ringer lactate in the management of acute blood loss has been advocated (Dudley *et al.*, 1968). Fluids should be warmed to 35–40°C before administration and although controversy surrounds the use of calcium, it is indicated if citrated blood is transfused at a rate exceeding 500 ml. in 5 minutes. Low molecular weight dextran has been considered to be more effective than plasma in restoring the peripheral blood flow and has a value in reducing blood viscosity. In extensive burns, saline or plasma are indicated where the haematocrit exceeds 55 per cent.

**Vasopressors and Vasodilators.** It has been widely held that the most important factor in improving peripheral blood flow in shock was raising systemic arterial pressure, usually by the administration of sympathomimetic amines with predominant alpha effects. This approach is now obsolete (*Lancet*, 1967). The administration of an alpha effective agent, such as nor-adrenaline, produces vasoconstriction in most vascular beds; this enhances the action of endogenous catecholamines, the levels of which are already high in shock. Although systemic arterial pressure is elevated, pulse pressure and tissue blood flow is reduced; the net effect is to enhance the existing shock.

Attention has been directed at drugs which block the action of adrenaline at alpha receptors. These include tolazoline, phentolamine and phenoxybenzamine, which, due to its longer action, has been most widely used in the treatment of shock. The dose recommended is 1 mg/Kg. body weight, given as an infusion over one hour (Nickerson, 1965). The overall effect is to produce vasodilatation. Systemic arterial pressure falls and the use of alpha adrenergic blocking agents *must be accompanied by adequate fluid replacement*, of which the central venous pressure is the best guide. This is maintained at 12–15 cm. H$_2$O. If circulating volume is maintained and dilatation of the microcirculation has occurred, a systemic pressure of 70 mm. Hg. is adequate to support tissue perfusion. Lillehei (1965) recommends the use of alpha adrenergic blocking agents in cases of shock which do not respond to blood replacement and digitalization.

Isoprenaline, predominantly a beta effective agent, is of value in maintaining cardiac output. The combination of isoprenaline and phenoxybenzamine has been shown to be effective treatment of endotoxic shock in dogs, and has been recommended for use in man (Lillehei *et al.*, 1964).

**Steroids.** The use of large doses of steroids has been advocated in the treatment of shock unresponsive to fluid replacement. An initial dose of 50 mg/Kg. body weight of cortisol intravenously has been recommended (Bloch *et al.*, 1966). The benefit may be due to a positive inotropic action or an adrenolytic effect, as it is unrelated to impaired steroid production which is very high in shock.

**Antibiotics.** Antibiotics are of value in shock associated with infection. Shock is most frequently seen in Gram negative septicaemia, but unfortunately the drug sensitivities are variable. Regimes recommended include the use of chloramphenicol and novobiocin and of tetracycline alone or in combination with chloramphenicol and penicillin. Where septicaemia due to staphylococcus pyogenes is suspected, the use of benzylpenicillin and cloxacillin has been suggested.

**Bicarbonate.** Metabolic acidosis accompanies the peripheral stagnation of shock, and its correction, using sodium bicarbonate, has been recommended (MacLean, 1966).

**Oxygenation.** In shock, arterial oxygenation may be impaired by alveolar under-ventilation and venous admixture. This will aggravate the already inadequate tissue oxygen supply. It is essential to administer oxygen and to maintain adequate ventilation, using intermittent positive pressure ventilation if necessary. Hyperbaric oxygen has been shown to be of value in the experimental animal.

## INDUCED HYPOTENSION

Induced hypotension refers to the deliberate lowering of systemic arterial pressure during anaesthesia and surgery with the aim of reducing bleeding and facilitating surgery. Hypotension may be achieved by block of the sympathetic outflow in one of two ways:

(1) By high subarachnoid or extradural block (Griffiths and Gillies, 1948, Bromage, 1951), in this way blocking preganglionic sympathetic impulses.

(2) By the use of ganglionic blocking agents, either long acting, such as hexamethonium or pentolinium, or short acting, such as trimetaphan or homatropinium (Enderby, 1962).

The mechanisms by which arterial pressure is reduced using these techniques are probably complex resulting from both reduced peripheral resistance and also reduced cardiac output. Cardiac output may be reduced in a variety of ways during induced hypotension:

**(1) Reduced venous return.** Vasodilation produces venous pooling, reduced venous return, stroke volume and cardiac output.

**(2) Decreased myocardial contractility.** Sympathetic blockade, as well as producing vasodilation, also reduces myocardial sympathetic tone and myocardial contractility. Heart rate may also be decreased. Many anaesthetic agents, including halothane, directly decrease myocardial contractility.

Such mechanisms have been described in the human subject (Lynn *et al.*, 1952, Didier *et al.*, 1965, Theye and Tuohy, 1965) and in the experimental animal (Beck, 1958).

Further control of systemic arterial pressure and cardiac output may be obtained by:

**(1) Posture.** A head-up position will promote venous pooling in the lower body, with subsequent decrease in venous return and cardiac output. For each 2·5 cm. elevation above the level of the heart, local arterial pressure is reduced by 2 mm. Hg.; this not only has important implications as far as the cerebral circulation is concerned, but stresses the surgical importance of maintaining the site of operation uppermost. This ensures local arterial hypotension and adequate venous drainage.

**(2) Intermittent positive pressure ventilation.** This technique may produce a raised mean intrathoracic pressure and this will reduce effective ventricular filling pressure and with it cardiac output. However, intermittent positive pressure ventilation is of value in compensating for the large increase in physiological dead space encountered during induced hypotension (q.v.).

**(3) Adjuvants.** In some patients, particularly young adults, it often proves impossible to establish hypotension. Repeated doses of a ganglionic blocking agent fail to reduce arterial pressure and are accompanied by a tachycardia. This phenomenon has been explained in a variety of ways. It may follow sensitization of the peripheral vascular system to circulating catecholamines. Tachycardia may follow hypotension via the baroreceptor mechanism (Marey's Law) and if stroke volume is maintained then cardiac output may be increased. As such a condition is unlikely to be due to incomplete ganglionic blockade it is of little value to administer increasing doses of ganglionic blocking agents or to use a different blocking agent to achieve hypotension. Several techniques have been suggested to overcome this difficulty:

(1) Such an outcome is less likely to follow the use of a large loading dose of a ganglionic blocking agent; however, this is contra-indicated in many patients.

(2) If tachycardia is to be avoided, atropine may be omitted as a premedicant and gallamine should not be used.

(3) Procaine amide has been used to reduce tachycardia, but the drug is a direct myocardial depressant and interferes with the conduction mechanism of the heart.

(4) Guanethidine has been used with success, but has the disadvantage of being a long acting drug; its effects may last 48 hours into the post-operative period.

(5) More recently propranalol has been used in doses of 1–2 mg. intravenously (Hellewell & Potts, 1966, Hewitt *et al.*, 1967). This beta adrenergic blocking agent reduces heart rate, and may give rise to profound bradycardia in the non-atropinized, anaesthetized patient; it also decreases myocardial oxygen requirements and may decrease cardiac output by a negative inotropic effect.

(6) Halothane is probably the most commonly used adjuvant to hypotensive anaesthesia. Halothane depresses cardiac output and the sympathetic response to hypotension. It does not itself increase plasma catecholamine levels.

## BLOOD FLOW AND INDUCED HYPOTENSION

Although cardiac output may be reduced during induced hypotension, this does not constitute shock. As already described shock is a complex disorder affecting the pumping ability of the heart, peripheral vascular resistance, microcirculatory mechanisms, blood volume regulation and blood rheology and coagulability. In induced hypotension, unlike shock, it appears that tissue and organ blood flow may remain adequate.

Referring once more to the expression

$$F = \frac{\Delta P}{R}$$

it can be seen that the difference between shock and induced hypotension is that in the former resistance is increased and in the later decreased, although in both overall flow (cardiac output) may be reduced. Thus for the same arterial pressure regional tissue flow will be higher in induced hypotension.

### Myocardial blood flow

Coronary perfusion decreases in direct relation to mean arterial pressure. Fortunately, myocardial work and oxygen consumption fall in parallel with the fall in arterial pressure and cardiac output, and on this basis it seems that coronary perfusion remains adequate during induced hypotension. Rollason & Hough (1959) found no electrocardiographic evidence of permanent myocardial damage following induced hypotension with ganglionic blocking agents, although some 40 per cent of cases showed evidence of transient myocardial ischaemia.

### Cerebral blood flow

A major consideration in induced hypotension is the adequacy of cerebral blood flow and oxygenation . Cerebral blood flow may be given by the general expression

$$F = \frac{\Delta P}{R}$$

where in this specific case

$\Delta P$ = mean perfusing pressure
$R$ = cerebrovascular resistance

**Mean perfusing pressure.** This is dependent upon the difference between cerebral venous and arterial pressure. Due to alterations in hydrostatic pressures, both head-up and head-down tilts may reduce cerebral blood flow by reducing the mean perfusing pressure.

Present evidence suggests that at physiological levels, systemic arterial pressure plays little part in the control of cerebral blood flow (Lassen, 1959) and that auto regulation of cerebral blood flow occurs between mean systemic arterial pressures of 70 and 150 mmHg (Lassen, 1964). However, when systemic arterial pressure falls below a critical level, between 50 and 70 mmHg, it would appear to play a determinant role in cerebral blood flow, which declines (Finnerty et al., 1954; Lassen, 1959). At these pressure levels Harper and Glass (1965) were unable to demonstrate a constrictor response to hypocapnia in the dog, although Eckenhoff and his co-workers (1963) did demonstrate such a response. If this is so, the combination of hypotension and hyperventilation with hypocapnia would appear undesirable.

Many attempts have been made to lay down a safe systemic arterial pressure level during induced hypotension and these have varied from 30–80 mm.Hg. This is an impossibility as pressure is only one facet of a many sided problem, and in most circumstances pressure is of less importance than flow.

**Cerebrovascular resistance.** This is dependent upon:

(1) Blood viscosity
(2) Cerebrospinal fluid pressure
(3) Vessel diameter
(4) Body temperature

The most important determinant is vessel diameter. Cerebral vascular diameter and resistance is altered by humoral and probably by neurogenic factors. Cerebral vasodilation occurs when mean arterial pressure is lowered, thus maintaining cerebral blood flow. Vasodilation also follows an increase in arterial carbon dioxide tension, a fall in oxygen tension and a fall in pH. Many anaesthetic agents, particularly inhalational agents such as halothane and trichlorethylene, also produce cerebral vasodilation.

The adequacy, or otherwise, of cerebral blood flow during induced hypotension has been studied by a variety of methods. Direct techniques have included assessment of radioactive Xenon clearance (Slack & Walther, 1963), electroencephalography and measurement of jugular bulb oxygen tensions (Eckenhoff et al., 1963). In this last study the lowest jugular oxygen tension observed was 27 mmHg. suggesting that cerebral oxygenation was adequate. Post-operative tests of cerebral function have included the application of flicker-fusion and psychometric testing.

All methods of measuring cerebral blood flow and cerebral oxygenation under conditions of clinical anaesthesia and hypotension are relatively crude. The results derived from such studies show that hypotension produces no change in cerebral function, or produces transient, slight and reversible signs of cerebral hypoxia. However, Little (1955 and 1956) reviewed records of nearly 30,000 hypotensive anaesthetics from many centres and found cerebral thrombosis and hypoxia to be blamed as a common cause of morbidity and mortality using this technique, particularly in association with the head-up position.

### Renal blood flow

Renal filtration decreases with a fall in arterial pressure, and below 70 mm. Hg. urine excretion ceases. Renal perfusion remains adequate to meet intrinsic metabolic demands, despite cessation of glomerular filtration, and in fact during hypotensive anaesthesia renal blood flow returns to control levels following initial depression. (Morris et al., 1953, Moyer et al., 1955).

### Hepatic blood flow

The liver derives 20 per cent of its blood supply from the hepatic artery and 80 per cent from the portal vein. Under conditions of both normovolaemic and hypovolaemic hypotension where overall flow is reduced, considerable desaturation occurs in the splanchnic circulation and the liver may become almost totally dependent upon hepatic artery blood flow. Should hepatic artery flow be inadequate, then hypoxia will occur. Bromage (1952) has described hepatic cyanosis during extradural block with arterial pressures of 45–60 mmHg.; this reverted to normal when the arterial pressure was raised using a pressor agent.

The effect of induced hypotension upon liver function has been but little studied. Greene and his co-workers (1954) found no correlation between hypotension and bromsulphthalein retention, and what changes did occur were similar to those found in patients undergoing normotensive general anaesthesia.

### PULMONARY BLOOD FLOW AND HYPOTENSION

In situations where reduced pulmonary blood flow and reduced pulmonary artery pressure are found, ventilation/perfusion inequalities may be anticipated. It is customary to divide distribution into two aspects. Firstly, the ventilation of relatively underperfused alveoli, which is quantified in terms of physiological dead space, and secondly the perfusion of relatively underventilated alveoli which is described in terms of alveolar to arterial oxygen tension gradient, venous admixture and physiological shunt.

There have been few measurements of venous admixture in shock. Both Freeman and Nunn (1963) and Gerst, Rattenborg and Holaday (1959) found reductions in venous admixture in bled dogs. Despite this, arterial oxygenation was reduced due to the admixture of grossly desaturated venous blood. In myocardial infarction with shock studies by McNichol and his co-workers (1964) and MacKenzie and his co-workers (1964) have shown moderate increases in alveolar to arterial oxygen tension differences and increased shunt ratios. These findings have been explained on the basis of atelectasis and pulmonary oedema.

Increases in physiological dead space have been found following haemorrhage in dogs (Gerst et al., 1959, Freeman and Nunn, 1963) and in man (Cournand et al., 1943). Increases have also been observed following myocardial infarction (McNichol et al., 1964). In shock, cardiac output and consequently pulmonary blood flow are reduced, while ventilation is maintained and often increased, and this situation is responsible for the increases in alveolar, and with it physiological dead space. Since these changes are accompanied by large increases in arterial to alveolar carbon dioxide tension gradients Gerst and his co-workers (1959) suggest that total collapse of certain pulmonary capillaries occurs rather than generalized pulmonary vascular constriction.

Hyperventilation occurs during rapid haemorrhage with an increase in respiratory rate. As haemorrhage proceeds, respiration becomes gasping, intermittent and alveolar ventilation declines. It has been suggested that the initial hyperventilation is due to the metabolic acidosis accompanying shock (Nunn 1966). The dead space changes in shock emphasize the necessity of oxygen therapy, the value of intermittent positive pressure ventilation and the need to avoid the use of respiratory depressants.

Increases in physiological dead space occur in anaesthetized patients rendered hypotensive by the use of ganglionic blocking agents (Eckenhoff et al. 1963). Dead space values amounting to 60–70 per cent of tidal volume have been recorded under induced hypotension, levels similar to those found in bled dogs.

The widespread use of induced hypotension as an aid to surgery has established the overall usefulness and safety of the technique. A better understanding of the physiological changes involved has led to awareness of the potential limitations and possible dangers that can occur when hypotension is induced in an uncontrolled or unphysiological manner.

## REFERENCES

Beck, L. (1958), "Effect of the Autonomic System on Arteriolar Tone in the Experimental Animal." *Circulation*, **17**, 798.
Bloch, J. H., Dietzman, R. H., Pierce, C. H. and Lillehei, R. C. (1966), "Theories of the Production of Shock," *Brit. J. Anaesth.*, **38**, 234.
Broder, G. and Weil, M. H. (1964), "Excess Lactate: An Index of Irreversibility of Shock in Human Patients," *Science*, **143**, 1457.
Bromage, P. R. (1951), "Vascular Hypotension in 107 Cases of Epidural Anaesthesia," *Anaesthesia*, **6**, 26.
Bromage, P. R. (1952), "Effect of Induced Vascular Hypotension on the Liver. Alterations in Appearance and Consistance," *Lancet*, **ii**, 10.
Cournand, A., Riley, R. L., Bradley, S. E., Breed, E. S., Nossle, R. P., Lawson, H. D., Gregersen, M. I. and Richards, D. W. (1943), "Studies of the Circulation in Clinical Shock," *Surgery*, **13**, 964.
Crowell, J. W. and Guyton, A. C. (1961), "Evidence Favouring a Cardiac Mechanism in Irreversible Haemorrhagic Shock," *Amer. J. Physiol.*, **201**, 5.
Crowell, J. W. and Smith, E. E. (1964), "Oxygen Deficit and Irreversible Haemorrhagic Shock," *Amer. J. Physiol.*, **216**, 313.
Didier, E. P., Clagget, O. T., Theye, R. A. (1965), "Cardiac Performance during Controlled Hypotension," *Anaesth. and Analges. Curr. Res.*, **44**, 379.
Dudley, H. A. F., Knight, R. J., McNeur, J. C. and Rosengarten, D. S. (1968), "Civilian Battle Casualties in South Vietnam," *Brit. J. Surg.*, **55**, 332.
Eckenhoff, J. E., Enderby, G. E. H., Larson, A., Edridge, A. and Judevine, D. E. (1963), "Pulmonary Gas Exchange during Deliberate Hypotension," *Brit. J. Anaesth.*, **35**, 750.
Eckenhoff, J. E., Enderby, G. E. H., Larson, A., Davies, R. and Judevine, D. E. (1963), "Human Cerebral Circulation during deliberate hypotension and head-up tilt. *J. Appl. Physiol.*, **18**, 1130.
Enderby, G. E. H. (1962), *Postgraduate Courses*, **71**, *First European Congress of Anaesthesiology*. Vienna: Weiner medizinischen Akademie.
Fine, J. (1954), *Bacterial Factor in Traumatic Shock*. Springfield: Thomas.
Finnerty, F. A., Witkin, L., and Fazekas, J. F. (1954), Cerebral haemodynamics during cerebral ischaemia induced by acute hypotension. *J. Clin. Invest.*, **33**, 1227.
Freeman, J. and Nunn, J. F. (1963), "Ventilation-perfusion Relationships after Haemorrhage," *Clin. Sci.*, **24**, 135.
Gerst, P. H., Rattenborg, C. and Holaday, D. A. (1959), "The Effects of Haemorrhage on Pulmonary Circulation and Respiratory Gas Exchange," *J. Clin. Invest.*, **38**, 524.
Greene, N. M., Bunker, J. P., Kerr, W. S., Von Felsinger, J. M., Keller, J. W. and Beecher, H. K. (1954), "Hypotensive Spinal Anaesthesia; Respiratory, Metabolic, Hepatic, Renal and Cerebral Effects," *Ann. Surg.*, **140**, 641.
Griffiths, H. W. C. and Gillies, J. (1948), "Thoraco-lumbar Splanchniectomy and Sympathectomy: Anaesthetic Procedure," *Anaesthesia*, **3**, 134.
Guyton, A. C. (1966), *Textbook of Medical Physiology*, p. 384. Philadelphia: Saunders.
Hardaway, R. M. (1963), "The Role of Intravascular Clotting in the Aetiology of Shock," *Ann. Surg.*, **155**, 3.
Harper, A. M. and Glass, H. I. (1965), Effect of alterations in arterial carbon dioxide tension on the blood flow through the cerebral cortex at normal and low arterial blood pressures, *J. Neurol. Neurosurg. Psychiat.*, **28**, 449.
Hellewell, J. and Potts, M. W. (1966), "Propranolol during Controlled Hypotension," *Brit. J. Anaesth.*, **38**, 794.
Hewitt, P. B., Lord, P. W. and Thornton, H. L. (1967), "Propranolol in Hypotensive Anaesthesia," *Anaesthesia*, **22**, 82.
*Lancet* (1967), **i**, 830.
Lassen, N. A. (1959), Cerebral blood flow and oxygen consumption in man, *Physiol. Rev.*, **39**, 183.
Lassen, N. A. (1964), Autoregulation of cerebral blood flow, *Circ. Res.*, **15**, 201.
Lillehei, R. C. (1965), In discussion of paper "Treatment of Experimental Cardiogenic Shock," by Bloch, J. H., Pierce, C. H., Manax, W. G. and Lillehei, R. C. *Surgery*, **58**, 213.
Lillehei, R. C., Longerbeam, J. K., Bloch, J. H. and Manax, W. G. (1964), "The Nature of Irreversible Shock," *Ann. Surg.*, **160**, 682.
Little, D. M. (1955), "Induced Hypotension during Anaesthesia and Surgery," *Anesthesiol.*, **16**, 320.
Little, D. M. (1956), *Controlled Hypotension in Anaesthesia and Surgery*. Springfield: Thomas.
Lynn, R. B., Sancetta, S. M., Simeone, F. A. and Scott, R. W. (1952), "Observations on the Circulation in High Spinal Anaesthesia," *Surgery*, **32**, 195.
MacKenzie, G. J., Taylor, S. H., Flenley, D. C., McDonald, A. H., Staunton, H. P. and Donald, K. W. (1964), "Circulatory and Respiratory Studies in Myocardial Infarction and Cardiogenic Shock," *Lancet*, **ii**, 825.
MacLean, L. D. (1966), "The Clinical Management of Shock," *Brit. J. Anaesth.*, **38**, 255.
McNichol, M. W., Kirby, B. J., Everest, M. S., Freedman, S. and Bhoola, K. D. (1964), "Circulatory and Respiratory Studies in Myocardial Infarction and Cardiogenic Shock," *Lancet*, **ii**, 1180.
Mellander, S. and Lewis, D. H. (1963), "Effect of Haemorrhagic Shock on the Reactivity of Resistance and Capacitance Vessels and on Capillary Filtration Transfer in Cat Skeletal Muscle," *Circulation Res.*, **13**, 105.
Morris, G. C., Moyer, J. H., Snyder, H. B. and Haynes, B. W. (1953), "Vascular Dynamics in Controlled Hypotension; Study of Cerebral and Renal Haemodynamics and Blood Volume Changes in Controlled Hypotension," *Ann. Surg.*, **138**, 706.
Moyer, J. H., Morris, G. C. and Seibert, R. A. (1955), "Renal Function during Controlled Hypotension with Hexamethonium and Following Norepinephrine," *Surg. Gynae. Obstet.*, **100**, 27.
Nickerson, M. (1965). In: *The Pharmacological Basis of Therapeutics*. (L. S. Goodman and A. Gilman, Eds.), 3rd Ed., p. 553. London: Macmillan.
Nunn, J. F. (1966). In: *Oxygen Measurements in Blood and Tissues*. (J. P. Payne and D. W. Hill, Eds.), p. 240. London: Churchill.

Rollason, W. N. and Hough, J. M. (1959), "Some Electrocardiographic Studies during Hypotensive Anaesthesia," *Brit. J. Anaesth.*, **31**, 66.

Slack, W. K. and Walther, W. W. (1963), "Cerebral Circulation Studies during Hypotensive Anaesthesia using Radioactive Xenon," *Lancet*, **i**, 1082.

Theye, R. A. and Tuohy, G. F. (1965), "Effect of Trimetaphan on Haemodynamics and Oxygen Consumption during Halothane Anaesthesia in Man," *Brit. J. Anaesth.*, **37**, 144.

Wiggers, C. J. and Werle, J. M. (1942), "Cardiac and Peripheral Resistance Factors as Determinants of Circulatory Failure in Haemorrhagic Shock," *Amer. J. Physiol.*, **136**, 421.

*CHAPTER 7*

# CIRCULATION IN THE TISSUES
## (The Microcirculation)

### I. A. SEWELL

Circulating blood provides a transport medium to facilitate the activities of the tissues. All living cells require external sources of nutriment at some stage in their metabolic activities, and those products of metabolism not required for further intracellular activity must be removed before their accumulation inhibits further vital biochemical changes. Furthermore, the metabolic products of one group of cells may be essential to the activities of a distant tissue: the speediest method of delivery will be by way of the circulation. Taking this view of circulatory function, it is apparent that the contents of the circulation must be in easy communication with the tissues it serves. For this reason, the circulation must not be considered as a closed circuit isolated from tissue activity, merely carrying blood or lymph. A knowledge of circulation at the tissue level is essential in all spheres of clinical studies. It is a scientific discipline which cuts across all the basic medical sciences. Recent advances in its exploration suggest that alterations in tissue vessel activity may be the basis of many pathological changes hitherto unsuspected of having a circulatory origin or basis. To the anaesthetist it is vital, since all his techniques will ultimately have profound effects on circulation at the tissue level.

## Integration of Tissue Activity by Circulating Fluid in the Intact Organism

Before we begin to discuss circulation at the active tissue level, we must consider such a local circulation in relation to the circulation as a whole (the general circulation). The latter has already been the subject of another part of this book (Chapter 2), where the role of the heart, arteries and veins in oxygen transport has been specifically outlined. For our present task it may be convenient to temporarily ignore the anatomical concepts of arteries and veins, and think instead of the circulation as channelled fluid flow having ready communication with both the inter- and intracellular fluids of the immediately surrounding tissues, even though the composition of this extra-circulatory fluid differs from that within the vessels.

This is a concept which is acceptable on hydrodynamic ground but may be difficult to appreciate if the traditional views of anatomy and physiology are too slavishly followed. For the purposes of discussion, we can also neglect for a while those factors extrinsic to the circulation, such as the pumping action of muscles and augmented negative intrathoracic pressure during inspiration, which nevertheless ensure its continuity. Cardiac activity is of fundamental importance to all circulatory activities. Traditionally, all discussions of circulatory phenomena begin with the heart. However, we are concerned with circulation in the tissues and it will therefore make the situation clearer if we begin with vessels at this level and then relate their activities to those of the great vessels and the heart itself.

### Influence of Cellular Activity on Fluid Flow

The immediate pathway into and from the cell is the surrounding interstitial fluid (Fig. 1). In fully integrated activity in the healthy organism, there is a constant stream of water across the cell membrane in both directions, with selection of solutes and colloids according to locally pertaining biophysical and biochemical states. Disturbance of water flow and of solute and colloidal selection will initiate pathological change. In theory, supply of nutriment and the transport of metabolites to distant sites could take place entirely through the medium of the interstitial fluid, since each cell in the body is in fluid continuity with all the rest. But, such a system provides only for integrated activity at its lowest level, as may be observed in the simplest three-layered animals. Fluid flow is assured, but its speed would be well below that optimal for the requirements of metabolic production in more complex animals such as the mammals.

Adjacent cells in normal tissues are so integrated in their activities that their fluid relations can be considered collectively (Fig. 2). Since they share a common fluid medium, inter-cell communication is possible via the immediate interstitial fluid. However, even in small organs (such as parathyroid tissue) the interstitial fluid

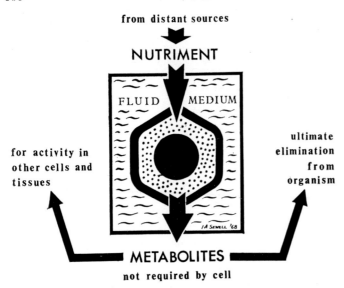

FIG. 1. Fluid relations of individual cells. Each cell of the body (excepting at certain sites such as the epidermis) is surrounded by interstitial fluid, providing pathways for cellular nutrient uptake and metabolic exit. The relationship between cell and its surrounding fluid is fundamental to all considerations of circulation in the tissues. In theory, all cells can communicate with one another by way of the interstitial fluid.

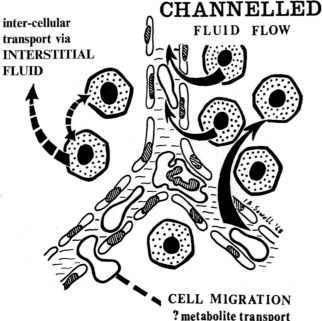

FIG. 2. Fluid relations in the tissues between active cell groups and channelled fluid flow. In active tissues, only adjacent cells rely on communication via the interstitial fluid. In the same tissue, channelled fluid flow provides more speedy communication between cells, this flow being influenced by both local biophysical change and general circulatory effects. Cellular transmigration between the fluid channels and the interstitial spaces may play some part in metabolic transport.

flow is inadequate for even local transport and biochemical communication. *In vivo* examination shows that fluid flow takes place via special channels, and relatively simple experiments demonstrate that the channelled flow is much faster than the movement of interstitial fluid. However, despite these differences, metabolites pass easily between channelled fluid and that between the cells under highly localized physiological influences. An additional

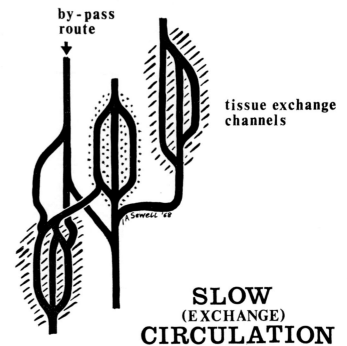

FIG. 3. The slow (exchange) circulation. Adjacent and distant tissues are in communication via channelled fluid flow and the interstitial fluid. The tissue channelled fluid flow is theoretically continuous throughout the organism. Communication between the fluid channels and the interstitial fluid is governed by cellular activity, these channels providing a 'service' activity. This concept also holds good for bypass channels, which take the channelled fluid flow past dormant or inactive tissues. The fluid channels facilitate 'exchange' and the flow in them is adjusted to meet local biophysical and biochemical requirements. In contrast to the 'general' circulation, flow in these exchange vessels has to be slow—hence the term used here.

phenomenon is the presence of cells within these fluid channels which will occasionally undergo transmigration, and it is quite possible that such cells may play an active part in the transport of metabolites between the circulation and the tissues.

### Slow (Exchange) Circulation

The fluid channels in a particular tissue are linked with those of other tissues (Fig. 3). Just as the interstitial fluid is in continuity throughout the complex organism, so are the simple fluid channels. This arrangement provides another, but more efficient, means of distant communication. The fluid flow in these channels is integrated with tissue activity, its rate and volume being modified by the demands of particular cell groups, and ultimately by both organ and tissue activity. These fluid channels in theory form a circulation on their own in the true sense of the term. Their basic activity is to facilitate the *exchange* of nutriments and metabolites at the tissue level. In a sense, this circulation can be viewed as providing a 'tissue service,' and can aptly be described as the *Slow* or *Exchange Circulation* (Fig. 4). Even so, such a transport system is as slow as its title suggests and could

communication is provided by the vessels seen at operation, even those just visible to the naked eye. The force propelling the fluid in them is provided by the pumping action of the heart and augmented by such mechanisms as muscular contraction, the inspiratory rise in negative intrathoracic pressure, and by gravity. The channels of the Slow (exchange) Circulation are connected to these larger vessels at particular intervals (Fig. 5).

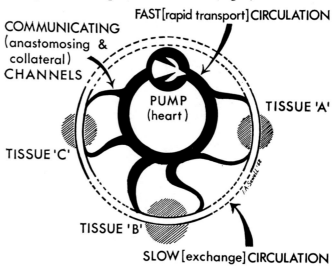

FIG. 5. Fast (Rapid Communication) Circulation. The diagram shows the connection between the channels of the *slow* (Exchange) *circulation* and those of the *fast* (Rapid Communication) *circulation* whereby the results of exchange between the tissue channelled fluid flow and the interstitial fluid are put into rapid communication with other widely separated tissues in the organism. The energy for the *fast circulation* is provided by the pumping mechanism of the heart augmented by such factors as muscle activity, respiration and gravity.

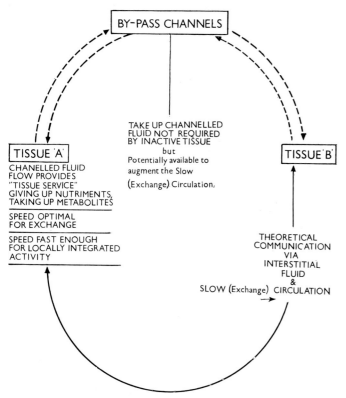

FIG. 4. The slow (exchange) circulation. In conjunction with Fig. 3, this flow diagram summarizes its relationship to, and dependence on, tissue activity at different sites, even though widely separated. The factors given under 'TISSUE A' apply equally well to 'TISSUE B'. The bypass function of the Slow Circulation acts as a regulating mechanism to ensure optimum speed of fluid flow for exchange and local communication in active tissues, by taking up excess of volume and flow rate over local requirements.

not adequately cope with all the demands of a rapidly acting complex organism such as man. It is fully represented in simple creatures where the circulation consists only of interconnecting fluid channels. The 'tissue service' aspect of the Slow (exchange) Circulation is often seen in experiments on the microcirculation when the local channelled fluid flow (the 'blood') is minimal during the resting phase of a tissue, the bulk of the blood bypassing this area.

## Fast (Rapid Communication) Circulation

Whereas components of the Slow (exchange) Circulation are intimately responsible for metabolic exchange in the tissues, fluid connection between widely separated tissues must be rapid for speedy integrated activity. Such rapid

## Tissue By-pass Channels

By macroscopic techniques alone—as Harvey fully appreciated—there are situations where the continuity of the visible vessels is in question. With the discovery of 'capillary networks' by Marcello Malpighi and others, it was naturally assumed that these microscopic structures were the missing link. It was further assumed that all the blood in the circulation found its way through these capillary networks. However, investigation has shown that a considerable volume of blood bypasses these capillaries (the fluid channels of the tissues). Again, if all the blood passed through the totally available capillary networks, then the circulation time as measured by currently used methods would be many times as long as normally found in clinical investigation. Thus, there exist certain channels in the circulation whereby the tissue circulation proper is completely bypassed. In recent years, these channels have acquired the term 'arteriovenous communications.' They are, in fact, the pickup and shedding points for connection with the Slow (exchange) Circulation. In investigations where microparticulate radio-contrast medium is used to demonstrate the finer vessels, it is these arteriovenous communications which are actually shown, since such contrast medium is not taken up by the true capillary networks.

## Integration of the Tissue and General Circulation

Thus, besides the Slow (exchange) Circulation, there exists a Fast (rapid transport) Circulation providing ready communication between all organs and tissues of the body. The Slow Circulation is connected to the Fast Circulation, tapping and returning quanta of blood as required for the varying activities of the tissues. There is a good deal of evidence to support the view that the constitution

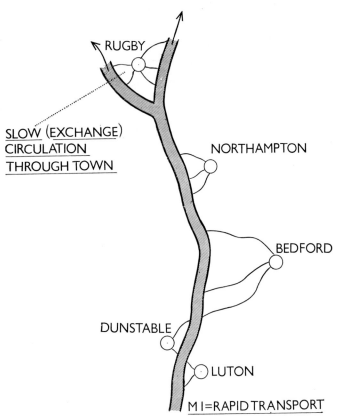

FIG. 6. The motorway system provides a good analogy with the components of the peripheral circulation. The motorway itself (as here illustrated by the M1) is equivalent to the *fast* (Rapid Transport) *circulation*, providing speedy communication over great distances, whereas roads through towns like Bedford, Northampton and Rugby represent the *slow* (Exchange) *circulation*, for these roads serve active centres and yet still communicate with the fast flow of the motorway.

of the blood in the two circulations differs, and this is probably related to the differing functions of transport and exchange. This concept of circulation is analogous to the Motorway System in which the motorways themselves provide rapid communication between regions but have facilities for traffic to leave and re-enter at points where this is destined for towns off the fast routes (Fig. 6). Once off the motorway, the traffic must slow down so that business can be transacted in the town, but when this is over, the traffic may progress rapidly to another part of the country by re-entering the motorway stream.

Close observation of the tissue circulation reveals a certain independence from the Fast Circulation but this is more apparent than real. The two circulations are closely integrated and interdependent and it is often difficult to be sure where the division lies.

## Structure of Microvessels

The channelled fluid flow of the body is contained within a continuous tubular system, the only cul-de-sacs being the lymphatic radicles. This system is lined throughout by a single layer of cells called the *Endothelium*. A basic knowledge of this structure provides the key to understanding the phenomena of circulation at the tissue level, for its differing properties at various sites contribute to the regulation of fluid, solute and particulate exchange across microvessel walls in accordance with the needs of each functioning tissue. This 'inner lining' of vessels may or may not be clothed with additional tissues. Such extra tissues modify the role of the various morphological components which are recognized as constituting the tissue microvessels. It is most important to note that neither structure nor size provide an adequate criterion for classification, since this is finally determined by function (*vide infra*).

### Endothelium

Our current knowledge of endothelium is largely based on electron microscopic studies, since the resolution obtained with transmitted light is generally too low for adequate visualization of such fine structure. Such knowledge remains incomplete because the techniques of electron microscopy do not permit direct in vivo study. **Varieties of Endothelium.** Although each organ and tissue appears to have its own type of endothelium, for our present purpose it is possible to classify this structure into 3 major groups (Fig. 7):

Group I: CONTINUOUS ENDOTHELIUM
in which there are no recognizable openings in the endothelial sheet.

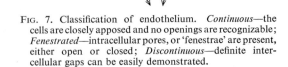

CONTINUOUS

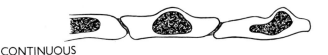

FENESTRATED

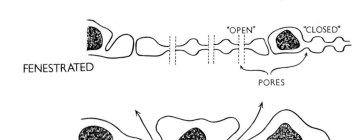

DISCONTINUOUS

FIG. 7. Classification of endothelium. *Continuous*—the cells are closely apposed and no openings are recognizable; *Fenestrated*—intracellular pores, or 'fenestrae' are present, either open or closed; *Discontinuous*—definite intercellular gaps can be easily demonstrated.

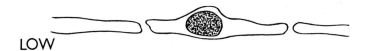

LOW

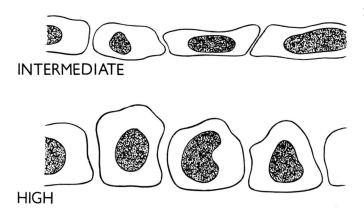

INTERMEDIATE

HIGH

FIG. 8. Changes in endothelial form. Electron microscope studies have shown variations from the low (pavement) form to the high (cubical) forms—as seen in the spleen. All grades of intermediate forms exist between these two, and these differences may be a reflection of functional changes, the microscope picking out a particular form at one moment in time.

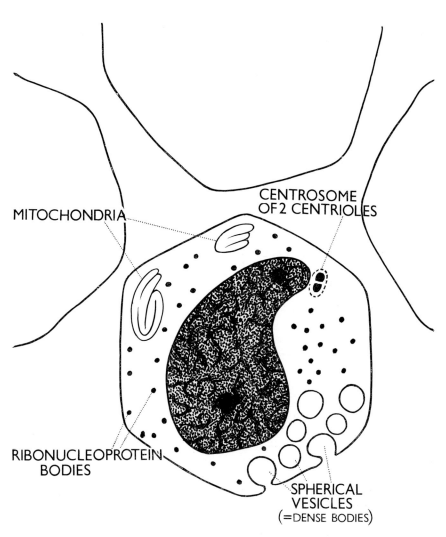

MITOCHONDRIA

CENTROSOME OF 2 CENTRIOLES

RIBONUCLEOPROTEIN BODIES

SPHERICAL VESICLES (=DENSE BODIES)

FIG. 9. Common characteristics of the endothelial cell. The diagram simply summarizes those ultrastructural features of the endothelial cell which assist in identification. Note that the nucleus is relatively large but that mitochondria are few. The centrosome consists of 2 centrioles usually situated close to one pole of the nucleus. The outstanding feature of endothelium is the presence of large numbers of dark-staining spherical vesicles, many of which are continuous with the cell envelope.

Group II: FENESTRATED ENDOTHELIUM
in which intracellular pores or 'fenestrae' are identifiable. These pores may be open or closed.

Group III: DISCONTINUOUS ENDOTHELIUM
where definite inter-cellular gaps can be demonstrated.

It is also possible to identify different endothelial cell morphologies, a factor employed in certain classifications. However, a changing shape may be associated with changes in function, the form recognized being that at the particular moment in time when the electron microscope study was undertaken. It is sufficient to appreciate that the endothelial cell may be flattened out (Low Endothelium), may be cubical in form (High Endothelium) or that several intermediate forms may be observed (Fig. 8). This has an analogy with the changes in the epithelial lining of the thyroid follicle during the various phases of normal glandular activity.

**Characteristics of Endothelial Cells.** Endothelial cells have many features in common (Fig. 9). When their intraluminal surface is examined, an hexagonal outline is usually noted. Their thickness varies from $0.01$ to $2-3\mu$, the bulging coinciding with the position of the nucleus. There are few mitochondria, 2 centrioles are common and small piles of cisterna can be identified. The endoplasmic reticulum is evenly distributed and ribonucleoproteins are enmeshed in it. Fat droplets are recognizable. So-called 'dense bodies' are frequently seen: these may result from pinocytosis or from intracellular particulate migration. The cytoplasmic matrix usually contains irregular bundles of fibrils, multivesicular bodies and a system of spherical vesicles. These spherical vesicles may occupy almost the whole of the intraluminar or even the whole of the tissue aspect of the cell and up to a third of its volume. It is probably of some functional importance that many of the spherical vesicles appear to be in close contact with the endothelial cell envelope: they often appear continuous with it.

**Intercellular Junctions (Fig. 10).** In both continuous and fenestrated endothelium, an intercellular junction can be demonstrated. It would appear to occur nearer the lumen of the vessel, and part appears to be an actual fusion of the plasma components of adjacent cell membranes, giving rise to the term 'tight junction.'

**Endothelial Basement Membrane.** Except for those with a discontinuous endothelium, vascular endothelium is supported by a basement membrane. Only in exceptional circumstances can this be identified by light microscopy and it has most probably never been observed in *in vivo* studies. Those workers who claim demonstration by P.A.-S staining have probably seen dye deposition on a surface, rather like paint clinging to a wall. The structure of the basement membrane is most likely to be collagen-based, a concept which has recently emerged from histochemical studies: previously it was considered to be a mucopolysaccharide. Proline, which is actually produced by endothelial cells, is currently considered to be the source of basement membrane collagen—not fibroblasts, as originally suggested.

At least 2 layers can be recognized in endothelial basement membranes (Fig. 11). Immediately adjacent to the endothelial cell there is an almost translucent zone (Subendothelial Lamina), and this is surrounded by a dense zone which lessens progressively in density, often blending with the matrix or intercellular substance of the surrounding tissues.

The basement membrane varies in its composition with different organs and tissues. It also splits to enclose extra-endothelial cells or pericytes and may also partially envelope smooth muscle cells of certain tissue microvessels. In general, it thickens with age and in certain disease processes.

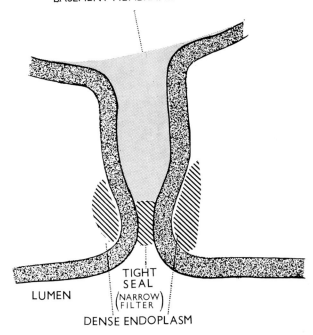

TRANSLUCENT (CLEAR) LAYER OF BASEMENT MEMBRANE

LUMEN

TIGHT SEAL (NARROW FILTER)

DENSE ENDOPLASM

Fig. 10. Endothelial intercellular junctions. Basically, the ectoplasm of adjacent endothelial cells is held together towards the lumen by a tight seal which is, in fact, a narrow filter. Commonly, the endoplasm in the vicinity of the tight seal is dense. The remaining gap between the cells is usually filled with the translucent zone of the basement membrane.

**The Pericytes**

Tissue microvessels are frequently characterized morphologically by cells outside the endothelial layer but lying within the substance of the basement membrane. These are known as pericytes and correspond to structures previously named Rouget Cells or Mural Cells. Apart from the nucleus, their structure is extremely delicate and it is doubtful whether they have ever been adequately defined by transmitted light microscopy, although Zimmerman in 1923, and Plenk in 1927, gave descriptions based on silver impregnation techniques which agree reasonably well with more recent electron microscopic findings.

Morphologically (Fig. 12), pericytes differ slightly in

structure according to their relation to various tissue microvessels, but such differences are only of interest to the ultracytologist. True capillary pericytes adhere to adjacent endothelial cell membranes through gaps in the basement membrane. In very vascular tissues, the processes of adjacent pericytes may connect one capillary with another.

Identification of pericytes may be difficult, even by the electron microscope, for they have many intracellular

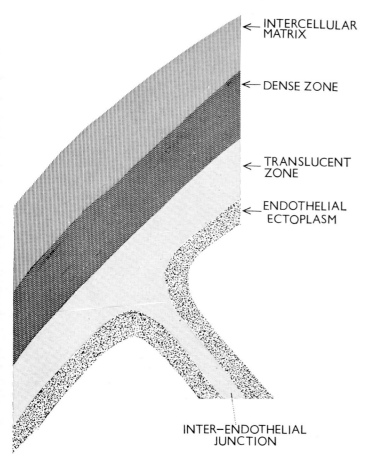

FIG. 11. Structure of the endothelial basement membrane. This consists of a translucent (sub-endothelial—laminal) zone which is continuous with the contraluminal part of the inter-endothelial junction. Outside this is a dense zone which blends with the matrix of the surrounding intercellular substance of the immediately adjacent tissues. The endothelial basement membrane splits to enclose immediately adjacent structures such as pericytes or smooth muscle cells.

features in common with both endothelial cells and vascular smooth muscle cells. However, Kuwabara and Cogan have used successful histochemical techniques and have demonstrated that the enzyme DPN-diaphorase is present only in pericytes. A further difficulty lies in the apparent resemblance between pericytes and fast-lodged leucocytes in the tissues, and other cells closely associated with the endothelium such as the podocytes of the renal glomerulus. Identification is made more difficult by the fact that such cells may also breach the microvessel lumen.

## The Capillary

So far as is currently known, the basic composite structure of the tissue microvessels is the capillary. This term was first used by Marcello Malpighi in 1661 to describe the 'hair-like' structures seen in various living preparations in which red corpuscles were observed in continuous movement. The term 'capillary' has been used in a variety of circumstances and senses. It is now

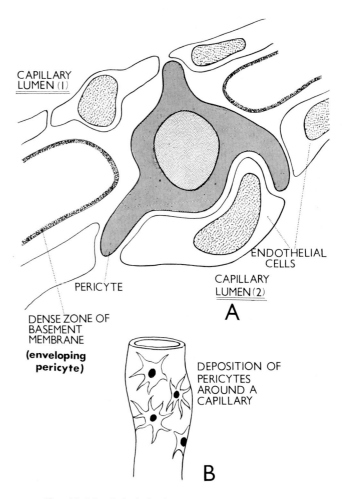

FIG. 12. Morphological relations of the pericytes. A. In very vascular tissues, the pericyte may connect the endothelium of adjacent capillaries, and its pseudopodia may become intraluminal. They are commonly surrounded by the dense zone of the endothelial basement membrane. B. Pericytes appear to 'cling' to microvessel walls like limpets to a rock, their pseudopodia often being in close contact with one another.

generally accepted that the term should be restricted to a structure which is nothing more than a simple endothelial tube and is sometimes clothed by a basement membrane (Fig. 13). Extra-endothelial cells are included provided they have an intimate and apparently functional connection with either the basement membrane or the endothelial sheet itself. Thus, the pericyte, the podocyte (renal glomerulus) and the glial cell (cerebral capillaries) are considered closely associated extra-endothelial cells in true capillaries, whereas smooth muscle cells, non-myelinated nerve endings and fibroblasts in close extra-endothelial association would automatically disqualify the composite structure from being considered a true capillary. Again, one cannot lay down qualifications as to size, since sinusoids with no more than endothelium and a basement membrane in their walls are now classified with the capillaries. In practice, the capillary is commonly of such a size that it will only just permit an erythrocyte to pass smoothly and will allow a leucocyte to pass with some deformation of the endothelial wall. Special *in vivo* preparations are required to make these distinctions, and

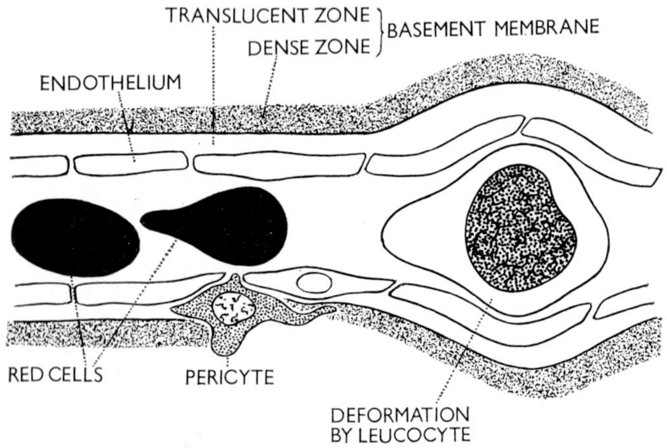

FIG. 13. The true capillary. The capillary is essentially a simple endothelial tube, the cells of which vary in character with different tissues: for simplicity low, continuous endothelium is shown here. Normally, red cells may just pass, but capillaries may be deformed by the passage of leucocytes. The basement membrane is shown with its dense zone splitting to enclose a pericyte.

commonly, the presence of the capillary can only be made out by the movement of intravascular cells. Such very thin preparations as the vascular membrane developed in the rabbit ear observation chamber (Sandison, 1924) and in the human skin bridge (Brånemark, 1963) require exploration of polarized light techniques before the capillary wall structure can be accurately identified. Unfortunately, the term capillary is still used as a generalization where, in fact, 'microvessel' is about as accurate as one can be. A good example of this is the clinical description of 'nail fold capillaries' for those microvessels in the posterior nail folds which are enclothed in muscle. It is also to be noted that no qualification is laid down with regard to diameter of a capillary, nor to direction of the blood flow, since the latter may occur in either direction according to local circumstances.

The 3 basic types of endothelium are, of course, represented in the capillaries of different tissues and organs, and are obviously subservient to different functions. Capillaries with a continuous endothelium (Group I) are found in striated muscle, in myocardium and in the smooth muscle of the reproductive tract and the digestive system. They are also found in brain substance. Capillaries with fenestrated endothelium (Group II) are identifiable

in highly active glandular tissue such as the endocrine organs, in the choroid plexus, and in the intestinal villi. The discontinuous endothelial-lined capillaries (Group III) occur in basically 'sinusoidal' tissues such as the liver, spleen and bone marrow: it is not unreasonable to suppose that there may be some connection here with the necessity for easy transit of cells between the microvessels and tissues, since these are the sites of reticulo-endothelial activity and also of numerical control of the free vascular population.

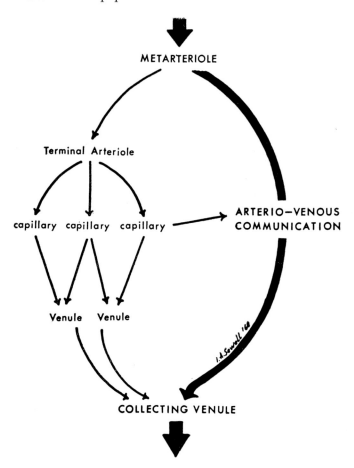

FIG. 14. Relation of the muscle-clothed microvessels to the capillaries. The diagram shows the general arrangement of the tissue microvessels on a functional basis. Only the capillaries (by definition) are not enclothed in muscle.

## Muscle-clothed Microvessels

Undoubtedly, the capillaries are the microvessels in most intimate contact with the active tissues. Their structure readily facilitates transmural exchange. Attention must now be paid to microvessels supplying capillaries and to those which drain them. In essence, they are capillaries with one or more muscle coats, and, like capillaries, have a variety of extra-endothelial structures in close association (Fig. 14). It is also convenient at this point to consider the structure of the tissue 'by-pass' vessels or arteriolo-venular communications (anastomoses) which divert blood past the true capillaries, since there are many similarities.

It is very difficult on structural grounds alone to distinguish between capillary-feeding, capillary-draining or capillary-bypass vessels, either *in vivo* or by transmitted light microscopy of fixed and stained preparations. Even electron microscopy has to be augmented by advanced histochemical techniques. It must be stressed that such terms as arteriole and venule are dependent on a functional interpretation (Fig. 14). This point is frequently neglected in accounts of tissue circulation and often leads to misunderstandings in interpretation.

**Arterioles.** In general, the term arteriole is confined to those muscle-clothed vessels which feed blood to an active tissue area, whether or not that blood actually finds its way through capillary networks. Arterioles are branches of arteries but must not be considered as terminal structures alone because they contribute to the bypass vessels as well as to capillary nets. Where the arteriole is seen to contribute to both capillaries and bypass vessels it is considered to be a metarteriole. By common usage (even if not strictly correct), a branch of a metarteriole solely supplying a capillary net may be spoken of as 'terminal'. In general descriptions and for most physiological considerations, qualification of the term 'arteriole' is usually superfluous.

**Venules.** The term venule describes those muscle-clothed endothelial tubes which either drain capillary networks or receive blood flow from arteriolo-venular communications (Fig. 14). A venule is considered to begin where the first muscle cell can be identified in its wall—often a matter of opinion in observations of *in vivo* preparations. Different authors use different terminology in describing venular structures, and until there is common agreement, the terms venule for the first part of the post-capillary tract and collecting venule for more distant structures would be considered quite adequate.

**Arteriolo-venular Communications.** These are vessels in which blood flow definitely bypasses the capillary networks, even though on occasion capillary networks can be observed to drain into these bypass channels. As with the venules, a plethora of terms may be found in the literature for their description and there is little foreseeable chance of any international agreement. The term 'arteriolo-venular communication' merely implies a direct connection between an arteriole and a venule whether or not a capillary drains into this vessel. It is a term of functional description. On semantic grounds, the term 'arteriovenous anastomosis' implies a direct connection between an artery and a vein: plenty of these can be found by standard anatomical techniques but they are well outside the immediate area of tissue circulation. However, this term 'arteriovenous anastomosis (-communication, -channel)' is frequently used where the term arteriolo-venular anastomosis should be used, and it must be left to the reader to interpret this as best he may.

Arteriolo-venular communications may be almost straight narrow channels in which the speed of flow is very rapid, they may be very tortuous and of varied calibre, or they may be of intermediate form. These varieties are peculiar to particular tissues and they are subject to the greatest variations in pathological changes.

**Extra-endothelial Structure of the Muscle-clothed Microvessels.** The basic composition of all these structures is the capillary ensheathed with muscle cells, arranged in one or more layers. At the transition point with the capillary, the muscle cells may be widely separated as a single

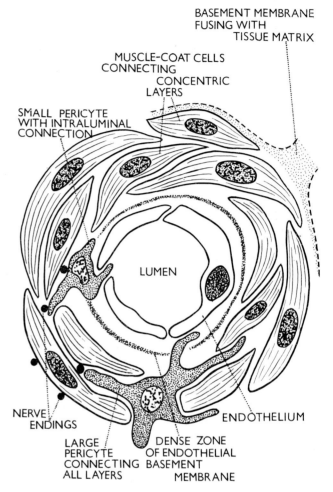

Fig. 15. Basic structure of the muscle-clothed microvessels. The core is the intravascular lumen which is immediately enclosed by endothelium. The dense zone of the endothelial basement membrane splits to enclose the pericytes and also becomes continuous with that of the muscle cells. The muscle cells constitute one or more layers around the endothelium, but the individual muscle cells may encroach on adjacent layers. Nerve endings occur in the muscle layers. Varieties of pericytes may occur in any part of the wall and may be in contact with the endothelium or with the cells of the immediately surrounding tissues. The basement membrane of the outer layer of muscle cells fuses with the matrix of adjacent tissue.

coat, but in the well-defined arteriole or venule the muscle cells are in close proximity to each other and are arranged in well-recognizable layers. Apart from the basement membrane surrounding the endothelial layer, each muscle coat also possesses a basement membrane, the most external of these blending with the matrix or intercellular substance of the immediately adjacent tissue. Special non-medullated nerve endings can be identified in the muscle layers, as are varieties of pericytes (Fig. 15).

As with endothelium, variations in structure of the

muscle-ensheathed microvessels are associated with particular tissues, and this is obviously determined by function. These variations range from dimensions of the smooth muscle cells, their arrangement and the number of layers, to incidence and distribution of non-myelinated nerve endings. Thus, in skeletal muscle, arteriolar muscle cell layers are seldom more than two in number and the cells are loosely arranged, but the incidence of nerve endings is very high. However, in the mesentery, three or more layers of muscle are common and the cells are closely knit, but nerve-endings tend to be widely separated. Arteriovenular communications are commonly seen to have tightly bound muscle layers with sparse basement membranes, and nerve-endings are concentrated at junctional sites. This list could be indefinitely extended.

The extra-endothelial layers of the venules do not appear to be so varied as the arterioles, but it should be mentioned that they have not so far been so extensively investigated. From published work, it seems that both endothelium and basement membrane have different histochemical properties from the capillaries they drain and that their muscle cells are more widely separated and consistently fewer in the number of layers as compared with arterioles of similar dimensions and in the same situation. These facts may account for the comparatively broader dimensions of venules when compared with the companion arterioles.

## Lymphatic Microvessels (The Lymphatics)

Much of what has been said of the structure of the blood-carrying tissue microvessels is also true of the tissue lymphatics. Thus, like the capillaries, lymphatic radicles are not readily visualized by transmitted light microscopy, and again, the results of recent electron microscopic investigations have given a slightly better understanding of structure and function, even though many facts await clarification.

The endothelium of the tissue lymphatics closely resembles the continuous (Group I) endothelium of the capillaries. Endothelial cytoplasm is very thin and the nuclei bulge prominently into the lymphatic lumen, which tends to be much larger than that of a comparable capillary. In addition to nuclear bulging lymphatic endothelium is characterized by intraluminar protrusion of flaps and pseudopodia, and by extra-endothelial projections into the surrounding connective tissue (Fig. 16). There are irregularities in the thickness and composition of the basement membrane, but it is much thinner than that of comparable capillaries. Collagen fibres are closely bound to the basement membrane but lymphatic pericytes have not been identified, those in association being considered to belong to adjacent blood microvessels. However, smooth muscle cells are found loosely applied to the lymphatic wall. The greatest difference from the capillaries appears to be at the intercellular junctions, which may be sinuous, broadly overlapping, or consisting of adhesion plates. Well-defined muscle layers may be found in lymphatics but these are usually in situations well away from any close association with tissue activity. Nerve endings have not been demonstrated with any certainty.

## Arrangement of Tissue Microvessels

The arrangement and continuity of tissue microvessels varies with particular tissues and organs and from species to species: our knowledge of this in the human is very far from complete. However, it is quite permissible to offer a generalized scheme, and, surprisingly enough, the results of investigations into tissue blood flow show that such a scheme can be applied to most situations. For our present purpose, the scheme has been considerably simplified, since, from a clinical point of view, no useful purpose is served by a more detailed consideration, nor by enumerating specific tissue and species differences.

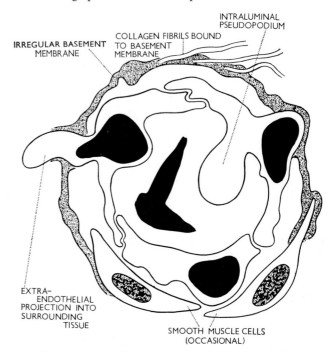

FIG. 16. Structural arrangements of tissue lymphatics. Lymphatic endothelium is characterized by prominent pseudopodia which project into the lumen and into the surrounding tissues. Endothelial nuclei tend to bulge into the lumen. The basement membrane is irregular and has collagen fibrils bound to it. Smooth muscle cells are seen occasionally and are but loosely bound to the basement membrane.

Most modern textbooks of physiology and those concerned specifically with peripheral circulation reproduce the microvessel maps devised by Zweifach and colleagues which are based on the most elegant studies of frog and rat mesenteries, but recent advances in our knowledge suggest that a fresh and more simplified approach is indicated. It is more convenient to consider oxygenated and nutriment-enriched blood approaching the tissue under study via a 'main' arteriole. Depending on tissue function at any particular moment, varying proportions will travel via particular metarterioles to arteriovenular communications and to terminal arterioles supplying individual capillary networks. The main arteriole may go on to contribute to an arterio-arteriolar collateral vessel or may become another connection with venous drainage, probably outside the boundaries of the tissue circulation proper.

The metarteriole gives off a terminal arteriole which supplies a particular capillary network. Commonly, 2 terminal arterioles may supply the same network. Some workers describe the last muscle cell of the terminal arteriole as the 'pre-capillary sphincter,' attributing to it powers of control over arteriolar flow into the capillary net. The capillary network itself may consist of many anastomosing vessels, the more peripheral ones joining to drain into simple venules, themselves draining into arteriolo-arteriolar anastomoses, arteriolo-venular anastomoses or into major collecting venules.

Lymphatic radicles appear in association with capillary networks, but there is no direct connection between them and the tissue microvessels just described.

From the foregoing simplified general description of the arrangement of the tissue microvessels it can be seen that many different pathways exist in the tissue circulation. Not all are in operation simultaneously, but their existence is one of the major factors contributing to the versatility and lability of the tissue circulation to meet changing demands.

### The Activities of Tissue Microvessels

At the beginning of this chapter, it was pointed out that the tissue microvessels provided a 'service' for the cells of the active tissues by way of the Slow (exchange) Circulation. Via connection with the Fast (rapid transport) Circulation, metabolic communication was assured between distant sites. The lability and versatility of the tissue microvessels to cope with ever changing demands of active tissues has already been stressed but it must be emphasized that these channels are not the sole factor, for in any study of tissue activity, the microvessels, their contents, the interstitial fluid and the active cells must all be taken together since each one of these depends upon the other for fully integrated activity. However, such a task is almost overwhelming because of its complexity, so that in this section we shall only be considering tissue activity from the microvascular aspect. Briefly, we shall be concerned with what is meant by 'Microcirculation,' transmural exchange, some basic facts about blood flow itself in microvessels, the blood reservoir function of microvessels, the significance of peripheral resistance, the principles operating in the control of local (tissue) fluid balance, and some comments on local cell migration.

### The Microcirculation

In just over a decade, a new term 'Microcirculation' has been introduced into the terminology of peripheral circulatory physiology. Enunciated by Fulton in 1954, it was meant to encompass our particular knowledge of very small blood vessels—a new term, in fact, for one of the oldest biological studies. Unfortunately, the good intentions implied in introducing a new and comprehensive term have been defeated by those who ignore the special relationship which exists between the microvessels and the general circulation, and this has resulted in a series of definitions based on vessel size and which ignore the all-important aspect of function. The very word 'Microcirculation' would appear to imply a microscopic circulation without reference to 'where' or 'how.' By relatively common usage, it is a term which is here to stay so that a practical appreciation must be made of its significance. From a functional point of view, we may consider that:

*The Microcirculation is that part of the cardiovascular and lymphatic systems in intimate contact with active tissues to facilitate metabolic exchange and promote the fully integrated activity of the whole organism.*

Thus, any component of the tissue microvessels directly concerned with transmural exchange and metabolite transfer at the level of tissue activity comes within the scope of this term. Since some of these structures can be seen by the well-trained naked eye it is difficult on occasion to define where the precise limits of the Microcirculation lie.

### Transmural Exchange

Until fairly recently, it was taught that metabolite exchange could only occur across the capillary wall and that this was largely determined by transmural pressure gradients, themselves influenced by hydrostatic pressures and osmotic differences. This is the classical concept of Starling. It certainly gives an easy explanation but does not stand up to searching investigation by up-to-date methods. We now know that there are many more factors to be considered than pressure and molecular attraction.

It is often stated that the object of transmural exchange is to achieve uniformity between the solutes of both serum and tissue fluid. There is really no logical reason for this and one cannot envisage it ever occurring, for the whole basis of cell life is constant change and this particularly applies at the tissue level. It is probably nearer the truth to say that exchange occurs to maintain solute concentration for specific activity. In consequence, no general statements will cover all the variations in transmural exchange but in a work of this nature it would be burdensome to list all the differences.

#### Endothelial Transport

We can probably best appreciate the basis of transmural exchange by considering the mechanisms which take place in the several components of the capillary wall. The only constant and unalterable factor is the endothelial tube, neglecting temporarily that this may be one of 3 main varieties. There are 3 pathways for the transfer of water, solutes and particulate matter (Fig. 17).

**Direct Transport.** The straightest of these pathways is directly across the endothelial wall, and if we accept the concept of capillary permeability as discussed by Chinard and his colleagues (1955), water and very small molecules can take this route without the presence of pre-existing endothelial pores. For water, permeability rates differ from tissue to tissue, and there is acceptable indirect evidence that this is also true of small molecules.

**Vesicle Transfer.** The second trans-endothelial route is by way of active 'vesicle transfer.' Particles are enclosed in fluid 'quanta' (sub-microscopic 'globes') at the cell surface and then engulfed. This corresponds to the 'cell-drinking' mechanism or pinocytosis, described by W. H. Lewis in 1931. However, these vesicles do not shrink within the endothelial cell, and they are discharged at its opposite surface, hence the term 'pinocytosis' is not really applicable in this situation. Moore and

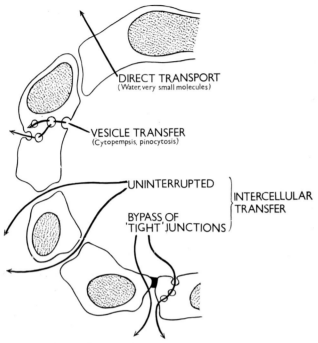

FIG. 17. Pathways in endothelial transport (Transmural Exchange). Three routes are available: direct transport across the endothelial cell (for water and very small molecules), vesicle transfer across the endothelial cell, or intercellular transfer, uninterruptedly between the cells of discontinuous endothelium or bypassing the tight junction by diffusion or vesicle transfer.

Ruska (1957) have suggested the term 'cytopempsis'—transmission by cell, cellular pumping, etc.—to describe this particular transportation phenomenon.

**Inter-cellular Transfer.** The third route is via the inter-cellular spaces, either by uninterrupted passage through capillary walls lined by discontinuous endothelium, by diffusion around tight sealed junctions until the inter-cellular gap is reached, or by vesicle transfer around tight junctions.

### 'Endocytosis'

Some evidence exists to support the view that transfer across the endothelial cell can also be effected by an active phagocytosis as distinct from 'cytopempsis,' although such phagocytosis is not the same as may occur with elements of the reticulo-endothelial system, such as the Küpffer cells of the liver. The phagocytic activity of the endothelium, or 'endocytosis' probably bears some relation to that seen in protozoa, whereby protein is adsorbed onto the cell membrane, which in turn is drawn towards the cytoplasm until the latter flows round it to produce a vesicle. It is important to note that adenosine

triphosphatase has been histochemically identified in such vesicles, and that this enzyme has been implicated in both sodium and potassium ion transport. It is frequently stated that solute transmigration is dependent on exact quantities of water of solution being transferred. No experiments are reported to confirm this, and in any case, both serum and tissue fluid are variable colloids so that inferences from simple osmotic phenomena may not be applicable.

A very active endocytosis may be observed in venules with large accumulations of intraluminal debris, especially following microthrombi formation.

### Transport Through Basement Membranes

Outside the endothelial lining of the capillary there may be either a basement membrane or an intercellular ground substance coincident with that of the immediately adjacent cells. Detailed studies of basement membranes have shown that this allows transmigration of water and small molecules of the order 80–100 Å in size. It is of some significance that transmigration of larger molecules has only been observed across capillaries with discontinuous endothelium, and that lymphatic radicles contain protein molecules of small size unless intercellular disruption of endothelium occurs, as in inflammation. However, the basement membrane structure varies considerably, and in theory the proline molecular model allows for considerable modifications in its spatial arrangements, a point of importance when considering the relative permeability of the basement membrane of some capillaries with a continuous endothelium to fairly large bodies such as chylomicrons. It must not be assumed that the basement membrane acts as a simple passive diffusible barrier, since there is considerable evidence suggesting an active selectivity at particular sites.

### The Possible Role of the Pericytes in Transmigration

Recent work has shown that the pericytes are actively phagocytic and that this phenomenon is very similar to endocytosis. This is not surprising, since pericytes have many features in common with endothelial cells. To some extent, pericytes are permeable to water and certain solutes. The precise role of the pericytes in transmural exchange is by no means clear. They are certainly not a major obstacle and it is quite possible that they may exert some regulatory influence although there is very little factual evidence in support of this hypothesis.

### Transmigration Across Muscle-clothed Microvessels

The basic facts about transmigration across endothelium and basement membrane can also be extended to muscle-clothed vessels such as arterioles and venules. Categoric statements that exchange does not take place across these structures should now be ignored. In 1930, Rous and colleagues showed that post-capillary venular structures were even more permeable than the preceding capillary and they could find no obstacle to transport in either the muscle cells or the basement membrane. Particulate carbon of the order 200–350 Å in size can infiltrate tissue microvessel walls to pass into the surrounding tissues and many of these particles show no evidence of migration either by phagocytosis or by endocytosis. In theory at least, it is possible that all the tissue microvessels offer facility for transmural exchange, but structural differences and selective activity of different cell and basement membranes directly influence the speed of this exchange. This idea has some support from the fact that the sole source of nourishment of a major arteriole is the blood in its lumen, albeit that the arteriole is many muscle coats thick.

### Hydrostatic and Osmotic Pressure Gradients

Since Starling's time, the general physiologist has explained transmural exchange across vascular membranes by considering hydrostatic and osmotic pressure gradients. Existence of these gradients is not doubted, but are they the cause or the effect of the specialized biological activity of particular vascular membranes? The convenient application of the behaviour of the semipermeable membrane when separating two dissimilarly osmotic liquids takes no account of the vital activity of the living endothelial cell. Mjano's experiments (1953) to verify the role of altering hydrostatic pressures in influencing fluid exchange have shown that this is independent of such mechanical force, at least at the level of tissue activity and in health. It would therefore appear that the role of purely mechanical forces in determining exchange across the vascular membrane may be considerably modified by local vital activity.

### Blood Flow in the Tissue Microvessels

Transmural exchange is in part dependent upon the characteristics of the blood flow in the tissue microvessels, but before discussing this factor it is important to re-orientate ourselves as to the general layout of these vessels and the reader is therefore referred back to the section of this chapter on Structure of Microvessels/Arrangement of Tissue Microvessels (p. 168). The capillary network, its supplying arterioles, draining venules and the arteriolo-venular by-pass vessels all contribute to a functional unit called 'The Microvascular Bed'. This is identical with the term "Capillary Bed" used by some authors, but this latter term is really a misnomer since other structures than capillaries are concerned in its composition.

### Factors Influencing Tissue Blood Flow (Fig. 18)

Undoubtedly, the prime factor at any site is the demand created by active cells for nutrient supply and the need to remove metabolites for the reasons given at the beginning of this chapter (p. 125). Increase in tissue activity results in an increase in local blood volume, and direct observation at suitable sites shows that a vast number of capillaries are under active perfusion. Conversely, during quiescence, the number of observable capillary nets is greatly decreased and the by-pass channels are prominent. In certain situations, such as active skeletal muscle, the increase in the fully perfused microvascular bed does not always coincide with the period of tissue activity and this may be delayed until the end of the contraction period.

**Calibre Changes.** Any change in blood flow is accompanied by changes in vessel calibre and this phenomenon is observable in all components of the microvascular bed. Calibre change is an active phenomenon in arterioles, venules and the arteriolo-venular channels, being mediated through smooth muscle in the vessel wall. In the capillaries, it is passive and is effected by alterations in the form

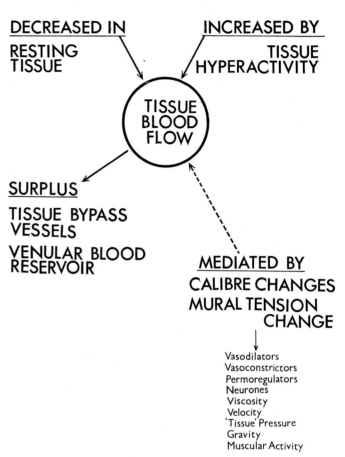

Fig. 18. Factors influencing tissue blood flow. The diagram summarizes the factors which alter blood flow through tissues. Total increase or decrease is a function of tissue activity, but where the tissues are inactive (e.g. during the resting phase in muscle), total blood flow may not be appreciably altered since the bypass vessels will take up a large proportion. Mediation of changes in blood flow is by calibre change and alterations in mural tension, both being influenced by biophysical and biochemical phenomena, as well as by nervous activity.

and size of the endothelial cells. It is therefore not strictly comparable with the activity of the smooth muscle of the other microvessels. The reader is warned against misinterpretation of the term 'capillary contraction' which is so frequently misused in descriptions of microvascular activity for the use of the term suggests an activity which would not appear to be possible. Changes in capillary calibre occur in the form of an intraluminar block or as passive distension due to increase in perfusion brought about by relaxation of the pre-capillary sphincter. Despite extensive studies using electron microscopy with histochemical techniques, the basis of these changes in capillaries is by no means clear.

Calibre changes in the muscle-clothed microvessels can be attributed to the action of chemical substances and to nervous activity, both of which are discussed in detail later. They may also be due to pressure differences in the general circulation and may arise from the necessity to modify the effect of the vis a tergo originating in cardiac activity. There is a fall in mean vascular pressure from between 100–120 mm. Hg. during systole at the aortic arch to zero over the last few cms. of the superior and inferior vena cava. This fall is slight until the tissues are

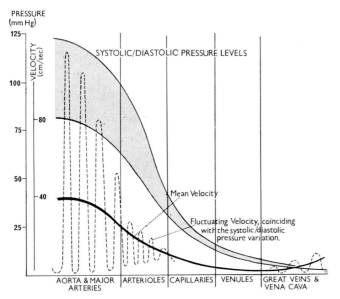

Fig. 19. Attainment of smooth blood flow for transmural exchange by resolution of pressure differences and alternating velocities. Differences between systolic and diastolic pressures are reduced as arteriolar peripheral resistance rises, and once through the microcirculatory beds, change in pressure is induced by changes in right heart filling. These later changes do not affect tissue circulation because the latter is protected by venular muscle contractility. The mean velocity falls steadily through the circulation, being lowest through the tissues (*slow* [Exchange] *circulation*) and rising again in the vena cava due to negative intrathoracic pressure. Mean velocity is the resultant vector of the wide variations in both systole and diastole during blood flow through the aorta and major arteries. This variation is produced again on very much smaller scale in blood flow through the great veins and vena cava.

reached and maintenance of the pressure level is due to the peripheral resistance created by arteriolar tone, an important factor which is discussed separately at a later stage in this chapter (p. 140) The vascular pressure is subjected to variations proportional to the systolic and diastolic pressure but the smooth blood flow essential for transmural exchange in the tissue circulation is ensured by variations in the arteriolar tone, which tends to buffer the vis a tergo, thus providing protection for the capillary nets (Fig. 19).

**Protection of Tissue Microvessels from Overdistension.** Quite apart from damping of the vis a tergo effect of cardiac activity by continuous variations in arteriolar tone, the microvessels (and especially the capillaries) are protected from over-distension and rupture by a relatively

simple principle originally deduced by Laplace from his studies of mechanics and hydrodynamics. In what is commonly known as the Law of Laplace, he stated that the distending pressure of a pliable hollow container is equal to the tension in its wall divided by its two principal radii of curvature at equilibrium, or

$$P = \frac{T}{R_1 + R_2}$$

In small blood vessels, including small portions of capillaries, $P$ = the transmural pressure (or pressure difference between the plasma stream and the interstitial fluid), $R_1$ may almost equal $R_2$, hence

$$P = T/R$$

Therefore, as the radius of a vessel is reduced in size, so the tension exerted by the wall to balance distension will fall proportionally. In a young healthy adult male, it has been calculated that aortic tension is of the order of 150,000 dynes/cm., tension in the vena cava about 20,000 dynes/cm., whereas in capillaries it may be only 15 dynes/cm. Even so, this distending pressure is exceeded in a number of disease processes, with consequent rupture of the vessel. However the rise in such distending pressures is very much higher than would be expected from calculations, and it is possible that other than mechanical factors are involved.

**The Role of Chemical Substances in Tissue Blood Flow**

The significance of the activities of various chemical substances on tissue blood vessels is of fundamental importance to anaesthetists, since the concentrations of naturally-occurring vaso-active substances may be altered in pathological states and by the administration of anaesthetic agents. Many anaesthetic agents themselves have profound influences on tissue microvessels, either by their direct action, or by altering the activities of naturally occurring substances. The central effects of anaesthetic agents may reduce the quantity of peripherally acting vaso-active substances released. The subject is an extensive one and can only be very briefly covered in a work of this nature. There is also room for much further research in this field. This section will therefore be concerned only with chemical substances known to have specific micro-vascular activity and with those agents likely to be encountered by the anaesthetist in his routine work.

In general terms, chemical substances act on tissue microvessels to produce either vasodilatation or vasoconstriction through their effects on the smooth muscle of the walls, or, they may alter endothelial permeability and morphology to produce intraluminar change and alteration in local transmural exchange. They may act as chemical mediators in neural transmission affecting the smooth muscle of microvessels, or, they may act on the tissue cells to alter the local biophysical and biochemical state, which in turn will affect local blood flow. Thus different actions may take place simultaneously with the same substance and it may be very difficult to elicit precise activity. Again, many substances which induce vaso-dilation as a primary action may also induce an increase in permeability. In some instances, this is out of all proportion to the increase in calibre, and it may be impossible to determine how much of this is due to direct action on the endothelium and the basement membrane.

**Locally Produced Vasodilators.** Certain substances acting on tissue microvessels have their origins in the tissues themselves. Dornhorst (1963) has shown that there is a widely distributed substance, a nonapeptide currently known as Bradykinin (also called kallidin 9) which has a specifically dilator action. The mechanism of its production is probably the conversion of alpha-2 globulin fractions of the serum derived from the decapeptide kallidin 10 by the kallikrein group of enzymes, with removal of the N-terminal lysine by aminopeptidase. Its precise source is not known, although it is found in high concentrations in sweat glands, salivary glands and the exocrine pancreas. It is also highly concentrated in the leucocytes found in traumatized tissue. It is slow-acting and appears to be most active in the period of quiescence following great activity: this is certainly true of skeletal muscle. It is unlikely to be the result of any oxidative process and its concentration is not inhibited by loss of sympathetic activity.

Tissue activity results in accumulations of carbonic acid and lactic acid, and when these are present in great excess as a result of severe local anoxia, vasodilatation will occur—with the result that tissue clearance of unwanted metabolites is expedited.

**Histamine.** Another substance originating in tissues is histamine. This is the decarboxylation derivative of the essential amino-acid histidine. It can be identified in all tissues but occurs in high concentrations in the skin and lungs. It occurs in rapidly rising concentrations at the sites of trauma and tissue destruction, and its general circulatory level rises progressively where there is rapid depletion of circulating blood volume as in bacteraemic shock and in severe burns. In dilution, it produces profound vasodilatation by specific activity on vascular smooth muscle, which leads to greatly increased perfusion of capillary nets. However, when given experimentally in higher concentration, a profound hypotension may follow, often completely cutting off local tissue perfusion. In laboratory rodents this may result in a rapid 'ischaemic' death, and it is thought to be responsible for renal necrosis in the crush syndrome and in human anaphylaxis. The precise mechanism of the ischaemia following concentrated histamine injection is not known.

Both the vasodilatation and ischaemia following histamine administration can be prevented by the pre-administration of antihistamines, which may account for some of the beneficial effects following the use of pro-methazine hydrochloride as a sedative prior to general anaesthesia.

Histamine will also produce increased endothelial permeability independent of its vasodilating effects.

**Endocrine Substances.** Present knowledge indicates that all the circulating hormones will indirectly induce increased perfusion at their target organs, but effects on non-target tissue may be varied and specific—e.g. oestrogenic sub-stances appear to inhibit blood flow through prostatic tissue transplants. Assessment of the general effects of most of the hormones for their specific action on tissue circulation are only scantily reported, but it is well-known that Vasopressin from the posterior pituitary lobe can produce an intense vasoconstriction, and it is considered very likely that thyroxine and its derivatives may act as general tissue vasodilators simultaneously with their effects as general tissue catalysts.

**Naturally-occurring Vasoconstrictive Agents.** Known naturally-occurring vasoconstrictor agents include sero-tonin (derived from platelet breakdown), angiotensin II (an octapeptide derived from alpha-2-globulin angio-tensinogen by the action of renin from the kidney), and the catechol amines adrenaline and noradrenaline. When locally applied, they produce intense vasoconstriction, and they can be extracted from vasoconstricted areas resulting from causes other than the application of chemical substances.

**Adrenaline and Noradrenaline.** Of all the chemical substances implicated in vasoactivity, both noradrenaline and adrenaline have received more attention than any others. Quite apart from their role in autonomic nervous activity, their direct effects have been studied in great detail and the resulting literature is vast. There follows a brief summary of well-established facts and the more important theories about both.

Adrenaline may act as both a vasodilator and a vaso-constrictor, the particular action depending upon site and mode of administration. When it acts as a vasodilator, there is a growing amount of evidence to suggest that it promotes the release of bradykinin-like substances. This would certainly fit in with recent suggestions by Burns that the alpha- and beta- responses of arterioles are due to activity by two separate substances rather than to different types of nerve fibre as suggested by Ahlquist. Adrenaline produces vasoconstriction in the skin, in muscle when given intra-arterially, in liver when given via the portal vein, and in the kidney. It produces vasodilatation in muscle, when given intravenously, in the liver following systemic administration, and in the brain (note 'adrena-line' headache following repeated use of this substance to relieve severe bronchospasm).

Noradrenaline is usually a vasoconstricting substance. This effect is well-marked in the skin, muscle, in the liver following portal vein infusion, kidney (though not as effective as adrenaline), the mucosa of the alimentary tract, and the brain. For these reasons, noradrenaline is a potentially dangerous substance when used therapeutically and its real usefulness is very limited. Probably, the only indication for administration is to prevent too profound an hypotension following removal of a phaeochromo-cytoma. Its use following generalized arteriolar dilatation due to general anaesthesia, and drug overdose should be restricted to those situations when the fall in venous return lowers cardiac output. Its indiscriminate use to counter hypotension may cause dangerous tissue ischaemia. Its most dangerous application has been to restore blood pressure in the hypovolaemic patient following haemorrhage at a time when the tissues are already severely ischaemic.

**Acetylcholine.** Quite apart from its role as a mediator in the autonomic control of the peripheral circulation, acetylcholine produces vasodilatation by direct action. However, unless perfusion of this substance is continuous, or eserine is given in conjunction, the effect is short-lived because of destruction by cholinesterase.

**Oxidase.** Some mention must be made of the effects of amine oxidase, even though very few and inconclusive studies have been carried out to determine its direct

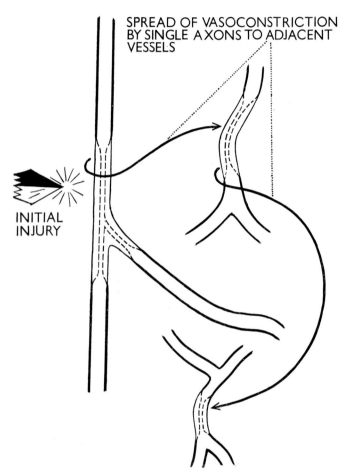

Fig. 20. Local axon reflex activity in microvascular beds: single axon reflexes. *Highly localized trauma may directly induce vasospasm. This local microvascular change may stimulate a local single axon reflex which may result in vasoactivity in the immediately surrounding microvessels. Initially, this is most commonly vasoconstriction but is later followed by vasodilatation.*

effects on tissue microvessels. This substance destroys both adrenaline and noradrenaline and therefore reverses the specific effects of both. It is present at all sites of normal noradrenaline release, destroying noradrenaline more quickly than adrenaline and making the effects of the latter appear more potent. Usually, the continued effects of both noradrenaline and adrenaline depend on continued perfusion, but when both are stopped after simultaneous perfusion, the adrenaline effect outlasts that of noradrenaline. This difference in apparent activity of the two catechol amines is abolished by sympathectomy, since this operation is followed by a profound reduction in

tissue amine oxidase levels, although this enzyme reappears in small amounts in about a month to 6 weeks. During this initial period, tissue blood vessel sensitivity is increased to direct application of both adrenaline and noradrenaline.

Amine oxidase activity is inhibited by ephedrine and similar substances, which would account for the reduced effect of the latter when perfused through recently sympathectomized tissues.

These remarks apply only to sympathectomy performed by actual nerve section or excision. We have no information, so far, as to amine oxidase levels and catechol amine sensitivity following 'chemical' sympathectomy using phenol or alcohol block techniques.

### Nervous Control and Influence in Tissue Microvessel Activity

The muscle-clothed microvessels are liberally supplied with nerve fibres but these have not been demonstrated in the capillary wall. These microvessels are immediately influenced by local reflex activity, but there is a considerably delayed effect when the central nervous system or the large peripheral nerves are involved, the final effects on the tissue vessels being secondary to changes induced in the general circulation. This is beautifully illustrated by the observations from the transparent chambers inserted in rabbits ears in which direct stimulation of the membrane microvessels produces immediate response, whereas stimulation of the nerves around the central artery of the ear causes a delayed effect. Tissue microvessels show an immediate response to the direct application of various chemical substances acting as peripheral mediators of the autonomic system, a subject which has just been discussed. There are clear differences between the responses of the microvessels of the limbs and viscera and those of the skin and muscle following nerve stimulation. The commonest clinical example of this is the overall vasospasm which occurs simultaneously in both the skin and splanchnic bed accompanying widespread vasodilatation is skeletal muscle as a response to the 'fight and flight' reflexes.

**Local Reflexes.** A good deal of the versatility and lability of the microvessels to meet changing tissue demands is vested in a complex system of local reflexes. Much speculation exists as to precise pathways, but only two of these can be demonstrated with any certainty (Fig. 20). The simplest of these is the Single Axon Reflex, in which local sensory stimulation in the microvascular bed is immediately mediated by non-medullated nerve fibres activating adjacent microvessels. This can be demonstrated by applying highly localized trauma with a fine needle electrode and then observing the immediate vasoconstriction of the nearest microvessels which rapidly spreads to adjacent vessels. If local nerve fibres are damaged in the process, then the time interval between repeated trauma and the vasoconstrictor response is considerable. This kind of experiment has been most elegantly recorded by Sanders using very high-speed cinephotomicrography.

Another local reflex of some significance is Antidromic Vasodilatation, in which stimulation of pain-sensitive areas such as the skin and superficial mucous membranes results in a profound localized vasodilatation at the site of stimulation. The impulse passes along centrifugal fibres in sensory nerves (Fig. 21), the pathway being distal to the posterior root ganglion (Lewis, 1927). It is only abolished after complete degeneration in the peripheral segment of the sensory nerve following section distal to the posterior root ganglion. Antidromic vasodilation accounts for the central flushing and consequent oedema in the Lewis Triple Response to locally applied trauma.

**Autonomic Nervous Influence on Tissue Microvessels.** Autonomic nervous control of the general circulation has an indirect influence on local blood flow, but its direct effect is probably limited to the actions of its chemical mediators. There is much speculation in this field and many traditional concepts do not stand the tests of searching investigation. Whatever the pathways and mechanisms involved, alterations in autonomic nervous activity have profound effects on tissue circulation, all of which are of profound importance.

In general, tissue microvessels are immediately influenced by post-ganglionic sympathetic activity, and certainly, post-ganglionic fibres can be demonstrated in microvessel walls. Increased sympathetic activity results in vasoconstriction of microvessels in skin, muscle (notably in the resting muscles during general exercise) and in the deep viscera. There is a well-established reciprocity of blood flow between skin and mucosa. Bearing in mind that a general rise in sympathetic activity results in overall increase in blood flow and velocity in the general circulation, these local vasoconstrictor effects must be sufficient to overcome the increased perfusing force presenting at the microcirculatory bed and can therefore be considered complementary to the sympathetic activity which ensures adequate perfusion in the most active tissues. Thus in muscle, immediately after exercise, there is prolonged vasodilatation following sympathetic stimulation, but this must not be confused with that due to local bradykinin release (previously discussed) which is independent of sympathetic activity. Sympathectomy results in abolition of vasoconstrictor tone and of responses to temperature changes: however, this effect decreases with time, although the degree varies with the site of the sympathectomy.

Unlike sympathetic activity, parasympathetic activity is almost universally vasodilator. This is particularly well illustrated in glands having a parasympathetic motor supply. This correlates well with the need for increased local perfusion during glandular activity. Local tissue perfusion in pelvic viscera is markedly increased following stimulation of the nervi erigentes (pelvic splanchnic nerves): e.g. perfusion of blood vessels in the broad ligament may be increased tenfold.

At higher levels (Fig. 22), the vasomotor centre influences tissue circulation via its pressor and depressor areas (older terminology vasoconstrictor and vasodilator centres). The pressor area produces widespread vasoconstriction when stimulated, whereas stimulation of the depressor area will reverse vasoconstriction but further stimulation is required before an active vasodilatation is induced.

## The Nature of Blood Flow in the Tissue Circulation

Direct observation of the tissue microvessels reveals that blood flow in them is not simple. Indeed, it is very far from being a column of fluid of uniform constitution advancing with identical speed in all parts. This particular aspect of blood flow constitutes a special part of the study of hydrodynamics known as *rheology*. Rheologists

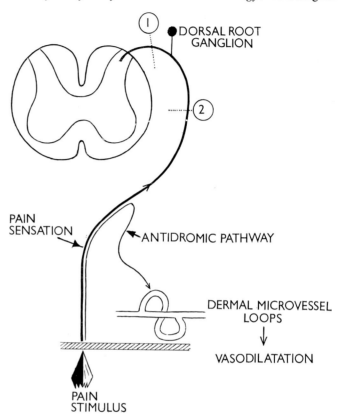

Fig. 21. Nerve pathways in the antidromic vasodilator response (After T. Lewis, 1927). Stimulation of pain-sensitive areas (skin, mucous membranes) result in the centripetal passage of pain sensations to the dorsal root ganglion and the posterior spinal columns. Simultaneously, an antidromic fibre is stimulated. This fibre turns back from the main pain pathway distal to the dorsal root ganglion to pass to the skin blood vessels in the stimulated area to produce an intense vasodilation. Section at (1) does not affect the antidromic response. Section at (2) only abolishes the response when there is complete degeneration of the peripheral segment of the sensory nerve.

have investigated the flow of blood in both large and small blood vessels in many different sites in the body, but apart from some generalizations, their findings show that the flow at the 'microvessel' level cannot be predicted, is very difficult to measure, and is subject to frequent changes in the same vessel, even when local conditions vary only slightly.

**Laminar and Turbulent Flow.** In some vessels such as arterioles and arteriolar-venular connections, where an observable portion is sufficiently long and straight, the flow appears to be 'streamlined.' That is to say, the very thin layer of fluid immediately adjacent to the vessel wall does not appear to move at all, whereas each concentric layer appears to be moving progressively faster. This is called *laminar flow*. Laminar flow will occur until a certain rate is reached, providing there are no obstructions to flow. This rate is known as the *critical velocity*, and

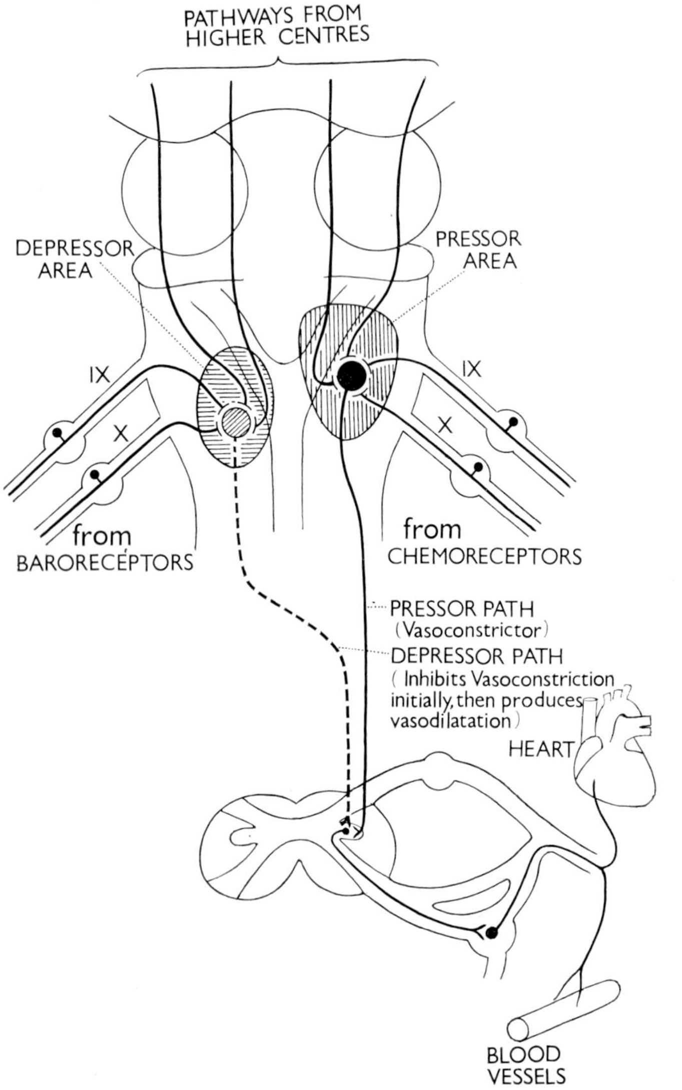

Close observation of the microvascular bed reveals that turbulent flow is very much more common than laminar flow. This is to be expected because vascular dichotomy is frequent, the blood in a variety of tributaries may enter at different speeds, peripheral cell migration is frequent

FIG. 22. Vasomotor centre influences on tissue circulation (After Uvnas, 1960). The vasomotor centre is situated in the hind brain, and consists of a pressor (activating) and depressor (inhibiting) area. Pressor fibres pass down in the antero-lateral columns of the spinal cord on the same side and pass out with the sympathetic outflow to target areas (heart and blood vessels) inducing vasoconstriction and augmented cardiac activity. Depressor fibres cross the midline extensively and travel with the pressor fibres at the lower levels. They inhibit vasoconstriction initially, but further depressor pathway stimulation may result in an active vasodilatation.

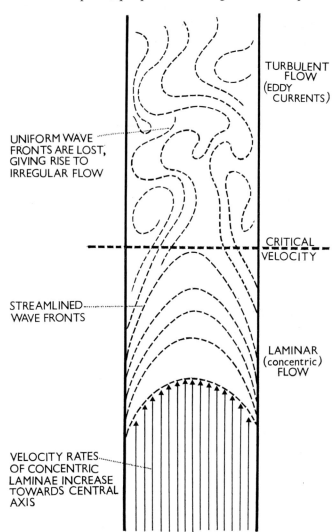

FIG. 23. Effects of changing velocity on flow characteristics. At low, uniform speed, laminar (concentric) flow occurs whereby the axial speed is high compared with the peripheral flow, producing a 'streamline' wave front. The summit of the parabola of this wave front increases in height as velocity increases until a critical velocity is reached. At this point, the uniform wave front is broken and the concentric layers of the advancing column form their own wave fronts independent of each other to produce turbulent flow. Turbulent flow is enhanced by calibre change or by alteration of the internal configuration of the vessel.

above this, eddy waves are set up and the stream becomes *turbulent* (Fig. 23).

In microvessels where laminar flow is in progress, the cellular constituents of the blood are confined to the central axis of flow. Laminar flow is lost whenever cells stray to the outer layers of the fluid column, e.g. where the microvessels branch.

(especially at junctions) and variations in calibre are common and often continuous. In capillaries, where both red and white cells are sometimes larger than the average lumen of the vessel, laminar flow is impossible and turbulence can be inferred even by the routine use of transmitted light microscopy. Turbulence does not appear to affect what might be called 'normal' flow, possibly because of the

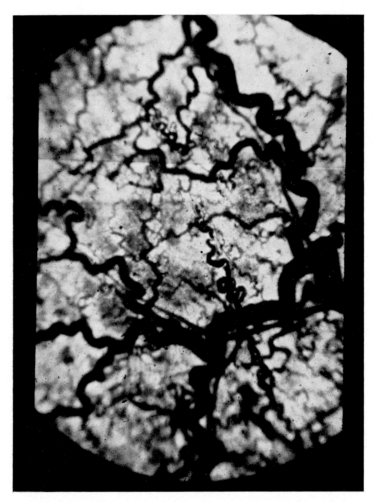

Fig. 25. Photomicrograph of a connective tissue microvascular bed showing the relatively high proportion of venous side vessels. Demonstrating that the arteriolar structures, are few in number. (Author's in vivo preparation of hamster cheek pouch wall membrane enclosed in a transparent tissue observation chamber for living microscopy: Sewell, 1966).

influence of local tissue activity and also because there is a possibility that the creation of a negative pressure phase may occur in front of each advancing cell, this sucking it forwards.

**Flow Velocity.** Rheologists speak of 'average velocity' when attempting to give some idea of the particular activity of a fluid system. In clinical studies, this has some application when we study circulation times by the injection of fluorescing substances or radio-active isotopes and calculating the time it takes for them to be identified at a distant site. At any given point in the circulation, average velocity is inversely proportional to the total cross-sectional area. Thus, it will be very high in the aorta and very low in the capillary nets. However, velocity in the tissue circulation is very much more variable than in the general circulation. So far as we know, this variability is a function of the very small calibre changes which are constantly taking place at the tissue level. These flow variations in active tissues are directly observable in certain types of experiment but it is extraordinarily difficult to measure them precisely.

The relationship between calibre change and blood flow rates can be forecast by a modification of the Poiseuille–Hagen formula for calculating resistance in long tubes through which fluid flows at a steady rate, where

$$R = \frac{8\eta L}{\pi r^4}$$

($R$ = resistance, $\eta$ = viscosity, $L$ = length of vessel, $r$ = radius)

By application, it can be calculated that blood flow in a very small vessel such as a major arteriole will be doubled by an increase in radius of about 16 per cent, or, doubling the radius reduces resistance to about 1/16. Hence, both blood flow and resistance are markedly affected by small calibre changes. A warning is given that the Poiseuille–Hagen formula can only be applied with great reservations in comparatively few situations in the microcirculatory bed because very few vessels are straight enough and long enough, and there is frequent calibre change.

**Viscosity.** Blood flow through the tissues is also governed by the characteristics of the blood itself, such as the viscosity, which in turn is influenced by the number of circulating cells and platelets. In theory, blood flow velocity is inversely proportional to the viscosity, but this only applies in major vessels, thus a changing haematocrit will affect blood flow in large vessels but it has very little influence on flow in microvessels, mainly because laminar flow is an inconstant feature. However, when the overall haematocrit is very low, striking changes may occur in tissue circulation. Peripheral resistance will fall and the phenomenon of *plasma skimming* may occur (Fig. 24). This can be seen in anaemias associated with bone marrow hypoplasia in which the very few red cells remain in the central axis of the larger vessels, and 'cell-free' plasma is 'skimmed off' into the tissue circulation thus giving rise to a local ischaemia.

**Blood Reservoir Function of the Tissue Circulation**

From direct observations of the tissues *in vivo*, various workers have estimated that 60–70 per cent of the blood volume lies in the venular structures (Fig. 25). At rest periods, the blood in the venules has been observed to re-circulate in these structures, and this locally confined circulation appears to extend to the collecting venules. This would agree well with measurement of different components of the circulating blood volume, where at least 50 per cent of the Fast (Rapid Transport) Circulation lies in the veins and another 16–20 per cent cannot be accounted

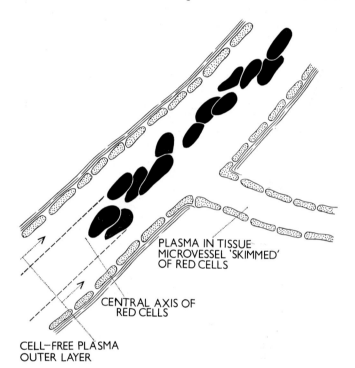

Fig. 24. 'Plasma skimming'. In red cell deficiency anaemias, peripheral resistance falls and the red cells flow in the centre of the stream, leaving a cell-free plasma outer layer. This outer layer is 'skimmed off' into the tissue microvessels thus inducing local tissue ischaemia.

for by measurement of the blood volume of the heart, major arteries and the arterioles. This 'pool' of relatively static blood is far from evenly distributed between the tissues, but *in toto*, provides a circulatory reserve which under quiescent conditions should not be regarded as a part of the active circulation. This 'capacitance' factor of the tissue circulation augments that of the great veins. The larger pools are to be found in the skin, splanchnic circulation, and in resting muscle. In humans, there are much smaller pools in the spleen, bone marrow and in active skeletal muscle.

**Re-distribution of Blood Reservoirs.** In an apparently contrary manner, the blood reservoirs are temporarily augmented by the increased perfusion of active tissues, but these local reserves are short-lived and are rapidly distributed. In general terms, blood reservoirs are depleted locally in conditions where greatly increased perfusion of active tissues at distant sites is required, and this is especially true where situations arise in which the integrity of the whole complex organism depends for survival on adequate perfusion of the really vital organs, such as the brain, the myocardium and the kidney. The triggering mechanisms for this re-distribution of the tissue blood reservoirs are complex and it is often difficult to isolate them individually. So far as we can tell (Fig. 26), the

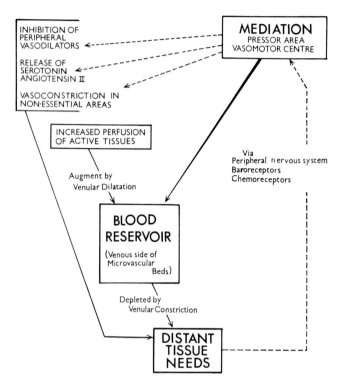

Fig. 26. Redistribution of blood reservoirs. In tissue circulation, the venular components and the bypass channels constitute a blood reservoir which can be diverted to distant sites in time of need. The peripheral baroreceptors and chemoreceptors are stimulated to act on the vasomotor centre whereby the pressor area initiates venular constriction to empty these reservoirs, vasoconstriction of arterioles in non-essential areas, inhibition of production of vasodilating agents (e.g. bradykinin and histamine), releases serotonin and angiotensin II, and augments endocrine activity (e.g. adrenals).

commonest combination is mediation through the pressor area of the vasomotor centre following transmission from the peripheral baroreceptors and chemoreceptors whereby venular vasoconstriction occurs. There is widespread closure of terminal arterioles in non-essential microvascular beds, endocrine activation (particularly adrenal glands) and arrested production of the widely distributed vasodilating agents such as bradykinin and histamine. Serotonin and angiotensin II may also be released.

## Peripheral Resistance

If one looks upon the venular structures of the microcirculatory bed as a part of the 'vascular capicitance of the circulation, then the arteriolar and arteriolo-venular components must be regarded as contributing the 'vascular resistance'. Peripheral resistance is derived from the arteriolar and arteriolo-venular tone at the tissue level. This tone is a prominent factor determining the lower level of the pressure in the circulation and is the major factor contributing to the maintenance of the diastolic pressure. There is considerable variation in peripheral resistance from tissue to tissue, due principally to the different demands of individual tissues for blood flow.

The significance of the peripheral resistance factor may be summarized as follows:

1. It protects the capillaries from great changes in circulation pressure by damping the oscillations of the arterial pulse. This damping mechanism is highly effective because oscillations are rarely seen in direct observations of the microvascular beds.

2. It ensures a constant blood flow at optimal speed for transmural exchange.

3. It constitutes the most important factor in determining mean arterial pressure.

4. It indirectly produces change in cardiac output to combat changes in mean arterial pressure. Thus, increased tissue demands, as in exercise, induce a fall in peripheral resistance and a rise in cardiac output.

5. By virtue of its effect on diastolic pressure, peripheral resistance determines the pulse pressure (difference between systolic and diastolic pressures). Since pulse pressure is one of the factors which determine local tissue perfusion, peripheral resistance serves to control the volume and speed of flow of blood in local tissue perfusion.

6. It determines changes in the distribution of local blood flow. This is illustrated by the relatively minor fall in peripheral resistance in active skeletal muscle increasing local blood flow twentyfold (as compared with only a fivefold increase in cardiac output) but completely shutting off blood flow in non-active areas by increasing the local peripheral resistance.

From the above, it can be seen that the control of peripheral resistance is one of the most important factors in circulatory regulation. Undoubtedly, one of the most important triggering mechanisms is the activity of tissues determining the demand for blood which is met initially by local changes in peripheral resistance. As demand rises, so variations in peripheral resistance spread, ultimately bringing about change in the whole of the circulation in many instances.

**Critical Closing Pressure.** This is the pressure at which flow ceases in tissue blood vessels. It is due to local increase in peripheral resistance, and available evidence shows that the principal site of action is the pre-capillary sphincter. Contraction of the pre-capillary sphincter is augmented by increases in local interstitial fluid pressure, resulting in such a local rise of tissue pressure (cells + interstitial fluid + peripheral resistance) that the force available to propel red cells through the capillaries is overcome. Local tissue perfusion cannot recur until the critical closing pressure is exceeded. It is important to note, however, that critical closing pressure is an integration of many factors and is not merely the force expended in the contraction of the pre-capillary sphincter.

## Local (Tissue) Fluid Balance

Clinicians are well-versed in the importance of maintaining the fluid balance in their patients in terms of fluid volume and its composition, but sometimes it is not fully appreciated that this balance is mediated through the tissue microvessels and that the mechanisms responsible are complex, vary from tissue to tissue and are subject to frequent changes. In humans there are many tissues which are beyond exploration by methods currently available for investigating the intact patient so that our knowledge is far from complete.

At the tissue level, the term 'Tissue Fluid Balance' implies the maintenance of a dynamic equilibrium between cellular, interstitial and circulating fluid to provide an ideal environment for both individual cell and integrated tissue activity as a contribution to the normal functions of the whole organism. The total fluid balance is therefore the sum of individual local tissue fluid balances, but even the most refined techniques for investigation of the total body fluid balance may give no indication of a local disorder. Thus, correction of total body fluid balance may not correct a local disturbance which may be a reflection of disintegration of the all-important tissue/interstitial fluid/microcirculatory harmony—a serious matter in a vital tissue, which if not corrected, may lead to irreversible change.

### Factors Known to Affect the Dynamic Equilibrium of Tissue Fluid (Fig. 27)

**Cell and Tissue Activity.** The demand for nutriment and the output of metabolites constantly alters the biophysical-biochemical state of both the intracellular and extracellular fluid, in turn affecting the activities of the microvessels. Increased metabolic activity results in local release of tissue vasodilators of the 'kinin' type.

**Alterations in Interstitial Fluid.** These may be independent, or additional to changes in local tissue activity. Augmented local tissue activity or cell break-down may result in the accumulation of osmotically active agents whose collective action may exceed the selective powers of the vascular membrane, turning it into a simple semipermeable membrane (or fully permeable in some cases), complying with the laws of osmotic action. Cell death on a large scale may induce gross increase in local collections of interstitial fluid, well seen in the early stages of peripheral gangrene.

**Disorders of Transmural Exchange.** Only a few of these have been fully explored. The commonest is the change in capillary net perfusion resulting from alterations in vasoactivity at the pre-capillary sphincter, with inhibition of this normal local compensating mechanism. Reduction in local capillary net perfusion reduces transmural exchange rates, and an increase in perfusion may lead to capillary rupture. There may be alterations in endothelial permeability and lack of the enzymes essential for selective transport.

**Variations in Local Blood Flow.** In addition to locally vasoactive agents such as the kinins and histamine, blood flow may be altered by abnormal reflex activity due to trauma, or as a result of severe exercise or hyperactivity of the tissue concerned. Local blood flow may also be altered by major increases in venous pressure due to gravity, heart failure, valvular incompetence, venous obstruction and over-transfusion.

**Characteristics of the Locally Circulating Blood.** So far as we can gather from experimental techniques available, changes in the blood itself have to be grossly abnormal before local tissue fluid balance is upset and plasma protein deficiency must be really low before peripheral oedema is manifest.

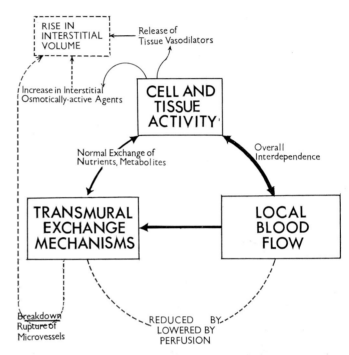

Fig. 27. Factors affecting the dynamic equilibrium of tissue fluid. In health, there is a complete integration between cell and tissue activity, transmural exchange mechanisms and the characteristics of local blood flow in maintaining dynamic equilibrium in the tissue fluid. Changes in any of these factors will bring about changes in the others and may precipitate an irreversible pathological process.

**Simple Diffusion.** The available evidence suggests that simple diffusion processes only apply to water and water-soluble substances (see section on Transmural Exchange) and that diffusion is simultaneous in both directions at similar rates unless there are gross differences between circulating and tissue fluids. Certainly, as far as water is concerned, these compartmental differences are corrected on a whole-body basis unless local tissue circulations are disordered. Provided renal function is normal, interstitial fluid increase is only temporary. If at a local level, the enzyme control of solute movement across the vascular membrane is lost, then relations between the interstitial and intravascular fluid will remain disturbed.

**Filtration Pressures.** This factor exists, but in the past, there has been a tendency to over-simplify this factor to one of simple hydrostatic pressure relationships. This situation is in fact more complex and may be considerably modified by selective ion transport and vesicle movement of colloids such as proteins. Experiments show that the hydrostatic pressure differences between the arteriolar and venular parts of the microvascular bed do not always result in flow from vessels to interstices at the arteriolar end, and inflow from tissues to vessel at the venular. Even the ultra-filtration factor in glomerular activity may not be simply hydrostatic as is commonly supposed.

### Local Cell Migration

Evidence is accumulating that normally intraluminar cells (the erythrocytes and the leucocytes) may have a significant role in nutriment and metabolite transport. The transmigration of these cells between the microvessels and the immediately surrounding tissues has been long recognized, although this phenomenon is usually associated with such pathological changes as inflammation in which endothelial permeability is disturbed. Attraction of cells from the blood stream into the interstitial spaces has been ascribed to 'chemotaxis' in which chemical agents are presumed to be liberated as a result of local pathological change. However, cellular transmigration can be observed *in vivo* in situations where there is no other evidence of a pathological change. In experimentally produced local ischaemia (e.g. local vasoconstriction due to adrenaline) the ensuing vasodilatation is often followed by a post-vasoconstrictive diapedesis. It is therefore not unreasonable to suppose that this red cell transmigration may well serve the purpose of augmenting interstitial oxygen supplies.

The presence of white cells in the tissue spaces is well-recognized in a number of pathological situations, quite apart from inflammation. Thus, in all varieties of the reaction to tissue transplantation (resulting in either rejection or grafting success), the non-phagocytic elements abound. Granted that these cells may be implicated in many of the aspects of the immune response and that in immuno-suppressive therapy their numbers are decreased, it must be remembered that these cells are enzyme-rich and that some of these enzymes are essential to both normal tissue metabolism and solute transport. On these grounds, it could be supposed that transmigration of certain white cells may be in support of active tissue enzyme systems.

Some remarkable *in vivo* cinephotomicrographic studies have shown that changes in microvessels associated with tissue damage are accompanied by adherence of vast numbers of white cells to the vessel wall. It has also been shown that this may occur whether or not transmigration of cells into the interstitial spaces follows. At this stage there is little or no evidence of increased vessel wall permeability. What, then, is the factor which induces this adherence in the first instance? Apart from local electrostatic changes at cell surfaces of both endothelium and adhering white cell, it is also possible that this phenomenon may be a reflection of a deficiency, in the immediately surrounding zone, of some enzyme or metabolite which may be carried by the involved white cell.

### Lymphatics

The lymphatic capillaries and the channels into which they drain are an integral component of tissue circulation. They assist in maintaining the dynamic equilibrium of interstitial fluid by adsorbing excess water and solute not taken up by the blood microvessels. Lymphatics appear to provide a preferential route for protein drainage, but recent work has shown that there is considerable exchange of protein between lymphatics and microvessels at all points, this being especially so at lymph nodes. The lymphatics provide the main drainage route for tissue leucocytes. Some tissues depend upon an efficient lymphatic flow for normal function: thus, urine concentration and the renal counter-current mechanism is dependent on normal lymphatic drainage from the kidney.

The lymphatics do not constitute a separate fluid circulation. They are blind radicles, endothelial cell-lined and draining ultimately into the great veins at the root of the neck. They provide an excellent example of the open-ended nature of the circulation, as indicated at the beginning of this chapter. Fluid flow in lymphatics depends on active transmigration from the interstitial fluid, the mechanisms being basically similar to those which operate across the vascular membrane.

### Formation of Lymph

Squire (1953) has produced an acceptable theory to account for one aspect of lymph formation. He suggests that the colloidal gel component of the interstitial ground substance attracts aqueous solutions to expand its volume. Increased volume of the gel sets up a 'swelling pressure' which resists removal of water against changes in blood microvessel hydrostatic pressure and to some extent, osmotic pressure changes. This theory can be extended and modified. There must come a point where the 'swelling pressure' of the interstitial space plus the increase in volume would inhibit normal fluid flow essential to the vital activity of the adjacent cells. The lymph radicle is initially empty and since the lymphatic endothelial ground substance is continuous with that of the interstices, it is quite possible that water and solutes are passed into the empty radicle, thus permitting local interstitial fluid flow.

There is little available evidence suggesting the precise nature of protein transmigration, but electron microscope studies infer that this may be due to selectivity at the lymphatic endothelium. In addition, protein transport may well be related to electrostatic attraction and to leucocyte transmigration. However, the protein exchange between the lymphatics and the microcirculation indicates that this view needs modification, possibly in relation to molecule size.

The composition of lymph varies considerably in different parts of the lymphatic drainage and from tissue to tissue. It appears to be related to tissue activity, proximity of lymph radicles to microvessels and to vascular endothelial permeability.

## Lymphatic Permeability

Lymphatic radicles are permeable to a wide variety of substances, notably proteins, chylomicrons, leucocytes, and also red cells. They are also permeable to bacteria and such foreign bodies as particulate carbon (either as Indian ink, graphite or specially prepared in colloidal solution). This permeability appears to be governed by endothelial selectivity and molecular size, because, although protein is exchanged with the microvessels, other substances are not, unless they have molecular weights of less than 3,000. Unexchanged substances are shed ultimately into the venous drainage. Certainly there is very little reverse transmigration once the lymphatic has acquired muscle and fibrous elements in its wall.

## Lymphatic Flow

The normal 24 hour lymph flow is of the order of 2–4 litres, which is considerably less than the fluid transfer across the vascular membrane. However, more than 50 per cent of the blood protein crosses the vascular membrane per 24 hours and this amount is returned via the lymphatics in the same time. This indicates that lymph flow is related to protein circulation and that its role in water and solute transport is a relatively minor one. Thus in heart failure, lymph drainage is not markedly increased, despite interstitial swelling.

Flow is assisted towards the great veins by a one-way valve system, augmented by skeletal muscular contraction, rises in intra-abdominal pressure and increases in negative intrathoracic pressure during inspiration.

Lymph flow is increased in all sites of increased tissue activity, only the central nervous system being excepted (there are no lymphatics as such). Various agents, known collectively as lymphagogues, stimulate lymph flow. These are similar to active vasodilating agents and those which increase capillary permeability. The muscular elements in the major lymphatics also increase flow: this has been observed in human groin lymphatics by Kinmonth and Taylor (1956) who showed that the increase in peristaltic waves induced lymph flow.

Lymph flow is reduced in all states of low blood perfusion, as in post-haemorrhagic hypovolaemia.

## REFERENCES

Ahlquist, R. P. (1948), "A Study of the Adrenotropic Receptors," *Amer., J. Physiol.*, **153**, 586–599.

Brånemark, P.-I., Aspegren, K. and Breine, U. (1964), "Microcirculatory Studies in Man by High Resolution Vital Microscopy," *Angiology*, **15**, 329–332.

Burn, J. H. (1961), "A New View of Adrenergic Nerve Fibres Explaining the Action of Reserpine, Bretylium and Guanethidine," *Brit. med. J.*, **1**, 1623–1627.

Chinard, F. P., Vosburgh, G. H. and Enns, T. (1955), "Transcapillary Exchange of Water and of other Substances in Certain Organs of the Dog," *Amer., J. Physiol.*, **183**, 221–234.

Dornhorst, A. C. (1963), "Hyperaemia Induced by Exercise and Ischaemia," *Brit. med. Bull.*, **19**, 137–140.

Kinmonth, J. B. and Taylor, G. W. (1956), "Spontaneous Rhythmic Contractility in Human Lymphatics," *J. Physiol.*, **133**, 3p.

Kuwabara, T. J. M. and Cogan, D. G. (1963), "Retinal Vascular Patterns: vi. Mural Cells of the Retinal Capillaries," *Arch. Ophthal., N.Y.*, **69**, 492–502.

Lewis, T. (1927), in *Blood Vessels of the Human Skin*, London: Shaw.

Lewis, W. H. (1931), "Pinocytosis," *Johns Hopk. Hosp. Bull.* **49**, 17–29.

Majno, G. (1963), "Ultrastructure of the Vascular Membrane," in *Handbook of Physiology*, ed. W. F. Hamilton and P. Dow, Sect. II, Vol. 3, Chap. 64, p. 2341. Washingston, D.C.: American Physiological Society.

Malpighi, M. (1661), "De pulmonibus. Observationes anatomicae, Bologna," from translation by Young, J. (1929), *Proc. roy. Soc. Med.* **23**, 7–10.

Moore, D. H. and Ruska, H. (1957), "Fine Structure of Capillaries and Small Arteries," *J. Biophys. Biochem. Cytol.*, **3**, 457–462.

Plenk, H. (1927), "Uber argyrophile Fasern (Gitterfasern) und ihre Bildungszellen," *Ergebn. Anat. EntwGesch.*, **27**, 302–412.

Rous, P., Gilding, P. and Smith, F. (1930), "The Gradient of Vascular Permeability," *J. exp. Med.*, **51**, 807–830.

Sandison, J. C. (1924), "A New Method for the Microscopic Study of Living Growing Tissues by the Introduction of a Transparent Chamber in the Rabbit's Ear," *Anat. Rec.*, **28**, 281–287.

Sewell, I. A. (1966), "Studies of the Microcirculation using Transparent Tissue Observation Chambers Inserted in the Hamster Cheek Pouch," *J. Anal.*, **100**, 839–856.

Squire, J. R. (1953), "The Nephrotic Syndrome," *Brit. med. J.* **2**, 1389–1399.

Uvn'as, B. (1960), "Central Cardiovascular Control." in *Handbook of Physiology*, Sect. I, Vol. 2, pp. 1131–1162, ed. H. W. Magoun and J. Field. Washington, D.C.: American Physiological Society.

Zimmermann, K. W. (1923), "Der feinere Bau der Blutcapillaren," *Z. Anat. EntwGesch.*, **69**, 29–109.

## FURTHER READING

Sewell, I. A. (1967), "Some Aspects of Human Microcirculation," Biomedical Engineering **2**, 68–77.

Weideman, Mary P. (1963), "Arteriovenous Pathways," in *Handbook of Physiology*, Sect. II, Vol. 2, Chapter 27, ed. W. F. Hamilton and P. Dow. Washingston, D.C.: American Physiological Society.

Zweifach, B. W. (1959), "The Microcirculation of the Blood," *Scientific American* (Jan., 1959).

# CHAPTER 8

# ELECTROCARDIOGRAPHY

## P. R. FLEMING

The torrent of sodium ions which pours across the myocardial cell membranes at the moment of depolarization is reflected in the inscription of the waves of the clinical electrocardiogram. Although much has been learnt, particularly in recent years, about the manner in which these two events are related, it must be admitted that much of clinical electrocardiography remains an empirical study. On this account many of the explanations given in this chapter of the "causes" of electrocardiographic phenomena are, at best, only partially correct. At worst, oversimplification and dogmatic statements have, regrettably, been found necessary from time to time.

### Electrical Activity of a Single Myocardial Cell

A micro-electrode placed within a *resting* myocardial cell records a potential of about −90 mv. with respect to the exterior of the cell. The cell membrane across which this "transmembrane potential" exists is only slightly permeable to sodium ions of which the extracellular concentration is some seven times the intracellular. Potassium, on the other hand, can cross the membrane more easily but despite this, the very high intracellular potassium concentration is maintained by the negative intracellular potential which restrains the efflux of the positively charged potassium ions. At the moment of excitation the membrane suddenly becomes permeable to sodium ions which, entering the cell, abolish and even reverse the transmembrane potential. The cell is then said to be depolarized. The intracellular potential rises to about +30 mv. relative to the exterior. This potential persists for about 200 m.sec. and then declines, slowly at first, and then more rapidly as the cell becomes repolarized with the expulsion of the sodium ions. The time course of these events is illustrated in Figure 1a, in which they are related to the events of the conventional electrocardiogram.

During electrical diastole the negative intracellular potential remains constant in the great majority of the myocardial cells. This is not the case with the cells of the pacemakers, actual or potential, which are found not only in the sino-atrial node but at various other sites in the atria and throughout the whole ventricular conducting system. In these so-called "automatic" cells a slow depolarization proceeds during diastole and, when the intracellular potential reaches about −60 mv., the threshold potential, rapid depolarization occurs (Fig. 1b). Clearly, the rate at which diastolic depolarization occurs and the levels of the threshold and resting potentials together determine the rate of discharge of any particular pacemaker cell. The effects of drugs and electrolytes on these variables have been studied extensively and related to the clinically observable effects of these substances. For example, a rapid fall in extracellular potassium concentration causes a reduction in the resting potential, contrary to the theoretical expectations, and increases the rate of diastolic depolarization; this effect is more marked in the automatic cells of the ventricular conducting system which thus tend to discharge more frequently. This change may be clinically manifest as ventricular ectopic beats or paroxysms of ventricular tachycardia. The effects of changes in extracellular calcium concentration which affect mainly the threshold potential, quinidine which reduces the rate of diastolic depolarization, hypoxia, changes in $P_{CO_2}$ and many other variables have been studied but space does not permit a detailed account of this work.

### Electrical Activity of Groups of Myocardial Cells

Depolarization spreads sequentially from cell to cell throughout the myocardium so that, at any moment during this process, the potential on the surface of those cells which have already been depolarized is negative relative to those still at rest. It is the sum of these potential differences between different parts of the myocardium which is recorded as the clinical electrocardiogram.

The effects of the passage of the wave of depolarization can be studied most simply as it occurs in a strip of myocardium. If such a strip is suspended in a bath of saline the changes in potential at various sites on the strip can be studied in relation to the constant potential of an electrode suspended in the saline at a theoretically infinite distance from the muscle (Fig. 2). In summary, a galvanometer connected to an electrode towards which the depolarization wave is travelling records a positive deflection; the peak of the positive deflection signals the passage of the wave beneath that electrode; a galvanometer connected to an electrode from which the wave is receding records a negative deflection (Fig. 3). In addition, other things being equal, the greater the mass of muscle through which the wave is passing the larger will the deflections be. In a strip of myocardium repolarization follows the same course as depolarization and, if the depolarization deflection is positive, is manifest as a negative deflection, broader and of lower amplitude than that of depolarization, but enclosing the same area (Fig. 4).

From these simple concepts it is possible to deduce the basic patterns of the clinical electrocardiogram. Before developing this theme, however, the terminology of the deflections of the electrocardiogram and the axes and polarity of the electrocardiographic leads in current use must be considered.

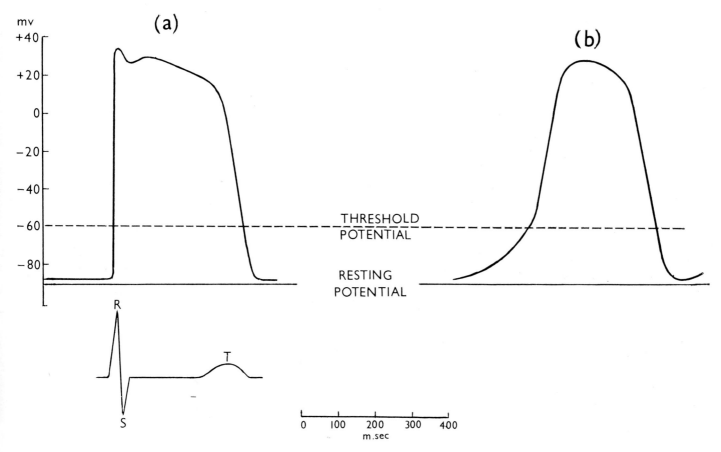

Fig. 1. Intracellular potential of (a) myocardial cell, and (b) "automatic" (pacemaker) cell during depolarization and repolarization.

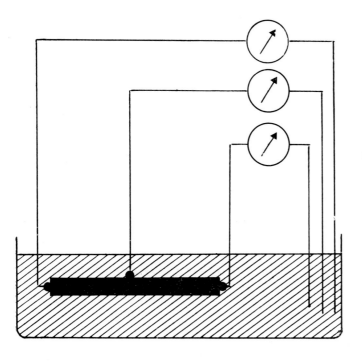

Fig. 2. Strip of myocardium suspended in bath of saline. Electrodes on the two ends and on the middle of the strip are connected via galvanometers to indifferent electrodes in the saline at a theoretically infinite distance from the myocardium.

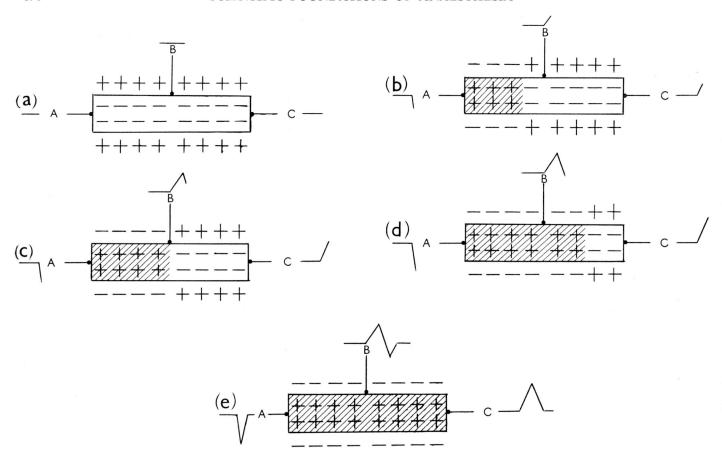

FIG. 3. Sequence of depolarization in a strip of myocardium, isolated as in Fig. 2. As the wave of depolarization spreads from left to right the intracellular potential becomes positive (hatched area). The complexes recorded from electrodes placed on the two ends (A and C) and on the middle (B) of the strip are shown. In (a) the whole strip is polarized (resting) and all the records are isoelectric. From electrode A a monophasic negative deflection is recorded as, throughout depolarization, the wave is receding. Similarly a monophasic positive deflection is recorded from electrode C. From electrode B a biphasic (+ −) deflection is recorded as the wave first approaches (b), passes beneath (c) and recedes from (d) the electrode. Depolarization is complete in (e).

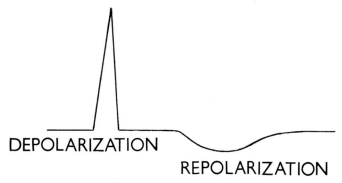

FIG. 4. Deflections recorded during theoretically "ideal" depolarization and repolarization of a myocardial strip. The deflection representing repolarization (T wave) is opposite in direction to that of depolarization but encloses an equal area.

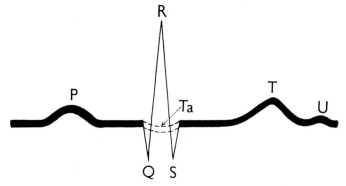

FIG. 5. The waves of the electrocardiogram (see text).

### The Waves of the Electrocardiogram (Fig. 5)

The first deflection of a normal electrocardiogram, the P wave, represents atrial depolarization. This is followed by the, usually iso-electric, P–R segment. The P–R interval is defined as the time from the beginning of the P wave to the first deflection of the QRS complex, whether positive or negative. Ventricular depolarization is manifested by the QRS complex of which the first deflection, *if it is negative*, is defined as the Q wave. All positive deflections are called R waves; a second R wave in any complex is denoted R[1]. Any negative deflection preceded by an R wave is called an S wave. A monophasic negative complex is described as QS.

The effects of repolarization of the atria are not always

seen in the electrocardiogram. The atrial T wave (Ta) is frequently lost in the QRS complex but may sometimes be visible as a deformity of the P–R segment. The T wave, which follows the normally iso-electric RS–T segment, represents ventricular repolarization and, contrary to theoretical considerations, is usually upright in man. The U wave is an inconstant small, usually positive, deflection closely following the T wave and will not be discussed further.

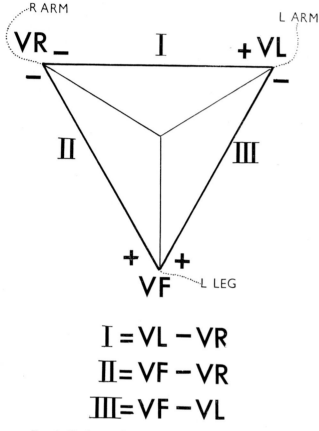

$$I = VL - VR$$
$$II = VF - VR$$
$$III = VF - VL$$

FIG. 6. Einthoven triangle illustrating the axes and polarity of the bipolar limb leads and the axes of the unipolar limb leads. The mathematical relationships between the bipolar and unipolar leads are also shown.

### Electrocardiographic Leads

The standard leads (I, II and III) are *bipolar*, recording the potential difference between two points on the body surface. The electrodes are placed on the limbs which can be regarded as extensions of the lead wires so that, effectively, the axis of Lead I (left arm positive; right arm negative) is horizontal. The axes of Leads II and III are conventionally regarded as completing the equilateral Einthoven triangle and the polarity shown in Fig. 6 should be carefully studied. It will be seen that the right arm terminal is always negative and the left leg always positive; the sign of the left arm terminal varies depending on whether it forms part of Lead I or Lead III.

*Unipolar* leads are also recorded from the limbs, designated VR (right arm), VL (left arm) and VF (left

leg). In these leads, the positive terminal is on the limb concerned and the negative, or indifferent, electrode is formed by uniting the connections from the two arms and the left leg. It can be shown that the potential of this *central terminal* does not vary significantly throughout the cardiac cycle and that the deflections in a unipolar lead represent essentially the potential changes at the positive electrode. The bipolar leads can be 'synthesized' therefore from the unipolar limb leads; Lead I, for example, represents the algebraic sum of the deflections in leads VL and VR. In practice, as the deflections in the unipolar

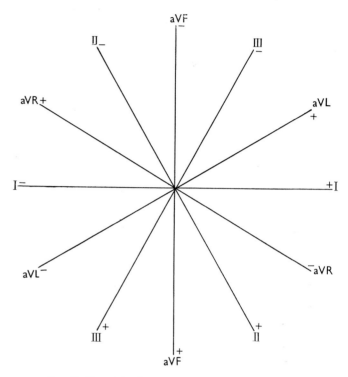

FIG. 7. Hexaxial reference system derived from Fig. 6 by displacing the lead axes so that they all intersect at the centre of the triangle. This does not alter the mathematical relationships between the leads. The directions of the axes, measured in degrees (*see* Fig. 8) should be noted. Thus the positive terminal of Lead I is at 0°, of Lead II at +60° and of Lead III at +120°. The positive terminals of Leads aVR, aVL and aVF are at −150° −30° and +90° respectively.

limb leads are often very small in amplitude, they are usually recorded as *augmented* leads (aVR, aVL, aVF). For this purpose the central terminal is formed from the two limb leads other than the one being recorded (e.g. for aVR, leads from the left arm and left leg form the central terminal). At the expense of slight loss of validity of the concept of unchanging potential of the central terminal, records of larger amplitude are obtained.

The axes of the unipolar limb leads run from the appropriate corner of the Einthoven triangle to its centre. It is sometimes convenient to redraw the axes of all the limb leads, bipolar and unipolar, to form a hexaxial reference system (Fig. 7). This is particularly useful when determining the electrical axis of the heart.

Six unipolar chest leads are usually recorded. The electrodes (positive terminals) are sited as follows:

V₁. 4th right intercostal space at the sternal border.
V₂. 4th left intercostal space at the sternal border.
V₃. Midway between V₂ and V₄.
V₄. 5th left intercostal space in mid-clavicular line.
V₅. In left anterior axillary line at the same *horizontal* level as V₄.
V₆. In left mid-axillary line at the same horizontal level as V₄ and V₅.

In all cases the indifferent electrode is provided by the central terminal, formed from the union of wires from the right arm, left arm and left leg, as in the unipolar limb leads. The axes of the chest leads run from the site of the electrode to the centre of the chest in an approximately horizontal plane. Less attention is paid to these axes than to those of the limb leads in routine electrocardiographic interpretation but they are important if the *vector* approach to electrocardiography is used.

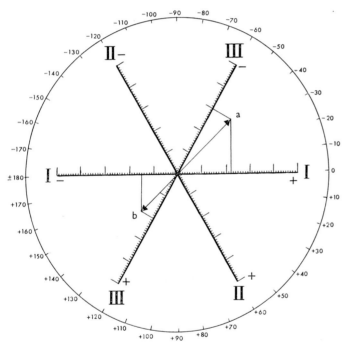

Fig. 8. Determination of the electrical axis on triaxial reference system. Any two of the standard leads can be used for this purpose. The algebraic sum of the deflections in each lead is plotted on the appropriate lead axis; perpendiculars are then drawn as shown and the electrical axis drawn from the centre of the reference system to the intersection of the perpendiculars. Two examples are shown: (a) if in Lead I the R wave is 25 mm. and the S wave 3 mm., the net deflection in this lead is +22 mm. If the net deflection in Lead III, similarly determined, is −30 mm., the electrical axis will be at −45° (= left axis deviation); (b) with a net deflection of −15 mm. in Lead I and of +20 mm. in Lead III, the electrical axis will be at +135° (= right axis deviation).
For the determination of the net deflections in the various leads, the algebraic sum of the *amplitude* of the deflections is usually sufficiently accurate. A more precise determination of the electrical axis requires the calculation of the *areas* bounded by the deflections; this process is time-consuming and, fortunately, rarely necessary.

## The Electrical Axis and the Vector Approach

Space does not permit a full account of the vector approach to electrocardiographic interpretation, although this approach is implicit in many sections of this chapter. It is probably the most intellectually satisfying method of studying electrocardiograms and is dealt with fully by Grant (1956). His book should be studied by all who aspire to higher things than 'rules of thumb'.

Mention must be made, however, of the *electrical axis* of the heart which is the frontal projection of the mean spatial vector. This can be regarded as a convenient means of summarizing the direction and magnitude of the deflections in the limb leads. The method of plotting the electrical axis is shown in Figure 8. It is recorded in degrees as shown and normally lies between 0° and +110°; axes within the range 0° to −30° are dubiously abnormal. Deviations from this range occur in many pathological conditions, notably intraventricular conduction defects and right ventricular hypertrophy, but considerable variations in the electrical axis can occur due to postural change, recumbency tending to cause left axis deviation. Changes also occur during thoracic surgery when the chest and, particularly, the pericardium are opened; such changes in axis must not be interpreted as significant changes in the electrical activity of the myocardium.

## Electrical Activity of the Atria

The wave of depolarization spreads across the atria from the sino-atrial node resulting in the inscription of the P wave. In addition, specialised inter-nodal tracts transmit the impulse to the atrio-ventricular node. Because the sino-atrial node is situated in the right atrium, this

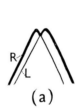
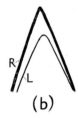
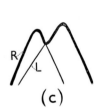

Fig. 9. Synthesis of the P wave in Lead II from right and left atrial components (R and L) in (a) normal, (b) right atrial hypertrophy, and (c) left atrial hypertrophy.

chamber is depolarized slightly before the left. In the frontal plane depolarization spreads caudally and towards the left, more or less parallel to the axis of Lead II. For this reason the tallest P waves are usually seen in this lead. The leftward trend produces upright P waves in Lead I; in Lead III the amplitude of P is smaller and it may be isoelectric or even negative.

Due to the slight delay in left atrial depolarization it may be possible to identify components from the two atria in the normal P wave (Fig. 9). A tiny notch may be visible on its peak but, more often, this is blurred to produce a smoothly rounded summit. The asynchronous depolarization is more easily seen in leads whose axes lie in the horizontal plane. Right atrial depolarization proceeds anteriorly whereas that of the left atrium is directed posteriorly. The two waves summate to produce a biphasic (+ −) deflection in, for example, $V_1$ (Fig. 10).

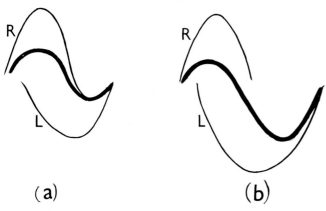

( a )                    ( b )

FIG. 10. Synthesis of the P wave in $V_1$ from right and left atrial components (R and L) in (a) normal, and (b) left atrial hypertrophy.

### Atrial Hypertrophy

Hypertrophy of an atrium, as of any other part of the myocardium, produces deflections of larger amplitude and longer duration than normal. In right atrial hypertrophy, the right atrial component of the P wave becomes taller and wider so that it completely overlaps the left atrial component (Fig. 9 and 11). The result is a tall, sharply peaked P wave seen best in Lead II. In left atrial hyper-

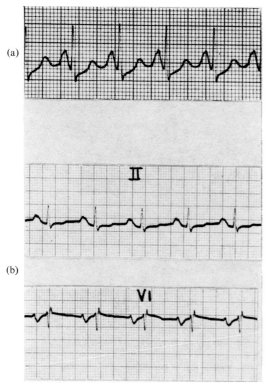

FIG. 11. (a) Lead II in severe pulmonary hypertension showing the sharply peaked P wave of right atrial hypertrophy. (b) Leads II and VI from a case of mitral stenosis showing the broad P wave with deep negative component in VI characteristic of left atrial hypertrophy.

trophy, on the other hand, the increase in amplitude and, particularly, in duration of the left atrial component causes widening of the whole P wave; the notch separating the two components becomes more clearly visible (Fig. 9 and 11). This pattern is often known as the *mitral* P wave from its common occurrence in mitral valve disease. This abnormality is well seen in Lead II but is even more striking in $V_1$ where the dominant, posteriorly directed, left atrial forces (vector) produce a deep wide negative deflection following the smaller positive right atrial component (Figs. 10 and 11). The conveniently M-shaped P wave in Mitral stenosis has not escaped the attention of the mnemonically minded and those who find logical thought distressing may prefer to use this aide-memoire.

The effects of abnormally sited pacemakers on the form of the P waves are discussed below in the section on Dysrhythmias.

### Electrical Activity of the Ventricles

Depolarization of the ventricles is more complex than that of the atria. The passage of the impulse from the atrio-ventricular node down the atrio-ventricular bundle and through the Purkinje network produces no electrical activity detectable in surface leads. It is the outward spread of depolarization from endocardium to epicardium which produces the QRS complex.

The first part of the ventricular myocardium to be depolarized is the interventricular septum. The left branch of the bundle conveys the impulse for this so that depolarization proceeds from left to right. Following this the two ventricles are depolarized more or less simultaneously. This process can be summarized as two waves: one, due to the right ventricular depolarization, proceeds forwards and slightly, to the right and another towards the left. Due to the greater mass of the left ventricle, the right ventricular forces are overwhelmed and the net effect is as of a single wave travelling towards the left.

The effects of these forces on leads facing the right ventricle ($V_1$ and $V_2$) and left ventricle ($V_5$ and $V_6$) are as follows (Fig. 12). The small rightward directed forces of septal depolarization produce a small positive deflection in $V_1$ and a small negative deflection in $V_6$. Following this the net leftward directed forces of depolarization of the main ventricular mass produce a deep S wave in $V_1$ and a tall R wave in $V_6$. The letters denoting waves of relatively low amplitude are usually printed in lower case so that the normal QRS pattern in $V_1$ would be described as rS and that in $V_6$ as qR (Fig. 13).

The net ventricular forces are directed not only towards the left but also caudally so that the qR pattern seen in $V_6$ is recorded in Leads I, II and aVL. The patterns seen in Leads III and aVF depend on the direction of the electrical axis and on whether the heart is electrically horizontal or vertical. The axis of Lead aVR is approximately at 180° to the electrical axis of the heart and hence, in this lead, a dominantly negative deflection is normally recorded; the P wave is, of course, also negative in this lead. Greater details on the effects of changes in the electrical axis should be sought in standard textbooks of electrocardiography.

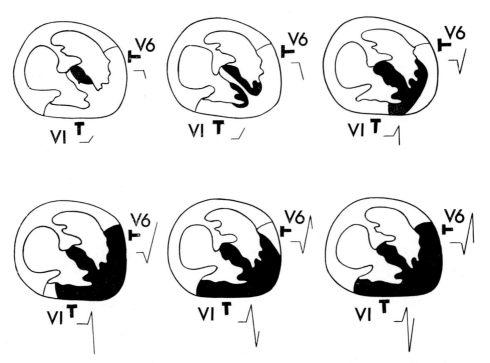

FIG. 12. Stages of ventricular depolarization, at intervals of approximately 15 m.sec., with resultant deflections in $V_1$ and $V_6$. In each drawing the shaded area represents depolarized myocardium.

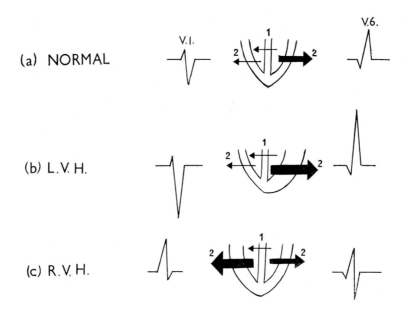

FIG. 13. Diagrammatic representation of ventricular depolarization in (a) normal, (b) left ventricular hypertrophy, and (c) right ventricular hypertrophy. In each case, septal depolarization (1), from left to right, is followed by simultaneous depolarization of the two ventricles (2). The magnitude of the forces is illustrated by the width of the appropriate arrows and the consequent patterns in $V_1$ and $V_6$ are shown.

The normal QRS patterns which have been described depend on a normal sequence of ventricular depolarization. In any situation in which this sequence is distorted, grossly abnormal QRS complexes are recorded. Such complexes are seen in bundle branch block or lesser degrees of aberrant ventricular conduction, ventricular ectopic beats and in some cases of complete heart block (*see* below).

In the presence of right ventricular hypertrophy the rightward and anteriorly directed forces of right ventricular depolarization may be dominant over those of the left ventricle. Taller R waves are, therefore, to be expected in $V_1$ and $V_2$ as the effect of right ventricular depolarization is added to that of the septum (Fig. 13c). An R wave in $V_1$ of greater amplitude than the S wave in that lead is most

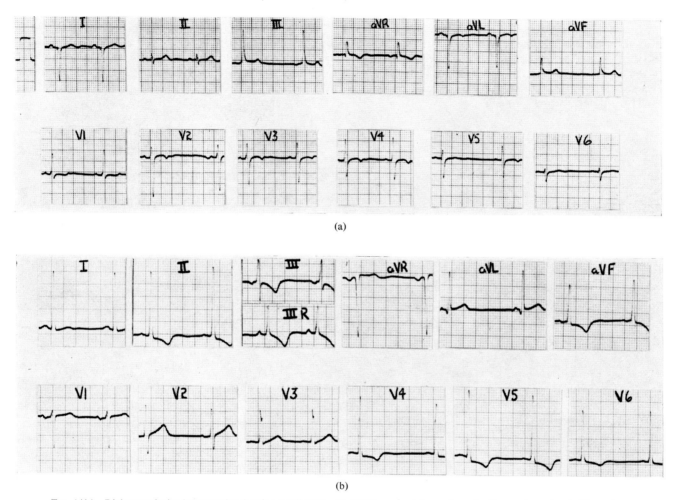

(a)

(b)

Fig. 14(a). Right ventricular hypertrophy showing a tall RVI with RS-T segment depression, also T wave inversion in $V_{2-4}$; there is right axis deviation (axis + 140°). (b) Left ventricular hypertrophy showing tall R waves with RS-T segment depression and T wave inversion in $V_{4-6}$. (Note that in both records the chest leads are recorded at half the normal standardization.)

### Ventricular Hypertrophy

The patterns produced by ventricular hypertrophy in the chest leads, and reflected in the limb leads, can now be deduced. If the left ventricle is hypertrophied the predominance of the leftward directed forces is even greater than normal so that very tall R waves in $V_5$ and $V_6$ and deep S waves in $V_1$ and $V_2$ are recorded (Fig. 13b). Conventionally left ventricular hypertrophy is regarded as probably present if the sum of the amplitudes of the R wave in $V_5$ or $V_6$ and the S wave in $V_1$ is greater than 3·5 mv (=35 mm with normal standardization of 1 cm = 1 mv); this rule is only approximately true and may not be valid in children or in thin-chested individuals.

commonly due to right ventricular hypertrophy; as will be seen, however, there are other conditions in which the R wave may be dominant in $V_1$.

Important changes are also often seen in the RS-T segments and the T waves in ventricular hypertrophy. In the leads in which the R wave is excessively tall the RS-T segment is depressed, with an upward convexity, and the T wave is inverted (Fig. 14). This is sometimes referred to as the *strain* pattern and this term is acceptable as long as it is remembered that it carries no precise physiological connotation. The mechanism is not clear but, most probably, such changes reflect relative ischaemia, the myocardium having, as it were, outgrown its blood supply.

Other changes produced by ventricular hypertrophy

include deviations of the electrical axis. Left ventricular hypertrophy is often associated with left axis deviation but such change in axis is usually due to a lesion of part of the left branch of the bundle of His and not to the hypertrophy itself. Right axis deviation is a more significant change and is an important piece of evidence in favour of right ventricular hypertrophy.

The classical electrocardiographic patterns of ventricular hypertrophy which have been described are most often seen when the ventricle is required to generate a high pressure as in aortic or pulmonary stenosis. This has been called the *systolic overload* pattern and differs somewhat from the changes recorded from a ventricle burdened by an increase in total stroke volume—the so-called *diastolic*

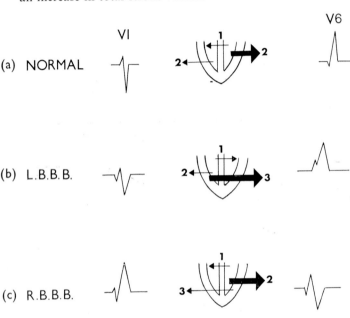

FIG. 15. Diagrammatic representation of ventricular depolarization in (a) normal and in (b) left and (c) right bundle branch block. The asynchronous depolarization (2 and 3) of the two ventricles should be noted.

*overload* pattern. Right ventricular diastolic overload is classically seen in atrial septal defect and is characterized by an $RR^1$ pattern of moderate amplitude in $V_1$ or even by right bundle branch block (*see* below). Diastolic overload of the left ventricle is produced by, for example, aortic incompetence and ventricular septal defect and, in these conditions, the pattern in the left ventricular leads consists of prominent Q waves, very tall R waves and tall upright T waves. In left ventricular systolic overload the Q wave is rather inconspicuous. The concept of systolic and diastolic overloading, with the implication that haemodynamic changes can be inferred from the electrocardiogram, is an attractive one. However, as so often in clinical electrocardiography, the correlation is by no means constant.

## Bundle Branch Block

If conduction is interrupted in one or other branch of the atrio-ventricular bundle the sequential spread of depolarization through the ventricle illustrated in Fig. 12

and 15a is distorted. The wave can reach the ventricle whose bundle branch is blocked only relatively slowly by spread through the myocardium from the other, normally depolarized, ventricle. Hence, prolongation of the duration of the QRS complex above its upper limit of 0·1 sec. is a cardinal feature of bundle branch block.

The characteristic changes in the QRS complexes can be deduced as follows (Fig. 15). The septum is, as has been shown, normally depolarized from left to right. In the presence of left bundle branch block, however, this cannot occur and septal depolarization can only proceed from right to left. This produces a small Q wave in $V_1$ and a small R in $V_6$. Depolarization of the right ventricle proceeds normally with the inscription of a small R in $V_1$ and a negative deflection (S wave) in $V_6$. It should be noticed that the presence of a septal Q wave in a left ventricular lead excludes left bundle branch block. Finally the left ventricle is depolarized slowly by intramyocardial spread and the final deflection of the QRS complex is a broad deep S in $V_1$ and a prominent secondary R wave ($R^1$) in $V_6$ (Fig. 16).

Similar considerations apply in right bundle branch block. Septal depolarization proceeds normally producing the usual $RV_1$ and $QV_6$. Normal left ventricular depolarization produces the expected S in $V_1$ and R in $V_6$ and the final, delayed, right ventricular depolarization is reflected in a tall secondary R in $V_1$ and a deep broad S in $V_6$ (Fig. 17). As always, the chest lead appearances in left and right bundle branch block are reflected in the appropriate limb leads.

More refined diagnosis of intraventricular conduction defects is also possible. The left branch of the bundle divides early in its course into anterior and posterior divisions and a block of either of these produces characteristic changes. If the anterior division is blocked (left anterior hemiblock) left ventricular depolarization takes place via the posterior division which lies somewhat inferior to the anterior division. The wave of depolarization therefore spreads upwards and to the left resulting in pathological left axis deviation (beyond $-30°$), (Fig. 17). Similarly, left posterior hemiblock, which is a much less common lesion, causes right axis deviation and may closely simulate right ventricular hypertrophy.

## Disorders of Rhythm

The term 'arrhythmia', although hallowed by tradition, is being displaced in cardiological literature by 'dysrhythmia'. The latter is undoubtedly more correct etymologically as 'arrhythmia' implies that *no* rhythm of any kind is present. The prefix 'dys' signifies 'a disorder of' and the term 'dysrhythmia' will be used in this chapter.

### Supraventricular Dysrhythmias

It is possible that most supraventricular dysrhythmias are due to the discharge of a focus of automatic cells sited somewhere in the atria. The occasional discharge of such a pacemaker produces ectopic beats. Progressively more rapid discharge causes supraventricular tachycardia, atrial flutter and atrial fibrillation. This must not, however, be taken as a denial of the concept of a *circus movement* as a cause of some at least of these dysrhythmias, particularly atrial flutter; it is postulated that a wave of depolarization courses rapidly round the atria at such a rate as to be self-perpetuating.

## Supraventricular Ectopic Beats

The position of the sino-atrial node, as has been shown, determines the direction of spread of the wave of depolarization across the atria. Clearly, therefore, the discharge and those due to discharge of the sino-atrial node should be regarded as evidence that it arises from an ectopic focus. Not only is the P wave of an atrial ectopic beat abnormal in configuration but it is also premature, appearing before the next sinus P wave would have been expected. These two features are the diagnostic signs of discharge of an atrial ectopic focus and are important in the recognition of supraventricular tachycardia as well as ectopic beats.

The conduction of a supraventricular ectopic beat to the ventricle must now be considered. If, for example, the

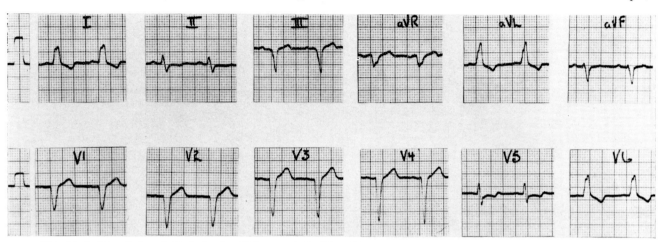

FIG. 16. Left bundle branch block showing RR$^1$ pattern in I, aVL and V$_6$. The T wave inversion in these leads is secondary to the conduction defect and is not, by itself, evidence of myocardial disease.

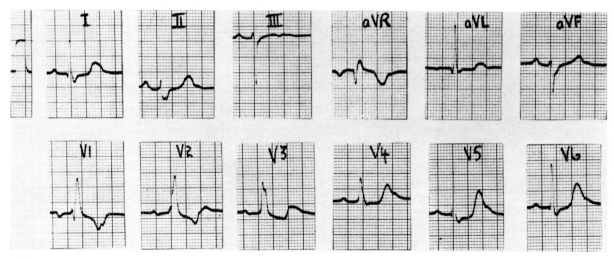

FIG. 17. Right bundle branch block and left anterior hemiblock with 2:1 atrioventricular block. The RR$^1$ pattern in V$_1$ with prolonged QRS should be noted, also the pathological left axis deviation (axis −70°). The small deflection in the ascending limb of the T wave in V$_1$ is a P wave (see Fig. 24).

of a focus situated elsewhere in the atria will cause depolarization to spread in an abnormal direction. The shape of the P wave will thus differ from normal to a degree depending on the site of the ectopic focus. If, for example, the focus is situated well to the left of the sino-atrial node, the axis of the P wave may point towards the right so that, in Lead I, the P wave will be negative. An abnormal configuration of the P wave, negative, biphasic or iso-electric, is, therefore, a cardinal feature of a supraventricular ectopic beat. The abnormality, in fact, may not be gross and any difference in shape between a particular P wave ectopic focus is low in the right atrium, near the atrio-ventricular node, abbreviation of the P-R interval might be expected and is, indeed, often seen. However, if the ectopic beat is very premature, the atrio-ventricular node and bundle may still be partially refractory and the P-R interval may be prolonged above the upper normal limit of 0·2 sec. Following a supraventricular ectopic beat, therefore, the P-R interval may be normal, prolonged or abbreviated. Similar considerations apply to more distal conduction. Most often the QRS complex following an ectopic P wave is normal in configuration implying normal conduction down the branches of the atrio-ventricular bundle. If, however, one or other branch of the bundle has not recovered from the previous beat the pattern of bundle branch block may be present following the supraventricular ectopic discharge. This phenomenon, known as aberrant ventricular conduction, must be carefully distinguished from the pattern of a ventricular ectopic beat which it closely resembles (*see* below). It is clear, however, that if the associated P wave can be clearly identified a supraventricular origin for the ectopic beat can be confidently diagnosed (Fig. 18).

of atrio-ventricular conduction can occur and, in particular, atrial tachycardia with partial atrio-ventricular block is an important manifestation of digitalis toxicity. Aberrant ventricular conduction causes particular difficulty; if it is present, it may be quite impossible to distinguish supraventricular tachycardia from ventricular as the abnormal P waves may be obscured by the abnormal QRS complexes and T waves. Only if the first beat of a paroxysm is recorded may it be possible to identify a P wave with certainty and be confident that the dysrhythmia is of supraventricular origin.

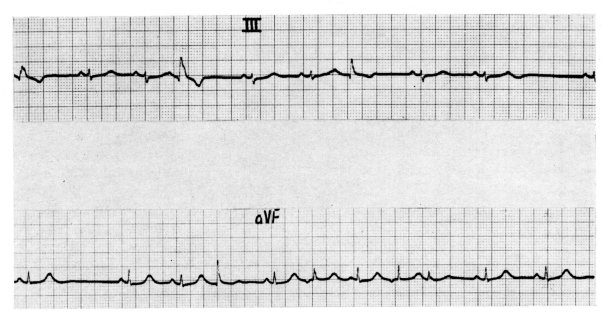

FIG. 18. Supraventricular ectopic beats with normal and aberrant ventricular conduction. The two strips were recorded immediately consecutively. In III the fourth and seventh complexes are supraventricular ectopic beats conducted with ventricular aberration; in each case a P wave can be identified preceding the QRS complex. In aVF the fourth beat also is almost certainly supraventricular in origin although a P wave cannot be identified with certainty. The sixth and eighth complexes are supraventricular ectopic beats with normal intraventricular conduction; note the inverted P.

An ectopic focus in or near the atrio-ventricular node may produce virtually simultaneous depolarization of the atria and ventricles. In this case the P wave may be incorporated in the QRS complex and appear to be absent; it may even occur after the QRS producing a terminal negative deflection which the unwary may regard as evidence of bundle branch block. Ectopic rhythms arising in this region are commonly called 'junctional'; the adjective 'nodal' has been superseded since it was realized that the main bundle of His is the site of the ectopic focus as, or more, often than the atrio-ventricular node itself.

### Supraventricular Tachycardia

An ectopic focus in the atria discharging at a rate of 150–200 per minute causes supraventricular tachycardia, which can be regarded as a series of supraventricular ectopic beats. The same considerations as have been discussed in relation to the latter apply also to supraventricular tachycardia. In diagnosis, the abnormal configuration of the P waves is important as also is the fact that the QRS complex is usually normal. Disturbances

### Atrial Flutter

In this condition the ectopic supraventricular focus discharges at a rate of about 250–350 per minute. Some degree of atrio-ventricular block is characteristic, 2:1 and 4:1 being common ratios. The QRS complexes are typically normal, although ventricular aberration can occur, and the diagnostic feature is the regularity of the P waves producing a characteristic 'saw-tooth' appearance of the base-line (Fig. 19).

### Atrial Fibrillation

If an ectopic atrial focus discharges at a rate of 500–600 per minute, the smooth spread of depolarization through the atria is disorganized and fragmented. Waves spread irregularly through the myocardium between groups of refractory cells so that the activity of the fibres is unco-ordinated. Waves impinge on the atrio-ventricular node in a random fashion and are conducted to the ventricles at a rate depending on the integrity of the atrio-ventricular bundle. The well-known total irregularity of the ventricular response is seen in the electrocardiogram as irregularly spaced QRS complexes. No definite P waves are seen but the baseline is deformed by rapid, low-voltage oscillations, best seen in Lead V₁ on account of its proximity to the right atrium. These are commonly known as 'f' waves. As in the case of other supraventricular dysrhythmias, aberrant ventricular conduction may occur, particularly if the ventricular rate is rapid. In the absence of P waves it may then be difficult to identify the QRS complexes as having their origin in a supraventricular focus (Fig. 20).

configuration of the QRS complex. This is because the wave of depolarization, spreading from a ventricular focus, can only reach the contra-lateral ventricle by travelling through the myocardium; hence the QRS pattern is very similar to that of bundle branch block. Indeed, study of the form of the QRS complex of a ventricular ectopic beat in several leads may allow an opinion on the site of the ectopic focus; it is clear that a focus in the right ventricle will produce a QRS complex resembling that of left bundle branch block. There is little point in this exercise, however,

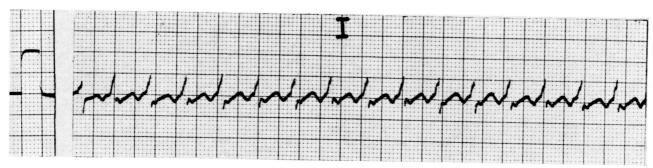

FIG. 19.  Atrial flutter with 2:1 atrio-ventricular block; the atrial rate is 334 and the ventricular 167 per minute.

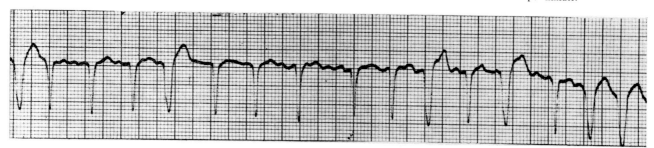

FIG. 20.  Atrial fibrillation with phasic aberrant ventricular conduction. Analysis of a longer record made it clear that the broad QRS complexes were not ventricular in origin.

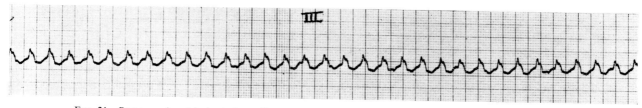

FIG. 21.  Paroxysmal ventricular tachycardia at a rate of 194 per minute. Certain distinction from supraventricular tachycardia with aberrant ventricular conduction is not possible although minor deflections of the base-line which may be *independent* P waves are visible.

During a paroxysm of supraventricular tachycardia RS-T depression and T wave inversion are common due to relative or absolute ischaemia. These changes may persist for many hours or days after the end of the paroxysm.

### Ventricular Dysrhythmias

The occasional discharge of an ectopic focus in a group of automatic cells in the ventricles produces ventricular ectopic beats. Progressively more rapid discharge causes ventricular tachycardia at faster and faster rates until, as in the atria, smoothly sequential depolarization is impossible and ventricular fibrillation ensues.

The cardinal diagnostic feature of a ventricular ectopic beat, apart from its prematurity, is the grossly bizarre

as the information is of virtually no clinical significance. As in bundle branch block the T waves are usually in the opposite direction to the main deflection of the QRS complex.

In *ventricular tachycardia* a series of QRS complexes, each resembling a ventricular ectopic beat, is seen; the rate varies markedly but may be more than 200 per minute (Fig. 21). The diagnosis is usually easy but the possible confusion with a supraventricular tachycardia with aberrant ventricular conduction must be remembered.

A variant of this dysrhythmia which may be seen particularly after myocardial infarction is *accelerated idioventricular rhythm*. In this condition the ventricles are the site of an ectopic focus which discharges much more slowly than in ventricular tachycardia but faster than the usual spontaneous rate of a ventricular focus as, for example, in complete heart block (Fig. 22).

A word must be said about so-called *ventricular flutter*. This term is used from time to time to describe ventricular tachycardia at an extremely fast rate but has nothing to commend it. Atrial flutter has a characteristic effect on the electrocardiogram but very rapid discharge of a ventricular focus has an effect qualitatively identical to that of a more moderate rate of discharge.

In *ventricular fibrillation* the identification of QRS

## Sino-atrial Block

In this condition the impulse generated in the sino-atrial node fails to reach the atrial myocardium. The consequent failure of depolarization of the atria and hence of the ventricles is manifested by complete absence of any electrical activity at a time when the next complex would have been expected. A complete cycle is therefore deleted. Following this long diastole the next beat may be a normal sinus beat but, at times, a focus in the atrio-ventricular node or ventricles discharges to produce a nodal or ventricular escape beat. Such escape beats are also seen in other

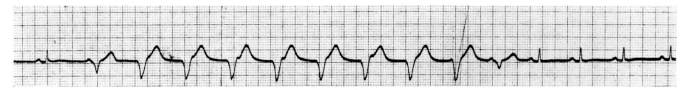

Fig. 22. Accelerated idioventricular rhythm for nine beats at a rate of about 80 per minute; the dysrhythmia is preceded and followed by sinus rhythm. P waves, independent of the QRS complexes, can be identified throughout nearly the whole of the record.

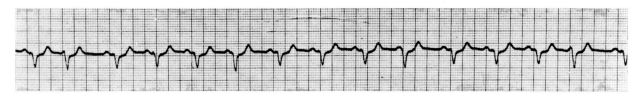

Fig. 23. Junctional parasystole. The second, sixth, tenth and fourteenth beats are ectopic with a constant inter-ectopic interval of 2.85 sec. Atrial depolarization is normal throughout as shown by the regular P waves deforming the QRS complexes of the ectopic beats although temporally unrelated to them.

complexes as such becomes impossible and they are replaced by very rapid deflections varying markedly in amplitude and configuration.

## Escape Rhythms and Parasystole

The dysrhythmias which have been discussed above are all classified as *extrasystolic* in type. There are two other situations in which the heart is driven by an ectopic pacemaker. One is the result of the failure of discharge of the sino-atrial node with an 'escape' of a lower pacemaker which may discharge once, or several times, at its own, usually slow, rate; thus one speaks of junctional or ventricular *escape rhythm*. Another ectopic rhythm requiring mention is *parasystole* in which an ectopic focus discharges regularly and 'captures' the ventricles whenever it finds them in a non-refractory state. The diagnosis of parasystole may be difficult but the essential feature is the occurrence of ectopic beats appearing at intervals which are all multiples of the cycle length of the ectopic focus (Fig. 23).

## Disorders of Conduction

Apart from bundle branch block which has already been discussed, conduction may be partially or completely interrupted within the sino-atrial node or in the main atrio-ventricular bundle.

situations in which diastole is intermittently prolonged; they are not infrequent during the bradycardia of the 'overshoot' phase following a Valsalva manoeuvre.

## Atrio-ventricular Block

Impairment of conduction of the impulse in the main atrio-ventricular bundle may be manifested as (a) prolongation of the P-R interval (1st degree a-v block), (b) failure of transmission of a proportion of the supraventricular impulses to the ventricles (2nd degree a-v block), or (c) total failure of the impulse to reach the ventricles which are stimulated by a pacemaker situated at one of a number of possible sites in the conducting system below the block (3rd degree a-v block, complete heart block). A recently developed technique whereby, by the use of an intracardiac electrode, the passage of the impulse along the bundle of His can be recorded is adding considerably to the understanding of conduction defects; space does not permit a full account of this interesting and valuable development.

First degree atrio-ventricular block requires no further discussion, the diagnosis depending on accurate measurement of the P-R interval. Of 2nd degree block two distinct types are recognized. Type I of mild degree is characterized by the Wenckebach phenomenon with progressive lengthening of the P-R interval from beat to beat until finally conduction is completely interrupted and a P wave is inscribed without an associated QRS complex. The cycle is then repeated so that, over a period of time, a fixed relationship between the number of P waves and of QRS complexes is present, e.g. 4:3, 5:4 atrio-ventricular block. In more severe cases a fixed 2:1 block occurs but this variety of partial atrio-ventricular block is characteristically transient and benign. In Type II partial atrio-ventricular block (Mobitz Type II) dropped beats occur as in Type I but without the previous progressive lengthening of the P-R interval; later a fixed 2:1 or 3:1 relationship develops and this may finally progress to complete heart block (Fig. 24).

In 3rd degree (complete) atrio-ventricular block there is complete dissociation between the atria and ventricles so that there is no simple mathematical ratio between the cycle lengths of the P waves and of the QRS complexes.

discharge and cause depolarization of the atria. As in complete heart block, the cycle lengths of the P waves and

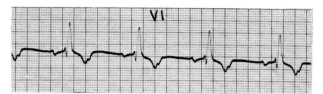

FIG. 24. 2:1 atrio-ventricular block. Every second atrial impulse is blocked, the P waves being superimposed on the T wave of the previous beat. Right bundle branch block is also present. (From the same case as Fig. 17.)

of the QRS complexes are unrelated but, in atrio-ventricular dissociation, the ventricular rate exceeds the atrial.

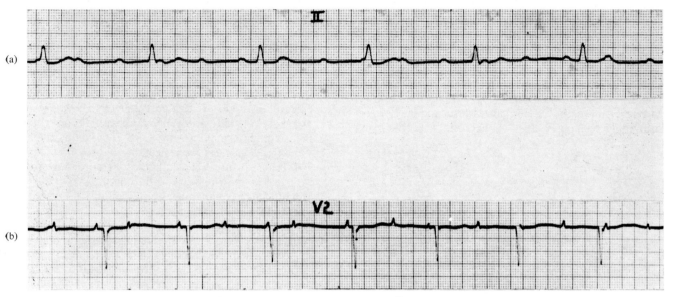

FIG. 25. Two cases of complete heart block. In (a) the pacemaker is in the right ventricular conducting system and the QRS complexes have the pattern of left bundle branch block. In (b) the ventricular pacemaker is situated in the atrio-ventricular junction and, as the ventricles are depolarized normally, the QRS complexes are normal in form.

The ventricular rate is usually of the order of 30–40 per minute except in congenital heart block in which it may be as high as 50 or 60. The form of the QRS complexes depends on the site of the ventricular pacemaker within the conducting system. If this is in the main bundle below the block, ventricular depolarization follows its usual sequence and the QRS complexes are normal. If, however, the pacemaker is situated in one or other bundle branch, depolarization of the corresponding ventricle will occur earlier than that of the other which can only be depolarized by a wave travelling through the myocardium. The QRS complexes will, therefore, closely resemble those of bundle branch block or ventricular ectopic beats (Fig. 25).

In complete heart block, as has been shown, the atrial and ventricular rhythms are dissociated. However, the term *atrio-ventricular dissociation* has come to acquire a special meaning. This term implies a situation in which the ventricles are driven by a pacemaker in the atrio-ventricular node or main bundle at a rate faster than that of the sino-atrial node which nevertheless continues to

The *Wolff-Parkinson-White syndrome* is a rare disorder of conduction in which an anomalous conduction pathway exists between the atria and the ventricles. The impulse travels down both the normal atrio-ventricular bundle and the anomalous pathway but more rapidly down the latter. The effects in the electrocardiogram include a short P-R interval and widening of the QRS complex, superficially resembling bundle branch block. This disorder is benign except that it is associated with a tendency to paroxysms of supraventricular tachycardia (Fig. 26).

## Myocardial Infarction and Ischaemia

Electrocardiography plays an extremely important part in the diagnosis of ischaemic heart disease. It must, however, be remembered that, occasionally, myocardial infarction and, quite commonly, angina may occur in the presence of a normal electrocardiogram. The electrocardiogram can confirm, but can never exclude, a diagnosis of ischaemic heart disease.

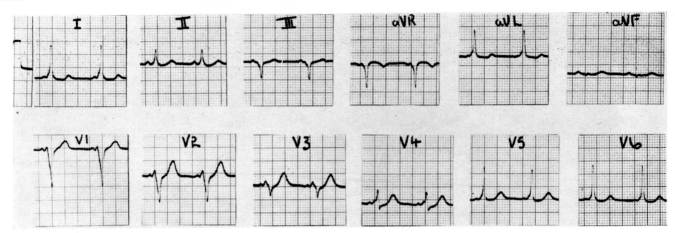

Fig. 26. Wolff-Parkinson-White syndrome. The characteristic 'delta' wave, preceding the R wave, is well seen in I, aVL, V₅ and ₆.

## Myocardial Infarction

An infarct in the myocardium can be considered schematically as concentric areas, from within outward, of necrosis, 'injury' and ischaemia (Fig. 27). In the necrotic area, irreversible pathological changes occur and the electrocardiographic changes due to necrosis are, likewise,

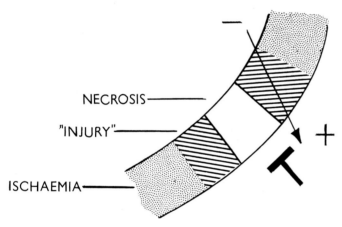

Fig. 27. Diagrammatic cross-section of infarct in wall of left ventricle. The arrow indicates the direction of spread of the normal wave of depolarization. An electrode indicated as facing the necrotic area records the negative intracavitary potential.

irreversible. The term 'injury' implies damage to the cells of sufficient severity to impair temporarily the functions of the cell membrane; these changes are potentially reversible as are the changes seen in the less severely damaged area of ischaemia surrounding the infarct.

The electrocardiographic changes due to necrosis can be understood if it is realised that dead tissue is electrically inert. An electrode placed over such an area will, therefore, record the potential changes occurring within the ventricular cavity. The term 'electrical window' has been used to describe the effect of a necrotic area and the concept that an electrode in this position 'sees' the intracavitary potential may be helpful. Almost all infarcts occur in the left ventricle and an electrode lying within that chamber would

record a monophasic QS deflection. This is because the waves of depolarization travel, in all directions, *away* from the ventricular cavity, either through the septum or through the mural myocardium from endocardium to epicardium. This is the potential change 'seen' by the external electrode through the 'electrical window' and hence the main abnormality in the QRS complex in myocardial infarction is a negative deflection—a prominent Q wave. This differs from the normal Q wave recorded over the left ventricle in both depth and duration. A Q wave whose amplitude is more than one-third that of the R wave in that lead and whose duration exceeds 0·04 sec. is almost always evidence of myocardial infarction. In terms of the vector concept of electrocardiographic interpretation the changes of necrosis can be described as a force (vector) pointing away from the necrotic area towards the centre of the heart during the first 0·04 sec. of the QRS complex. This approach to the problem will be found particularly helpful in the diagnosis of infarction in an unusual area of the myocardium, for example true posterior infarction (*see* below).

In the area of 'injury' surrounding the necrotic centre of the infarct, the damage to the cell membranes produces important electrical effects (Fig. 28). The maintenance of the negative intracellular potential and the relatively positive surface potential of the resting cell depends on the integrity of the membrane. If this is damaged, the transmembrane potential is abolished so that the external surface of the cell becomes relatively negative. A potential difference therefore appears between this region and the surface of neighbouring uninjured cells whose normal positive external charge has been maintained. As a result of this potential difference a current flows—the so-called *current of injury*. The electrocardiogram reflects changes, not of current but of potential and if it were possible to record from an electrode on a segment of myocardium at the moment of injury, the baseline would be seen to shift abruptly downwards as the external surface of the cells became negative (Fig. 28a). If depolarization were now to begin in the normal manner (Fig. 28b), the charge on the surface of the healthy cells would also become negative so that, when depolarization was complete, all the cells, healthy and injured, would have the same surface potential (Fig. 28c). As long as the myocardium is depolarized therefore the record would remain at its original 'baseline', the current of injury no longer flowing. Repolarization begins at the time of inscription of the T wave so that once again the 'baseline' would fall as the potential difference between healthy and injured muscle reappeared. In the clinical electrocardiogram these changes are seen as elevation of the RS-T segment, the only part of the whole cycle when the surfaces of healthy and injured cells are at the same potential.

RS-T segment elevation is an important sign of recent myocardial infarction and, like the Q wave, is recorded from electrodes facing the infarcted area. In vectorial terms, a force pointing towards the infarct is present during the inscription of the RS-T segment.

The ischaemia surrounding the injured area is responsible for the third cardinal sign of infarction, T wave inversion. In practice, this is not always seen in electrocardiograms recorded soon after the episode as the elevation of the terminal part of the RS-T segment 'cancels out' the tendency to negativity of the T wave. T wave inversion is a non-specific sign of infarction but the differentiation from, for example, left ventricular strain, can usually be made without difficulty. In the latter condition, using the vector concept, both the RS-T and T wave vectors point in the same direction—away from the left ventricle—producing RS-T depression as well as T wave inversion. In myocardial infarction, the T vector points away from the infarct and the RS-T vector towards it.

The evolution of the electrocardiographic changes of myocardial infarction as time passes may be of diagnostic importance and are of some value in determining the age of an infarct. Within a few days or, at most, a week or two, the RS-T segment becomes iso-electric. The loss of the vectorial forces pointing towards the infarct allows the oppositely directed T wave vector to become dominant so that deep T inversion appears at this time. Over the next few weeks the T wave may return towards normal, becoming iso-electric and, often, upright. The pathological

Q wave, however, reflecting irreversible necrosis, persists indefinitely as the 'tombstone' of the dead muscle.

The site of an infarct can be determined with some accuracy from the electrocardiogram. If the pathognomonic changes—pathological Q, RS-T elevation and subsequent T inversion—are seen in the chest leads and in Leads I and aVL, an *anterior* infarct can be diagnosed (Fig. 29). Greater precision may be possible if the abnormalities are restricted to fewer leads; *antero-septal* infarction, with changes in $V_{1-4}$, *antero-lateral* infarction, with changes in I, aVL and possibly $V_6$ only, are all recognized.

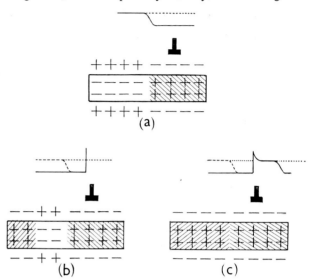

FIG. 28. Genesis of RS-T segment elevation due to myocardial injury. In (a) is shown the base-line shift due to the potential difference between polarized (resting) and injured muscle. In (b) and (c) the effect of depolarization of the healthy muscle is shown (*see* text for details).

Infarction of the diaphragmatic surface of the left ventricle was, for many years, known as *posterior* infarction, but recently this term has been replaced by *inferior* or *diaphragmatic* infarction. This change in terminology has been

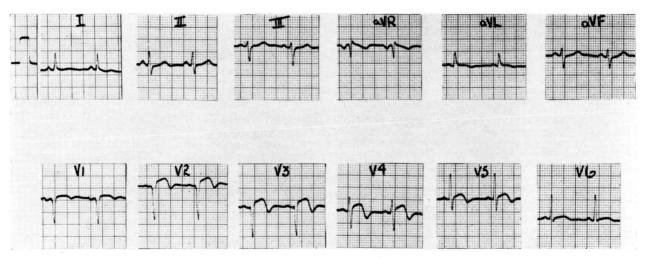

FIG. 29. Anteroseptal myocardial infarction. There is a pathological Q wave in $V_2$ and the typical RS-T segment elevation and T wave inversion are seen best in $V_{2-5}$.

necessitated by the recognition of infarction of the small area of left ventricle lying posteriorly, near the spine—the *true posterior* infarct. The changes of *inferior* infarction are seen in the leads whose axes run more or less vertically, i.e. Leads II, III and aVF (Fig. 30); occasionally changes may also be seen in V$_6$ in which case the infarction would be described as infero-lateral.

although in an opposite sense, from an electrode placed diametrically opposite to the infarct (Fig. 31). In practice, in lead V$_1$, tall broad R waves with RS-T depression and, subsequently, tall T waves can be recorded (Fig. 32). It must be remembered, however, that there are other causes, commoner than true posterior infarction, of tall R waves in V$_1$; these, of which right ventricular hypertrophy is the

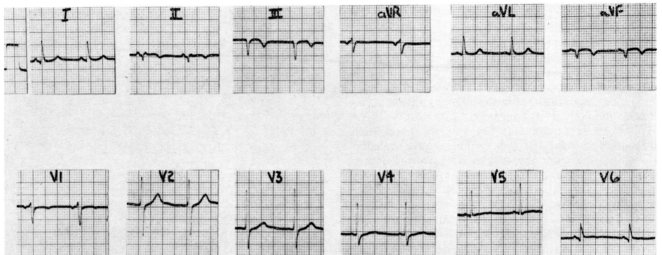

FIG. 30. Inferior (diaphragmatic) myocardial infarction. Pathological Q waves, RS-T segment elevation and T wave inversion are present in II, III and aVF.

The diagnosis of true posterior infarction is more difficult. If it were possible to place an electrode on or near this part of the myocardium there is no doubt that the characteristic changes would be seen. Such electrode placement is not routinely possible, however, and the

most important, must be excluded before infarction at this site can be diagnosed.

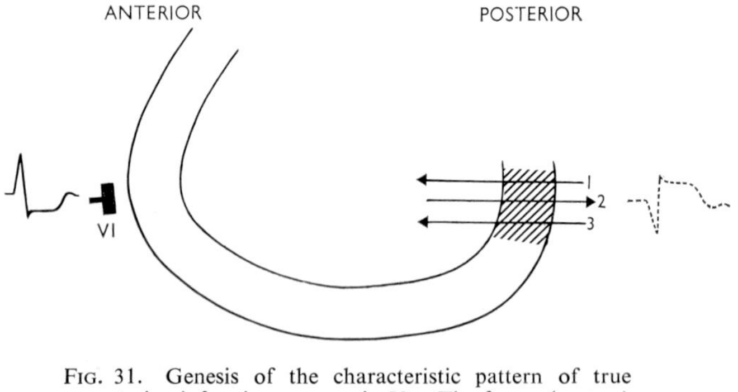

### Myocardial Ischaemia

Many changes may be seen in the electrocardiogram as a result of ischaemia. Probably the most important of these is depression of the RS-T segment; this is believed to be due to transient injury to the subendocardial myocardium. Great care is needed, however, in the interpretation of such changes as parts of the RS-T segment may be depressed in other circumstances. For example, depression of the *junction* between the QRS complex and the RS-T segment is, usually, of no pathological significance (Fig. 33); the changes produced by digitalis (*see* below) must also be distinguished. The characteristic pattern seen in ischaemia is depression of the whole of the RS-T segment, the so-called *plane* depression (Fig. 33) and even this should be disregarded unless it is at least 1 mm below the baseline. T wave inversion also is seen as a result of ischaemia but, as has been indicated, this abnormality is so non-specific as to reduce its reliability as precise diagnostic evidence.

An electrocardiogram recorded after exercise may be of diagnostic value but requires very careful interpretation. Space does not permit a more detailed account of this nor of the more subtle ischaemic changes which may be seen in the resting electrocardiogram. It must be emphasized, in any case, that the most important element in the diagnosis of myocardial ischaemia is a carefully taken history.

ANTERIOR                              POSTERIOR

VI

FIG. 31. Genesis of the characteristic pattern of true posterior infarction as seen in V$_1$. The forces (vectors) associated with infarction have three components: (1) a force during the first 0·04 sec. of the QRS complex directed away from the infarct towards the centre of the heart (Q wave); (2) a force directed towards the epicardial surface of the infarct during the inscription of the RS-T segment and (3) a force directed away from the infarct during repolarization (inverted T wave). These forces are recorded in V$_1$ as a "mirror-image" of the classical pattern of infarction.

diagnosis rests on an understanding of the vectorial changes of infarction. These can be summarized as a force pointing away from the infarct during the first 0·04 sec. of the QRS (the pathological Q wave), a force directed towards the infarct as long as the myocardium is depolarized (RS-T elevation) and deviation of the T vector away from the infarct. Clearly it should be possible to record these forces,

### Effects of Drugs and Electrolytes

Many drugs can produce changes in the electrocardiogram. Of these, by far the most commonly seen are those due to *digitalis*. The RS-T segment is depressed in a characteristic manner, sloping downwards from its iso-electric junction with the QRS complex (Fig. 33). This sign is almost invariable if the patient has been on digitalis for more than a few days and should not be regarded as evidence of toxicity. Another very common feature is shortening of the Q-T interval.* Overdosage with digitalis and increased sensitivity to this drug, as occurs in the presence of hypokalaemia, are manifested by many electrocardiographic abnormalities. Atrial and ventricular ectopic beats are common, the latter often occurring regularly after each sinus beat to produce one of the varieties of pulsus bigeminus or 'coupled beats'. Ectopic supraventricular or ventricular tachycardias can occur and atrial tachycardia with partial atrioventricular block is particularly characteristic of digitalis toxicity. In addition to these manifestations

complex occurs and, with extremely high potassium levels, it may merge with the T wave producing a bizarre double-

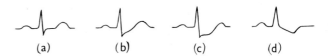

(a)    (b)    (c)    (d)

Fig. 33. Configuration of (a) the normal RS–T segment compared with (b) junctional depression, usually of no pathological significance, (c) "plane" depression, characteristic of ischaemia, and (d) the typical "digitalis effect".

peaked complex. The P waves are often absent. In the presence of *hypokalaemia* the first electrocardiographic change is prominence of the, usually inconspicuous, U

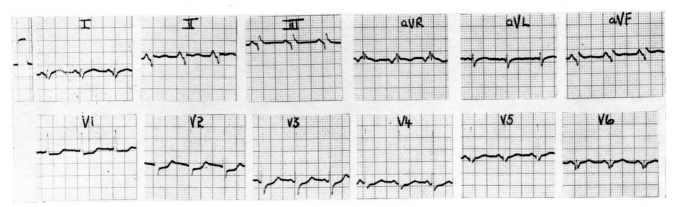

Fig. 32. Postero-inferior myocardial infarction. Pathological Q waves are present in II, III and aVF and tall R waves with RS-T segment depression are seen in $V_{1-3}$.

of increased myocardial irritability evidence of impaired conduction may be found. All degrees of atrio-ventricular block may be seen, complete heart block being evidence of very serious intoxication. Many, if not all, of the electrocardiographic changes produced by digitalis can be reversed by the administration of potassium. This is, however, not necessarily the treatment of choice for digitalis intoxication.

Evidence of serious toxicity appears much more readily in the electrocardiogram as a result of *quinidine* than of digitalis. The most constant feature is prolongation of the Q-T interval. Slurring and widening of the QRS complex also occurs with widening of the T wave which may become inverted. Marked change in the duration of the QRS complex is an absolute indication for discontinuing quinidine therapy, as asystole or ventricular fibrillation may occur without further warning.

It is probable that changes in the concentrations of all the plasma electrolytes, including hydrogen, can produce electrocardiographic changes. Of these, those produced by changes in potassium and calcium are the best known and most significant. *Hyperkalaemia* causes the T waves to become tall and peaked; later widening of the QRS

wave. Later, the amplitude of the T wave is reduced and the RS-T segment depressed. If the serum potassium is very low the T wave may be iso-electric and the prominent U wave may be misinterpreted as a T wave following a grossly prolonged RS-T segment.

The effects of changes in the serum ionized *calcium* are mainly seen as changes in the duration of the Q-T interval; hypocalcaemia causes prolongation and hypercalcaemia abbreviation so that at very high levels of serum calcium the T wave 'takes off' from the QRS complex.

### Conclusion

This chapter is intended as a brief account of what must pass, at the present time, as the scientific basis of electrocardiography. It is not in any sense exhaustive and, for the benefit of those who wish to extend their knowledge of the subject, a brief bibliography is appended.

### Select Bibliography

Goldman, M. J. (1967), *Principles of Clinical Electrocardiography*, 6th edition. Oxford: Blackwell.

This is a relatively inexpensive book which can be used for reference by all except those concerned with the minutiae of the subject. It is very well illustrated and contains a useful list of references.

* For methods of correcting the Q-T interval for heart rate, standard works on electrocardiography should be consulted.

Schamroth, L. (1966), *An Introduction to Electrocardiography*, 3rd edition. Oxford: Blackwell.

One of the best of the shorter texts on the subject and well worth reading in full.

Grant, R. P. (1957), *Clinical Electrocardiography*. New York: McGraw-Hill.

A brilliant account of the vector approach to electrocardiographic interpretation. It is not a textbook of vectorcardiography, a subject which, at present, is best left to the experts, but an account of a method of study which is both intellectually stimulating and clinically valuable.

Many other textbooks on electrocardiography are, of course, available. Most of these are sound and some are exhaustive. Those referred to above, however, are thoroughly reliable and have proved their worth in the author's personal experience.

*SECTION II*

**PHYSIOLOGICAL BASIS OF THE SCIENCE OF ANAESTHESIA**

*B. RESPIRATION*

# CHAPTER 1

# CENTRAL CONTROL OF RESPIRATION

S. J. G. SEMPLE AND J. R. CAMERON

## INTRODUCTION

Respiratory control of blood pH, $P_{CO_2}$ and $P_{O_2}$ is an important homeostatic mechanism. The role of pH, $P_{CO_2}$ and $P_{O_2}$ as factors controlling the level of ventilation has been studied in detail since early workers demonstrated the respiratory responses to hypoxia and acidosis. One of the most controversial aspects of this subject has been the nature of the $P_{CO_2}$/pH stimulus to ventilation and its site of action. Denervation of the known arterial chemoreceptors does not abolish the respiratory response to the inhalation of $CO_2$. It would appear that receptors in the central nervous system (CNS) govern this response. Considerable doubt has existed concerning the site of the receptors and whether their response to $CO_2$ is more closely related to changes in the cerebrospinal fluid (CSF) than to changes in arterial or venous blood.

It is the purpose of this review to discuss the relationship between the 'computing' elements of the medullary control mechanism and the central chemoreceptor, and to develop the view that this receptor responds to pH changes in the CSF/brain ECF compartment. During steady states it appears that brain ECF is in equilibrium with CSF in the ventricular cavities. The acid-base control of the brain ECF/CSF compartment is, therefore, of paramount importance in determining the activity of the central chemoreceptor. The factors which are involved in this control and the contribution of ionic exchanges between CSF, brain (ECF and ICF) and blood will be discussed. In chronic acidosis and alkalosis the relative contribution of the peripheral and central chemoreceptors is in some doubt. This relationship will be considered in as far as changes in the peripheral chemoreceptor drive will change the response of the central mechanism.

## 1. Central Control of Rhythmic Breathing

The chemical control of respiration is imposed on the CNS mechanisms which generate rhythmic breathing. Many other afferent stimuli, which may not be chemical in nature, can affect this intrinsic rhythmicity. The influence of noise and emotional disturbances on the respiratory response to a chemical stimulus will be readily appreciated by anyone who has investigated the control of breathing in man. The central control of respiration is modified by the action of the peripheral chemoreceptors (Dejours, 1962), by the action of the vagus nerves (Guz *et al.*, 1966) and possibly by afferent stimuli from muscles (Campbell, 1966) and joints (Newsom Davis, 1967). The interaction

of these mechanical and chemical stimuli may be important in determining the abnormalities of breathing in disease (Clark, 1968).

Our knowledge of the organization of the central respiratory control mechanisms is largely derived from a correlation of the results of action potential recording, electrical stimulation and of ablation of areas of the CNS in animals. The medulla alone is capable of maintaining rhythmic breathing but it is gasping—a short inspiratory effort terminating abruptly. Eupnoea, defined as rhythmic, continuous inspiratory and expiratory movement without perceptible halt at any phase of the cycle, requires an intact pons.

Neurones showing bursts of activity in phase with respiratory movement are referred to as respiratory neurones and are found in the medulla and pons. There is intermingling of inspiratory and expiratory neurones in the medulla but the former are more predominant in the ventral part of the reticular formation and the latter are predominant in the dorsal part. There is good evidence that inspiratory and expiratory neurones are not only excitatory but may exert reciprocal inhibition on each other. The activity of the respiratory neurones is affected by nearby neurones which may not be respiratory.

The respiratory neurones in the pons are necessary for eupnoea; they are thought to facilitate the smooth transition from inspiration to expiration and vice versa. Such respiratory neurones are found in the upper part of the pons (pneumotaxic area) and in the middle and lower pons (apneustic area). The neurones in the pneumotaxic area have no intrinsic rhythmic activity of their own but ablation of this area leads to respiratory slowing and apneusis; the latter term describes the type of breathing in which respiration stops in full inspiration. Stimulation of the pneumotaxic area leads to an increase in ventilation accompanied by an increase in rate. The pneumotaxic area probably inhibits the lower apneustic area and prevents the apneusis which would occur with uncontrolled activity of the apneustic area. Ablation both of the pneumotaxic and apneustic areas abolishes apneusis which is replaced by the gasping type of respiration described earlier for the medulla.

So far we have been concerned with those structures in the CNS concerned with the co-ordination of rhythmic breathing but there are other regions of the CNS which influence respiration. Stimulation of the reticular activating system in the mid-brain by electrical stimulation, by arousal from sleep or by $CO_2$ will increase respiration. Sleep and anaesthetics lead to a reduced activity of the reticular activating system and decreased respiratory activity. Ablation of this area in animals leads not only to a reduction in ventilation but a reduced responsiveness to $CO_2$. Finally there are several areas of the cortex in man and animals which, when stimulated, will alter respiration.

A change in $P_{CO_2}$ could influence the discharge of the central respiratory neurones in a variety of ways. First, the discharge could be affected by afferent stimuli from the peripheral chemoreceptors; this undoubtedly occurs, as will be discussed later, but cannot be responsible for the full respiratory response to a rise or fall in $P_{CO_2}$. Second, a change in $P_{CO_2}$ might directly affect the respiratory neurones; the resulting change in ventilation could be due to stimulation of excitatory neurones or depression of inhibitory neurones. Third, a change in $P_{CO_2}$ at the chemo-sensitive area in the medulla may stimulate or depress non-respiratory neurones or chemoreceptors which could influence the activity of respiratory neurones lying at a greater depth from the surface of the medulla. At present it is not known whether the central chemical drive to ventilation arises from a direct effect on respiratory neurones, or, an indirect effect through non-respiratory neurones or chemoreceptors. It is, of course, possible that both mechanisms operate.

The experimental evidence of Mitchell *et al.* (1963) suggests that the central chemical control of respiration is due to acid-base changes around or within non-respiratory neurones or chemoreceptors lying about 200 microns below the surface of the chemosensitive area in the medulla. The evidence for this view rests largely on the speed with which respiration changes when the composition of the fluid over the surface of the medulla is changed. Pledgets, soaked in saline equilibrated with 100 per cent $CO_2$, exert an almost immediate respiratory effect. Pappenheimer *et al.* (1965) have challenged this interpretation on the basis of the speed with which ions can diffuse through the ECF of brain from the surface. This diffusion might be sufficiently rapid for changes in acid-base composition of the fluid at the surface of the medulla to exert a direct effect on respiratory neurones lying deep in the medulla. This controversy has been considered in greater detail in Section 3.

## 2. The Location of the Central Chemoreceptor

The exact location of the central chemosensitive elements has been attempted by many techniques. Although these receptors have been functionally characterized there has, as yet, been no histological identification of a chemoreceptor equivalent to the carotid body. Neither has there been any satisfactory delineation of the relationship between the neurones of the respiratory centres in the medullary reticular formation and the chemosensitive elements.

Comroe (1943) studied the central control of respiration by using micropipettes to inject various solutions into the electrically defined medullary respiratory centres. It was found that the rate and depth of breathing were most often increased by injections of $NaHCO_3$. Localized changes in $P_{CO_2}$ and pH appeared to produce respiratory stimulation. These experiments provided direct evidence that the neurones of the respiratory centres were involved in the

central chemosensitive response. Kim and Carpenter (1961) have thrown doubt on the interpretation of such experiments. They demonstrated that injections into the region of the respiratory centre were by no means a specific stimulant of respiration. In addition to respiratory effects there was evidence of a general, non-specific excitation of the medullary reticular formation. They postulated that these generalized effects could be due to changes in the ionization of $Ca^{++}$ around neurones. Injection of citrate or calcium chelating agents into this area produced excitatory effects, which were abolished on addition of $CaCl_2$ to the injectate. It seems that the direct demonstration of respiratory centre chemosensitivity by the method of micro-injection is complicated by the secondary changes which occur in the environment of the respiratory neurones on injection of the test solution. Since all neurones are sensitive to such changes (particularly of $Ca^{++}$ or $K^+$) these experiments do not conclusively indicate the presence of specifically chemosensitive elements in the region of the respiratory centre.

Leusen (1954a and b) established that changes in the composition of the CSF could influence ventilation. This work led to a new search for central chemosensors in relation to the CSF. Again many areas have been defined which are functionally active, but there has been no histological evidence of a true chemoreceptor area. Loeschcke and his co-workers have contributed extensively to this investigation and have defined various sites for the postulated receptors. All these areas were situated outside the classical respiratory centres. Several possible sites for the receptors were defined, including the choroid plexus, the floor of the fourth ventricle and a localized area in the lateral recesses of the fourth ventricle (*see* Loeschcke, 1965 for review). It had been previously suggested (Mitchell *et al.*, 1960) that the receptor area was to be found in the region of the area postrema. It is tempting to assign an important specialized function to this area in view of its apparent morphological differentiation. The area postrema projects into the fourth ventricle and is remarkable for a lack of neuronal elements and a high degree of vascularity. The ready penetration of dyes and drugs into this area which do not pass into other parts of the CNS has been taken to indicate an absence of the blood-brain barrier. Florez and Borison (1967) have shown that ablation of the area postrema does not change the response to inhaled $CO_2$. Localized vascular perfusion of this area has not revealed a respiratory response to changes in the $P_{CO_2}$, pH or $[HCO_3^-]$ of the perfusate (W. S. Yamamoto, personal communication).

Mitchell *et al.* (1963) investigated the chemosensitivity of the surface of the brain stem of anaesthetized cats. They defined a localized, chemosensitive area on the ventro-lateral surface of the medulla near the roots of the VIIth, IXth and Xth cranial nerves (see Fig. 1). Their techniques included local perfusion of various areas, or direct application of small pledgets of filter paper equilibrated with $CO_2$ or soaked in the various test solutions. Respiration was stimulated by application of pledgets or solutions with a high $P_{CO_2}$ or low pH, and by nicotine and acetyl choline. Respiration was depressed by a low $P_{CO_2}$, procaine, lobeline, sodium cyanide and local cooling. They concluded that the receptors were localized, since responses were obtained only in certain well-defined areas, and superficial, since the response occurred extremely rapidly. Blocking of this receptor area with procaine regularly produced apnoea in animals whose peripheral chemoreceptors had been denervated; it was deduced that these receptors

Apnoea also resulted in the decerebrate unanaesthetized preparation after procaine block if there had been severe haemorrhage. Central chemosensitivity cannot therefore be explained in terms of one receptor area. It appears probable that in addition to the area described by Mitchell *et al.* (1963), there are other chemosensitive elements deeper in the brain tissue.

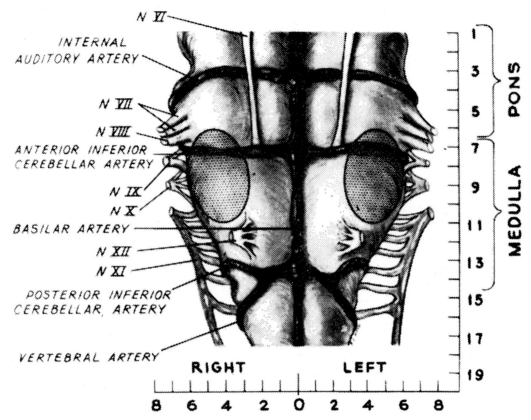

Fig. 1. Ventral view of cat medulla and pons. The stippled areas represent the superficial chemosensitive regions. Stereotaxic co-ordinates are in millimetres. (From Severinghaus *et al.*, 1963. Reproduced by kind permission of the authors and the editors of *J. appl. Physiol.*)

accounted wholly for the central respiratory chemosensitivity.

Pappenheimer and his colleagues (*see* Pappenheimer, 1965 for review) had found that during ventriculo-cisternal perfusion of conscious goats with a mock CSF of varying [$HCO_3^-$], respiration did not appear to be solely determined by the pH of the CSF in the large cavities. The central chemoreceptor behaved not as though situated in the CSF, but rather as though placed deep in the brain, at some point in a diffusion pathway between blood and CSF. There is therefore, a discrepancy in these views. Cozine and Ngai (1967) have confirmed the existence of the chemoreceptor area defined by Mitchell *et al.* (1963). They found, however, that in decerebrate, unanaesthetized, chemoreceptor odenervated animals a reduced response to $CO_2$ persisted after procaine block of this area. It would appear therefore, that there are other chemosensitive elements and this area does not represent the sole central chemoreceptor. When the animal was given chloralose (the anaesthetic used by Mitchell *et al.*, 1963), apnoea always followed procaine block.

### 3. Central Respiratory Response to Changes in $P_{CO_2}$/pH

Early experiments showed that hyperventilation occurred in response to inhalation of $CO_2$, or administration of acids. In 1911, Winterstein produced his first reaction theory in which he related all respiratory stimuli to arterial pH. It became rapidly apparent that such a unitarian view of respiratory control could not explain all the observed facts. Hooker, Wilson and Connett (1917) perfused the isolated medulla of dogs and showed that for a given change in arterial pH, $CO_2$ produced a greater respiratory effect than hydrochloric or lactic acids. Scott (1918) found that in decerebrate, unanaesthetized cats made alkalotic with sodium carbonate, breathing correlated with arterial $P_{CO_2}$ and not pH. It was therefore suggested that $CO_2$ had some specific respiratory effect which could not be accounted for solely in terms of pH.

The specific action of $CO_2$ as a respiratory stimulant was elucidated by the classic experiments of Jacobs (1920a and b), who showed how $CO_2$ might act on the interior of plant and animal cells. Jacobs observed that a saturated solution of $CO_2$ was more toxic to tadpoles and protozoa than other acid solutions of the same pH. Even when sufficient $HCO_3^-$ was added to the $CO_2$ solution to make it alkaline, the toxic effect was not diminished. He observed that with flagellated protozoa containing intracellular contractile structures, $CO_2$ appeared to act on the intracellular mechanisms causing little injury to the flagellae, whereas mineral acids did the opposite. He postulated that the special property of $CO_2$ as a respiratory stimulant was its diffusibility across membranes and into cells. This view was confirmed by experiments using the flowers of symphytum peregrinum, the petals of which are pink in an acid solution and blue in an alkaline solution. When placed in a $CO_2$ solution made alkaline with $NaHCO_3$, the petal turned pink demonstrating the ability of $CO_2$ to cause an intracellular acidosis even in an alkaline solution.

The concept that the diffusibility of $CO_2$ and its ability to enter cells could produce a paradoxical change in the pH of fluids separated from blood by a membrane found ready acceptance. The existence of a blood-brain barrier was already recognized. Collip and Backus (1920) showed that intravenous infusion of $NaHCO_3$ had no immediate effect on the CSF $HCO_3^-$. Both Gesell (1923) and Winterstein (1921) formulated theories relating the control of ventilation to the pH in the central chemoreceptor. Inhalation of $CO_2$ would produce pH changes which were rapidly reflected centrally, whereas the diffusion of other acids and $HCO_3^-$ into the CNS would be restricted. Confirmation for these ideas was provided by simultaneous, continuous measurement of blood and CSF pH (Gesell and Hertzmann, 1926). Arterial, venous and CSF pH were recorded during the administration of $CO_2$ or $NaHCO_3$. During $CO_2$ breathing arterial, venous and CSF pH all became acid, $NaHCO_3$, however, produced an alkalosis in arterial and venous blood, but an acidosis in the CSF. Cestan, Sendrail and Lasalle (1925) compared the effect of respiratory and metabolic acidosis on CSF pH. CSF pH changes were found to depend on the mode of acidification; during respiratory acidosis CSF pH fell, after i.v. infusion of HCl there was no change in CSF pH. It became clear that changes in blood pH were not an indication of changes occurring in the environment of the central chemoreceptor; such a guide might be obtained from measurements made on the CSF. Leusen (1954a and b) in a series of classic studies investigated the effect of changes in CSF $P_{CO_2}$ and pH on ventilation. He used the technique of ventriculo-cisternal perfusion to perfuse the ventricles of anaesthetized dogs with a mock CSF of varying composition. An increase in $P_{CO_2}$ and a fall in pH of the perfusing fluid produced an increase in respiration. It was therefore firmly established that acid base changes in the CSF could be of primary importance in the chemical control of breathing.

If the central chemoreceptors responded to acid-base changes in CSF it became important to investigate the CSF response to chronic acidosis and alkalosis. Many workers confirmed that in chronic metabolic acidosis and alkalosis CSF pH appeared to remain within the limits of normality (Bradley and Semple, 1962; Mitchell et al., 1965; Posner, Swanson and Plum, 1965). It must be emphasized that the changes in CSF pH are small compared to those in blood. Consequently the scatter of such measurements is large when compared to the small changes observed. Since it is so poorly buffered, pH measurements on CSF are technically difficult.

Bradley, Semple and Spencer (1965) and Coxon and Swanson (1965) studied the time course of equilibration of $CO_2$ between blood, brain and CSF. Bradley et al. measured the changes in cisternal CSF $P_{CO_2}$ in man during $CO_2$ administration; from their results they predicted that the rise in cisternal $P_{CO_2}$ would be complete only after 30 min. Coxon and Swanson using [14]C-labelled $HCO_3^-$ found that exchange of $CO_2$ was more rapid between blood and brain than between blood and CSF. Isotopic equilibrium between the $CO_2$ of blood and CSF would be reached in cats in about 9 min. The central component of the respiratory response to $CO_2$ would therefore be relatively slow. This provided an explanation for the observation that following $CO_2$ administration and after hyperventilation, ventilation does not reach a new steady state until 20–30 min. have passed.

The adaptation to altitude had been a problem for many theories of respiratory regulation. No satisfactory explanation had been found for the observation that chronic exposure to altitude resulted in a greater increase in

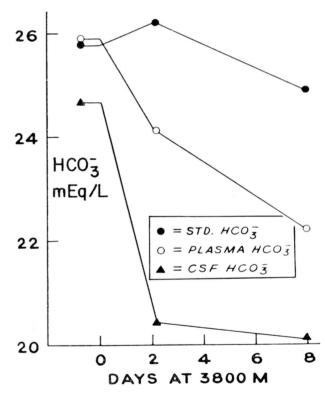

FIG. 2. Changes in blood and CSF [$HCO_3^-$] during acclimatization to altitude. The fall in CSF [$HCO_3^-$] is greater and more rapid than that in plasma. The standard $HCO_3^-$ in plasma is the [$HCO_3^-$] of plasma equilibrated at a $P_{CO_2}$ of 40 mm. Hg. (From Severinghaus et al., 1963. Reproduced by kind permission of the authors and the editors of J. appl. Physiol.)

ventilation than acute exposure, and that correction of altitude hypoxia did not result in an immediate abolition of hyperventilation. Severinghaus *et al.* (1963) investigated the changes occurring in CSF pH during the adaption to altitude. Exposure to altitude hypoxia leads to hyperventilation with a consequent reduction in arterial $P_{CO_2}$ and a rise in pH. The renal excretion of $HCO_3^-$ will produce a slow return of blood pH towards normal. The initial hyperventilation causes a rise in CSF pH and a fall in CSF $P_{CO_2}$. This results in a decrease in the activity of the medullary chemoreceptor which 'opposes' the anoxic drive from the peripheral chemoreceptor. In the 48 hr. after ascent to altitude it was observed that the CSF $HCO_3^-$ fell, so that CSF pH returned to normal (*see* Fig. 2). When the CSF pH was again normal, the anoxic drive would no longer be opposed centrally and ventilation would therefore increase. The fall in CSF $HCO_3^-$ was greater and occurred more rapidly than could be accounted for by the renal correction of plasma $HCO_3^-$. To confirm this, Severinghaus (1964) showed that even if plasma $HCO_3^-$ was kept constant during altitude acclimatization by ingestion of $HCO_3$, the fall in CSF $HCO_3$ was not abolished. To explain these findings it was postulated that a process of active transport across the blood-CSF barrier existed, which was capable of reducing CSF $HCO_3^-$ and thereby returning CSF pH to normal. This introduced the concept that CSF pH was actively regulated.

It appeared that under all conditions of acid-base disturbance, CSF pH was regulated to within normal limits of 7·30–7·36 (Mitchell *et al.*, 1965), *see* Fig. 3. Control of

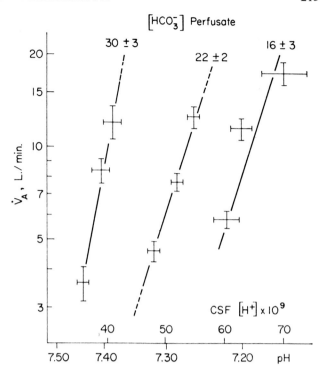

Fig. 4. Ventilatory responses to $CO_2$ inhalation for normal goats during ventriculo-cisternal perfusion with 30, 22 and 16 mEq./l. [$HCO_3^-$]. Crosses represent means and standard error from 75 steady-state periods in six goats. (From Pappenheimer, 1965. Reproduced by kind permission of the author and the editors of *Harvey Lect.*)

CSF pH was possible only between certain limits of arterial pH (Mitchell *et al.*, 1964). Below an arterial pH of 7·3 or above 7·5 the control of CSF pH was no longer perfect. If CSF pH remains constant, so must that part of the respiratory drive originating in the medullary chemoreceptor. Changes in ventilation in chronic metabolic acidosis and alkalosis (blood pH being between 7·3–7·5) must result from changes in the activity of the peripheral chemoreceptors. This view of the control of ventilation has been comprehensively presented (Mitchell, 1966); it may be said to rest on three main points. First, in chronic acid-base derangements CSF pH is maintained within the normal range, provided arterial pH lies between 7·3 and 7·5. Second, under these circumstances ventilation is controlled by the peripheral chemoreceptors, and third, all medullary chemosensitivity may be attributed to the area defined on the ventro-lateral surface.

The work of Pappenheimer and his colleagues has led to a reappraisal of the changes in CSF pH in chronic acid-base disturbances. The application of a perfected form of ventriculo-cisternal perfusion to conscious goats provided evidence of the remarkable sensitivity of the central chemoreceptor to a small change in CSF pH. Prior to this work relatively large changes were required during ventriculo-cisternal perfusion to produce respiratory effects in anaesthetized animals (Leusen, 1954a). Pappenheimer *et al.* (1965) demonstrated that small changes in the [$HCO_3^-$] and pH of the fluid perfusing the ventricles produced large changes in the resting ventilation and $CO_2$ response of

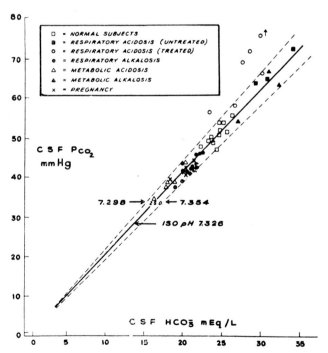

Fig. 3. Relationship between CSF $P_{CO_2}$ and [$HCO_3^-$] in normal subjects and patients with abnormal acid-base balance. Central iso pH line represents normal mean CSF pH (7·326); outer lines indicate 2 SD from the mean. (From Mitchell *et al.*, 1965. Reproduced by kind permission of the authors and the editors of *J. appl. Physiol.*)

conscious goats. The extremes of ventilation measured in these goats (4–18 l./min.) were associated with a CSF pH change of only 0·1 unit. Their results also showed that ventilation was not a single function of CSF pH. For any given CSF pH ventilation varied with the CSF [HCO$_3^-$], see Figure 4. This observation led to the conclusion that ventilation was not determined by the pH of the CSF in the ventricular cavities, and that an entirely superficial chemoreceptor as postulated by Mitchell *et al.* (1963) was unlikely. During ventriculo-cisternal perfusion

with plasma [HCO$_3^-$] (*see* Fig. 6). During acidosis the CSF [HCO$_3^-$] was 5 m. mols. greater than plasma [HCO$_3^-$] while in alkalosis it was 18 m. mols. less. The exchange of [HCO$_3^-$] between CSF and blood was again studied during ventriculo-cisternal perfusion with fluids of varying [HCO$_3^-$]. It was found that there was no net flux of [HCO$_3^-$] across the ependyma when the perfusing fluid maintained the same gradient between blood and CSF as observed in the chronic states. Zero net flux during such a perfusion may be interpreted as indicating the absence

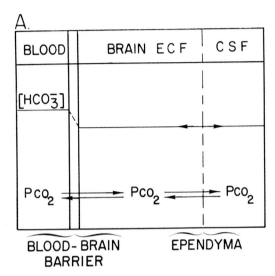
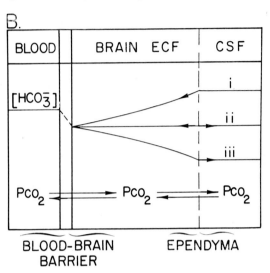

FIG. 5. A diagrammatic representation of concentration gradients for HCO$_3^-$ between cerebral capillary blood, brain ECF and CSF during: (*a*) Normal steady state conditions (no ventriculo-cisternal perfusion). Blood, brain ECF and CSF P$_{CO_2}$ are equal. Plasma [HCO$_3^-$] is higher than that in brain ECF or CSF. Brain ECF and CSF [HCO$_3^-$] and pH are equal. (*b*) Ventriculo-cisternal perfusion with artificial CSF of varying [HCO$_3^-$]. (i) Perfusion with high HCO$_3^-$ CSF. There is a net flux of HCO$_3^-$ out of CSF across the ependyma. (ii) Perfusion with a normal HCO$_3^-$ CSF. There is no net flux across the ependyma. (iii) Perfusion with low HCO$_3^-$ CSF. There is a net flux of HCO$_3^-$ into CSF across the ependyma. During these unsteady states (i and iii) there will be a concentration gradient for HCO$_3^-$ through brain ECF. Since P$_{CO_2}$ is constant through brain ECF this will result in a pH gradient also.

with an artificial CSF of varying [HCO$_3^-$] it was observed that a net flux of [HCO$_3^-$] occurred across the ependymal linings of the ventricles. The possible concentration gradients for [HCO$_3^-$] in blood, brain ECF and CSF are considered in Figure 5. During perfusion with a CSF of normal [HCO$_3^-$] (6 mM below that of plasma) there was zero net flux across the ependyma. This HCO$_3^-$ gradient between plasma and CSF seemed likely to be maintained by active transport either at the cerebral capillary-glial membrane (the probable blood-brain barrier) or at the ependymal linings of the ventricles. During ventriculo-cisternal perfusion with fluids of varying [HCO$_3^-$] a concentration gradient would be produced in brain ECF It was possible to find a point in this concentration gradient where ventilation became a linear function of the calculated interstitial pH for either position of the HCO$_3^-$ pump. To test these hypotheses concerning the position of the HCO$_3^-$ pump, Fencl, Miller and Pappenheimer (1966) studied a situation where the HCO$_3^-$ distribution ratio between CSF and plasma was altered chronically and naturally, that is during chronic metabolic acidosis alkalosis in conscious goats. Contrary to previous findings CSF pH varied slightly but continuously

of a concentration gradient through brain interstitial fluid. A plot of ventilation against arterial pH showed the normal shift of the response curve to the left in acidosis and to the right in alkalosis. When a similar plot was made against cisternal CSF pH, ventilation was a single function of pH. It was argued, therefore that since there was zero net flux of HCO$_3^-$ at the observed resting concentration gradient, CSF and brain ECF must, in these chronic states, be in equilibrium as regards pH and [HCO$_3^-$]. Ventilation will become a single function not only of CSF, but of brain ECF pH. The HCO$_3^-$ pump appeared therefore to be placed at the blood-brain barrier. Had the HCO$_3^-$ pump been placed at the ventricular ependyma, ventilation would not have been a single function of CSF pH during acidosis and alkalosis. To confirm these views Fencl *et al.* (1966) plotted ventilation against pH from two sets of data; first, the CSF pH during chronic acidosis and alkalosis and second, the calculated interstitial pH during perfusion with fluids of varying [HCO$_3^-$] and inhalation of CO$_2$. Ventilation was a single function of both sets of pH data; the respiratory chemoreceptor would therefore seem to be in brain ECF and during chronic acid-base derangements CSF and brain ECF were in equilibrium.

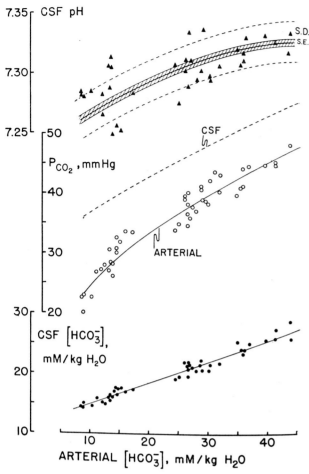

FIG. 6. [HCO₃⁻], pH and P_CO₂ in CSF and blood during chronic metabolic acidosis and alkalosis in goats. CSF pH varies continuously with plasma [HCO₃⁻]. Data obtained from five conscious goats breathing air. (From Fencl *et al.*, 1966. Reproduced by kind permission of the authors and the editors of *Am. J. Physiol.*)

This work has been dealt with at length since its implications are of extreme importance for the control of ventilation during all types of acid-base imbalance. The main conclusions arising from this work on the conscious goat are:

1. CSF pH varies with plasma [HCO₃⁻]. It is not controlled within normal limits during chronic metabolic acidosis and alkalosis.

2. The small changes observed in CSF pH during these chronic states could account for the changes in ventilation. There is, therefore, no necessity to postulate a role for the peripheral chemoreceptors.

3. The medullary chemoreceptor does not appear to be superficially placed with regard to CSF, but behaves as though situated in brain ECF.

4. During chronic metabolic acidosis and alkalosis ventricular CSF and brain ECF appear to be in equilibrium as regards pH and [HCO₃⁻] (since jugular venous P_CO₂ is equal to cisternal CSF P_CO₂, there is no gradient for P_CO₂).

This work is of exceptional value since all measurements were made on conscious animals. The small changes in CSF pH which produced extremes of ventilation in these

goats lay within the scatter of previous CSF pH measurements. Fencl *et al.* (1966) abstracted data from the literature and showed that a CSF pH derived from measured CSF [HCO₃⁻] and a calculated jugular venous P_CO₂ varied continuously with arterial [HCO₃⁻]. The view that CSF pH was completely controlled had arisen from an underestimate of the sensitivity of the medullary chemoreceptor and the scatter of pH measurements when compared with the small changes observed.

Pontén and Siesjö (1967) have confirmed that in chronic metabolic acidosis and alkalosis in rats, CSF pH varied continuously with that of plasma. Although CSF [HCO₃⁻] was linearly related to plasma [HCO₃⁻], the changes were only 35 per cent of those in plasma. The findings on the conscious goat have been confirmed in man by Fencl, Vale and Broch (1968). In chronic metabolic acidosis and alkalosis ventilation was a single function of lumbar CSF pH breathing air and CO₂ mixtures up to 6 per cent CO₂.

It would seem reasonable to conclude that CSF pH is controlled within narrower limits than arterial pH, but this control is not perfect. In comparing changes in the acid-base balance of blood, brain ECF and CSF, it is important to remember that equilibrium will be reached at different rates in each compartment. For this reason, data which do not apply to a steady state may be extremely difficult to interpret. Arterial pH, brain ECF pH, cisternal and lumbar CSF pH all change at different rates; therefore the selection of the time and site of sampling during a changing state may be critical in the interpretation of the results. Fisher and Christianson (1963) showed that lumbar CSF P_CO₂, changes lagged 10–20 min. behind those in cisternal CSF in man. Robin *et al.* (1958) showed that in acute metabolic alkalosis or acidosis CSF pH may move in the opposite direction to blood pH. As suggested by Pappenheimer (1965) these paradoxical changes may depend on the different rates of equilibration of HCO₃⁻ in brain ECF and CSF. A change in plasma [HCO₃⁻] may cause a relatively rapid change in brain ECF [HCO₃⁻]; if the respiratory chemoreceptor is in brain ECF this will produce a new level of ventilation and a change in P_CO₂. The change in P_CO₂ will result in stabilization of the pH in brain ECF at the new [HCO₃⁻]. The P_CO₂ will also change rapidly in CSF where the [HCO₃⁻] has not yet changed. CSF pH will therefore move paradoxically in the opposite direction to that of the plasma because of this delay in equilibration between brain ECF and CSF HCO₃⁻ will continue to diffuse passively into CSF until the entire CSF/brain ECF compartment is in equilibrium; CSF will then return from its paradoxical change within the [HCO₃⁻] becomes appropriate to the new P_CO₂. Changes in CSF composition may only be considered to represent changes in ECF during steady states.

The position regarding the central chemoreceptor is complex. It does not seem that a receptor placed superficially with regard to CSF can explain all the findings; nor can the area on the ventro-lateral surface of the medulla described by Mitchell *et al.* (1963) and confirmed by Cozine and Ngai (1967) be disregarded. Even if there is more than one receptor area it is clear that in steady states the central component of the chemical drive is determined by the pH in this compartment. During changing states, however, the situation will be complicated by the presence of concentration gradients for $HCO_3^-$ and pH between brain ECF and CSF. Ventricular CSF is, in all probability, not entirely homogeneous. For these reasons it is important to consider the nature of the exchanges between blood, brain and CSF and the contribution of these exchanges to the stability of CSF pH.

### 4. The Control of CSF pH

CSF pH is controlled within narrow limits; what mechanisms contribute to this control? From the preceding section it is clear that a respiratory receptor in the CSF/brain ECF compartment, sensitive to changes in pH will confer stability on CSF pH by producing appropriate changes in $P_{CO_2}$. This mechanism will not explain the observed stability of CSF pH in respiratory acidosis or alkalosis. It is necessary, therefore, to consider the contribution of two other mechanisms; first, that of variations in cerebral blood flow (CBF) and second, the role of ionic exchanges between blood, brain (ICF and ECF) and CSF. Such exchanges may take place by means of active or passive processes.

(i) **Changes in CBF.** The increase in CBF which is observed with increasing $P_{CO_2}$ will tend to reduce the brain a-v $P_{CO_2}$ difference. Since cisternal CSF is in equilibrium with jugular venous $P_{CO_2}$ (Bradley and Semple, 1962), this will tend to limit $P_{CO_2}$ changes in CSF and brain. A rise in CBF will reduce the $P_{CO_2}$ difference between CSF and blood, whereas a fall in CBF will increase this $P_{CO_2}$ gradient. How changes in $P_{CO_2}$ control CBF has been a matter of some controversy. It appears likely that brain ECF pH, or the ECF pH adjacent to arterioles may be the critical factor (Severinghaus, 1965a; Skinhøj, 1966; Betz and Heuser, 1967). If this is so, the control of CBF and ventilation may be interrelated by brain ECF pH and form a single homeostatic mechanism to limit pH changes in the environment of the brain. In respiratory alkalosis, for example, a fall in arterial, brain and ECF $P_{CO_2}$ will lead to a reduction in CBF and a fall in ventilation. Both changes tend to limit the rise in brain and CSF pH.

(ii) **Active and passive transfer between blood, brain and CSF.** The CSF is secreted by the choroid plexus although it is possible that fluid is secreted at other sites. Pollay and Curl (1967) have shown that during perfusion of the aqueduct of Sylvius (where there is no choroid plexus) a gain of fluid by the perfusate may be demonstrated. Bering and Sato (1963) showed by separate perfusion of the ventricles and subarachnoid space of dogs that up to 40 per cent of the CSF appeared to be secreted extra-ventricularly. This complicates the simple view that CSF is formed only in the choroid plexus, flows through the ventricles to the subarachnoid space, where it is absorbed through the arachnoid villi. Since the contribution of fluid secreted outside the choroid plexus is obscure, this simple view will be accepted for the purpose of this review. During its passage through the ventricular cavities CSF may be modified by equilibration with brain

ECF by exchanges across the blood-brain or blood-CSF barriers or by exchanges with brain ICF.

There is firm evidence that the secretion of the choroid plexus is formed by an active process, and that it is not a simple dialysate of plasma. Ames, Sakanoue and Endo (1964) collected the choroid plexus secretion and showed that it differed slightly but significantly from a plasma ultra-filtrate in the rabbit. Comparison of cisternal CSF with such an ultra-filtrate revealed that in its passage through the ventricles CSF had become even further removed from a simple dialysate. Ames, Higashi and Nesbett (1965) found that the $[K^+]$ of the choroid plexus secretions remained relatively constant in spite of imposed fluctuations in plasma $[K^+]$. It appears that CSF $[K^+]$ is controlled during the formation process. Unfortunately there are no available data on the $[HCO_3^-]$ or pH of the secretion, so that it is not known to what degree the control of CSF pH is effected during the formation process.

During its passage through the ventricles CSF attains equilibrium with brain ECF provided steady state conditions exist. The ventricular ependyma appears to present no diffusional barrier to small ions or even to molecules as large as inulin (Rall, Oppelt and Patlak, 1962). Exchanges between brain ICF and CSF or between brain ECF and CSF take place through the narrow extra-cellular clefts. Nicholls and Kuffler (1964) have shown that $K^+$, $Na^+$ and sucrose may move through the extra-cellular clefts of the leech CNS at speeds consistent with free diffusion. Rapid exchanges may well be expected between brain and CSF. Cohen, Gerschenfeld and Kuffler (1968) have estimated the $[K^+]$ in the ECF of the optic nerve in the amphibian Necturus; this was achieved by using the membrane potential of a glial cell as an index of the extracellular $[K^+]$ (the cell was used as a $K^+$ electrode). They found that brain ECF $[K^+]$ was equal to that in the CSF, and that both were similarly controlled when plasma $[K^+]$ was changed. This confirms directly that ionic equilibrium exists between CSF and brain ECF and supports the deductions of Fencl et al. (1966) regarding pH and $[HCO_3^-]$. The composition of the brain ECF/CSF compartment may be influenced by exchanges with blood across the blood-brain barrier, or by exchanges with brain ICF. The relative contribution of these two mechanisms represents one of the most complex aspects of this subject.

The distribution of ions between blood and CSF cannot be explained on the basis of a simple Donnan equilibrium. In order to study the distribution further it is essential to measure any potential difference that may exist between the two fluids. Under normal circumstances CSF is 4 mV positive to blood (Held, Fencl and Pappenheimer, 1964; Severinghaus, 1965b). Consideration of the electro-chemical gradients for the various ions between plasma and CSF shows that only $Ca^{++}$ and $Cl^-$ approach passive distribution (Held et al., 1964). $Na^+$ and $Mg^{++}$ appear to be transported from blood to CSF, while $K^+$ and $HCO_3^-$ are transported from CSF to blood. The CSF-blood potential was found to vary with blood pH; the CSF becoming more positive as blood pH fell.

It has been postulated that this might represent a mechanism which would stabilize CSF pH, since in acidosis the increased positivity of the CSF would increase the passage $HCO_3^-$ into the CSF.

Both Severinghaus (1965b) and Pappenheimer (1965) attribute changes in the CSF [$HCO_3^-$] to active transport across the blood-brain barrier. Siesjö and Pontén (1966) produced evidence that such changes might be explained by exchanges between brain ECF and ICF. During chronic metabolic acidosis and alkalosis in rats there were changes in CSF [$HCO_3^-$]; derivation of intracellular [$HCO_3^-$] revealed that the changes in this compartment were in the opposite direction to those in the CSF. They postulated that CSF [$HCO_3^-$] was adjusted by a redistribution between brain ECF and ICF, rather than transport across the blood-brain barrier.

The importance of exchanges between brain and CSF is emphasized by the finding that during respiratory alkalosis there is an increase in CSF lactate concentration (Leusen and Demeester, 1966). The increase in CSF lactate occurs independently of changes in blood lactate and correlates well with an increase in brain lactate. It seems probable that it occurs as a result of cerebral hypoxia during hyper-ventilation. In respiratory alkalosis there is a fall in CBF and this may be sufficiently severe, when $P_{CO_2}$ falls to values of about 20 mm. Hg, to produce tissue hypoxia. This observation throws doubt on the hypothesis (Severinghaus et al., 1963) that the fall in CSF [$HCO_3^-$] during altitude acclimatization is due to transport of $HCO_3^-$ across the blood-brain barrier, since the accumulation of lactate could account for the fall in [$HCO_3^-$]. Cotev, Cullen and Severinghaus (1968) investigated the changes in brain ECF pH and [$HCO_3^-$] in anaesthetized dogs while hypoxia was induced at a normal and low $P_{CO_2}$. It was found that the fall in ECF [$HCO_3^-$] was similar whether the $P_{CO_2}$ was held constant or allowed to fall. In profound hypoxia the CSF became acidotic and there was no evidence of pH regulation. It was presumed that the fall in ECF [$HCO_3^-$] in the dogs with a constant $P_{CO_2}$ was due to $H^+$ diffusion into the ECF from an intracellular lactic acidosis. It is clear that changes in CSF [$HCO_3^-$] during acidosis and alkalosis cannot be entirely attributed to CSF/plasma exchanges. The role of exchanges between brain and CSF are not at this time fully understood. Until new evidence accumulates it must be assumed that the control of CSF pH results from complex interchanges between CSF and plasma and between brain ICF and the brain ECF/CSF compartment.

## 5. Aortic and Carotid Chemoreceptors

Changes in pulmonary ventilation due to alterations in $PA_{O_2}$ are mediated through the peripheral chemoreceptors. Only when the $PA_{O_2}$ rises above about 170 mm. Hg is there no detectable chemical drive to ventilation from the $PA_{O_2}$. The proportion of the total chemical drive to ventilation when breathing air arising from a $P_{O_2}$ stimulus has been estimated to be about 10 per cent in man (Dejours et al., 1958; Downes and Lambertsen, 1966), though this is probably an underestimate (Dejours, 1962). Electrophysiological studies have shown that changes in arterial $P_{O_2}$, $P_{CO_2}$ and pH will all stimulate the peripheral chemoreceptors (Dejours, 1962; Comroe, 1964). The quantitative assessment of the effect of these stimuli on respiration in the intact animal is difficult and complex. Two experimental techniques have been used to evaluate the contribution of the peripheral chemoreceptors to the total chemical drive to respiration. Firstly the effect on ventilation of denervating the carotid and aortic chemoreceptors may be investigated in animals. Using this technique the respiratory response to hypoxia and $CO_2$ may be measured both before and after denervation, as well as the resting ventilation breathing air. Second, the immediate respiratory effects of changes in the $P_{CO_2}$ or $P_{O_2}$ of the inhaled gas can be measured in animals and man. The alterations in ventilation during the first few seconds after such a change are presumed to reflect changes in peripheral chemoreceptor activity; later alterations in ventilation are attributed to the activation of central mechanisms. Both experimental techniques are unsatisfactory; carotid sinus denervation may interfere with other reflexes, and, in acute experiments dissection and manipulation of tissues may change the blood supply and environment of the chemoreceptors, thereby altering their discharge before denervation (Comroe, 1964; Paintal, 1968). The second test is indirect and based on assumptions which cannot be rigorously tested. It is not surprising therefore that the results from such experiments are inexact and often contradictory. Although it is not possible to consider the results in detail here, it is our view that the peripheral chemoreceptors make a significant contribution to the chemical drive to respiration in man when breathing air, $CO_2$ mixtures with 21 per cent $O_2$ or gas mixtures of low $O_2$ content.

There is no detectable drive to ventilation from the peripheral chemoreceptors in man when the arterial $P_{CO_2}$ is normal and the $PA_{O_2}$ over 200 mm. Hg. This is also true for animals although Hesser (1949) found a very small drop in ventilation after "cold block" of the sinus nerve in anaesthetized dogs breathing a high $O_2$ mixture. When $PA_{O_2}$ is below 170 mm. Hg a peripheral chemoreceptor drive from $P_{CO_2}$ becomes detectable. This is probably because interaction occurs between $P_{O_2}$ and $P_{CO_2}$ as stimuli to breathing, this interaction being more than additive (Cunningham, Patrick and Lloyd, 1964). The multiplicative component of the combined stimulus may arise at the peripheral chemoreceptors or centrally in the medulla (Torrance, 1968). Breathing air, the combined stimulus to the peripheral chemoreceptors from $O_2$ and $CO_2$ has been estimated to be between 24 per cent (Fitzgerald et al., 1964) in the anaesthetized dog and 30 per cent (Dejours, 1962) in conscious dogs.

The contribution of the peripheral chemoreceptors to the increase in ventilation produced by the administration of $CO_2$ in 21 per cent $O_2$ (balance nitrogen) is more difficult to assess quantitatively. Gesell, Lapides and Levin (1940) and Hesser (1949) concluded from their experiments on anaesthetized dogs that the peripheral chemoreflex drive was only appreciable when the inspired $CO_2$ concentration was 3 per cent or less; at 6 per cent $CO_2$ the chemoreflex drive was entirely central. This was not the finding of

Bouverot *et al.* (1965) in unanaesthetized dogs; following chemodenervation the respiratory response to the administration of 3 per cent and 5 per cent $CO_2$ for 4 min. was considerably reduced. Following chemodenervation, however, the animals were hypercapnic when breathing air; it is known that chronic hypercapnia reduces the respiratory sensitivity to $CO_2$. This loss of $CO_2$ sensitivity is almost certainly due to a change in the central response to $CO_2$, so that the contribution of the peripheral chemoreceptors in these experiments cannot be assessed with certainty. Both Bernards, Dejours and Lacaisse (1966) and Lambertsen, Gelfand and Kemp (1965) have analysed in man the respiratory changes at the start and end of $CO_2$ administration in terms of the interplay of a fast chemoreceptor ventilatory drive and of a delayed central ventilatory drive. Lambertsen *et al.* (1965) have estimated, from the fall in ventilation immediately after the cessation of 5 per cent $CO_2$ administration, that the contribution of the peripheral chemoreceptors is 12 per cent of the total chemical drive to ventilation.

These experimental results suggest that the contribution of the peripheral chemoreceptors to the control of ventilation in man and animals breathing air is appreciable. The emphasis placed in this section on the role of the peripheral chemoreceptors might be considered to be at variance with the postulate of Fencl *et al.* (1966) that the small change in CSF pH during chronic states of acid-base imbalance could account for the observed changes in ventilation, no role of the peripheral chemoreceptors being envisaged. This work dealt with chronic states and does not exclude a significant contribution from the peripheral chemoreceptors in acute acid-base disturbances. Alternatively, if the views of Mitchell (1966) are accepted, the peripheral chemoreceptors play an important role in the control of breathing in acute and chronic acid-base derangements.

The most important role of the peripheral chemoreceptors in the regulation of respiration is that of a fine and rapidly acting control mechanism. Small and rapid changes in arterial $P_{CO_2}$ are less likely to be attenuated in transmission from blood to the site of chemical excitation in the carotid sinus, than in transmission to the corresponding site in the medulla. In metabolic acid-base disturbances stimulation of breathing due to changes in plasma $[HCO_3^-]$ and hence pH, is likely to be slower than in respiratory disturbances because of the delay in movement of $HCO_3^-$ between blood and brain ECF. However, pH changes in the ECF of the carotid sinus in metabolic disturbances may well be much faster than in the medulla and complete after about 1 hour (Hornbein and Roos, 1963). Thus in all acid-base disturbances, whether respiratory or metabolic, the immediate changes in respiration may be due primarily to alterations in peripheral chemoreceptor activity.

## 6. Clinical Application in Anaesthesia

The effect of changes in $PA_{CO_2}$ on the cerebral blood flow and the composition of the CSF may be of clinical importance to the anaesthetist in his choice of inspired gases and in determining the level of ventilation, and hence $P_{CO_2}$, to be maintained during anaesthesia.

Hyperventilation for several hours may lead to reduction in the $[HCO_3^-]$ of the CSF secondary to the fall in $P_{CO_2}$. Following anaesthesia, when the $P_{CO_2}$ rises, the CSF will be more acid for any given $P_{CO_2}$ because of the reduced $[HCO_3^-]$. The central chemical drive would be greater, for any $P_{CO_2}$, than before anaesthesia and might help to maintain pulmonary ventilation at a higher level postoperatively until the $[HCO_3^-]$ of the CSF returns to its normal concentration. Hyperventilation may lead to cerebral hypoxia even when the inspired concentration of $O_2$ is high (Cohen, Alexander and Wollman, 1968; Betz, Pickerodt and Weidner, 1968; Granholm, Lukjanova and Siesjö, 1968). The further reduction in CSF $[HCO_3^-]$ due to lactic acid production by the hypoxic brain might further enhance the postoperative chemical drive to breathing. Against this advantage must be weighed the possible damage due to cerebral hypoxia which might be of special importance in the elderly with cerebrovascular disease. The harmful effects of a reduction in cerebral blood flow might be avoided however by the use of an anaesthetic agent such as halothane which is known to produce a considerable decrease in cerebrovascular resistance (Alexander *et al.*, 1964).

Relative hypoventilation during anaesthesia with a high inspired $O_2$ concentration would avoid the dangers of cerebral hypoxia. However, a high $P_{CO_2}$ might lead to a rise in $[HCO_3^-]$ of the CSF and thus to a decreased chemical drive to breathing after anaesthesia.

The choice of anaesthetic agents, inspired gas concentration and the level of ventilation will depend on many other factors not considered in this discussion. This chapter has been concerned with some of the factors concerned with the physiology of the CSF, cerebral blood flow and brain metabolism which are of importance to the anaesthetist.

## REFERENCES

Alexander, S. C., Wollman, H., Cohen, P. J., Chase, P. E. and Behar, M. (1964), "Cerebrovascular Response to $P_{A CO_2}$ during Halothane Anaesthesia in Man," *J. appl. Physiol.*, **19**, 561–565.

Ames, A., Higashi, K. and Nesbett, F. B. (1965), "Relation of Potassium Concentration in Choroid Plexus Fluid to that in Plasma," *J. Physiol. (Lond.)*, **181**, 506–515.

Ames, A., Sakanoue, M. and Endo, S. (1964), "Na, K, Ca, Mg and Cl Concentrations in Choroid Plexus Fluid and Cisternal Fluid Compared with Plasma Ultrafiltrate," *J. Neurophysiol.*, **27**, 672–681.

Bering, E. A. and Sato, O. (1963), "Hydrocephalus: Changes in Formation and Absorption of Cerebrospinal Fluid within the Cerebral Ventricles," *J. Neurosurg.*, **20**, 1050–1063.

Bernards, J. A., Dejours, P. and Lacaisse, A. (1966), "Ventilatory Effects in Man of Breathing Successively $CO_2$-free, $CO_2$-enriched and $CO_2$-free Mixtures with Low, Normal or High Oxygen Concentration," *Resp. Physiol.*, **1**, 390–397.

Betz, E. and Heuser, D. (1967), "Cerebral Cortical Blood Flow During Changes of Acid-base Equilibrium of the Brain," *J. appl. Physiol.*, **23**, 726–733.

Betz, E., Pickerodt, V. and Weidner, A. (1968), "Respiratory Alkalosis: Effect on C.B.F., $PO_2$ and Acid/base Relations in Cerebral Cortex with a Note on Water Content," *Scand. J. Lab. & Clin. Invest.*, Suppl. 102, IVD.

Bouverot, P., Flandrois, R., Puccinelli, R. and Dejours, P. (1965), "Étude du role des chémorécepteurs artériels dans la régulation de la respiration pulmonaire chez le chien éveillé," *Arch. int. Pharmacodyn.*, **157**, 253–271.

Bradley, R. D. and Semple, S. J. G. (1962), "A Comparison of Certain

Acid-base Characteristics of Arterial Blood, Jugular Venous Blood and Cerebrospinal Fluid in Man, and the Effect on them of some Acute and Chronic Acid-base Disturbances," *J. Physiol.*, (*Lond.*), 160, 381–391.

Bradley, R. D., Semple, S. J. G. and Spencer, G. T. (1965), "Rate of Change of Carbon Dioxide Tension in Arterial Blood, Jugular Venous Blood and Cisternal Cerebrospinal Fluid on Carbon Dioxide Administration," *J. Physiol.* (*Lond.*), 179, 442–455.

Campbell, E. J. M. (1966), "The Relationship of the Sensation of Breathlessness to the Act of Breathing," in *Breathlessness*, ed. Howell, J. B. L. and Campbell, E. J. M., pp. 55–64. Oxford: Blackwell.

Cestan, R., Sendrail, M. and Lasalle, H. (1925), "Les modifications de l'équilibre acide-base du liquide céphalorachidien, dans les acidoses expérimentales," *C.R. Soc. Biol., Paris*, 93, 475–478.

Clark, T. J. H. (1968), "The Ventilatory Response to $CO_2$ in Chronic Airways Obstruction Measured by a Rebreathing Method," *Clin. Sci.*, 34, 559–568.

Cohen, P. J., Alexander, S. C. and Wollman, H. (1968), "Effects of Hypocarbia and of Hypoxia with Normocarbia on Cerebral Blood Flow and Metabolism in Man," *Scand. J. Lab. & Clin. Invest.*, Suppl. 102, IVA.

Cohen, M. W., Gerschenfeld, H. M. and Kuffler, S. W. (1968), "Ionic Environment of Neurones and Glial Cells in the Brain of an Amphibian," *J. Physiol.* (*Lond.*), 197, 363–380.

Collip, J. B. and Backus, P. L. (1920), "The Alkali Reserve of the Blood Plasma, Spinal Fluid and Lymph," *Amer. J. Physiol.*, 51, 551–567.

Comroe, J. H. (1943), "The Effects of Direct and Electrical Stimulation of the Respiratory Center in the Cat," *Amer. J. Physiol.*, 139, 490–498.

Comroe, J. H. (1964), "The Peripheral Chemoreceptors," in *Handbook of Physiology*, Section 3, Respiration 1, ed. Fenn, W. O. and Rahn, H. Chap. 23. Washington, D.C.: American Physiological Society.

Cotev, S., Cullen, D. and Severinghaus, J. W. (1968), "Cerebral E.C.F. Acidosis Induced by Hypoxia at Normal and Low $P_{CO_2}$," *Scand. J. Lab. & Clin. Invest.*, Suppl. 102, IIIE.

Coxon, R. V. and Swanson, A. G. (1965), "Movement of [$^{14}$C] Bicarbonate from Blood to Cerebrospinal Fluid and Brain," *J. Physiol.* (*Lond.*), 181, 712–727.

Cozine, R. A. and Ngai, S. H. (1967), "Medullary Surface Chemoreceptors and Regulation of Respiration in the Cat," *J. appl. Physiol.*, 22, 117–121.

Cunningham, D. J. C., Patrick, J. M. and Lloyd, B. B. (1964), "The Respiratory Response of Man to Hypoxia," in *Oxygen in the Animal Organism*, ed. Dickens, F. and Neil, E., pp. 277–291. Oxford: Pergamon.

Dejours, P. (1962), "Chemoreflexes in Breathing," *Physiol. Rev.*, 42, 335–358.

Dejours, P., Labrousse, Y., Raynaud, J., Girard, F. and Teillac, A. (1958), "Stimulus oxygène de la ventilation au repos et au cours de l'exercise musculaire, à basse altitude (50 m.) chez l'homme," *Revue fr. Étud. Clin. biol.*, 3, 105–123.

Downes, J. J. and Lambertsen, C. J. (1966), "Dynamic Characteristics of Ventilatory Depression in Man on Abrupt Administration of $O_2$," *J. appl. Physiol.*, 21, 447–453.

Fencl, V., Miller, T. B. and Pappenheimer, J. R. (1966), "Studies on the Respiratory Response to Disturbances of Acid-base Balance, with Deductions Concerning the Ionic Composition of Cerebral Interstitial Fluid," *Amer. J. Physiol.*, 210, 459–472.

Fencl, V., Vale, J. R. and Broch, J. R. (1968), "Cerebral Blood Flow and Pulmonary Ventilation in Metabolic Acidosis and Alkalosis," *Scand. J. Lab. & Clin. Invest.*, Suppl. 102, VIIIB.

Fisher, V. J. and Christianson, L. C. (1963), "Cerebrospinal Fluid Acid-base Balance during a Changing Ventilatory State in Man," *J. appl. Physiol.*, 18, 712–716.

Fitzgerald, R. S., Zajtchuk, J. T., Penman, R. W. B. and Perkins, J. F. (1964), "Ventilatory Response to Transient Perfusion of Carotid Chemoreceptors," *Amer. J. Physiol.*, 207, 1305–1313.

Florez, J. and Borison, H. L. (1967), "Tidal Volume in $CO_2$ Regulation; Peripheral Denervations and Ablation of Area Postrema," *Amer. J. Physiol.*, 212, 985–991.

Gesell, R. (1923), "On the Chemical Regulation of Respiration, 1. The Regulation of Respiration with Special Reference to the Metabolism of the Respiratory Center and the Coördination of the Dual Function of Hemoglobin," *Amer. J. Physiol.*, 66, 5–49.

Gesell, R. and Hertzmann, A. B. (1926), "The Regulation of Respiration, IV. Tissue Acidity, Blood Acidity and Pulmonary Ventilation. A study of the effects of semipermeability of membranes and the buffering action of tissues with the continuous method of recording changes in acidity," *Amer. J. Physiol.*, 78, 610–629.

Gesell, R., Lapides, J. and Levin, M. (1940), "The Interaction of Central and Peripheral Chemical Control of Breathing," *Amer. J. Physiol.*, 130, 155–170.

Granholm, L., Lukjanova, L. and Siesjö, B. (1968), "Evidence of Cerebral Hypoxia in Pronounced Hyperventilation," *Scand. J. Lab. & Clin. Invest.*, Suppl. 102, IVC.

Guz, A., Noble, M. I. M., Widdicombe, J. G., Trenchard, D. and Mushin, W. W. (1966), "The Effect of Bilateral Block of Vagus and Glossopharyngeal Nerves on the Ventilatory Response to $CO_2$ of Conscious Man," *Resp. Physiol.*, 1, 206–210.

Held, D., Fencl, V. and Pappenheimer, J. R. (1964), "Electrical Potential of Cerebrospinal Fluid," *J. Neurophysiol.*, 27, 942–959.

Hesser, C. M. (1949), "Central and Chemoreflex Components in the Respiratory Activity during Acid-base Displacements in the Blood," *Acta physiol. Scand.*, 18, Suppl. 64.

Hooker, D. R., Wilson, D. W. and Connett, H. (1917), "The Perfusion of the Mammalian Medulla; the Effect of Carbon Dioxide and Other Substances on the Respiratory and Cardiovascular Centers," *Amer. J. Physiol.*, 43, 351–361.

Hornbein, T. F. and Roos, A. (1963), "Specificity of H ion Concentration as a Carotid Chemoreceptor Stimulus," *J. appl. Physiol.*, 18, 580–584.

Jacobs, M. H. (1920a), "To What Extent are the Physiological Effects of Carbon Dioxide due to Hydrogen Ions?" *Amer. J. Physiol.*, 51, 321–331.

Jacobs, M. H. (1920b), "The Production of Intracellular Acidity by Neutral and Alkaline Solutions containing Carbon Dioxide," *Amer. J. Physiol.*, 53, 457–463.

Kim, J. K. and Carpenter, F. G. (1961), "Excitation of Medullary Neurons by Chemical Agents," *Amer. J. Physiol.*, 201, 1187–1190.

Lambertsen, C. J., Gelfand, R. and Kemp, R. A. (1965), "Dynamic Response Characteristics of Several $CO_2$-reactive Components of the Respiratory Control System," in *Cerebrospinal Fluid and the Regulation of Ventilation*, ed. Brooks, C. McC., Kao, F. F. and Lloyd, B. B., pp. 211–240. Oxford: Blackwell.

Leusen, I. (1954a), "Chemosensitivity of the Respiratory Center. Influence of $CO_2$ in the Cerebral Ventricles on Respiration," *Amer. J. Physiol.*, 176, 39–44.

Leusen, I. (1954b), "Chemosensitivity of the Respiratory Center. Influence of Changes in the $H^+$ and total Buffer Concentrations in the Cerebral Ventricles on Respiration," *Amer. J. Physiol.*, 176, 45–51.

Leusen, I. and Demeester, G. (1966), "Lactate and Pyruvate in the Brain of Rats during Hyperventilation," *Arch. Int. Physiol. Biochem.*, 74, 25–34.

Loeschcke, H. H. (1965) "A Concept of the Role of Intracranial Chemosensitivity in Respiratory Control," in *Cerebrospinal Fluid and the Regulation of Ventilation*, ed. Brooks, C. McC., Kao, F. F. and Lloyd, B. B. pp. 183–207. Oxford: Blackwell.

Mitchell, R. A. (1966), "Cerebrospinal Fluid and the Regulation of Respiration," in *Advances in Respiratory Physiology*, ed. Caro, C. G., pp. 1–47. London: Arnold.

Mitchell, R. A., Bainton, C. R., Severinghaus, J. W. and Edelist, G. (1964), "Respiratory Response and C.S.F. pH during Disturbances in Blood Acid-base Balance in Awake Dogs with Denervated Aortic and Carotid Bodies," *Physiologist*, 7, 208.

Mitchell, R. A., Carman, C. T., Severinghaus, J. W., Richardson, B. W., Singer, M. M. and Shnider, S. (1965), "Stability of Cerebrospinal Fluid pH in Chronic Acid-base Disturbances in Blood," *J. appl. Physiol.*, 20, 443–452.

Mitchell, R. A., Loeschcke, H. H., Massion, W. H. and Severinghaus, J. W. (1963), "Respiratory Responses Mediated through Superficial Chemosensitive Area on the Medulla," *J. appl. Physiol.*, 18, 523–533.

Mitchell, R. A., Massion, W. H., Carman, C. T. and Severinghaus, J. W. (1960), "Fourth Ventricle Respiratory Chemosensitivity and the Area Postrema," *Fed. Proc.*, **19**, 374.

Newsom Davis, J. (1967), "Contribution of Somatic Receptors in the Chest Wall to Detection of Added Inspiratory Airway Resistance," *Clin. Sci.*, **33**, 249–260.

Nicholls, J. G. and Kuffler, S. W. (1964), "Extracellular Space as a Pathway for Exchange between Blood and Neurons in the Central Nervous System of the Leech: Ionic Composition of Glial Cells and Neurons," *J. Neurophysiol.*, **27**, 645–671.

Paintal, A. S. (1968), "The Possible Influence of the External Environment on the Responses of Chemoreceptors," in *Arterial Chemoreceptors*, ed. Torrance, R. W., pp. 149–151. Oxford: Blackwell.

Pappenheimer, J. R. (1965), "The Ionic Composition of Cerebral Extracellular Fluid and its Relation to Control of Breathing," *Harvey Lect.*, Ser. 61, 71–94.

Pappenheimer, J. R., Fencl, V., Heisey, S. R. and Held, D. (1965), "Role of Cerebral Fluids in Control of Respiration as Studied in Unanaesthetized Goats," *Amer. J. Physiol.*, **208**, 436–450.

Pollay, M. and Curl, F. (1967), "Secretion of Cerebrospinal Fluid by the Ventricular Ependyma of the Rabbit," *Amer. J. Physiol.*, **213**, 1031–1038.

Pontén, U. and Siesjö, B. K. (1967), "Acid-base Relations in Arterial Blood and Cerebrospinal Fluid of the Unanaesthetized Rat," *Acta physiol. Scand.*, **71**, 89–95.

Posner, J. B., Swanson, A. G. and Plum, F. (1965), "Acid-base Balance in Cerebrospinal Fluid," *Arch. Neurol.*, **12**, 479–496.

Rall, D. P., Oppelt, W. W. and Patlak, C. S. (1962), "Extracellular Space of Brain as Determined by Diffusion of Inulin from the Ventricular System," *Life Sciences*, **1**, 43–48.

Robin, E. D., Whaley, R. D., Crump, C. H., Bickelmann, A. G. and

Travis, D. M. (1958), "Acid-base Relations between Spinal Fluid and Arterial Blood with Special Reference to Control of Ventilation," *J. appl. Physiol.*, **13**, 385–392.

Scott, R. W. (1918), "The Significance of Undissociated Carbon Dioxide in Respiration," *Amer. J. Physiol.*, **47**, 43–59.

Severinghaus, J. W. (1964), "Active Transport Regulation of C.S.F. H+ with Altitude Acclimatization Hypocapnia Despite Alkalization," *Fed. Proc.*, **23**, 259.

Severinghaus, J. W. (1965a), "Role of Cerebrospinal Fluid pH in Normalization of Cerebral Blood Flow in Chronic Hypocapnia," *Acta neurol. Scand.*, Suppl. 14, 116–120.

Severinghaus, J. W. (1965b), "Electrochemical Gradients for Hydrogen and Bicarbonate Ions Across the Blood-C.S.F. Barrier in Response to Acid-base Balance Changes," in *Cerebrospinal Fluid and the Regulation of Ventilation*, ed. Brooks, C. McC., Kao, F. F. and Lloyd, B. B., pp. 247–258. Oxford: Blackwell.

Severinghaus, J. W., Mitchell, R. A., Richardson, B. W. and Singer, M. M. (1963), "Respiratory Control at High Altitude Suggesting Active Transport Regulation of C.S.F. pH," *J. appl. Physiol.*, **18**, 1156–1166.

Siesjö, B. K. and Pontén, U. (1966), "Acid-base Changes in the Brain in Non-respiratory Acidosis and Alkalosis," *Expl. Brain Res.*, **2**, 176–190.

Skinhøj, E. (1966), "Regulation of Cerebral Blood Flow as a Single Function of the Interstitial pH in the Brain," *Acta neurol. Scand.*, **42**, 604–607.

Torrance, R. W. (1968), "Prolegomena," in *Arterial Chemoreceptors*, ed. Torrance, R. W., pp. 1–40. Oxford: Blackwell.

Winterstein, H. (1911), "Die Regulierung der Atmung durch das Blut " *Pflügers Arch. ges. Physiol.* **138**, 167–184.

Winterstein H. (1921), "Die Reaktionstheorie der Atmungsregulation," *Pflügers Arch. ges. Physiol.*, **187**, 293–298.

*CHAPTER 2*

# THE MECHANICS OF VENTILATION

## M. K. SYKES

The ventilation of the lungs is determined by the activity of the respiratory centre and by the balance of forces acting across the lungs and chest wall; the latter aspect forms the subject of this chapter.

The *transpulmonary gradient*, that is the pressure difference from the alveoli to the pleural space, influences lung size. An increase in this gradient increases the lung volume. Similarly the *transmural gradient*, the pressure difference from the pleural space to the outside of the chest wall when muscle tone is absent, determines the expansion of the thoracic cage.

The forces opposing deformation of the thorax are determined by the static and dynamic properties of the lungs, airways and the chest wall. The static, or elastic, component is described by the relation between the applied force (change in pressure gradient) and the displacement produced (change in volume). This relationship, which is independent of time, is known as the *compliance*:

$$\text{compliance (l. per cm. } H_2O)$$
$$= \frac{\text{change in volume (litres)}}{\text{change in pressure gradient (cm. } H_2O)}$$

The dynamic, or non-elastic, component, is defined by the relation between the applied force (pressure gradient) and the rate of displacement (volume flow rate):

$$\text{non-elastic resistance (cm. } H_2O \text{ per litre per second)}$$
$$= \frac{\text{pressure gradient (cm. } H_2O)}{\text{rate of volume change (l. per second)}}$$

Since this relation involves a rate of change it is obviously time dependent.

## STATIC PROPERTIES

*Lungs.* The retractive forces which tend to cause collapse of the lung are the elasticity of the lung parenchyma and the liquid-gas interface in the alveolus. In the normal lung the surface tension forces generated at this interface are minimized by the presence of a complex lipo-protein known as surfactant: as a result the contribution of each component to the total retractive force is approximately the same.

When the lungs are removed from the thorax they contract to a volume which is well below the residual volume (i.e. the volume reached after a maximal expiration in the intact chest). A transpulmonary pressure gradient of 2–3 cm. $H_2O$ must therefore exist at the residual volume to maintain the lungs at this degree of expansion. To expand

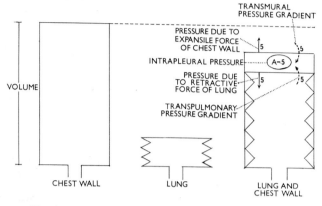

FIG. 1. Pressure gradients across lung and chest wall at the resting expiratory position (FRC). The resting position of the isolated lung and chest wall are also shown. Pressures in cm. $H_2O$. A = atmospheric pressure so that A-5 = 5 cm. $H_2O$ below atmospheric pressure.

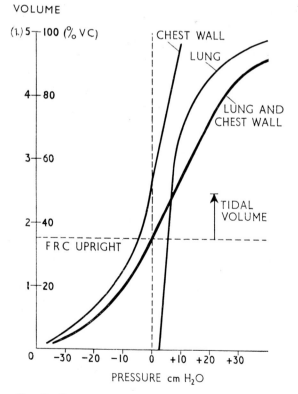

FIG. 2. Pressure-volume diagram of lungs, chest wall and lung-chest wall combination in erect position. A transpulmonary pressure gradient of 5 cm. $H_2O$ is required to inflate the lung to the resting expiratory level (FRC). This is balanced by an equal and opposite pressure gradient across the chest wall. The transthoracic pressure gradient at this position is zero. As the chest is expanded the transpulmonary and transthoracic gradients increase whilst the transmural gradient decreases towards zero, reaches zero at its own resting expiratory position and then increases.

the lungs to the normal resting expiratory position (functional residual capacity) this gradient must be increased (Figures 1 and 2). Over most of the range of lung expansion encountered in the intact chest the volume increment which results from unit pressure change across the lung (i.e. the compliance) is constant and equal to about 0·2 l./cm. $H_2O$. However at the upper limit of chest expansion smaller volume changes result from given increments of pressure. This reduction in lung compliance governs the upper limit of the vital capacity in the normal person.

*Airways.* The airways form an integral part of the lung structure and expand, both in length and diameter, in proportion to the rest of the lung parenchyma.

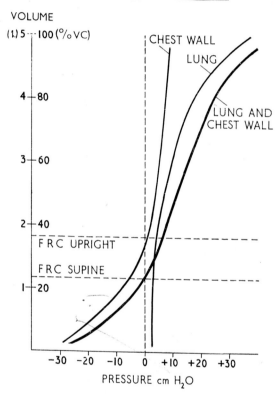

FIG. 3. Pressure-volume diagram of lungs, chest wall and lung-chest wall combination in supine position. The weight of the abdominal contents causes a shift of the chest wall pressure/volume plot and a reduction in FRC.

*Chest Wall.* The mobile portions of the chest wall are the rib cage and diaphragm. Throughout most of the range of chest movement in the upright position the compliance of the chest wall is constant and approximately equal to that of the lungs, i.e. 0·2 l. per cm. $H_2O$. However, below the resting expiratory level the pressure/volume plot becomes curved, smaller changes in volume resulting from unit changes of pressure. It is this factor which largely governs the volume of air left in the lungs of a normal patient after a maximal expiration.

In the mid-range of lung inflation the pressure/volume relationships of the lung and chest wall are reasonably linear and of approximately equal magnitude. To expand the thorax by 0·2 l. it is necessary to apply a pressure gradient of 1 cm. $H_2O$ across the lung and 1 cm. $H_2O$ across the chest wall. The compliance of the thorax is therefore

$$\frac{0 \cdot 2}{1 + 1} = 0 \cdot 1 \, \text{l./cm. } H_2O \quad \text{i.e.} \quad \frac{1}{C_T} = \frac{1}{C_{CW}} + \frac{1}{C_L}$$

where $C_T$ = total thoracic compliance

$C_{CW}$ = chest wall compliance

$C_L$ = lung compliance

As already mentioned the pressure/volume relationships of lung and chest wall are not linear at the extremes of lung volume. This leads to alinearity in the pressure/volume plot for the complete thorax (Figure 2). Although this is not of any clinical importance, since the greatest alinearity is outside the normal tidal volume range, it does lead to difficulties when comparing compliance values obtained by different authors. For example, the value obtained at a pressure of 30 cm. $H_2O$ will be less than one obtained at 10 or 5 cm. $H_2O$.

### Factors Determining the Normal Resting Expiratory Position of the Thorax

*Upright.* From Figure 2 it can be seen that at the normal resting expiratory position there is a transpulmonary pressure gradient of 5 cm. $H_2O$ tending to hold the lung inflated. If the respiratory muscles are relaxed this gradient must be balanced by an equal and opposite gradient

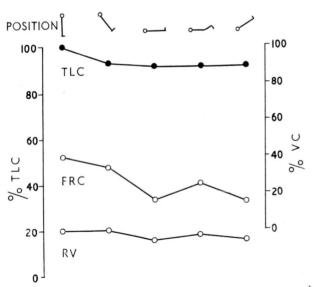

FIG. 4. Alterations in total lung capacity (TLC), vital capacity (VC), functional residual capacity (FRC) and residual volume (RV) with posture. Data from Agostini and Mead (1964).

across the chest wall. Such a gradient is developed by the natural elasticity of the chest wall as it is pulled inwards from its own resting position. Since the transmural gradient at the point of balance must equal the transpulmonary gradient (5 cm. $H_2O$), and since the chest wall compliance is 0.2 l./cm. $H_2O$, it can be calculated that the

chest wall must be $0.2 \times 5 = 1.0$ l. below its own resting position when it is pulled inwards by the lungs. (This is equivalent to a change of position from 55 per cent to 35 per cent of the vital capacity.) At the resting position, therefore, there is an intra-pleural pressure 5 cm. $H_2O$ below atmospheric pressure and there are transpulmonary and transmural gradients of 5 cm. $H_2O$ maintaining the balance between the retractive force of the lung and the expansile force of the chest wall.

Since the resting expiratory position is determined by the point at which the opposing pressure gradients across the lungs and chest wall are in balance it follows that any alteration in compliance of either lungs or chest wall will alter the resting expiratory position. Thus if lung compliance is reduced, for example by atelectasis, the pressure gradient required to maintain a given lung volume will be increased. The point of balance will therefore only be achieved at a lower lung volume: this will predispose to further atelectasis. On the other hand if lung compliance is increased, as in emphysema or old age, the lung retractive force will be decreased and the resting expiratory level will be greater than normal.

*Supine.* In the upright position the chest is relatively little affected by the weight of the abdominal contents or chest wall. However as the subject changes to a more recumbent position the gravitational effects of abdomen and chest wall become more important.

The major effects are due to the pressure exerted by the abdominal contents on the diaphragm. At the end of expiration there is negligible electrical activity in the muscle of the diaphragm and its position is determined by the pressure gradient between the abdominal and pleural cavities. Mechanically, the abdomen behaves like a bag containing fluid and, in the upright position, there is a gradient of pressure from the top to the bottom of the abdomen. The level at which this pressure equals atmospheric depends on the equilibrium between the elastic forces of the abdominal wall and thorax, and the gravitational force of the abdominal contents. At the resting end-expiratory position in the standing posture the zero point lies about 4 cm. below the dome of the diaphragm. When the subject is supine the zero level corresponds with the ventral wall of the abdomen. The weight of the abdominal contents thus supplements the retractive force of the lung and the diaphragm rises into the chest. The final point of balance is then determined by the elasticity of the diaphragm itself. In the prone position the zero point corresponds with the dorsal abdominal wall whilst in the lateral position it is mid-way between the two sides. These changes in the gravitational effects of the abdominal contents are chiefly responsible for the alterations in functional residual capacity (FRC) with posture (Figures 2, 3 and 4). Further changes may be induced by alterations in intra-abdominal pressure due to air, fluid, tumour or external pressure.

### Pressure Gradients During Inflation of the Lungs

Since the full significance of a pressure/volume diagram is often difficult to comprehend a further diagram (Figure

5) has been included to illustrate the changes in pressure gradient during inflation of the lungs.

Figure 5d illustrates the resting expiratory position of the lung-chest wall combination. To hold the lung expanded at this volume a pressure gradient of 5 cm. $H_2O$ across the lung is required. The retractive force generated by the lung is balanced by the expansile force generated by the elasticity of the chest wall when this is below its own normal resting level. The pressure gradient across the chest wall is therefore 5 cm. $H_2O$ and the intrapleural pressure is 5 cm. $H_2O$ below atmospheric pressure. If the compliance of the chest wall is 0·1 l./cm. $H_2O$ the

force must distend both lung and chest wall. For example at a tidal volume of 750 ml. (Fig. 5a) the transpulmonary gradient is $5 + \frac{750}{100} = 12.5$ cm. $H_2O$ and the transmural gradient is $\frac{250}{100} = 2.5$ cm. $H_2O$. The force produced by the inspiratory muscles must therefore be equivalent to a total pressure gradient of 15 cm. $H_2O$.

Similar considerations apply to the use of positive pressure ventilation (Figs. 5e, f, g). However, since the pressure inside the alveoli now becomes positive with respect to atmospheric, the intrapleural pressure becomes

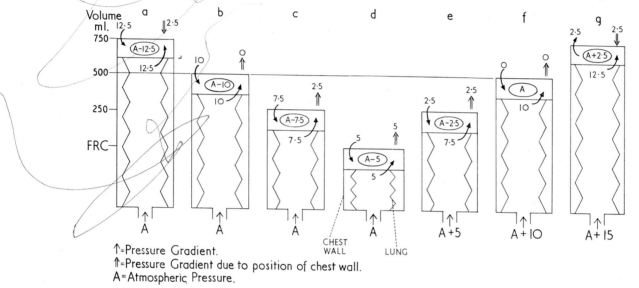

↑ =Pressure Gradient.
⇑ =Pressure Gradient due to position of chest wall.
A =Atmospheric Pressure.

FIG. 5. Pressure gradients during expansion of the thorax with spontaneous ventilation (a, b, c), at FRC (d) and during IPPV (e, f, g). Lung compliance and chest wall compliance assumed to equal 0·1 l./cm. $H_2O$.

thoracic cage will occupy a position which is 500 ml. below its own natural resting position.

When inspiration occurs the inspiratory muscles exert a force on the chest wall which then expands. After 250 ml. of air have been drawn into the lungs (Fig. 5c) the transpulmonary pressure gradient must have increased by $\frac{250}{100} = 2.5$ cm. $H_2O$. The total gradient therefore equals 7·5 cm. $H_2O$ and the intrapleural pressure must be 7·5 cm. $H_2O$ below atmospheric. Since the chest wall is now only 250 ml. below its own resting volume the pressure gradient due to the chest wall elasticity must be reduced to 2·5 cm. $H_2O$. The inspiratory muscles must therefore be exerting a force equivalent to a pressure gradient of $7.5 - 2.5 = 5$ cm. $H_2O$.

When 500 ml. of air has been drawn into the chest (Fig. 5b) the transpulmonary pressure gradient must be $5 + \frac{500}{100} = 10$ cm. $H_2O$. At this degree of expansion the chest wall is at its normal resting position. All the inspiratory muscle force (equivalent to 10 cm. $H_2O$) must therefore be exerted against the lung. When the chest is inflated to volumes above this level, however, the inflating

less negative with inspiration, then equals atmospheric and finally becomes positive with respect to atmospheric.

**Airway Closure**

So far it has been assumed that the intrapleural pressure is the same throughout the pleural cavity. However it is now known that there is a gradient of pressure from the top to the bottom of the pleural space (Daly and Bondurant, 1963). This fact is of great importance for it not only determines the variation in alveolar size from the top to the bottom of the lung (Glazier et al., 1966) but it also affects the regional distribution of ventilation and blood flow (Kaneko et al., 1966). Of greater importance to the anaesthetist is the recognition that this gradient of pleural pressure may lead to airway closure and collapse of alveoli at the base of the lung (Milic-Emili, Henderson and Kaneko, 1968).

The gradient of pleural pressure can best be understood by imagining the lung as a bag with semi-fluid contents anchored by the hilum. The effect of gravity on the contents would cause the bag to bulge outwards at the bottom and inwards at the top. Similar gravitational forces acting on the lung would therefore tend to create a greater subatmospheric pressure at the top of the pleural space than at the bottom. The magnitude of this pressure gradient will depend on the density of the lung. Since the lung is about one quarter of the density of water the gradient of pleural pressure (in cm. $H_2O$) will be about one quarter of the lung height (in cm.). Thus if the height of the lung in the upright position is 30 cm., the gradient of pleural pressure will be $\frac{30}{4} = 7.5$ cm. $H_2O$. At the end of a normal expiration the pressure at the top of the pleural space will therefore be about 10 cm. $H_2O$ below atmospheric whereas the pressure at the bottom of the space will only be 2.5 cm. $H_2O$ below atmospheric (Fig. 6a). During a normal inspiration the pressure gradient between alveoli

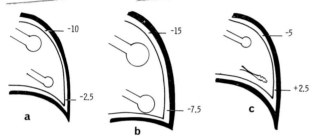

FIG. 6. Pleural pressures at top and bottom of lung in erect posture

(a) at FRC
(b) at end-inspiration
(c) during expiration towards residual volume. Airway closure has occurred at the base of the lung in "c".

and pleural space increases by 5 cm. $H_2O$ so that the pressures now become 15 and 7.5 cm. $H_2O$ below atmospheric (Fig. 6b). As the patient expires below the normal resting expiratory level the pressures in the pleural space approximate more closely to atmospheric although the gradient of pressure from the top to the bottom of the space remains the same. If expiration is continued towards residual volume the pressure at the bottom of the pleural space may become greater than atmospheric. The normal gradient of pressure holding the airways open is thus abolished and airway closure may occur (Fig. 6c).

In young adults with normal lungs the pleural pressure at the bottom of the space only becomes greater than atmospheric at lung volumes which are close to residual volume. As the patient ages the lung volume at which airways begin to close (the closing volume) increases until by the age of 65 years, most patients will have some closed airways at the resting expiratory position even though they are in the erect posture (Fig. 7). At the age of 40–45 years the closing volume is less than the FRC in seated or standing subjects but equal to or greater than the reduced FRC found in the same subject in the supine position. Because the head-down position causes still greater reductions in FRC the closing volume exceeds FRC at an even earlier age in this position (Craig, Wahba and Don, 1971).

The increase in closing volume with age is believed to be associated with the gradual loss of elastic fibres in the ageing lung. These changes also lead to an increase in lung compliance with age and therefore to an increase in residual volume and FRC (Fig. 7). It is now known that smoking

increases closing volume at a given age as does obesity or a rapid infusion of fluid and it is probable that a number of other factors will be found to affect it (Collins 1973).

It seems likely that airway closure associated with age and body position accounts for the increased alveolar-arterial $O_2$ tension difference in elderly patients before

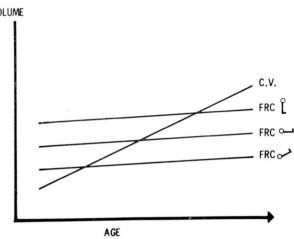

FIG. 7. Relation of closing volume (C.V.) and functional residual capacity (FRC) to age. The increase in FRC with age is much less than the increase in C.V. FRC is lower in the supine ( ⟋ ) or head down ( ⟋ ) positions than in the erect position. ( ⟋ ).

operations (Leblanc, Ruff and Milic-Emili, 1970). However the induction of anaesthesia has also been shown to reduce FRC (Laws, 1968) and Don et al., (1970) have shown that the magnitude of FRC reduction is related to the weight/height ratio of the patient (Fig. 8). Hence the reduction in FRC is likely to be greater in short, fat patients than in their leaner colleagues. This observation ties up with the greater fall in lung compliance in fat patients on induction of anaesthesia observed by Gold and Helrich (1965a).

## DYNAMIC PROPERTIES

The force required to overcome the various *elastic* resistances to inflation is solely dependent on the compliance and volume displacement and is not affected by the time taken to effect the change in volume. The force required to overcome the *non-elastic* resistances, however, depends on the rate of change of volume of the lung.

The major non-elastic resistances are the frictional resistance to flow in the airways and the viscous resistance of the lungs and chest wall. Small quantities of energy are also used to overcome inertia and to impart kinetic energy to the gases moved: however these are so small that they will be ignored.

### Viscous Resistance

The tissue viscous resistance of the lungs accounts for 20–30 per cent of the total lung non-elastic resistance under normal conditions of respiration. This factor is small and relatively constant and will therefore not be discussed further (Marshall and Dubois, 1956a and b).

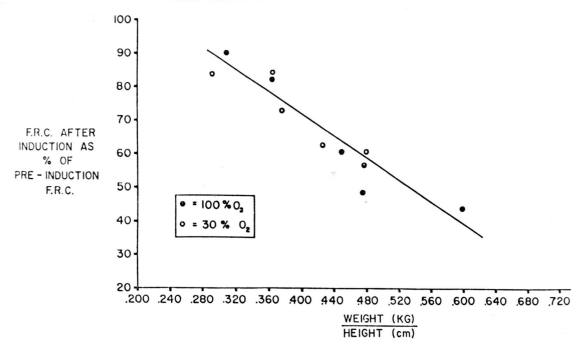

FIG. 8. Reduction in functional residual capacity (FRC) after induction of anaesthesia related to weight/height ratio. (Reproduced from Don *et al.* (1970) *Anesthesiology*, **32**, 521.)

## Airway Resistance

Resistance to airflow normally accounts for 70–80 per cent of the total non-elastic resistance of the lungs. It depends on the characteristics of the airway and the rate and pattern of airflow. There are three main patterns of airflow:

*Laminar* flow occurs when the gas passes down parallel-sided tubes at less than a certain critical velocity. With laminar flow the pressure drop down the tube is proportional to the flow rate and may be calculated from the equation derived by Poiseuille:

$$P = \frac{\dot{V} \times 8\,l. \times \mu}{\pi r^4 \times 980}$$

where $P$ = pressure drop (in cm. $H_2O$)
$\dot{V}$ = volume flow rate (in ml./sec.)
$l$ = length of tube (in cm.)
$r$ = radius or tube (in cm.)
$\mu$ = viscosity (in poises)

When flow exceeds the critical velocity it becomes turbulent. The velocity at which this occurs may be calculated by determining Reynold's number ($N$) from the equation:

$$N = \frac{2\rho\dot{V}}{\pi r \mu}$$

where $\rho$ is the density of the gas.

Turbulent flow occurs when $N$ exceeds 2,000. However this type of calculation can only be applied to smooth tubes with parallel sides. Small variations in the diameter of the lumen or branching often cause turbulence in airways at much lower flow rates than would be expected from theoretical calculations.

The significant feaure of turbulent flow is that the pressure drop along the airway is no longer *directly proportional to flow rate* but is proportional to the *square of flow rate* according to the equation:

$$P = \frac{\dot{V}^2 f\,l.}{4\pi^2 r^5}$$

where $f$ is a friction factor which depends on the roughness of the tube wall and on Reynold's number.

A third type of flow (*orifice* flow) occurs at constrictions such as the larynx. In these situations the pressure drop is also proportional to the square of flow rate but density replaces viscosity as the important factor in the numerator. This explains why a low density gas such as helium diminishes the resistance in severe obstructions to the upper airway.

Since the total cross-sectional area of the airways increases as branching occurs the velocity of air flow decreases; laminar flow is therefore chiefly confined to the airways below the main bronchi. Orifice flow occurs at the larynx and flow in the trachea is turbulent during most of the respiratory cycle. From the above equations it can be seen that many factors may affect the pressure drop down the airways during respiration. However it is obvious that variations in diameter of the smaller bronchi and bronchioles are critical and that the pressure drop along the airways is intimately related to flow rate. Since flow rate during inspiration follows an approximately sinusoidal pattern it is to be expected that the curve representing pressure drop along the airways will also have a roughly sinusoidal shape (Fig. 9). During expiration there is a sudden increase in flow to a peak followed by an exponential decline in flow rate. Narrowing of the airways during expiration somewhat modifies the shape of the pressure gradient overcoming airway resistance but the general pattern closely follows the shape of the flow velocity curve.

To sum up: The pressure gradients developed during inflation and deflation of the thorax overcome two types

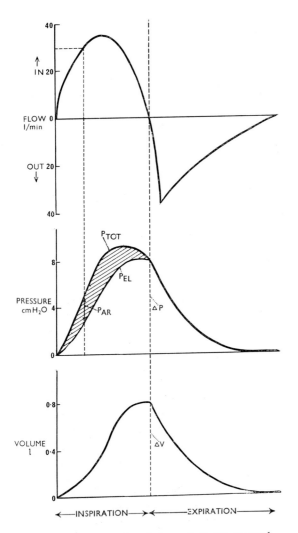

FIG. 9. Inspiratory and expiratory flow rate, transpulmonary pressure and volume in lung during one respiratory cycle. Dynamic compliance is measured by relating $\Delta V$ to $\Delta P$ at the point of inspiratory-expiratory flow reversal since airway resistance is zero when flow is zero and all the pressure gradient is exerted against the elastic component. The line ($P_{EL}$) shows the proportion of the total inflation pressure ($P_{TOT}$) which overcomes the elastic resistance during inflation. The remainder of the pressure gradient (shaded) shows the pressure which overcomes the non-elastic component ($P_{AR}$).

of resistance—elastic and non-elastic. The pressure gradient required to overcome the elastic resistance is proportional to the change in lung volume and may be plotted if the compliance and change in volume are known (Fig. 9). The remainder of the pressure gradient overcomes non-elastic resistance. The energy used in overcoming non-elastic resistance is roughly proportional to flow rate during most of the respiratory cycle.

## DYNAMIC COMPLIANCE: TIME CONSTANTS

So far, the static and dynamic properties of the chest have been discussed in complete isolation. However it is obvious that if only a finite time is available for alveolar filling then the degree of filling must be affected by the duration of inspiration. For simplicity in this analysis it is assumed that the pressure gradient at the mouth is suddenly increased to a fixed value and that this pressure is maintained at a constant level during inflation of the lungs. The pressure gradient for alveolar filling (i.e. atmospheric minus alveolar pressure) will thus be maximal initially but will decline as the alveolus fills and the retractive force increases. Filling will cease when the pressure

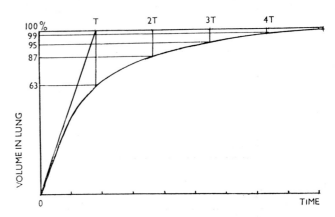

FIG. 10. Exponential pattern of filling of lung in response to constant applied pressure. The slight change in airway resistance during inspiration is ignored.

resulting from the retractive force balances the applied pressure. The rate at which the alveolus fills will also be affected by the resistance in the airways leading to that alveolus. As the lungs expand the airways lengthen and widen. The reduction in resistance caused by widening of the airways during inspiration predominates over the increase in resistance due to their elongation and therefore airway resistance decreases somewhat as the lung expands. However the pressure gradient available to overcome this resistance (mouth pressure minus alveolar pressure) decreases as the lung inflates. The rate of filling therefore declines in an approximately exponential manner (Fig. 10). An exponential curve can be described mathematically by utilizing its time constant. This is the time that it would take to complete a given change if the initial rate of change were maintained.

One can calculate the time-constant ($T$) for the lungs from the equation:

$$T = C \times R$$

where $C$ = compliance in 1./cm. $H_2O$, $R$ = airway resistance in cm. $H_2O/1./sec.$

$$= 0.1 \times 2 = \underline{0.2} \text{ sec.}$$

From this it can be calculated that filling of the alveoli should be 95 per cent complete in $3T = 0.6$ seconds.

If this equation is now applied to individual alveolar

units it becomes apparent that the time taken to fill such a unit will increase as airway resistance increases: however it will also increase as compliance increases, since a greater volume of air will be transfered into a more compliant alveolus before the retractive force equals the applied pressure. The compliance of individual alveoli differs from top to bottom of the lung and the resistance of individual airways will vary widely depending on their length and calibre. Furthermore, as already mentioned, pleural pressure varies with the height of each part of the lung. It is therefore likely that there will be a wide scatter of time constants throughout the lung. At average rates of respiration in the normal lung it appears that filling of individual alveolar units is almost complete at the end of inspiration. However, during fast respiratory rates in normal lungs (above 60 breaths/min.) it seems likely that equilibrium is not always obtained in the time available. A number of alveoli will thus be incompletely filled and ventilation/perfusion inequality will be increased. In abnormal lungs there is a wide spread of time-constants. This leads to marked abnormalities of distribution even at normal respiratory rates and dynamic compliance becomes lower than static compliance.

# THE MEASUREMENT OF THE MECHANICAL PROPERTIES OF THE CHEST

## Static Compliance

In the patient who can breathe spontaneously static lung compliance is determined by recording the mouth to oesophageal pressure gradient while the patient holds his breath after inspiring a measured volume of gas from a spirometer. The measurement is repeated at a number of different volumes and the compliance is calculated from the slope of the pressure/volume plot so obtained. During the period of breath-holding the pressure gradient falls due to stress relaxation (p. 230) and to the displacement of blood from the lungs. The readings of pressure are accordingly taken after about 15 seconds or when there is a satisfactory plateau. At this point air flow is zero so that mouth pressure may be taken to be equal to alveolar pressure.

Total thoracic compliance is more difficult to measure since it is difficult to eliminate inspiratory muscle tone in the conscious patient. Measurements have been made in trained subjects by recording the static pressures at the mouth after the subject has inspired various volumes from a spirometer and then relaxed against a shutter with an open glottis. However the validity of the method is doubtful. Similar criticisms may be levelled at measurements of chest wall compliance made in the spontaneously breathing patient since these are obtained by subtracting measurements of lung compliance from total thoracic compliance.

In the apnoeic or paralysed patient respiratory muscle tone is abolished. The measurement of lung, chest wall and total thoracic compliance is therefore easily achieved by measuring the appropriate pressure gradient when the lungs have been inflated to known volumes by the application of positive pressure to the mouth or sub-

atmospheric pressure to the outside of the chest (tank ventilator). The lungs can either be inflated by pressure from a reservoir bag and the inflation pressure and expired volume recorded, or else a known volume of air can be insufflated from a large syringe and the pressure recorded after a fixed interval.

## Dynamic compliance

The dynamic compliance of the lungs is obtained by recording pressure, flow and volume traces during spontaneous ventilation (Fig. 9). Flow is recorded by pneumotachograph and the volume measured by integration of the flow rate or by a recording spirometer. Compliance is measured by relating the inspired volume to the transpulmonary pressure gradient at the point of zero air-

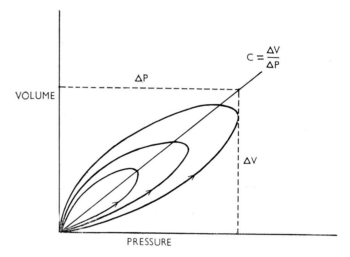

FIG. 11. Pressure-volume loops recorded during successive inspirations at increasing volumes. Compliance is calculated from the slope of the line joining the points of maximum volume.

flow at the height of inspiration. Since the intra-oesophageal pressure is subject to interference from cardiac pulsations compliance is usually calculated over 6–10 cycles and the mean taken.

Dynamic compliance can also be obtained from a series of pressure-volume loops recorded on an oscilloscope or $X$–$Y$ recorder (Fig. 11) or by a subtraction technique utilizing pressure flow-loops (Fig. 12).

Total thoracic compliance can be determined during spontaneous ventilation by relating the change of end-expiratory volume to the change in end-expiratory pressure produced by breathing against a resistance or or by adding weights to the bell of a spirometer from which the subject breathes. Again some degree of training is necessary to ensure that the subject relaxes his respiratory muscles at the end of expiration. Allowance must also be made for the change in water level in the water seal in the spirometer due to the change of pressure inside the bell.

## Non-elastic Resistance

Since the dimensions of the airway vary with lung volume and since the proportions of turbulent and laminar flow vary with flow rate it is not possible to quote a value for non-elastic resistance which is applicable throughout the full range of respiratory activity. However, in most patients, non-elastic resistance is reasonably linear at flow rates up to 0·5 l./second and therefore resistance values are usually quoted in cm. $H_2O/1/second$ as measured at a flow rate of 0·5 l./second.

When making this measurement the first requirement is to separate the pressure gradient exerted against elastic recoil from the total pressure gradient measured. This may be done in a number of ways.

**1. Subtraction Techniques.** Pressure, flow and volume traces are recorded during spontaneous or controlled

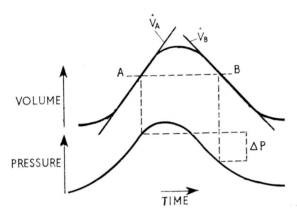

Fig. 12. Simplified method of determining resistance from volume and pressure traces. Flow rates ($\dot{V}_A$ and $\dot{V}_B$) are determined by drawing tangents to the curves at A and B.

$$Resistance = \frac{\Delta P}{\dot{V}_A + \dot{V}_B}.$$

ventilation (Fig. 9). Compliance is first calculated from the relation of volume and pressure at the point of zero air flow at the height of inspiration. A suitable point during inspiration is then selected (e.g. when flow rate equals 0·5 l./second) and the pressure gradient overcoming elastic recoil is calculated from the volume inspired and the compliance. By subtracting this pressure gradient from the total pressure at this point the pressure gradient overcoming non-elastic resistance can be calculated. This is then related to the air flow to give total non-elastic resistance. The resistance value obtained depends on which pressure gradient is recorded. If the transpulmonary gradient is used the resistance measured will be airway resistance plus lung tissue resistance. If the transthoracic gradient is recorded chest wall tissue resistance will be included.

A simplified, but less accurate method utilizing continuous volume and pressure curves is illustrated in Figure 12. Two points A and B are chosen at the same lung volume during inspiration and expiration. Since the lung volume is the same the pressure overcoming elastic recoil will be the same. The difference in pressure between the points therefore represents the sum of the pressures exerted against non-elastic resistance during inspiration and expiration. Flow is determined from the slopes of the volume curves and resistance is then obtained by dividing the pressure difference by the sum of the flow rates at A and B.

The subtraction of elastic pressure from the total pressure gradient can also be accomplished electrically. A signal proportional to flow is displayed on the y-axis of an oscilloscope and the total pressure gradient is displayed on the x-axis. A pressure flow loop results (Fig. 13). A signal proportional to volume is now subtracted from the pressure signal on the x-axis. The proportion of the volume signal which is subtracted is then increased: this causes the pressure-flow loop to narrow until it finally

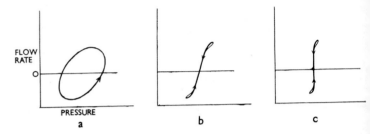

Fig. 13. Measurement of mechanics by subtraction method using pressure-flow loops.

(a) Pressure-flow loop. (b) The same after the subtraction of increasing proportions of the volume signal from the pressure signal on the x-axis. When the loop becomes flattened to a straight line the only pressure signal displayed on the x-axis is that due to non-elastic resistance. Resistance can therefore be calculated from the relationship between pressure and flow. (c) A signal proportional to flow rate is now subtracted from the x-axis until the line becomes vertical, indicating that there is now no pressure signal on the x-axis. The reading on the potentiometer controlling the proportion of the volume signal subtracted in (b) can be calibrated to give a direct reading of compliance and the reading on the potentiometer controlling the proportion of the flow signal subtracted in (c) can be calibrated to give a direct reading of resistance (Miller and Simmons, 1960).

becomes a straight line. At this point the only pressure signal left on the x-axis is that exerted against non-elastic resistance and the slope of the pressure-flow plot indicates the non-elastic resistance. By calibrating the potentiometers used in this device and carrying the subtraction technique one stage further it is possible to obtain direct readings of compliance and non-elastic resistance (Miller and Simmons, 1960).

**2. Interrupter technique.** Another method of determining non-elastic resistance utilizes a shutter which rapidly interrupts the airflow at the mouth for periods of 0·1 seconds. When this technique was originally proposed it was assumed that at the moment of interruption the airflow would be reduced to zero and mouth pressure would equal alveolar pressure. By recording the flow rates and pressures before and after the interruptions it was thought that a pressure-flow plot could be constructed which would yield a value for airway resistance. It is now known that the technique yields a value closer to total non-elastic resistance since a true equilibrium between mouth and alveolar pressure cannot be achieved when the lung is moving.

**3. Plethysmographic technique.** This is now the standard by which all other methods are judged. The subject is seated in a closed box and pants through a tube connecting the box with the outside. The airflow can be measured at the mouth with a pneumotachograph and mouth pressure can be measured by a pressure transducer. Alveolar pressure is derived indirectly by applying Boyle's Law to the volume of gas contained in the lungs. This volume of gas is determined by measuring the change in mouth pressure and change in thoracic volume (box pressure) when the patient pants against a closed shutter in the mouthpiece. When the patient pants through the open mouthpiece the difference in volume flow recorded at the mouth and in the box must be due to the change in alveolar pressure compressing and expanding the volume of gas in the lungs. Since the latter is known the change in alveolar pressure can be calculated. The panting procedure is adopted so that the humidity and temperature of the gas in the pneumotachograph remains constant.

**4. Measurements from single inspirations or expirations.** A simple clinical method of estimating changes in airway resistance is to measure the airflow rate during a maximal inspiration or expiration. Since a maximal inspiratory effort is more difficult to achieve than a maximal expiration, the latter is most commonly used. Although the pattern of expiratory flow rate is determined by both expiratory muscle force and airway resistance it is the variation in resistance which predominantly affects flow rate. A number of indices of expiratory flow have been proposed. The most common are the following:

(a) *Timed expiratory volume.* The volume of air expired during 0·75 or 1 second is measured with a spirometer having minimal inertia. This measurement is best related to the vital capacity, more than 70 per cent of the vital capacity being expired in 0·75 seconds if the airway resistance is normal.

(b) *Mid-expiratory flow rate.* Expiratory flow rate is usually very high at the commencement of expiration (when the bronchi are maximally dilated) and very slow at the end of expiration. A measurement of flow rate which ignores the first and last quarters of the expiration is therefore often used.

(c) *Peak-expiratory flow rate.* This can be measured with a peak flowmeter (Wright and McKerrow, 1959). This instrument is very portable but the measurement is much more dependent on muscular activity and is therefore not so reliable as a measure of airway resistance as are the other measures listed.

(d) *Exponential methods.* During anaesthesia similar measurements can be made by inflating the lung artificially and then allowing it to deflate naturally. It is found that the pattern of flow is roughly exponential. By utilizing the known properties of an exponential curve one can calculate various indices of airway resistance (Newman *et al.*, 1959, Bodman, 1963 and Bergman, 1968).

(e) *Constant flow techniques.* These are illustrated by the method described by Don and Robson (1965). Air is forced into the lungs at a constant, known rate for 0·75–1·0 seconds and the pressure at the mouth is recorded.

The increase in pressure at the mouth when flow commences yields a value for airway resistance whilst the difference between the pressure before and after the lung inflation, together with the volume of gas insufflated into the lung, yields the static compliance.

## VARIATIONS IN COMPLIANCE

The force required to extend a piece of elastic 10 cm. long by 1 cm. will be much greater than that required to extend a similar piece of elastic 100 cm. long by the same amount. In other words the measure of elasticity used (in this case increase in length per unit of force) must be related to the initial length. In the same way compliance depends not only on the elasticity of the lung tissue but also on the initial volume of the lung before it is stretched. It is therefore necessary to determine whether an alteration in compliance represents a change in the elasticity of the lung tissue itself or whether it is due to a change in initial lung volume. Since lung compliance is related most closely to functional residual capacity (Marshall, 1957):

$$C_L(\text{l./cm. H}_2\text{O}) = 0.05 \times \text{FRC (l.)}$$

it has been proposed that the best method of eliminating the effects of a change in lung volume is to determine the specific compliance:

$$\text{Specific compliance} = \frac{C_L(\text{l./cm. H}_2\text{O})}{\text{FRC (l.)}}$$

The normal value is 0·05 and the range is 0·038–0·070 l./cm. $H_2O/l$.

This measure provides a useful method of comparing compliance in patients of different age and size. For example, although the compliance of the lungs of newborn babies of 3·5 Kg. body weight is approximately 5 ml./cm. $H_2O$, this does not compare on a weight basis with adult values of compliance. However, the FRC of newborn infants is about $2\frac{1}{2}$ times smaller than would be expected from adult values scaled down according to body weight. When specific compliance is calculated with an FRC value of 95 ml. the result is 0·053 l./cm. $H_2O/l$. FRC, which is in agreement with the adult figures.

As already mentioned FRC is reduced in the supine, prone, lateral and Trendelenberg positions, and this leads to corresponding reductions in compliance. A reduction in the number of aerated alveoli due to atelectasis, consolidation or oedema will also reduce compliance. Changes in compliance due to an alteration in the elastic properties of the lung parenchyma are relatively uncommon, and difficult to separate from the changes due to an altered FRC unless the latter is measured. For example, compliance is greatly reduced in the respiratory distress syndrome of the newborn. This is due partly to the absence of surfactant which allows unmodified surface tension forces to act, but is also associated with the atelectasis which results. Fibrosis provides another example: this decreases tissue elasticity but also causes alveolar destruction. Pulmonary congestion also decreases compliance, mainly because the raised left atrial pressure increases intrathoracic blood volume and so decreases initial lung volume.

Another important consideration in interpreting changes in compliance is the volume history of the lungs. Thus, if a lung is inflated with equal increments of volume and then deflated in a similar manner it is found that the pressure gradient generated by a given lung volume is less during deflation than inflation. This phenomenon is termed hysteresis or stress-relaxation and is attributed to the recruitment of additional alveoli during the expansion of the lung. Similarly it has been observed that compliance increases after hyperinflation of the lung and then gradually decreases when the original tidal volume is resumed.

### Anaesthesia

Changes in compliance associated with anaesthesia must be considered in relation to posture, anaesthetic agents, intermittent positive pressure ventilation (IPPV) and duration of anaesthesia.

**Posture.** (Table 1). The effect of posture on FRC and the consequent reduction in compliance has already been

TABLE 1

FALL IN TOTAL THORACIC COMPLIANCE WITH POSTURE (VALUES
EXPRESSED AS PER CENT OF SUPINE CONTROL)
(Data of Safar and Aguto–Escarraga, 1959)

| | |
|---|---|
| Supine control | 100 |
| Lithotomy | 102 |
| Head up 20° | 118 |
| Head down 20° | 82 |
| Gall-bladder support | 91 |
| Prone | 78 |
| Prone and jack-knife | 75 |
| Prone and head down | 64 |
| Lateral | 94 |
| Kidney support | 83 |

mentioned. Lim and Luft (1959), for example, found that FRC decreased from about 3·7 to 2·5 litres on changing from the erect standing to the supine position whilst lung compliance fell from 0·19 to 0·14 l./cm. $H_2O$. Attinger, Monroe and Segal (1956) found that lung compliance fell from 0·19 l./cm. $H_2O$ sitting to 0·14 l./cm. $H_2O$ supine and 0·15 l./cm. $H_2O$ prone. Lynch, Brand and Levy (1959) found a decrease in static total thoracic compliance in the supine position and a further decrease in the prone position. These changes were particularly marked in patients with severe scoliosis.

Posner, Brody and Ravin (1965) also found a decrease in lung compliance in the prone position whilst Potgieter (1959) demonstrated a reduction in compliance in the dependent lung in the lateral nephrectomy position.

The effects of external pressure due to surgeons, retractors, packs and tight bandages must also be considered (Safar and Aguto–Escarraga, 1959). Finally it must be remembered that gravitational effects may be magnified by the presence of obesity. Naimark and Cherniak (1960), for example, showed in the very obese that chest wall compliance was a third of normal and that the excess weight on the chest wall caused a marked reduction in total thoracic compliance in the supine position.

### Anaesthetic Agents

The difficulties in interpreting intraoesophageal pressure measurements in the supine position and variations due to the volume history of the lungs have made it difficult to draw sound conclusions concerning the effect of anaesthetic agents on lung compliance.

Some of the earliest observations comparing measurements on the same patients in the conscious and anaesthetized state were those of Nims, Conner and Comroe (1955). These authors measured total thoracic compliance and observed a fall from 0·099 to 0·056 l./cm. $H_2O$ in patients anaesthetized with a number of different agents and rendered apnoeic by hyperventilation or a depolarizing relaxant. They felt that there was some doubt about the validity of the relaxation-pressure method used to measure total thoracic compliance in the conscious state but could see no reason to doubt the measurements made during anaesthesia. Wu, Miller and Luhn (1956) found a reduction in lung compliance from 0·128 to 0·080 l./cm. $H_2O$ during anaesthesia with spontaneous ventilation and drew attention to the possible role of an alteration in intrathoracic blood volume as the cause of this change. In 1957 Howell and Peckett investigated 12 patients with a static method and a further 15 patients with a method using slow cyclical inflation of the lungs. With both these methods the values for lung and chest wall compliance were lower than described by other workers for conscious patients, the mean values being 0·084 and 0·174 l./cm. $H_2O$ respectively. These authors studied 4 supine subjects before and after the induction of thiopentone-relaxant anaesthesia. The mean value for lung compliance fell from 0·154 l./cm. $H_2O$ to 0·109 l./cm $H_2O$ although there was little change in FRC following either the thiopentone or relaxant. After reviewing a number of possible causes for the reduction in compliance these authors postulated that the changes might be due to an alteration in the distribution of ventilation. Butler and Smith (1957) also found a reduction in static lung compliance of about 25 per cent after induction of anaesthesia with thiopentone and a relaxant, but noted little change in chest wall compliance. These authors found an average fall in FRC of 177 ml. in 10 patients after administration of scoline but they pointed out that the continual change in lung volume due to gas exchange made the change in FRC difficult to assess.

Contrary findings were reported in 1957 by Foster, Heaf and Semple. These authors studied dynamic lung compliance before and after induction of anaesthesia in 10 patients. There was no change in compliance in 5 patients, an increase in 4 patients and a fall in only 1 patient.

In 1958 Bromage found total thoracic compliance to average 0·070 l./cm. $H_2O$ after induction of anaesthesia with thiopentone and a relaxant. He noted that whereas the induction of a high extradual block did not alter compliance in normal patients it produced an increase in patients with severe chronic bronchitis. Bromage also noted that the reduction in total thoracic compliance which occurred with surgical stimulation under light thiopentone relaxant anaesthesia was abolished by extra-dural block. Bromage further demonstrated a reduction in compliance after ether-induced coughing or aspiration of the trachea.

Safar and Aguto–Escarraga (1959) found a reduction in total thoracic compliance during cyclopropane anaesthesia (a finding hinted at by Price et al., 1951) but they found no evidence of any change in compliance after the administration of d-tubocurarine. This was contrary to experience in dogs where d-tubocurarine produced a marked fall in compliance (Safar and Bachman, 1956). Safar and Aguto-Escarraga also noted that hypoventilation led to a decrease in compliance whereas with hyperventilation total thoracic compliance was unchanged or even increased.

Further studies during spontaneous ventilation were reported in 1965(a) by Gold and Helrich. These authors found that dynamic lung compliance in the supine position decreased from an average of 0·12 l./cm. $H_2O$ to 0·08 l./cm. $H_2O$ after thiopentone, nitrous oxide and halothane anaesthesia. This fall in lung compliance (33 per cent) was associated with a 50 per cent reduction in tidal volume. The fall in compliance was less in patients who were lightly anaesthetized and there was only a 17 per cent fall in compliance in those who were anaesthetized with halothane and nitrous oxide without a thiopentone induction. The fall in compliance did not occur in asthenic individuals but there was no difference in the percentage fall between normal and fat patients. A change from spontaneous to controlled ventilation caused a further fall in compliance which averaged 24 per cent. These findings were corroborated in a second study (Gold, Han and Helrich, 1966).

Comparative values before and after anaesthesia have not been reported in children. Richards and Bachman (1961) and Nightingale and Richards (1965) noted similar values for compliance whether suxamethonium or d-tubocurarine was used for relaxation. Reynolds and Etsten (1966) found that both static and dynamic compliance averaged 2–3 ml./cm. $H_2O$ in neonates and that chest wall compliance was very high (22 ml./cm. $H_2O$). These findings have been confirmed by Lunn (1967).

It thus seems to be established without doubt that there is a fall in lung compliance after the induction of anaesthesia. Recent measurements by Laws (1968) suggest that there is a reduction of FRC during anaesthesia but to date no measurements of specific compliance have been made before and after anaesthesia. Although there are many possible explanations for this reduction in compliance it seems most likely that the changes are due to alterations in the distribution of pulmonary blood volume or to terminal airway closure. The latter may be caused by changes in FRC or alterations of the mechanical forces in the lung.

## IPPV

Opie, Spalding and Stott (1959) found that dynamic lung compliance fell as soon as partially paralysed patients were changed from spontaneous to mechanical ventilation. Emerson, Torres and Lyons (1960) found that there was no significant difference between normal spontaneous ventilation, hyperventilation or intermittent positive pressure breathing with a Bird ventilator. In 1962(a) Watson reported an increase in dynamic lung compliance when patients with respiratory weakness were changed from mechanical ventilation to spontaneous and in 1966 Grenvik reported similar findings in patients 24 hours after operation. Further observations by Watson (1962b) showed that dynamic compliance during mechanical ventilation was reduced by a short inspiratory period (less than 1 second) and by a sub-atmospheric expiratory phase, that there was a slight increase in compliance if a +5 cm. $H_2O$ end-expiratory pressure was applied and that compliance was not affected by the shape of the inspiratory pressure curve.

### Duration of Anaesthesia

The dependence of compliance on the volume history of the lungs has already been emphasized. It was the observations of Mead and Collier (1959) in dogs and Ferris and Pollard (1960) in humans that showed that shallow tidal volumes that decreased the compliance which could be reversed by maximal inflations. This is a manifestation of the stress-relaxation or hysteresis noted by Bernstein (1957) and Butler (1957). Egbert, Laver and Bendixen (1963) studied changes in total thoracic compliance during anaesthesia and noted that this rose from a mean of 35·6 ml./cm. $H_2O$ to 42·8 ml./cm. $H_2O$ after a series of deep breaths and then fell within 5–10 minutes to a mean of 36·1 ml./cm. $H_2O$. In this, and a number of other studies on the changes in alveolar-arterial oxygen tension differences with time, Bendixen and his colleagues stressed that the changes in compliance were closely related to the volume history of the lungs. It was suggested that the tidal volume necessary to prevent progressive falls in compliance was about 7 ml./Kg. body weight in patients with normal lungs: at a respiratory frequency of 20/minute this produced a mean arterial $P_{CO_2}$ of 27 mm. Hg. To overcome the problem of decreasing compliance in patients respiring at lower tidal volumes it was suggested that deep breaths should be given every 5–10 minutes. A number of subsequent studies have thrown some doubt on the general applicability of these conclusions. Thus Fletcher and Barber (1966) found no change in dynamic lung compliance during spontaneous breathing in normal subjects and Panday and Nunn (1968) found no change in alveolar-arterial oxygen tension difference under similar conditions during anaesthesia. Colgan and Whang (1968) were also unable to find any fall in lung compliance or increase in intrapulmonary shunting with nembutal, methoxyflurane and halothane anaesthesia in dogs and humans. During controlled ventilation Judd and King (1967) found that if the lungs were hyperinflated and the tidal volume then maintained at normal levels by mechanical ventilation, the most rapid fall in compliance occurred during the first minute after the hyperinflation. After 15 minutes the lung compliance was decreased by 29 per cent compared with the value obtained just after hyper-inflation but thereafter they could detect no change even if the ventilation was continued for up to 3 hours. These findings are supported by the absence of change of alveolar-arterial oxygen tension differences noted by Askrog *et al.* (1964) and Lumley, Morgan and Sykes (1969). Since there are a number of differences in the premedication, anaesthesia and type of ventilation used in these studies it would seem wise to use the maximum tidal ventilation compatible with a normal arterial $P_{CO_2}$ and to utilize every opportunity to re-expand the lungs. This is particularly important after the patient has been in a position which reduces FRC: it should also be carried out after coughing, intubation and the aspiration of secretions.

## VARIATIONS IN AIRWAY RESISTANCE

The diameter of the airways depends on body size, on the pressure gradients holding them open, on the thickness of the bronchial mucosa and on the degree of bronchomotor tone.

**Body Size.** Above a functional residual capacity of 2·5 litres, body size does not appear to affect airway resistance, the normal value being 1–3 cm. $H_2O$/l./second at 0·5 l./second flow rate. Below an FRC of 2·5 l. airway resistance increases as body size falls (Helliesen *et al.*, 1958, Cook *et al.*, 1958). In neonates the average resistance is 0·03 cm. $H_2O$/ml./second.

**Pressure Gradients.** In the thorax, the trachea and main bronchi are exposed to the gradient of pressure between the atmosphere and the intrapleural space. The airways within the lung are exposed to a similar gradient of pressure due to the elasticity of lung tissue. An increase in this gradient during inspiration therefore widens the airways whilst the converse occurs during expiration. Similarly any factor which alters the retractive pressure of the lung will alter the diameter of the airways. At any given lung volume the airways will thus tend to be larger in patients with fibrosis or atelectasis and smaller in patients with emphysema.

**Bronchial Mucosa.** Small changes in the calibre of the smaller airways lead to marked changes in resistance. The presence of secretions or an increase in thickness of the mucosa are thus very common causes of an increased airway resistance. Little is known about the changes in the thickness of the bronchial mucosa resulting from physiological or pathological stimuli but it is probable that such variations play an important part in the changes of airway resistance due to posture or alterations in pulmonary blood volume. Certainly in patients with pulmonary oedema the mucosa is often extremely congested and oedematous and on occasions the author has noted almost complete occlusion of the main bronchi on bronchoscopic examination.

**Bronchial Muscle Tone.** Bronchial muscle tone is under the control of the autonomic system; bronchi are constricted by parasympathetic activity and dilated by sympathetic stimulation. Drugs produce similar effects. Thus isoprenaline, adrenaline, atropine and ganglion blocking drugs such as hexamethonium produce bronchodilatation whilst histamine, acetylcholine and irritant gases cause bronchoconstriction and an increase in airways resistance. An increase in smooth muscle contraction is probably the predominant cause of the increased airway resistance in asthma where resistance may increase to 20–50 cm. $H_2O$/l./second.

In addition to the causes already mentioned it must be remembered that increases in airway resistance will occur when there are localized obstructions to airflow (foreign body, tumour, extrinsic pressure), and that bypassing the upper airways by a tracheostomy may lower the total airway resistance.

### Anaesthesia

The three factors which are most likely to affect airway resistance during anaesthesia are airway obstruction or the use of artificial airways, changes in the alveolar gas tensions and drugs used in premedication and anaesthesia.

**The Airway.** In the normal patient 20–30 per cent of the airway resistance is incurred above the cricoid cartilage. Obstruction at the larynx or above may greatly increase airway resistance which may not be alleviated by the passage of an airway. Thus Gold and Helrich (1965b) found that the induction of anaesthesia with thiopentone, nitrous oxide and either halothane or methoxyflurane resulted in an average increase in resistance of 123 per cent over control values. When an oropharyngeal airway was inserted the resistance was 55 per cent above control values, whilst the insertion of an oral endotracheal tube reduced the resistance to 18 per cent below the control values. Wu, Miller and Luhn (1956) also noted that airway resistance could usually be kept within normal limits by the passage of an endotracheal tube.

**Alveolar Gas Tensions.** In man hypocapnia has been shown to cause bronchoconstriction by a central effect mediated by the vagus. Changes in alveolar oxygen tension seem to produce variable effects on airway resistance.

**Drugs.** Of the drugs used in premedication only atropine produces a marked reduction in airway resistance. Morphine tends to increase airway resistance, whilst pethidine and the barbiturates produce little change.

There are very few studies which demonstrate changes in airway resistance associated with specific anaesthetic agents in man. Values for airway resistance are approximately double those quoted for normal patients (i.e. they range from 5–9 cm. $H_2O$/l./second) and there does not seem to be a marked difference between the inhalation agents used. The only relaxant shown to alter airway resistance is d-tubocurarine. This was shown to decrease airway resistance slightly in 7 out of 23 patients studied (Westgate *et al.*, 1962).

## CONCLUSIONS

It will be apparent that the changes in the mechanics of breathing associated with anaesthesia can be due to a multiplicity of causes. The variations encountered between normal patients are large and the variations due to pathological changes are sometimes great enough seriously to impair ventilation. However respiratory failure rarely arises from a low compliance alone: it is nearly always due to a combination of low compliance with a high airway resistance and to the retention of secretions and central respiratory depression from drugs or toxaemia. Whatever the cause it is obvious that the most important factor in the prevention of respiratory failure is the maintenance of optimal mechanical function in the lungs. This can be accomplished by removal of secretions, re-expansion of all areas of atelectasis and bronchodilatation. Although detailed measurements of respiratory mechanics are seldom made in clinical practice a great deal can be learned from such simple tests as the vital capacity and forced expiratory volume. The application of these tests, and the interpretation of the pressures and volumes measured during mechanical ventilation, are within the province of every anaesthetist and should be closely integrated into clinical practice.

## REFERENCES

Agostini, E. and Mead, J. (1964), "Statics of the Respiratory System," In: *Handbook of Physiology-Respiration*, Vol. 1, p. 387. Washington D.C. American Physiological Society.

Askrog, V. F., Pender, J. W., Smith, T. C. and Eckenhoff, J. E. (1964), "Changes in Respiratory Dead Space During Halothane, Cyclopropane and Nitrous Oxide Anesthesia," *Anesthesiology*, **25**, 342.

Attinger, E. O., Monroe, R. G. and Segal, M. S. (1956), "The Mechanics of Breathing in Different Body Positions. I. In Normal Subjects," *J. clin. Invest.*, **35**, 904.

Bergman, N. A. (1968), "Properties of Passive Exhalations in Anesthetized Subjects," *Anesthesiology*, **30**, 378.

Bernstein, L. (1957), "The Elastic Pressure-volume curves of the Lungs and Thorax of the Living Rabbit," *J. Physiol. Lond.*, **138**, 473.

Bodman, R. I. (1963), "Clinical Applications of Pulmonary Function Tests," *Anaesthesia*, **18**, 355.

Bromage, P. R. (1958), "Total Respiratory Compliance in Anaesthetized Subjects and Modifications Produced by Noxious Stimuli," *Clin. Sci.*, **17**, 217.

Butler, J. (1957), "The Adaptation of the Relaxed Lungs and Chest Wall to Changes in Volume," *Clin. Sci.*, **16**, 421.

Butler, J. and Smith, B. H. (1957), "Pressure-volume Relationships of the Chest in the Completely Relaxed Anaesthetized Patient," *Clin. Sci.*, **16**, 125.

Colgan, F. J. and Whang, T. B. (1968), "Anesthesia and atelectasis," *Anesthesiology*, **29**, 917.

Collins, J. V. (1973) Closing Volume—A Test of Small Airway Function? *Brit. J. Dis. Chst*, **67**, 1.

Cook, C. D., Helliesen, P. J. and Agathon, S. (1958), "Relation Between Mechanics of Respiration, Lung Size and Body Size from Birth to Young Adulthood," *J. appl. Physiol.*, **13**, 349.

Craig, D. B., Wahba, W. M. and Don, H. H. (1971), "Airway Closure and Lung Volumes in Surgical Positions," *Canad. Anes-Soc. J.*, **18**, 92.

Daly, W. J. and Bondurant, S. (1963), "Direct Measurement of Respiratory Pleural Pressure Changes in Normal Man," *J. appl. Physiol.* **18**, 513.

Don, H. F. and Robson, J. G. (1965), "The Mechanics of the Respiratory System during Anesthesia," *Anesthesiology*, **26**, 168.

Don, H. F., Wahba, M., Cuadrado, L. and Kelkar, K. (1970), "The Effects of Anesthesia and 100 per cent Oxygen on the Functional Residual Capacity of the Lungs," *Anesthesiology*, **32**, 521.

Egbert, L. D., Laver, M. B. and Bendixen, H. H. (1963), "Intermittent Deep Breaths and Compliance During Anesthesia in Man," *Anesthesiology*, **24**, 57.

Emerson, P. A., Torres, G. E. and Lyons, H. A. (1960), "The Effect of Intermittent Positive Pressure Breathing on the Lung Compliance and Intrapulmonary Mixing of Gases," *Thorax*, **15**, 124.

Ferris, B. G., Jr. and Pollard, D. S. (1960), "Effect of Deep and Quiet Breathing on Pulmonary Compliance in Man," *J. clin. Invest.*, **39**, 143.

Fletcher, G. and Barber, J. L. (1966), "Lung mechanics and Physiologic Shunt during Spontaneous Breathing in Normal Subjects," *Anesthesiology*, **27**, 638.

Foster, C. A., Heaf, P. J. D. and Semple, S. J. G. (1957), "Compliance of the Lung in Anesthetized Paralysed Subjects," *J. appl. Physiol.*, **11**, 383.

Glazier, J. B., Hughes, J. M. B., Maloney, J. E., Pain, M. C. F. and West, J. B. (1966), "Decreasing Alveolar Size from Apex to Base in the Upright Lung," *Lancet*, **2**, 203.

Gold, M. I. and Helrich, M. (1965a), "Pulmonary Compliance during Anesthesia," *Anesthesiology*, **26**, 281.

Gold, M. I. and Helrich, M. (1965b), "Mechanics of Breathing during Anesthesia: 2. The Influence of Airway Adequacy," *Anesthesiology*, **26**, 751.

Gold, M. I., Han, Y. H. and Helrich, M. (1966), "Pulmonary Mechanics During Anesthesia: III. Influence of Intermittent Positive Pressure and Relation to Blood Gases," *Anesth. Analg. Curr. Res.* **45**, 631.

Grenvik, Å. (1966), "Respiratory, Circulatory and Metabolic Effects of Respirator Treatment," *Acta Anaesthesiologica Scand.* Suppl. XIX.

Helliesen, P. J., Cook, C. D., Friedlander, L., Agathon, S. (1958), "Studies of Respiratory Physiology in Children. I: Mechanics of Respiration and Lung Volumes in 85 Normal Children 5 to 17 Years of Age," *Pediatrics (Springfield)*, **22**, 80.

Howell, J. B. L. and Peckett, B. W. (1957), "Studies of the Elastic Properties of the Thorax of Supine Anaesthetized Paralysed Human Subjects," *J. Physiol., Lond.*, **136**, 1.

Judd, B. C. and King, B. D. (1967), "Human Lung Compliance During Prolonged Positive Pressure Ventilation," *Anesthesiology*, **28**, 257.

Kaneko, K., Milic-Emili, J., Dolovich, M. B., Dawson, A. and Bates, D. V. (1966), "Regional Distribution of Ventilation and Perfusion as a Function of Body Position," *J. appl. Physiol.*, **21**, 767.

Laws, A. K., (1968), "Effects of Induction of Anaesthesia and Muscle Paralysis on Functional Residual Capacity of the Lungs," *Canad. Anaes. Soc. J.*, **15**, 4, 325.

Leblanc, P., Ruff, F. and Milic-Emili, J. (1970). "Effects of Age and Body Position on 'Airway Closure' in Man," *J. appl. Physiol.*, **28**, 448.

Lim, T. P. K. and Luft, U. C. (1959), "Alterations in Lung Compliance and Functional Residual Capacity with Posture," *J. appl. Physiol.*, **14**, 164.

Lumley, J., Morgan, M. and Sykes, M. K. (1969), "Changes in Arterial Oxygenation and Physiological Dead Space Under Anaesthesia," *Brit. J. Anaesth.*, **41**, 279.

Lunn, J. N. (1967), "Measurements of Compliance in Apnoeic Anaesthetized Infants," *Anaesthesia*, **23**, 175.

Lynch, S., Brand, L. and Levy, A. (1959), "Changes in lung-thorax compliance during orthopedic surgery," *Anesthesiology*, **20**, 278.

Marshall, R. (1957), "The Physical Properties of the Lungs, in Relation to the Subdivisions of Lung Volume," *Clin. Sci.*, **16**, 507.

Marshall, R. and Dubois, A. B. (1956a), "The Measurement of the Viscous Resistance of the Lung Tissues in Normal Man," *Clin. Sci.*, **15**, 161.

Marshall, R. and Dubois, A. B. (1956b), "The Viscous Resistance of Lung Tissue in Patients with Pulmonary Disease," *Clin. Sci.*, **15**, 473.

Mead, J. and Collier, C. (1959), "Relation of Volume History of Lungs to Respiratory Mechanics in Anesthetized Dogs," *J. appl. Physiol.*, **14**, 669.

Milic-Emili, J., Henderson, J. A. M. and Kaneko, K. (1968), "Regional Distribution of Pulmonary Ventilation." In: *Form and Function in the Human Lung*. Ed. G. Cumming and L. B. Hunt. Edinburgh: E. & S. Livingstone.

Miller, J. H. and Simmons, D. H. (1960), "Rapid Determination of Dynamic Pulmonary Compliance and Resistance," *J. appl. Physiol.*, **15**, 967.

Naimark, A. and Cherniack, R. M. (1960), "Compliance of the Respiratory System and its Components in Health and Obesity," *J. appl. Physiol.*, **15**, 377.

Newman, H. C., Campbell, E. J. M. and Dinnick, O. P. (1959), "A Simple Method of Measuring the Compliance and the Non-elastic Resistance of the Chest During Anaesthesia," *Brit. J. Anaesth.*, **31**, 282.

Nightingale, D. A. and Richards, C. C. (1965), "Volume-pressure Relations of the Respiratory System of Curarized Infants," *Anesthesiology*, **26**, 710.

Nims, R. G., Conner, E. H. and Comroe, J. H. Jr. (1955), "The Compliance of the Human Thorax in Anesthetized Patients," *J. clin. Invest.*, **34**, 744.

Opie, L. H., Spalding, J. M. K. and Stott, F. D. (1959), "Mechanical Properties of the Chest During Intermittent Positive-Pressure Respiration," *Lancet*, **1**, 545.

Panday, J. and Nunn, J. F. (1968), "Failure to Demonstrate Progressive Falls of Arterial $P_{O_2}$ During Anaesthesia," *Anaesthesia*, **23**, 38.

Posner, A., Brody, D. and Ravin, M. (1965), "Effect of Prone Position with Constant Volume Ventilation on $Pa_{O_2}$ in Man," *Anesth. Analg. curr. Res.*, **44**, 435.

Potgieter, S. V. (1959), "Atelectasis: Its Evolution during Upper Urinary Tract Surgery," *Brit. J. Anaesth.*, **31**, 472.

Price, H. L., King, B. D., Elder, J. D., Libien, B. H. and Dripps, R. D. (1951), "Circulatory Effects of Raised Airway Pressure During Cyclopropane Anesthesia in Man," *J. clin. Invest.*, **30**, 1243.

Reynolds, R. N. and Etsten, B. E. (1966), "Mechanics of Respiration in Apneic Anesthetized Infants," *Anesthesiology*, **27**, 13.

Richards, C. C. and Bachman, L. (1961), "Lung and Chest Wall Compliance of Apneic Paralysed Infants," *J. clin. Invest.*, **40**, 273.

Safar, P. and Aguto-Escarraga, L. (1959), "Compliance in Apneic Anesthetized Adults," *Anesthesiology*, **20**, 283.

Safar, P. and Bachman, L. (1956), "Compliance of the Lungs and Thorax in Dogs Under the Influence of Muscle Relaxants," *Anesthesiology*, **17**, 334.

Watson, W. E. (1962a), "Observations on the Dynamic Lung Compliance of Patients with Respiratory Weakness Receiving Intermittent Positive Pressure Respiration," *Brit. J. Anaesth.*, **34**, 690.

Watson, W. E. (1962b), "Some Observations on Dynamic Lung Compliance During Intermittent Positive Pressure Respiration," *Brit. J. Anaesth.*, **34**, 153.

Westgate, H. D., Gordon, J. R., Van Bergen, F. H. (1962), "Changes in Airway Resistance following Intravenously Administered d-tubocurarine," *Anesthesiology*, **23**, 65.

Wright, B. M. and McKerrow, C. B. (1959), "Maximum Forced Expiratory Flow Rate as a Measure of Ventilatory Capacity: with a Description of a New Portable Instrument for Measuring It," *Brit. med. J.*, **2**, 1041.

Wu, N., Miller, W. F. and Luhn, N. R. (1956), "Studies of Breathing in Anesthesia," *Anesthesiology*, **17**, 696.

---

*CHAPTER* 3

# VENTILATION-PERFUSION RELATIONSHIPS

JOHN B. WEST

The prime function of the lung is to exchange gas between the inspired air and the venous blood. It is clear at the outset therefore that if a given part of the lung receives either no inspired gas or no mixed venous blood, gas exchange cannot occur there at all. It is also true that if the amounts of ventilation and blood flow are poorly matched in the different regions, gas exchange becomes inefficient. The serious effects of mismatch of ventilation and blood flow have only been fully appreciated in the last few years, and it is now recognized that the commonest cause of hypoxemia and hypercarbia in lung disease is uneven ventilation and blood flow.

## Alveolar Ventilation

Not all the gas which is inspired reaches the alveoli where gas exchange occurs. For example, if the tidal volume is 500 ml., only some 350 ml. gets to the alveoli because approximately 150 ml. remains in the bronchi and is exhaled with the next breath. Since the bronchi are not provided with pulmonary capillaries, gas exchange cannot occur within them and they constitute a *dead space*.

The volume of fresh gas entering the alveoli per minute is known as the alveolar ventilation. The normal value is in the region of 5 litres per minute.

The alveolar gas is in a constant state of agitation because of molecular diffusion and as a result the whole volume is available for gas exchange at any time. Indeed, it is now believed that the gas only reaches the alveoli because of the rapid diffusion process within the airways. This is because ordinary bulk flow (like water flowing down a river) only carries the inspired molecules to the terminal or respiratory bronchioles. The rest of the distance to the alveoli is then accomplished by random diffusion. For this reason, large particles such as dust or aerosol droplets which diffuse very slowly often fail to penetrate to the alveoli and are deposited in the small airways.

## Distribution of Ventilation

It is now known that during spontaneous respiration, the dependent regions of the lung are better ventilated than the upper zones. This is true whether the subject is seated upright, or is lying in the supine, prone, or lateral positions.

By contrast, if the subject breathes at an abnormally low

lung volume, the distribution of ventilation is reversed; that is, the superior regions of the lung ventilate well, but the dependent zones are poorly ventilated or indeed no fresh gas may reach them at all. This reversed pattern of ventilation is also seen in older persons even at normal lung volumes and also in patients with chronic obstructive lung disease.

The difference in distribution is shown clearly when a normal subject breathes in slowly in steps from residual volume. At first, all the inspired gas enters the upper zones and the lower regions do not ventilate at all. However, after a certain lung volume has been passed, the lower

small decrease in pleural pressure during inspiration will cause a larger increase in volume of the basal alveoli than at the apex. For both these reasons the basal regions are normally better ventilated than those at the apex.

Figure 1(B) shows that the situation is changed dramatically at very low lung volumes. At residual volume, for example, the pleural pressure at the base of the upright lung actually exceeds atmospheric pressure. Thus this lung is not being expanded but is being compressed under these conditions. For this reason a small decrease in pleural pressure will result in good ventilation of the lung apex but no ventilation of the base. Only when the pleural

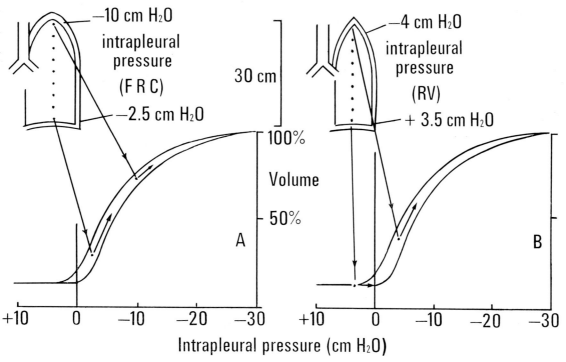

FIG. 1. Diagram to explain the distribution of ventilation in the normal upright lung. 1(A) shows that at normal lung volumes, the base is better ventilated than the apex because the basal alveoli have a smaller resting volume and a larger increase in volume than those at the apex. 1(B) shows that at residual volume, the basal alveoli do not receive any gas during a small inspiration and that only the apex is ventilated.

regions receive most of the gas and this pattern is maintained up to maximal volumes.

### Cause of the Distribution of Ventilation

The pressure in the intrapleural space is normally negative (less than atmospheric) in order to keep the lung expanded. However, recent measurements show that the pleural pressure is less negative at the base of the upright lung than it is at the top. This is not particularly surprising because the lung has weight and in order to support it, the pressure below it must be greater than the pressure above.

It is possible to explain the normal distribution of ventilation on the basis of these regional differences in pleural pressure. Figure 1(A) shows that at normal lung volumes, because the expanding pressure at the base of the lung is smaller than that at the apex, the resting volume of the alveoli at the base is small. Furthermore, because of the curved shape of the pressure-volume curve of the lung, a

pressure at the base of the lung goes below atmospheric pressure does the base of the lung begin to ventilate.

### Regional Difference in Alveoli Size

Figure 1 implies differences in the resting volume of the alveoli between the apex and base of the lung. Figure 2 shows the results of direct histological measurements of the relative size of the alveoli down the lung of a dog in the upright (head up) position. These measurements were made after fixing the lungs *in situ* by freezing the animal. Note that the alveoli at the apex are about four times larger by volume than those at the base. Furthermore, most of the change in volume occurs over the upper regions of the lung. Presumably a similar pattern occurs in man.

These striking differences in alveolar size and the pattern of ventilation associated with them have important implications in various clinical situations. For example, the small alveoli at the base are relatively unstable and tend to collapse. Since these regions are the best perfused, the impairment of gas exchange may then be severe. The reduced ventilation of the dependent regions at low lung

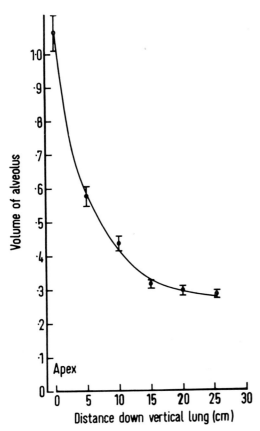

FIG. 2. Differences in alveolar size down the lungs of upright (head up) dogs. Note that the alveoli at the base are about four times smaller by volume than those at the apex.

volumes is important in obesity which causes a low lung volume or following abdominal surgery when the diaphragm may be elevated. These dangers are particularly important in patients with chronic bronchitis and emphysema where even at normal lung volumes the bases are often poorly ventilated.

## Pulmonary Blood Flow

Since the total output of the right heart goes through the lungs, the pulmonary blood flow is equal to the cardiac output, that is some five or six litres per minute. However, the actual volume of blood in the capillaries is probably less than 100 ml. This small figure contrasts with the volume of gas in the alveoli which is two to three litres. However, it is of interest that in spite of the very different volumes of blood and gas undergoing gas exchange in the alveoli at any moment, the volume of fresh gas entering the alveoli per minute, that is the alveolar ventilation, and the volume of blood flow are both approximately the same. Thus the normal ratio of alveolar ventilation to pulmonary blood flow is approximately one.

## Distribution of Pulmonary Blood Flow

In the normal upright lung, blood flow per unit volume decreases rapidly from bottom to top, reaching very low values at the apex (Fig. 3). This pattern is affected by change of posture and exercise. When the subject lies supine, the apical and basal blood flows become the same, but the posterior (dependent) part of the lung has a higher blood flow than the anterior region. In the lateral position,

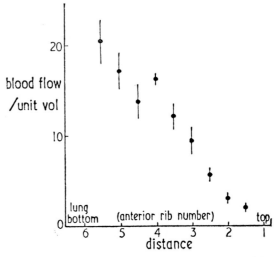

FIG. 3. Distribution of blood flow in the normal upright lung as measured with radioactive carbon dioxide. Note that blood flow decreases rapidly from bottom to top reaching very low values at the apex.

the dependent regions again are best perfused. On exercise in the upright position, both apical and basal blood flows increase so that the proportion of the total flow going to the apex rises.

Changes in lung volume affect the distribution of blood flow just as they do the distribution of ventilation. At low lung volumes, a zone of decreased blood flow is seen at the bottom of the lung, and indeed at residual volume this area of increased vascular resistance spreads up the lung until the apical blood flow actually exceeds basal flow.

## Cause of the Distribution of Blood Flow

The uneven distribution of blood flow is caused by the hydrostatic pressure differences within the lung. The pulmonary circulation is unique in that air and blood are separated by a very thin delicate membrane over a vertical distance of some 30 centimetres and consequently the hydrostatic effect of this large column of blood determines the calibre of the small vessels.

Figure 4 shows the importance of the relative magnitudes of the pulmonary arterial, alveolar, and venous pressures. There may be a *zone 1* at the top of the lung where pulmonary arterial pressure is less than alveolar pressure (normally atmospheric). The reason why the pulmonary arterial pressure is low here is the hydrostatic gradient within the pulmonary arterial tree. If arterial pressure is less than alveolar, this part of the lung is unperfused presumably because the delicate pulmonary capillaries are directly exposed to alveolar pressure and collapse when the pressure outside them exceeds the pressure inside. Indeed, histological examination of lung rapidly frozen under these conditions shows collapsed bloodless capillaries. It should be emphasized that in the normal lung, the pulmonary arterial pressure is just sufficient to raise blood to the top. However, if the arterial pressure is reduced as in haemorrhage, oligemic shock, or exposure to acceleration, or if the alveolar pressure is raised as in positive pressure ventilation, then an unperfused zone may be present. This constitutes an alveolar dead space and is useless for gas exchange.

Further down the lung in *zone 2*, pulmonary arterial pressure exceeds alveolar pressure and alveolar exceeds venous pressure. Here it has been shown that blood flow depends on the difference between arterial and alveolar pressure. This is known as the vascular waterfall or

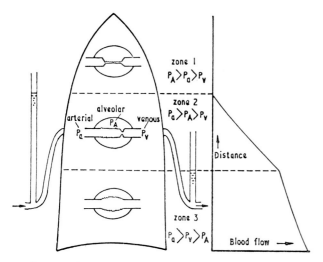

Fig. 4. Diagram to explain the distribution of blood flow according to the relative magnitude of the pulmonary arterial, alveolar and venous pressures. See text for details.

Starling resistor effect and is caused by a collapse developing in the thin walled capillaries. Consequently, since arterial pressure increases down the zone but alveolar pressure is constant, blood flow increases down the zone.

In *zone 3*, venous pressure exceeds alveolar pressure, the collapsible vessels are held open, and flow is determined in the ordinary way by the arterial-venous pressure difference. The reason why blood flow increases in this zone is that the pressure inside the vessels is increasing whereas the pressure outside is constant and therefore the calibre of the vessels gets larger. It has been shown in quick frozen lungs that the diameter of the pulmonary capillaries increases down this zone.

The cause of the zone of reduced blood flow at the base of the normal lung at low lung volumes can be ascribed to the larger pulmonary blood vessel. These are held open by the expansion of the lung much as the bronchi are. Consequently, at the base of the lung where the parenchyma is poorly expanded (Fig. 2), the larger blood vessels have a small calibre and thus cause an area of increased vascular resistance.

## Ventilation-Perfusion Ratio

Because blood flow increases more rapidly than ventilation from the top to the bottom of the upright lung, the ventilation perfusion ratio has a high value at the apex and a low value at the base of the lung. The key importance of this ratio is more easily understood if we consider a simple model of the lung (Fig. 5). In this model powdered dye is poured in (analogous to the addition of oxygen by ventilation), and the dye is removed by a flow of water corresponding to the blood flow. What determines the concentration of dye in the alveolar compartment (and

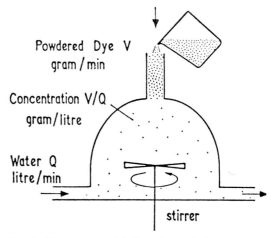

Fig. 5. Diagram to explain how the ventilation-perfusion ratio determines the concentration of gas in any lung region. In this analogy, dye is poured into a vessel through which water is pumped. See text for details.

thus the effluent blood) under steady state conditions? Intuitively it can be seen that both the rate at which the dye is poured in, and the rate at which the water is pumped through the model determine the concentration of dye. In fact, if the dye is poured in at the rate of $V$ gm. per minute, and water is pumped through at the rate of $Q$ litres per minute, the concentration of dye under steady state conditions is given by $V/Q$ grams per litre. In exactly the same way the concentration (or partial pressure) of oxygen in the alveolar gas is given by the ratio of ventilation to blood flow. This ratio also determines the concentrations of carbon dioxide and nitrogen or any other gas under steady state conditions.

## Regional Differences in Gas Exchange

Since the ventilation-perfusion ratio decreases down the upright lung and because this ratio determines the gas exchange which occurs in any region, it follows that regional differences in gas exchange must occur. Figure 6 shows that the alveolar oxygen tension is calculated to change by more than 40 mm. Hg between the apex and the base of the upright lung. The tension is high at the top of the lung because the ventilation-perfusion ratio is high there, and therefore the amount of oxygen being added by ventilation is large by comparison with the amount which is being removed by the blood flow. Again the carbon dioxide tension varies by more than 10 mm. Hg. In this case, the high ventilation-perfusion ratio means that a relatively large amount of carbon dioxide is removed compared with the small amount coming in via the blood flow.

Appreciable differences in the gas contents of the blood draining from different regions of the lung can also be seen. Note that the apex contributes relatively little to oxygen uptake because of its low blood flow, though on exercise when the proportion of blood flow to the apex increases, it carries more of the load.

### Overall Gas Exchange

Although these differences in ventilation-perfusion ratio cause large changes in regional gas exchange, their effects

the result that the arterial oxygen tension is depressed, and the carbon dioxide tension is raised.

There is an additional reason why the arterial oxygen tension is reduced by ventilation-perfusion ratio inequality. While the oxygen content of blood draining from alveoli with a low ventilation-perfusion ratio is always abnormally low, alveoli with a high ventilation-perfusion ratio are not able to oxygenate their blood much more than normal alveoli. This is because the blood is normally almost fully saturated with oxygen owing to the shape of the oxygen dissociation curve. This additional reason does not apply to carbon dioxide.

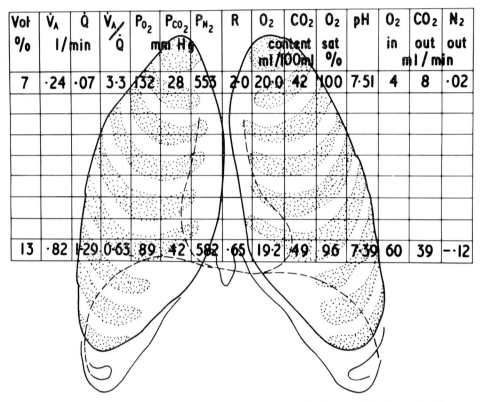

| Vol % | $\dot{V}_A$ l/min | $\dot{Q}$ | $\dot{V}_A/\dot{Q}$ | $P_{O_2}$ | $P_{CO_2}$ mm Hg | $P_{N_2}$ | R | $O_2$ content ml/100ml | $CO_2$ | $O_2$ sat % | pH | $O_2$ in | $CO_2$ out ml/min | $N_2$ out |
|---|---|---|---|---|---|---|---|---|---|---|---|---|---|---|
| 7 | ·24 | ·07 | 3·3 | 132 | 28 | 553 | 2·0 | 20·0 | 42 | 100 | 7·51 | 4 | 8 | ·02 |
| 13 | ·82 | 1·29 | 0·63 | 89 | 42 | 582 | ·65 | 19·2 | 49 | 96 | 7·39 | 60 | 39 | –·12 |

FIG. 6. Regional differences in gas exchange down the normal upright lung resulting from the differences in the ventilation-perfusion ratio. The lung is divided into nine imaginary slices but only the values for the top and bottom regions are shown.

on overall gas exchange are of much greater physiological and clinical importance. It can be shown that a lung with uneven ventilation and blood flow is less efficient at transferring gas either from air to blood or vice versa, than an homogeneous lung. The reason for this impairment of gas exchange in the normal lung can be seen by referring to Figure 6. This shows that the base of the lung is much more important than the apex in determining the arterial blood composition because it contributes most of the blood. However, the base has a low oxygen tension (because of its low ventilation-perfusion ratio). Thus inevitably the arterial oxygen tension is depressed because it is loaded with less well oxygenated blood. For the same reason, the carbon dioxide tension in the blood is elevated. It is as if the presence of uneven ventilation-perfusion ratios sets up a barrier between the gas and the blood with

In the normal lung, the effects of uneven ventilation-perfusion ratios on overall gas exchange are trivial; the arterial oxygen tension is reduced by a few mm. Hg and the carbon dioxide tension is raised by less than 1 mm. Hg. Both these liabilities can be met by the lung increasing its total ventilation and thus its overall ventilation-perfusion ratio. Indeed, the level of overall ventilation is normally set by the respiratory centre via the arterial carbon dioxide tension. Thus, if uneven ventilation-perfusion ratios elevate the arterial carbon dioxide tension, this is brought back by the increased respiratory drive and the consequently higher overall ventilation.

In the diseased lung, the effects of ventilation-perfusion ratio inequality on gas transfer may be very severe because the degree of uneven ventilation and blood flow is far greater than in the normal lung. The arterial oxygen tension may be depressed by 50 or more mm. Hg and in practice no amount of increased ventilation can return it to its normal level. The carbon dioxide tension, however, is often brought down by an increase in total ventilation though sometimes this is not possible and hypercarbia develops.

### Measurement of Ventilation-Perfusion Inequality

Unfortunately, in the abnormal lung, it is usually not possible to map out the distribution of ventilation and blood flow as can be done in the normal lung using radio-active gas techniques (Fig. 6). This is because most of the inequality is at the alveolar level and thus great variation occurs within individual counting fields. The best method of measuring ventilation-perfusion inequality in these instances is by the analysis of expired gas and arterial blood.

We saw in Figure 6 that the arterial oxygen tension is depressed in the presence of ventilation-perfusion ratio inequality because it is loaded with less well oxygenated blood from the well perfused lung base. By contrast, the expired alveolar gas receives a disproportionately high contribution from the apex where the oxygen tension is high. An alveolar-arterial oxygen difference therefore develops, and the magnitude of this difference is a measure of the amount of ventilation-perfusion ratio inequality.

While arterial blood can be collected by puncture, a representative sample of mixed alveolar gas is often impossible to obtain in the diseased lung because of its disturbed pattern of emptying. An alternative is to collect all the expired gas (including the dead space from the bronchi) using a valve-box and a large bag or spirometer and calculate what is called the *ideal alveolar oxygen tension*. This is the value which the alveolar gas would have in the absence of ventilation-perfusion ratio inequality. This calculation is made using the arterial carbon dioxide tension and the alveolar gas equation.

The oxygen tension difference between ideal alveolar gas and arterial blood chiefly reflects those alveoli with an abnormally *low* ventilation-perfusion ratio, that is the alveoli which are overperfused in relation to their ventilation. These alveoli cause the hypoxemia and their presence has the same effect as the admixture of some venous blood with arterial blood. Indeed, it is possible to express their contribution as if a certain proportion of the venous blood bypassed the lung altogether and was then added to the arterial blood. This is called *venous admixture* or wasted blood flow and is calculated from the oxygen tension difference between ideal alveolar gas and arterial blood. Normally, calculated venous admixture is less than 5 per cent of the pulmonary blood flow, but it may rise to 30 per cent or higher in the presence of severe ventilation-perfusion ratio inequality.

The alveoli with an abnormally *high* ventilation-perfusion ratio, that is those which are over-ventilated in relation to their perfusion, mainly affect carbon dioxide elimination. They behave as if a certain proportion of the inspired gas bypassed the alveoli altogether, that is as if the dead space were increased in size thus resulting in wasted ventilation. Their contribution can be calculated from the carbon dioxide tension of arterial blood and mixed expired gas using the Bohr equation. This gives a value for the *physiologic dead space* which includes not only the volume of the bronchi, but also the so-called alveolar dead space attributable to the over-ventilated alveoli. Normally the physiologic dead space is less than 30 per cent of the tidal volume at rest, but it may rise to 50 per cent or more in the presence of severe disease.

### FURTHER READING

Rahn, H. and Farhi, L. E. (1964), "Ventilation, Perfusion and Gas Exchange—The $V_A/Q$ Concept," in *Handbook of Physiology*, Section 3, Vol. 1, 735–765, ed. by W. O. Fenn and H. Rahn. Washington: American Physiological Society.

West, J. B. (1970), *Ventilation/Blood Flow and Gas Exchange* 2nd edn. Oxford: Blackwell Scientific Publications.

*CHAPTER* 4

# RESPIRATORY FUNCTION TESTS

ANDREW THORNTON

The primary function of the lungs is gas exchange, the elimination of carbon dioxide, added to the blood as a result of tissue metabolism, and the oxygenation of blood returning to the tissues.

The arterial oxygen saturation ($Sa_{O_2}$), and oxygen tension ($Pa_{O_2}$) in a subject with normal lungs, breathing air at sea level, are 95%, or greater, and approximately 100 mm. Hg. respectively. The arterial carbon dioxide tension is 40 mm. Hg. (*see* Figs. 1 and 2). These values are maintained within a relatively narrow range by the remark-

ably sensitive respiratory centre, which can rapidly readjust the rate and depth of ventilation in response to demands put upon it.

It follows that measurement of the tension of respiratory gases in the blood leaving the lungs might be logically regarded as the most significant test of pulmonary function. However, because of the existence of a very considerable 'pulmonary reserve', and because of the mechanisms which readjust ventilation and perfusion, arterial gas tensions may remain within normal limits, even under the stress

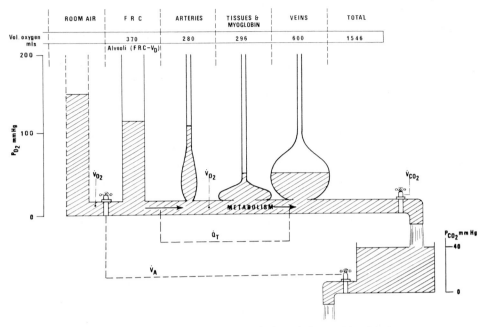

| | ROOM AIR | FRC | ARTERIES | TISSUES & MYOGLOBIN | VEINS | TOTAL |
|---|---|---|---|---|---|---|
| Vol. oxygen mls | | 370 | 280 | 296 | 600 | 1546 |

FIG. 1.  Body stores for oxygen and carbon dioxide.  (After Farhi and Rahn, 1955.)

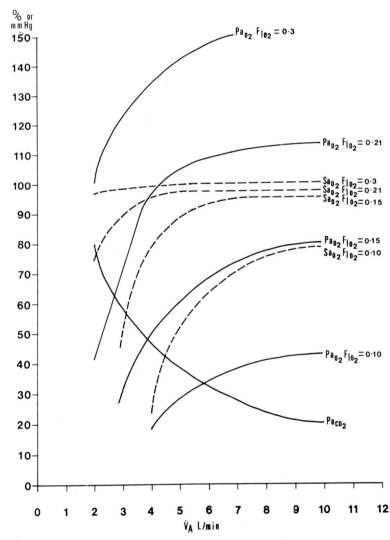

FIG. 2.  Relationship between alveolar ventilation ($V_A$) and arterial blood gases for varying concentrations of inspired oxygen.

of exercise, despite the presence of extensive disease of the lungs.

For these various reasons, measurement of properties of the lung, such as size (or volume), ventilatory ability (vital capacity, maximum breathing capacity), can often give a much more complete picture of the state of the lung in disease than can be gained from a study of arterial blood gas measurement alone.

## Lung Volumes (*see* Fig. 3)

If the gas containing parts of the lung are compared with a homely fire-side bellows, then the maximal excursion of the bellows can be considered to represent the *vital capacity*.

The vital capacity can be measured using apparatus employed for the determination of tidal volume. However, instruments which rely on the rotation of a vane in the stream of humidified expired air (e.g. Wright anemometer) (*see* p. 75), may prove to be inaccurate and may indeed be damaged by forced expiration. The vital capacity may be measured using the conventional Benedict-Roth type of spirometer if measurements are made without a forced expiration. However, as has been pointed out, the measurement of vital capacity against time (the *timed vital capacity* or TVC—*forced vital capacity* or FVC), is a more valuable determination. Under these latter circumstances it is essential that the measuring device has the appropriate

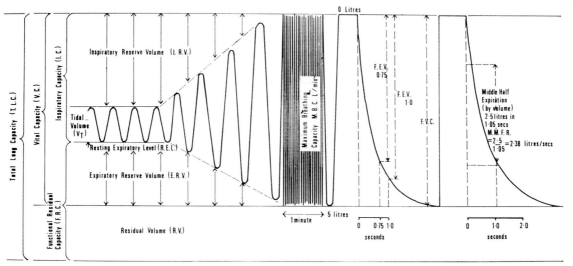

FIG. 3.   'Static' and 'Dynamic' lung volumes.

The *total lung capacity* is that amount of air which is contained in the bellows, when as much air as possible has been sucked in. The volume of air remaining in the bellows when they have been fully squeezed, and when no further air will flow, can be regarded as the *residual volume*. However, what is of importance to the individual attempting to kindle a fire is not only the size of the bellows in his hands, but his ability to shift the air in and out of the bellows as quickly as possible. Likewise the *maximum breathing capacity* (MBC) of the lungs depends not only on the size of the respiratory excursion, as indicated by the vital capacity (maximal stroke volume), but also on the rate at which the lungs can be ventilated. The latter is largely determined by the resistance to airflow in the respiratory passages.

Thus vital capacity determinations carried out without reference to the time it takes to empty the lungs give us only limited information with regard to the presence, for instance, of obstructive airway disease. For, given enough time, the patient with obstructive airway disease may deliver a normal vital capacity.

## Measurement of Lung Volumes

The performance of measuring devices used for the estimation of tidal volumes is discussed elsewhere (Chapter 5, p. 71). The spirometer is usually sufficiently accurate for the purpose of measuring this aspect of respiratory function. (Fig. 4).

frequency response and resonance characteristics and for this reason the Benedict-Roth type spirometer is unsuitable. Bernstein, D'Silva and Mendel (1952) have laid down the specifications for such apparatus and these requirements are incorporated in most of the apparatus used today (*see* Fig. 4). McKerrow *et al.* (1960) have devised a spirometer for the measurement of the timed vital capacity which is reasonably portable. However, the more recently introduced wedge type spirometers have increased in popularity ['McDermott': (Collins *et al.*, 1964), 'Vitalor': (McKerrow and Edwards, 1961): 'Vitalograph'] as their portability is even greater. When measuring the forced vital capacity, the patient is placed in a seated or standing position. A nose clip is applied and the large bore mouthpiece of the spirometer inserted. Care is taken to avoid leaks in the system. The rotation of the recording drum is started. The patient is exhorted to take in as deep a breath as possible and then to expire as hard and fast as possible. It is customary to take this test three times, retaining the best result. The young patient with normal airways and no respiratory obstruction will forcibly expire over 85 per cent of the forced vital capacity in one second.

$$\frac{\text{Forced expiratory volume in one second (FEV}_{1 \cdot 0})}{\text{Forced vital capacity (FVC)}} \times 100 = \begin{array}{l} \text{Forced} \\ \text{expiratory} \\ \text{ratio} \\ \text{(FER) per} \\ \text{cent} \end{array}$$

Where the fixed time for the forced expiratory volume measurement is 0·75 sec. the corresponding abbreviation is $FEV_{0.75}$. The $FEV_{0.75}$ correlates closely with the *maximum ventilatory volume* (MVV) at a respiratory frequency of 40 breaths per minute ($MVV_{40}$). If the $FEV_{0.75}$ is multiplied by 40 or the $FEV_{1.0}$ by 30, an approximation of the maximum breathing capacity (Indirect MBC) can be obtained. Another measure of ventilatory capacity is the *maximum expiratory flow rate* (MEFR) obtained by measuring the time to expire the first litre after a maximal inspiration (having discarded the initial 200 ml of expirate) (*see* Fig. 3). Alternatively

rate below 0·6 litres/second. On the other hand 80 per cent of patients who can extinguish a lighted match held 6 in. from the mouth are likely to have a maximal breathing capacity in excess of 60 litres/minute.

The DeBono whistle (DeBono, 1963) is an extremely simple item of apparatus. The patient blows down a wide-bore tube at the end of which is a whistle. In the side of the tube is an adjustable leak hole. The whistle shows when the rate of airflow through the whistle exceeds a certain value. The subject whose expiratory flow rate is to be measured is asked to fill his lungs, close his lips around the mouthpiece, and exhale as rapidly as possible. The size

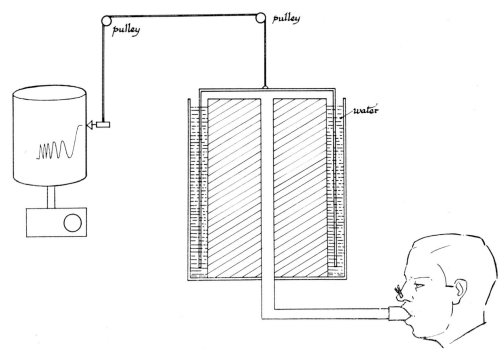

Fig. 4. Spirometer for measuring dynamic lung volumes. (After Bernstein, D'Silva and Mendel, 1952.)

the maximum mid expiratory flow rate (MMFR—time taken to expire the middle half of expiration) may be used (*see* Fig. 3). There is probably little to choose between the $FEV_{0.75}$, $FEV_{1.0}$, and MMFR as laboratory screening methods. The measurement of *peak expiratory flow rate* (PEFR) using the Wright Peak Flow Meter is another measurement of a single expirate, and the method carries the great advantage of being simple with a portable instrument. Both the PEFR and MEFR show greater variability in results compared with the other single breath tests.

### DeBono Whistle and Snider Match Test

Both these methods give an indication of the ability to shift air and are useful bed-side tests which require the minimum of equipment. The Snider match test has been shown to be of considerable value in the preoperative assessment of patients (Ravin, 1964). A patient who is unable to extinguish a lighted match held 3 in. from the open mouth is likely to have a ·maximal breathing capacity under 40 litres/minute or a maximal mid expiratory flow

of the leak hole is increased stage by stage until a maximal expiratory effort cannot effect a whistle. The expiratory flow rate is then read off the calibration on the instrument.

### Maximum Breathing Capacity (MBC)

This is the maximum volume of air that a subject can breathe per minute. Like the vital capacity it can be measured with a spirometer, or alternatively the expired gas can be collected over a measured period of time in a Douglas bag or Tissot spirometer. The Warring Ventube can also be used for this measurement (Warring and Siemsen, 1957). Motivation to ensure maximal effort, muscular force and endurance are often lacking in patients with severe disability and for this reason the measurement is often made over 15 or 30 seconds, or the value is derived indirectly from a single breath FEV (indirect MBC). As maximal ventilatory ability is dependent upon breathing frequency it is customary to breath at some pre-determined rate set against a metronome. Under these circumstances, where for instance the breathing frequency is 80 breaths per minute, the MBC is designated $MVV_{80}$. If the rate is not specified then the rate used voluntarily by the subject (e.g. 50 b.p.m.) is denoted $MVV_{F50}$.

### Response to Antispasmodic Mucolytic and Antibiotic Therapy

The timed vital capacity and its associated volumes, the PFR, and the maximum breathing capacity are valuable measurements in the assessment of the degree of reversibility of airway obstruction. Comparisons of these measurements before, during, and after therapy are useful guides as to the progress of the disease process and the response to therapy. Where airways obstruction is demonstrated by one of these tests, it is customary practice to administer an inhalational anti-spasmodic and repeat the test to assess reversibility of the airways obstruction.

The forced vital capacity is reduced and unaffected in restrictive lung disease (e.g. ankylosing spondylitis).

### Exercise Ventilation

Shortness of breath (dyspnoea) is the major disabling symptom in chronic pulmonary disease. The subjective estimate of dyspnoea has shown a relationship to reductions in MVV. Dyspnoea develops either when there is a decrease in MVV, when there is an increase in ventilation required for given exercise, or when both of these takes place. Hugh Jones (1952) has devised a dyspnoeic index relating standardized exercise ventilation to MVV.

### Ventilatory Response to Carbon Dioxide and Oxygen

In patients with gross pulmonary disease the ventilatory response to carbon dioxide or increased oxygen in the inspired gas, may be disturbed.

**Carbon Dioxide.** In emphysema, as the disease process increases in severity compensating increase in ventilation becomes impossible and alveolar hypoventilation ensues, resulting in further hypoxaemia and carbon dioxide retention. The ventilatory response to carbon dioxide is characteristically reduced. Though not routinely used as a test of pulmonary function the carbon dioxide challenge gives useful information on the integrity of the respiratory centre and respiratory drive. A steady state or rebreathing method may be used (Clark, 1968). The normal $\Delta\dot{V}_E / \Delta P_{CO_2}$ is of the order of 2·5 l./min./mm. $P_{CO_2}$.

**Oxygen.** Patients who rely on hypoxaemia as a drive for ventilation, will respond to the inhalation of 100% oxygen by a fall in ventilation, with a consequent rise in $Pa_{CO_2}$ which may further stimulate ventilation. The controlled administration of oxygen with observation of the ventilatory response is a useful guide to the use of oxygen therapy.

### Inspiratory and Expiratory Capacity

These volumes can be determined from an analysis of the normal spirogram (see Fig. 3).

### Residual Volume and Functional Residual Capacity

These volumes are normally determined from the *resting expiratory level* (REL) (*see* Fig. 3). The volume remaining in the lungs after the expiration of a normal relaxed tidal volume being the functional residual capacity (FRC). There are two principal methods for the determination of FRC:

(a) Gas dilution:

      1. Closed Circuit.
      2. Open Circuit.

(b) Body Plethysmograph (Boyle's Law: $P \times V = k$)

The gas dilution method measures the gas volume occupying the ventilated parts of the lung. The closed circuit method most widely used employs the rebreathing of a known volume of gas which is relatively insoluble in blood helium). The closed circuit permits carbon dioxide absorption, whilst allowing for adequate oxygenation of the patient. Rebreathing proceeds until equilibrium of helium concentration between lungs and spirometer occurs. Helium concentration is usually monitored using a katharometer (*see* p. 94). The unknown lung volume (FRC) is then calculated on the principle that the concentration of the initial quality of helium will fall in inverse proportion to the volume in which it is placed (FRC).

$$FRC = \frac{V \, (He_1 - He_2)}{He_2} \text{ litres (B.T.P.S.)}$$

where V is the volume of gas in the circuit.

    $He_1 =$ initial concentration of helium
    $He_2 =$ final concentration of helium

The functional residual capacity (FRC) can also be determined by monitoring the nitrogen concentration using a nitrogen meter (*see* p. 90), whilst rebreathing oxygen in a closed circuit. Under these circumstances, allowance has to be made for the entry into the circuit of nitrogen lost from the blood. If a patient is given nitrogen-free oxygen to breathe and the exhaled gas is collected in a Douglas bag or Tissot spirometer until the concentration of nitrogen in alveolar gas falls to 2%, the functional residual capacity can again be determined. Due allowance must again be made for the loss of nitrogen from the blood during the duration of the investigation. This method (open circuit method) is usually carried out using a nitrogen meter, but a simple Haldane gas analyser (*see* p. 85) is all that is really necessary.

$$FRC = \frac{(V_E + V_{DS}) \, (F_{E_{N_2}} - F_{I_{N_2}})}{F_{A_{1N_2}} - F_{A_{2N_2}}}$$

where $V_E$ = volume of expired gas (for measuring devices, *see* p. 76).

    $V_{DS}$ = volume of dead space of collecting system.

    $\left.\begin{matrix} F_{E_{N_2}} \\ F_{I_{N_2}} \end{matrix}\right\}$ Fractional concentration of nitrogen in expired and inspired gas respectively.

    $\left.\begin{matrix} F_{A_{1N_2}} \\ F_{A_{2N_2}} \end{matrix}\right\}$ Fractional concentrations of nitrogen in alveolar gas before and at the end of the period of oxygen breathing.

The Body Plethysmograph (Dubois *et al.*, 1956) has in recent years become a standard tool for the determination of thoracic lung volumes. The patient is seated in a transparent air-tight chamber (*see* Fig. 5), and the pressure of the air contained in a box is continuously monitored as the patient breathes through a pneumotachograph (*see* p. 73). By means of an airway interrupter, and the simultaneous measurement of airway pressure, and by the application of Boyle's Law the thoracic gas volume can be determined. The application of this method also permits the determination of airway resistance.

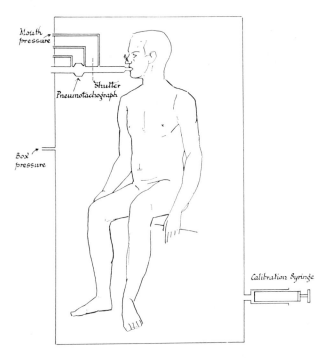

FIG. 5. Body Plethysmograph.

**Interpretation of Results**

It is important to stress that all measurements of lung volumes should be carried out with the patient consistently in the same posture. Alteration of the position of the patient from test to test and from time to time will invalidate the results. All volumes (except $CO_2$ production and oxygen consumption) must be corrected to body temperature and pressure, saturated with water vapour (BTPS). Serial measurements of vital capacity and residual volume over months or years undertaken with these provisos may be of value in assessing the progress of a disease process or a response to therapy.

Normal individuals of similar age, sex and stature may deviate as much as ±20 per cent from the predicted values (*see* Figs. 6a–6f). Owing to the wide range of normal values an alteration of vital capacity or residual volume must be large to be considered significant. Thus their measurement cannot be of aid, as an isolated single determination in the direction of subtle or moderate change.

The resting expiratory level (REL) (Fig. 3) is determined by two forces which at this level of lung inflation are equal and opposite (the elastic force of the thoracic cage to expand is counter-balanced by an equal and opposite force of the lungs to collapse). The volume of air contained

NORMAL LUNG FUNCTION

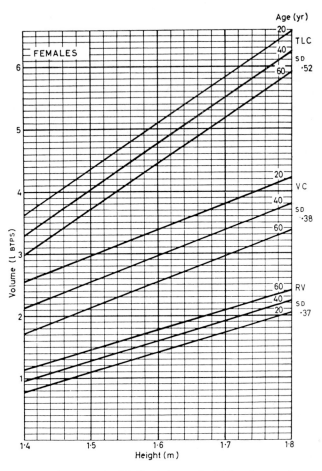

Total lung capacity (TLC), vital capacity (VC) and residual volume (RV) in normal adult females

Fig. 6(a). Predicted values for lung volumes (Cotes, 1965).

in the lungs in this mechanically neutral position is the functional residual capacity (FRC). It is into this latter volume that the tidal volume ($V_T$) is diluted. Most anaesthetists will be familiar with the prolongation of induction of anaesthesia associated with the administration of an inhalational agent to a patient with emphysema. In emphysema of the lung, loss of elasticity gives rise to hyperinflation, increased FRC and raised REL, which are associated with the characteristic barrel shaped chest and hyper-resonance.

**Compliance and Resistance**

Reduction in expiratory and inspiratory flow rate is found in *Obstructive Respiratory Disease*. Such increased airway resistance can be detected by a reduced timed

LUNG VOLUMES IN MALES

VENTILATORY CAPACITY IN MALES

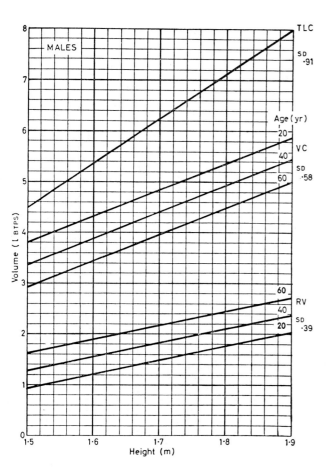

Total lung capacity (TLC), vital capacity (VC) and residual volume (RV) in normal adult males (Cotes, 1965).

FIG. 6(b)

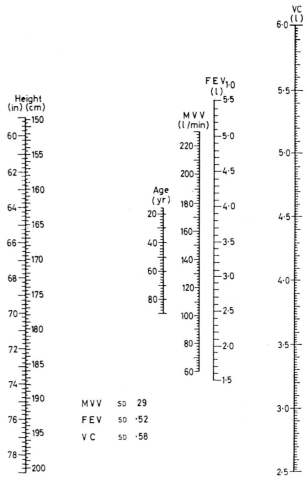

Nomogram relating indices of ventilatory capacity to weight and height for normal adult males.  (Cotes, 1965).

FIG. 6(c)

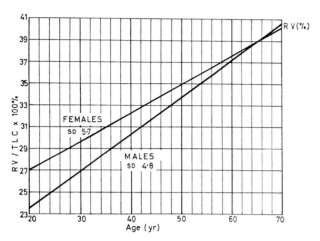

Residual volume as a percentage of total lung capacity (RV%) in normal adults of both sexes (Cotes, 1965).

FIG. 6(d)

**NORMAL LUNG FUNCTION**

**EXPIRATORY PEAK FLOW RATE**

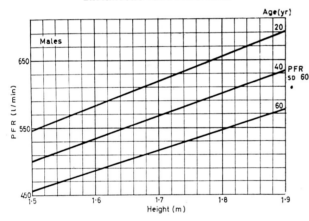

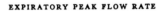

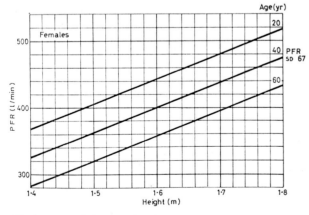

Expiratory peak flow rate (PFR) in normal adults of both sexes (Cotes, 1965).

FIG. 6(e)

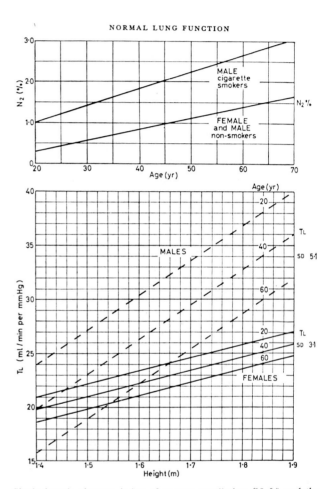

Single breath nitrogen index of uneven ventilation ($N_2$%) and the transfer factor (diffusing capacity of the lung, $Tl$ or $Dl$) in normal adults of both sexes (Cotes, 1965).

FIG. 6(f)

vital capacity and reduced maximal breathing capacity vide supra). However, more precise measurement of airway resistance can be carried out. The pressure volume diagram of the lung (*see* Fig. 7) enables the concepts of *compliance* and *resistance* to be considered. In order to produce such a trace it is necessary to monitor continuously the change in subatmospheric pressure within the pleural 'cavity', simultaneously with the associated change in the lung volume as the patient breathes. It has been shown that the intra-oesophageal pressure change closely follows the pressure change that occurs within the pleural

volume change per unit pressure change is what is called the *static lung compliance*.

$$\text{Compliance} = \frac{\Delta V}{\Delta P}$$

i.e. at point B compliance $= \dfrac{1000 \text{ ml}}{-5 \text{ cm. } H_2O}$

$$= 0 \cdot 200 \text{ litres/cm. } H_2O$$

The normal value for pulmonary compliance averages $0 \cdot 165$ litres/cm. $H_2O$. There is a definite relationship

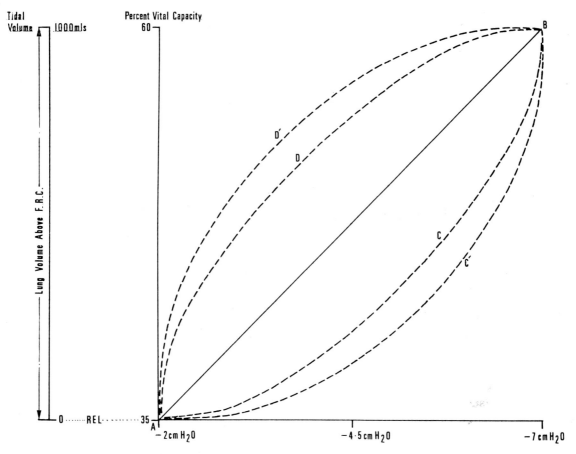

FIG. 7. Pressure (intrapleural) plotted against tidal volume (per cent vital capacity).

cavity. The position and size of the oesophageal balloon chosen for detecting this pressure change are however critical. A flexible rubber balloon, 10 cms. long and 1 cm. diameter is secured over the terminal portion of a polyethylene tube into which several holes have been made. After the tube has been swallowed and positioned behind the heart the system is filled with 0·5 ml. air and connected to an electromanometer. The electrical signals proportional to the variables transduced are fed into the X and Y axes of a cathode ray oscilloscope or XY recorder. Considering Fig. 7, if the change in negative pressure within the chest is plotted against the volume change associated with the patient taking a breath, the line AB can be produced (if the values are determined when airflow is zero). The

between the size of the lungs and their compliance. For a given change in intrapleural pressure, the small lung changes its volume less than the large lung. In a new born infant with a vital capacity of 140 mls. the compliance calculated over a tidal volume of 15 mls. is 0·0005 litres/cm. $H_2O$. In adults the best correlation is between compliance and functional residual capacity:

$$\text{Compliance (l/cm. } H_2O) = 0 \cdot 05 \times \text{FRC (litres)}$$

If the pressure change is monitored during breathing the characteristic pressure/volume loop is described (Fig. 7) ACBD. The area bounded by the loop astride the line AB represents the work (i.e. volume × pressure) done by the respiratory muscles against resistance and inertia (non-elastic resistance) during inspiration and expiration. The faster the breathing rate or the greater the airway obstruction, the more the loop tends to move away from the line AB, i.e. the lines AB'C and BD'A *dynamic compliance*).

The resistance to air movement (plus a small element of tissue resistance) can be calculated from the pressure/volume loop, and is the difference between the static (no airflow) and dynamic (airflow) intrapleural pressure, being that necessary to overcome resistance to a given flowrate. Normal values for airway resistance during quiet breathing at rest lie around 2 cm. $H_2O$/litre/second. Normally between 30 and 40 per cent of the total work of breathing is used in overcoming non-elastic resistances of which most is due to airflow, and the remainder is work against elastic forces. In obstructive respiratory disease the work of breathing against airway resistance amounts to 60–70 per cent.

Largely on account of the difficulty of obtaining an acceptable degree of reproducibility with the technique employing an oesophageal balloon, and, the associated unpleasantness for the patient, other methods tend now to be employed for measuring airway resistance.

### Interrupter Method

A rotating shutter which occludes the airway for alternate periods of 0·05 second is placed in series with a resistance and a pneumotachograph through which the patient breathes. The pressure at the mouthpiece is recorded both when the shutter is open and when it is closed. The pressure ($P_1$) when the airway is not occluded taken at the mouth is a measure of the airflow through the apparatus. The pressure ($P_2$) when the airway is occluded represents the pressure (alveolar) required to overcome the resistance of the airway.

$$\text{Airway resistance} \atop \text{cm. } H_2O\text{/litre/second} = \frac{P_2 - P_1}{P_1} \times f$$

where f is a factor correcting for the resistance of the apparatus.

A modification of this principle of airway interruption has been employed in the paralysed patient (Don and Robson, 1965). A variation on this method is the use of an oscillating pressure within the airway as the patient breathes (Tanabe *et al.*, 1965; Goldman *et al.*, 1970). Though relatively simple the principle of airway interruption tends to become increasingly inaccurate as the airway resistance increases.

### Plethysmograph

The principle of this method for the determination of thoracic lung volume has been described (*see* p. 244, Fig. 5). If a patient is placed in a closed plethysmograph and the pressure within the box is monitored, there should be no change in pressure within the box if there was no resistance to the passage of air through the patients airways. For, as the thoracic cage moves outwards at one and the same time the air so displaced would enter the patients lungs. However, because of airway resistance, the pressure within the box fluctuates. During inspiration the expansion of the thoracic cage temporarily lowers the pressure in the alveoli and raises it in the box. The relationship between box pressure (BoxP) and alveolar pressure ($P_A$) is an inverse one. The box pressure (Box $P_1$) may be taken as an index of alveolar pressure ($P_{A_1}$). If the patient pants against a closed shutter, because there is no airflow, the pressure ($P_{A_1}$) is uniform throughout the whole respiratory tract, and so may be measured at the mouthpiece. The patient then repeats the procedure of panting gently and shallowly through the pneumotachograph ($\dot{V}$) at flow rates up to 0·5 litres/second, with the shutter open and the box pressure is again recorded (BoxP₂). The airway resistance is then determined using the relationship:

$$\text{A.W.R.} = \frac{\Delta P_{A_1}}{\Delta P \text{Box}_1} \times \frac{\Delta P \text{Box}_2}{\dot{V}} \text{ cm. } H_2O\text{/litre/second.}$$

### Distribution of Inspired Air

Normally the inspired air is distributed almost equally in time and volume to all alveoli. However, patchy variations of elasticity within the lung and varying degrees of obstruction of smaller airways may give rise to both overventilation and underventilation of some areas of the lung. If either of these circumstances is not precisely matched by a coincident readjustment of pulmonary blood flow, ventilation/perfusion inequality will result and this will predispose to hypoxaemia (vide infra).

Methods are available whereby it is possible to study with relative simplicity this maldistribution of inspired air, whereas precise studies of maldistribution of perfusion have so far defied all attempts other than bv using expensive and sophisticated methods.

Methods available:

1. Pulmonary nitrogen washout. Becklake lung clearance index.
2. Single breath analysis of alveolar nitrogen.
3. Closed circuit helium.

The nitrogen meter is a rapid response instrument, which depends for its function on the characteristic spectral discharge when nitrogen is exposed to a subatmospheric pressure and a high direct current voltage (*see* p. 90). Using this instrument, it is possible to follow the nitrogen concentration breath by breath.

### Pulmonary Nitrogen Washout

Using this technique the patient breathes 100 per cent oxygen and the alveolar nitrogen concentration is monitored continuously. In the subject with normal lungs the alveolar nitrogen is less than 2·5 per cent after 7 minutes of oxygen breathing. An alveolar nitrogen concentration greater than 2·5 per cent indicates non-uniform distribution. The Becklake Lung Clearance Index is a more precise way of expressing this process:

$$\text{Lung clearance index} = \frac{\text{volume of oxygen inspired to lower alveolar nitrogen to 2 per cent}}{\text{FRC}}$$

(Normal range 5·0–9·0)

If the alveolar nitrogen concentration during washout is plotted on semi-log paper against the number of breaths, it is possible to analyse the 'curve' and to divide it into two or more exponentials representing well-ventilated and poorly ventilated parts of the lung. This latter method, however, is not usually applied to routine assessment of lung function.

### Single-breath Analysis of Expired Nitrogen

If a patient is allowed to inhale a measured volume of oxygen and then the exhaled gas is continuously monitored a trace similar to that shown in Fig. 8 may be produced. If at the same time the exhaled volume is monitored an analysis of the changing nitrogen concentration can be carried out. The last gas into the lung is the last gas out, and as this gas was 100 per cent oxygen the nitrogen meter

between lung and a spirometer containing an inert relatively insoluble gas such as helium, is a function of uniform distribution of gas in the lung. The number of breaths which are completed by the subject up to the time when the concentration of helium in the apparatus has fallen to within 10 per cent of its equilibrium value is the usual index taken. Subjects with a normal lung achieve this state within 15–30 breaths whilst in subjects in whom the distribution of inspired gas is uneven a large number of breaths is required. It is important to obtain control values for comparison as the size, mixing efficiency of the closed circuit and the response time of the Katharometer influence the results.

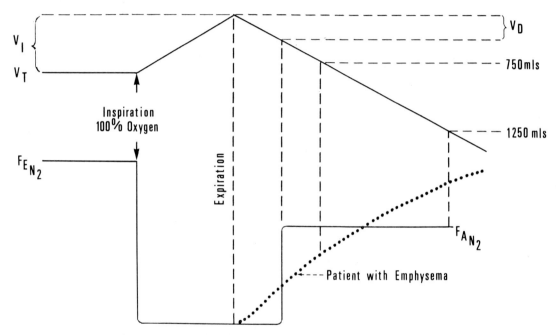

Fig. 8. Nitrogen concentration of expired gas following inspiration of 100 per cent oxygen.

registers zero until alveolar gas (which has been diluted with 100 per cent oxygen) passes the sampling point. At this point the nitrogen concentration rises abruptly and then remains stabilised so that the concentration changes less than 1·5 per cent over 750 to 1250 mls. of expirate in a subject with healthy lungs. The volume of gas exhaled from the commencement of expiration to the mid-point of the rise in nitrogen concentration to its plateau can be regarded as fairly close measure of the anatomical dead space. (The volume of gas that occupies that part of the tracheo-bronchial tree and upper respiratory passages which does not participate in gaseous exchange.)

In patients with distribution abnormalities the initial rapid rise is less marked and the nitrogen concentration continues to rise without reaching a plateau, and the change in nitrogen concentration may reach 10 per cent over the 500 ml. of gas expired between 750 and 1250 ml. of expirate.

### Closed Circuit Helium

This method operates on the principle that the rate at which gaseous equilibrium is attained, with rebreathing,

### Ventilation/Perfusion Relationships *(see ch. 3 p. 234.)*

Hypoventilation of alveoli in relation to blood flow gives rise to an increased 'venous-admixture', whilst hyperventilation in relation to blood flow gives rise to an increased 'dead-space effect'. Normally the relationship between ventilation and perfusion for the lung as a whole gives a ratio of ventilation perfusion of 0·8. This represents a composite of varying ventilation perfusion ratios throughout the lung.

**Dead-space Effect.** In the normal healthy lung the anatomical dead space represents the overall dead space. However, in conditions where there is an overall increase of ventilation in relationship to perfusion an alveolar dead space is created. The sum of anatomical and alveolar dead spaces is what is called the physiological dead space. The physiological dead space normally does not exceed 30 per cent of the tidal volume ($V_D/V_T = 0.3$). However, with increasing age and in conditions such as emphysema the value may approach 70 per cent.

The physiological dead space is determined by the use

of Bohr's equation substituting arterial carbon dioxide pressure for alveolar carbon dioxide pressure. Thus:

$$V_D/V_T = \frac{Pa_{CO_2} - P\overline{E}_{CO_2}}{Pa_{CO_2}}$$

where $Pa_{CO_2}$ = arterial $CO_2$ tension.

$P\overline{E}_{CO_2}$ = mixed expired $CO_2$ tension.

This ratio can be readily obtained by taking an arterial sample whilst expired gas is collected in a Douglas bag for subsequent analysis of mixed expired carbon dioxide concentration (tension).

### Venous Admixture

The pressure of oxygen in alveolar gas is calculated from the respiratory exchange ratio (R) or

$$\frac{\dot{V}_{CO_2}}{\dot{V}_{O_2}} = \frac{\text{Carbon dioxide production}}{\text{Oxygen consumption}}$$

and the carbon dioxide pressure of alveolar air, which in turn varies inversely with alveolar ventilation. Using this relationship it is possible to obtain the ideal alveolar oxygen tension ($P_{Ao_2}$):

$$P_{Ao_2} = P_{Io_2} - P_{Aco_2} \left[ F_{Io_2} + \frac{1 - F_{Io_2}}{R} \right]$$

where $P_{Io_2}$ = Inspired oxygen tension

$P_{Ao_2}$ = Alveolar carbon dioxide tension

$F_{Io_2}$ = Inspired oxygen concentration

a modification of this equation allows the $P_{Ao_2}$ to be determined during an 'unsteady state' such as pertains during the administration of inhalational anaesthetic agents:

$$P_{Ao_2} = P_{Io_2} - Pa_{co_2} \left[ \frac{P_{Io_2} - P\overline{E}_{o_2}}{P\overline{E}_{co_2}} \right]$$

When the inspired oxygen concentration is 100 per cent the alveolar oxygen tension can be determined from the relationship:

$$P_{Ao_2} = P_{Io_2} - Pa_{co_2}$$

### Alveolar-arterial Gradients

The normal difference between alveolar $P_{O_2}$ and arterial $P_{O_2}$ in a subject breathing air is 10 mm. Hg. In the normal individual most of the 10 mm. Hg. oxygen tension difference is due to anatomical shunts (bronchial veins to pulmonary veins: anterior cardiac and Thebesian veins to left ventricle). An increase in this gradient can be due to a number of factors:

1. Venous admixture due to anatomical shunts.
2. Venous admixture due to low ventilation/perfusion ratios (*see* p. 235).
3. Limitation to diffusion of oxygen across the alveolar-capillary membrane.
4. Lower mixed venous oxygen content due to one or a combination of:

    a. Excessive oxygen extraction at the periphery.

    b. Poor cardiac output.
    c. Low haemoglobin (low oxygen carrying capacity).

The alveolar-arterial oxygen tension difference during oxygen breathing is mainly due to venous admixture arising from anatomical shunts.

The alveolar-arterial nitrogen tension gradient in normal subjects is 2 or 3 mm. Hg. In patients in whom the range of ventilation perfusion ratios is increased the difference may exceed 20 mm. Hg. (i.e. patients with regions under-ventilated and over-perfused). This method requires measurement of the nitrogen tension in the alveolar (nitrogen meter or mass spectrometer), and arterial blood, subcutaneous tissues or urine. The arterial-alveolar carbon dioxide tension gradient is mainly due to over-ventilation and underperfusion of alveoli (*see* physiological dead space).

### Shunts

The administration of 100 per cent oxygen will correct arterial oxygen desaturation due to venous-admixture arising from ventilation/perfusion inequality, and from an 'alveolar-capillary' diffusion defect. The oxygen desaturation due to an anatomical shunt will only be corrected by the administration of 100 per cent oxygen if the shunt is less than 30 per cent of cardiac output and the mixed venous content is not less than 17·5 vols per cent. Partition of the venous-admixture into components due to an anatomical shunt and ventilation/perfusion inequality can be done by administering 100 per cent oxygen. Most of the difference between the tension of oxygen in the mixed alveolar gas and systemic blood is then due to admixture with venous blood which has either by-passed the lung (anatomical shunt) or perfused alveoli which are not ventilated. The anatomical shunt can be calculated using the relationship:

$$Qs/Q_T = \frac{C\dot{c}_{o_2} - Ca_{o_2}}{C\dot{c}_{o_2} - C\overline{V}_{o_2}}$$

where arterial oxygen content ($Ca_{o_2}$) =
$$Pa_{o_2} \times 0.00301 + Hb \times 1.34 \times Sa_{o_2}$$
end pulmonary capillary oxygen content ($C\dot{c}_{o_2}$) =
$$P_{Ao_2} \times 0.00301 + Hb \times 1.34$$
mixed venous oxygen content ($C\overline{V}_{o_2}$) =
$$P\overline{V}_{o_2} \times 0.00301 + Hb \times 1.34 \times S\overline{V}_{o_2}$$

mixed venous samples are taken from a catheter placed in the pulmonary artery. For the reasons given under 4 above it is not reliable to assume that the mixed venous-arterial oxygen content difference is constant (i.e. 5 vols. per cent).

The separate function of right and left lung can be studied using endobronchial tubes (e.g. Carlen's catheter). Information on individual lobes can be obtained using Argon flow probes and a mass spectrometer (Hugh-Jones and West, 1960).

The recent introduction of techniques employing isotopes has permitted detailed analysis of the distribution of pulmonary ventilation and perfusion on a regional basis. Xenon-133 which is relatively insoluble in blood can be inhaled and the rate of disappearance from the field of counting taken as a function of the alveoli in question. Xenon-133 can also be dissolved in saline and injected intravenously, the activity under the counter then being a measure of perfusion of that zone. For carbon dioxide labelled with oxygen-15 the clearance of the isotope from the field of counting is a function of the rate of blood flow. For labelled carbon monoxide both the rate of transfer into the pulmonary capillary and the rate of blood flow are important. Nunn and his colleagues (Hulands *et al.*, 1970) have employed xenon-133 to study the spread of ventilation perfusion ratios under anaesthesia. For further details of these techniques the reader is referred to the work of West (1965).

## Gas Transfer Across Alveolar/Capillary Membrane

The overall transfer of gas from the alveoli to the blood is a complex process and depends not only on the diffusion characteristics of the lung membrane, and the inter-relationship of distribution of ventilation and perfusion, but also, in the case of oxygen and carbon monoxide on the rate at which the gas combines with haemoglobin.

The term diffusing capacity is perhaps more appropriately applied to the actual process of diffusion across the membrane which separates the alveolus from the pulmonary capillary blood, whereas the *transfer factor* ($T_L$) described the whole process. The physical definition of *diffusing capacity* is more straightforward. The volume of gas diffusing across the alveolar/capillary membrane per unit time is dependent upon the relationship:

$$\text{Volume of gas diffusing per unit time} \propto \text{Diffusing capacity of the gas} \times \text{Pressure gradient}$$

where the diffusing capacity of the gas is proportional to:

$$\frac{\text{Surface area of membrane}}{\text{Thickness of membrane}} \times \frac{\text{Aqeous solubility}}{\sqrt{MW}}$$

Thus the diffusing capacity of oxygen ($D_{O_2}$) can be defined as the number of millilitres of oxygen that diffuse across the alveolar/capillary membrane per mm. Hg. per minute:

$$D_{O_2} = \frac{\dot{V}_{O_2}}{\overline{P}_{A_{O_2}} - \overline{P}_{C_{O_2}}}$$

There is, however, no acceptable method for the measurement of $D_{O_2}$, as to-date, there has been no way of obtaining the mean capillary oxygenation ($\overline{P}_{C_{O_2}}$) despite various attempts to derive this quantity indirectly.

However the transfer factor for carbon monoxide can be calculated using the relationship:

$$D_{CO} = \frac{\dot{V}_{CO}}{\overline{P}_{A_{CO}} - \overline{P}_{C_{CO}}}$$

Because of the great affinity of carbon monoxide for haemoglobin (250 × as great as $O_2$) and the low capillary value the mean back tension of CO can be represented by the mixed venous CO tension ($P_{V_{CO}}$), which is effectively zero when low concentrations of carbon monoxide are breathed.

The relationship:

$$\frac{1}{Tl} = \frac{1}{D_m} + \frac{1}{a\dot{Q} + \theta.Vc}$$

describes the process of gas transfer within the lung.

where Tl = Transfer factor = rate of uptake of gas from alveoli in ml./min./mm. Hg.
$D_m$ = Diffusing capacity of the alveolar/capillary membrane in ml. STPD/min./mm. Hg. gradient.
a = is the solubility of the gas at 37°C in ml. STPD per ml. blood/per mm. Hg.
a = $\alpha/760$ where $\alpha$ = bunsen solubility co-efficient.
$\theta$ = rate of combination of gas with blood in ml. STPD/ml./mm. Hg.
$\dot{Q}$ = cardiac output in mls.
Vc = volume in mls. of blood in alveolar capillaries.

For gas which do not combine with haemoglobin $\theta$ is zero.

$D_m$ is large compared with $a\dot{Q}$.
$1/D_m$ is very small in relation to $1/a\dot{Q}$.
The transfer factor therefore simplifies to $a\dot{Q}$

At the time when the term diffusing capacity was introduced it was thought that the rate of combination of oxygen or carbon monoxide with haemoglobin was so quick that the factor $\theta$ was neglected. The rate of combination CO is slower than $O_2$, the rate also reduced when $O_2$ saturation haemoglobin high. However, that rate at which the gas leaves the alveolus by combining with the haemoglobin in the capillary is fast relative to the rate at which it is removed by blood flow. $a\dot{Q}$ is therefore small compared with $\theta Vc$. $\frac{1}{Tl}$ becomes $\frac{1}{D_m} + \frac{1}{\theta Vc}$.

The magnitude of the transfer factor is therefore determined not only by the diffusion characteristics of the lung membrane but also by the rate at which carbon monoxide combines with haemoglobin in the pulmonary capillaries. Perfusion thus plays a relatively small part in the estimate of transfer factor for CO but the technique does however permit an estimate to be made of pulmonary capillary BV (approximately 100 ml.).

## Methods

The concentration of carbon monoxide in the alveoli and the rate of uptake into the blood per minute are estimated by steady-state or single-breath methods. The mixed venous carbon monoxide tension can be derived using a re-breathing method. Carbon monoxide concentration in gas mixtures can be estimated using an Infra-Red Analyser (*see* p. 89).

## Steady State Method

Low concentrations of carbon monoxide are breathed for several minutes. The uptake of carbon monoxide is determined from a knowledge of the inspired and expired concentrations. The tension of carbon monoxide in alveolar gas is obtained from the relationship:

$$P_{A_{CO}} = P_{I_{CO}} - (P_{I_{CO}} - P_{\bar{E}_{CO}}) \times (P_{A_{CO_2}}/P_{\bar{E}_{CO_2}})$$

$P_{A_{CO_2}}$ is determined either by analysis of arterial blood ($Pa_{CO_2}$) (where it is only safe to assume that $P_{A_{CO_2}} = Pa_{CO_2}$ when the range of $V_{A/Qc}$ ratios is not wide), by end-tidal sampling, or by the re-breathing method).

### Single-breath Method

This method consists in inspiring a small concentration of carbon monoxide (0·3 per cent) together with 2–12 per cent helium after emptying the lungs to residual volume. The volume inspired is to the full inspiratory position (i.e. vital capacity). The breath is held for 10 seconds and the expired gas is collected at the same time an alveolar sample is obtained. The initial dilution of the gas in the lung is obtained by comparing the concentration of helium in the inspired gas with that in the alveolar sample. The alveolar concentration of carbon monoxide at the start of breath-holding can also be derived from this as the degree of dilution of carbon monoxide is the same as that of helium. The final concentration of alveolar carbon monoxide at the end of breath-holding is obtained from the end-tidal sample. The capillary blood concentration of carbon monoxide is assumed to be zero. From a knowledge of the carbon monoxide consumption the diffusing capacity for carbon monoxide can be determined.

### Fractional Carbon Monoxide Uptake

Though not measuring diffusion directly this method indicates how much surface area is available for diffusion. The method has the advantage of simplicity. 0·15 per cent carbon monoxide is breathed on an open circuit for 2 minutes.

$$\frac{\text{Fractional}}{\text{CO uptake}} = \frac{\text{Volume CO taken up by body}}{\text{Volume of CO inspired}} \times 100$$

(Normal value (resting) 50–60 per cent)

### Factors Affecting Transfer Factor

($T_L$) The transfer factor has a mean value of 20–38 ml./min./mm. Hg.

Factors increasing:    Increases with size subject.
Higher for males than females.
Increases with exercise.
Increases with depth inspiration.
Increases in polycythaemia.
Increases in change of posture from upright to head-down.

Factors decreasing:    Increasing age.
Inhalation high concentrations oxygen.
Diseases lung parenchyma.

### Factors Affecting Resistance of Membrane to Diffusion ($1/D_m$)

Factors decreasing:    Decrease in thickness membrane.
Increase in surface area.

Large lung volumes.
Pulm. lymphangitic carcinoma.
Hanan-Rich syndromes.
Miliary tuberculosis.
Beryllosis.
Scleroderma asbestosis.
Interstitial oedema.
Pulm. congestion.

Factors increasing:    Increase in thickness, alveolar membrane.
Sarcoidosis.
Pulmonary granulomatoses.
Reduction in surface area.
Loss of lung parenchyma, e.g. emphysema.
Age.
Includes disorders of ventilation/perfusion.

In mitral stenosis there is reduction in diffusion across the membrane but this is offset by an increase in the volume of the pulmonary capillaries and therefore the transfer factor tends to stay the same.

### Factors Affecting Volume of Blood in Pulmonary (Vc)

The volume of blood in the pulmonary capillaries is about 60 ml. (upright).

Increase:    With exercise.
With rise in pulmonary venous pressure (mitral stenosis).
Some types of congenital heart disease.

Decrease:    When blood is diverted elsewhere—meals, skin vasodilation.
Late stages chronic lung disease, i.e. when pulmonary hypertension is established.
With age.

The $D_{CO}$ correlates best with body surface area:
$$D_{CO} \text{ (rest)} = \text{Body surface area (m}^2\text{)} \times 18·85 - 6·8 \pm 3·92 \text{ SE.}$$

### Blood Gases

It has been pointed out that because of the considerable ability of the lung to compensate for disturbance in lung function, blood gases may remain within normal limits despite significant changes in lung function. Changes in $Pa_{CO_2}$ are governed by the relationship:

$$Pa_{CO_2} \propto \frac{\dot{V}_{CO_2}}{\dot{V}_A}$$

A reduction by half in alveolar ventilation (normal level of 4 litres/min.) (see Fig. 2) will, for a given level of carbon dioxide production ($\dot{V}_{CO_2}$) double the $Pa_{CO_2}$. The $Pa_{CO_2}$ is therefore a sensitive measure of the adequacy of alveolar ventilation (carbon dioxide elimination). Provided that no abnormal venous admixture exists such a fall in alveolar ventilation in a subject breathing air is unlikely to result in a great fall in $Sa_{O_2}$ (see Fig. 2). The $Pa_{O_2}$, however, falls considerably and should a further reduction in alveolar occur the $Sa_{O_2}$ will fall precipitously. Impairment of diffusing capacity is unlikely to result in a measurable reduction of $Pa_{O_2}$ provided that a normal $P_{A_{O_2}}$ is maintained and the patient is in a resting state. Venous admixture (*see* p. 250) will however have profound effects upon arterial oxygenation.

## REFERENCES

Bernstein, L., D'Silva, J. L. and Mendel, D. (1952), "The Effect of the Rate of Breathing on Maximum Breathing Capacity Determined with a New Spirometer," *Thorax*, **7**, 255.

De Bono, E. F. (1963), "A Whistle for Testing Lung Function," *Lancet*, **2**, 1146.

Clark, T. J. H. (1968), "The Ventilatory Response of Carbon Dioxide in Chronic Airways Obstruction Measured by a Rebreathing Method." *Clinical Science*, **34**, 559.

Collins, M. M., McDermott, M. and McDermott, T. J. (1964), "Bellows Spirometer and Transistor Timer for the Measurement of Forced Expiratory Volume and Vital Capacity," *J. Physiol.* (*Lond.*), **172**, 39.

Cotes, J. E. (1965), *Lung Function*. Oxford: Blackwell.

Don, H. F. and Robson, J. G. (1965), "The Mechanics of the Respiratory System during Anesthesia," *Anesthesiology*, **26**, 168.

Dubois, A. B., Botelho, S. Y., Bedell, G. N., Marshall, R. and Comroe, J. H. (1956), "A Rapid Plethysmographic Method for Measuring Thoracic Gas Volume," *J. clin. Invest.*, **35**, 322.

Farhi, L. E. and Rahn, H. (1955), "Gas Stores of the Body and the Unsteady State," *J. appl. Physiol.*, **7**, 472.

Goldman, M., Knudson, R. J., Mead, J., Peterson, N., Schwaber, J. R. and Wohl, M. E. (1970), "A Simplified Measurement of Respiratory Resistance by Forced Oscillation," *J. appl. Physiol.*, **28**, 113.

Hugh-Jones, P. and Lambert, A. V. (1952), "A Simple Standard Exercise Test and its Use for Measuring Exercise Dyspnoea," *Brit. med. J.*, **1**, 65.

Hugh-Jones, P. and West, J. B. (1960), "Detection of Bronchial and Arterial Obstruction by Continuous Gas Analysis from Individual Lobes and Segments of the Lung," *Thorax*, **15**, 154.

Hulands, G. H., Greene, R., Iliff, L. D. and Nunn, J. F. (1970), "Influence of Anaesthesia on the Regional Distribution of Perfusion and Ventilation in the Lung," *Clin. Sci.*, **38**, 451.

McKerrow, C. B., McDermott, M. and Gilson, J. C. (1960), "A Spirometer for Measuring the Forced Expiratory Volume with a Simple Calibrating Device," *Lancet*, **1**, 149.

McKerrow, C. B. and Edwards, P. (1961), "The McKesson Vitalor," *J. Amer. med. Assn.*, **177**, 865.

Ravin, M. B. (1964), "The Match Test as an Aid to Preoperative Pulmonary Evaluation," *Anesthesiology*, **25**, 391.

Tanabe, G., Takahashi, H., Fujimoto, K., Yamabayashi, H., Ichinosawa, A., Tonomura, S. and Tani, H. (1965), "The Measurement of Respiratory Resistance by Oscillation Technique," *Ann. Resp. Center. Adult Dis.*, **5**, 83. Japan: Osaka.

Warring, F. C. and Siemsen, J. K. (1957), "A Convenient Method for Measuring Ventilation based upon the Venturi Principle," *Amer. Rev. Tuberc.*, **75**, 303.

West, J. B. (1965), "*Ventilation Blood Flow and Gas Exchange*. Oxford: Blackwell.

*CHAPTER 5*

# OXYGEN THERAPY AT AMBIENT PRESSURE

### JULIAN M. LEIGH

Oxygen fulfils its metabolic role at the mitochondrial level. The inspired oxygen tension represents the highest value in a descending sequence of oxygen tensions concerned with delivering oxygen to this site (Figure 1).

```
INSPIRED        e.g. 150   ↓
    ALVEOLAR          103   ↓
        ARTERIAL          100   ↓
            CAPILLARY          51   ↓
                MITOCHONDRIAL    1–10 mm Hg
```

FIG. 1. The oxygen cascade, with examples of oxygen tension at each stage. Note how small is the mitochondrial tension.

Various factors operate at each stage in this 'oxygen cascade' to reduce oxygen tension. Should the inspired tension be low or the gradient at any stage be steeper than usual, it may be combated by raising the inspired oxygen tension and thus raising the driving pressure at the beginning of the cascade.

In general, the further down the cascade is the lesion to be treated, then the higher the inspired oxygen tension that is necessary. Campbell (1965) has computed the increases in oxygen content of arterial blood per 1 per cent rise in inspired oxygen concentration, for lesions at different sites (Table 1).

TABLE 1

CHANGES IN OXYGEN CONTENT OF ARTERIAL BLOOD FOR DEFECTS AFFECTING OXYGENATION
(Based on Campbell, 1965)

| Lesion | Changes in $O_2$ content per 1% rise in inspired oxygen concentration |
|---|---|
| Low inspired $O_2$ concentration | 3·0  ml/100 ml |
| Decreased alveolar ventilation | 3·0  ml/100 ml |
| Venous admixture | 0·02 ml/100 ml |
| Low haemoglobin | 0·04 ml/100 ml |
| CO haemoglobinaemia | 0·03 ml/100 ml |
| Met haemoglobinaemia | 0·03 ml/100 ml |
| Low cardiac output | 0·03 ml/100 ml |
| Poisoning of cell enzymes | 0·03 ml/100 ml |

### The Concept of Tissue Oxygen Availability

It is very useful to consider the total quantity of oxygen which is theoretically available to the tissues per minute. This concept was first developed by Richards (1943) and further elaborated by Freeman and Nunn (1963). It is simply the product of arterial oxygen content and cardiac output per minute ($\dot{Q}$):

Available oxygen/minute

$$= (\text{haemoglobin content} + \text{plasma content}) \times \dot{Q}$$

This expression may be fully formulated as:

Available $O_2$/min =

$$\left( \frac{1 \cdot 39 \times Hb \times Sa_{O_2}}{100} + 0 \cdot 003 \times Pa_{O_2} \right) \times \frac{\dot{Q}\,ml}{100}$$

where,

1·39 = oxygen capacity of haemoglobin in ml/g calculated for a molecular weight of haemoglobin of 64,458.

Hb = measured haemoglobin content in g/100 ml of whole blood.

$Sa_{O_2}$ = percentage oxygen saturation of the haemoglobin in arterial blood.

0·003 = ml of oxygen dissolved in the plasma of 100 ml of whole blood/mm Hg applied oxygen tension.

$Pa_{O_2}$ = measured arterial oxygen tension in mm Hg

Consideration of some real values further helps to highlight the usefulness of this concept, e.g.

available $O_2$/min.

$$= \left( \frac{1 \cdot 39 \times 14 \cdot 5 \times 97 \cdot 5}{100} + 0 \cdot 003 \times 100 \right) \times \frac{5,000}{100}$$
$$= (19 \cdot 7 + 0 \cdot 3) \times 50$$
$$= 985 + 15$$
$$= 1,000 \text{ ml/ min}$$

Notice how small is the plasma contribution relative to that from haemoglobin, due to the properties of the haemoglobin dissociation curve.

Suppose the patient under consideration has an oxygen consumption of 250 ml/min. Then his 'coefficient of utilization' of oxygen will be,

$$\frac{250}{1,000} \text{ or } 25 \text{ per cent}$$

Now, suppose we chose some values of haemoglobin and cardiac output which are lower, but by no means unreasonable, and at the same time permit the arterial oxygen tension to fall to 60 mm Hg (91 per cent saturation); then,

available $O_2$/min.

$$= \left( \frac{1 \cdot 39 \times 10 \times 91}{100} + 0 \cdot 003 \times 60 \right) \times \frac{3,000}{100}$$
$$= (12 \cdot 65 + 0 \cdot 18) \times 30$$
$$= 379 \cdot 5 + 5 \cdot 4$$
$$= 385 \text{ ml/min}$$

If we still assume an oxygen consumption of 250 ml/min then the 'coefficient of utilization' of oxygen has become

$$\frac{250}{385} \text{ or } 65 \text{ per cent.}$$

It is now obvious that the safety margins are considerably reduced. A further loss of haemoglobin, fall in cardiac output or increase in oxygen consumption, e.g., due to shivering, would place this patient in jeopardy. Such a state of affairs is not uncommon in the early post-operative phase.

Furthermore, where there is a high coefficient of utilization of oxygen, more tissues will be relatively hypoxic necessitating anaerobic glycolysis and thus producing metabolic acidosis. The latter will move the oxyhaemoglobin dissociation curve to the right, i.e., a higher oxygen tension will then be required to produce the same percentage oxygen saturation of haemoglobin. Also, acidosis has a deleterious effect on cardiac contractility and thus on cardiac output. Acidosis therefore has an extremely adverse effect on oxygen availability and may constitute part of a vicious spiral with fatal consequences, if untreated.

A full appreciation of the concepts embodied in the oxygen availability expression and in the 'coefficient of utilization' of oxygen is an invaluable aid to patient management. The relevant points may be summarized:

**Factors Reducing Oxygen Availability**

    (i) Low arterial oxygen content

$$\text{low } Sa_{O_2} \begin{cases} \text{low } Pa_{O_2} \\ \text{acidosis} \end{cases}$$

$$\text{low haemoglobin} \begin{cases} \text{anaemia} \\ \text{CO Hb} \\ \text{Met Hb} \end{cases}$$

    (ii) Low cardiac output

**Factors Increasing Oxygen Requirement** (raising the coefficient of utilization)

    (i) Shivering

    (ii) Oxygen cost of increased ventilatory effort or tachycardia

    (iii) Hyperpyrexia.

**Measures to Increase Oxygen Availability**

    (i) Raise arterial oxygen tension.

    (ii) Raise haemoglobin content.

    (iii) Alleviate acidosis.

    (iv) Increase cardiac output.

**Measures to Reduce Oxygen Requirements**

    (i) Paralysis and I.P.P.V.

    (ii) Digitalization.

    (iii) Prevention of hyperthermia.

    (iv) In extreme circumstances induction of hypothermia, e.g., at 30°C oxygen requirement is 40 per cent of normal.

## Shifts of the Oxygen Dissociation Curve

Shifts of the oxyhaemoglobin dissociation curve make no difference to *oxygen loading*, provided that the arterial point is on the flat-top segment—once the arterial point is on the steep segment then oxygen loading is adversely affected by a right shift, as already indicated. Conversely, since oxygen unloading always tends to be on the steep segment, a right shift favours oxygen delivery to the tissues as the haemoglobin is capable of unloading more oxygen at a given $P_{O_2}$. The position of the steep segment thus reflects the affinity of oxygen for haemoglobin.

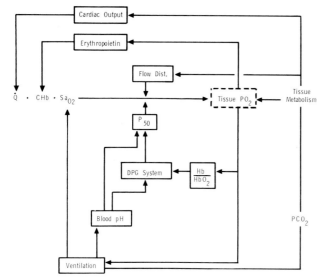

Fig. 2. Factors concerned in tissue oxygen supply. Modified from Finch and Lenfant (1972).

It has become fashionable to describe the position of the dissociation curve in terms of a single co-ordinate, *viz.*, the tension at which 50 per cent saturation of the haemoglobin occurs—*the $P_{50}$*—which has a normal value of 26·5 mm. Hg. Thus an increase in $P_{50}$ indicates a low affinity of haemoglobin for oxygen.

### Factors Which Increase $P_{50}$

These are (i) An increase in $[H^+]$.

(ii) An increase in the intracellular organic phosphate ester 2, 3—diphosphoglycerate (DPG) which is generated by the anaerobic glycolytic pathway. DPG, binds to haemoglobin and reduces its affinity for oxygen. The level of DPG is increased by a fall in intracellular pH and increasing levels of reduced haemoglobin. Thus, increasing oxygen extraction from the erythrocyte favours the production of DPG, and further enhances oxygen release.

All the factors which are concerned in tissue oxygen supply are summarized diagrammatically in Figure 2.

## Oxygen Therapy

The object of oxygen therapy is to raise tissue oxygen tension. The only route is the arterial blood. Except for patients on cardio-pulmonary by-pass, the only access to the arterial blood is via the alveolar-capillary membrane and thence via the inspired gas mixture. Adequate alveolar ventilation is therefore a necessary prerequisite.

A rise in inspired oxygen tension may be achieved either,

(i) by raising inspired oxygen concentration ($F_{I_{O_2}}$),

(ii) by raising the total atmospheric pressure and thus secondarily affecting $P_{I_{O_2}}$, or

(iii) both the above.

The latter two constitute hyperbaric oxygenation (*see* Chapter 6). This account refers to category (i). It specifically relates to spontaneously ventilating nonanaesthetized patients at ambient atmospheric pressure.

Oxygen therapy is achieved by the application of suitable apparatus to the patient and this chapter deals with the resultant effects on the gas phase. It is not intended to review the history, indications or physiological effects of oxygen therapy. For the historical aspects, the reader is referred to Barach (1962); for the rationale of oxygen therapy to Flenley (1967) and Saltzman (1967); for a lengthy review on the whole subject to Hedley-Whyte and Winter (1967) and for current concepts in oxygen transport to Finch and Lenfant (1972).

## Basic Requirements

The basic requirements for oxygen therapy equipment were stated by Barach and Eckman (1941) as:

1. Control over oxygen percentage of the inspired gas.

2. Prevention of excessive accumulation of carbon dioxide.

3. Elimination of resistance to breathing.

4. Efficiency and economy in the use of oxygen.

5. Adaptability of the apparatus for helium and oxygen therapy—to which one might add, over a quarter of a century later, adaptability for administration of gases or vapours for analgesia.

Many devices in current use were not in fact designed to meet these requirements. However, awareness of the performance characteristics of the various devices enables more appropriate selection in a given clinical situation.

With devices which operate on the air admixture principle, the inspired oxygen concentration achieved by a particular oxygen flow may be affected by a variety of factors which differ from patient to patient resulting in *between patient* variation of inspired oxygen concentrations. While the likely range of oxygen concentrations to be expected for a given oxygen flow may be stated by the manufacturer or obtained from the literature, the gas phase performance of such a device in a particular patient under specific clinical conditions cannot necessarily be predicted. Furthermore, since the flow and time characteristics of ventilation are not necessarily constant in a specific patient, there is more *within patient* variation of inspired oxygen concentration from breath to breath than is widely appreciated.

## User Demands

The minimum 'user demands' asked of any oxygen therapy system must be: *what is the inspired oxygen concentration?* and *what is the inspired carbon dioxide concentration?* The latter is influenced by that part of the previous expirate which is reinhaled, i.e., the functional apparatus dead space.

These primary considerations are influenced by both patient and device factors. The important patient factors are the inspiratory flow rate and the duration of the expiratory pause. The device factors are physical volume, oxygen flow rate and vent resistance where appropriate.

## Ventilatory Flow

An appreciation of the flow pattern of spontaneous ventilation is important when considering the interaction of these various factors. Figure 3 shows the flow pattern

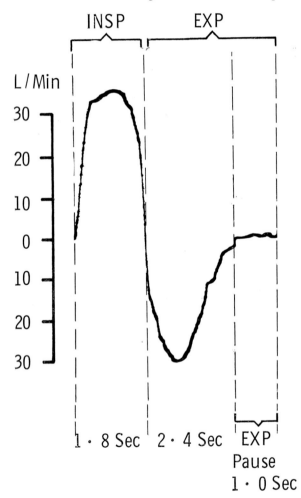

FIG. 3. One respiratory cycle from the pneumotachograph of a resting healthy male subject.

obtained with a pneumotachograph, of one respiratory cycle of a resting healthy subject. Inspiratory flow is sinusoidal. Expiratory flow reaches a peak in a similar time but then decreases more slowly. There are three time intervals during each cycle, viz., inspiratory time, expiratory time and expiratory pause time. The latter is

characterized by 'no flow'. Figure 4a is from the same tracing. This may be contrasted with Figure 4b which is from the same subject following exertion. Note the increase in peak inspiratory flow rate and the reduction in inspiratory and expiratory time, with the virtual absence of an expiratory pause. The significance of these changes will be apparent as the discussion progresses.

### The Evaluation of Oxygen Performance

A method for the analysis of performance in the gas phase during clinical oxygen therapy has been developed by Leigh (1970). This technique involves measurement of $P_{CO_2}$ and $P_{O_2}$ in discrete samples of expired gas. If the patient-device system has a constant performance then a graph plot of the co-ordinate points will give a straight line (the gas exchange ratio or R line) with minimal scatter (Fig. 5). The intercept of this line on the oxygen axis, i.e., where the carbon dioxide tension is zero, is the inspired oxygen tension of the patient-device system. If there is between patient variation, then in different patients receiving the same flow from the same mask, R lines with different intercepts will be produced. If there is within patient variation then the scatter will increase due to there being a breath to breath variation of R line intercept.

### Methods of Oxygen Therapy

The methods of giving oxygen therapy to spontaneously breathing conscious patients may be subdivided into *fixed performance* and *variable performance* systems. The former will give a controlled oxygen concentration independent of patient factors. The latter constitute air/oxygen admixture systems in which oxygen is supplied at a rate much less than inspiratory flow rate; performance is thus dependent upon their interrelationship with the patient. Figure 6 shows a comparison between a fixed performance system (35 per cent Ventimask) and a variable performance system (M.C. mask) in five subjects of varying build.

Not all the patient and device factors, indicated above, are operative in all the systems which are available for oxygen therapy. It is first necessary to classify fully the mode of operation of the various systems and then consider the role of the operative factors in each case. The classification is based on the technique of expired gas analysis outlined above and is given together with examples of devices in current use in British practice.

### Classification of Devices

A. **Fixed Performance Systems:** Independent of patient factors

    (i) *High Flow*—Ventimasks.
    (ii) *Low Flow*—Anaesthetic circuits.

B. **Variable Performance Systems:** Patient dependent

    (i) *No capacity system*: Inspired oxygen subject to between patient variation: oxygen catheters or nasal cannulae at *low* oxygen flows.

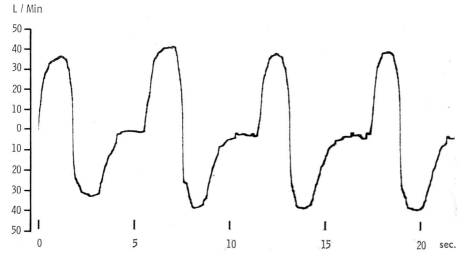

FIG. 4a. Pneumotachograph of a resting healthy subject.

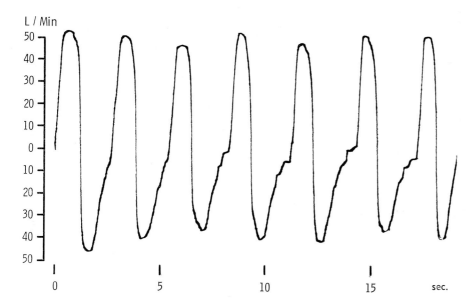

FIG. 4b. Pneumotachograph of the same subject in a 'breathless' state. Note the increase in peak inspiratory flow rate and [the decrease in the time intervals.

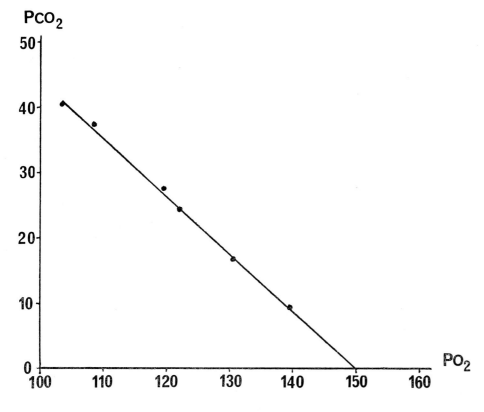

FIG. 5. Example of a gas R line drawn as the result of analysis of discrete samples of expirate, from separate breaths, with the subject breathing air. The intercept on the oxygen axis is 150 mm Hg, which is the $P_{O_2}$ of air.

(ii) *Capacity system*: Inspired oxygen subject to both between and within patient variation.

    (a) *Small capacity system*:

        1. For $O_2$ *only*—catheters or cannulae at *higher* $O_2$ flows.

        2. For *both* $O_2$ *and* $CO_2$ (i.e. with rebreathing)—M.C., Harris and Edinburgh masks.

    (b) *Large capacity system*:

        For *both* $O_2$ *and* $CO_2$ (i.e. with rebreathing)—Pneumask Polymask, Oxyaire, BLB and Portogen.

        Oxygen tent and incubator.

### Fixed Performance Systems

The fixed performance devices, when used in the proper manner, supply the predetermined oxygen concentration irrespective of the characteristics of the patient's ventilation.

As inspiratory flow is sinusoidal in character, a fixed concentration system must be capable of delivering the chosen mixture at a rate equal to or greater than peak inspiratory flow rate. When breathing from an anaesthetic circuit this criterion is satisfied since any flow can be met by collapse of the reservoir bag during inspiration. If there were no reservoir bag in a circuit, the fresh gas inflow would have to be greater than or equal to inspiratory flow at all times in order to ensure fixed performance. This state of affairs is precisely that which occurs with the Ventimasks. With anaesthetic circuits, volume demands by the patient are met by collection of gas in the reservoir bag during expiration. Any desired mixture can be given by this technique, but anaesthetic circuits are impractical for clinical oxygen therapy in conscious patients.

Although the high flow system is much less economical, it has distinct advantages, viz., rebreathing is minimized and so is the need for a tight fit to the face.

The high flow system with a variable venturi could be used to provide any required mixture without rebreathing, but the disadvantage would be the expense, especially when giving high oxygen concentrations from cylinder sources.

Ventimasks have been investigated by Bethune and Collis (1967a) and when oxygen is given at the proper flow rate, functional apparatus dead space is eliminated. Anaesthetic circuits have only been mentioned for completeness since it is with them that anaesthetists habitually give oxygen mixtures. Their functional dead space characteristics are, however, more complex (*see* page 505).

### Variable Performance Systems

These may give 21–100 per cent oxygen depending upon the interrelationship of oxygen flow, device factors and patient factors.

**No Capacity System.** With nasal or naso-pharyngeal delivery at low oxygen flows, there is not sufficient storage of oxygen in the airway during the expiratory pause to significantly affect the next inspiration. Enrichment is

then a pure function of inspiratory flow rate and oxygen flow rate.

In an air/oxygen mixture the total quantity of oxygen present is the sum of:

$$\text{Vol } O_2 \text{ from air} + \text{Vol } O_2 \text{ added}$$

and the concentration of oxygen ($F_{I_{O_2}}$) in the mixture is given by the ratio of that volume to the total volume:

$$\frac{\text{Vol } O_2 \text{ from air} + \text{Vol } O_2 \text{ added}}{\text{Vol air} + \text{Vol } O_2}$$

therefore

$$F_{I_{O_2}} = \frac{(\text{Vol air} \times 0\cdot2093) + (\text{Vol } O_2 \times 1\cdot0)}{\text{Vol air} + \text{Vol } O_2} \quad \text{(i)}$$

where $0\cdot2093$ and $1\cdot0$ are the fractional concentrations of oxygen in air and pure oxygen, respectively.

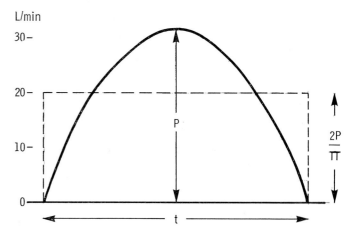

FIG. 6. Inspiratory flow wave-form. The area of the rectangle bounded by the broken line is the same as that of the sinusoid and is equal to the inspired volume.

During inspiration tidal volume is acquired as the integral of flow and time. As inspiratory flow is sinusoidal in character (Fig. 6) the relation between volume and flow rate is stated by,

$$\text{Vol} = \frac{2Pt}{\pi}$$

where $P$ is peak flow and $t$ is time; or in words—the area of the sinusoid is equal to the area of the rectangle of peak flow rate times $2/\pi$ and with the same time base.

In a system where enrichment only occurs during inspiration $F_{I_{O_2}}$ will be given by,

$$\frac{\text{Flow of } O_2 \text{ from air} + \text{flow of } O_2 \text{ added}}{\text{total flow}}$$

By substitution this expression becomes,

$$F_{I_{O_2}} = \frac{\left(\dfrac{2P}{\pi} - O_2 \text{ flow}\right) \times 0\cdot2093 + O_2 \text{ flow}}{\dfrac{2P}{\pi}}$$

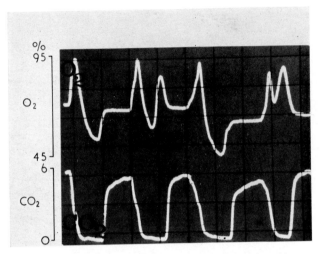

FIG. 8. Tidal $O_2$ and $CO_2$ measured at the lips with rapid response gas analysers during breathing with an M.C. mask at 10 1/min. There are four inspirations with four fairly typical $CO_2$ wave forms, but note that each of the $O_2$ wave forms rises at the beginning of inspiration towards 100 per cent but falls *within the same inspiration* towards 21 per cent as the inspired flow rate exceeds that of the oxygen inflow. The peak swings *during inspiration* vary from 45–95 per cent and the five end-tidal plateaux show a variation in oxygen concentration of 10 per cent (70 mm. Hg. approx.).

Which simplifies to,

$$F_{IO_2} = 0.2093 + 1.242 \left( \frac{O_2 \text{ flow}}{P} \right) \qquad \text{(ii)}$$

i.e., oxygen concentration is dependent upon peak flow and added oxygen flow and is independent of the duration of inspiration.

As we are considering a system in which the oxgyen flow is small compared to $P$ the breath to breath difference in $F_{IO_2}$ is not marked. A given subject in a steady state therefore receives a reasonably constant $F_{IO_2}$, given by equation (ii). However, since average peak inspiratory flow rates vary from patient to patient, depending upon physical build and state of the airways, etc., between patient variation in $F_{IO_2}$ occurs.

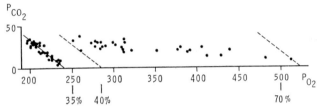

FIG. 7. Comparison between fixed performance and variable performance systems. The $O_2/CO_2$ diagram shows the analysis of separate samples of expiratory gas during the evaluation in five subjects (range of heights 159–196 cm.; range of weights 58·5–87·5 kg.) of a 35 per cent ventimask—left hand side—and an M.C. mask at 5 l./min. The possible scatter of inspired concentrations with the latter device is indicated by the broken 'R' lines and ranges from 40–73 per cent.

Since there is no imposed apparatus dead space, re-breathing of carbon dioxide does not occur. In fact the patient's physiological dead space is reduced at all flows (Bethune and Collis, 1967b).

The *oxygen capacity system* is an entirely functional description of nasal and nasopharyngeal delivery at higher oxygen flows. At these flows significant storage of oxygen in the airway occurs during the expiratory pause. However, since the expiratory pause is variable in length a variable volume of oxygen accumulates. Furthermore, as oxygen flow rate increases relative to peak inspiratory flow rate, breath to breath variation in peak flow rate has a more significant effect upon the inspired oxygen concentration. Thus, within patient variation is added to between patient variation. However, the effects of within patient variation are not as marked with these devices as with the large capacity devices.

The flow at which a no capacity system becomes an oxygen capacity system will of course vary from patient to patient but is of the order of 2–3 litres/minute.

**Small Capacity System for Oxygen and Carbon Dioxide**

Here apparatus dead space is added in the form of a mask shell. This allows for rebreathing of carbon dioxide and oxygen. While some economy of expired oxygen is achieved some of the fresh oxygen flow is lost through the vent. These masks thus do not provide a quantitative improvement in performance over the previous devices, which deliver oxygen directly into the airway. However, at high flows, they are much more comfortable.

During inspiration the mask, the volume of which is small relative to tidal volume, empties first *in series* with inspired air so that higher oxygen concentrations are inhaled at the beginning of each inspiration. Figure 8 clearly shows this effect. The performance of these masks is subject to between patient variation at low flows and both between and within patient variation at high flows (Fig. 9), in a similar manner to the oxygen capacity system.

**Rebreathing and Apparatus Dead Space**

Functional apparatus dead space is not the same as the physical volume of the apparatus, being equal to that part of the previous expirate which is re-inhaled. Its value depends upon similar factors to the inspired oxygen concentration and is therefore subject to a similar kind of variation.

It is very important to realize that patients may respond to imposed apparatus dead space by increasing their alveolar ventilation and thus overcoming its effect; or conversely, its imposition may be akin to increasing asphyxia in patients with incipient or actual respiratory failure.

There is, as yet, no accurate quantitative method for measuring tidal volume when wearing an oxygen therapy device, nor is it possible to collect mixed expired gas. Thus functional dead space cannot be measured clinically.

During clinical oxygen therapy, the only reliable estimate of rebreathing would be the continuous presence of carbon dioxide during the end-inspiratory phase of a continuous carbon dioxide trace (e.g., obtained by infra-red analysis). A rise in end-tidal or arterial carbon dioxide tension might also occur if there were insufficient compensation by an increase in alveolar ventilation. However, these could also be the result of respiratory depression from some other cause.

This important aspect of oxygen therapy has been well covered by Cotes (1956), Kory *et al.* (1962), and Bethune and Collis (1967a, b). In particular, the latter authors, using either a model patient-device system or a subject trained to breathe at a constant tidal volume, have elegantly demonstrated the dead space characteristics of the devices under such idealized circumstances.

The following points are of importance and functional dead space or rebreathing will be increased when:

(a) physical volume of the device is large
(b) flow of oxygen delivered is low;
(c) expiratory pause is short;
(d) inspiratory resistance of the vent is high (the mask is a good fit).

The vent resistance is a function, not only of the cross sectional area of the vent which is placed in the mask deliberately by the designer but also, of that leak area which is added by a poor fit to the face. This latter may be a potent cause of variation in performance.

**Large Capacity System**

These devices are characterized by the presence of a rebreathing bag (or reservoir bag in the case of the Porto-gen mask). The Pneumask and Polymask are simply rebreathing bags, while the remainder consist of mask shell plus bag. The Portogen mask has a one-way valve between bag and mask. All these devices have a large volume which empties *in parallel* with inspired air. Inspired oxygen has three sources, viz. fresh oxygen flow which continues throughout the ventilatory cycle; expired gas trapped in the dead space, and air coming through the total vent.

Since expired tidal volume is not constant, the quality of the expirate, i.e., the reciprocally related quantities of carbon dioxide and oxygen may vary from breath to breath.

rate. However, a patient with respiratory depression would not be at such a disadvantage with this system.

### Oxygen Tent and Incubator

The *oxygen tent* is a large capacity system in which the patient is enclosed. The build up of oxygen concentration within a tent is an exponential function. However, since both the tent capacity and the leakage are relatively large, the exponential has a long time constant. Only the most elaborately constructed oxygen tents are capable of

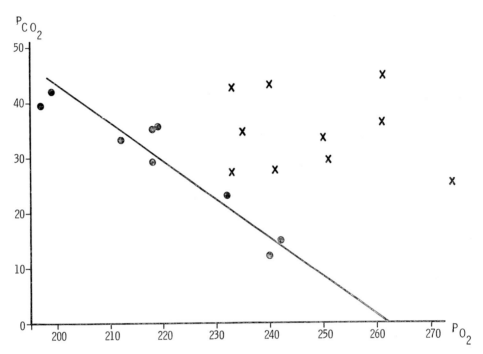

FIG. 9. Oxygen flow 4 litres (●) and 8 litres (×) in the same subject using an Edinburgh mask. The change in flow from 4 litres to 8 litres per minute shows up the effect of within patient variation as an increase in scatter of the $O_2/CO_2$ co-ordinate points.

The concentrations in the bag just before expiration thus depend upon the quality of the previous expirate, expiratory pause time and the loss of fresh oxygen flow from leaks. The ratio of gas volume taken from the bag to air volume taken through the total vent depends upon the relative flow resistances. The latter will vary with the distending pressure in the bag throughout inspiration. Since the times, volumes, flows and resistances vary, the performance of the devices in this group is exceedingly variable from breath to breath, even in the steady state (Figs. 10 and 11). It follows that the larger the capacity of the system, the greater is the effect produced by within patient variation of inspired oxygen values.

With the large capacity system it is not too difficult to predict that the shorter the expiratory pause time and the larger the expiratory flow, the less oxygen the patient will get and the more carbon dioxide. In other words, the more the patient requires oxygen therapy, the less well the device will perform at a given oxygen flow rate. 'Breathless' patients should therefore have a high oxygen flow

achieving oxygen concentrations of 50 per cent. This has its advantage, of course, in that carbon dioxide build up is equally limited.

Access to the patient is restricted, so that patient care and oxygen therapy may conflict since the oxygen concentration falls rapidly to ambient on opening the tent. The risk of fire is greatest with this method.

The oxygen tent should be reserved for children who will not tolerate an oxygen mask or catheter. For infants, an *incubator* not only constitutes the only possible method of continuous oxygen therapy but provides a controlled environment in respect of humidity and temperature. Oxygen and carbon dioxide build up is dependent upon the same factors as in the oxygen tent.

In neonatal resuscitation oxygen can only be given by mask or endotracheal tube. Oxygen by intragastric tube may dangerously raise intragastric pressure and only that which leaks back up the oesophagus can contribute to raising the inspired oxygen concentration. Oxygen by glass funnel is ineffective.

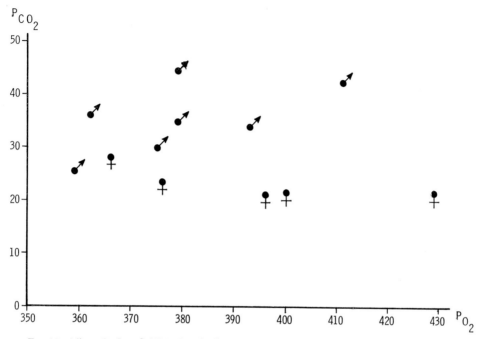

FIG. 10. 4 litres $O_2$ flow ♀ (65 Kg.) and 8 litres $O_2$ flow ♂ (82 Kg.) using the Pneumask. This plot demonstrates both within and between patient variation since the female gets approximately the same average enrichment as the male but is receiving only half the oxygen flow.

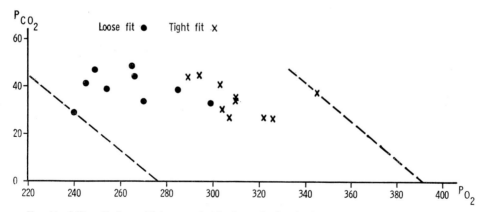

FIG. 11. 2 litres $O_2$ flow with loose and tight fit to the face in the same subject using the Oxyaire mask. This plot shows the additional within patient variation produced by alteration of the total vent resistance. The variation of inspired oxygen is indicated by the broken R lines and is equal to 110 mm Hg (15·5 per cent $O_2$).

Tables 2–4 summarize the characteristics of the variable performance systems.

TABLE 2

NO CAPACITY SYSTEM

$F_{IO_2}$ subject to between patient variation.
Dead space of patient diminished

|  |  | $F_{IO_2}$ |
|---|---|---|
| Peak insp. flow | + | ↓ |
|  | − | ↑ |
| Oxygen flow | + | ↑ |
|  | − | ↓ |

TABLE 3

OXYGEN CAPACITY SYSTEM

$F_{IO_2}$ subject to both between and within patient variation.
Dead space of patient further diminished

|  |  | $F_{IO_2}$ |
|---|---|---|
| Peak insp. flow | + | ↓ |
|  | − | ↑ |
| Oxygen flow | + | ↑ |
|  | − | ↓ |
| Exp. pause time | + | ↑ |
|  | − | ↓ |

TABLE 4

CAPACITY SYSTEMS WITH REBREATHING

$F_{IO_2}$ and $F_{ICO_2}$ subject to both between and within patient variation

|  |  | $F_{IO_2}$ | $F_{ICO_2}$ |
|---|---|---|---|
| Physical volume | + | ↑ | ↑ |
|  | − | ↓ | ↓ |
| Oxygen flow | + | ↑ | ↓ |
|  | − | ↓ | ↑ |
| Vent resistance | + | ↑ | ↑ |
|  | − | ↓ | ↓ |
| Exp. pause time | + | ↑ | ↓ |
|  | − | ↓ | ↑ |
| Insp. flow rate | + | ↓ | ↑ |
|  | − | ↑ | ↓ |

## Conclusions

Consideration of the factors influencing oxygen availability and oxygen requirement enables a rational approach to oxygen therapy to be adopted.

While it may be argued that what matters to the patient is his resultant arterial oxygen tension, the clinical value of this measurement is severely limited unless it is considered in relation to inspired or ideal alveolar oxygen tension. Since the ideal alveolar oxygen tension depends on inspired oxygen tension and cannot be derived without it, accurate knowledge of and control over inspired oxygen tension should be a fundamental prerequisite of oxygen therapy.

The Ventimasks provide a constant controlled inspired oxygen tension between 24 and 40 per cent without imposing functional apparatus dead space. One can have very little idea of the precise performance of any other device, particularly as capacity and oxygen flows increase.

It would be advantageous if oxygen therapy above 40 per cent could be administered by carefully controlling the dose delivered with the apparatus selected. This is particularly important since the risks of possible toxic effects incurred by the over-administration of oxygen may be just as important as not giving enough.

The latter concepts have been introduced into the management of patients on ventilators (Pontoppidan and Berry, 1967). As yet there is no commercially available device for giving accurate oxygen concentrations above 40 per cent to spontaneously breathing patients.

## REFERENCES

Barach, A. L. and Eckman, M. (1941), "A Physiologically Controlled Oxygen Mask Apparatus," *Anestheiology*, **2**, 421.

Barach, A. L. (1962), "Symposium—Inhalational Therapy. Historical Background," *Anesthesiology*, **23**, 407.

Bethune, D. W. and Collis, J. M. (1967a), "The Evaluation of Oxygen Masks. A Mechanical Method," *Anaesthesia*, **22**, 43.

Bethune, D. W. and Collis, J. M. (1967b), "The Evaluation of Oxygen Therapy Equipment. Experimental Study of Various Devices on the Human Subject," *Thorax*, **22**, 221.

Campbell, E. J. M. (1965), "Methods of Oxygen Administration in Respiratory Failure," *Ann. N.Y. Acad. Sci.*, **121**, 861.

Cotes, J. E. (1956), "Reassessment of Value of Oxygen Masks that Permit Rebreathing," *Brit. Med. J.*, **1**, 269.

Finch, C. A. and Lenfant, C. (1972), "Oxygen Transport in Man," *New Eng. J. Med.*, **286**, 407.

Flenley, D. C. (1967), "The Rationale of Oxygen Therapy," *Lancet*, **1**, 270.

Freeman, J. and Nunn, J. F. (1963), "Ventilation-perfusion Relationships after Haemorrhage," *Clin. Sci.*, **24**, 135.

Hedley-Whyte, J. and Winter, P. M. (1967), "Oxygen Therapy," *Clin. Pharm. and Therapy.*, **8**, 697.

Kory, R. C., Bergmann, J. C., Sweet, R. D. and Smith, J. R. (1962), "Comparative Evaluation of Oxygen Therapy Techniques," *J. Am. Med. Assoc.*, **179**, 767.

Leigh, J. M. (1970), "Variation in performance of oxygen therapy devices," *Anaesthesia*, **25**, 210.

Pontoppidan, H. and Berry, P. R. (1967), "Regulation of the Inspired Oxygen Concentration during Artificial Ventilation," *J. Am. Med. Assoc.*, **201**, 11.

Richards, D. W. (1943–44), "The Circulation in Traumatic Shock in Man," *Harvey Lect.*, Series 39, 217.

Saltzman, H. A. (1967), "Rational Normobaric and Hyperbaric Oxygen Therapy," *Annals Int. Med.*, **67**, 843.

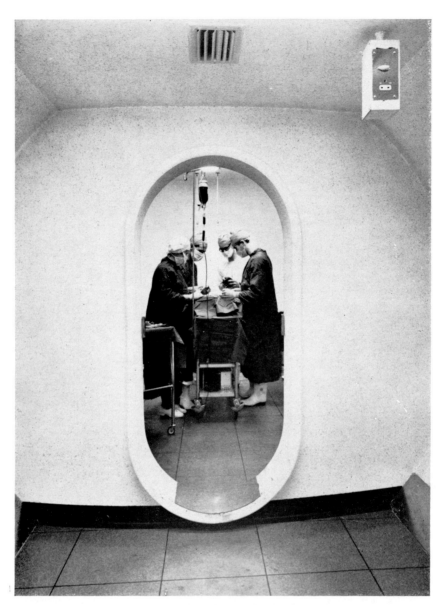

Fig. 1. Hyperbaric operating chamber
(*courtesy of Normalair Ltd., Yeovil*).

# CHAPTER 6

# HYPERBARIC OXYGEN

JOHN THURSTON

### Introduction

Hyperbaric oxygen therapy is defined as treatment with oxygen administered above atmospheric pressure. The actual pressure or tension present is the partial pressure of oxygen or $P_{O_2}$. In pure oxygen this is the same as the total ambient pressure whereas in air it corresponds to one-fifth of the total pressure.

The pressure can be effected either in a large walk-in chamber (Figs. 1 and 2) which can hold several people together with large equipment, or the smaller, individual, single patient chamber. The large chambers are supplied with compressed air which all in the chamber must breath, only the patient breathing pure oxygen from a cylinder by face mask. In the single patient chamber, only pure compressed oxygen is used. In medical practice, hyperbaric oxygen is given in pressures up to three atmospheres absolute (A.T.A.). This gives an inspired $P_{O_2}$ of 1520 mm. Hg. at 2 A.T.A. (760 mm. Hg. $\times$ 2), and 2280 mm. Hg. at 3 A.T.A. (760 mm. Hg. $\times$ 3). On an engineers' pressure gauge, where atmospheric pressure reads 0 pounds per square inch (p.s.i.), 2 atmospheres absolute is 15 p.s.i. and 3 is 30 p.s.i. (These readings are taken at sea level and take no account of water vapour pressure.)

### History

The administration of oxygen at higher than normal pressure has interested physiologists ever since they discovered the basic need of living organisms for oxygen. Early research was founded on the premise that if oxygen was essential for life, then giving more of it might provide some sort of benefit. In the last century many studies were performed, mainly using compressed air, on various aspects of animal and plant metabolism, and on the human body, both in health and disease. The early experimenters not only ran into technical difficulties with compression and decompression but also the problem of obtaining consistent results. This was because the nitrogen in air had its own separate effects, as also did the rising carbon dioxide concentration that occured in inadequately ventilated chambers. Nevertheless, the application of compressed air, even to sick human subjects, was promising and clinical use was started on quite a large scale around 1850, especially on the Continent of Europe. The striking feature, however, was the lack of any scientific rationale and the treatment was recommended for virtually any disease. As a result the hyperbaric centres became progressively more spa-like.

In the last fifty years accurate research into hyperbaric oxygen has been carried out as a result of the development of deep sea diving and of the problems associated with the use of submarines. The period leading up to and including the second world war was particularly fertile. The current interest started around 1956 and by coincidence at three separate centres simultaneously. In Glasgow work was started on its use in several different clinical conditions and in Amsterdam, Boerema used hyperbaric conditions to lengthen the safe period of circulatory arrest in cardiac surgery. In London, Churchill–Davidson started using hyperbaric oxygen in conjunction with deep X-ray therapy. As more clinical work was performed the physiology was better understood and, the usefulness of hyperbaric oxygen in a number of clinical conditions was investigated. As it was only necessary to give the high oxygen concentration to the patient alone, small one-man chambers were constructed. Provided there was no question of surgery being performed, and if no bulky equipment or research apparatus was needed when a walk-in pressurized operating suite would be required, the individual chamber was found to be a practicable, simpler and cheaper method of administering hyperbaric oxygen.

### Physiology

The benefits of hyperbaric oxygen follow from its effect on the absorption and transport of the gas. The higher the $P_{O_2}$ of the inspired gas the higher the arterial $P_{O_2}$ in a roughly linear relationship. The higher the arterial $P_{O_2}$ the higher the actual amount of oxygen carried physically dissolved in the arterial blood.

Oxygen is not very soluble in water, and with a normal $P_{AO_2}$ of 100 mm Hg, arterial blood at atmospheric pressure contains only 0·3 ml. blood in simple solution per 100 ml. of blood. 100 ml. of saturated blood carries about 19·5 ml. of oxygen combined with haemoglobin at the same $P_{AO_2}$. This, together with 0·3 ml. of oxygen dissolved in the plasma, constitutes the oxygen 'content' of arterial blood, expressed also as 19·8 'volumes per cent'. Thus the oxygen content of arterial blood is largely dependent on the haemoglobin content at normal atmospheric pressure. When hyperbaric oxygen is inhaled the haemoglobin cannot increase its oxygen load because it is already fully saturated and as the $P_{O_2}$ rises the oxygen content rises only by further simple solution in the plasma, in a fixed ratio of about 2·3 ml. per 100 ml. of blood per atmospheric pressure (760 mm). At twice atmospheric pressure, for example, (2 A.T.A.) the inhaled $P_{O_2}$ is $760 \times 2 = 1520$ mm Hg. At this $P_{O_2}$ the oxygen content is 20 ml as oxy-haemoglobin, plus $2·3 \times 2 = 4·6$ ml. physically dissolved giving a total of about 24 ml/100 ml. blood. In practice the $P_{AO_2}$ is always lower than the inhaled value, because the $CO_2$ and water vapour pressure constitute about 100 mm. of the 1520 mm. total pressure in the alveoli and further reductions due to imperfect ventilation–perfusion ratios and an alveolar-arterial oxygen gradient occur. To meet normal tissue oxygen requirements, 6 ml. of oxygen are abstracted from each 100 ml. of arterial blood, leaving 14 ml. of oxygen in every 100 ml. of mixed venous blood returning to the right atrium. Under hyperbaric conditions, at 3 A.T.A. where an extra $2\cdot3 \times 3 = 6\cdot9$ ml. of oxygen are dissolved in the plasma, this is sufficient to meet the normal oxygen requirement of the body without drawing on the haemoglobin oxygen and so the venous blood returns with the haemoglobin still fully saturated.

At 3 A.T.A. oxygen will be physically dissolved in the body water to an extent of about 7 ml. per 100 ml. In a 70 Kg. adult with a 50 litre body water, this would create a potential oxygen reservoir of $7 \times 500 = 3,500$ ml. of oxygen. Not all of this would be available for meeting the overall body needs for oxygen, but it would theoretically allow a period of total oxygen deprivation of 15 minutes. In a patient breathing room air, the principal oxygen reservoir is the oxygen carried by haemoglobin. At 1 A.T.A. oxygen, the oxygen in the lungs (F.R.V.) becomes quantitatively important, whilst at 3 A.T.A. the physically dissolved oxygen in the body water constitutes the largest oxygen reserve. The most important physiological advantage to be gained from hyperbaric oxygen therapy is the ability of tissues to survive temporary circulatory and respiratory arrest, due to the increased oxygen reservoir in the body fluids.

Hyperbaric oxygen affects the physiological state in several ways. It causes increasing constriction of arterioles, with a corresponding rise in systemic vascular resistance. There is thus a reduction in peripheral blood flow, and a rise in mean arterial blood pressure. The heart, if in normal sinus rhythm, slows slightly, this being an effect which can be abolished by atropine. The combined result of oxygen at 2–3 atmospheres absolute, is a small reduction of cardiac output, with the stroke volume and cardiac work remaining approximately unchanged. Perfusion has been measured in several organs under hyperbaric oxygen, and blood flow is reduced by the vasoconstriction in the kidneys and brain, causing a 20–30 per cent reduction in the blood flow at 2 A.T.A. Although the local circulation to various organs is reduced the arterial blood is so hyperoxygenated that the $P_{O_2}$ in the tissues supplied actually increases due to the higher content of dissolved oxygen. It has been shown that if the $P_{CO_2}$ in the brain is allowed to rise the arterial constriction is overcome and the flow increases. With normal ventilation, however, the arterial blood gases, apart from the oxygen, are not significantly changed, and the pH stays at the normal level.

## Hypoxia

Where hypoxia exists, tissue metabolism becomes impaired, and metabolic acidosis occurs. Hyperbaric oxygen has the ability not only to combat the hypoxaemia, but to reverse the acidosis by correcting the hypoxic metabolism at tissue level. When hyperbaric oxygen is inspired, increased oxygen can be carried in solution, even

when ventilatory efficiency and cardiac output are decreased, oxygen is available to the tissues, providing there is some local perfusion. The higher the $P_{O_2}$ in the arterial blood, the greater the diffusion gradient out of the capillaries. This gradient is largest in the tissues which are most hypoxic. This is particularly important when the blood supply to a damaged tissue is reduced, as with a myocardial infarct.

## Clinical Application

There are two methods of treating patients in hyperbaric oxygen. One method is to employ a large pressure chamber, usually the size of a small room, where the patient and attendant staff are placed. The room contains any equipment that may be required, and there is often space for the treatment of more than one patient if necessary. Surgery may be performed under hyperbaric conditions in which case the chamber is fitted out like an operating theatre. The chamber can be divided into two parts, so that staff or patients can enter or leave the main room by being compressed or decompressed in the subsidiary room, without altering the pressure in the main compartment. Similar smaller air locks enable items needed during surgery to be passed to and from the hyperbaric operating theatre.

These walk-in chambers contain air and the pressure within is raised by pumping in more air until the required pressure is obtained. Inside the chamber normal activities continue, and anaesthesia by the usual techniques presents little difficulty using normal anaesthetic apparatus.

The increased ambient pressure in these chambers causes a progressive increase in the density of all gases and this will effect the accuracy of the rotameter settings. McDowall (1964) has demonstrated that the rotameters behave as predicted according to the relationship

$F_x = F_0 \times \rho_0/\rho_x$
$F_x$ = actual flow at $x$ atmospheric pressure
$F_0$ = flow reading at $x$ atmospheres
$\rho_0$ = density of gas at pressure at which calibration was made
$\rho_x$ = density of gas at $x$ atmospheric pressure

He also demonstrated an increase in the halothane concentration delivered from a Fluotec vaporizer at 2 A.T.A. This effect was most marked at low concentration settings.

Under hyperbaric conditions the cuff of an endotracheal tube should be inflated with water rather than air. This is necessary as the cuff will tend to expand during decompression if it has been filled with air and may cause rupture of the trachea. Ventilation of the chamber is usually by a non-return valve and an open circuit. When the treatment is completed, the compressed air is released very slowly to avoid decompression sickness. Because of the length of time needed for safe decompression, the treatment sessions are made as long as possible. Slow decompression is essential due to the presence of nitrogen in the compressed air, which because of its poor solubility, may cause bubble emboli. The oxygen itself does not necessitate slow decompression. Although there is little difference in the

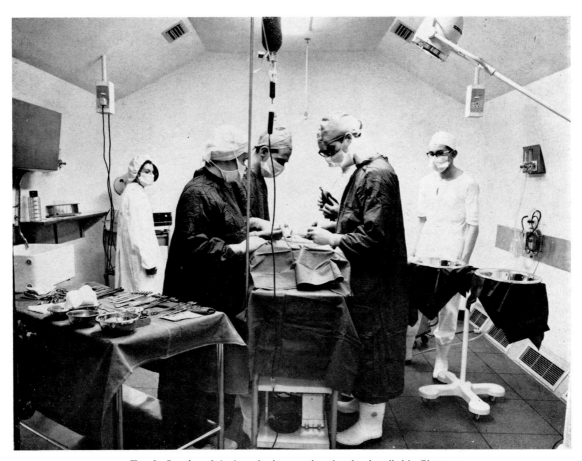

Fig. 2. Interior of the hyperbaric operating chamber installed in Glasgow.

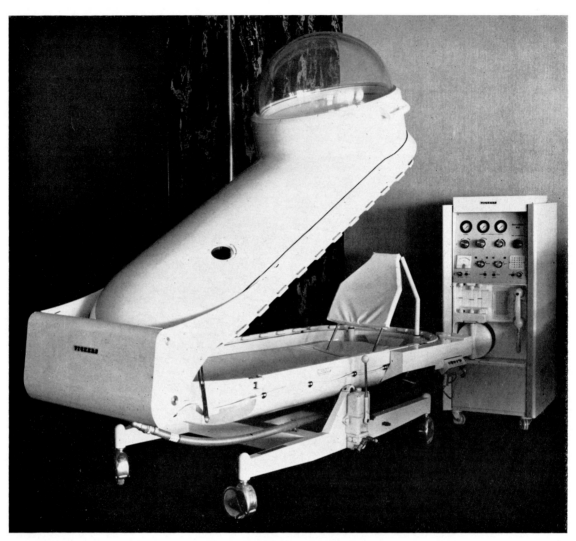

Fig. 3. Individual oxygen chamber
(*courtesy of Vickers Ltd.*).

chances of a fire *starting* in compressed air or oxygen, there is a better chance of extinguishing it in the former.

The second method of using hyperbaric oxygen employs a pressure chamber designed to contain the patient alone. This type of apparatus is normally pressurized with pure oxygen. The most widely used design, the Vickers Medical Hyperbaric Bed (Fig. 3) is basically a bed surrounded by a metal and transparent plastic case. The upper half hinges upwards and the patient can remain in the bed and be nursed in the same way as with an oxygen tent. The oxygen is used in closed circuit, enabling its temperature and humidity to be controlled, while carbon dioxide is removed, and only the minimum amount of additional oxygen is required. Various other facilities are available. Any probe that is needed for patient monitoring can be used in the hyperbaric bed, the wire passing through the base of the bed to the exterior, via a pressure seal. Tissue $P_{O_2}$ levels, and skin temperature, can thus be measured. The patient can also be maintained on positive pressure ventilation should it be indicated and the patient's blood pressure can be taken from outside the chamber, the cuff being inflated by the use of pure oxygen.

### Conditions treated with Hyperbaric Oxygen

Four absolute indications for the use of hyperbaric oxygen have now become established.

1. Carbon monoxide poisoning. Hyperbaric oxygen keeps the patient alive on dissolved oxygen at a time when his haemoglobin is not available for combination with oxygen. It also increases the rate of dissociation of carboxyhaemoglobin. A single therapy at 3 A.T.A. is usually curative and is always preferable to the traditional administration of 95 per cent $O_2$ and 5 per cent $CO_2$.

2. Air embolism. This may occur when catheters are introduced into the left side of the heart, or at cardiac surgery. At hyperbaric pressures the air is redissolved.

3. Gas gangrene. Infection with Clostridium perfringens, an anaerobe, is usually dramatically halted by hyperbaric oxygen. The toxic, pyrexial, confused, hypotensive and haemolysing patient becomes rapidly better after 5–7 treatments given over 2–3 days. This is usually given before ablative surgery nowadays and obviates the need for anti-gas gangrene serum and even penicillin.

4. The 'bends' or Caisson disease. Compression in hyperbaric oxygen will relieve the symptoms and sequelae of this condition.

Hyperbaric oxygen has in addition been used successfully in nearly all branches of medicine. In particular any condition in which local tissue flow is reduced may benefit. Thus patients with peripheral vascular disease, diabetic or rheumatoid arteritis and Raynaud's disease have all been seen to improve.

In Buffalo, New York, Dr. Winter and his colleagues have shown an improvement in patients with senile dementia treated with hyperbaric oxygen compared with matched controls.

A controlled series of patients treated with hyperbaric oxygen following acute myocardial infarction has shown a reduction in mortality in the treated group. Patients with heart failure, cardiogenic shock, heart block or a history of previous myocardial infarction all have a lower mortality than those in the control group.

Hyperbaric oxygen has been used in the treatment of pressure sores, in the prevention of sickle cell crises and also bacteriostatically in chronic infection by aerobic organisms, such as occurs in chronic osteomyelitis.

Hyperbaric oxygen has also been used as an adjunct to radio therapy. The rationale for this combination is that cancer cells are least resistant to ionising rays when fully oxygenated. Ordinarily, at the centre of ischaemic tumours, the cells are almost dormant and relatively immune to the therapeutic beam. Hyperbaric oxygen compensates for the poor blood supply by increasing the oxygen tension and thus restoring the radio-sensitivity of the malignant tissue.

### Toxicity and Hazards

Oxygen toxicity, the subject of much research, has been found to be of negligible importance when humans are exposed to pressures up to 2 A.T.A. for periods of several hours. Between 2 and 3 A.T.A. if the exposure is restricted to two hours at a time, with pure oxygen, there is a small incidence of side effects. These consist of feelings of vague discomfort and apprehension, numbness of extremities, muscle twitching and, finally, convulsions. The latter should not occur if close supervision is maintained, As soon as the premonitory signs are observed, the pressure should be allowed to fall slowly to 7 p.s.i. (0·5 A.T.A.) below the existing level and this will usually prevent further trouble. If a fit does occur, decompression must be completed rapidly unless the patient is in a walk-in chamber where embolism may occur. If this is accomplished there are usually no permanent sequelae.

When compressed air is being used, rather than pure oxygen, nitrogen bubble emboli can cause the 'bends' and other variations of decompression sickness. If this occurs re-compression is required, followed by a very slow decompression.

Long-term side effects are insignificant with pure oxygen. These are manifest as parasthesae of the extremeties and are only likely to occur when a long course of treatment is being given for a chronic condition.

With compressed air the most serious long term hazard is avascular bone necrosis. This can cause fractures of long bones. It may occur after prolonged exposures to high pressures. At levels up to 3 A.T.A. the risk of developing this condition is minimal. It is probably the result of nitrogen bubbles forming during too rapid decompression. The remaining hazard is the risk of fire. If precautions are taken, the risk of a fire starting in a hyperbaric chamber is negligible. The actual high pressure does not of itself make a fire more likely, but if a spark or a flame is formed there is obviously a great risk of it spreading to neighbouring materials. If this happens in compressed air, the resulting fire can be extinguished with water. In pure oxygen, combustion is extremely rapid, and for practical purposes prevention of fire is the only feasible policy. This is carried out by preventing the humidity falling below 60 per cent to reduce static sparking, and by keeping all electrical devices out of the chamber if they are connected to high voltage sources.

## REFERENCES AND FURTHER READING

"Hyperbaric Medicine" (1966), The Proceedings of the Third International Conference (Brown and Cox, Ed.).

"Hyperbaric Oxygen" (1965), The Proceedings of the Second International Conference (Ledingham, Ed.).

McDowall, D. G. (1964), "Anaesthesia in a Pressure Chamber." *Anaesthesia*, **19**, 321.

Proceedings of the 4th International Congress on Hyperbaric Medicine (J. Wada and T. Iwa, Eds.), 1970. Tokyo: Igaku Shoin Ltd.

# CHAPTER 7

# ARTIFICIAL VENTILATION

## H. B. FAIRLEY

A wide variety of techniques have been devised for the maintenance of ventilation in the absence of satisfactory spontaneous breathing. Each has the common objective of producing an intermittent pressure differential across the lungs and airway and, consequently, the first section of this chapter will consider aspects of the mechanics of breathing relevant to artificial ventilation.

As a corollary to the mechanics of artificial ventilation, there are changes in the haemodynamics of venous return, of cardiac output and of the pulmonary circulation and its distribution, as well as changes in the distribution of inspired air to the various regions of the lung. Thus, the next two sections will consider the effects of artificial

create a larger pressure gradient than is required to move the same volume of air during spontaneous breathing. This is primarily related to a reduction in *lung compliance*. Typical values are shown in Table 1.

*Chest wall compliance* varies with the degree of muscle paralysis. It is usually greater than the lung compliance in paralysed patients. For example, Smith and Spalding (1959) demonstrated a lung compliance of approximately 53 ml./cm.$H_2O$ and a chest wall compliance of 110 ml./cm.$H_2O$.

Paradoxically, *non-elastic resistance* is lower during I.P.P. ventilation. This is partly due to by-passing the upper airway but, even when this consideration is excluded,

TABLE 1

| Reference | Dynamic Compliance ml./cm.$H_2O$ | | Comment |
|---|---|---|---|
| | Spontaneous | I.P.P. | |
| Opie *et al.*, (1959) | 209 | | Supine conscious volunteers |
| | | 52 | Conscious paralysed patients |
| Gold and Helrich, (1965) | 107 | | Supine awake normal patients |
| | 83 | | Lightly anaesthetized patients |
| | | 62 | Lightly anaesthetized patients |
| Watson (1962) B | | | |
| Spalding and Smith, (1963) | 120 | 65 | Partially paralysed conscious patients |

ventilation on haemodynamics and on ventilation/perfusion relationships. Some consideration will also be given to problems of measurement during artificial ventilation.

This chapter will concern itself primarily with the physiological changes occurring during intermittent positive pressure (I.P.P.) and positive-negative pressure (P.N.P.) breathing, since these are the forms of artificial ventilation most commonly used by anaesthetists. Those wishing to read previous reviews are referred to those of Watrous *et al.* (1950), Whittenberger (1955), Pierce and Vandam (1962), Spalding and Smith (1963), Whittenberger (1962) and Elam (1965), the last two being particularly useful for those interested in the field of resuscitation.

### Mechanics of Artificial Ventilation

During normal spontaneous breathing, the force of the respiratory muscles generates a pressure gradient sufficient to overcome the elastic recoil of the lungs and chest wall, the resistance of the airways to airflow and the frictional resistance between each tissue component of the lung and chest wall. Normal values for these components are quoted in Chapter 2.

During artificial ventilation, it is usually necessary to

the non-elastic resistance of the lungs themselves may be lower during I.P.P. ventilation (Opie *et al.*, 1959). However, the contribution of non-elastic resistance, to the actual pressure gradients required during I.P.P. ventilation, can only be considered in terms of specific flow rates since the relationship between pressure and flow is non-linear. Thus, this aspect of the mechanics of I.P.P. ventilation is very much a function of the ventilatory pattern.

A pressure-cycled ventilator, set at rapid flows, may cycle relatively early in inspiration—increasing the delivered volume only when inspiratory flow is reduced, since the peak pressure will then be related to elastic recoil rather than to air flow resistance.

Figures are not available, comparing the pressures required to overcome the *non-elastic resistance of the chest wall*, during I.P.P. ventilation and spontaneous breathing. However, during the former, this represents only a fraction of the total non-elastic resistance (less than 20 per cent in our own series).

The cause of the low lung compliance found during I.P.P. ventilation has yet to be determined. Among the most popular of the theories is the possibility that there is an inherent maldistribution of air during I.P.P. due to the different distribution of pulmonary deformation forces in this method of breathing. If this were the case, tidal volumes would overexpand some areas of lung while others less exposed to these forces (e.g. peripheral areas) would remain relatively underventilated. As a consequence,

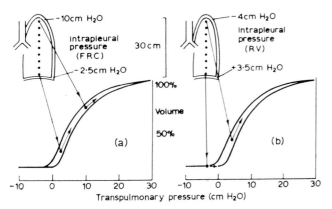

FIG. 1. Compliance curves of apex and base of lung in erect position, at (a) functional residual capacity, (b) residual volume. Note that compliance falls if tidal ventilation occurs in over-inflated areas, large pressures being necessary to move a given volume. (From J. B. West, *Advances in Respiratory Physiology*, Ed. by C. G. Caro, Arnold, 1966 and J. Milic-Emili, *Fed. Proc.* **23**, 117).

the end-inspiratory pressure would be that of over-inflation, the pressure-volume relationship moving up the compliance curve towards the relatively flat portion at total regional lung capacity (Fig. 1).

This theory is compatible with the finding that the alveolar dead space increases during I.P.P. ventilation (see below).

A second possible cause of the low compliance is that resting lung volume (FRC) is reduced in the absence of normal spontaneous breathing (Mead and Collier, 1959). It has been suggested that intermittent deep breaths are the mechanism employed in spontaneous breathing, to prevent alveolar collapse, and that their absence in I.P.P. ventilation permits a reduction in lung volume. Evidence for this is somewhat inconclusive, although the finding that compliance changes almost immediately, when I.P.P. is changed to spontaneous breathing (Watson, 1961) (Spalding and Smith, 1963) suggests that atelectasis is not the only factor. However, a fall in FRC has been demonstrated within minutes of the onset of respiratory paralysis (Laws, 1968) and this possibility cannot be excluded.

It has been suggested that atelectasis may occur progressively during the course of I.P.P. ventilation and that this may be avoided by the intermittent application of large inflations, simulating normal spontaneous ventilation (Egbert *et al.*, 1963). Certainly, this progression may occur with low tidal volumes (Hedley-Whyte *et al.*, 1965) but with larger tidal volumes this is not usually a problem.

A third possibility, occasionally mentioned, is that I.P.P. may produce a reduction in surface tension, possibly due to mechanical interference with cells producing surfactant. While there is evidence that this may occur with gross overdistension, it has been shown not to occur during prolonged I.P.P. with normal tidal volumes (Greenfield *et al.*, 1964).

## Airway Closure

Airway closure has been demonstrated to occur when the pressure outside peripheral airways exceeds that inside. In normal individuals, this occurs when regional lung volume falls below the normal resting position, i.e., when FRC approaches residual volume (Sutherland *et al.*, 1968) (Fig. 2).

This is usually present to some degree at the lung bases in the upright position and posteriorly in the supine position. The main consequences of this are the resulting venous admixture effect and the possibility of absorption atelectasis. Since this is a feature of any reduction in FRC and of low terminal airway pressures, relative to their surroundings, the application of a negative phase appears hazardous. Evidence of narrowed airways under such circumstances has already been obtained by Lynch *et al.* (1959) and by Galloon and Rosen (1965).

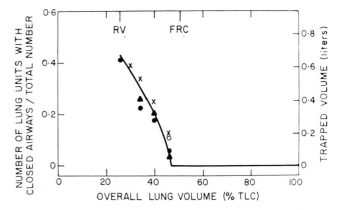

FIG. 2. Estimate of proportion of alveoli behind closed airways, obtained by Xenon washout in seated subjects, during lung deflation from total lung capacity. Airways begin to close at approximately 46 per cent TLC, nearly half the lung being involved at residual volume. (From Sutherland, J. B. (1968), *J. Appl. Physiol.*, **25**, 566.)

## Haemodynamic Effects of I.P.P.

An important mechanical distinction between I.P.P. ventilation and spontaneous breathing is that, although the pressure gradient produced during inspiration is positive at the upper airway relative to the pleural cavity in both instances, this is effected by increasing the upper airway pressure first during I.P.P., and by lowering the pleural pressure first during spontaneous breathing. Thus, regardless of whether greater pressure differentials are necessary during I.P.P. *mean intrathoracic pressure* will be higher than during spontaneous breathing. This has the effect of raising central venous pressure, thereby reducing the pressure gradient between the peripheral and central veins. Venous return is impeded.

Cournand *et al.* (1948) have established that this effect may be minimized by employing a rapid inflation, permitting quick deflation and maintaining an *inspiration/ expiration time ratio* less than 1:1. In the conscious subjects which they studied, no important effect on cardiac output resulted when such a pattern was used. More recently Prys-Roberts *et al.* (1967), studying patients anaesthetized with nitrous oxide and using an inspiration/expiration ratio of 1:2, were unable to demonstrate any consistent change in cardiac output when mean inflation pressure was altered. Thus, of Cournand's recommendations, the inspiration/expiration ratio seems the more important.

The relationships between airway pressure, inspiration/expiration ratio and blood flow in systemic great veins, pulmonary and arterial circulations have been studied by Morgan et al. (1966), at constant arterial $P_{CO_2}$, using dogs with implanted flow meters (Fig. 3). Caval flow

There is disagreement as to whether the venous capacity vessels change their distensibility (Watson, 1962; Blair et al., 1959), although this may relate to the time course of the two studies, since Watson noted that the response of the capacity vessels wore off gradually over a two to three minute period. Certainly, it is known that venous and arteriolar tone may be influenced by anaesthetic agents and, consequently, the effects of I.P.P. ventilation in the anaesthetized and unanaesthtized may differ in magnitude. Similarly, when the peripheral venous system is already constricted as a result of hypovolaemia,

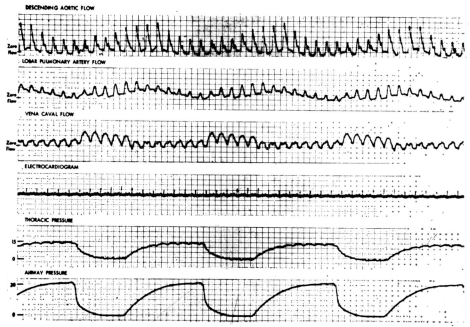

FIG. 3. Relative changes in flow in great vessels throughout I.P.P. ventilation cycle. From anaesthetized dog. (Morgan et al. (1966), *Anesthesiology*, **27**, 584.)

fell as airway pressure rose, followed by a reduction in pulmonary artery and aortic flow. On release of airway pressure, caval flow started to increase within one heart beat, pulmonary flow one beat later and aortic flow followed after the next beat. However, peak pulmonary artery flow was not regained until end-expiration, with peak aortic flow two beats later.

Various investigators, including Maloney et al. (1953) and Hubay et al. (1954) have demonstrated that the reduction in mean intrathoracic pressure produced by *P.N.P. ventilation* will increase cardiac output when compared with I.P.P. ventilation. However, in view of the demonstrated efficiency of a low inspiration/expiration ratio and the possible hazard of airway closure, a negative phase is probably not to be recommended.

In normal individuals, compensation for the increase in intrathoracic pressure produced by I.P.P. is said to be brought about by an increase in *peripheral venous tone* (Watson et al., 1962; Guyton, 1963; Blair et al., 1959), and it is known that systemic arteriolar constriction also occurs when intrathoracic pressure is raised (Lee, Matthews and Sharpey-Shafer, 1954).

the normal degree of compensation may not be possible. Watson et al. (1962) suggest this may also be the case when normal sympathetic pathways are impaired, as in patients with polyneuritis or high spinal cord transection.

Clearly, there is a balance to be struck between mean intrathoracic pressure, blood volume and peripheral venous tone, alteration in any one being capable of influencing venous return and therefore cardiac output.

Under certain circumstances, intermittent positive pressure ventilation may improve cardiac output. In addition to occasions when it is used as a resuscitative measure, I.P.P. has been shown to improve cardiac output in patients with cardiac disease. Maloney and Whittenberger (1957) feel this may be due to the reduction in venous filling of a failing heart, permitting it to function on a more advantageous part of the Starling curve. Spencer et al. (1959) and Gilston (1962) have both demonstrated improvements in post-cardiac surgery patients. Damman et al. (1963) found a fall in cardiac index in post-cardiac surgical patients when ventilated by I.P.P., but the fall correlated well with the associated reduction in work of breathing. The detailed mechanisms involved are not clear and a generalization is probably inappropriate.

Distinct from the effects on cardiac output produced by changes in intrathoracic pressure, any change in *arterial carbon dioxide tension* resulting from I.P.P. ventilation will produce a change in cardiac output. This has been demonstrated in anaesthetized man by Prys-Roberts *et al.* (1968) (Fig. 4), and in dogs by Morgan *et al.* (1967). Both cardiac output and stroke volume are reduced as $P_{CO_2}$ falls and this is independent of associated changes in intrathoracic pressure.

Although changes in cardiac output relate best to the reduction in venous return, there are associated changes

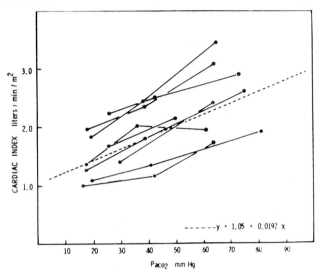

Fig. 4. Changes in cardiac index at differing levels of $P_{aCO_2}$ in anaesthetized man during passive ventilation. Lines join values from each patient. (Prys-Roberts *et al.* (1968), *J. Appl. Physiol.*, **25**, 80.)

in *pulmonary vascular resistance* and flow which may be of particular importance in ventilating patients with pulmonary disease.

Pulmonary blood flow depends on the inter-relationship between pulmonary artery, pulmonary venous and alveolar pressures. Since there is an abnormally high alveolar pressure at peak inflation, it is to be expected that pulmonary capillary flow will be impaired. The situation is likely to be most exaggerated at peak inspiratory pressures, when venous return and therefore pulmonary artery flow is reduced. Presumably, the uppermost parts of the lung will be most affected and an enlarged physiological dead space might be anticipated (see below).

Roos *et al.* (1961) have examined the inter-relationship between pressures in the pulmonary artery, pulmonary vein, pleural cavity and alveoli and their influence on pulmonary vascular resistance in the dog. When I.P.P. was applied, pulmonary vascular resistance rose. In man, pulmonary artery pressure rises with each inflation phase. Thomas *et al.* (1961) have demonstrated a fall in pulmonary vascular resistance when excised lung is inflated to approximately 50 per cent of total lung capacity (TLC), resistance increasing again as lung is inflated further. Presumably the high resistances at the lowest lung volumes

are due to pulmonary vascular collapse. Kira and Kukushima (1968) have shown that the rise in pulmonary vascular resistance as lung is inflated towards TLC is less if intravascular pressure is maintained at a high level. Lopez-Muniz *et al.* (1968) have demonstrated that the critical closing pressure of pulmonary vessels changes with $P_{CO_2}$ and with pH—acidity causing earlier closure.

Two other effects of intrathoracic pressure change should be mentioned. Sieker *et al.* (1964) and Salem *et al.* (1964) found that there was a diuretic response to lowering intrathoracic pressure. Pace-Floridia and Galinda (1968) have reported the onset of ventricular bigeminae with the introduction of a negative phase and its abolition by changing to I.P.P. ventilation—independent of blood gas change.

### Ventilation/Perfusion Inequalities

It is generally agreed that intermittent positive pressure ventilation is less efficient than spontaneous breathing, in achieving an optimal relative distribution of alveolar ventilation and pulmonary capillary blood flow.

An increase in physiological dead space is a constant finding during intermittent positive pressure ventilation and, although less consistently reported, there is frequently an increased venous admixture effect.

The aetiology of these findings is probably inter-related with the factors already described as being possible causes of low dynamic lung compliance and increased pulmonary vascular resistance.

### Dead Space Effect

The increase in dead space to tidal volume ratio ($V_D/V_T$) first demonstrated by Campbell *et al.* (1958) has been confirmed repeatedly. The aetiology has been reviewed in a most careful study by Cooper (1967), who found $V_D/V_T$ to vary in ventilated anaesthetized subjects from approximately 0·4 to 0·7, compared to the more usual value for spontaneous ventilation of <0·3 (Fig. 5). He demonstrated an increase in relation to *abnormalities in pulmonary status*, *age* and the higher *respiratory frequencies*. His values approximated $V_D/V_T$

per cent $= 33 + \dfrac{\text{Age}}{3}$, in patients with normal lungs. The

dead space volume did not bear a constant relationship to tidal volume, $V_D/V_T$ falling as tidal volume increased.

The reason for the increased dead space in individuals with normal lungs is uncertain. It has been demonstrated that it is predominantly at the alveolar level and there is some evidence that it may be related to *maldistribution of air*, as suggested by the associated low dynamic compliance. However, Bergman (1963) was unable to demonstrate impaired distribution when comparing I.P.P. with spontaneous ventilation, although this may have been due to the selected range of *inspiratory flow rates*, since Watson (1961) and Fairley and Blenkarn (1966) have shown an increase in $V_D/V_T$ when inspired volumes are delivered rapidly—possibly due to small variations in regional ventilatory time constants being amplified by the inspiratory flow exceeding the critical velocity, at the smaller of various parallel airways.

It is conceivable that $V_D/V_T$ changes related to inspiratory flow rate may also be $P_{CO_2}$ dependent although this has yet to be investigated. Newhouse *et al.* and Don and Robson (1965) have demonstrated $P_{CO_2}$ to be one of the factors influencing airway resistance, the latter rising at low $P_{CO_2}$. Thus, maldistribution may be more likely to occur at low $P_{CO_2}$ levels. However, since pulmonary capillary closure occurs most easily in an acid

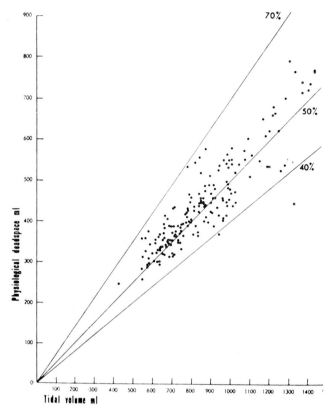

FIG. 5. Values for $V_D/V_T$ from anaesthetized patients during passive ventilation. (From Cooper, E. A. (1967), *Anaesthesia*, **22**, 199.)

environment, there may be a homeostatic mechanism directing pulmonary blood flow to the better ventilated alveoli.

A more attractive concept of the cause of increased dead space during I.P.P. ventilation, is that the high end-inspiratory alveolar pressures produce an *intermittent closure of pulmonary capillaries*. This would be most exaggerated in the uppermost alveoli—a situation likely to be worsened in haemorrhage, as demonstrated by Gerst *et al.* (1959). There is no direct evidence that this occurs during I.P.P., although the inter-relationship between alveolar and pulmonary vascular pressures is well recognized in normal spontaneous breathing. If this theory is correct, the most unfavourable situation would be the rapidly delivered inspiration, producing regional overinflation and pulmonary capillary blanching at peak inflation, then a rapid return to end-expiration without waiting for redistribution of air and blood to occur. Under such circumstances, ventilation would be maximal when blood flow was least available.

Bergman (1963) has demonstrated in dogs that *high mean pressures* in inspiration (as distinct from high peak pressures) produce the lowest alveolar-arterial $P_{O_2}$ gradients. Unfortunately, he was unable to reproduce these findings in man (1967), although he confirmed that slow inspiration gives the lowest $V_D/V_T$ values.

There is an apparent contradiction here, if one believes that the enlarged alveolar dead space is produced by closing of pulmonary capillaries at peak inflation pressure. However, it would be entirely possible to produce a high mean pressure without alveolar pressure at any time exceeding the critical closing pressure of the pulmonary capillaries.

Various authors have suggested that the increase in $V_D/V_T$ in persons with healthy lungs may be a reflection of an overall reduction in *pulmonary artery blood flow*, secondary to the reduced venous return. Suwa *et al.* (1966) have demonstrated that $V_D/V_T$ bears an inverse correlation to cardiac index, in anaesthetized dogs receiving I.P.P. ventilation.

The exact explanation for this increased $V_D/V_T$ is unknown, but it seems likely that critical closing pressure could be exceeded in any alveoli preferentially ventilated due to differences in air distribution. This would be most prevalent in uppermost alveoli, which would be more deprived of blood flow, for gravitational reasons, and would be exaggerated when right ventricular output fell. Presumably, a high mean pressure on inflation (e.g. by a slow inspiratory flow or zero flow at end-inspiration) permits a more nearly optimal distribution of air, critical closing pressure then being exceeded in fewer alveoli.

It should be noted at this point that there is a direct conflict between the ideal inspiratory wave form, from the haemodynamic standpoint, and that required to minimize the dead space effect. Fortunately, there is sufficient latitude under normal circumstances that this does not create a problem. The common practical limitation, in patients with cardio-pulmonary disease and particularly those with air trapping, is that of maintaining a slow inspiration and an inspiration/expiration ratio less than 1:1, while providing an adequate minute volume.

## Venous Admixture Effect

Changes in venous admixture effect during I.P.P. ventilation are less constant and depend on multiple variables. Campbell *et al.* (1958) were unable to demonstrate an increase in alveolar-arterial oxygen difference ($Aa\Delta o_2$) in anaesthetized ventilated patients, although this has not been the experience of others. Fairley and Blenkarn (1966) found no change in $Aa\Delta o_2$ due to *changes in inspiratory flow rate*, in anaesthetized normal individuals, although all values were high. Bendixen *et al.* (1963) demonstrated an increase during controlled ventilation and related this to the circumstances producing a progressive fall in compliance demonstrated by Egbert *et al.* (1963). However, the proposition that physiological shunt necessarily increases progressively during anaesthesia with spontaneous respiration and with controlled ventilation has not been confirmed. Panday and Nunn (1968) and Norlander *et al.* (1968) were unable to demonstrate this change. Nunn *et al.* (1965) found no consistent trends, although arterial oxygen tension tended to fall in the older patients. When this occurred, high sustained inflation pressures, sufficient to impair systemic arterial pressure, were required to restore arterial oxygen tension levels. Laver *et al.* (1966) have shown that, when atelectasis is produced intentionally by airway suction, physiological shunt may be minimized by using *large tidal volumes.* Hedley-Whyte *et al.* (1965) found a progressive change in $Aa\Delta O_2$ which is dependent upon tidal volume. When the latter was less than 7 ml./kg. the gradient tended to increase. (However, tidal volumes as high as 12 ml./kg. may be necessary to prevent this increase in the majority of instances.) This study was on a limited number of cases, under unusual anaesthesia circumstances, and should be repeated.

Nunn *et al.* (1965) have demonstrated increased physiological shunting at low *resting lung volume* and it is now recognized that airway closure occurs under such circumstances (Sutherland *et al.*, 1968). Thus, it is to be expected that methods of artificial ventilation working below FRC will be less effective in oxygenating the patient. This would include chest compression techniques and certain patterns of PNP ventilation.

Conversely, techniques which increase FRC may minimize physiological shunting and the studies of Frumin *et al.* (1959) and Cheney *et al.* (1967)—employing an expiratory resistance—demonstrated a reduction in $Aa\Delta O_2$ under such circumstances, although the actual volume of the FRC was not measured and, in the latter study, improvement did not occur until the resistance was removed—suggesting an added cardiovascular effect.

Fairley and Blenkarn (1966) have pointed out that, while certain I.P.P. patterns may assist in maintaining open alveoli, a negative feed back on the $Aa\Delta O_2$ may occur should cardiac output fall and the shunted mixed venous blood become more desaturated as a consequence.

### Respiratory Failure

In patients receiving mechanical ventilation for respiratory failure, Pontoppidan *et al.* (1965) have demonstrated an increase in $Aa\Delta O_2$ and $V_D/V_T$ with poor correlation between the two variables. They also noted that $V_D/V_T$ was highest when the ratio of tidal volume to peak inspiratory pressure was low. Using volume constant ventilation, peak inspiratory pressure may, of course, occur at end-inspiration or in mid-inspiration at the point of peak inspiratory flow. When the latter is the case, it may be due either to the use of rapid inspiratory flow rates, to the presence of a high airway resistance or to a combination of both. Consequently, Pontoppidan's finding that dead space varies directly with inspiratory pressure may point either to uneven distribution at rapid inspiratory flows, with resulting overdistension of certain alveoli or to pulmonary capillary closure at high end-inspiratory pressures.

### The Optimum Ventilatory Pattern

There is now ample evidence that, in patients with normal lungs, large tidal volumes are useful in minimizing physiological shunt. Volumes as high as 12 ml./kg. may be appropriate (Hedley-Whyte *et al.*, 1964, 1965). However, when the lung is grossly diseased and there are diffuse regional reductions in compliance, this may result in gross over-inflation of the more normal regions, causing an increased $V_D/V_T$—a possible explanation of Pontoppidan's findings (1965)—and this may also produce an increase in surface tension by a reduction of surfactant (Greenfield *et al.*, 1964).

The pattern of delivery of the tidal volume is probably unimportant, although the flow rate should not be excessive or $V_D/V_T$ will rise. Consequently, a relatively slow flow and a resulting high mean pressure may be useful. Norlander *et al.* (1968) have suggested that their failure to demonstrate a falling compliance or an increasing physiological shunt, as anaesthesia progresses, is due to the favourable wave form generated by the Engström ventilator (accelerating inspiratory flow and a period of zero flow at end-inspiration). However, the only experimental support for this is from a mechanical analogue with which Herzog and Norlander (1968) were able to demonstrate the effects of different wave forms on air distribution. Two airway-alveoli units with differing ventilatory time constants were shown to ventilate more evenly with the Engström ventilator than with a machine generating a constant gas flow. This model did not consider pulmonary blood flow, but probably confirms the in-vivo findings of Bergman (1963), to the effect that high mean intrathoracic pressures provide the lowest alveolar-arterial gradients.

A negative phase in expiration is to be avoided, in order to minimize airway closure. If cardiac output is not to be depressed, expiration should be at least as long as inspiration, and overinflation should be avoided.

### Mechanical Dead Space

A problem which arises, in using large tidal volumes in a patient in whom eucapnia is to be maintained, is the necessary slow ventilatory frequency. This may be of the order of 6, 7, or 8/min. depending on the magnitude of the physiological dead space. Changes in frequency of 1/min. may produce alterations in arterial $P_{CO_2}$ of several mm.Hg. When this is found to be the case, it may be more practical to raise the ventilatory frequency and to add mechanical dead space. Suwa and Bendixen (1968) have demonstrated that this may require to be larger than one might expect, from calculations assuming a given added volume of mechanical dead space to be equivalent to increasing anatomical dead space by the same volume, particularly in patients who already have an alveolar dead space.

### Measurement of Expired Gas During I.P.P.

Various of the features of I.P.P. ventilation introduce potential measurement inaccuracies in the measurement of expired gas.

Since gases are compressed in the lungs and ventilator circuit at end-inspiration, volumes collected during expiration will include a "compression volume." If the volume and valving characteristics of the particular ventilator are known, a correction factor may be employed. Various nomograms have been devised for this purpose (Engström and Herzog, 1959; Engström, 1962; Saklad and Paliotta, 1968; Haddad and Richards, 1968).

When expired gas is to be collected for analysis, contamination with inspired gas from the "compression volume" must be avoided, and an efficient non-return valve at the tracheostomy is most important. A suitable valve has been devised by Berry and Pontoppidan (1968).

When expired gas volume is to be measured for clinical purposes, a variety of devices will suffice—recognizing that the accuracy of gas meters and anemometers is flow-dependent. Continuous use of such meters is to be avoided since the humidity of the expired air eventually produces corrosion. In our experience this occurs even in silicone-coated meters, although a small heating coil may overcome the problem. Accurate volume measurements are better derived from the collection of expired gas over several minutes. This may then be put through a gas meter at a steady and defined flow rate.

Grenvik and Hedstrand (1966) have pointed out errors, related to compression and gas composition which may arise in pneumotachography during I.P.P. ventilation, and have suggested correction factors.

Herzog and Norlander (1968) have designed a switch valve, permitting the easy introduction of a pneumotachograph head into a ventilator circuit without any tubing disconnection.

When mechanical dead space is to be added, as a means of raising $P_{A_{CO_2}}$ while maintaining constant tidal volume and frequency, Suwa *et al.* (1968) have constructed a nomogram indicating the added mechanical dead space required to produce a $P_{A_{CO_2}}$ of 40 mm. Hg.

## Summary

Intermittent positive pressure ventilation is characterized physiologically by a reduction in dynamic lung compliance and in airway resistance and a raised mean intrathoracic pressure and $V_D/V_T$ ratio. Under certain circumstances it may produce a reduction in venous return and in cardiac output and an increase in physiological shunting. The reduction in venous return is usually minimized by an increase in peripheral venous tone paralleling the rise in intrathoracic pressure. This peripheral venoconstriction may be prevented by disease or by pharmacological agents, or offset by hypovolaemia.

The optimum ventilatory pattern is one with large tidal volumes, delivered moderately slowly and followed by an expiratory pause of at least equal length. If normal arterial carbon dioxide tension is required, this may dictate very slow respiratory frequencies or the addition of mechanical dead space.

## REFERENCES

Bendixen, H. H., Hedley-Whyte, J. and Laver, M. B. (1963), "Impaired Oxygenation in Surgical Patients During General Anesthesia with Controlled Ventilation," *New Eng. J. Med.*, **269**, 991.

Bergman, N. A. (1963), "Effect of Different Pressure Breathing Patterns on Alveolar-Arterial Gradients in Dogs," *J. Appl. Physiol.*, **18**, 1049.

Bergman, N. A. (1963), "Distribution of Inspired Gas During Anesthesia and Artificial Ventilation," *J. Appl. Physiol.*, **18**, 1085.

Bergman, N. A. (1967), "Effects of Varying Respiratory Wave Forms on Gas Exchange," *Anesthesiology*, **28**, 390.

Berry, P. R. and Pontoppidan, H. (1968), "A Non-Return Valve for Continuous Use with the Emerson Post-Operative Ventilator," *Anesthesiology*, **29**, 828.

Blair, D. E., Glover, W. E. and Kidd, B. S. L. (1959), "The Effect of Continuous Positive and Negative Pressure Breathing upon the Resistance and Capacity Blood Vessels of the Human Forearm and Hand," *Clin. Sci.*, **18**, 9.

Campbell, E. J. M., Nunn, J. F. and Peckett, B. W. (1958), "A Comparison of Artificial Ventilation and Spontaneous Respiration with Particular Reference to Ventilation—Blood Flow Relationships," *Brit. J. Anaesth.*, **30**, 166.

Cheney, F. W., Hornbein, T. F. and Crawford, E. W. (1967), "The Effect of Expiratory Resistance on the Blood Gas Tensions of Anesthetised Patients," *Anesthesiology*, **28**, 670.

Cooper, E. A. (1967), "Physiological Dead Space in Passive Ventilation," *Anaesthesia*, **22**, 90 and 199.

Cournand, A., Motley, H. L., Werko, L. and Richards, D. W. Jr. (1948), "Physiological Studies of the Effect of Intermittent Positive Pressure Breathing on Cardiac Output in Man," *Am. J. Physiol.*, **152**, 162.

Dammann, J. F., Thung, N., Christlieb, I. I., Littlefield, J. B. and Muller, W. H. (1963), "The Management of the Severely Ill Patient Following Open Heart Surgery," *J. Thorac. and C. V. Surg.*, **45**, 80.

Don, H. F. and Robson, J. G. (1965), "The Mechanics of the Respiratory System during Anesthesia," *Anesthesiology*, **26**, 168.

Egbert, L. D., Laver, M. B. and Bendixen, H. H. (1963), "Intermittent Deep Breaths and Compliance During Anaesthesia in Man," *Anesthesiology*, **24**, 57.

Elam, J. O. (1965), "Respiratory and Circulatory Resuscitation," Handbook of Physiology. Section 3, Respiration 2: 1265. Amer. Physiol. Soc.

Engström, C.-G. and Herzog, P. (1959), "Ventilation Nomogram for Practical Use with the Engström Respirator," *Acta Chir. Scand.* Suppl. **245**, 37.

Engström, C.-G., Herzog, P., Norlander, O. P. and Swensson, S. A. (1962), "Ventilation Nomogram for the Newborn and Small Children to be Used with the Engström Respirator," *Acta Anaesth. Scandinav.*, **6**, 175.

Fairley, H. B. and Blenkarn, G. D. (1966), "Effect on Pulmonary Gas Exchange of Variations in Inspiratory Flow Rate During Intermittent Positive Pressure Ventilation," *Brit. J. Anaesth.*, **38**, 320.

Frumin, M. J., Bergman, N. A., Holaday, D., Rackow, H. and Salanitre, E. (1959), "Alveolar-Arterial $O_2$ Differences During Artificial Respiration in Man," *J. Appl. Physiol.*, **14**, 694.

Galloon, S. and Rosen, N. (1965), "Changes in Airway Resistance and Alveolar Trapping with Positive-Negative Ventilation," *Anaesthesia*, **20**, 429.

Gerst, P. H., Rattenborg, C. and Holaday, D. A. (1959), "The Effects of Hemorrhage on Pulmonary Circulation and Respiratory Gas Exchange," *J. Clin. Invest.*, **38**, 524.

Gilston, A. (1962), "The Management of Respiratory Distress Following Cardio Thoracic Surgery," *Thorax*, **17**, 139

Gold, M. I. and Helrich, M. (1965), "Pulmonary Compliance During Anesthesia," *Anesthesiology*, **26**, 281.

Greenfield, L. J., Ebert, P. A. and Benson, D. W. (1964), "Effect of Positive Pressure Ventilation on Surface Tension Properties of Lung Extracts," *Anesthesiology*, **25**, 312.

Grenvik, A. and Hedstrand, H. (1966), "The Reliability of Pneumotachography in Respirator Ventilation," *Acta Anaesth. Scandinav.*, **10**, 157.

Guyton, A. C. (1963), "Circulatory Physiology: Cardiac Output and its Regulation," P. 383 Saunders.

Haddad, C. and Richards, C. C. (1968), "Mechanical Ventilation of Infants: Significance and Elimination of Ventilator Compression Volume," *Anesthesiology*, **29**, 345.

Hedley-Whyte, J., Laver, M. B. and Bendixen, H. H. (1964), "The Effect of Changes in Tidal Ventilation on Physiologic Shunting," *Am. J. Physiol.*, **206**, 891.

Hedley-Whyte, J., Pontoppidan, H., Laver, M. B., Hallowell, P. and Bendixen, H. H. (1965), "Arterial Oxygenation During Hypothermia," *Anesthesiology*, **26**, 595.

Herzog, P. and Norlander, O. P. (1968), "Distribution of Alveolar Volumes with Different Types of Positive Pressure Gas-Flow Patterns," *Opuscula Medica*, **13**, 3.

Hubay, C. A., Waltz, R. C., Brecher, G. A., Praglin, J. and Hingson, R. A. (1954), "Circulatory Dynamics of Venous Return During Positive-Negative Pressure Respiration," *Anesthesiology*, **15**, 445.

Kira, S. and Hukushima, Y. (1968), "Effect of Negative-Pressure Inflation on Pulmonary Vascular Flow," *J. Appl. Physiol.*, **25**, 42.

Laver, M. B., Löfström, B., Heitmann, H. and Pontoppidan, H. (1966), "Dead Space During Controlled Ventilation," *Anesthesiology*, **27**, 220.

Laws, A. K. (1968), "Effects of Induction of Anaesthesia and Muscle Paralysis on Functional Residual Capacity of the Lungs," *Canad. Anaesth. Soc. J.*, **15**, 325.

Lee, G. de J., Matthews, M. B. and Sharpey-Shafer, E. P. (1954), "The Effect of the Valsalva Manoeuvre on the Systemic and Arterial Pressure in Man," *Brit. Heart J.*, **16**, 311.

Lopez-Muniz, R., Stephens, N. L., Bromberger-Barnea, B., Permutt, S. and Riley, R. L. (1968), "Critical Closure of Pulmonary Vessels Analyzed in Terms of Starling Resistor Model," *J. Appl. Physiol.*, **24**, 625.

Lynch, S., Levy, A. and Ellis, K. (1959), "Effects of Alternating Positive and Negative Endotracheal Pressures on the Caliber of Bronchi," *Anesthesiology*, **20**, 325.

Maloney, J. V., Elam, J. O., Handford, S. W., Balla, G. A., Eastwood, D. W., Brown, E. S. and Tenpas, R. H. (1953), "Importance of Negative Pressure Phase in Mechanical Respirators," *J. Amer. Med. Assn.*, **152**, 212.

Maloney, J. V. and Whittenberger, J. L. (1957), "The Direct Effects of Pressure Breathing on the Circulation," *Ann. N.Y. Acad. Sci.*, **66**, 931.

Mead, J. and Collier, C. (1959), "Relation of Volume History of Lungs to Respiratory Mechanics in Anesthetized Dogs," *J. Appl. Physiol.*, **14**, 669.

Morgan, B. C., Martin, W. E., Hornbein, T. F., Crawford, E. W. and Guntheroth, W. G. (1966), "Hemodynamic Effects of Intermittent Positive Pressure Ventilation," *Anesthesiology*, **27**, 584.

Morgan, B. L., Crawford, E. W., Hornbein, T. F., Martin, W. E. and Guntheroth, W. G. (1967), "Hemodynamic Effects of Changes in Arterial Carbon Dioxide Tension During Intermittent Positive Pressure Ventilation," *Anesthesiology*, **28**, 866.

Newhouse, M. T., Becklake, M. R., Maklem, P. I. and McGregor, M. (1964), "Effect of Alterations in End Tidal $CO_2$ Tension on Flow Resistance," *J. Appl. Physiol.*, **19**, 745.

Norlander, O., Herzog, P., Nordèn, I., Hossli, G., Schaer, H. and Gattiker, R. (1968), "Compliance and Airway Resistance During Anaesthesia with Controlled Ventilation," *Acta. Anaesth. Scandinav.*, **12**, 136.

Nunn, J. F., Coleman, A. J., Sachithanandan, T., Bergman, N. A. and Laws, J. W. (1965). "Hypoxaemia and Atelectasis Produced by Forced Expiration," *Brit. J. Anaesth.*, **37**, 3.

Nunn, J. F., Bergman, N. A. and Coleman, A. J. (1965), "Factors Influencing the Arterial Oxygen Tension During Anaesthesia with Artificial Ventilation," *Brit. J. Anaesth.*, **37**, 898.

Opie, L. H., Spalding, J. M. K. and Stott, F. D. (1959), "Mechanical Properties of the Chest during Intermittent Positive Pressure Respiration," *Lancet*, **1**, 545.

Pace-Floridia, A. and Galindo, A. (1968), "Cardiac Arrhythmia Induced by Negative Phase in Artificial Ventilation," *Anesthesiology*, **29**, 382.

Panday, J. and Nunn, J. F. (1968), "Failure to Demonstrate Progressive Falls of Arterial $P_{O_2}$ During Anaesthesia," *Anaesthesia*, **23**, 38.

Pierce, E. C. Jr. and Vandam, L. D. (1962), "Intermittent Positive Pressure Breathing," *Anesthesiology*, **23**, 478.

Pontoppidan, H., Hedley-Whyte, J., Bendixen, H. H., Laver, M. B. and Radford, E. P. Jr. (1965), "Ventilation and Oxygen Requirements During Prolonged Artificial Ventilation in Patients with Respiratory Failure," *New Eng. J. Med.*, **273**, 401.

Prys-Roberts, C., Kelman, G. R., Greenbaum, R. and Robinson, R. H. (1967), "Circulatory Influences of Artificial Ventilation During Nitrous Oxide Anaesthesia in Man. II. Results: The Relative Influence of Mean Intrathoracic Pressure and Arterial Carbon Dioxide Tension," *Brit. J. Anaesth.*, **39**, 533.

Prys-Roberts, C., Kelman, G. R., Greenbaum, R., Kain, M. L. and Bay, J. (1968), "Hemodynamics and Alveolar-Arterial $P_{O_2}$ Differences at Varying $P_{A_{CO_2}}$ in Anesthetized Man," *J. Appl. Physiol.*, **25**, 80.

Roos, A., Thomas, L. J. Jr., Nagel, E. L. and Prommas, D. C. (1961), "Pulmonary Vascular Resistance as Determined by Lung Inflation and Vascular Pressures," *J. Appl. Physiol.*, **16**, 77.

Saklad, M. and Paliotta, J. (1968), "A Nomogram for the Correction of Needed Gases During Artificial Ventilation," *Anesthesiology*, **29**, 150.

Salem, M. R., Ginsberg, D., Rattenborg, C. C. and Holaday, D. A. (1964), "The Effect of Continuous Positive and Negative Pressure Breathing on the Urine Formation," *Fed. Proc.*, **23**, 362.

Sieker, H. O., Gauer, O. H. and Henry, J. P. (1954), "The Effect of Continuous Negative Pressure Breathing on Water and Electrolyte Excretion by the Human Kidney," *J. Clin. Invest.*, **33**, 572.

Smith, A. C. and Spalding, J. M. K. (1959), "Intermittent Positive Pressure Respiration. Some Physiological Observations," *Proc. Royl Soc. Med.*, **52**, 661.

Spalding, J. M. K. and Smith, A. C. (1963), "Clinical Practice and Physiology of Artificial Respiration," Blackwell.

Spencer, F. C., Benson, D. W., Liu, W. C. and Bahnson, H. T. (1959), "Use of a Mechanical Respirator in the Management of Respiratory or Pulmonary Disease," *J. Thorac. Surg.*, **38**, 758.

Sutherland, P. W., Katsura, T. and Milic-Emili, J. (1968), "Previous Volume History of the Lung and Regional Distribution of Gas," *J. Appl. Physiol.*, **25**, 566.

Suwa, K. and Bendixen, H. H. (1968), "Change in $P_{A_{CO_2}}$ with Mechanical Dead Space During Artificial Ventilation," *J. Appl. Physiol.*, **24**, 556.

Suwa, J., Geffin, B., Pontoppidan, H. and Bendixen, H. H. (1968), "A Nomogram for Dead Space Requirement During Prolonged Artificial Ventilation," *Anesthesiology*, **29**, 1206.

Suwa, K., Hedley-Whyte, J. and Bendixen, H. H. (1966), "Circulation and Physiologic Dead Space Changes on Controlling the Ventilation of Dogs," *J. Appl. Physiol.*, **21**, 1855.

Thomas, L. J. Jr., Griffo, Z. J. and Roos, A. (1961), "Effect of Negative Pressure Inflation of the Lung on Pulmonary Vascular Resistance," *J. Appl. Physiol.*, **16**, 451.

Watrous, W. G., Davis, F. E. and Anderson, B. M. (1950), "Manually Assisted and Controlled Respiration: Its Use During Inhalation Anesthesia for the Maintenance of a Near-Normal Physiologic State—A Review," *Anesthesiology*, **11**, 538, 661 and **12**, 33.

Watson, W. E. (1961), "Physiology of Artificial Respiration," Thesis submitted to Oxford University.

Watson, W. E. (1962), A. "Some Observations on Dynamic Lung Compliance During Intermittent Positive Pressure Respiration," *Brit. J. Anaesth.*, **34**, 153.

Watson, W. E. (1962), B. "Observations on the Dynamic Lung Compliance of Patients with Respiratory Weakness Receiving Intermittent Positive Pressure Respiration," *Brit. J. Anaesth.*, **34**, 690.

Watson, W. E. (1962), C. "Venous Distensibility of the Hand During Valsalva's Manoeuvre," *Brit. Heart J.*, **24**, 26.

Watson, W. E., Smith, A. C. and Spalding, J. M. K. (1962), "Transmural Central Venous Pressure During Intermittent Positive Pressure Respiration," *Brit. J. Anaesth.*, **34**, 278.

Whittenberger, J. L. (1955), "Artificial Respiration," *Physiol. Rev.*, **35**, 611.

Whittenberger, J. L. (Ed.), (1962), *Artificial Respiration, Theory and Applicatons*, Harper and Row.

# CHAPTER 1

# PLASMA MEMBRANE PHYSIOLOGY

## E. A. SCHWARTZ

Living membranes are dynamic, complex structures endowed with a selective chemical reactivity. Although a general theory of membrane physiology does not exist, biomembranes do possess common properties. Our purpose is to discover a general notion of their nature. For simplicity, we shall consider only the plasmalemma and artificial membrane models and infer an understanding from a limited number of special cases. We shall proceed first to build a barrier separating two aqueous phases and then add behavioural specificity.

Artificial membranes can be formed by painting a suitable mixture of phospholipid across an aperature separating two aqueous volumes. The barrier forms instantly. Living membranes are probably similar spontaneous phase aggregations. If the fresh water amoeba is manipulated into a water-air interface, surface tension disperses the membrane, allowing the granular cytoplasmic contents to diffuse away from the nucleus. If then the cell remnant, including nucleus and contractile vacuole, is quickly buried in the aqueous phase, surface films successively appear and dissolve. The membrane reforms by coalescence of these foci of spontaneous reaggregation. Complete recovery of the amoeba ensues. The 'instructions' for aggregation are intermolecular forces stabilizing molecular organization into lamellae.

Artificial films are molecular bilayers with apposing hydrophobic parts forming a central sheet. The hydrophobic region is a barrier to ion diffusion. Accordingly, they behave as lipid and have an extremely low ion permeability. Permeability to ions can be improved with specific additives to mimic biomembrane behaviour. Valinomycin is a peptide which dissolves in lipid bilayers creating an increased permeability to potassium. The increased translocation of $K^+$ occurs at the locus of solvated valinomycin. A similar $K^+$ permeability exists for many animal cells. Biomembranes probably contain analogous permeability-inducing proteins. But these living 'holes' are plastic and readily deformed by environmental change.

Lamellar aggregation into bilayers does not require a fixed ratio of a specific set of molecular constituents. For example, the composition of membranes from the bacteria *Mycoplasma laidlawii*, which can be harvested and re-aggregated, vary with the culture media. The membrane aggregates from available molecules with suitable hydrophobic and hydrophilic parts. It should be expected that pharmacologic agents of the appropriate structure might also dissolve in membranes. This might be true of volatile anaesthetics and is the basis of several theories of anaesthetic action. By dissolving into and stressing the general membrane structure they would simultaneously alter several membrane functions. Diethyl ether in pharmacologic concentration applied to the squid axon inhibits impulse conduction and ATP mediated $Na^+$ extrusion (*see* below). Simultaneous effect on these two discrete functions may be due to a general alteration of membrane structure.

A membrane barrier can separate two aqueous phases with different ionic composition. To transfer electric charge across the membrane requires work which can be calculated from the Goldman constant field equation:

$$V = \frac{RT}{F} \log \frac{(P_K K_0 + P_{Na} Na_0 + P_{Cl} Cl_i)}{(P_K K_i + P_{Na} Na_i + P_{Cl} Cl_0)}$$

$V$ = emf
$R$ = gas constant
$F$ = Faraday's constant
$T$ = temp A°
$Na_0$; $K_0$; $Cl_0$ = extracellular concentration
$Na_i$; $K_i$; $Cl_i$ = intracellular concentration
$P_K$, $P_{Na}$, $P_{Cl}$ = permability of appropriate ion species
at 37°C, $\frac{RT}{F} = 61·5$ mV.

As a first approximation $P_{Na}$ and $P_{Cl}$ may frequently be taken as zero at the resting potential to yield the Nernst equation:

$$V = \frac{RT}{F} \log \frac{K_0}{K_i}$$

Many cells approximate the Nernst potential over a limited range of ion concentration. But there are exceptions. The membrane potential of the squid axolemma does not follow the Nernst equation with a change in internal $K^+$ concentration (Fig. 1). Although the membrane is in part a passive diffusion barrier, its structure and permeability depend upon the ion environment.

'Plastic' macromolecules dissolved in membranes can frequently undergo a change of configuration or state of aggregation. Transitions which effect electrical properties are usually described in the 'black box' terms of an equivalent circuit. The significance of this as a description by analogy should be understood. A non-biological example is the description of piezoelectric crystals such as quartz. These crystals are deformed by a potential field. Conversely, mechanical distortion dislocates electric charge and modifies current flow equivalent to a circuit containing resistance, capacity, and inductance. In this electromechanical system, the inductance is determined by the mass of the crystal, the capacity by its elasticity, and the resistance by frictional losses. It must be kept in mind that an equivalent circuit is only a description by analogy.

The most complete equivalent circuit description of bioelectric behaviour has been determined for the propagating impulse of the squid giant axon. The conductance change is composed of an initial, inward depolarizing fast ion current, (f.i.c.) and a later, outward repolarizing slow ion current (s.i.c.). These currents should not be identified with any one specific ion but with the underlying molecular reorganization. In the squid axon, the f.i.c. is predominantly associated with sodium ions. However, the f.i.c. 'gate' is not infinitely selective. The ratios of

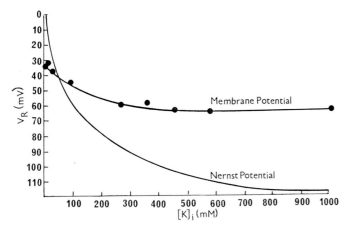

FIG. 1. The change of membrane potential with internal potassium concentration is compared with the predicted value from the Nernst potential. The resting membrane potential is plotted in millivolts as ordinate against internal potassium concentration as abscissa. Axons were bathed in artificial sea water containing 10 mM potassium. The internal solution was established by perfusion of an appropriate concentration of $K_2SO_4$. Sucrose was added sufficient to maintain isotonicity. (Data from Narahashi, *J. Physiol.*, **169**, 91 (1963); Adelman and Gilbert, *J. Cell Comp. Physiol.* **64**, 423 (1964); Adelman and Fok, *J. Cell. Comp. Physiol.* **64**, 429 (1964)).

selectivity for $Li^+:Na^+:K^+:Rb^+:Cs^+$ are $1\cdot1:1:1/12:$ $1/40:1/61$ from which it is seen that the f.i.c. gate actually uses $Li^+$ better than $Na^+$. The s.i.c. is usually considered to be predominately associated with potassium ion. However, the fraction of current transferred by potassium ion in the s.i.c. is a function of resting membrane potential. At least part of the variable remainder of the s.i.c. is carried by inward-moving chloride. The specific set of ion selectivity ratios found in the squid axon should not be expected in other cells. There are examples where different ratios and even different ions carry the principal current fraction. These transients are best considered in terms of structural changes rather than the resultant ion currents. But the former are experimentally less accessible and thus poorly understood. The equivalent circuit describes only part of the events of impulse conduction. There are also changes in heat, birefringence, and fluorescence. The impulse is a momentary molecular reorganization of the membrane which may be studied by observing changes in several parameters.

The ion selective current transients traverse the membrane at distinct molecular sites. Evidence derived from

voltage clamp of the squid axon suggests that there are no more than 100 f.i.c. 'channels'/$\mu^2$ axon surface. In lobster axons, it has been estimated that 13 molecules of the specific poison tetrodotoxin/$\mu^2$ axon surface can block the f.i.c. With an estimate of 50 'channels'/$\mu^2$ and the experimental flux of $5 \times 10^{-12}$ mole/cm²-impulse, each molecular site would translocate 600 ions per impulse.

Lipid bilayers can be modified to imitate the ion translocation of action potentials. Alamethicin, a cyclic peptide similar to valinomycin, imparts this ability. The kinetics of current onset indicate a molecular configuration or aggregation change which allows a current transient.

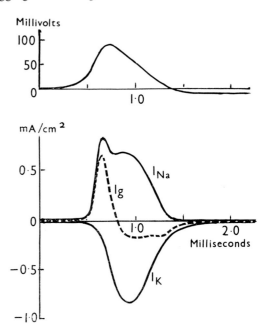

FIG. 2. The deviation of the propagated action potential from the resting potential is compared with the predominately sodium f.i.c. ($I_{Na}$), the predominately potassium s.i.c. ($I_K$) and the net ion current ($I_g$). Positive indicates inward current.

The similarity between electric behaviour in modified lipid bilayers and biological membranes remains to be determined. An important difference is the non-selective current in bilayers in contrast to the ion selective f.i.c. and s.i.c. in biological membranes.

During the impulse, internal $K^+$ is interchanged with external $Na^+$, there is an influx of NaCl and a small flux of other ions including $Ca^{+2}$. These changes must be reversed in order to maintain a constant internal and external milieu. The cell must also maintain the proper concentration of sugars, amino acids, steroids, fats and other small biomolecules. The accumulation and expulsion of small molecules, apart from diffusional flow, occurs at specialized membrane sites requiring metabolic support. An ubiquitous principle of biology is the use of the hydrolysis of ATP for driving unfavourable reactions. Membrane enzymology has begun with the study of the $Na^+$ translocating unit. A crude membrane extract of Na–K stimulated ATPase is identified with this system.

A partial summary of ion flux in the squid axon is given

in Table 1. Na⁺ efflux has been best studied. An ouabain sensitive Na⁺ efflux is non-stoichiometrically coupled to a K⁺ influx. With increasing internal Na⁺ the exchange ratio of K⁺ influx: Na⁺ efflux decreases and teleologically unprofitable Na⁺–Na⁺ exchange increases.

An ouabain insensitive Na⁺ efflux in squid nerve is in part coupled to Ca$^{+2}$ influx (Table 1). This Na⁺–Ca$^{+2}$

TABLE 1

THE EFFECT OF OUABAIN AND CYANIDE ON ION FLUX IN THE GIANT AXON OF THE SQUID, *Loligo forbesii* (OR *L. pealii*, INDICATED BY *) Normal values are the best experimental values. Values in parenthesis are the 'passive' flux in ATP depleted axons; ↓ indicates a greater than 10 per cent decrease from control value; n.e. indicates no effect. Active flux is indicated by metabolic support sensitive to cyanide.

| | Na⁺ | | K⁺ | | Cl⁻ | | HPO₄⁻/PO₄$^{-2}$ | Ca$^{+2}$ |
|---|---|---|---|---|---|---|---|---|
| | Efflux | Influx | Efflux | Influx | Efflux | Influx | Influx | Influx |
| Normal Value (10⁻¹² M./cm.² sec.) | 56(1·3*) | 19(4·3) | 38 | 24 | 21 | 0·02 | 0·15 | |
| Ouabain | ↓ | ↓ | | n.e. | | ↓ | n.e. | |
| Cyanide | ↓ | ↓ | n.e. | ↓ | n.e. | ↓ | | |

exchange is enhanced by a raised internal Na⁺. This may explain the cardiotonic action of cardiac glycosides. Ouabain, in therapeutic doses, seems to have no direct effect on Ca$^{+2}$ efflux itself, but inhibits Na⁺–K⁺ exchange and increases internal Na⁺ concentration. If heart muscle behaves like squid nerve, a rise in internal Na⁺ would promote Ca$^{+2}$ influx. Ouabain would therefore be expected to have a secondary effect on Ca$^{+2}$ influx. Since muscle contraction is elicited by Ca$^{+2}$ released from a sarcoplasmic pool during impulse invasion, an increased sarcoplasmic pool of Ca$^{+2}$ would be expected to increase the efficiency of excitation-contraction coupling.

A relatively greater loss of ionic gradients occurs per impulse in small diameter processes with a large surface-to-volume ratio. As a result, the highest metabolic rate and oxygen consumption occurs in dendritic processes. These areas are the most sensitive to anoxia and metabolic inhibition and might be depolarized while the soma shows little change. Fluctuation in the composition of the internal milieu in small diameter processes might overwhelm the ability of the active transport system to maintain a steady state.

It has been a fortunate experimental coincidence that bioelectric and metabolically-supported ion transport can be studied independently in the squid axon. However, in other cells, the ion flux supported by metabolism may yield a transmembrane potential difference. Metabolically supported transport may contribute to the membrane

potential and excitation threshold. Certain neurons of the marine gastropod *Aplysia* are hyperpolarized by a rise in internal Na⁺ or a rise in the O₂ in the bathing medium and depolarized by K⁺-free medium or the specific transport poison ouabain. Metabolically-supported ion transport can yield a transmembrane potential if influx is not perfectly balanced against efflux, yielding a net charge transfer.

The membrane density of active macro-molecules dissolved in the membrane may be affected by neighbouring cells. Normal frog sartorius muscle fibres have a peak acetylcholine sensitivity at the neuro-muscular endplate and an extra-junctional reduced sensitivity over the remainder of the fibre surface. In denervated muscle, the extra-junctional sensitivity is increased while the maximum sensitivity at the endplate is not greatly affected. (The activity of cholinesterase at the endplate is coincidently decreased.) Increased acetylcholine sensitivity occurs in muscle fibres having one innervated and one denervated endplate and cannot be attributed to a cessation of activity. Nor is it due to the presence of transmitter, since denervated muscle fibres bathed in acetylcholine also develop increased sensitivity. It appears that the motor neuron exerts an inhibiting influence on the acetylcholine-sensitivity of the extra-junctional membrane (and maintains the cholinesterase activity of the junctional membrane). The difference in acetylcholine sensitivity between fast and slow muscles is determined by the type of innervation and is not a property inherent in the muscle fibre. Presumably a product of the motor neuron other than transmitter suppresses the extra-junctional density of a macromolecular receptor, possibly by influencing the control of receptor synthesis or degradation.

The surface of a single cell is heterogeneous and organized into micro patches of specialized activity. Synaptic areas are obvious specializations. There are also areas of low resistance sensitive to electrotonic invasion acting as trigger zones, of selective transport giving polarized function relative to visceral lumens or canaliculi, of selective contact and migration inhibition, determining an overall geometry and tissue structure. Within the spontaneously forming membrane substructure, an assembly of enzymes and macromolecules are organized in space. The cueing mechanisms for this spatial separation are unknown. Great problems remain in our understanding of membrane physiology. As experiment progresses, we shall discover membrane diseases and integrate membrane physiology into an understanding of animal behaviour. For this to proceed, we must constantly enlarge and condense the very simple notions presented here.

## REFERENCES

Caldwell, P. C. (1968), "Factors Governing Movement and Distribution of Inorganic Ions in Nerve and Muscle," *Physiol. Rev.*, **48**, 1.

Lehninger, A. L. (1968), "The Neuronal Membrane," *Proc. Nat. Acad. Sci. (U.S.A.)*, **60**, 1069.

Miledi, R. (1962), "Induction of Receptors." In: *Ciba Found. Symp. Enzymes and Drug Action*, pp. 220.

Rothfield, L. and Finkelstein, A. (1968), "Membrane Biochemistry," *Ann. Rev. Biochem.*, **37**, 463.

Siekevitz, P. (1972), "Biological Membranes: The Dynamics of their Organization," *Ann. Rev. Physiol.*, **34**, 117–140.

Skou, J. C. (1965), "Enzymatic Basis for Active Transport of Na$^+$ and K$^+$ across Cell Membranes," *Physiol. Rev.*, **45**, 596.

For an introduction to current experimental work, the reader may consult the indexes of *J. Physiol. (Lond.)* and *J. Gen. Physiol.*

*CHAPTER* 2

# APPROACHES TO A THEORY OF ANAESTHETIC ACTION

J. J. KENDIG and J. R. TRUDELL

## GENERAL INTRODUCTION

Historically, the approaches to a comprehensive theory of anaesthesia have evolved from two very different directions. Clinicians have probed the observable states of narcosis in man, while neuro physiologists have succeeded in directing their observations to single neurons. On the other hand, biochemists have studied the intimate details of the effects of anaesthetics in model systems including olive oil, phospholipid bilayers, and erythrocyte membranes. The clinician and neurophysiologist observe many physiologic effects of the anaesthetic but are unable to describe them on a molecular level. The biochemist, in turn, describes the way in which an anaesthetic molecule affects lipid molecules in a bilayer, but is unable to establish the necessary correspondence between a bilayer and the central nervous system.

A survey of compounds which produce anaesthesia includes large molecules like the steroids, small volatile agents such as chloroform, and chemically inert monoatomic agents like xenon. This would suggest that there must be very many different ways of producing anaesthesia. The varying amounts of narcosis, excitation, depression, and convulsive activity caused by minor substituent changes in the morphine alkaloids implies an extraordinary sensitivity and complexity in the organism's response to these drugs. Yet what is known about the phenomenon of nerve conduction allows for only a few points of intervention, certainly not as many as the number of different anaesthetics. Most of the regulatory systems in the body are elegant in their simplicity. Therefore it seems most unlikely that a separate response is provided for each isomer of every drug. Thus one is forced to think in terms of unifying theories which hopefully will accommodate most drugs and responses.

To date, work on the theories of anaesthesia divides readily into two facets. The inductive approach compiles and analyses many experimental data points such as anaesthetic solubilities in olive oil, vapour pressures, boiling points, and dipole moments, continually searching for the elusive link between structure and function. On the other hand, nearly enough is now known about membrane structure and nerve transmission to justify the proposal of deductive theories of anaesthetic action. In the succeeding three sections we will discuss both approaches to a theory of anaesthesia, beginning with the inductive accumulation of facts.

Bridging the gap between clinical observation and the atomic model system is a fundamental goal of anaesthesia research. When such is realized, a review such as this one will flow smoothly from considerations of model systems to discussions of anaesthetics in patients. Until such time, however, one must consider the subject in its two parts. Let us first consider anaesthetics in model systems, and then anaesthetics in living cells and nervous systems.

## I. MOLECULAR BASIS OF ANAESTHESIA IN MODEL SYSTEMS

Undoubtedly, a discussion of model systems must begin with the pioneering work of Meyer (1899) and Overton (1901). These investigators made the observation that the potency of anaesthetics correlated remarkably well with their water to olive oil partition coefficients. Thus olive oil became the first model for the central nervous system. Recent work by Eger (1969) (Fig. 1) and Miller (1967) has shown that this correlation, established seven decades ago, is still the best available. In these studies the authors included compounds such as xenon, nitrogen, nitrous oxide and fluorosulfur compounds, as well as the common inhalation anaesthetics. Other workers have improved on this early model system. Ferguson (1939) improved the potency-oil solubility correlation by suggesting that the thermodynamic activity of an anaesthetic in a hydrocarbon phase should be substituted for its concentration. Mullins (1954) proposed that the most important property of an inhalation anaesthetic was not its dipole moment, its ability to create or destroy hydrogen bonds, or its stereochemistry, but rather it was simply the element of volume that the anaesthetic occupied in the hydrocarbon phase.

Although a pure hydrocarbon phase provided the first good correlation with anaesthetic potency, anaesthetic action in other phases and sites has been proposed. For example, Pauling (1961) and Miller (1961) proposed that anaesthetics might act by forming hydrates and disrupting the hydration layer which surrounds membranes and membrane-associated proteins. On the other hand, Featherstone and Muehlbacher (1963) have observed that anaesthetics are capable of associating directly with proteins. Several additional theories have been proposed; however, most experimental evidence supports a primary anaesthetic action in a lipid phase. For example, Lever *et al.* (1971) have used thermodynamic principles to calculate that the solubility parameter ($\delta$) of the region in which anaesthetics act is $9 \pm 1$; this is close to that of a hydrocarbon phase (benzene $\delta = 9 \cdot 2$).

Fortunately it is possible to prepare nerve models which are much more like real nerves than is olive oil. Two of

lipids may be synthesized with precisely known hydrocarbon chain lengths and unsaturation. This allows the formation of bilayers of various thickness and internal fluidity. By appropriate selection of the head group the bilayer may be made to have a net surface charge or dipole. It has recently become possible to incorporate functional proteins into synthetic bilayers (Hong and Hubbell, 1972). Thus one can now reproducibly construct a nerve membrane model with exactly known lipid constitution containing single, well-defined proteins of known concentration.

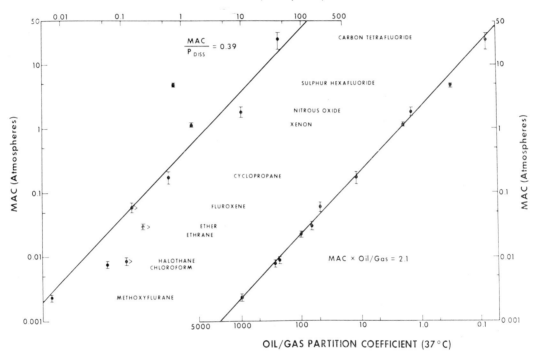

FIG. 1. These graphs permit a visual comparison of the correlation of MAC with hydrate dissociation pressure (left graph, upper scale) and lipid solubility (right graph, lower scale). If the data followed the correlation: MAC/hydrate dissociation pressure equals a constant or MAC × oil/gas partition coefficient equals a constant, then the data should lie along the 45°-angle slopes as indicated. (Eger, Lundgren, Miller and Stevens, 1969).

these model systems are erythrocyte cell membranes and phospholipid bilayer vesicles. The erythrocyte may be haemolysed and washed, leaving only the cell membrane, called an erythrocyte ghost. Used in either the intact or ghost form, the erythrocyte provides a naturally formed, protein-containing lipid membrane. Phospholipid vesicle bilayers are prepared by dissolving the desired phospholipid in water and sonicating the solution. The ultrasonic energy thus provided allows the phospholipids to reassemble in their minimum energy configuration. This is a double-layered sphere with phosphate head groups exposed to water on the inside and outside of the sphere's shell and the phospholipid's hydrocarbon chains meeting at the center of the sphere wall, forming a hydrophobic central region. One advantage of the synthetic phospholipid bilayer is the great degree of control the researcher has over its physical and chemical characteristics. Phospho-

The application of many forms of spectroscopy and analysis to these model systems has been most fruitful. Only a few examples of membrane model research will be mentioned here; the significance of the work will be discussed in a later section. For instance, Seeman and co-workers (Seeman, 1972) have established extensive correlations between anaesthetic concentration and cell membrane expansion as well as with membrane hydraulic permeability. Papahadjopoulous (1970) has studied the effect of anaesthetics and calcium ion on the passive leak rate of potassium ions through a membrane. Trauble and Haynes (1971) have used X-ray diffraction data and dilatometer measurements to formulate a model of membrane surface area expansion related to phase transition-induced disorder. Eisenman *et al.* (1973) have investigated the effect of phospholipid membrane surface charge, anaesthetic concentration and divalent cation concentration on the conductance of monovalent ions through a membrane.

Trudell *et al.* (1973a) have recently used the technique of electron spin resonance to demonstrate that the inhalation anaesthetics, halothane and methoxyflurane, increase molecular motion in phospholipid bilayers in a concentration-dependent manner (Fig. 2). These increases in membrane fluidity take place at anaesthetic concentrations approaching clinical anaesthesia and similar to those producing anaesthesia in a nerve membrane and are compatible with those predicted by Meyer and Overton, i.e. 30–60 m.moles/l. of lipid.

thesia *in vivo*. Secondly, the close agreement of this phenomenon produced in the pure lipid to that produced in intact animal systems lends support to the theory that anaesthesia is first produced in the lipid phase. These data also suggest that pressure reversal occurs in the lipid rather than in the protein regions of nerve membranes. The authors interpret the results as indicating that the inhalation anaesthetics increase the motion of the hydrocarbon chains of the nerve membrane bilayer. This is consistent with the anaesthetic-induced increase in membrane surface area described by Seeman (1972) and increased bilayer mobility found by Metcalfe *et al.* (1968) with proton relaxation

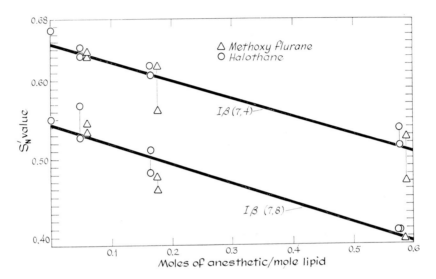

Fig. 2. Change in the order parameter ($S_N'$) of spin labels $I\beta(7,8)$ in phospholipid vesicles containing varying amounts of halothane and methoxyfluorane. Bilayer order decreases and fluidity increases with increasing anaesthetic concentration (Trudell, Hubbell and Cohen, 1973).

The above experimental approach has been applied in a further test of whether lipid regions are the primary site of anaesthesia. It is known that the effects of anaesthetics in luminous bacteria, newts, tadpoles and mice are reversed by application of 150–200 atmospheres of helium or of hydrostatic pressure (Johnson and Flagler, 1951; Eger *et al.*, 1969; Johnson and Miller, 1970). If pressure reversal of anaesthesia occurs in intact nerve systems, then all theories of anaesthesia must accommodate this phenomenon, and nerve membrane model systems must demonstrate it as well. Electron spin resonance studies on spin-labelled phospholipid bilayers demonstrate that the disorder induced by the inhalation anaesthetic halothane in spin-labelled phospholipid vesicles is also reversed by increased pressures of helium (Trudell *et al.*, 1973b).

The demonstration of pressure reversal of inhalation anaesthetic-induced disorder in phospholipid vesicles allows two conclusions. First, phospholipid vesicles would appear to be good models with which to define the primary site of action of anaesthetic, in so far as the disorder is produced within the vesicles at clinical concentrations of anaesthetics and the disorder is reversed at increased helium pressures similar to those which produce reversal of anaes-

experiments. It would seem that the application of high pressures of helium decreases the surface area, forces the chains together, and decreases their motion. The small anaesthetic molecule which induces this disorder was shown not to be excluded from the membrane under conditions of pressure reversal; rather the hydrocarbon chains were reordered around the perturbing molecule (Trudell *et al.*, 1973c).

As will be discussed in greater detail subsequently, a theoretical approach to anaesthetic action is made difficult by the lack of knowledge as to which component of nerve action is inhibited during clinical anaesthesia. Despite the lack of neurophysiological information, it is possible to make some generalizations about the mechanisms of anaesthesia. The experimental work discussed above supports a lipid region as the primary site of action of inhalation anaesthetics. In addition recent work by Kendig *et al.* (1973) with the two stereoisomers of halothane has shown a lack of stereospecificity of anaesthetic action such as might be expected at a protein binding site. Moreover, the extreme range of molecules which produce anaesthesia, from xenon to steroids, makes a protein binding site an unlikely primary site of anaesthetic action. However, proteins are surely the best candidates for those nerve components which control sodium and potassium permeability, control neurotransmitter release and reception, and mediate the relationships between chemical and electrical events in nerve cell membranes.

A recent paper by Trudell, Hubbell and Cohen (1973a) postulated a means of communicating the presence of an anaesthetic in a nerve lipid phase to protein subunits. It is known that there are membrane proteins of highly hydrophobic nature which are 'solvated' by the hydrocarbon chains of an organized lipid structure, presumably a bilayer (Singer and Nicolson, 1972). The solute-solvent relationship of membrane proteins to membrane phospholipids has been clearly demonstrated in the case of rhodopsin in the rod outer segment membranes (Cone, 1971) and in the proteins of the erythrocyte membrane (Bretscher, 1971). It is well known that the configuration of a water-soluble protein is highly dependent on solvent conditions, such as pH and ionic strength, and that such changes dramatically alter enzyme turnover rate. The resonance experiments cited above (Trudell, Hubbell and Cohen, 1973a and b; Metcalfe, Seeman and Burgen, 1968) demonstrate that membrane internal viscosity is altered by anaesthetics. It is then possible that this viscosity change would alter the function of membrane solvated proteins in a manner analogous to that of water solvated enzymes.

Nerve functional proteins may be thought of as operating in a milieu of optimum polarity and viscosity. Any alteration in these characteristics of the proteins' environment due to the presence of drugs, the application of pressure, or change in temperature would inhibit nerve transmission. Once the balance is altered by anaesthesia, any antagonist, such as pressure, which restores this optimum, would tend to restore nerve conduction.

## II. BASIS OF ANAESTHESIA IN NERVE CELLS

It is not easy to transfer insight gained in relatively simple model systems to the more complex level of the actual nerve cell. However the evidence outlined above, in support of the proposition that anaesthetics exert their primary effect on lipid mobility and thus secondarily on membrane protein conformation, raises a number of promising possibilities. Much work has been done on the probable roles of membrane proteins in nerve cell activity, and although much remains to be done there are clear indications of the direction for future research. There are three main possibilities for anaesthetic interference with nerve cell function via changes in protein conformation.

### Nerve Function Inhibition

#### Inhibition of Active Transport

As has been described above, several membrane enzymes require the environment of their normally associated lipids to be fully active. The ability of nerve cells to conduct impulses, and to respond with appropriate electrical potential changes to the arrival of chemical transmitter molecules at their sub-synaptic areas, is dependent on the maintenance of a difference in electrical potential between the inside and the outside of the cell. The electrical potential difference or resting potential that exists across all nerve cell membranes is ultimately a function of the transmembrane active transport of small inorganic ions, particularly sodium, against an electrochemical gradient. The activity of the enzyme most closely associated with this metabolically dependent process is sodium-potassium dependent ATP-ase. The way in which anaesthetic distortion of membrane lipids could prevent the normal function of such an enzyme has been described above. Experimentally, anaesthetics have been shown to inhibit this particular ATP-ase *in vitro* (Israel and Salazar, 1967). Furthermore, anaesthetics of all kinds inhibit active transport of sodium in several kinds of excitable tissue (Andersen, 1966; Schwartz, 1968), either directly by an action on the enzyme or more remotely by depressing oxidative metabolism (Quastel and Wheatley, 1932). The relationship between these phenomena and anaesthesia has been intensively debated, and a central role for depression of active transport has heretofore been rejected on two grounds. First, in the squid giant axon, the preparation used for much of the basic work in neurophysiology, it is possible to poison the cell with metabolic inhibitors without short term impairment of either the resting potential or the ability of the axon to conduct impulses (Hodgkin and Keynes, 1955). Second, depression of oxygen consumption appears to be more a consequence than a cause of central nervous system depression (Michenfelder, Van Dyke and Theye, 1970). Several considerations, however, prevent complete exclusion of this possibility at the moment. The squid axon is atypical in that it is a giant cell with a large ionic reserve and a resting potential relatively free from immediate dependence on active ion transport. It has been suggested that small-diameter preterminal areas of fibers in the central nervous system would respond much more rapidly to inhibition of active transport, since a few impulses could quickly bring about a relatively large change in the intracellular sodium and potassium concentrations (Mullins, 1971). Also, many cells have now been shown to have a portion of their resting potential directly dependent on and controlled by an electrogenic form of active transport (Locke and Solomon, 1967; Rang and Ritchie, 1968). Alteration of pump activity in this type of cell brings about a very rapid alteration of resting potential. Finally, metabolic inhibition, instead of directly altering resting potential by allowing the sodium gradient to fall, may rather exert its main effect through a secondary alteration of membrane permeability. This mechanism is discussed in more detail below.

### Changes in Membrane Resting Permeability

A second way in which anaesthetics may disrupt cell function is by changing the selective permeability of the membrane to particular ion species. One possible molecular basis for a permeability change might be the secondary distortion of proteins referred to above. The presence of anaesthetics in the lipid might alter the configuration of proteins which extend through the membrane and act as selective channels for ions of a particular species. The demonstration that anaesthetic-induced changes in lipid bilayers can indeed increase the carrier-mediated potassium permeability of the latter offers another mechanism (Johnson and Bangham, 1967). A third possibility arises from the demonstration that metabolic inhibitors such as dinitrophenol may have as their predominant effect an increase in internal calcium ion concentration, and a resultant increase in membrane potassium conductance in a number of cell types (Godfraind et al., 1971). An increase in potassium conductance in actual nerve cells would increase membrane resting potential and thus move the resting potential farther from the cell's threshold for excitation. The experimental evidence on the applicability of this phenomenon to nerve cells is unfortunately of a conflicting nature. Aplysia cell bodies respond to a number of types of anaesthetics and related drugs with membrane hyperpolarization and consequent decrease in excitability (Chalazonitis, 1967; Sato et al., 1967; Levitan and Barker, 1972). The basis for the hyperpolarization in this preparation has been shown to be a selective increase in potassium permeability (Sato et al., 1967). However, anaesthetics produce no consistent change in resting potential or membrane conductance in other cell types. Peripheral axons respond to general anaesthetics with depolarization as conduction is blocked (Paton and Speden, 1965). Central motor neurons have been reported to display no consistent resting potential changes in response to ether or to barbiturates (Somjen and Gill, 1963). Therefore at present there appears to be an imperfect correspondence between any unitary change in the selective permeability of model systems and the actual responses of a variety of excitable cells.

### Inhibition of Electrogenesis

The remaining possibility is a derangement of the trigger mechanisms which normally alter membrane characteristics in response to a stimulus. These include the event which alters axonal membrane sodium permeability and thus initiates the conducted action potential; the changes at nerve terminal membranes which lead to release of transmitter in response to an arriving impulse; and the graded changes in selective permeability or electrogenic ion pump activity by which the chemosensitive subsynaptic membrane responds to its appropriate transmitter.

The probability that anaesthetics act primarily by blocking conduction has been accepted as a working hypothesis by a number of investigators (Mullins, 1971; Seeman, 1972). It is certain that local anaesthetics as used clinically do this. All anaesthetic agents will act as local anaesthetics in the sense that at high enough concentrations they will block axonal conduction. The order in which they do so agrees well with their lipid solubility and with their potency in producing general anaesthesia.

The initial event in the generation of the conducted action potential is not yet completely understood. In response to a stimulus which consists of a sudden decrease in the membrane resting potential (depolarization) the membrane for a brief time increases its selective permeability to sodium. The triggering event in the membrane may be an unblocking of sodium-selective channels by a change in protein conformation. There is some evidence that calcium ion is involved in this process (Triggle, 1972). The suggestion has been made that anaesthetics may 'stabilize' membranes by preventing a shift in calcium ion from the membrane (Seeman, 1972).

Much less is known about the membrane changes involved in transmitter release and in the electrogenic response to transmitter at the postsynaptic membrane. The necessity for calcium in both processes may offer an encouraging link to anaesthetic effects on resting membrane permeability and on the generation of the action potential (Triggle, 1972), in that in all three cases anaesthetics may exert their action by blocking normal $Ca^{++}$ movement. As will be discussed below, postsynaptic electrogenesis in response to chemical transmitters is a very diverse phenomenon; in the best-known type of synaptic transmission, exemplified by the postjunctional membrane in neuromuscular transmission, there is a depolarizing conductance increase to $Na^+$ and $K^+$. The same possibilities for anaesthetic interference apply as in the blockade of conduction. That is, anaesthetics may distort the proteins that form ion-selective channels, or may prevent the type of protein conformational change that in turn alters permeability.

### Site of Action of Anaesthetics at the Nerve Cell

Having explored the ways in which anaesthetic-induced changes in lipid mobility may secondarily alter nerve cell functions by altering protein structure or by preventing protein activity, it is necessary to examine the evidence for a unitary action of anaesthetics at the cellular level. Is there one nerve cell function interrupted by all anaesthetics at their respective anaesthetic concentrations? The choice lies between axonal impulse conduction, or some step in the process of synaptic transmission (Fig. 3).

### Blockade of Impulse Conduction

The ways in which impulse conduction can be blocked have been outlined above: they include blockade of the initial sodium conductance shift, alterations in passive permeability which prevent the membrane from reaching its threshold, and alterations in active transport leading to a decline in the resting potential. As mentioned above, all anaesthetics do block conduction. The major drawback to acceptance of conduction block as the site of anaesthesia is the fact that in peripheral axons, where most of the experimental work has been carried out, the anaesthetic concentrations required to block conduction are much greater than those required to bring about general anaesthesia. On the other hand, two considerations weaken this objection: first, as suggested above, small-diameter neurons in the CNS may have a much lower safety factor than large-diameter peripheral neurons, and thus may require a much smaller disturbance to interrupt conduction. Second, there is a little-explored possibility that axonal membranes may be specialized. If this is the case, the membranes of some neurons may be inherently more sensitive to anaesthetics than those of others. An important piece of evidence which supports conduction block as the site of anaesthesia is that it can apparently be reversed by high pressure (Spyropoulos, 1957); as indicated above, pressure reversal is a powerful criterion which must be satisfied by any theory of anaesthetic action.

Blockade of conduction thus remains a strong contender for a possible site of anaesthetic action on nerve cell function. It is a tempting hypothesis because much is known about the events in conduction, allowing a more thorough explanation for the molecular basis of anaesthesia than any other site presently offers, and because it provides a mechanism for anaesthesia which potentially includes all agents.

calcium-independent subsequent steps in transmitter release (Quastel et al., 1970).

Many anaesthetics also depress the response of the membrane to a given amount of transmitter (Thesleff, 1956; Bloom et al., 1965). Although it is easy to see how a postulated primary action of anaesthetics on membrane lipids might distort membrane receptors and thus alter transmitter–receptor interactions, there is as yet no evidence that this is what actually occurs. The diversity of anaesthetic molecular structure argues against a direct

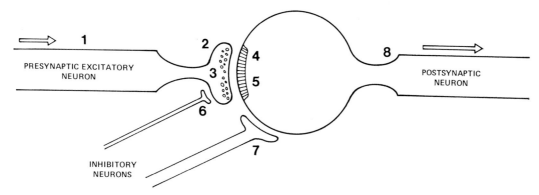

FIG. 3. Possible sites of anaesthetic action in nerve cells. Arrows indicate the direction of impulse traffic. **1.** Conduction of the action potential. All anaesthetic agents block conduction, but at higher concentrations than those at which they block synaptic transmission. **2.** $Ca^{++}$—dependent depolarization-secretion coupling and **3,** subsequent $Ca^{++}$—independent steps in transmitter release. Several agents (barbiturates and alcohols) decrease the amount of ACh released from presynaptic terminals in sympathetic ganglia. At the neuromuscular junction these agents increase $Ca^{++}$—independent spontaneous transmitter release. Therefore **2,** $Ca^{++}$—dependent depolarization—secretion coupling is the probable site of anaesthetic inhibition of transmitter release. **4.** Transmitter-receptor interaction. Volatile agents and barbiturates depress the postsynaptic response at the neuromuscular junction and in the central nervous system. The diversity of anaesthetic molecular structures makes a direct action of anaesthetics on the receptor unlikely; however a secondary effect on receptor proteins through derangement of their lipid environment is possible. **5.** Electrogenesis in the subsynaptic membrane. There is as yet little evidence about anaesthetic alterations in subsynaptic membrane function. **6 and 7,** pre- and post-synaptic inhibition, may be selectively enhanced by barbiturates which may thus indirectly depress excitability. **8.** Initiation of the impulse in the postsynaptic neuron. Ether and barbiturates increase the threshold level of depolarization necessary for impulse generation in spinal cord neurons.

## Alteration of Synaptic Transmission

The alternative possibilities are all included in the category of synaptic transmission, and they are much more diverse (Fig. 3). The main evidence for synaptic transmission rather than conduction as the site of anaesthesia is that anaesthetics block transmission across a synapse at concentrations lower than those at which they depress conduction (Larrabee and Pasternak, 1952).

Within the process of synaptic transmission there are numerous processes subject to anaesthetic action. First is the possibility that conduction is being blocked at some point near the presynaptic terminal that has a lower safety factor than the main axon, where conduction is usually monitored. This has been shown not to be the case both in spinal neurons (Somjen, 1963) and at the neuromuscular junction (Karis, Gissen and Nastuk, 1967), where impulse invasion of the terminals remains unchanged at concentrations of anaesthetics which depress synaptic and neuromuscular transmission. The second step, transmitter release, is depressed by several agents (Matthews and Quilliam, 1964). Anaesthetics probably inhibit the calcium-dependent process of depolarization-secretion coupling, since at least some agents actually potentiate the

action on the receptor proteins themselves. The remaining possibility is that anaesthetics interfere with some subsequent step in chemical electrogenesis. The process of synaptic electrogenesis is as yet poorly understood. Subsynaptic membranes are widely diverse. Some respond to the appropriate transmitter with a depolarizing conductance increase to sodium and potassium. At many inhibitory synapses the response is a stabilizing conductance increase to potassium and chloride ions. Some synapses may show a depolarizing excitatory conductance decrease to potassium (Krnjevic et al., 1971). For yet others there is evidence for a hyperpolarizing increase in the rate of active ion transport (Siggins et al., 1969). Anaesthetics have not been tested at all these types of synapse. Of those agents which have been tested, most can depress an excitatory response to iontophoresis of putative transmitter (Thesleff, 1956; Bloom et al., 1965). Barbiturates are capable of increasing the magnitude of inhibitory responses (Eccles et al., 1963; Larson and Major, 1970). It is too soon to say whether any one of these actions on any particular type of synapse is a probable a mechanism of anaesthesia.

In summary, there is evidence for synaptic transmission

as a site for anaesthetic action on the ground of sensitivity of the process to anaesthetics, but the diversity of anaesthetic effects militates against this as a unitary mechanism for anaesthesia. In addition, pressure reversibility has not yet been demonstrated for any anaesthetic effect on synaptic transmission.

## III. ANAESTHESIA IN THE BRAIN

The difficulties of projecting from one level to the next higher level of organization are nowhere more clearly apparent than in the consideration of anaesthetic effects on the brain. If it is difficult to pinpoint the site of anaesthesia in the single nerve cell, at least the number of possibilities is known and restricted. In the intact brain, with its large populations of specialized neurons, the number of ways in which anaesthetics may disrupt the orderly patterns of activity which maintain the conscious state becomes very large. The probability that all anaesthetics do so in the same way, that there is a unitary mechanism of anaesthesia at the level of the organized central nervous system, becomes correspondingly small.

### Definition of Anaesthesia

In spite of decades of research and speculation the nature of anaesthetic disruption of brain function is still so poorly understood that a rational attack on the problem is difficult to design. Recently, however, one of the major stumbling blocks to coherent studies of anaesthesia at this level has been removed with the acceptance of MAC as a definition of an anaesthetic endpoint. MAC was originally stated to be the minimum alveolar anaesthetic concentration necessary to prevent movement of 50 per cent of subjects in response to a controlled painful stimulus such as tail clamp or skin incision (Eger et al., 1965). For inhalation agents, MAC thus provides a completely operational definition of anaesthesia or anaesthetic endpoint in terms of an $ED_{50}$. By converting from alveolar to serum concentration, MAC can also be made to apply to intravenous agents.

The provision of an endpoint defined as the abolition of a response to a stimulus of a certain intensity has several advantages. It is simple to determine and is a clinically relevant definition of anaesthesia. Furthermore, it leads directly to the formulation of experimental questions. Thus we can determine how a strong stimulus arouses the unanaesthetized animal, and then ask how and where anaesthetics disrupt the arousal mechanism.

### The Arousal System

The classical lesion work of Moruzzi, Magoun and others demonstrated that in the acute animal, apparently normal wakefulness occurs if the brainstem reticular formation is left connected to the cerebrum, and that the animal can be aroused by stimulating the reticular formation directly. Conversely, the animal with a section through the midbrain reticular formation is comatose and cannot be aroused by sensory stimulation mediated through lemniscal pathways (Moruzzi, 1972). Thus it appears that consciousness depends on input from the ascending reticular formation

to the cerebrum. Furthermore, the work of French, Verzeano and Magoun (1953) established that reticular system evoked potentials were blocked at a lower concentration of anaesthetics than cortical evoked potentials, and thus it appeared reasonable to assume that anaesthetics produce unresponsiveness by blocking reticular formation processing of sensory input to the cortex. This remains the most widely accepted view of the essential central action of anaesthetics.

Two pieces of more recent experimental evidence may alter this concept, although their significance with respect to anaesthesia remains to be evaluated. The first is that in the chronic preparation (as opposed to the acute), consciousness, as estimated by a desynchronized EEG is possible even without the midbrain reticular formation, with the posterior hypothalamus apparently able to maintain wakefulness in the cerebrum without input from the more caudal reticular formation (Genovesi et al., 1956). The second is the finding that for at least some anaesthetics, changes can be noted in the pattern of cortical activity before there are changes in the activity of reticular formation neurons (Darbinjan et al., 1971).

If it is still accepted as a working hypothesis that anaesthesia corresponds to blockade of the reticular formation, the basis for the latter's special sensitivity to anaesthetics remains to be established. It was at one time proposed that the multiplicity of synaptic connections in the reticular formation rendered it vulnerable, on the assumption that there was a finite chance of failure of transmission at each synapse and that therefore the chance of successful transmission was diminished as the number of synapses increased (Bárány, 1947). However, it has been demonstrated that in the spinal cord polysynaptic pathways are not necessarily more sensitive to anaesthetics than are monosynaptic (de Jong et al., 1968). It therefore seems advisable to look for some more specific property of the reticular formation or of its constituent neurons as an explanation for its sensitivity to anaesthetics. The proposal has been made that anaesthetics specifically depress a cholinergic system of neurons within the reticular formation (Krnjevic, 1967).

### Consciousness and its Disruption

The parallels between anaesthesia and sleep have led to some fruitful research. However, it is questionable to what extent the analogy between the two states is a valid one, since the patterns of cortical activity observed with anaesthetics do not correspond closely to any of the patterns of sleep. Furthermore, the cortical EEG is different for different anaesthetics (Hosick et al., 1971). A particular problem is that some agents not only do not simply depress cortical activity, but as in the case of enflurane (Ēthrane), produce a pattern strongly reminiscent of convulsant activity (Joas and Stevens, 1969). All the EEG patterns seen in anaesthesia differ from those associated with normal consciousness; however it is unclear whether these EEG manifestations are essential parts of the anaesthetic state or are essentially side effects unrelated to anaesthesia. Phrased somewhat differently, the question is whether all anaesthetics have a single action that leads to loss of responsiveness, or whether anaesthesia corresponds to a number of different possible CNS states ranging from extreme cortical depression through something resembling seizure activity.

## IV. SUMMARY

At the molecular level the initial event in anaesthesia is becoming fairly well established. The long-known and still good correlation of potency and lipid solubility, with the more recent ESR evidence on the effects of anaesthetics on lipids, supports the hypothesis that anaesthetics enter the lipid bilayer of the nerve cell membrane and disorder it. From this basis it is a reasonable speculation that in a disordered lipid environment some membrane proteins cease to function normally.

The nerve cell event, if there is a single event disrupted by anaesthesia, remains undecided. On balance, because of its universality and pressure reversibility, conduction block appears to be the strongest candidate for a mechanism of anaesthesia at the cellular level. Finally, at the level of the central nervous system, blockade of the reticular formation remains acceptable as a unitary mechanism of anaesthesia, but with a number of important problems remaining to be solved.

## ACKNOWLEDGMENTS

This work was supported by NIH Program Project Grant No. GM 12527.

We wish to express our sincere appreciation to Dr. Ellis N. Cohen for reading the manuscript and offering many helpful suggestions.

## REFERENCES

Andersen, N. B. (1966), "Effect of General Anesthetics on Sodium Transport in the Isolated Toad Bladder," *Anesthesiology*, **27**, 304.

Barnay, E. H. (1947), "A Theoretical Note Concerning the Action of Drugs on the Central Nervous System," *Arch. int. Pharmacodyn.*, **75**, 222.

Bloom, F. E., Costa, E. and Salmoiraghi, G. C. (1965), "Anesthesia and the Responsiveness of Individual Neurons of the Caudate Nucleus of the Cat to Acetylcholine, Norepinephrine and Dopamine Administered by Microelectrophoresis," *J. Pharmacol Exp. Therap.*, **150**, 244.

Bretscher, M. (1971), "A Major Protein which Spans the Human Erythrocyte Membrane," *J. Mol. Biol.*, **59**, 351.

Chalazonitis, N. (1967), "Effects of Anesthetics on Neural Mechanisms," *Anesthesiology*, **28**, 111.

Cone, R. A. (1971), "Relaxation Times of Rhodopsin Detected by Photodichroism," *Biophys. Soc. Abstr.*, **II**, 246A.

Darbinjan, T. M., Golvchinsky, V. B. and Plehotkina, S. I. (1971), "The Effects of Anesthetics on Reticular and Cortical Activity," *Anesthesiology*, **34**, 219.

de Jong, R. H., Robles, R., Corbin, R. W. and Nance, R. A. (1968), "Effect of Inhalation Anesthetics on Monosynaptic and Polysynaptic Transmission in the Spinal Cord," *J. Pharmacol Exp. Therap.*, **162**, 326.

Eccles, J. C., Schmidt, R. and Willis, W. D. (1963), "Pharmacological Studies on Presynaptic Inhibition," *J. Physiol. (Lond.)*, **168**, 500.

Eger, E. I., Lundgren, C., Miller, S. L. and Stevens, W. C. (1969), "Anesthetic Potencies of Sulfur Hexafluoride, Carbon Tetrafluoride, Chloroform and Ēthrane in Dogs; Correlation with the Hydrate and Lipid Theories of Anesthetic Action," *Anesthesiology*, **30**, 129.

Eger, E. I., Saidman, L. J. and Brandstater, B. (1965), "Minimum Alveolar Anesthetic Concentration: A Standard of Anesthetic Potency," *Anesthesiology*, **26**, 756.

Eisenman, G., Szabo, G., Ciani, S., McLaughlin, S. and Krasne, S. (1973), "Ion Binding and Ion Transport Produced by Neutral Lipid-Soluble Molecules," in *Progress in Surface and Membrane Science*, Vol. 6 (J. F. Danielli, M. D. Rosenberg and D. A. Cadenhead, Eds.). New York: Academic Press.

Featherstone, R. M. and Muelbacher, C. A. (1963), "The Current Role of Inert Gases in the Search for Anesthesia Mechanisms," *Pharmacol. Rev.*, **15**, 97.

French, J. D., Verzeano, M. and Magoun, H. W. (1953), "A Neural Basis of the Anesthetic State,' *Arch. Neurol. Psychiat.*, **69**, 519.

Ferguson, J. (1939), "The Use of Chemical Potentials as Indices of Toxicity," *Proc. R. Soc. Biol.*, **127**, 387.

Genovesi, V., Moruzzi, G., Palestini, M., Rossi, G. F. and Zanchetti, A. (1956), "EEG and Behavioral Patterns Following Lesions of the Mesencephalic Reticular Formation in Chronic Cats with Implanted Electrodes," Abstr. *Comm. 20th Int. Physiol. Congr.*, Brussels, 335.

Godfraind, J. M., Kawamura, H., Krnjevic, K. and Pumain, R. (1971), "Actions of Dinitrophenol and some other Metabolic Inhibitors on Cortical Neurones," *J. Physiol.*, **215**, 199.

Hodgkin, A. L. and Keynes, R. D. (1955), "Active Transport of Cations in Giant Axons from Sepia and Loligo," *J. Physiol.*, **128**, 28.

Hong, K. and Hubbell, W. L. (1972), "Preparation and Properties of Phospholipid Bilayers Containing Rhodopsin," *Proc. Nat. Acad. Sci. (U.S.A.)*, **69**, 2617.

Hosick, E. C., Clark, D. L., Adam, N. and Rosner, B. S. (1971), "Neurophysiological Effects of Different Anesthetics in Conscious Man," *J. Appl. Physiol.*, **31**, 892.

Israel, Y. and Salazar, 1. (1967), "Inhibition of Brain Microsomal Adenosine Triphosphatases by General Depressants," *Arch. Biochem. Biophys.*, **122**, 310.

Joas, T. A. and Stevens, W. C. (1969), "Convulsive Properties of Ēthrane, Fluroxene, Halothane and Chloroform Anesthesia," *Anesthesiology*, **30**, 343.

Johnson, F. H. and Flagler, E. A. (1951), "Hydrostatic Pressure Reversal of Narcosis in Tadpoles," *Science*, **112**, 91.

Johnson, S. M. and Bangham, A. D. (1969), "The Action of Anesthetics on Phospholipid Membranes," *Biochim. Biophys. Acta*, **193**, 92.

Johnson, S. M. and Miller, K. W. (1970), "Antagonism of Pressure and Anesthesia," *Nature*, **228**, 75.

Karis, J. H., Gissen, A. J. and Nastuk, W. L. (1967), "The Effect of Volatile Anesthetic Agents on Neuromuscular Transmission," *Anesthesiology*, **28**, 128.

Kendig, J. J., Trudell, J. R. and Cohen, E. N. (1973), "Halothane Stereoisomers: Lack of Stereospecificity in Two Model Systems," *Anesthesiology*. In press.

Krnjevic, K. (1967), "Chemical Transmission and Cortical Arousal," *Anesthesiology*, **28**, 100.

Krnjevic, K., Pumain, R. and Reynaud, L. (1971), "The Mechanism of Excitation by Acetylcholine in the Cerebral Cortex," *J. Physiol.*, **215**, 247.

Larrabee, M. G. and Pasternak, J. M. (1952), "Selective Action of Anesthetics on Synapses and Axons in Mammalian Sympathetic Ganglia," *J. Neurophysiol.*, **15**, 91.

Larson, M. D. and Major, M. A. (1970), "The Effect of Hexobarbital on the Duration of the Recurrent IPSP in Cat Motorneurons," *Brain Res.*, **21**, 309.

Levitan, H. and Barker, J. L. (1972), "Membrane Permeability: Cation Selectivity Reversibly Altered by Salicylate," *Science*, **178**, 63.

Locke, S. and Solomon, H. C. (1967), "Relation of Resting Potential of Rat Gastrocnemius and Soleus Muscles to Innervation, Activity, and the Na-K Pump," *J. Exp. Zool.*, **166**, 377.

Matthews, E. K. and Quilliam, J. P. (1964), "Effects of Central Depressant Drugs Upon Acetylcholine Release," *Brit. J. Pharmacol.*, **22**, 415.

Metcalfe, J. C., Seeman, P. and Burgen, A. S. V. (1968), "The Proton Relaxation of Benzyl Alcohol in Erythrocyte Membranes," *Mol. Pharmacol.*, **4**, 87.

Meyer, H. H. (1899), *Arch. Pharmacol. Exp. Pathol.*, **42**, 109.

Michenfelder, J. D., Van Dyke, R. Z. and Theye, R. A. (1970), "The Effects of Anesthetic Agents and Techniques on Canine Cerebral ATP and Lactate Levels," *Anesthesiology*, **33**, 315.

Miller, K. W., Paton, W. D. M. and Smith, E. B. (1967), "The Anesthetic Pressures of Certain Fluorine-Containing Gases," *Brit. J. Anaesth.*, **39**, 910.

Miller, K. W., Paton, W. D. M., Smith, E. B. and Smith, L. A. (1971), "Physicochemical Approaches to the Mode of Action of General Anesthetics," *Anesthesiology*, **36**, 339.

Miller, S. L. (1961), "A Theory of Gaseous Anesthetics," *Proc. nat. Acad. Sci. (U.S.A.)*, **47**, 1515.

Moruzzi, G. (1972), "The Sleep Walking Cycle," *Ergebn. Physiol.*, **64**, 1.

Mullins, L. J. (1954), "Some Physical Mechanisms in Narcosis," *Chem. Rev.*, **54**, 289.

Mullins, L. J. (1971), "Anesthetics," in *Handbook of Neurochemistry*, Vol. 6 (A. Lajtha, Ed.). New York: Plenum Press.

Overton, E. (1901), *Studien über Die Narkose*. Jena: Fisher.

Papahadjopoulous, D. (1970), "Antagonistic Effects of $CaF_2$ and Local Anesthetics on the Permeability of Phosphatidyl Serine Vesicles," *Biochim. Biophys. Acta*, **211**, 467.

Paton, W. D. M. and Speden, R. M. (1965), "Uptake of Anesthetics and their Action on the Central Nervous System," *Brit. med. Bull.*, **21**, 44.

Pauling, L. (1961), "A Molecular Theory of Anesthesia," *Science*, **134**, 15.

Quastel, D. M. J., Hackett, J. T. and Cooke, J. D. (1970), "Calcium: Is it Required for Transmitter Secretion?", *Science*, **172**, 1034.

Quastel, J. H. and Wheatley, A. H. M. (1932), "Narcosis and Oxidations of the Brain," *Proc. roy. Soc. Lond.*, **112**, 60.

Rang, H. P. and Ritchie, J. M. (1968), "On the Electrogenic Sodium Pump in Mammalian Non-myelinated Nerve Fibers and its Activation by Various External Cations," *J. Physiol. (Lond.)*, **196**, 183.

Sato, M., Austin, G. M. and Yai, H. (1967), "Increase in Permeability of the Postsynaptic Membrane to Potassium Produced by 'Nembutal'," *Nature*, **215**, 1506.

Schwartz, E. A. (1968), "Effect of Diethyl Ether on Sodium Efflux from Squid Axons," *Currents Mod. Biol.*, **2**, 1.

Seeman, P. (1972), "The Membrane Action of Anesthetics and Tranquilizers," *Pharmacol. Rev.*, **24**, 583.

Siggins, G. R., Hoffer, B. J. and Bloom, F. E. (1969), "Cyclic Adenosine Monophosphate: Possible Mediator for Norepinephrine Effects on Cerebral Purkinje Cells," *Science*, **165**, 1018.

Singer, S. W. and Nicolson, G. L. (1972), "The Fluid Mosaic Model of the Structure of Cell Membranes," *Science*, **175**, 720.

Somjen, G. (1963), "The Effect of Ether and Thiopental on Spinal Presynaptic Terminals," *J. Pharmacol.*, **140**, 396.

Somjen, G. and Gill, M. (1963), "The Mechanism of the Blockade of Synaptic Transmission in the Mammalian Spinal Cord by Diethyl Ether and by Thiopental," *J. Pharmacol Exp. Therap.*, **140**, 19.

Spyropoulos, C. S. (1957), "The Effects of Hydrostatic Pressure upon the Normal and Narcotized Nerve," *J. Gen. Physiol.*, **40**, 849.

Thesleff, S. (1956), "The Effect of Anesthetic Agents on Skeletal Muscle Membrane," *Acta Physiol. Scand.*, **37**, 335.

Trauble, H. and Haynes, D. H. (1971), "The Volume Change in Lipid Bilayer Lamellae at the Crystalline-Liquid Crystalline Phase Transition," *Chem. Phys. Lipids*, **7**, 324.

Triggle, D. J. (1972), "Effects of Calcium on Excitable Membranes and Neurotransmitter Action," in *Progress in Surface and Membrane Science*, Vol. 5 (J. F. Danielli, M. D. Rosenberg and D. A. Cadenhead, Eds.). New York: Academic Press.

Trudell, J. R., Hubbell, W. L. and Cohen, E. N. (1973a), "The Effect of Two Inhalation Anesthetics on the Order of Spin-Labelled Phospholipid Vesicles," *Biochim. Biophys. Acta*, **291**, 321.

Trudell, J. R., Hubbell, W. L. and Cohen, E. N. (1973b), "Pressure Reversal of Inhalation Anesthetic-Induced Disorder in Spin-Labelled Phospholipid Vesicles," *Biochim. Biophys. Acta*, **291**, 328.

Trudell, J. R., Hubbell, W. L., Cohen, E. N. and Kendig, J. J. (1973), "Pressure Reversal of Anesthesia: The Extent of Small-Molecule Exclusion from Spin-Labeled Phospholipid Model Membranes," *Anesthesiology*, **38**, 207.

*CHAPTER* 3

# NEUROMUSCULAR TRANSMISSION

## J. P. PAYNE

The physiological mechanisms involved in neuromuscular transmission have been demonstrated almost entirely by pharmacological experiment; indeed there is no better example in the whole of physiology of the interdependence of the two disciplines. Of all the drugs involved curare has made the greatest impact; originally as the crude vegetable extract used by South American Indians to poison their arrow-heads, and latterly as the highly purified version in clinical use today.

The first published account of the arrow poison used by the South American Indians appeared within 25 years of the discovery of the New World but although the growth of the literature on the subject was extensive during the next 300 years it was not until the beginning of the nineteenth century that the mode and site of action of curare was investigated systematically.

The scientific evaluation began with Brodie's observation (1811) that when the lungs of curarized guinea pigs were inflated with oxygen the dark colour of the blood reaching the lungs was replaced by a healthier red colour. For the purpose of inflation Brodie used a gum bottle and showed, by bubbling the contents through lime water, that carbon dioxide accumulated in the bottle in proportion to the duration of the paralysis. Presumably because of this accumulation of carbon dioxide the guinea pigs failed to survive and in further experiments Brodie adopted the twin-bellows system described by John Hunter in 1776 to inflate the lungs of cats apparently dead from the effects of curare. By this means he demonstrated that the use of artificial respiration throughout the period of paralysis was sufficient to sustain life until spontaneous breathing returned, and concluded that the action of curare was to suspend temporarily the function of the brain. It was nearly another 50 years before Claude Bernard carried out the experiments which proved conclusively that the action of curare was peripheral and not central as Brodie had supposed. But Bernard's experiments had far greater implications; by demonstrating that the junction between the nerve endings and the muscle fibres had peculiar properties he established neuromuscular transmission as a separate physiological entity.

Bernard's experiments involved the exposure and ligation of the blood supply to one lower limb in a pithed but otherwise intact frog. This was followed by the intraperitoneal injection of curare whereupon all the muscles in the body became paralysed except those deprived of their blood supply. But when a stimulus was applied directly to the muscles of the paralysed lower limbs a reflex movement resulted in the unaffected limb. From this Bernard concluded that an intact blood supply is necessary for the distribution of curare in the body, that conduction in motor nerves is unaffected by the presence of curare, and that sensory nerve conduction and spinal cord transmission are not abolished by curare. The experiment was then extended; both sciatic nerves were tied as far proximally as possible, divided close to the vertebral column and mobilized so that they could be stimulated by the same electrode. When the stimulus was applied a contraction was elicited in the muscles deprived of their blood supply but not in the curarized muscles which however responded to direct stimulation. Bernard concluded that curare has no direct effect either on muscle or nerve and must therefore act at the junction between them.

The simplicity and logic of Bernard's experiments have not been surpassed by more modern methods; they still offer not only a convenient means of testing new drugs for neuromuscular blocking properties but also a simple, effective and inexpensive method for instructing students.

The therapeutic possibilities of curare were soon recognized and already by 1858 it had been used to treat tetanus; although it is only within recent years that its place in the management of this disease has been assured. Other diseases in which its use was less justified included hydrophobia, epilepsy and chorea. The history of these early clinical endeavours has been described by McIntyre in his monograph entitled "Curare" (McIntyre 1947).

Unfortunately the early assessment of the action of curare was complicated by the fact that crude curare contained a number of different alkaloids of similar pharmacological properties with the results that different extracts had a variable potency making standard dosage impossible. The unreliability of the curare preparations led to a search for compounds with a more dependable action and in 1868 Crum Brown and Fraser, after making the important observation that a wide range of quaternary salts possessed a curare-like action, attempted and succeeded in making partial synthesis of curarizing agents. The apparent affinity of these quaternary ammonium compounds for the motor end plate was later to be of significant value in the elucidation of the mechanisms of neuromuscular transmission.

Although Claude Bernard established the specific properties of the neuromuscular junction the precise mechanisms of transmission had not then been demonstrated and as late as 1934 Sir Henry Dale in arguing the case for the chemical transmission of nervous effects was able to say,

"I think I am right in supposing that the prevalent conception of the excitation of a voluntary muscle fibre by a nervous impulse assumes that the wave of physico-chemical disturbance, propagated along the nerve fibre as the nervous impulse, passes directly to the muscle fibre and there excites contraction as it is further propagated."

The first suggestion that nervous impulses might be transmitted by the release of a specific chemical stimulant was made in 1904 by T. R. Elliott. In an attempt to explain the close relationship between the actions of adrenaline and those of sympathetic nerves he proposed that the nerves might release adrenaline at their endings. This idea was taken up by W. E. Dixon who further proposed that parasympathetic nerves also could produce their effects by the release of a chemical transmitter. At that time no chemical substance was known in the body with actions similar to those produced by parasympathetic stimulation but Dixon managed to show that an extract from a dog's heart removed under vagal inhibition would a slow a frog's heart rate and that this bradycardia was atropine-sensitive. He was not however able to identify it further, but suggested that it might be muscarine.

In 1914 the chance discovery of acetylcholine as a constituent of a sample of ergot and therefore as a product of nature caused Sir Henry Dale to make a detailed study of its properties and led to the discovery of its muscarinic and nicotinic properties. The possible physiological significance of acetylcholine became apparent when Dale drew attention to the fact that it reproduced the various effects of parasympathetic nerves in the same way that adrenaline simulated the effects of sympathetic stimulation.

The outbreak of war diverted the attention of Dale and his colleagues to work more directly concerned with the national emergency, and it was not until 1921 that Otto Loewi produced convincing evidence that the vagus nerve exerted its effect on the frog's heart by releasing an inhibitor substance. In a simple yet elegant experiment he showed that when the fluid contained in a heart during vagal stimulation was transferred to a second heart the vagal effects were reproduced. He showed that the substance concerned had properties corresponding in every respect to acetylcholine and that it was rapidly destroyed by an esterase present in the heart muscle which could be inhibited by physostigmine. This latter observation was later to prove important in the identification of cholinergic nerves.

Subsequently, as the evidence accumulated Loewi's fundamental discovery was extended from the vagus nerve to the rest of the parasympathetic system and it was only a matter of time before the possibility of a similar mechanism operating at the neuromuscular junction was considered. Until this time the electrical theory of the propagation of excitation across synaptic and myoneural junctions was predominant and as late as 1933 Loewi himself expressed the view that chemical transmission was unlikely to apply to the nerve endings in striated muscle. In contrast, in the same year Lord Adrian wrote "It is by no means certain that the humoral transmission of the vagal effect differs in kind from the transmission of activity from motor nerve to striated muscle. An exciting substance liberated at a nerve ending but destroyed within a few thousandths of a second would have little chance of spreading by diffusion and would account well enough for the known properties of the nerve ending. It is equally likely that the more direct kinds of transmission depend, as in nerve fibre, on electric forces disturbing the balanced reactions of surface membranes."

Twelve months later Dale and Feldberg obtained the first evidence in support of a chemical transmission mechanism at motor nerve endings in voluntary muscle, for this purpose they stimulated the motor nerve supply to the perfused tongue of a cat and extracted from the perfusate a substance possessing all the properties of acetylcholine. Thereafter in a series of carefully planned experiments Dale and his colleagues established the facts on which the chemical transmission theory is based.

First, it was shown that when the motor nerve to perfused voluntary muscle was stimulated acetylcholine appeared in the venous effluent but when the nerve stimulation ceased to produce a muscle contraction acetylcholine disappeared from the effluent. This suggested that acetylcholine was necessary to produce the muscle contraction when the nerve was stimulated; but the possibility had to be excluded that it was derived from the muscle itself as a by-product of the contractile process, or that it had been trapped in the extracellular fluid and expressed mechanically when the muscle contracted. Accordingly, a normally innervated muscle was stimulated directly and acetylcholine was immediately detected in the venous outflow; a similar result was obtained when a muscle deprived only of its autonomic nerve supply was stimulated. However when a muscle completely denervated by degeneration was stimulated no acetylcholine could be detected in the perfusate even when the muscle contracted vigorously. Thus it was clear that the production of acetylcholine was not a necessary component of muscle contraction; its presence after direct stimulation of normal muscle could be explained by the fact that it has proved impossible to effectively stimulate a muscle without at the same time stimulating the motor nerve endings in its substance.

It remained therefore only to test the effects of motor nerve stimulation in the complete absence of muscular contractions, and the availability of curare provided this opportunity. The experiments were carried out on the perfused tongue of a cat. The hypoglossal nerve was stimulated before and after curarization and the venous effluent collected. The appearance of acetylcholine in the effluent during curarization demonstrated conclusively that its production was not directly or indirectly due to the contraction of the muscle fibres.

From these experiments Dale and his colleagues concluded that either acetylcholine sensitized the effector cell to enable the direct transmission of the propagated disturbance in the nerve fibre or more likely that its liberation at the nerve ending caused a direct stimulation of the effector cells, initiating an essentially new propagated wave of excitation in the muscle fibre.

The case in favour of chemical transmission was strengthened by the knowledge that acetylcholine and an enzyme, choline acetylase, capable of its rapid synthesis are to be found along the length of motor but not sensory nerves and that a second enzyme, 'true' cholinesterase, capable of the rapid destruction of acetylcholine is to be found in high concentrations at the nerve endings under the muscle membrane.

Convincing proof that acetylcholine was the chemical substance intervening between nerve and muscle came in a second series of experiments by Dale and his colleagues (Brown, Dale and Feldberg, 1936) on the reactions of normal mammalian muscle to acetylcholine and eserine. In these experiments it was shown firstly that the close intra-arterial injection of acetylcholine caused a contraction of muscle not substantially different from that obtained by stimulation of the motor nerve, and that this response was abolished by curare but was not affected by atropine. Secondly, it was shown that when eserine, a powerful anticholinesterase was injected intravenously into a spinal cat the response to a maximal nerve volley was changed from a simple twitch to a repetitive response like a brief tetanus. This modification of the response by eserine is only explicable if it is accepted that the transmission of excitation from nerve to muscle occurs through the mediation of acetylcholine. Further support for this view was obtained when it was shown that when a close intra-arterial injection of acetylcholine was made in the presence of eserine the response was intensified.

As a result of the efforts of Dale and his colleagues and subsequent workers the pattern of events in the chemical transmission of nervous impulses across the neuromuscular junction has been reasonably well defined. Figures 1 and 2 illustrate the anatomical details of this region. The motor nerve supply to muscle reaches it as a myelinated axon which divides into branches to supply from 5 to 300 muscle fibres. As the nerve branch approaches the muscle fibre it loses its myelin sheath and further sub-divides to form fine terminations, about 100 microns long which lie in grooves on the surface of the muscle. But even in this position the nerve endings are prevented from making direct contact with muscle fibres by the presence of fine membranes on both nerve and muscle. The pre-synaptic membrane ensheathes the nerve endings and is separated from the muscle membrane by a minute but distinct extracellular gap which in turn is partitioned by a basement membrane. In the vicinity of the nerve endings the muscle membrane becomes highly specialized to form the post-synaptic membrane, arranged in a series of regular folds about one micron deep. These folds in which cholinesterase is now known to be concentrated run into the muscle at right angles to the direction of the nerve endings.

Acetylcholine is synthesized in the nerve terminal by the action of the enzyme, choline acetyltransferase, on choline after its absorption from the surrounding extracellular fluid. The choline itself is derived from the hydrolysis of acetylcholine by cholinesterase. This reaction serves two purposes, the rapid termination of the action of acetylcholine on the post-synaptic membrane, and the provision of fresh supplies of choline for resynthesis. Once formed, acetylcholine is stored in the nerve terminal as separate small pockets or quanta; about 200,000 of these, enough to respond to several thousand impulses can be stored, but only a fraction, sufficient for a few impulses, is immediately

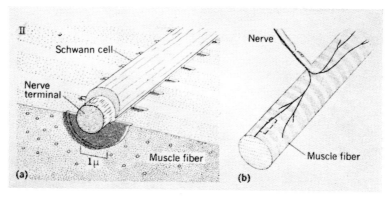

Fig. 1(a) and (b). Anatomy of the end plate region. (Birks, Huxley and Katz (1960),
*J. Physiol.*, **150**, 134.)

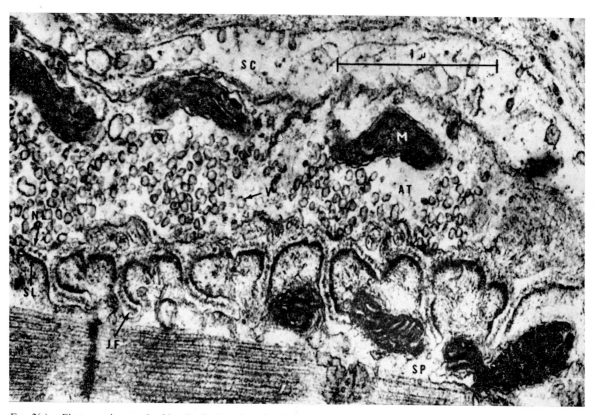

Fig. 2(a).  Electron micrograph of longitudinal section of end plate region.  (Birks, Huxley and Katz (1960), *J. Physiol.*, **150**, 134.)

AT—Axon terminal
SC—Schwann cell
M—Mitochondria
NL—Neurolemma
SL—Sarcolemma
SP—Junctional fold
V—Vesicles
MF—Myofilaments

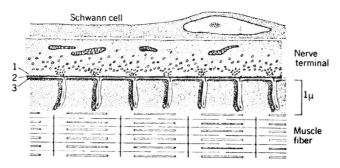

Fig. 2(b).  Schematic legend for Fig. 2(a).

available. When an impulse reaches the nerve terminal some of the readily available acetylcholine is released. During repetitive nerve stimulation the fraction of this readily available pool released by an individual impulse is determined by the amount present at the time of stimulation, by the amount of previous activity and by the calcium ion concentration; a reduction in the number of calcium ions reduces the transmitter availability. The rate at which the release of acetylcholine can continue is determined by the extent to which its mobilization from the main store can keep pace with its utilization.

The precise mechanism of acetylcholine release is not known but once released it diffuses across the extracellular gap to the post-synaptic membrane where it combines with the receptor sites located on the outer surface of the end-plate, the highly specialized section of the membrane situated immediately opposite the nerve endings. The temporary combination of acetylcholine with the receptor evokes an electrical change; the resting potential of the end plate becomes less negative and if it reaches a "critical threshold" it becomes self reinforcing and produces an action potential on the surface of the adjacent membrane causing the muscle fibre to contract. The force of the contraction depends on the number of motor units excited.

The mechanism responsible for the end-plate potential and that causing the action potential are fundamentally different. The end-plate potential which is non-propagated is evoked by the specific action of acetylcholine on the receptor and once this has occurred, acetylcholine, which is destroyed within a few milliseconds of its release by the cholinesterase present at the end-plate has no further part to play in the subsequent muscle activity.

The action potential is brought about by an increase in membrane permeability resulting in a rapid influx of sodium ions and a loss of potassium ions across the cell membrane. In a normal resting cell the interior has a negative charge of 90 mV in relation to the outside. This resting potential of $-90$ mV is due to the imbalance of sodium and potassium ion concentrations on either side of the cell membrane and is maintained by the sodium pump with the expenditure of energy (see Nernst equation, Chapter 1, p. 277).

The resting potential is potassium dependent but excitability depends on the sodium concentration in the extracellular environment and experimentally is quickly and reversibly abolished by the withdrawal of sodium ions from the extracellular fluid. At the normal resting potential the ability of sodium to penetrate the membrane is very limited but for some reason not yet explained sodium permeability is markedly increased when the resting potential is lowered by the action of acetylcholine. As a result positively charged sodium ions flow into the muscle cells and the membrane potential falls further towards zero and eventually overshoots so that the inside of the cell becomes positive relative to the external surface of the membrane. The membrane potential difference at the crest of the action potential and the rate of ascent of the muscle spike are both directly related to the sodium concentration. It is the propagation of this process, known as depolarization, over the whole surface of the muscle membrane that elicits the muscle contraction.

The unequal distribution of ions and the maintenance of the potential difference between the interior and exterior of the cell are functions of the metabolic activity of the cell. Even in the resting cell, energy is needed to drive the mechanisms concerned with expelling sodium which has leaked into the cell and with preserving the normal partition of potassium between the inside and outside of the cell. But the main expenditure of energy occurs during the process of recovery when the depolarized membrane has to be repolarized in readiness for the next stimulus. During activity, although there is a greatly increased flow of sodium and potassium ions, this occurs in the direction of the concentration gradients and lasts for less than one millisecond; consequently very little energy is needed to effect the change in distribution. During repolarization however the situation is different; to effect the restoration of the original resting state the extrusion of sodium and the uptake of potassium ions must take place against the concentration gradient over a longer period of time. Thus a relatively large amount of energy, considerably in excess of that needed to maintain the resting state, is required to bring about recovery after depolarization.

Although the controversy about electrical or chemical transmission at the neuromuscular junction has been largely resolved in favour of a chemical mechanism there are still those who cling to a modified form of the electrical theory. However the action of curare and the action of cholinesterase inhibitors in converting a single twitch to a repetitive response after a supra-maximal stimulus is difficult to explain on such a theory. More remarkable is the fact that the arguments used previously by the protagonists of the electrical theory to refute the idea of chemical transmission have now been used to destroy the concept of electrical transmission. It was argued, for instance, that the transmission process was too rapid to be of a chemical nature; it has now been shown that the latent period between the arrival of the impulse at the motor end-plate and the initiation of the action potential is too long to be explained on an electrical basis. Similarly the presence of an electric current at the motor nerve endings at one time favoured the electrical theory but it is now known that the amount of current available is insufficient to stimulate the relatively massive fibre whose end-plate has an electrical excitability not substantially different from the rest of the fibre. Perhaps the weaknesses of the electrical theory of transmission at the neuromuscular junction were summarized most effectively by Katz (1966) when he remarked "It is clear that the structural discontinuity at this synapse renders the possibility of any electric cable transfer extremely unlikely; even if there were protoplasmic continuity, the impedances of nerve terminals and muscle fibres are so badly 'mismatched' that one can hardly conceive of a system less suitably designed for electrical transmission of signals."

Interference with neuromuscular function will occur if the release of acetylcholine at the nerve endings is inhibited, if acetylcholine already released is prevented from occupying the receptors at the motor end-plate or if the excitability of the muscle membrane in the vicinity of the motor end-plate is reduced. Experimentally, neuromuscular block has been established in each of these three ways and similar types of block have been demonstrated in clinical practice. Before discussing the different types of interference with neuromuscular transmission observed clinically some of the commoner techniques used for the investigation of neuromuscular function will be described. Assessment of neuromuscular function in the experimental animal is not difficult and many techniques have been described for this purpose.

Perhaps the most useful of the simpler methods is the rabbit head-drop test devised by Holaday for assessing the potency of new blocking agents. An aqueous solution of the substance under test is injected into a rabbit-ear vein in doses of 0·1 ml. every second until the point is reached at which the rabbit can no longer support its head. The advantages of this method are not confined to pharmacology; it could also be used in forensic practice to detect the presence of curare-like substances in body fluids.

A more elaborate rest for potency was introduced by Garcia de Jalon in 1947 who utilized the ability of the neuromuscular blocking drugs to antagonize the acetyl-choline-induced contracture of the isolated frog rectus. The rectus abdominis muscle of a frog is carefully dissected and immersed in a water-bath containing 4 ml. of aerated frog-Ringer solution. One end of the muscle is fixed to a suitable lever recording on a smoked drum. The bath is drained and re-filled with a further 4 ml. of Ringer solution containing the drug under test which is allowed to remain in contact with the muscle for a fixed period. At the end of this time a suitable dose of acetylcholine is added and the resulting contracture recorded. After one minute the recording is discontinued, the bath is emptied and the Ringer solution replaced. The cycle is then repeated. In the original method the various operations in the assay cycle were carried out by hand but this practice often led to errors. For this reason an automatic bio-assay apparatus has been devised by Boura, Mongar and Schild (1954) to control the timing of the stages of the cycle.

In addition to its use in the direct assay of curare-like preparations this method has been exploited by Kalow (1954) to study the influence of pH on ionization and biological activity of tubocurarine, by Crawford and Gardiner (1956) to determine the ability of certain neuromuscular blocking drugs to cross the human placental barrier, and by Payne and Webb (1962) to investigate the ability of serum from jaundiced patients to modify the action of neuromuscular blocking agents.

An alternative but equally effective method of investigating neuromuscular block is by means of the isolated phrenic nerve-diaphragm preparation in the rat, first described by Edith Bulbring (1946).

For a more general analysis of the pharmacology of relaxant drugs whole animal studies are required and the sciatic nerve-anterior tibialis muscle preparation in the intact cat (Brown, 1938) offers one of the more convenient methods of evaluation. The sciatic nerve is exposed through a longitudinal incision on the posterior aspect of the thigh, crushed as far proximally as possible and ligated; its medial division is treated likewise. The tendon of the anterior tibialis muscle is avulsed from its insertion and attached to a flat steel spring myograph recording on smoked paper. The stimulus is a square wave pulse of 0·5 m.sec. duration and with a strength of 1–3 volts applied at regular intervals of about 0·1 Hz. to the sciatic nerve through shielded platinum electrodes. Sometimes the soleus or gastronemius muscle is used either separately or simultaneously with the tibialis anterior muscle.

For more sophisticated analysis both surface and intra-cellular electrodes have been developed and are often used in conjunction with the electron microscope. Unfortunately the highly specialized nature of these techniques virtually places them beyond the scope of the ordinary investigator and makes them the prerogative of the neurophysiologist.

In man the assessment of neuromuscular function is sometimes handicapped by ethical considerations of risk and trauma that do not necessarily apply in the experimental animal.

Perhaps the first attempt at the quantitative assessment of neuromuscular function in man was made in 1932 by Ranyard West who endeavoured to use curare for the relief of certain spastic states. To assess the value of his treatment he devised a simple apparatus to measure the force required to extend the leg at the knee joint in a seated patient before and after the injection of curare. For this purpose a board of suitable dimensions was applied to the exterior surface of the thigh so that it overlapped the knee joint. A second board hinged to its under-surface was suspended along the anterior aspect of the leg. Extension was applied by means of a spring balance tied to the ankle. The degree of extension was determined by measuring the angle between the boards. Assessment was based on the force required to produce a given degree of extension as indicated on the balance.

Despite the pioneering efforts of a few dedicated clinicians like West, neuromuscular function remained largely of academic interest, until, during World War II, Griffiths and Johnson (1942) were persuaded to use curare to reduce the tone of abdominal muscles during surgery. This single step was to revolutionize anaesthesia once the war was over but its impact was to spread far beyond. Physiologists resurrected old interests in neuromuscular function, chemists and pharmacologists saw the possibilities of other neuromuscular blocking drugs with fewer disadvantages than the relatively crude curare preparations and the pharmaceutical industry began to concentrate many of its resources on the task of synthesizing new compounds.

The advent of neuromuscular blocking drugs saw the introduction of new techniques for their quantitative assessment and, perhaps for the first time, a general awareness of the need for precise measurement in clinical medicine.

In 1948 the use of decamethonium as a neuromuscular blocking agent was proposed by Paton and Zaimis on the basis of animal experiments and with Organe (1949) they studied the effects of this drug on ventilation and muscle tone in conscious volunteers. Almost simultaneously, in

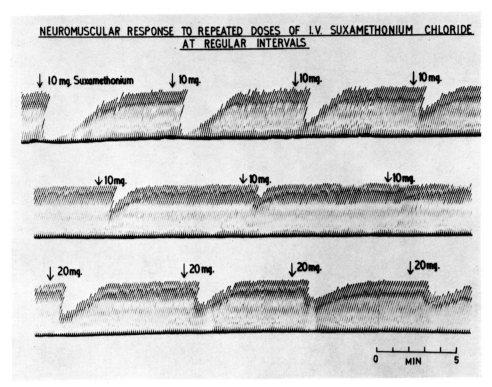

FIG. 3. Effect of repeated doses of suxamethonium. Recording the 'twitches' of two medial fingers following stimulation of ulnar nerve. (Payne and Holmdahl (1959), *Brit. J. Anaesth.*, **31**, 341.)

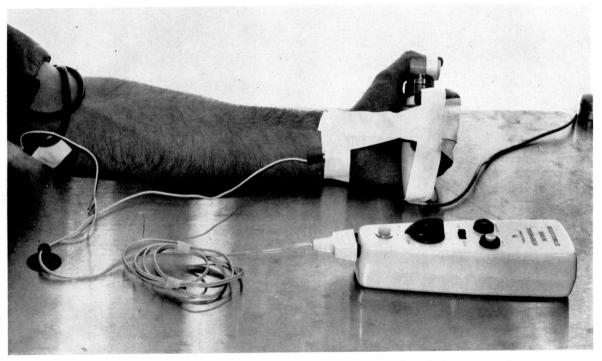

FIG. 4. Quantitative measurement of neuromuscular block using a Statham force-displacement transducer.

the first studies carried out in this country on gallamine, another new relaxant, Mushin and his colleagues (1949) used a dynamometer to measure the power to flex the fingers in volunteers before and after the intravenous injection of the drug. At the same time they measured the contractile force of the rectus abdominis muscles by means of a spring-loaded pad applied directly over the anterior abdominal wall. Three years later Bodman (1952) compared two new curarizing compounds with tubocurarine by measuring the effect of the drugs on the hand-grip of conscious volunteers. In Bodman's method the strength of the hand grip was assessed by compressing a rubber bulb filled with water and connected to a mercury manometer. The relative incompressibility of the water enabled the mercury column to be raised by a single compression whereupon a reading was taken. Intervals of two minutes were needed between compressions to avoid fatigue effects.

Such methods had the disadvantage that the evidence for interference with neuromuscular transmission was essentially presumptive; no attempt was made to correlate muscle weakness with nervous activity. In addition, these tests that depended on voluntary control could only be carried out on conscious volunteers. Thus there was a need for more precise and more specific methods of measuring neuromuscular block, both in the conscious volunteer and in the anaesthetized patient, and these were soon forthcoming. In 1955 Mapleson and Mushin described a method which involved measuring the tension developed by the contractions of the small muscles of the thumb when sub-maximal tetanic stimuli were applied to the median nerve at the wrist by means of a surface 'multiwick' electrode. Poulsen and Hougs also stimulated the median nerve when they studied the effects of some curarizing substances on conscious volunteers. Another convenient method was that employed by Payne and Holmdahl (1959) to study the effects of repeated and continuous injections of suxamethonium in anaesthetized man. For this purpose a supra-maximal stimulus, provided by a square-wave pulse of 0·5 m.sec. duration at 70–100 volts, was applied through a surface electrode placed over the ulnar nerve in the region of the elbow joint. The resultant twitches of the two medial fingers connected through a pivot to a steel spring myograph were recorded on a rotating drum (Fig. 3). A more accurate method measuring the contraction of the adductor pollicis muscle of the thumb following supra-maximal stimulation of the ulnar nerve at the elbow and wrist, has been described by Katz (1965). A development of this technique using a Statham force transducer mounted in a bicycle handle grip is illustrated in Fig. 4 (Tyrrell, 1969).

A more sophisticated and possibly more elegant technique for the analysis of neuromuscular transmission is that employed by Desmedt (1957) for the study of the transmission mechanism in myasthenic patients. After blocking the ulnar nerve at the elbow with lignocaine it was stimulated supra-maximally at the wrist twenty times per second. The electrical response of the adductor pollicis muscle elicited with belly-tendon surface electrodes was recorded on a cathode-ray oscillograph and photo-graphed together with the isometric contractions recorded with a strain-gauge myograph.

The value of electromyography in the assessment of neuromuscular transmission in man was first realized by Harvey and Masland who described its use in 1941. The technique is based on the fact that when muscle fibres contract a muscle action potential is set up, and provided that the temperature and the initial muscle tension are maintained reasonably constant, a quantitative relationship exists between the voltage of the action potential and the number of fibres stimulated. Thus, such a voltage can measure the extent of neuromuscular activity. In man any accessible nerve-muscle combination can be used, but as with mechanical recording the small muscles of the hand supplied by the ulnar nerve have proved convenient. With the arm placed in supination on a padded board and held in position by broad straps on the forearm, wrist and fingers to prevent movement, two recording electrodes are placed in position, one on the thenar eminence and the other a short distance away on the proximal phalanx of the thumb. A stimulating electrode is placed close to the ulnar nerve usually at the elbow and an earth lead more distally anywhere on the forearm. For recording concentric needle electrodes are probably the most satisfactory but occasionally if the patient is conscious, surface electrodes held in position with collodion are more suitable.

Although more convenient, spirometry offers a less satisfactory and less specific method of studying the action of neuromuscular blocking agents. A recording spirometer of the Benedict Roth type is suitable and its value is enhanced if it is used in combination with recording pneumographs (Mushin et al., 1949; Unna et al., 1950).

Spirometry presents no particular problem during anaesthesia if a closed system of administration is employed since the spirometer can be substituted for the reservoir bag of the anaesthetic circuit and records made directly. But if a Magill attachment with partial rebreathing is in use then direct records are not possible without considerable modifications of the apparatus. Satisfactory tracings however can be obtained indirectly if the reservoir bag of the Magill attachment is inserted through the neck of a sealed aspirating bottle which is connected by wide-bore tubing to the spirometer (Brennan, 1956).

With the physiological characteristics of neuromuscular function reasonably well-defined and suitable techniques of measurement available, the pharmacological approach seemed straightforward. However, as new blocking agents were developed it became clear that the apparently simple process of neuromuscular transmission was far more complex than had been anticipated.

As already indicated pharmacological interference with neuromuscular transmission can occur by inhibiting the release of acetylcholine, by preventing its combination with specific receptors at the motor end-plate, or by reducing the sensitivity of the muscle membrane to the spread of electrical excitation.

Failure of acetylcholine release at nerve endings may be due to inadequate synthesis and storage or to its defective mobilization. These processes are disturbed by the drug hemicholinium which blocks the synthesis of acetylcholine from choline, by procaine-like local anaesthetic drugs, certain antibiotics of the kanamycin or neomycin group, by botulinus toxin, or by abnormal ionic conditions such as a low concentration of calcium or a high concentration of magnesium. From the clinical aspect this type of block is relatively unimportant but the possibility exists that future neuromuscular blocking agents with this particular action will be synthesized. Interference with neuromuscular transmission by preventing the combination of acetylcholine with its receptors at the motor end-plate is the main property of the curare alkaloids. Originally these alkaloids were impure extracts that needed to be tested by biological assay but after Harold King had established the chemical structure of tubocurarine during 1935 and subsequent years, a uniformly active, pure, natural alkaloid sufficiently specific for clinical use was obtained. Tubocurarine and the more recently synthesized compounds like gallamine, alcurorium and pancuronium owe their effect to their ability to compete with acetylcholine for the receptor sites on the post-junctional membrane. Evidence for such competition has been obtained from every striated muscle in which it has been sought. The effect is envisaged as a competition between acetylcholine and tubocurarine for the receptors, and the extent to which the tubocurarine-receptor reaction suppresses the acetylcholine-receptor combination is determined by the respective ECF levels of the two compounds according to the Law of Mass Action. The higher the concentration of tubocurarine the less effective is transmission since the tubocurarine-receptor combination, unlike that of acetylcholine, does not provoke an end-plate potential; nor does it change the membrane permeability, as a result no propagated action potential is developed and the muscle remains inactive. On the same basis, however, it is possible to antagonize the action of tubocurarine and other competitive blocking agents by prolonging the action of acetylcholine or by promoting its increased secretion. In clinical practice as well as in the pharmacological laboratory the intravenous administration of an anticholinesterase such as neostigmine will prevent the hydrolysis of acetylcholine thereby allowing it to accumulate. An increase in both the potassium and the calcium ion concentration will also raise the acetylcholine level in the vicinity of the end-plate.

Tubocurarine's ability to provide muscle relaxation during surgery stimulated a search for other agents, free from its side-effects of ganglion block and histamine release. The quaternary groupings in the curare molecule had already attracted attention and the search was concentrated on the polymethylene bistrimethyl-ammonium series which incorporate within their structure the same groupings. As a result decamethonium was introduced by Barlow and Ing, and by Paton and Zaimis in 1948.

There were however fundamental differences between decamethonium and the curare drugs in their mechanism of action. Decamethonium interferes with neuromuscular transmission by reducing the sensitivity of the muscle membrane to the spread of electrical excitation. In contrast with the competitive block of tubocurarine, this type of agent causes a specific depolarization of the post-junctional membrane at the motor end-plate exactly analogous to that produced by acetylcholine. But unlike acetylcholine, which lasts only for a few thousandths of a second, the depolarization persists and spreads to the immediately adjacent regions of the muscle membrane.

If the action of acetylcholine is made to persist by the injection of a large dose into a muscle or by the administration of anticholinesterase there will follow neuromuscular block with the same characteristics as that due to decamethonium. Clinically neuromuscular block with acetylcholine is not practicable but suxamethonium, which can be regarded structurally as two molecules of acetylcholine united through their acetyl groups has become established as the most useful of the depolarizing neuromuscular blocking agents.

The main advantage of suxamethonium is its brevity of action due to its rapid destruction by the enzyme, plasma cholinesterase. If a more prolonged action is needed a continuous intravenous infusion can be used. It was soon noticed however that particularly after large doses, the action of suxamethonium could sometimes be antagonized by neostigmine and this combined with evidence that decamethonium could, with lapse of time, change its action to one resembling tubocurarine, suggested that the action of the depolarizing drugs was more complex than originally supposed.

It has long been established that depolarization block, due to the action of decamethonium, suxamethonium, or acetylcholine, is associated with a major change of permeability at the depolarized end-plate with a simultaneous efflux of potassium and a loss of the trans-membrane ionic gradient. Gradually, as the metabolic processes in the cell tend to restore the gradient, the depolarization block is ended. More recent work however has shown that if the depolarizing drugs continue to act a 'desensitization' block develops; although the ionic gradient across the membrane is re-established and the end-plate potential tends to approach its resting state the excitable membrane becomes progressively less responsive to the action of the depolarizing drugs and neuromuscular block persists. Why this should be so is not clear. This shift from depolarization block to desensitization block has also been described as a move from phase I to phase II block. Desensitization block is sometimes described as dual block. It is probable that the occurrence of progressive desensitization block after prolonged exposure to depolarizing muscle relaxants, underlies the phenomenon of tachyphylaxis (Fig. 3).

Apart from emphasizing the complexity of the neuromuscular blocking action of the so-called depolarizing drugs the introduction of suxamethonium into clinical practice also drew attention to the occurrence of inherited differences in serum cholinesterase formation. This arose when it was discovered that certain patients unduly sensitive to suxamethonium had an apparent defect in their serum cholinesterase also present in some of their otherwise normal relatives. On the basis of the dibucaine (cinchocaine) inhibition test, which measures the ability of dibucaine to inhibit serum cholinesterase activity, it was established that three genetically determined cholinesterase phenotypes exist. Dibucaine produces approximately an 80 per cent inhibition of the activity of serum cholinesterase from normal individuals, about 62 per cent inhibition in a second group amounting to 3 per cent of the population and not more than 16 per cent inhibition in a very rare third group of abnormal individuals possibly of the order of 1 in 5000 of the population.

The current theory suggests that mutation of the gene responsible for human serum cholinesterase has occurred and that now two allelic genes are distributed in the population. These in turn have given rise to the three phenotypes just mentioned. The first and third are homozygous and represent the distribution of the normal and abnormal gene respectively; the intermediate group is heterozygous and carries both genes. Only the third phenotype gives rise to serious clinical difficulties.

Undue sensitivity to relaxant-drugs is not confined to those patients given suxamethonium. Tubocurarine has also been implicated in several categories of patients. Soon after it had been introduced into clinical practice it was noticed that patients suffering from myasthenia gravis were remarkably sensitive to small doses. The etiology of the disease is still not understood but it clearly involves a disturbance of transmission at the neuromuscular junction. The distribution of muscle weakness is variable and subject to remission but it most often affects the cranial and bulbar muscles and the small muscles of the hand. Myasthenic patients respond to anticholinesterases, and neostigmine combined with atropine forms the basis for the routine treatment of the disease. Such patients are not sensitive to decamethonium or suxamethonium; they may indeed be resistant or even temporarily strengthened. This tolerance of myasthenic patients to depolarizing drugs forms the basis for the post-synaptic hypothesis of the disease process.

The balance of evidence however favours a pre-synaptic mechanism. The results obtained from electro-physiological studies on myasthenic patients indicate that during repetitive excitation the action potentials and muscle contractions gradually wane. Furthermore if a brief tetanus is applied, the muscles exhibit post-activation exhaustion in response to single test shocks at short intervals, as witnessed by a marked fall in action potential and strength of contraction after a brief period of facilitation. This pattern is unlike that seen in partially curarized muscles but is almost identical with that obtained in muscles treated with hemicholinium, which blocks neuromuscular transmission by interfering with the uptake of choline necessary for the synthesis of acetylcholine in the nerve endings. The post-activation exhaustion phenomenon is characteristic and suggests that some disturbance of the normal presynaptic mechanisms is a fundamental component of the disease.

A pattern of readily induced fatigue and muscle weakness not unlike that found in myasthenia gravis has been described in patients with malignant disease, especially of the lung. As in myasthenia gravis, these patients are markedly sensitive to tubocurarine but some have also shown sensitivity to depolarizing drugs which can be reversed by anticholinesterases, even though the anti-cholinesterases have little effect on the muscle weakness itself. This myasthenic syndrome, tends to disappear after surgical removal of the tumour much in the same way as improvement sometimes follows the removal of the thymus or thyroid gland in myasthenic patients.

Premature and new-born infants make up the remaining group of patients who are markedly sensitive to tubocurarine. On the basis of electromyographic studies it has been shown that the pattern of neuromuscular transmission is different in these infants from that in normal adults but is not unlike that in myasthenic patients. Remarkably large doses of suxamethonium are readily tolerated and block, when it occurs, is reversed by cholinesterase inhibitors.

Treatment with cholinesterase inhibitors raises its own problems which, in the case of neostigmine and the other relatively short-acting drugs, are to some extent self-limiting. When poisoning occurs it shows, in addition to the characteristic effects of parasympathetic stimulation, a depolarizing type of neuromuscular block due to the accumulation of acetylcholine. The main problem however lies with the phosphorus cholinesterase inhibitors which produce a more or less irreversible inhibition by phosphorylating the enzyme. These anticholinesterases have little or no role as therapeutic agents but they are widely used as insecticides and accidental exposure in the factory or in agricultural use may induce severe intoxication. Moreover their prolonged toxicity lends itself to exploitation in the field of chemical warfare. Surprisingly low concentrations of these phosphoryl compounds can activate the cholinesterase enzymes for many days and with the lipoid soluble agents symptoms of central nervous system involvement such as insomnia, confusion, hallucinations and paraesthesia are superimposed on the signs of cholinesterase inactivation. Those potentially dangerous are respiratory obstruction due to secretions or bronchospasm, respiratory failure from weakness of respiratory muscles and circulatory failure with hypotension and bradycardia. Except for the neuromuscular blocking effect, atropine in large doses is a good antidote and together with artificial ventilation, frequent aspiration of secretions and support for the circulation, has formed the basis of treatment. Recently more powerful antidotes such as pyridine-2 aldoxime methiodide (PAM) have been developed. Such compounds reactivate the cholinesterases and are particularly effective in relieving neuromuscular block, an effect which runs parallel with the regeneration of the serum cholinesterase.

This chapter has outlined the development of knowledge about neuromuscular transmission from the early recognition that the neuromuscular junction possesses special properties to the present recognition of the influence of such factors as drugs, disease and heredity. The overall mechanisms concerned with neuromuscular function are now reasonably well defined but there are deficiencies in our knowledge at certain levels. For example, the detailed mechanisms involved in ionic shift and acetylcholine mobilization have still to be identified though there is little doubt that with the elegant and sophisticated techniques now available their definition is only a matter of time.

# REFERENCES

Adrian, E. D. (1933), "The All-or-nothing Reaction," *Ergebn. d. Physiologie*, 35, 744.

Barlow, R. B. and Ing, H. R. (1948), "Curare-like Action of Polymethylene Bisquaternary Ammonium Salts," *Nature*, 161, 718.

Bernard, C. (1851), "Action de Curare et de la Nicotine sur le systeme Nerveux et sur le systeme Musculaire," *Compt. rend. Soc. biol.*, 2, 195.

Bodman, R. I. (1952), "Two New Curarizing Agents in Man," *Brit. J. Pharmacol.*, 7, 409.

Boura, A., Mongar, J. L. and Schild, H. O. (1954), "Improved Automatic Apparatus for Pharmacological Assays on Isolated Preparations," *Brit. J. Pharmacol.*, 9, 24.

Brennan, H. J. (1956), "Dual Action of Suxamethonium Chloride," *Brit. J. Anaesth.*, 28, 159.

Brodie, B. C. (1811), "Experiments and Observations on the Different Modes in which Death is Produced by Certain Vegetable Poisons," *Phil. Trans. Roy. Soc.*, 101, 194.

Brodie, B. C. (1812), "Further Experiments and Observations on the Action of Poisons on the Animal System," *Phil. Trans. Roy. Soc.*, 102, 205.

Brown, G. L. (1938), "Preparation of the Tibialis Anterior (Cat) for Closed Arterial Injection," *J. Physiol.*, 92, 23P.

Brown, G. L., Dale, H. H. and Feldberg, W. (1936), "Reactions of Normal Mammalian Muscle to Acetylcholine and to Eserine," *J. Physiol.*, 87, 394.

Bulbring, E. (1946), "Observations on the Isolated Phrenic Nerve Diaphragm Preparation of the Rat," *Brit. J. Pharmacol.*, 1, 38.

Crawford, J. S. and Gardiner, J. E. (1956), "Some Aspects of Obstetric Anaesthesia, Part II. The Use of Relaxant Drugs," *Brit. J. Anaesth.*, 28, 154.

Crum Brown, A. and Fraser, T. R. (1868), "On the Connection between Chemical Constitution and Physiological Action," *Trans. Roy. Soc. Edin.*, 25, 151.

Dale, H. H. (1914), "The Action of Certain Esters and Ethers of Choline and their Relation to Muscarine," *J. Pharmacol. Exp. Ther.*, 6, 147.

Dale, H. H. (1934), "Chemical Transmission of Effects of Nerve Impulses," *Brit. med. J.*, i, 835.

Dale, H. H. and Feldberg, W. (1934), "Chemical Transmission at Motor Nerve Endings in Voluntary Muscle," *J. Physiol.*, 81, 39P.

Desmedt, J. E. (1957), "Nature of the Defect of Neuromuscular Transmission in Myasthenic Patients Post Tetanic Exhaustion," *Nature*, 179, 156.

Dixon, W. E. (1905), "The Selective Action of Cocaine on Nerve Fibres," *J. Physiol.*, 32, 87.

Elliott, T. R. (1904), "On the Action of Adrenaline," *J. Physiol.*, 31, 20–21P.

Garcia de Jalon, P. (1947), "Simple Biological Assay of Curare Preparations," *Quart. J. Pharm.*, 20, 28.

Griffiths, H. R. and Johnson, G. E. (1942), "The Use of Curare in General Anaesthesia," *Anesthesiology*, 3, 418.

Harvey, A. M. and Masland, R. L. (1941), "A Method for the Study of Neuromuscular Transmission in Human Subjects," *Bull. Johns Hopk. Hosp.*, 68, 81.

Kalow, W. (1954), "The Influence of pH on the Ionization and Biological Activity of d-Tubocurarine," *J. Pharmacol.*, 110, 433.

Katz, R. L. (1965), "Comparison of Electrical and Mechanical Recording of Spontaneous and Evoked Muscle Activity," *Anesthesiology*, 26, 204.

Katz, R. L. (1966), "Neuromuscular Effects of Diethyl Ether and its Interaction with Succinylcholine and d-Tubocurarine," *Anesthesiology*, 27, 52.

King, H. (1935), "Curare Alkaloids: 1. Tubocurarine," *J. Chem. Soc.*, 1381.

Loewi, O. (1921), "Uber humorale ubertragbarkeit der herznervenwirkung," *Pflueger Arch. Ges. Physiol.*, 189, 239.

Loewi, O. (1933), "Humoral Transmission of Nervous Impulses," Harvey Lecture, 1932–1933.

McIntyre, A. R. (1947), *Curare*. Chicago, Illinois: University of Chicago Press.

Mapleson, W. W. and Mushin, W. W. (1955), "Relaxant Action in Man; Experimental Study; Results with Intravenous Gallamine Triethiodide," *Anaesthesia*, 10, 379.

Mushin, W. W., Wien, R., Mason, D. F. J. and Langston, G. T. (1949), "Curare-like Actions of tri-(Diethylamino-ethoxy) Benzene Triethyliodide," *Lancet*, i, 726.

Organe, G., Paton, W. D. M. and Zaimis, E. J. (1949), "Preliminary Trials of Bistrimethyl Ammonium Decane and Pentane Diiodide (C.10 and C.5) in Man," *Lancet*, i, 21.

Paton, W. D. M. and Zaimis, E. J. (1948), "Clinical Potentialities of Certain Bisquaternary Salts Causing Neuromuscular and Ganglionic Block," *Nature*, 162, 810.

Payne, J. P. and Holmdahl, M. (1959), "The Effect of Repeated Doses of Suxamethonium in Man," *Brit. J. Anaesth.*, 31, 341.

Payne, J. P. and Webb, Carolyn (1962), "The Effect of Serum from Jaundiced Patients on the Activity of Neuromuscular Blocking Agents," *Brit. J. Anaesth.*, 34, 863.

Poulsen, H., and Hougs, W. (1957), "The Effect of some Curarizing Drugs in Unanaesthetized Man. 1," *Acta anaesth. Scandinav.*, 1, 15.

Tyrrell, M. F. (1969), "The Measurement of the Force of Thumb Adduction," *Anesthesia*, 24, 626.

Unna, K. R., Pelikan, E. W., Macfarlane, D. W., Cazort, R. J., Sadove, M. S., Nelson, J. T. and Drucker, A. P. (1950), "Evaluation of Curarizing Drugs in Man," *J. Pharmacol.*, 98, 318.

Varney, R. F., Linegar, C. R. and Holaday, H. A. (1949), "The Assay of Curare by the Rabbit Head Drop Method," *J. Pharmacol.*, 97, 72.

West, R. (1932), "Curare in Man," *Proc. Roy. Soc. Med.*, 25, 1107.

# CHAPTER 4

# PAIN: THEORY AND MANAGEMENT

JORDAN KATZ, R. D. MILLER and R. R. JOHNSTON

## SECTION 1

### Anatomical Pathways

The approach of most anaesthetists and surgeons to the treatment of pain has been based on interruption of nervous impulses in the central or peripheral nervous system. Recent neurophysiological information of pain pathways suggests that in addition to interruption of the nervous impulse, stimulation of these same nerve fibres may result in pain relief. The following chapter traces the classical anatomical pathways of pain from the peripheral into the central nervous system and provides the foundation for discussion of current theories of pain. In addition to more established methods of pain relief the last section will discuss some of these newer treatments based on these theories of pain.

**A. Peripheral Receptors.** Pain receptors in skin, periosteum, arterial walls, and joint surfaces are usually free nerve endings. Specificity of these nerve endings has been recently elaborated upon (Iggo, 1960). However, morphologists state that the definition of a specific pain ending or receptor is far from established (Miller, 1967). Such a definition awaits further correlation between structure, function, and sensory mechanisms.

**B. Transmission and Peripheral Nerves.** Both A and C fibres transmit painful impulses to the spinal cord. The gamma and delta fibres of the A-grouping, transmit impulses at velocities from 5 to 40 metres/second, while C fibre transmission is at a rate of 0·5 to 2 metres/second. The importance of the difference in velocities and function between A and C fibres will become more apparent when the 'gate control' theory of pain is discussed. All pain fibres enter the cord via the dorsal rootlets.

**C. Transmission in the Cord** (Fig. 1). Upon entering the cord, the pain fibres may project cephalad for 1–6 segments in Lissauer's tract and, eventually anastomose with second order neurones in the posterior horns of the grey matter. The majority of second order neurones cross, via the anterior commissure of the cord, to the contralateral spinalthalamic tract where they ascend to the ventro-basal nuclei of the thalamus. When entering the cord, some large rapidly conducting A fibres send branches not only to the substantia gelatinosa, but long branches in the posterior columns directly to the dorsal column nuclei in the medulla. The second order neurones from these fibres form the medial lemniscal system which also ascends to the thalamus. Fibres carrying C-responses have been located in the fasciculus proprius bilaterally as well as in the posterior commissure (Shealy et al., 1966). Therefore, pain sensations can ascend in both lateral funiculi as well as the posterior columns.

There are other ascending pathways—the spinal reticular,

spinal mesocephalic and paleospinalthalamic tracts (the paramedial system) which arborize in areas of the reticular formation in the limbic midbrain and medial thalamic regions.

The thalamus is the main relay station in the pain pathway. It sends third order neurones to such diffuse areas as the frontal lobe, red nucleus and areas of the parietal cerebral and somatosensory cortex. This somesthetic cortex has been anatomically and physiologically divided into two areas. Area 1 appears to be primarily

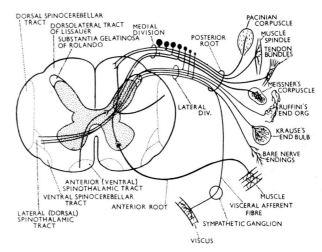

FIG. 1. Diagram showing transmission of nervous impulses from peripheral receptors to the spinal cord. (*Bonica*, 1953, p. 40.)

involved with a definite spatially represented receptor system for touch, vibratory, kinesthetic and pressure sensations (the functions of the medial lemniscal system), whereas Area II probably receives the bulk of the input originating in the spinolthalamic projections.

Additional fibres from the limbic midbrain and thalamic reticular formation find their way to the limbic forebrain structures (hippocampus and amygdala), hypothalamus and frontal cortex (Nauta, 1958). In addition to ascending transmission from the cord and integration among systems in the brain, numerous different pathways return information from the cortex and thalamus to spinal cord neurones. These pathways allow modification of the peripheral sensory input to the cord.

## SECTION 2

### Theories of Pain

The following sections will describe briefly several theories of pain, upon which most of the currently available therapies are based.

**A. The specificity theory** states that there is a progression of the painful stimulus from a specific pain receptor to a specific pain centre in the brain. The simplicity of such a concept has been attractive to clinicians and many diagnostic and therapeutic regimes are based on interrupting this neuropathway. The theory, however, is incomplete and can be challenged at many levels. For example, the existence of a specific pain receptor has never been established. As early as the turn of the century, Sherrington (1906) questioned the specificity of a pain receptor. This theory suggests that because this receptor is specific, any stimulation will elicit 'pain'. Yet certain stimuli, ordinarily non-painful, such as gentle touch, may result in severe pain in

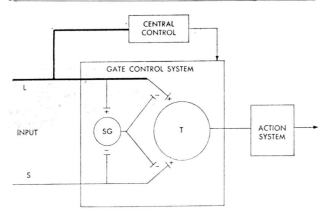

FIG. 2. Schematic diagram of the gate control theory of pain mechanisms: L, the large-diameter fibres; S, the small-diameter fibres. The fibres project to the substantia gelatinosa (SG) and first central transmission (T) cells. The inhibitory effect exerted by SG on the afferent fibre terminals is increased by activity in L fibres and decreased by activity in S fibers. The central control trigger is represented by a line running from the large-fibre system to the central control mechanisms; these mechanisms, in turn, project back to the gate control system. The T cells project to the entry cells of the action system. + = excitation; − = inhibition. (Melzack and Wall, *Science*, 1965.)

some circumstances such as occurs with herpes zoster neuralgia. Similarly, pressure, vibration, itching, and many other non-noxious stimuli can produce pain under given conditions (Livingston, 1943). Many classes of pain, i.e., phantom limb, obviously are not linked to a specific receptor. In addition, all of the neuro-destructive procedures designed to interrupt the pain pathway, have incidences of failure. Finally, pain by definition, is a subjective sensation. A 'pain centre' could not explain the vast and many times unpredictable responses that people have to apparently similar stimuli (Beecher, 1959).

**B. Central Summation.** Theories based on central summation or pattern recognition have been expounded upon ever since the late 19th century (Goldscheider, 1894). Pattern theories discard specificity of fibre endings and claim that pain results from intense stimulation of multiple receptors (Weddell, 1955). The quality of these neurone impulses, as perceived by the conscious mind, are determined by certain spatial temporal relationships.

The theories which are based on central summation tend to minimize the importance of the nature of the peripheral stimulation. Livingston (1943) proposed that intense

noxious or pathological stimuli activate internuncial pools in the spinal cord which may thus be triggered by what under ordinary circumstances would be a non-noxious impulse. The resulting neural discharges are then interpreted by the conscious brain as pain. A control system, modifying the input and thereby preventing summation from occurring has been postulated (Bishop, 1959; Noordenbos, 1959). Chronic pain is, therefore, hypothetized as occurring when the modulating system is ineffective. The combined input modification and central summation are helpful in explaining various types of pain, for example, causalgia and phantom limb.

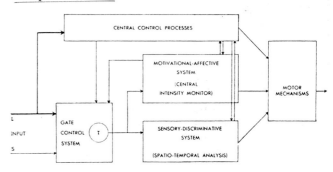

FIG. 3. Conceptual model of the sensory, motivational, and central control determinants of pain. The output of the T cells of the gate control system projects to the sensory-discriminative system (via neospinothalamic fibres) and the motivational-affective system (via the paramedial ascending system.) The central control trigger (comprising the dorsal-column and dorsolateral projection systems) is represented by a line running from the large fibre system to central control processes; these, in turn, project back to the gate control system, and to the sensory-discriminative and motivational-affective systems. All three systems interact with one another, and project to the motor system. (Casey, K. L. and Melzack, R., "Mural Mechanisms of Pain: A Conceptual Model in New Concepts in Pain and Its Clinical Management," edited by E. Leong Way, F. A. Davis, *Philadelphia*, 1967, Chap. 3, p. 18.)

**C. The gate control theory** of pain, as proposed by Melzack and Wall (1965) tries to correlate physiological and psychological data. For simplicity this theory can be considered as two mutually antagonistic systems of nerves (Figs. 2 and 3). 'Pain' results when there is an increase of small fibre relative to large fibre activation. When a critical level of discharge of small fibres is attained, the response—a complex course of events referred to as 'pain'—is activated. More specifically Melzack and Wall propose that there is a 'gate' which 'opens' and 'closes' to increase or decrease stimulation of the 'action system' —the complex process of pain. This 'gate theory' consists of three important features. First, the cells of the substantia gelatinosa (SG) in the dorsal spinal cord act as the 'gate' or modulator of information travelling in large and small fibres from the periphery to the target cells (T cells). Second, these target cells summate all input from the 'gate' in the spinal cord and information descending from the higher centres in the brain. Once a critical level is reached, the T cells stimulate the action systems. Third, as alluded to earlier, large rapidly conducting fibres entering the cord send fibres via the dorsal columns to the higher centres, which return information to the gate control system. The latter may represent impulses descending from cortex, thalamus, etc. and account for the 'psychic' influence on pain. The SG and T cells independently receive impulses from the large and small fibres (Fig. 2). Melzack and Wall believe the small myelinated fibres and unmyelinated C fibres are tonically active and account for the normal input to the 'gate'. The large and small fibres both stimulate the T cells. The cells of the SG are *stimulated* by large fibres and *inhibited* by small fibres (Fig. 2). The peripheral input to the T cells is thus a result of direct stimulation by large and small fibres, modulation by the cells of the SG and a negative or positive feedback of the large and small fibres respectively. The interrelationship among the SG, T cells and central control mechanisms determine whether the 'action system' is activated and 'pain' is felt. Melzack and Wall postulate that the gate is held 'open' by a constant firing of the tonically active C fibres. A new stimulus will increase small as well as large fibre activity, but since more larger fibres are inactive without stimulation, there will be a proportionately greater number of large fibres activated. These large fibres initially increase firing of T cells but as a result of the negative feedback, via stimulation of SG by the large fibres, the gate becomes relatively 'closed'. With prolonged stimulation, the large fibres 'adapt' and results in a relative increase in small fibre activity which rapidly increases firing of the T cells to a critical level. Again for simplicity, it can be thought that relative increases in large fibre stimulation decrease pain whereas increases in small fibre activity increase pain. By blocking small fibre activity or increasing large fibre activity, pain might be alleviated.

The 'action system' is the response of the individual to pain. Melzack and Wall emphasized that pain is not a single modality, but a process of several responses which result in involvement of the motor system, autonomic system, recall of previous experiences, etc. This complicated response ultimately results from the relationship of the transmission of the large and small fibres to the spinal cord 'gate' and the input to the gate from the higher centres. It is important to recognize these interrelationships to understand some recent advances in pain treatment (Fig. 4).

Two of the major components of the 'gate theory' have been challenged. The physiological activity of the cells of the substantia gelatinosa 'the gate cells' is unproven. Secondly, the constant activity of the small fibres has been questioned.

## SECTION 3

### Therapy

**Introductory Remarks.** Fear, anxiety, and apprehension always accompany pain and involve not only the patient but also his immediate family and friends. Unfortunately, many times the doctor reacts to the anxiety producing situation in a nonobjective way. He may either over-treat the symptom without pursuing the aetiology or, more frequently and especially in the patient with chronic

pain, he may reject the patient's complaint as functional. All too often the patient is labelled as neurotic or an over-reactor early in the course of his illness. This stigma may influence the objectiveness of future examinations.

A recent case can be used as an example. A 24-year-old male was referred with the following history: in good

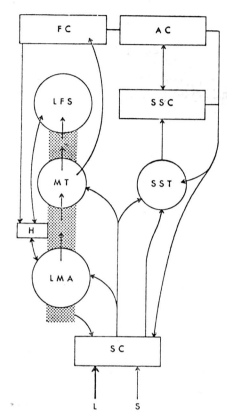

FIG. 4. Schematic diagram of the anatomical foundation of the proposed pain model. On the right: thalamic and neo-cortical structures subserving discriminative capacity. On the left: reticular and limbic systems subserving mo-tivational-affective functions. Ascending pathways from the spinal cord (SC) are: (1) the dorsal column-lemniscal and dorsolateral tracts (right ascending arrow) projecting to the somatosensory thalamus (SST) and cortex (SSC), and (2) the anterolateral pathway (left ascending arrow) to the somatosensory thalamus via the neospinothalamic tract, and to the reticular formation (strippled area), the limbic midbrain area (LMA) and medial thalamus (MT) via the paramedial ascending system. Descending path-ways to spinal cord originate in somatosensory and associated cortical areas (AC) and in the reticular forma-tion. Polysynaptic and reciprocal relationships in limbic and reticular systems are indicated. Other abbreviations: FC—frontal cortex; LFS—limbic forebrain structures (hippocampus, septum, amygdala, and associated cortex); H—hypothalamus.

general health until six months previously when working as a labourer in a sheet metal factory he developed dis-comfort in the right groin. A small inguinal hernia was detected and repaired surgically. The patient recovered uneventfully until approximately one month post surgery when the groin pain, albeit of different character, re-turned. Several visits to the surgeon did not reveal any recurrence of the hernia nor obvious reason for the pain. After visits to a neurologist, psychiatrist, and a second surgeon, it was assumed that the patient was malingering: there was some question of his not liking his job, he was receiving unemployment compensation, and his family was pampering him. The patient was sent to an anaesthetist for confirmation of the diagnosis of neurosis. A series of placebo (saline) and local anaesthetic nerve blocks elicited convincing evidence of the organic nature of the pain and a diagnosis of ilio-inguinal and/or ilio-hypogastric nerve entrapment or neuroma was made. Subsequent surgery discovered a neuroma of the ilio-inguinal nerve which was excised with lasting relief from symptoms.

Approaching the patient in pain must be done with the utmost of delicacy and compassion. The medical history should be reviewed in detail, with particular emphasis to the onset of precipitating events related to the pain. Description of the type of pain, i.e., sharp, dull ache, boring, etc., often helps in the determination of an aetiology. Care must be taken to ascertain prior diagnostic or therapeutic regimes to which the patient was exposed. Finally a complete clinical history and physical examination should be made and proper laboratory tests should be undertaken.

In the more complicated cases, a multi-disciplinary approach is often advantageous. In essence, this involves the case presentation to a panel of experts interested in the management of pain. This panel could include a neurosurgeon, neurologist, radiotherapist, psychiatrist, anaesthetist, and the referring physician. The patient's history is reviewed and the various modalities of diagnosis and therapy evaluated. Such an approach saves the patient many weeks of consultation. In addition, members of the panel are continually alerted to advances in other disciplines. Once a decision on therapy is reached, the individual physician-patient relationship is established. One cannot overemphasize the necessity of this relationship before attempting to treat the patient.

The anatomical and theoretical considerations presented are the basis for current therapeutic approaches. It is beyond the scope of this chapter to go into any one approach in detail. Some forms of treatment—drug therapy, destructive neurosurgical procedures, radiotherapy, psychotherapy and physiotherapy will not be discussed.

**A. Acute Pain.** The management of acute pain develops around the management of the basic aetiology. If the precipitating cause is known and treatable, for example incision and drainage of an abscess, the pain will go as a matter of course. Certain pathological conditions have short periods of pain associated with them (i.e., fractured ribs). Relief of pain in these situations is an end in itself. Most of the time, these acute conditions can be treated by drugs. Often, nerve blocks with local anaesthetics are effective adjuvants to therapy, especially with patients whose pain is too intense to be adequately controlled by drugs, or in whom drugs might be contra-indicated.

Several principles apply when a course of nerve blocks is contemplated for any indication.

1. Thorough knowledge of the neuroanatomy involved is essential. The possible anatomical variations in any one patient must also be borne in mind. The introduction into clinical practice of inexpensive and portable nerve stimulators with needle electrodes through which nerves can be accurately located and injected should help diminish the incidence of unsuccessful blocks.

2. Familiarity with toxic dose ranges of local anaesthetics used is necessary. One must always bear in mind that a toxic dose range is relative, depending upon the individual patient. A 70 kg. man, who may accept an injection of 500 mg. of a local anaesthetic agent when healthy, might show toxic symptoms with a much lower dose when shocked, febrile or hypovolaemic. The nerve stimulator helps in limiting the dose by accurate placement of the needle tip.

3. Be prepared to treat untoward reactions to local anaesthetics. Proper equipment for resuscitation should be immediately available. The recovery room or room adjacent to an operating suite with well trained nursing personnel may serve as optimal location to perform nerve blocks if large clinical practices are involved.

4. Use the simplest block that will give the desired results. For example, most pain associated with fractured ribs can be handled with intercostal nerve injections using the appropriate ribs as landmarks rather than resorting to paravertebral injections with their higher incidence of technical difficulties and complications.

5. Explain the procedure to the patient. For essentially all block procedures, the cooperation of the patient is necessary. If the patient has some minimal understanding of the procedure to be undertaken, he usually will assist in any way directed. Symptoms of common unwanted sequelae (i.e., a pneumothorax after an intercostal block) should be explained in general terms. The patient is instructed to keep the supervising physician aware of any onset or progression of symptoms secondary to the block. In the technically more difficult blocks, use whatever accessory equipment is needed, e.g. radiologic confirmation of needle placement, or muscle responses evoked with a nerve stimulator.

The reader is referred to the standard texts (Bonica, 1953; Moore, 1967; Adriani, 1967) for details of individual nerve block procedures.

**B. Chronic Pain.** The management of the patient with chronic pain is perhaps one of the most challenging situations with which a clinician is faced. Although pain may signal a pathologic condition, it serves no useful function and in its chronic and intractable form, a useful purpose may be a destructive disease in itself. The physician should then use the entire gamut of therapy available to stop this unnecessary suffering. Patients with chronic pain problems fall into two general categories: (1) those in whom the underlying disease, if any, is unclear, and (2) those with definitely established pathology, for example, cancer. The therapeutic approach to both groups differs.

In the patient referred with either minimal pathology or no known pathology but with complaints of constant pain, the diagnosis must be reviewed before embarking on a course of therapy. Occasionally, an underlying aetiology is uncovered and medical treatment can be instituted. In the case where the etiology is obscure, one must endeavour to determine whether the pain is organic or functional. In our clinic, a patient usually receives a random series of placebo (saline) and local anaesthetic injections. Results of these injections are quantitated by a second physician who remains unaware of the type of block. Placebo blocks are essential since pain improvement will result in a small number of patients with any treatment. Assuming that pain exists and is unmanageable by the non-narcotic analgesics or a combination of such drugs with tranquillizers, the patient undergoes a series of local anaesthetic blocks or has a block with a longer lasting agent to be discussed below. The rationale of repeated anaesthetic blocks is not easily explained by previously discussed theories. Success with repeated blocks is usually attributed to interruption of the pain 'cycle'. The pain cycle is thought to relate to the concept that initial pain produces skeletal muscle spasm, vaso-spasm, and other autonomic disturbances which then result in additional noxious stimuli to nerves. This vicious cycle may be interrupted by a series of nerve blocks and result in permanent pain relief. Clinical experience with a newer longer acting local anaesthetic bupivacaine suggested that a single nerve block may produce prolonged relief in a large percentage of patients (Hannington-Kiff, 1971). Results such as those support the concept that interruption of a 'pain cycle' is effective treatment of chronic pain. At least this approach has less inherent problems than many other drugs to be discussed and may be attempted initially.

If no permanent relief is obtained, but diagnostic blocks with local anaesthetics are successful, blocks with longer lasting agents may be indicated. Although these agents are exceedingly helpful, they may result in other more devastating problems. Thus it is incumbent upon the physician to emphasize these problems to the patient. The more common agents—alcohol, phenol, and ammonium compounds will be discussed below.

1. Ethyl alcohol, in many concentrations, has been used successfully for prolonged nerve blocks. Once in contact with the nerve, destruction of both axons and myelin sheaths occur. When using higher concentrations of alcohol (above 50 per cent), fibre size does not influence this neurolytic effect. All fibres that come into contact with the alcohol will be destroyed. Based on a review of available reports, concentrations below 50 per cent may affect only sensory fibres (Bonica, 1953). However, pathological confirmation for this is sketchy, and experimental evidence with other neurolytic agents (see below) also questions this assumption. When using the alcohol, tissue diffusion is minimal and precise location of the needle tip is necessary. The occurrence of alcohol neuritis, probably due to incomplete neurolysis, emphasizes the need for accurate needle placement.

Although many clinicians have been successful in immediately following diagnostic local anaesthetic blocks with alcohol injections, the author does not support this. When feasible, the permanent blocks should be done at a separate sitting for several reasons: (1) inability to determine displacement of the needle tip after the original injection, (2) parathesias are impossible to elicit, (3) dilution of the alcohol, and (4) since most commonly used local anaesthetics diffuse widely through the tissues, a successful diagnostic block does not equate with precise needle location.

Clinically, alcohol has been used for blocks of both the autonomic and somatic nervous system. The duration of effect has varied from days to years. In the average, however, relief can be expected from two to six months. Return of symptoms is probably due to regeneration of neural elements, and, therefore, repeated injections may be successful.

Alcohol neuritis is the most common complication of incomplete peripheral nerve blocks and occurs in approximately 28 per cent of patients (Bonica, 1953). It usually occurs in the more technically difficult nerve blocks or secondary to spillage of the agent on the somatic fibres. Most times the neuritis is mild and treatment is conservative, i.e. rest and analgesics. Alcoholic neuritis may be sever enough to warrant repeated alcohol blocks to complete the neurolysis or surgery (neurectomy or rhizotomy).

Alcohol neuritis however, is a rare sequel to intrathecal injection. One author (J.K.) has had one such case. During a mid-thoracic subarachnoid alcohol injection, a small volume of alcohol probably entered the epidural space. However, the resulting neuritis lasted for only eight hours. The major complication of sub-arachnoid injections is unwanted paresis of peripheral muscles, urinary bladder, and/or rectal sphincter. The reported incidence of these complications is under 10 per cent (Kuzucu et al., 1966). The majority of unwanted pareses decline with time. However, permanent sequelae of this type are known.

2. Phenol. Phenol probably acts similarly to alcohol. Extensive studies in our own laboratory (J.K.) and in others indicate that phenol, in concentrations as low as one per cent, destroys the nerve tissue with which it comes into contact. There is no sparing of fibres by size (Knott et al., 1968; Smith, 1964; Nathan et al., 1965). Phenol solutions of from 5–10 per cent have been used primarily to obtain long lasting sympathetic blockade and for intrathecal injections. If combined with glycerine, iodophendylate (Myodil) or like substances, the spread of the drug is limited. When used in such combinations, some authors believe a localized and profound block with less complications (compared to alcohol) will result (Mark et al., 1962). Since the phenol and glycerine mixtures are hyperbaric, the positioning of the patient for subarachnoid injections is just opposite to that of alcohol. This means that the painful side will be down, which in some cases is a disadvantage.

Excellent results have been obtained with both alcohol and phenol. The choice essentially depends on personal experience and the particular positioning problems with an individual patient. Aqueous solutions of phenol (usually 6 per cent) have been used successfully for peripheral nerve blocks. The possibility of neuritis exists here as with alcohol.

3. Ammonium sulphate. In 1931, Judovic produced relief of neuralgia-like symptoms by use of an extract from the pitcher plant. It was subsequently discovered that the ammonium ion was the active agent, and after promising clinical trials (Judovic et al., 1944) compounds

containing low concentrations of ammonium sulphate were marketed. Experience in many clinics did not substantiate the effectiveness of this compound in relieving pain and widespread use did not occur. Within the last decade reports from Scandinavia (Dam, 1965) using a mixture of 20 per cent ammonium sulphate (0·75 per cent was used in the original report) with equal volumes of mepivacaine, have been encouraging. Multiple acute and chronic conditions—cicatricial pain, neuralgia, myositis, etc.—have been treated successfully by series of injections of the mepivacaine—ammonium sulphate mixture. More recent work has suggested additional benefits for this compound. Wright *et al.* successfully treated intractible coccydynia with 15 per cent ammonium chloride producing pain relief for one month to two years in 10 of 12 patients (Wright, 1971). Most importantly no adverse sequalae resulted from this treatment. Miller *et al.* have used ten per cent ammonium sulphate in one per cent lidocaine for intercostal nerve blocks for treatment of post thoracotomy pain, herpes zoster neuralgia and costochondritis. Sixty per cent of patients received immediate relief lasting from four to twenty-four weeks (Miller *et al.*, 1973). Again no sequalae such as neuritis seen with alcohol or phenol has resulted with either ammonium sulphate or chloride. An important point with use of this compound is that patients must be told their pain may be worse for 24 to 48 hours following the injection. Again perhaps the main advantage in use of ammonium compounds rather than alcohol or phenol is the relative safety. No recent data are available on the use of ammonium sulphate intrathecally.

Since most patients with chronic pain are usually taking narcotics, it would be advantageous to decrease or eliminate their usage once pain is relieved. The following scheme has been used successfully by the author (J.K.) in many instances where high doses of narcotics have been taken prior to nerve block. The narcotic is continued at the same dosage for 24–48 hours after successful block. Dosage is halved for the next 48 hours and then substitution made with a weaker narcotic and/or a weaker narcotic-tranquillizer combination. The weaker narcotic is withdrawn over a period of days and the tranquillizer dosage is either increased or left unchanged. The patient is usually discharged with a maintenance dose of tranquillizers.

## SECTION 4

### Newer Approaches to Pain Relief

Newer therapeutic approaches to pain relief are being introduced into clinical medicine. The following section will briefly describe several of these which appear promising. The reader is referred to the references for a more complete discussion.

One of the theoretical possibilities of the 'gate theory' is that stimulation of larger diameter fibres would via the described negative feed-back mechanism, close the 'gate.' This in turn would decrease other 'painful stimuli' arising in the periphery by preventing the 'critical level' of the T cells being reached and thus removing the interpretation of 'pain'. Wall and Sweet (1967), report on attempted pain relief in eight patients by electrically stimulating the larger fibres of peripheral nerves in painful extremities. In four of the eight patients, pain relief lasted up to 30 minutes after the stimulus was discontinued. The authors explained this prolonged relief by assuming that the artificially generated large axon impulses effectively closed the gate and it took a certain period of time for the spontaneous activity in the smaller fibres to 'reopen' the gate. Additional cases have been described (Shealy *et al.*, 1967).

Using segmental and medullary recording sites to record prolonged after discharge (PSAD) as an indication of a painful response (Collins *et al.*, 1958), Shealy *et al.* (1967) stimulated the dorsal columns of the cord in cats via an implanted electrode. Normally painful stimuli (i.e. intense heat to the point of tissue damage) did not appear to disturb the animal. PSAD in the animal was eliminated.

This same concept has been successfully used to relieve pain in patients (Shealy *et al.*, 1970) (Hosabuchi, 1972). By implanting electrodes over the dorsal columns of the spinal cord, patients can stimulate their own posterior columns when pain occurs. The electrodes are connected to a radio receiver, implanted subcutaneously. It is activated transcutaneously by an external battery powered radio transmitter. Presumably, stimulation of the large fibres 'closes the gate'. By stimulation of the large fibres, small fibre input is inhibited which then prevents the response of the action system or 'pain'. A patient can then perform normal daily functions while the cord is being stimulated with electrical impulses. This technique requires a laminectomy and placement of the electrodes and radio receiver. Consequently major surgery is necessary for a procedure which is not without failure. Accordingly, Hosabuchi *et al.* (1972), advocates percutaneous dorsal column stimulation in awake patients prior to placement of the 'neuropacemaker'. He suggests that this procedure will 'educate' patients as to the sensation they may experience with stimulation and predict the efficacy of the device. These preliminary attempts to relieve pain via stimulation of large fibres should be encouraging to clinicians; at present one can only speculate as to the future of such methods of treatment.

Another method of eliminating chronic pain has been by irrigation of the subarachnoid space with either hypothermic, hyper or hypo-osmolar solutions. The rationale for this treatment is based on a differential effect of hypothermic solutions on C and A fibres (Hitchcock, 1967). Unmyelinated C fibres subserving pain were supposedly selectively interrupted since other sensations and motor functions were not lost. This explanation is questionable since conduction in larger A fibres is blocked sooner than that in C fibres during hypothermia (Lundberg, 1948). Hitchcock (1969) later obtained similar pain relief with hyperosmolar solutions (osmolarity = 3500). King and Jewett (1972), have subsequently demonstrated a differential blockade of C and A fibres with hyper and hypotonic solutions in the cat. With hypothermia they found no persistent block of C fibres and no potentiation of the block with hypertonic saline. The mechanism of the differential blockade is not proven, but may relate to changes in water content of nerve fibres exposed to nonphysiologic osmolar solutions. Because they are smaller and unmyelinated, C fibres are more susceptible to these solutions than the larger myelinated A fibres. Pain relief with placement of cold intrathecal saline may be due to increased osmolarity of the supernatant which is created by cooling normal saline in ice. Furthermore a cold saline wash alone probaly does not lower CSF temperature sufficiently to produce a conduction block (Battista, 1971).

Injection of these solutions results in pain relief of variable duration with few sequalae. Patients retain motor function and other sensations except pain. The technique is simple, but painful, and requires either spinal or general anaesthesia. Although definite mechanisms are still speculative, initial results in patients suggest that irrigation of the subarachnoid space with hyper and hypotonic solutions in the treatment of chronic pain has definite promise.

One newer and more innocuous method of pain relief is cerebrospinal fluid (CSF) barbotage. This technique involves repeated withdrawal and reinjection of CSF. Relief of chronic intractable pain from two days to three months follows. The explanation for this relief is unknown, but Lloyd et al. (1972) reported subsequent peripheral degeneration of spinal cord, possible secondary to local pressure effects on the cord. As no pain is elicited by this technique, its simplicity exceeds that of saline and water injections. Consequently it may prove to be a helpful adjunct to the treatment of intractable pain.

In summary, most available methods in the treatment of pain still involve the anatomical interruption of the pain pathways. However, new approaches based on expanding neurophysiological data are appearing.

## REFERENCES

Adriani, J. (1967), "Labat's Regional Anesthesia," *Techniques and Clinical Application*, 3rd Ed. Philadelphia: W. B. Saunders.

Battista, Arthur, F. (1971), "Subarachnoid Cold Saline Wash for Pain Relief," *Arch. of Surg.*, **103**, 672–675.

Beecher, H. K. (1959), "Measurement of Subjective Responses." New York: Oxford University Press.

Bishop, G. H. (1959), "The Relation Between Nerve Fiber Size and Sensory Modality: Phylogenetic Implications of the Afferent Innervation of the Cortex," *J. Nervous and Mental Diseases*, **128**, 89.

Bonica, J. J. (1953), "The Management of Pain." Philadelphia: Lea and Febiger.

Bonica, J. J. (1959), "Clinical Applications of Diagnostic and Therapeutic Nerve Blocks," p. 16. Springfield: Charles C. Thomas.

Collins, W. F. and Randt, C. T. (1958), "Evoked Central Nervous System Activity Relating to Peripheral Unmyelinated or 'C' Fibers in Cat," *J. Neurophysiology*, **21**, 345.

Dam, W. H. (1965), "Therapeutic Blocks," *Acta Chir. Scand.*, Suppl., **343**, 89.

Hannington-Kiff, J. G. (1971), "Treatment of Intractable Pain by Bupivacaine Nerve-Block," *Lancet*, **2**, 1392–1394.

Hay, R. C., Yonezawa, T. and Derrick, W. S. (1959), "Control of Intractable Pain in Advanced Cancer by Subarachnoid Alcohol Block," *JAMA*, **169**, 1315.

Hitchcock, E. (1967), "Hypothermic Subarachnoid Irrigation for Intractable Pain," *Lancet*, **1**; 1133.

Hitchcock, E. (1969), "Osmotic Neuralgia for Intractable Facial Pain," *Lancet*, **1**, 434–435.

Hosabuchi, Y., Adams, J. and Weinstein, P. (1972), "Preliminary Percutaneous Dorsal Column Stimulation Prior to Permanent Implantation," *J. of Neurosurg.*, **37**, 242–245.

Jewett, D. and King, J., "Conduction Block of Monkey Dorsal Rootlets by Water and Hypertonic Saline," *Lancet*, in press.

Judovic, B. and Bates, W. (1944), "Segmental Neuralgia in Painful Syndromes." Philadelphia: F. A. Davies Co.

King, J., Jewett, D. and Sundberg, H. (1972), "Differential Blockade of Cat Dorsal Root C Fibres by Various Chloride Solutions," **36**, 569–583.

Knott, L. W., Katz, J. and Rubinstein, L. J. (1968), "The Separate and Combined Effects of Phenol, Hyaluronidase and Dimethyl Sulfoxide on the Sciatic Nerve of the Rat; I. Acute Studies," *Arch. Phys. Med. Rehab.*, **49**, 100.

Kuzucu, E. Y., Derrick, W. S. and Wilber, S. A. (1966), "Control of Intractable Pain with Subarachnoid Alcohol Block," *JAMA*, **195**, 541.

Livingston, W. K. (1959), "Pain Mechanisms." New York.

Lloyd, J., Hughes, J. and Davis-Jones, G. (1972), "Relief of Severe Intractable Pain by Barbotage of Cerebrospinal Fluid," *Lancet*, **1**, 354–355.

Lundberg, A. (1948), "Potassium and the Differential Thermosensitivity of Membrane Potential: Spike and Negative after Potential in Mammalian A and C Fibers," *Acta Physiol. Scand.*, **15** (suppl. 50), 1–67.

Mark, V. H., White, J. C., Zervas, N. T., Ervin, F. R. and Richardson, E. P. (1962), "Intrathecal Use of Phenol for the Relief of Chronic Severe Pain," *New Engl. J. Med.*, **267**, 589.

Melzack, R. and Wall, P. D. (1965), "Pain Mechanisms: a New Theory," *Science*, **150**, 971.

Moore, D. C. (1967), *Regional Block*, 4th Edn. Springfield: Charles C. Thomas.

Miller, M. R. (1967), "Pain: Morphologic Aspects"; in *New Concepts in Pain and Its Clinical Management*, Chapter 2, p. 7. (E. Leong Way, Ed.). Philadelphia: F. A. Davis.

Miller, R. D. and Hosabuchi, Y. (1973), "Treatment of Intercostal Neuralgia with Ammonium Sulphate (in preparation)."

Nathan, P. W., Sears, T. A. and Smith, M. C. (1965), "Effects of Phenol Solutions on the Nerve Roots of the Cat: an Electrophysiological and Histological Study," *Neurol. Sci.*, **2**, 7.

Nauta, W. J. H. (1958), "Hippocampal Projections and Related Neural Pathways to the Midbrain in the Cat," *Brain*, **81**, 319.

Noordenbos, W. (1959), *Pain*. Amsterdam: Elsevier.

Shealy, C. N., Tyner, C. F. and Taslitz, N. (1966), "Physiological Evidence of Bilateral Spinal Projections of Pain Fibers in Cats and Monkeys," *J. Neurosurg.*, **24**, 708.

Shealy, C. N., Taslitz, N., Mortimer, J. T. and Becker, D. P. (1967), "Electrical Inhibition of Pain: Experimental Evaluation," *Anes. Analg. Current Res.*, **46**, 299.

Shealy, C. N., Mortimer, J. T. and Reswick, J. B. (1967), "Electrical Inhibition of Pain by Stimulation of the Dorsal Columns." Preliminary Clinical Report, *Anes. Analg. Current Res.*, **46**, 489.

Shealy, C. N., Mortimer, J. T. and Hogfors, N. R. (1970), "Dorsal Column Electroanalgesia," *J. Neurosurg.*, **32**, 560–564.

Sherrington, C. S. (1906), *The Integrative Actions of the Central Nervous System*. London: Constable.

Smith, M. C. (1964), "Histologic Findings Following Intrathecal Injections of Phenol Solutions for Relief of Pain," *Brit. J. Anaesth.*, **36**, 387.

Wall, P. D. and Sweet, W. H. (1967), "Temporary Abolition of Pain in Man," *Science*, **155**, 108.

Weddell, G. (1955), "Somesthesis and the Chemical Senses," *Ann. Rev. Psychol.*, **6**, 119.

Wright, B. D. (1971), "Treatment of Intractable Coccydynia by Transsacral Ammonium Chloride Injection," *Cur. res. Anaes. and Anal.*, **50**, 519–525.

*CHAPTER 5*

# ANAESTHESIA AND ENDOCRINE SECRETION

## R. A. MILLAR

Increased endocrine activity in relation to anaesthesia and surgery is commonly regarded as a manifestation of 'stress', which like 'shock' is a term used freely, but often without accurate definition. Physical stress appears to imply either that physiological responses are stretched toward their limits (as in exercise) or that abnormal stimuli have been imposed (as during anaesthesia and surgery). At present these two arbitrary categories can seldom be separated, and the crucial question as to whether, or when a functional response assumes pathological implications has not been answered adequately; this also applies to psychological factors. Such aspects will not be discussed here, the term stress will be avoided where possible, and an attempt will be made to survey the changes in endocrine secretion reported to have a direct relation to anaesthetic agents.

## MEASUREMENT

A historical feature in the development of improved methods of measurement of hormones in body fluids, particularly plasma, is that normal levels become progressively lower as the sensitivity and specificity of techniques increase. At present, several methods approach their limits of sensitivity at a plasma concentration currently acknowledged to be normal; while it is justifiable to accept increases in concentration above this level, scepticism should be shown toward reported reductions below normal. Also, some plasma hormone determinations do not distinguish unbound (active) from protein-bound (inactive) portions, and provide no information on tissue utilization, conjugation or on re-uptake after release (of catecholamines by sympathetic nerves, for example). There may be daily variation in the circulating level of endocrines, as shown by plasma corticosteroids, which are highest in the morning and may fall by as much as 75 per cent by late evening; such variations may be partially disrupted not only by endocrine pathology but also in certain psychiatric conditions, cardiovascular disease, and other medical illness (Doig *et al.*, 1966; Knapp, Keane and Wright, 1967; Connolly and Wills, 1967; Jacobs and Nabarro, 1969). Plasma corticosteroid levels may also be lower in infancy, and altered during pregnancy and in women taking oral contraceptives. These, and perhaps many other currently unknown factors, may influence the accurate assessment of hormonal function in relation to anaesthesia and surgery.

It is worth emphasis, also, that the number of well controlled studies in the field of anaesthesia and endocrine secretion is small, that many publications have emanated from too few sources, and that in some instances the confirmation required to ease the reviewer's task is lacking.

### Plasma Catecholamines

Prior to about 1956, the differential estimation of plasma noradrenaline and adrenaline could be accomplished by paper chromatography and bioassay, successful use of which was highly restricted (Holzbauer and Vogt, 1954). Over many preceding years, chemical techniques had been showing a steady slow improvement in specificity and sensitivity, yet the results obtained were often dubious. The introduction of the trihydroxyindole method was a significant advance (Euler and Floding, 1955); various modifications of these fluorimetric techniques have been described (Vendsalu, 1960), although they remain specialized research tools which require critical attention if reliable measurements on peripheral plasma are to be obtained (Callingham, 1972). Since 1955, however, investigations relating the cardiovascular actions of individual anaesthetics to their effects on sympathoadrenal activity have been based on the apparently successful measurement of plasma adrenaline and noradrenaline in the dog and man.

Recently, attention has been focussed on factors which could affect the accuracy of plasma catecholamine measurements (Carruthers *et al.*, 1970).

### Adrenocortical Hormones

Assessment of adrenocortical function has been attempted by a variety of methods, some of which, such as the measurement of circulating eosinophils or the determination of urinary 17-oxosteroids (17-ketosteroids) are insufficiently specific. The interested reader is referred to reviews by Prunty (1967) and James and Landon (1968). In relation to anaesthesia and surgery, the most common measurement has been that of 'plasma 17-hydroxycorticosteroids' (17OHCS) by the methods of Silber and Porter (1957), or Mattingly (1962); these measure mainly plasma cortisol, together with small amounts of 11-deoxycortisol or of corticosterone respectively. Prunty (1967) notes that 'the nomenclature of these methods for determining plasma steroids is not satisfactorily settled', but favours the fluorescence method of Mattingly, defining the values as 'plasma corticosteroids', with normal levels averaging 14·7 $\mu$g./100 ml. He makes the additional relevant comment: 'The interpretation of plasma 17-hydroxycorticosteroids and of plasma corticosteroids needs to be made with caution. They give information only at a specific moment of time, and are particularly liable to be elevated in agitated subjects. . . . It is now common knowledge that adrenocortical activity is increased, sometimes to a surprising degree, in agitated patients and those subjected to general anaesthesia and surgery.'

Radiochemical techniques have recently been used to separate free and protein-bound cortisol in plasma (Hamanaka *et al.*, 1970).

## ACTH

Measurements of ACTH during anaesthesia in man have been reported (Oyama *et al.*, 1968b) using a bioassay method in which the adrenal output of corticosterone in response to ACTH in hypophysectomized rats is measured fluorimetrically (Lipscomb and Nelson, 1962). Radio-immunoassay techniques have also been employed (Newsome and Rose, 1971).

### Thyroid Hormone

The effects on thyroid function of surgery, and more rarely of anaesthesia, have been assessed from changes in the circulating level of total and protein-bound iodine (indicative of altered thyroxine output by the gland), following oral or intravenous administration of anaesthetic drugs (Greene and Goldenberg, 1959; Johnston, 1964; Oyama *et al.*, 1969c, d).

### Preanaesthetic Measurements

While it is to be expected, according to the 'fight or flight' concept of Cannon (1929), that plasma adrenaline or noradrenaline concentrations would be raised in a proportion of patients awaiting surgery, this has not been demonstrated; in part, this is because the resting levels lie close to or below the current level of detection. Euler (1964) has discussed the quantitative measurement of 'stress' by means of catecholamine analysis; the available evidence from urinary excretion suggests that changes in arterial pressure or body posture are associated with a raised output of noradrenaline, whereas the adrenaline secretion is more closely related to emotional disturbances. In a recent investigation, only 4 of 30 patients studied were shown to have an increased urinary catecholamine output in the preoperative period (Martinez, Euler and Norlander, 1966). Such findings suggest that there is less apprehension in most surgical patients than, for example, in aircraft flying (Euler and Lundberg, 1954), paratroop training (Bloom, Euler and Frankenhauser, 1963), or simulated space flight (Ulvedal, Smith and Welch, 1963).

As indicated by the comment by Prunty (1967) quoted above, most experienced investigators of adrenocortical function consider emotional stress to be a powerful stimulus to cortical secretion. Some years ago, it was deduced from measurements made before and after college boat races, long-distance running, and in students presenting clinical cases or theses, that psychological factors were more important in causing adrenocortical stimulation than was muscular work in trained persons (Hill *et al.*, 1956; *Lancet*, 1956; Euler *et al.*, 1959). In accord with other stressful situations (Hetzel *et al.*, 1955), there are data which may suggest an increase in adrenocortical activity in preoperative surgical and dental patients (Franksson and Gemzell, 1955; Price, Thaler and Mason, 1957; Han and Brown, 1961; Shannon, Isbell and Szmyd, 1963). These findings

were variable, were obtained in a variety of environments, and were not confirmed when plasma corticosteroids were measured in specific relation to anaesthesia (Virtue, Helmreich and Gainza, 1957; Hammond *et al.*, 1958). Indeed, Vandam and Moore (1960) concluded that 'preoperative anxiety is not a major stimulus to adrenal cortical secretion'. However, the information may rather suggest (in accord with current clinical observation) that only a minority of surgical patients show marked anxiety preoperatively. In one study prior to herniorrhaphy, plasma corticosteroids were increased in proportion to the waiting period before operation (Bursten and Russ, 1965). Other workers have described raised levels in non-surgical patients in the first few days after admission to hospital, this being more marked in obviously anxious individuals (Friedman, 1965). Unpremedicated patients awaiting spinal analgesia have also shown raised plasma cortisol levels (Oyama and Matsuki, 1970a).

In a recent investigation on healthy volunteers, Utting and Whitford (1972) established convincingly that plasma cortisol (at 8.00 a.m.) was significantly increased after moderate sleep deprivation on the previous night. This finding, and factors such as the normal diurnal variation, emphasize the degree of precision required if the relatively small changes in endocrine secretion induced by some drugs are to be defined with accuracy.

It has been claimed that suggestions of fear to hypnotized subjects can elevate plasma corticosteroid concentrations (Persky *et al.*, 1956; Black and Friedman, 1965), and that hypnotic suggestion can limit the adrenocortical response provoked by ischaemic pain (Black and Friedman, 1968).

### Preanaesthetic Medication

The influence of premedication on the circulating levels of hormones, and in modifying the endocrine responses to anaesthesia and surgery, is difficult to assess from published data.

No alteration in urinary catecholamine excretion was detected after the administration of morphine, hyoscine, pentobarbitone, or atropine to preoperative patients (Martinez, Euler and Norlander, 1966).

Plasma corticosteroid levels may be lowered as a result of sedation, for example with pentobarbitone (Siker, Lipschitz and Klein, 1956). But in other investigations applied more specifically to surgical patients such effects were not obvious; for example, in the study of Hammond *et al.* (1958), 'normal' plasma measurements were reported in all but one of 29 patients premedicated with barbiturates and atropine or hyoscine, with or without opiates. No effect of premedicant drugs could be isolated in another, more complicated, situation (Nishioka, Levy and Dobkin, 1968). In 1960, Vandam and Moore commented as follows: 'In general it seems safe to conclude that the role of small quantities of preanaesthetic medication is not a very significant one in the assessment of the adrenal cortical response to anaesthesia'. This opinion now seems to require modification.

Oyama *et al.* (1968c) compared plasma corticosteroid levels in the same patients before and after premedication with pentobarbitone 50–100 mg., pethidine 35 mg. and atropine 0·5 mg. and showed a significant reduction from an average of 18·2 μg./100 ml. to a level of 14·0 μg./ml. after drug administration. This was confirmed in another study by the same workers (Oyama *et al.*, 1968d), and by others (Plumpton, Besser and Cole, 1969a).

Morphine was found to reduce plasma ACTH concentration in healthy human subjects, provided that nausea did not occur (this produced elevated levels), although it did not prevent adrenocortical responsiveness to ACTH (McDonald *et al.*, 1959), or presumably to surgical trauma. The investigators mentioned above (Oyama *et al.*, 1968b), using the same premedication, considered that the plasma ACTH levels after drug administration were normal, in confirmation perhaps of a previous report in which details of the drugs used were not given (Cooper and Nelson, 1962). Orally administered pentobarbitone, diazepam or nitrazepam were found to reduce preoperative rises in plasma cortisol (Oyama *et al.*, 1969a, b). However, the levels after intramuscular pethidine alone (in large doses of 2 mg./kg.) were significantly above those measured without medication at the same time on the previous day (Oyama *et al.*, 1969e). By comparison, the use of smaller doses of pethidine, with droperidol, for neuroleptanaesthesia, did not significantly increase plasma cortisol (Oyama and Takiguchi, 1970b).

## ANAESTHETIC AGENTS

### Intravenous Barbiturates

Significant changes in plasma adrenaline or noradrenaline concentrations have not been shown to accompany administration of intravenous thiopentone in man (Price *et al.*, 1959), while induction doses in the dog have neither raised the circulating levels nor prevented subsequent increases caused by other anaesthetic agents, or by haemorrhage or hypercarbia (Millar, 1960; Millar and Morris, 1960, 1961a, b). Nevertheless, both thiopentone and pentobarbitone can be readily shown to reduce preganglionic sympathetic discharge when this is recorded directly in animals (Millar *et al.*, 1970); the effect is sufficiently dramatic to suggest that failure to demonstrate changes in plasma catecholamines may result from insensitive assay methods or from variations in response to a given dose in different species.

The evidence available also fails to show any marked effect of intravenous thiopentone on plasma corticosteroid concentration in man (Virtue, Helmreich and Gainza, 1957; Hammond *et al.*, 1958; Oyama *et al.*, 1969c). This has been supported by more direct measurement on adrenal venous plasma in man (Hume and Bell, 1958) and in the dog given pentobarbitone (Hume, 1958). Although it was suggested that pentobarbitone decreases ACTH secretion in the rat (Royce and Sayers, 1958) and that barbiturates can reduce the adrenocortical responses to 'stress' (Ronzoni, 1950) and to hypothermia (Ganong, Bernhard and McMurrey, 1955; Kaada, Setekleiv and Skang, 1959), the many measurements of plasma corticosteroids made in surgical patients do not indicate that barbiturates in clinical dosage suppress the adrenocortical

response to surgery (Brunt and Ganong, 1963). Anaesthetic techniques involving thiopentone and nitrous oxide have not been shown to evoke any rise in the peripheral plasma levels (Virtue, Helmreich and Gainza, 1957; Hammond *et al.*, 1958; Oyama *et al.*, 1969c). This also applies to propanidid (Oyama *et al.*, 1970), whereas plasma cortisol was found to increase significantly after intravenous injection of ketamine (Oyama, Matsumoto and Kudo, 1970) and of gamma-hydroxybutyrate. None of these intravenous anaesthetics suppresses the endocrine response to surgical stimuli.

In one report serum thyroxine did not change significantly after thiopentone administration (Oyama *et al.*, 1969c); however, modification of the method of measurement has now suggested that serum thyroxine levels are lowered during thiopentone, nitrous oxide, tubocurarine anaesthesia (Oyama *et al.*, 1969d).

### Diethyl Ether

As previously indicated by much indirect evidence (see Price, 1960), the concentration of plasma catecholamines is increased during ether anaesthesia in man (Price *et al.*, 1959; Millar and Morris, 1961b). While agreement continues that plasma noradrenaline is mainly involved (Black *et al.*, 1969), significant increases in adrenaline were also measured in man by one group of workers (Millar and Morris, 1961b); during surgery, adrenaline was further raised without much more change in plasma noradrenaline  It was shown that bilateral adrenalectomy abolished the pronounced rise in plasma adrenaline evoked by ether in intact dogs, leaving a more erratic elevation in noradrenaline; removal of the adrenal medullary response also reduced the pronounced metabolic acidosis caused by ether in intact dogs. Thus, extra-adrenal sources of noradrenaline are in part contributing to the elevated plasma levels during ether anaesthesia, and their contribution probably becomes greater at high $PaCO_2$. When arterial pressure was lowered by haemorrhage during ether anaesthesia, also in the dog, there was a prompt rise in plasma adrenaline (Millar and Morris, 1961b).

The investigations described seem to suggest a catecholamine response to ether which is predominantly adrenal in the dog (Hume, 1958) and extra-adrenal in man; but it remains curious if sympathetic stimulation sufficient to release measurable amounts of noradrenaline from postganglionic nerve endings in man is without influence on the adrenal medulla.

Ether administration is associated with pronounced adrenocortical stimulation, and is used as a standard 'stress' in small animals by laboratory workers. In view of the overall consistency of the published data (Virtue, Helmreich and Gainza, 1957; Hammond *et al.*, 1958; Suzuki, Yamashita and Mitamura, 1959; Greene and Goldenberg, 1959; Oyama *et al.*, 1968b, 1969c), an increase in plasma corticosteroids can be accepted as a feature of ether anaesthesia in man. Early studies assumed that this was probably attributable to increased ACTH liberation; this one factor has now been confirmed (Oyama *et al.*, 1968b), the intermittent release of large amounts of ACTH being associated with a more gradual rise in plasma corticosteroids, which were restored two hours after terminating anaesthesia. There is some evidence to suggest that diethyl ether raises the serum thyroxine level (Oyama *et al.*, 1969c, d; this effect persisted for at least 24 hours, and was considered to be hepatic in origin (Oyama, Shibata and Matsuki, 1969).

### Cyclopropane

Plasma noradrenaline (not adrenaline) was reported to increase during cyclopropane anaesthesia in man, at normal $PaCO_2$ (Price *et al.*, 1959). Similar, if more erratic, results were obtained in another less well controlled clinical study (Millar and Morris, 1961b), in which rises in total catecholamines (adrenaline + noradrenaline) were measured in association with cyclopropane anaesthesia and surgery. Since the noradrenaline response occurred in adrenalectomized patients, and was abolished in one subject by high spinal anaesthesia, apparently it represented release from sympathetic nerves or other extra-adrenal areas (Price *et al.*, 1959).

However, it was reported later that in the dog the major response to cyclopropane involved adrenaline (Price *et al.*, 1963); and in other experiments on this species no increase in plasma noradrenaline was measured during ventilation with cyclopropane, the circulating adrenaline concentration being increased to a small although significant degree (Millar and Morris, 1961b). In the latter study acute respiratory acidosis caused pronounced elevations in both catecholamines during cyclopropane administration, and in man hypercarbia raised plasma noradrenaline to a greater extent in the presence of cyclopropane than in the conscious state (Price *et al.*, 1960).

These findings suggest that cyclopropane causes pronounced sympathetic activation which may be discrete or widespread. Direct recording of preganglionic sympathetic discharge in the rabbit and cat leaves no doubt that excitation of 'central' sympathetic neurones is a feature of cyclopropane anaesthesia (Millar and Biscoe, 1965; Price *et al.*, 1969). It remains unexplained, however (and requires further confirmation), why noradrenaline rather than adrenaline might be predominantly released in man, while the reverse may occur in at least one other species.

Increases in plasma corticosteroids occurred in one human volunteer anaesthetized without surgery (Hammond *et al.*, 1958); a similar effect was thought to occur during surgery in patients anaesthetized with this agent (Sandberg *et al.*, 1954). In another investigation, no changes were established during cyclopropane administration, but in this series the actions of ether also seemed erratic (Virtue, Helmreich and Gainza, 1957). Thus, there are insufficient measurements to permit a definite conclusion, although most reviewers consider that cyclopropane resembles diethyl ether in elevating plasma corticosteroids (Vandam and Moore, 1960; Brunt and Ganong, 1963).

Many studies have been directed toward the assessment of the functional importance of sympathetic activation in opposing cardiovascular depression by general anaesthetics,

exemplified by the investigations applied to dogs given diethyl ether by Brewster, Isaacs and Wainø-Andersen (1953) and the many measurements during cyclopropane anaesthesia in man by Price and co-workers (*see* Price, 1960, 1967). The question still awaits a definite answer, although it seems an unlikely possibility that increased plasma hormone concentrations reflect a physiologically purposeful attempt to counteract, quantitatively, direct cardiovascular end-organ depression by general anaesthetics.

### Halothane

No increases in plasma noradrenaline or adrenaline have been reported during halothane administration at normal or reduced $PaCO_2$ and in the absence of surgery. The data, obtained both in the dog (Millar and Morris, 1960) and in man (Price *et al.*, 1959; Millar and Morris, 1961b) do not exclude the possibility that small increases or reductions in circulating catecholamine concentrations may occur, since the 'normal' levels already extend the sensitivity of these methods to their limit. Small increases in plasma adrenaline, of statistical significance, were measured during surgery in patients anaesthetized with halothane (Millar and Morris, 1961b).

Since arterial hypotension is a frequent accompaniment to its use, it has been the common clinical impression that halothane should exert a blocking action on central autonomic function (Price, Linde and Morse, 1963). However, marked rises in plasma catecholamine levels were measured in dogs ventilated with 2 per cent halothane and subjected to hypercarbia or haemorrhage (Millar and Morris, 1960). In man, also, the average increase in plasma noradrenaline and adrenaline in response to elevated $PaCO_2$ during halothane administration, although below that measured in the presence of cyclopropane, was at least as high as that detected in the conscious state (Price *et al.*, 1960). In addition, preganglionic nerve recording indicates that the arterial hypotension evoked by halothane is not primarily dependent on suppression of efferent sympathetic activity (Millar and Biscoe, 1965, Millar *et al.*, 1969).

The small variations in sympathetic activity recorded when 70 per cent nitrous oxide is substituted for nitrogen in laboratory animals (Millar and Biscoe, unpublished observations) suggest that nitrous oxide is unlikely to cause measurable changes in circulating catecholamines. On the other hand, with a background anaesthetic of chloralose in cats, preganglionic sympathetic discharge usually increased when nitrous oxide replaced nitrogen during concurrent administration of halothane or other volatile agents (Millar *et al.*, 1969, 1970), while it was reported that plasma noradrenaline was raised by the addition of nitrous oxide to halothane (Smith *et al.*, 1970).

Information on the effect of halothane on adrenocortical function also is less than definitive. Oyama *et al.* (1968c) have recently studied plasma corticosteroid levels before and during administration of 0·5–1·0 per cent halothane concentrations in 50 per cent nitrous oxide/oxygen to premedicated patients in whom the control levels averaged 14·0 $\mu$g./100 ml. Very small, statistically insignificant rises were measured after 15 minutes of halothane following induction with thiopentone. When thiopentone was omitted, however, there were significant increases averaging 6·7 $\mu$g./100 ml. after 30 minutes of halothane administration. During surgery, plasma corticosteroids increased further to about 27·0 $\mu$g./100 ml. and the levels were even higher in the early postoperative period. It is just possible that these findings may have been influenced by intermittent succinylcholine injections. Previously, small and statistically insignificant rises had been described during halothane anaesthesia preceded by thiopentone and d-tubocurarine injections (Lewis, 1963), while urinary estimations suggested that the adrenocortical response to surgery was not suppressed by this anaesthetic (Stark, 1966). A recent report (Nishioka, Levy and Dobkin, 1968), that the increase in plasma corticosteroids in response to injection of a synthetic (ACTH-like) adrenocortical stimulant was reduced during halothane anaesthesia, awaits further confirmation. At present, there is no convincing evidence that the adrenocortical response to surgical trauma is depressed by halothane. It has been suggested that serum thyroxine levels are increased during halothane administration without surgery (Oyama et al., 1969d).

### Methoxyflurane

No change in plasma adrenaline or noradrenaline levels was measured when dogs were ventilated with methoxyflurane at normal $PaCO_2$ (Millar and Morris, 1961a), but recent work has reported that this anaesthetic reduced adrenal venous catecholamine concentration without changing the peripheral plasma level (Li, Shaul and Etsten, 1968). If this finding is difficult to assess in the absence of adrenal blood flow measurements, it may underline the various inadequacies of peripheral plasma determinations discussed earlier. Erratic, statistically insignificant changes in plasma corticosteroids were measured after 30 minutes of methoxyflurane anaesthesia in man, whereas there were abrupt elevations within 5 minutes of surgical incision (Oyama et al., 1968d).

Small but significant reductions in plasma cortisol have been described after 30 minutes administration of the halogenated ether, enflurane (Oyama, Matsuki and Kudo, 1972).

### Spinal Analgesia

Provided a sufficiently high level is achieved, spinal analgesia presumably abolishes catecholamine responses to general anaesthetic agents, as suggested in the case of cyclopropane (Price et al., 1959).

No detectable effect on adrenocortical secretion of injection of local analgesic has been reported in a very limited study (Hammond et al., 1958). Adequate spinal or epidural analgesia has been found to prevent the adrenocortical response to surgery, but only while blockade lasts (Virtue, Helmreich and Gainza, 1957; Hammond et al., 1958; Hume and Bell, 1958; Moore, 1959). In paraplegic patients, also, it has been said that the adrenocortical response to trauma is delayed or reduced (Hume, Bell and

Bartter, 1962). Johnston (1964), however, described brisk elevations in plasma corticosteroids during inguinal herniorrhaphy under spinal analgesia, and considered the responses no different from those to surgery under general anaesthesia.

It is of interest also that in three patients with complete spinal cord transections at C 6–7, in whom no anaesthesia was needed for superficial surgery, a substantial adrenocortical response was measured (Osborn et al., 1962). Such evidence may suggest that adrenocortical activation could occur neurogenically at spinal cord level. The most recent data infer that spinal analgesia for lower abdominal operations limits, but does not necessarily abolish, adrenocortical activation during surgery; however, the patients were unpremedicated, and showed varying degrees of preoperative arousal (Oyama and Matsuki, 1970a). The findings were similar in patients undergoing Caesarian section (Matsuki and Oyama, 1972).

There may be some change in thyroid function during surgery under spinal anaesthesia (Greene and Goldenberg, 1959; Oyama and Matsuki, 1971).

### OTHER INFLUENCES

#### Hypothermia

There is probably an increased production and secretion of catecholamines in response to cold; in animals, this may involve mainly noradrenaline from adrenergic nerves and adrenaline from the adrenal medulla (see Leduc, 1961). Contrary to such enhanced sympathetic responses, a depressant effect of hypothermia on adrenocortical function was suggested by Khalil (1954), and was supported in man by measurement of plasma and urinary corticosteroids (Bernhard et al., 1956; Swan, Jenkins and Helmreich, 1957); there was no further change in the levels during surgical operation. In adrenal venous plasma of the dog (Egdahl, Nelson and Hume, 1955) hypothermia was associated with a reduced corticosteroid output, which persisted when ACTH was infused; however, adrenal blood flow was also greatly reduced.

Similar findings in one patient (Hume and Bell, 1958) may confirm that there is a decline in synthesis of adrenal cortical hormones, a failure to respond maximally to ACTH, and a decreased metabolism of corticosteroids (Hume and Egdahl, 1959a). The findings are not consistent, however, as shown by one report in which unchanged corticosteroid levels in peripheral blood were measured during prolonged hypothermia and the response to ACTH was maintained (Barlow, Spurr and Bowe, 1959). Also, from measurements of urinary 17-ketosteroid excretion in dogs cooled to 26 °C for 72 hours it was deduced that adrenocortical output during hypothermia (pentobarbitone anaesthesia but no surgery) was near normal, but that enormous increases in steroid excretion occurred during rewarming (Macphee, Gray and Davies, 1958).

#### Hypotension and Haemorrhage

In the dog, haemorrhagic hypotension raises plasma adrenaline (Millar and Benfey, 1958), while hypovolaemia, with or without arterial hypotension, increases plasma corticosteroid levels (Gann and Egdahl, 1965). The adrenocortical responses also accompany hypotension due to trimetaphan or hexamethonium, possible mechanisms of action having been discussed in relation to peripheral receptors and the renin-angiotensin system (Gann and Egdahl, 1965).

### Carbon Dioxide and pH

There is ample evidence from animal experiments that plasma catecholamines increase in proportion to acute rises in arterial $P_{CO_2}$ (Morris and Millar, 1962a), while a similar if not identical response to non-respiratory acidaemia (Morris and Millar, 1962b) appears to be confirmed by recent work (Nahas *et al.*, 1967). It has also been noted that the sympathetic neurohumoral response to hypercarbia remains pronounced in the presence of general anaesthetics such as thiopentone, cyclopropane, diethyl ether, halothane and methoxyflurane (Millar and Morris, 1960, 1961a, b). Carbon dioxide also increases adrenocortical activity in experimental animals, apparently largely due to pituitary activation (*see* Tenney, 1960); pH change may also be important (Richards, 1957). In conscious human subjects, plasma adrenaline, noradrenaline, and corticosteroids increased during inspiration of 7–14 per cent $CO_2$ (Sechzer *et al.*, 1960).

The somewhat gross acute disturbances in $PaCO_2$ and pH induced by most animal investigators leave little doubt that the endocrine changes evoked by the central nervous and local systemic actions of acidaemia are complex and widespread; similarly diffuse effects of acute hypoxaemia and asphyxia are to be expected. It is in the assessment of less pronounced disturbances and their physiological compensation that evidence is more scanty. Recent laboratory experiments have suggested that an initial rise in plasma corticosteroids, catecholamines, and free fatty acids may subside as compensation to chronic hypercarbia occurs (Schaefer, McCabe and Withers, 1968).

### Antidiuretic Hormone

The reduction in urine volume long known to be associated with ether anaesthesia (Pringle, Maunsell and Pringle, 1905) suggested the possibility of ADH liberation by certain inhalation anaesthetics. Such an action by ether was deduced indirectly by several investigators (*see* Rothballer, 1956). There is also indirect evidence of ADH secretion in response to afferent stimuli and to the administration of various drugs including anaesthetics (Dudley *et al.*, 1954). Other factors to be considered may include pain, emotion, haemorrhage, and continuous positive pressure breathing (*see* Deutsch, Goldberg and Dripps, 1966); while a raised inspired $P_{CO_2}$ was said to inhibit ADH release (Barbour *et al.*, 1953; Valtin, Wilson and Tenney, 1959), the opposite conclusion was drawn from recent experiments (Philbin, Baratz and Patterson, 1970).

Antidiuretic hormone has been assayed directly in blood withdrawn from patients before, during and after various major surgical procedures (Moran *et al.*, 1964). Many

individuals showed slightly raised preoperative levels, possibly related to overnight fluid restriction especially if accompanied by gastric suction. Such elevations could be lowered by fluid administration following induction of anaesthesia with halothane, methoxyflurane, nitrous oxide, or thiopentone.

The ADH level was increased only slightly by anaesthesia alone, and to a small extent by skin incision, the latter effect being blocked by regional analgesia. Pronounced elevations occurred in association with visceral traction in the abdomen; these subsided during intestinal anastomosis but increased again on closure of the abdominal wall. The results showed some variability, but were thought to be related to the magnitude of the surgical procedure. ADH levels were also increased in neurosurgical patients, during cardiopulmonary bypass and in association with hypothermia and rewarming. The increases subsided to normal over 2–5 days postoperatively, and were not affected by deliberate overhydration.

Oyama and Kimura (1970) have reported a sharp but brief increase in plasma ADH after induction of anaesthesia with diethyl ether, followed by a more marked rise after the start of surgery.

In contrast to these (rare) findings obtained by direct assay, it has been suggested from renal function studies that ADH is released following induction of anaesthesia with halothane (Deutsch, Goldberg and Dripps, 1966; Deutsch *et al.*, 1966).

### Carbohydrate and Fat Metabolism

For many years it has been accepted that rises in blood (or plasma) glucose can accompany administration of inhalation anaesthetics, notably diethyl ether (Oyama and Takazawa, 1971b). That this historical evidence has recently been questioned (Clarke, 1970) suggests that the changes associated with modern anaesthetic techniques are probably small. However, there seems to be no doubt about surgically-induced hyperglycaemia, which is greater during intra-abdominal operations than with surface procedures (Clarke, Johnston and Sheridan, 1970), and is evident during all types of general anaesthesia. From one laboratory, the rises in blood glucose associated with lower abdominal surgery during spinal blockade were much smaller (Oyama and Matsuki, 1970b) than those measured during miscellaneous operations in which diethyl ether was used (Oyama and Takazawa, 1971b).

It is known that the rise in blood glucose in response to an intravenous glucose tolerance test is greater during anaesthesia and surgery than under control conditions (Dundee, 1956; Greene, 1963; Cervenko and Greene, 1967). Many 'diabetogenic' factors may be implicated such as the release of cortisol, ACTH, catecholamines, thyrotropic hormone, or human growth hormone, any or all of which could be secreted in increased amounts in association with anaesthetic administration or trauma. Abnormal glucose tolerance tests have now been reported in patients subjected to general surgical operations, cardiopulmonary by-pass, and after myocardial infarction, the disorder being attributed to a delay or partial failure in the insulin response to a glucose load (Allison, Tomlin and Chamberlain, 1969; Allison, 1971; *see* Johnston, 1967). During haemorrhagic hypotension (60 mm. Hg.) in baboons sedated with phencyclidine, serum insulin failed to rise in association with the hyperglycaemia which occurred (Moss *et al.*, 1970).

Recent additional measurements of plasma insulin (*see* Marks, 1969) during surgical procedures, from another two laboratories, have shown no change when anaesthesia was with thiopentone and nitrous oxide (Clarke, Johnston and Sheridan, 1970; Oyama, Takiguchi and Kudo, 1971), by spinal blockade (Oyama and Matsuki, 1970b), or with halothane (Oyama and Takazawa, 1971a), while variable reductions accompanied surgery with diethyl ether anaesthesia (Oyama and Takazawa, 1971b). However, it has also been reported that ether elevates the levels of both blood glucose and plasma insulin (Yoshimura, Kodama and Yoshitake, 1971). In one study, neuroleptanaesthesia before surgery was associated with significant increases in blood glucose and plasma insulin (Oyama and Takiguchi, 1970a).

A fall in the plasma level of free fatty acids (FFA) should normally accompany elevations of blood glucose (and insulin), while a rise in FFA could result from increased sympathetic activity (*see* Pawan, 1971). Allison, Tomlin and Chamberlain (1969) found that while the FFA and blood glucose levels were little affected by induction of anaesthesia, they were significantly increased by the transfer of patients from ward to operating room. Their study also showed that glucose infusion during surgery failed to reduce the FFA level. Cooperman (1970), on the other hand, described a normal FFA response to glucose infusion in surgical patients anaesthetized with cyclopropane. Although most workers have reported insignificantly changed FFA levels during surgical anaesthesia with various methods, including diethyl ether (Oyama and Takazawa, 1971b), the thiopentone-nitrous oxide-relaxant technique (Oyama, Takiguchi and Kudo, 1971; Allison, Tomlin and Chamberlain, 1969), spinal analgesia (Oyama and Matsuki, 1970b), and neuroleptanaesthesia (Oyama and Takiguchi, 1970a), elevations have been measured during surgery with cyclopropane and halothane anaesthesia, while in the same study diethyl ether caused no change (Cooperman, 1970).

The level of human growth hormone is elevated by surgical stimulation (Schalch, 1967); confirmation of this appears in several recent papers from one laboratory, where it was also found that the levels before surgery were unaffected by the thiopentone, nitrous oxide, relaxant sequence (Oyama, Takiguchi and Kudo, 1971), but were significantly increased when the techniques were based on methoxyflurane (Oyama and Takazawa, 1970), diethyl ether (Oyama and Takazawa, 1971b), or neuroleptanalgesia (Oyama and Takiguchi, 1970a).

The available information just presented can be seen to be inconsistent and based on differing studies from only a few sources. The overall conclusion is that major surgery induces a temporary diabetic-like state of glucose intolerance, and that the effects of individual anaesthetic agents on carbohydrate and fat metabolism are less striking but

probably not negligible. It is a matter of interesting speculation whether some of the data reported could have been affected by diurnal variations in glucose tolerance (Jarrett *et al.*, 1972), and by the impairment which has been measured after a few days' bed rest (Lipman *et al.*, 1972). Sympathetic nerve endings are stated to be numerous in the Islets of Langerhans and may terminate at the insulin-producing $\beta$ cells, while vagal stimulation releases insulin (*see* Marks and Samols, 1968). Thus, neurogenic stimuli are probably of prime importance in these disturbances associated with trauma and anaesthesia.

The proposition that high plasma free fatty acid levels are associated with an increased incidence of cardiac dysrhythmias in patients with myocardial infarction deserves mention because of a possible relevance to anaesthesia (Oliver, Kurien and Greenwood, 1968), but it remains controversial (Opie *et al.*, 1971), as do implications of the elevation in FFA level produced by heparin administration (Russo *et al.*, 1970).

### Renin-angiotensin-aldosterone System

The revival of interest in renin in recent years has underlined the possibility that this system could play a significant role in cardiovascular regulation in the surgical patient (renin released from the renal juxtaglomerular apparatus interacts with renin plasma substrate to form angiotensin I, which is converted in the pulmonary circuit to the active angiotensin II). Angiotensin itself has circulatory actions which may be related to the release of catecholamines, and in addition it stimulates aldosterone secretion (*see* Brown *et al.*, 1968). The likelihood 'that renin, angiotensin, and aldosterone are participants in a hormonal system involved in electrolyte homeostasis and blood pressure control' (Laragh, 1967), is apparent from the following factors which have been shown to increase renin secretion; a fall in renal perfusion pressure; a reduction in blood volume; sodium depletion (and adrenal insufficiency); stimulation of the renal nerves; most oedema syndromes; change from the recumbent to upright position; and ureteral obstruction (Tobian, 1967). Such influences have yet to be studied in the anaesthetized patient, while the possibility of interactions between renin, angiotensin and the sympathetic nervous system has of course been neglected in previous assessments of the mechanisms underlying the 'hyperdynamic' cardiovascular actions of anaesthetics such as cyclopropane and ether. Information may accrue as refined techniques of assay become available.

A recent publication mentioned a threefold rise in blood renin activity in dogs anaesthetized with pentobarbitone, adding that 'similar increases were found in anaesthetized humans' (Granger, Boucher and Genest, 1967). An increase in serum renin activity during hypoxia in man has been attributed to associated cardiovascular changes rather than to a direct effect (Tuffley *et al.*, 1970).

It may be of future interest that infusion of certain prostaglandins increases heart rate and lowers arterial pressure; the former response, and coincident mobilization of free fatty acids, apparently involves the sympathetic nervous system (Bergstrom, 1967).

## Abnormal Endocrine States

While long-continued corticosteroid therapy is known to suppress adrenocortical activity and cause adrenal atrophy (Prunty, 1967), the possible dangers in the anaesthetized patient may have been exaggerated, since in many cases the plasma corticosteroid levels are said to return to normal 48 hours after stopping systemic administration (Robinson, Mattingly and Cope, 1962). The question is considered in two recent publications which suggest the use of intramuscular hydrocortisone hemisuccinate as a supplement for major surgery, but consider this to be unnecessary if previous steroid administration ceased more than two months previously (Plumpton, Besser and Cole, 1969a, b). Intravenous supplements; before and during operation only, have been considered adequate in many cases (Brooke, 1967). No doubt the risks are greatest when systemic therapy has been intense, following removal of adrenal tumours, and in patients with pituitary or hypothalamic malfunction due to trauma or space-occupying lesions.

It is likely, when betamethasone is given in the treatment of cerebral oedema, that plasma cortisol will be low and unresponsive (Lines, Loder and Millar, 1971).

Much consideration has been given previously to anaesthesia in patients with phaechromocytoma; many or all general (Benfey and Millar, 1957) and regional (Bromage and Millar, 1958) techniques seem to be associated with the massive discharge of adrenal medullary catecholamines, usually and perhaps surprisingly without drastic consequences provided that anti-adrenergic therapy is used. Methoxyflurane has received recent recommendation as a result of the successful management of 16 patients (Crout and Brown, 1969).

Myoxoedema, if untreated, is said to increase the risk of cardiovascular collapse during anaesthesia (Abbott, 1967).

## Surgery and other Trauma

In the practical rather than experimental context, the endocrine response to surgical trauma cannot be dissociated from effects of anaesthetic agents, and is of greater consistency and magnitude. The surgical aspects have been reviewed many times (Moore, 1959; Hume and Egdahl, 1959a; Johnston, 1964; Johnston, 1967) and require only brief mention here.

The principal metabolic changes after injury (Kinney, 1967) which have been appreciated to an extent for more than a century, are an increased urinary, nitrogen and potassium excretion together with a reduced water and sodium output.

During major operations, plasma cortisol concentration rises quickly, reaches a peak level after about 5–6 hours, and returns towards normal within about 12 hours postoperatively. Increases may persist for several days after major surgery (Plumpton, Besser and Cole, 1969a). The urinary 17-oxogenic steroids (including cortisol and metabolites) are raised for 3–4 days postoperatively. While these findings relate in part to effects on conjugation they are mainly a result of increased production rates. The aldosterone output in urine was stated to be increased (Hume, Bell and Bartter, 1962), a finding supported from indirect investigation based on aldosterone blocking agents (Johnston, 1964). Thyroid hormone is also involved (Goldenberg, Hayes and Greene, 1959; Johnston, 1964).

One group has described a rise, during and after surgery, in the normally very low level of corticosterone in human plasma (Hamanaka et al., 1970).

It seems certain that the endocrine responses to surgery are mediated neurogenically (Hume, 1953; Hume and Egdahl, 1959b). Visceral traction in the abdomen is a powerful stimulus to secretion of ADH and ACTH. Presumably, the splanchnic nerves and abdominal vagus are important afferent pathways, but circulating ADH levels can also be influenced by sudden changes in left atrial pressure mediated through vagal afferents (Shu'ayb, Moran and Zimmerman, 1965). Abdominal trauma also appears to stimulate renin secretion (McKenzie, Ryan and Lee, 1967). It may still be questioned, perhaps, whether a 'wound hormone' could participate in widespread endocrine responses to injury. That painful and other strong afferent stimulation principally determine the magnitude of the endocrine response is supported by the recent finding that increases in plasma cortisol were smaller and more erratic during neurosurgical than during abdominal operations (Lines, Loder and Millar, 1971).

Since administration of ACTH or cortisol causes identical changes to those caused by surgical operations, it is easy but probably too simple to attribute the metabolic response to surgery entirely to such endocrine effects. Johnston (1964) has summarized the evidence against such a primary correlation: that totally adrenalectomized or hypophysectomized patients can be maintained on the same dosage of cortisone before and after further surgical operations; that a reduced metabolic and a normal adrenocortical response to surgery occurs in patients with gross malnutrition and wasting; and that anabolic steroids can diminish the metabolic response without altering the adrenocortical effects.

## COMMENT

The information on which the foregoing review is based is sparse in several important areas. However, there are indications already that individual anaesthetic agents may evoke a characteristic pattern of endocrine response. This is most obvious in the case of diethyl ether, which causes widespread stimulation of endocrine activity. The current belief, in regard to the mechanisms involved, is that adrenaline or noradrenaline do not themselves directly increase adrenocortical activity in man or the dog—although evidence has been published that adrenaline releases ACTH (see Hodges, Jones and Stockham, 1968). The following comment was made in a review of some years ago (Ramey and Goldstein, 1957), 'It would be difficult to describe a stressful situation resulting in increased steroid output from the adrenal cortex which would not simultaneously affect the autonomic nervous system'. The stresses referred to include haemorrhage, cold, heat, fever, infections, fear, burns, dehydration, and insulin hypoglycaemia. The same writers also emphasized that the adrenal steroids and sympathetic neurohormones appeared to act as a functional unit physiologically. It may be unwise, however, to apply such a concept to all the varied forms of stress encountered in the surgical patient. It is uncertain, for example, whether the sympathetic neurohormones are necessarily involved in those primary disturbances in fluid and electrolyte balance to which the adrenal steroids, and more particularly aldosterone, respond. In general, it is preferable to avoid the term 'stress' and to define the actual disorder with as much precision as available information permits.

The mechanism whereby anaesthetics like ether stimulate endocrine secretion is also likely to be neurogenic, and the time relationship of adrenocortical responses seems consistent with this view. Thus, liberation of ACTH from the anterior pituitary is said to occur within 15 seconds of 'stressful' stimulation (Vandam and Moore, 1960), the adrenal steroid output is raised within 2–3 minutes thereafter, and the peak response is reached after 7–10 minutes. ACTH also increases aldosterone secretion (Ganong, Biglieri and Mulrow, 1966). The stimulus to ACTH liberation is mediated through the hypothalamus; in this area, therefore, neuronal excitation caused directly or indirectly by anaesthetic agents could be a cause of pituitary activation; effects also may be exerted on the 'short' and 'long' feedback mechanisms operating at and above hypothalamic level (Mess and Martini, 1968). So far, seizure-like discharge patterns have been recorded during ether anaesthesia (Domino and Ueki, 1959), and some recent work suggests that a proportion of posterolateral ('sympathetic') hypothalamic neurones can increase their discharge rate during cyclopropane administration, even in deep anaesthesia when the cortical E.E.G. is suppressed (Millar and Silver, 1971). Further work may show, therefore, that sympathetic arousal and pituitary activation by general anaesthetics both depend on effects exerted on the hypothalamus, where certain cells are also known to be activated by carbon dioxide (Cross and Silver, 1963).

It is difficult to comment on the possible functional significance of endocrine responses to anaesthetic agents in relation to the general welfare of the surgical patient. At present, there is insufficient evidence to suggest whether the postoperative course is smoother when the anaesthetic is one which evokes minimal changes in plasma hormone levels, whether such responses to anaesthetics bear any close relation to physiological needs or are mere pharmacological accidents, or to consider whether it would be either beneficial or harmful to patients to modify deliberately the endocrine response to surgery by means of specific anaesthetic agents or other drugs. There is an obvious need for further studies based on direct and reliable methods of analysis.

## REFERENCES

Abbott, T. R. (1967), "Anaesthesia in Untreated Myxoedema," *Brit. J. Anaesth.*, **39**, 510.

Allison, S. P. (1971), "Changes in Insulin Secretion During Open Heart Surgery," *Brit. J. Anaesth.*, **43**, 138.

Allison, S. P., Tomlin, P. J. and Chamberlain, M. J. (1969), "Some Effects of Anaesthesia and Surgery on Carbohydrate and Fat Metabolism," *Brit. J. Anaesth.*, **41**, 588.

Barbour, A., Bull, G. M., Evans, B. M., Hughes-Jones, N. C. and Logothetopoulos, J. (1953), "Effect of Breathing 5 to 7 per cent Carbon Dioxide on Urine Flow and Mineral Excretion," *Clin. Sci.*, **12**, 1.

Barlow, G., Spurr, G. B. and Bowe, R. L. (1959), "Circulating Levels of 17-hydroxycorticosteroid in Prolonged Hypothermia," *J. appl. Physiol.*, **14**, 777.

Benfey, B. G. and Millar, R. A. (1957), "Catecholamines in Blood, Urine and Tumour in a Patient with Phaeochromocytoma," *Canad. med. Ass. J.*, **77**, 701.

Bergstrom, S. (1967), "Prostaglandins: Members of a New Hormonal System," *Science*, **157**, 382.

Bernhard, W. F., McMurrey, J. D., Ganong, W. F. and Lenningham, R. (1956), "Effect of Hypothermia on Peripheral Serum Levels of Free 17-hydroxycorticoids in Dog and Man," *Ann. Surg.*, **143**, 210.

Black, G. W., McArdle, L., McCullough, H. and Unni, V. K. N. (1969), "Circulating Catecholamines and some Cardiovascular, Respiratory, Metabolic and Pupillary Responses during Diethyl Ether Anaesthesia," *Anaesthesia*, **24**, 168.

Black, S. and Friedman, M. (1965), "Adrenal Function and the Inhibition of Allergic Responses under Hypnosis," *Brit. Med. J.*, **1**, 562.

Black, S. and Friedman, M. (1968), "Effects of Emotion and Pain on Adrenocortical Function Investigated by Hypnosis," *Brit. Med. J.*, **1**, 477.

Bloom, G., Euler, U. S. von and Frankenhauser, M. (1963), "Catecholamine Excretion and Personality Traits in Paratroop Trainees," *Acta Physiol. Scand.*, **58**, 77.

Brewster, W. R. Jr., Issaacs, J. P. and Wainø-Andersen, T. (1953), Depressant Effect of Ether on the Myocardium of the Dog and its Modification by Reflex Release of Epinephrine and Norepinephrine," *Amer. J. Physiol.*, **175**, 399.

Bromage, P. R. and Millar, R. A. (1958), "Epidural Blockade and Circulating Catecholamine Levels in a Child with Phaeochromocytoma," *Canad. Anaesth. Soc. J.*, **5**, 282.

Brooke, B. N. (1967), "Acute Adrenal Dysfunction," *Brit. J. Surg.*, **54**, 489.

Brown, J. J., Fraser, R., Lever, A. F. and Robertson, J. I. S. (1968), "Renin and Angiotensin in the Control of Water and Electrolyte Balance; Relation to Aldosterone." Chapter 9 in: *Recent Advances in Endocrinology*, 8th edition (V. H. T. James, Ed.). London: Churchill.

Brunt, E. E. van and Ganong, W. F. (1963), "The Effects of Preanesthetic Medication, Anesthesia and Hypothermia on the Endocrine Response to Injury," *Anesthesiology*, **24**, 500.

Bursten, B. and Russ, J. J. (1965), "Preoperative Psychological State and Corticosteroid Levels of Surgical Patients," *Psychosom. Med.*, **27**, 309.

Callingham, B. A. (1972), "Catecholamines in Blood," *Pharm. J.*, **208**, 77.

Cannon, W. B. (1929), *Bodily Changes in Pain, Hunger, Fear and Rage*. New York: Appleton.

Carruthers, M., Taggart, P., Conway, N., Bates, D. and Somerville, W. (1970), "Validity of Plasma—Catecholamine Estimations," *Lancet*, **2**, 62.

Cervenko, F. W. and Greene, N. M. (1967), "Effect of Cyclopropane Anesthesia on Glucose Assimilation Coefficient of Man," *Anesthesiology*, **28**, 914.

Clarke, R. S. J. (1970), "The Hyperglycaemic Response to Different Types of Surgery and Anaesthesia," *Brit. J. Anaesth.*, **42**, 45.

Clarke, R. S. J., Johnston, Hilary and Sheridan, B. (1970), "The Influence of Anaesthesia and Surgery on Plasma Cortisol, Insulin and Free Fatty Acids," *Brit. J. Anaesth.*, **42**, 295.

Connolly, C. K. and Wills, M. R. (1967), "Plasma Cortisol Levels in Heart Failure," *Brit. Med. J.*, **2**, 25.

Cooper, C. E. and Nelson, D. H. (1962), "ACTH Levels in Plasma in Preoperative and Surgically Stressed Patients," *J. clin. Invest.*, **41**, 1599.

Cooperman, L. H. (1970), "Plasma Free Fatty Acid Levels During

General Anaesthesia and Operation in Man," *Brit. J. Anaesth.*, **42**, 131.

Cross, B. A. and Silver, I. A. (1963), "Unit Activity in the Hypothalamus and the Sympathetic Response to Hypoxia and Hypercapnia," *Exp. Neurol.*, **7**, 375.

Crout, J. R. and Brown, B. R. (1969), "Anesthetic Management of Pheochromocytoma. The Value of Phenoxybenzamine and Methoxyflurane," *Anesthesiology*, **30**, 29.

Deutsch, S., Goldberg, M. and Dripps, R. D. (1966), "Postoperative Hyponatremia with the Inappropriate Release of Antidiuretic Hormone," *Anesthesiology*, **27**, 250.

Deutsch, S., Goldberg, M., Stephen, G. W. and Wu, W-H. (1966), "Effects of Halothane Anesthesia on Renal Function in Normal Man," *Anesthesiology*, **27**, 793.

Doig, R. J., Mummery, R. V., Willis, M. R. and Elkes, A. (1966), "Plasma Cortisol Levels in Depression," *Brit. J. Psychiat.*, **112**, 1263.

Domino, E. F. and Ueki, S. (1959), "Differential Effects of General Anesthetics on Spontaneous Electrical Activity of Neocortical and Rhinencephalic Brain Systems of the Dog," *J. Pharmacol. exp. Ther.*, **127**, 288.

Dudley, H. F., Boling, E. A., Le Quesne, L. P. and Moore, F. D. (1954), "Studies on Antidiuresis in Surgery: Effects of Anesthesia, Surgery, and Posterior Pituitary Antidiuretic Hormone on Water Metabolism in Man," *Ann. Surg.*, **140**, 354.

Dundee, J. W. (1956), "Effect of Thiopentone on Blood Sugar and Glucose Tolerance," *Brit. J. Pharmacol.*, **11**, 458.

Egdahl, R. H., Nelson, D. H. and Hume, D. M. (1955), "Adrenal Cortical Function in Hypothermia," *Surg. Gynec. Obstet.*, **101**, 715.

Euler, U. S. von (1964), "Quantitation of Stress by Catecholamine Analysis," *Clin. Pharmacol. Ther.*, **5**, 398.

Euler, U. S. von and Floding, L. (1955), "Fluorimetric Estimation of Noradrenaline and Adrenaline in Urine," *Acta physiol. Scand. Suppl.*, 118, **33**, 57.

Euler, U. S. von, Gemzell, C. A., Levi, L. and Strom, G. (1959), "Cortical and Medullary Adrenal Activity in Emotional Stress," *Acta Endocrin. (Copenhagen)*, **30**, 567.

Euler, U. S. von and Lundberg, U. (1954), "Effect of Flying on the Epinephrine Excretion in Air Force Personnel," *J. appl. Physiol.*, **6**, 551.

Franksson, C. and Gemzell, C. A. (1955), "Adrenocortical Activity in the Preoperative Period," *J. Clin. Endocr.*, **15**, 1069.

Friedman, S. (1965), "Plasma Hydroxycorticosteroids in Pathological and Physiological States in Man," M.D. Thesis, Univ. of Witwatersrand.

Gann, D. S. and Egdahl, R. H. (1965), "Responses of Adrenal Corticosteroid Secretion to Hypotension and Hypovolemia," *J. Clin. Invest.*, **44**, 1.

Ganong, W. F., Bernhard, W. F. and McMurrey, J. D. (1955), "Effect of Hypothermia on Output of 17-hydroxycorticoids from Adrenal Vein in Dog," *Surgery*, **38**, 506.

Ganong, W. F., Biglieri, E. G. and Mulrow, P. J. (1966), "Mechanisms Regulating Adrenocortical Secretion of Aldosterone and Glucocorticoids," *Recent Progress in Hormone Research*, **22**, 381. London: Academic Press.

Goldenberg, I. S., Hayes, M. A. and Greene, N. M. (1959), "Endocrine Responses to Operative Procedures," *Ann. Surg.*, **150**, 196.

Granger, P., Boucher, R. and Genest, J. (1967), "Note on the Preparation of Renin Substrate," *Can. J. Physiol. Pharmacol.*, **45**, 921.

Greene, N. M. (1963), "Inhalation Anesthetics and Carbohydrate Metabolism." Baltimore: Williams and Wilkins.

Greene, N. M. and Goldenberg, I. S. (1959), "The Effect of Anesthesia on Thyroid Activity in Humans," *Anesthesiology*, **20**, 125.

Hamanaka, Y., Manabe, H., Tanaka, H., Monden, Y., Uozumi, T. and Matsumoto, K. (1970), "Effects of Surgery on Plasma Levels of Cortisol, Corticosterone and Non-Protein-Bound Cortisol," *Acta endocr. (Kbh.)*, **64**, 439.

Hammond, W. G., Vandam, L. D., Davis, J. M., Carter, R. D., Ball, M. R. and Moore, F. D. (1958), "Studies in Surgical Endocrinology: Anesthetic Agents as Stimuli to changes in Corticosteroids and Metabolism," *Ann. Surg.*, **148**, 199.

Han, Y. H. and Brown, E. S. (1961), "Pituitary Blockage by Meperidine in Man," *Anesthesiology*, **22**, 909.

Hetzel, B. S., Schottstaedt, W. W., Grace, W. J. and Wolff, H. G. (1955), "Changes in Urinary 17-hydroxycorticosteroid Excretion during Stressful Life Experiences in Man," *J. Clin. Endocrinol.*, **15**, 1057.

Hill, S. R., Goutz, F. C., Fox, H. M., Murawski, B. J., Krakauer, L. J., Reinsenstein, R. W., Gray, S. J., Reddy, W. J., Hedberg, S. E., Marc, J. R. St. and Thorn, G. W. (1956), "Studies on Adrenocortical and Psychological Response to Stress in Man," *Arch. intern. Med.*, **97**, 269.

Hodges, J. R., Jones, M. T. and Stockham, M. A. (1968), "Control of Corticotrophin Secretion," Chapter 2 in: *Handbook of Experimental Pharmacology*, Vol. XIV/3 (H. W. Deane and B. L. Rubin, Eds.). New York: Springer-Verlag.

Holzbauer, M. and Vogt, M. (1954), "The Concentration of Adrenaline in the Peripheral Blood during Insulin Hypoglycaemia," *Brit. J. Pharmacol.*, **9**, 249.

Hume, D. M. (1953), "Neuro-endocrine Response to Injury: Present Status of Problem," *Ann. Surg.*, **138**, 548.

Hume, D. M. (1958), "Secretion of Epinephrine, Norepinephrine and Corticosteroids in Adrenal Venous Blood of the Dog Following Single and Repeated Trauma," *Surg. Forum*, **8**, 111.

Hume, D. M. and Bell, C. C., Jr. (1958), "The Secretion of Epinephrine, Norepinephrine, and Corticosteroid in the Adrenal Venous Blood of the Human," *Surg. Forum*, **9**, 6.

Hume, D. M., Bell, C. C. and Bartter, F. (1962), "Direct Measurement of Adrenal Secretion during Operative Trauma and Convalescence," *Surgery*, **52**, 174.

Hume, D. M. and Egdahl, R. H. (1959a), "Effect of Hypothermia and Cold Exposure on Adrenal Cortical and Medullary Secretion," *Ann. N. Y. Acad. Sci.*, **80**, 435.

Hume, D. M. and Egdahl, R. H. (1959b), "The Importance of the Brain in the Endocrine Response to Injury," *Ann. Surg.*, **150**, 697.

Jacobs, H. S. and Nabarro, J. D. N. (1969), "Plasma 11-hydroxycorticosteroid and Growth Hormone Levels in Acute Medical Illnesses," *Brit. med. J.*, **2**, 595.

James, V. H. T. and Landon, J. (1968), "Control of Corticosteroid Secretion—Current Views and Methods of Assessment." Chapter 2 in: *Recent Advances in Endocrinology*. 8th Edition (V. H. T. James, Ed.). London: Churchill.

Jarrett, R. J., Baker, I. A., Keen, H. and Oakley, N. W. (1972), "Diurnal Variation in Oral Glucose Tolerance: Blood Sugar and Plasma Insulin Levels Morning, Afternoon, and Evening," *Brit. Med. J.*, **1**, 199.

Johnston, I. D. A. (1964), "Endocrine Aspects of Metabolic Response to Surgical Operation," *Ann. Roy. Coll. Surg., Engl.*, **35**, 270.

Johnston, I. D. A. (1967), "The Role of the Endocrine Glands in the Metabolic Response to Operation," *Brit. J. Surg.*, **54**, 438.

Kaada, B. R., Setekleiv, J. and Skang, O. E. (1959), "Effects of Barbiturates and Nitrous Oxide on Level of 17-OH-steroids and Eosinophil Cells in Cat," *Acta pharmacol. (Kbh.)*, **16**, 87.

Khalil, H. H. (1954), "Effect of Hypothermia on Hypothalamic-pituitary Response to Stress," *Brit. med. J.*, **2**, 733.

Kinney, J. M. (1967), "The Effect of Injury on Metabolism," *Brit. J. Surg.*, **54**, 435.

Knapp, M. S., Keane, P. M. and Wright, J. G. (1967), "Circadian Rhythm of Plasma 11-hydroxycorticosteroids in Depressive Illness, Congestive Heart Failure, and Cushing's Syndrome," *Brit. med. J.*, **2**, 27.

*Lancet* (1956), "Annotation: Adrenocortical Function in Physiological Stress," **1**, 1056.

Laragh, J. H. (1967), "Renin, Angiotensin, Aldosterone and Hormonal Regulation of Arterial Pressure and Salt Balance," *Fed. Proc.*, **26**, 39.

Leduc, J. (1961), "Catecholamine Production and Release on Exposure and Acclimatization to Cold," *Acta physiol. Scand.*, **53**, suppl. 183.

Lewis, R. N. (1963), "Plasma Hydrocortisone Concentrations in Relation to Anaesthesia and Surgery," *Brit. J. Anaesth.*, **35**, 84.

Li, T-H., Shaul, M. S. and Etsten, B. E. (1968), "Decreased Adrenal Venous Catecholamine Concentrations During Methoxyflurane Anesthesia," *Anesthesiology*, **29**, 1145.

Lines, J. G., Loder, R. E. and Millar, R. A. (1971), "Plasma Cortisol

Responses During Neurosurgery and Abdominal Operations," *Brit. J. Anaesth.*, **43**, 1136.

Lipman, R. L., Raskin, P., Love, T., Triebwasser, J., Lecocq, F. R. and Schnure, J. J. (1972), "Glucose Intolerance During Decreased Physical Activity in Man," *Diabetes*, **21**, 101.

Lipscomb, H. S. and Nelson, D. H. (1962), "A Sensitive Biologic Assay for ACTH," *Endocrinology*, **71**, 13.

MacPhee, I. W., Gray, T. C. and Davies, S. (1958), "Effect of Hypothermia on the Adrenocortical Response to Operation," *Lancet*, **2**, 1196.

Marks, V. (1969), "The Immunoassay of Insulin and Glucagon," *Brit. J. Hosp. Med.*, **2**, 1103.

Marks, V. and Samols, E. (1968), "Glucose Homeostasis." Chapter 4 in: *Recent Advances in Endocrinology*, Eighth Edition (V.H.T. James, Ed.). London: Churchill.

Martinez, L. R., Euler, C. von and Norlander, O. P. (1966), 'The Sedative Effect of Premedication as Measured by Catecholamine Excretion," *Brit. J. Anaesth.*, **38**, 780.

Matsuki, A. and Oyama, T. (1972), "Thyroid—adrenocortical relationship During Caesarian Section and Minor Surgery Under Spinal Anaesthesia," *Der Anaesthesist*, **21**, 122.

Mattingly, D. (1962), "A Simple Fluorimetric Method for the Estimation of Free 11-hydroxycorticoids in Human Plasma," *J. clin. Path.*, **15**, 374.

McDonald, R. K., Evans, F. T., Weise, V. K. and Patrick, R. W. (1959), "Effect of Morphine and Nalorphine on Plasma Hydrocortisone Levels in Man," *J. Pharmacol. exp. Ther.*, **125**, 241.

McKenzie, J. K., Ryan, J. W. and Lee, M. R. (1967), "Effect of Laparotomy on Plasma Renin Activity in the Rabbit," *Nature*, **215**, 542.

Mess, B. and Martini, L. (1968), "The Central Nervous System and the Secretion of Anterior Pituitary Trophic Hormones." Chapter 1 in: *Recent Advances in Endocrinology*, Eighth Edition (V. H. T. James, Ed.). London: Churchill.

Millar, R. A. (1956), "The Fluorimetric Estimation of Adrenaline and Noradrenaline." M.D. Thesis, University of Edinburgh.

Millar, R. A. (1960), "Plasma Adrenaline and Noradrenaline during Diffusion Respiration," *J. Physiol.*, **150**, 79.

Millar, R. A. and Benfey, B. G. (1958), "The Fluorimetric Estimation of Adrenaline and Noradrenaline during Haemorrhagic Hypotension," *Brit. J. Anaesth.*, **30**, 159.

Millar, R. A. and Biscoe, T. J. (1965), "Preganglionic Sympathetic Activity and the Effects of Inhalation Anaesthetics," *Brit. J. Anaesth.*, **37**, 804.

Millar, R. A. and Morris, M. E. (1960), "Induced Sympathetic Stimulation during Halothane Anaesthesia," *Canad. Anaesth. Soc. J.*, **7**, 423.

Millar, R. A. and Morris, M. E. (1961a), "A Study of Methoxyflurane Anaesthesia," *Canad. Anaesth. Soc. J.*, **8**, 210.

Millar, R. A. and Morris, M. E. (1961b), "Sympatho-adrenal Responses during General Anaesthesia in the Dog and Man," *Canad. Anaesth. Soc. J.*, **8**, 356.

Millar, R. A. and Silver, I. A. (1971), "Excitation of Certain Posterolateral Hypothalamic Units by Cyclopropane and Ether," *Brit. J. Pharmacol.*, **42**, 315.

Millar, R. A., Warden, J. C., Cooperman, L. H. and Price, H. L. (1969), "Central Sympathetic Discharge and Mean Arterial Pressure During Halothane Anesthesia," *Brit. J. Anaesth.*, **41**, 918.

Millar, R. A., Warden, J. C., Cooperman, L. H. and Price, H. L. (1970), "Further Studies of Sympathetic Actions of Anaesthetics in Intact and Spinal Animals," *Brit. J. Anesth.*, **47**, 366.

Moore, F. D. (1959). *Metabolic Care of the Surgical Patient*. Philadelphia: Saunders.

Moran, W. H., Miltenberger, F. W., Shuayb, W. A. and Zimmerman, B. (1964), "The Relationship of Antidiuretic Hormone to Surgical Stress," *Surgery*, **56**, 99.

Morris, M. E. and Millar, R. A. (1962a), "Blood pH/plasma Catecholamine Relationships: Respiratory Acidosis," *Brit. J. Anaesth.*, **34**, 672.

Morris, M. E. and Millar, R. A. (1962b), "Blood pH/plasma Catecholamine Relationships: Non-respiratory Acidosis," *Brit. J. Anaesth.*, **34**, 682.

Moss, C. S., Cerchio, C. M., Siegel, D. C., Popovichi, P. A. and

Butler, E. (1970), "Serum Insulin Response in Hemorrhagic Shock in Baboons," *Surgery*, **68**, 34.

Nahas, G. G., Zagury, D., Milhaud, A., Manger, W. M. and Pappas, G. D. (1967), "Acidemia and Catecholamine Output of the Isolated Canine Adrenal Gland," *Amer. J. Physiol.*, **213**, 1186.

Newsome, H. H. and Rose, J. C. (1971), "The Response of Human Adrenocorticotrophic Hormone and Growth Hormone to Surgical Stress," *J. Clin. Endocr.*, **33**, 481.

Nishioka, K., Levy, A. A. and Dobkin, A. B. (1968), "Effect of Halothane and Methoxyflurane Anaesthesia on Plasma Cortisol Concentration in Relation to Major Surgery," *Canad. Anaesth. Soc. J.*, **15**, 441.

Oliver, M. F., Kurien, V. A. and Greenwood, T. W. (1968), "Relation Between Serum-Free-Fatty-Acids and Arrhythmias and Death After Acute Myocardial Infarction," *Lancet*, **1**, 710.

Opie, L. H., Norris, R. M., Thomas, M., Holland, A. J., Owen, P. and Van Noorden, S. (1971), "Failure of High Concentrations of Circulating Free Fatty Acids to Provoke Arrhythmias in Experimental Myocardial Infarction," *Lancet*, **1**, 818.

Osborn, W., Schoenberg, H. M., Murphy, J. J., Erdman, W. J. (3rd) and Young, G. D. (1962), "Adrenal Function in Patients with Lesions High in the Spinal Cord," *J. Urol. (Baltimore)*, **88**, 1.

Oyama, T. and Kimura, K. (1970), "Plasma Levels of Antidiuretic Hormone in Man During Diethyl Ether Anaesthesia and Surgery," *Canad. Anaesth. Soc. J.*, **17**, 495.

Oyama, T., Kimura, K., Takazawa, T. and Takiguchi, H. (1969a), "An Objective Evaluation of Tranquillizers as Preanaesthetic Medication: Effect on Adrenocortical Function," *Canad. Anaesth. Soc. J.*, **16**, 209.

Oyama, T., Kimura, K., Takazawa, T., Takiguchi, M. and Shibata, S. (1970), "Effects of Propanidid on Plasma Cortisol Concentration in Man," *Anesth. Analg. Curr. Res.*, **49**, 39.

Oyama, T., Kudo, T., Shibata, S. and Matsumoto, F. (1968a), "Effects of Gamma-Hydroxybutyrate on Plasma Hydrocortisone Concentration in Man," *Anesth. Analg. Curr. Res.*, **47**, 350.

Oyama, T. and Matsuki, A. (1970a), "Plasma Levels of Cortisol in Man During Spinal Anaesthesia and Surgery," *Canad. Anaesth. Soc. J.*, **17**, 234.

Oyama, T. and Matsuki, A. (1970b), "Effects of Spinal Anaesthesia and Surgery on Carbohydrate and Fat Metabolism in Man," *Brit. J. Anaesth.*, **42**, 723.

Oyama, T. and Matsuki, A. (1971), "Serum Levels of Thyroxine in Man During Spinal Anaesthesia and Surgery," *Anesth. Analg. Curr. Res.*, **50**, 309.

Oyama, T., Matsuki, A. and Kudo, M. (1972), "Effect of Ethrane Anaesthesia and Surgical Operation on Adrenocortical Function," *Canad. Anaesth. Soc. J.*, **19**, 394.

Oyama, T., Matsumoto, F. and Kudo, T. (1970), "Effects of Ketamine on Adrenocortical Function in Man," *Canad. Anaesth. Soc. J.*, **49**, 697.

Oyama, T., Saito, T., Isomatsu, T., Samejima, N., Uemura, T. and Arimura, A. (1968b), "Plasma Levels of ACTH and Cortisol in Man during Diethyl Ether Anesthesia and Surgery," *Anesthesiology*, **29**, 559.

Oyama, T., Shibata, S., Kimura, K. and Takazawa, T. (1969b), "An Objective Evaluation of Pentobarbital as Preanaesthetic Medication: Effect on Adrenocortical Function," *Anesth. Analg. Curr. Res.*, **47**, 48.

Oyama, T., Shibata, S. and Matsuki, A. (1969), "Thyroxine Distribution during Ether and Thiopental Anaesthesia in Man," *Anesth. Analg. Curr. Res.*, **48**, 1.

Oyama, T., Shibata, S., Matsuki, A. and Kudo, T. (1969c), "Thyroid-adrenocortical Responses to Anaesthesia in Man," *Anaesthesia*, **24**, 19.

Oyama, T., Shibata, S., Matsuki, A. and Kudo, T. (1969d), "Serum Endogenous Thyroxine Levels in Man during Anaesthesia and Surgery," *Brit. J. Anaesth.*, **41**, 103.

Oyama, T., Shibata, S., Matsumoto, F. and Kudo, T. (1968c), "Effects of Halothane Anaesthesia and Surgery on Adrenocortical Function in Man," *Canad. Anaesth. Soc. J.*, **15**, 258.

Oyama, T., Shibata, S., Matsumoto, F., Matsuki, A., Kimura, K., Takazawa, T. and Kudo, T. (1968d), "Adrenocortical Function

Related to Methoxyflurane Anaesthesia and Surgery in Man," *Canad. Anaesth. Soc. J.*, **15**, 362.

Oyama, T. and Takazawa, T. (1970), "Effect of Methoxyflurane Anaesthesia and Surgery on Human Growth Hormone and Insulin Levels in Plasma," *Can. Anaesth. Soc. J.*, **17**, 347.

Oyama, T. and Takazawa, T. (1971a), "Effects of Halothane Anaesthesia and Surgery on Human Growth Hormone and Insulin Levels in Plasma," *Brit. J. Anaesth.*, **43**, 573.

Oyama, T. and Takazawa, T. (1971b), "Effects of Diethyl Ether Anaesthesia and Surgery on Carbohydrate and Fat Metabolism in Man," *Canad. Anaesth. Soc. J.*, **18**, 51.

Oyama, T. and Takiguchi, M. (1970a), "Effects of Neurolept-anaesthesia on Plasma Levels of Growth Hormone and Insulin," *Brit. J. Anaesth.*, **42**, 1105.

Oyama, T. and Takiguchi, M. (1970b), "Effect of Neurolept-anaesthesia on Adrenocortical Function in Man," *Brit. J. Anaesth.*, **42**, 425.

Oyama, T., Takiguchi, M. and Kudo, T. (1971), "Metabolic Effects of Anaesthesia: Effect of Thiopentone-Nitrous Oxide Anaesthesia on Human Growth Hormone and Insulin Levels in Plasma," *Canad. Anaesth. Soc. J.*, **18**, 442.

Oyama, T., Takiguchi, M., Takazawa, T. and Kimura, K. (1969e), "Effect of Meperidine on Adrenocortical Function in Man," *Canad. Anaesth. Soc. J.*, **16**, 282.

Pawan, C. L. S. (1971), "Metabolism of Adipose Tissue," *Brit. J. Hosp. Med.*, **4**, 686.

Persky, H., Grinker, R. R., Hamburg, D. A., Fabshin, M. A., Korchin, S. J., Basowitz, H. and Chevalier, J. A. (1956), "Adrenal Cortical Function in Anxious Human Subjects," *Arch. Neurol. (Chic.)*, **76**, 549.

Philbin, D. M., Baratz, R. A., and Patterson, R. W. (1970) "The effect of carbon dioxide on plasma antidiuretic hormone levels during intermittent positive-pressure breathing." *Anesthesiology*, **33**, 345.

Plumpton, F. S., Besser, G. M. and Cole, P. V. (1969a), "Corticosteroid Treatment and Surgery. 1. An Investigation of the Indications for Steroid Cover," *Anaesthesia*, **24**, 3.

Plumpton, F. S., Besser, G. M. and Cole, P. V. (1969b), "Corticosteroid Treatment and Surgery. 2. The Management of Steroid Cover," *Anaesthesia*, **24**, 12.

Price, D. B., Thaler, M. and Mason, J. W. (1957), "Preoperative Emotional State and Adrenocortical Activity," *Arch. Neurol. (Chic.)*, **77**, 646.

Price, H. L. (1960), "General Anesthesia and Circulatory Homeostasis," *Physiol. Rev.*, **40**, 187.

Price, H. L. (1967), *Circulation During Anesthesia and Operation*. Springfield: Thomas.

Price, H. L., Cook, W. A. Jr., Deutsch, S., Linde, H. W., Mishalove, R. D. and Morse, H. T. (1963), "Hemodynamic and Central Nervous Actions of Cyclopropane in the Dog," *Anesthesiology*, **24**, 1.

Price, H. L., Linde, H. W., Jones, R. E., Black, G. W. and Price, M. L. (1959), "Sympatho-adrenal Responses to General Anesthesia in Man and their Relation to Hemodynamics," *Anesthesiology*, **20**, 563.

Price, H. L., Linde, H. W. and Morse, H. T. (1963), "Central Nervous Actions of Halothane Affecting the Systemic Circulation," *Anesthesiology*, **24**, 770.

Price, H. L., Lurie, A. A., Black, G. W., Sechzer, P. H., Linde, H. W. and Price, M. L. (1960), "Modification by General Anesthetics (Cyclopropane and Halothane) of Circulatory and Sympathoadrenal Responses to Respiratory Acidosis," *Ann. Surg.*, **152**, 1071.

Price, H. L., Warden, J. C., Cooperman, L. H. and Millar, R. A. (1969), "Central Sympathetic Excitation caused by Cyclopropane," *Anesthesiology*, **30**, 426.

Pringle, H., Maunsell, C. B. and Pringle, S. (1905), "Clinical Effects of Ether Anaesthesia on Renal Activity," *Brit. med. J.*, **2**, 542.

Prunty, F. T. G. (1967), "Current Techniques for the Assessment of Adrenocortical Function and their Interpretation." Chapter 9, in: *Modern Trends in Endocrinology* 3 (H. Gardiner-Hill, Ed.). London: Butterworth.

Ramey, E. R. and Goldstein, M. S. (1957), "The Adrenal Cortex and the Sympathetic Nervous System," *Physiol. Rev.*, **37**, 155.

Richards, J. B. (1957), "Effects of Altered Acid-base Balance on Adrenocortical Function in Anesthetized Dogs," *Amer. J. Physiol.*, **188**, 7.

Robinson, B. H., Mattingly, D. and Cope, C. L. (1962), "Adrenal Function after Prolonged Corticosteroid Therapy," *Brit. med. J.*, **1**, 1579.

Ronzoni, E. (1950), "Sodium Pentobarbital Anesthesia and Response of Adrenal Cortex to Stress," *Amer. J. Physiol.*, **160**, 499.

Rothballer, A. B. (1956), "Neurosecretory Response to Stress, Anaesthesia, Adrenalectomy and Adrenal Demedullation in the Rat," *Acta neuroveg. (Wien)*, **13**, 179.

Royce, P. C. and Sayers, G. (1958), "Blood ACTH: Effects of Ether, Pentobarbital, Epinephrine and Pain," *Endocrinology*, **63**, 794.

Russo, J. V., Friesinger, G. C., Margolis, S. and Ross, R. S. (1970), "Heparin and Ventricular Arrhythmias after Myocardial Infarction," *Lancet*, **2**, 1271.

Sandberg, A. A., Eik-Nes, K., Samuels, L. T. and Tyler, F. H. (1954), "Effects of Surgery on Blood Levels and Metabolism of 17-hydroxycorticosteroids in Man," *J. clin. Invest.*, **33**, 1509.

Sapira, J. I., Klaniecki, T. and Rizk, M. (1971), "Modified Fluorimetric Method for Determining Plasma Catecholamines," *Clin. Chem.*, **17**, 486.

Schaefer, K. E., McCabe, N. and Withers, J. (1968), "Stress Response in Chronic Hypercapnia," *Amer. J. Physiol.*, **214**, 543.

Schalch, D. S. (1967), "The Influence of Physical Stress and Exercise on GH and Insulin Secretion in Man," *J. Lab. Clin. Med.*, **69**, 256.

Sechzer, P. H., Egbert, L. D., Linde, H. W., Cooper, D. Y., Dripps, R. D. and Price, H. L. (1960), "Effect of $CO_2$ Inhalation on Arterial Pressure, E.C.G. and Plasma Catecholamines and 17-OH Corticosteroids in Normal Man," *J. appl. Physiol.*, **15**, 454.

Shannon, I. L., Isbell, G. M. and Szmyd, L. (1963), "Stress in Dental Patients. V. Effect of Time of Day on Adrenocortical Response to Oral Surgery," *J. oral Surg.*, **21**, 101.

Shu'ayb, W. A., Moran, W. H. Jr. and Zimmerman, Z. (1965), "Studies of the Mechanism of Antidiuretic Hormone Secretion and the Post-commissurotomy Dilutional Syndrome," *Ann. Surg.*, **162**, 690.

Siker, E. S., Lipschitz, E. and Klein, R. (1956), "Effect of Pre-anaesthetic Medications on Blood Level of 17-hydroxycorticosteroids," *Ann. Surg.*, **143**, 88.

Silber, R. H. and Porter, C. C. (1957), "Determination of 17,21-dihydroxy-20-ketosteroids in Urine and Plasma." In: *Methods of Biochemical Analysis* (D. Glick, Ed.), Vol. 4, p. 139. New York: Interscience.

Smith, N. Ty., Eger, E. I. (2nd), Stoelting, R. K., Whayne, T. F., Cullen, D. and Kadis, L. B. (1970), "The Cardiovascular and Sympathomimetic Responses to the Addition of Nitrous Oxide to Halothane in Man," *Anesthesiology*, **32**, 410.

Smith, N. Ty., Eger, E. I. (2nd), Whitcher, C. E., Stoelting, R. K. and Whayne, T. F. (1968), "The Circulatory Effects of the Addition of Nitrous Oxide to Halothane Anesthesia in Man," *Anesthesiology*, **29**, 212.

Stark, G. (1966), "Der Einfluss der Narkose auf die Ausscheidung von Aldosteron, cortisone und Cortisol Sowie Natrium und Kalium," *Der Anaesthesist*, **15**, 1, 4.

Suzuki, T., Yamashita, K. and Mitamura, T. (1959), "Effect of Ether Anesthesia on 17-hydroxycorticosteroid Secretion in Dogs," *Amer. J. Physiol.*, **197**, 1261.

Swan, H., Jenkins, D. and Helmreich, M. L. (1957), "Adrenal Cortical Response to Surgery: Changes in Plasma and Urinary Corticosteroid Levels during Hypothermia in Man," *Surgery*, **42**, 202.

Tenney, S. M. (1960), "The Effect of Carbon Dioxide on Neuro-humoral and Endocrine Mechanisms," *Anesthesiology*, **21**, 674.

Tobian, L. (1967), "Renin Release and its Role in Renal Function and the Control of Salt Balance and Arterial Pressure," *Fed. Proc.*, **26**, 48.

Tuffley, R. E., Rubinstein, D., Slater, J. D. H. and Williams, E. S. (1970), "Serum Renin Activity during Exposure to Hypoxia," *J. Endocr.*, **48**, 497.

Ulvedal, F., Smith, W. R. and Welch, B. E. (1963), "Steroid and

Catecholamine Studies on Pilots during Prolonged Experiments in a Space Cabin Simulator," *J. appl. Physiol.*, **18**, 1257.

Utting, J. E. and Whitford, J. H. W. (1972), "Assessment of Premedicant Drugs Using Measurements of plasma Cortisol," *Brit. J. Anaesth.*, **44**, 43.

Valtin, H., Wilson, I. D. and Tenney, S. M. (1959), "Carbon Dioxide Diuresis, with Special Reference to Role of the Left Atrial Stretch Receptor Mechanism," *J. appl. Physiol.*, **14**, 844.

Vandam, L. D. and Moore, F. D. (1960), "Adrenocortical Mechanisms Related to Anesthesia," *Anesthesiology*, **21**, 531.

Vendsalu, A. (1960), "Studies on Adrenaline and Noradrenaline in Human Plasma," *Acta Physiol. scand.*, **49**, Suppl. 173.

Virtue, R. W., Helmreich, M. L. and Gainza, E. (1957), "The Adrenal Cortical Response to Surgery: the Effect of Anesthesia on Plasma 17-hydroxycorticosteroid Levels," *Surgery*, **41**, 549.

Yoshimura, N., Kodama, K. and Yoshitake, J. (1971), "Carbohydrate Metabolism and Insulin Release during Ether and Halothane Anaesthesia," *Brit. J. Anaesth.*, **43**, 1022.

SECTION II

# PHYSIOLOGICAL BASIS OF THE SCIENCE OF ANAESTHESIA

## D. METABOLIC PROCESSES

# ANAESTHESIA AND THE KIDNEYS

## LAVINIA LOUGHRIDGE

The kidneys, like the liver, regularly suffer a considerable reduction in their blood supply during anaesthesia. Such is the reserve of renal function in the normal, however, that this temporary decrease in blood flow seldom presents any clinical problem; but where there is established parenchymal disease of the kidneys, the haemodynamic changes induced by anaesthesia may have critical effects upon function.

The particular problems of anaesthesia and surgery in the presence of advanced renal disease have been highlighted by the advent of kidney transplant surgery. These problems include specific aspects of the biochemical disorder created by failing renal function and recognition of the hazards of diminished renal excretion of anaesthetic agents.

The effects of anaesthesia upon renal haemodynamics in the normal patient, nephrotoxicity of anaesthetic drugs and the problems of anaesthesia in established disease of the kidneys will be discussed.

## The Kidneys

### Effects of Anaesthesia on the Normal Kidney

Some reduction in urine volume with retention of both water and sodium are commonly observed in patients in the post-anaesthetic, post-surgical period. These changes are spontaneously reversible and usually resolve within 1–3 days. The incidence of serious renal damage following anaesthesia and surgery is low. Amongst operations which carry a special risk to the kidney, surgery for relief of obstructive jaundice, particularly in the elderly, is of considerable importance. This vulnerability of the kidneys to ischaemic insult in the presence of obstructive jaundice underlies the term 'hepato-renal syndrome' introduced by Boyce and McFetridge (1935) to describe deaths due to renal failure following cholecystectomy. The heavily 'jaundiced kidney' is unduly susceptible to the effects of renal circulatory changes induced by anaesthesia and surgery. Other procedures not infrequently complicated by renal failure include prolonged heart surgery with cardio-pulmonary bypass, surgery of the abdominal aorta and extensive intra-abdominal procedures with a high risk of peritonitis. Acute post-surgical renal failure usually takes the form of potentially reversible ischaemic tubular necrosis; much more rarely, symmetrical cortical necrosis may occur carrying an unfavourable prognosis for significant recovery of renal function.

The kidneys together have a blood flow comparable to that of the liver, between 1,100 1,200 ml. per min., or 20–25 per cent of the total cardiac output. The final urine is the result of three processes, glomerular filtration, tubular reabsorption and tubular secretion. Final concentration of urine takes place in the distal tubule under the influence of antidiuretic hormone (ADH).

In assessing the effects of anaesthesia upon renal function, parameters customarily measured include urine volume and electrolyte content, glomerular filtration rate (GFR) based on renal clearance of either infused inulin or endogenous creatinine, and effective renal plasma flow (ERPF) measured by clearance of infused para-amino-hippurate. Blood urea is a relatively insensitive test of renal function; the level does not usually rise over the arbitrary maximum normal value of 45 mg per 100 ml until the GFR has falen bellow 30–40 ml per minute.

The effects of a number of pre-anaesthetic and anaesthetic agents upon renal function and haemodynamics have been studied in man with and without subsequent surgery, and the results are summarized below.

### Pethidine and Morphine

These drugs cause significant reduction of GFR and ERPF with diminished urine flow and increased urinary concentrations of sodium, potassium and chloride. The total electrolyte output is reduced despite increase in concentration. Reduction in potassium excretion parallels the fall in GFR while the excretion of sodium and chloride is disproportionately reduced (Habif *et al.*, 1951). The antidiuretic effect of pethidine and morphine occurring without increase in total solute excretion has been attributed to the observed fall in GFR and rate of solute excretion rather than to the release of ADH. Reduction in GFR and ERPF has in turn been interpreted as evidence of intra-renal vaso-constriction in the absence of any significant measured fall in systemic blood pressure.

### Atropine

Atropine may cause increased excretion of sodium without change in urine volume (Walker *et al.*, 1955).

### Promazine and Chlorpromazine

Both drugs cause diminished release of antidiuretic hormone with increased flow of a more dilute urine (Parrish and Levine, 1956).

### Cyclopropane

A sharp fall in GFR and ERPF and output of water and electrolytes occurs immediately or shortly after induction of anaesthesia with cyclopropane (Habif *et al.*, 1951). The fall in ERPF takes place despite a moderate rise in systemic arterial pressure, implying intra-renal vasoconstriction. Urine flow is considerably reduced, urinary concentration of infused inulin increases, but the concentrations of sodium and chloride fall to very low levels, indicating increased tubular reabsorption of water and electrolytes. In these studies, subsequent surgical procedures, often major in extent, appeared to have no additional effect upon renal haemodynamics. When cyclopropane administration is discontinued, GFR and ERPF return rapidly to control levels despite a fall in systemic blood pressure at this stage.

## Ether

The effect of ether anaesthesia upon renal haemodynamics is qualitatively similar but less profound (Habif *et al.*, 1951).

## Thiopentone

Similar changes occur in subjects anaesthetized with a thiopentone-nitrous oxide technique.

In patients receiving preliminary pethidine, the renal responses to cyclopropane, ether or thiopentone are not affected.

## Halothane

Halothane anaesthesia regularly causes a fall in urine flow, sodium excretion, GFR and ERPF (Mazze *et al.*, 1963). Measured changes in potassium excretion are inconstant. While a moderate fall in blood pressure is a feature of deep anaesthesia (delivered halothane concentration of 1·2–3 per cent) in these studies, the renal functional changes in both light (delivered concentration of 0·5–1 per cent) and deep anaesthesia are basically the same.

## Methoxyflurane

The renal effects of administration of this agent are discussed in a later section.

The remarkably constant changes in renal haemodynamics caused by each of the general anaesthetic agents have been attributed to renal vasoconstriction as part of a protective homeostatic mechanism to ensure adequate blood flow to brain and heart. This is supported by the observation of a simultaneous reduction in the splanchnic circulation as measured by effective hepatic blood flow using the bromsulphthalein method (Habif *et al.*, 1951). Miles and de Wardener (1952) showed direct evidence of renal vasoconstriction in dogs anaesthetized with ether and cyclopropane. The similarity of renal responses to different agents and their rapid resolution following cessation of anaesthesia may be taken as evidence against a *local* direct effect of a drug upon the renal circulation. A possible role of increased circulating catecholamines has been invoked in the case of ether and cyclopropane anaesthesia (Papper *et al.*, 1964) but it is known that halothane does not stimulate catecholamine release.

## Spinal Analgesia

The effect of spinal analgesia upon renal blood flow depends directly upon its effect on systemic blood pressure (Papper *et al.*, 1950).

## Clinical Significance of Anaesthetic-induced Changes in Renal Haemodynamics

Most patients undergoing anaesthesia and surgery suffer no ill effects from the renal circulatory changes described, and this is to be expected if the reserve renal function is good. In the elderly, however, where functional reserve is impaired and in those with established parenchymal renal disease, for example chronic glomerulonephritis or chronic pyelonephritis, a significant but usually temporary further rise in blood urea is often observed in the post-operative period. In such subjects an important factor in addition to anaesthetic-induced renal vasoconstriction is routine pre-operative restriction of fluid intake, an innocuous deprivation in those with normal kidneys but a well-recognized hazard to the patient with established renal disease.

The overall incidence of acute oliguric renal failure after surgery is low. In the majority of instances, it can be assumed that the kidneys were previously normal. 'Oliguria' in an adult implies a 24-hour urine output consistently below 400 ml., a much more severe reduction in volume than the 'normal post-operative' urinary suppression. The types of surgical procedure most prone to lead to this renal catastrophe have already been described and such factors as excessive prolongation of operation and anaesthesia, blood loss and hypoxia must contribute to a critical lowering of renal blood flow with resultant hypoxic or ischaemic changes seen in 'acute tubular necrosis'. The histological changes in the kidney occurring in post-operative acute renal failure do not differ from those seen in tubular necrosis from other causes such as septic abortion, myocardial infarction with severe hypotension and, multiple injuries with extensive skeletal muscle damage. The factor common to all of these is prolonged renal hypoxia or ischaemia. The renal lesion is potentially recoverable provided that the patient can be protected by conservative means and by dialysis, from the biochemical hazards of azotaemia, hyperkalaemia and metabolic acidosis, until diuresis supervenes. Conservative measures include severe restriction of fluid, sodium and potassium intake, moderate, rather than total, restriction of protein and early oral administration of an ion-exchange resin to prevent hyperkalaemia. Dialysis, either by the peritoneal route (if the surgical situation permits) or by an artificial kidney, is indicated when the blood urea has reached 200 mg. per 100 ml. or serum potassium has risen above 6 milli-equivalents per litre despite prophylactic resin. The duration of oliguria in post-surgical acute renal failure may be as long as 2–3 weeks.

While reduction of renal blood flow is almost certainly the *initial* insult leading to tubular necrosis, persistence of oliguria for a period of weeks thereafter is less readily explained. Renal blood flow returns to at least one third of normal, days or weeks, before diuresis occurs. Histological restoration of tubular epithelium on renal biopsy also occurs significantly earlier than the onset of diuresis. Persistent blockage of distal tubular lumina by casts derived from cellular débris, myoglobin (as in renal failure associated with muscle necrosis), or haemoglobin (as in renal failure due to intravascular haemolysis) may be an important factor delaying diuresis despite restoration of renal blood flow. In support of this is the abruptness and rapidity of diuresis when it occurs and the presence, on urine microscopy, at this time of unusually broad tubular casts, suggesting their origin in the distal nephron. These observations are relevant to the prophylactic administration of osmotic diuretics during surgery and anaesthesia to reduce the incidence of post-operative renal failure.

### Use of Intravenous Mannitol during Anaesthesia and Surgery

Hypertonic mannitol is a more effective osmotic diuretic than urea since none is reabsorbed by the renal tubules. There is considerable experimental evidence and increasing clinical enthusiasm for the beneficial effects of timely mannitol in preventing the development of 'organic' or parenchymal, as opposed to 'functional' or circulatory, renal failure in particularly dangerous surgical situations. Surgery of the abdominal aorta is extremely hazardous to the kidneys even when the aorta is clamped *below* the renal arteries, presumably due to reno-vascular spasm. The administration of a 20 per cent solution of mannitol intravenously to one group of patients undergoing abdominal aortic surgery has been shown to cause an increase in urine flow at all stages as compared with control patients who received no mannitol (Barry *et al.*, 1961). In addition, the treated subjects avoided the severe depression of renal plasma flow and glomerular filtration rate which regularly occurs when the aorta is clamped below the renal arteries. The protective effect of mannitol upon renal function and survival in the presence of obstructive jaundice in the rat has also been demonstrated (Dawson, 1964). Clinical experience supports the view that prophylactic mannitol reduces the renal hazard in patients undergoing surgery for obstructive jaundice.

The mechanism of action of mannitol in preventing renal damage during surgery is in dispute. It has been shown in experimental haemorrhagic hypotension in the dog or cat that 10–12 per cent mannitol is capable of preventing total anuria at very low levels of arterial blood pressure with corresponding gross reduction in glomerular filtration rate. In a further group of animals, mannitol (in a 30 per cent solution) was delayed until total anuria had developed and resulted in a significant recovery of urine flow with proportionately less improvement in glomerular filtration rate. It appears, therefore, that in haemorrhagic hypotension, mannitol restores glomerular filtration rate to some degree, possibly by reduction in afferent arteriolar vasoconstriction. The relatively greater increase in urine flow

compared with GFR may be a true manifestation of the osmotic diuretic action of mannitol (Peters and Brunner, 1963). Clinical experience has shown that mannitol is ineffective after renal failure has passed through the brief interval between 'functional' and 'organic' stages, marked by the development of histologically visible changes in the kidney. That mannitol may be of great value during this initial period has been emphasized by Barry and Malloy (1962) who advocate giving mannitol as an intravenous infusion of 12·5 G. in a 25 per cent solution over a 3-hour period to all patients up to 48 hours post-operatively where there is reduced urine flow and reduced urine concentration. If flow increases on this regime, a continuous infusion is indicated until diuresis is well established. The benefit of mannitol at this apparently late stage may lie in maintaining intra-luminal tubular volume and pressure, discouraging interstitial renal oedema and resultant tubular compression. In addition, the induced large urine flow may prevent the formation of casts and tubular blockage. The supposed effect of mannitol in reducing intra-renal vasoconstriction has been attributed to inhibition of renin release from the juxta-glomerular apparatus by the passage through the adjacent macula densa part of the renal tubule of urine of low sodium concentration, characteristic of an osmotic diuresis (Thurau, 1964).

Whatever its precise action the indications for prophylactic mannitol during anaesthesia for surgery of particular categories are clear. A careful trial up to 48 hours post-operatively in patients showing suppression of output and progressive decrease in osmolality is also justified.

### Nephrotoxic Effects of Anaesthetic Drugs

Evidence of serious nephrotoxicity due to anaesthetic agents is infrequent. Carbon tetrachloride is a well-recognized cause of severe but reversible acute renal failure due to a 'toxic' tubular necrosis and there have been occasional references to kidney damage from the clinically related compound chloroform. Barbiturates in overdosage may lead to acute renal failure from 'ischaemic' tubular necrosis resulting from a profound fall in systemic blood pressure.

Renal failure associated with muscle-necrosis and myoglobinuria complicating poisoning with a combination of alcohol and barbiturate has been reported; the muscle damage being due to pressure necrosis occurring in a neglected deeply comatose subject.

Acute renal failure has been described following an abnormal reaction to the depolarizing muscle relaxant succinylcholine (Bennike and Jarnum, 1964). A 29-year old male developed vigorous generalized muscle contractions immediately following the administration of 100 mg. of succinylcholine. Anaesthesia was terminated before any surgery could be attempted but blood urea rose sharply despite a moderately well-maintained urine volume, a finding not incompatible with a renal lesion of tubular necrosis type. The patient recovered and a history was later elicited of repeated episodes of painful swelling of the thighs since the age of 14 years. A muscle biopsy from the thigh showed acute severe degenerative changes. In retrospect this appears to have been a case of idiopathic paroxysmal myoglobinuria, a rare disease in which known precipitants of attacks include alcohol, barbiturates and exercise. Abnormal muscular reactions to succinylcholine have been the subject of several recent reports. The typical clinical picture is one of generalized severe muscle spasms beginning almost immediately after succinylcholine administration and of such severity that cessation of anaesthesia is always indicated. Affected subjects complain of muscle soreness for several days thereafter. Myoglobinuria has been demonstrated in most cases but this is usually a transitory finding.

Renal damage following abnormal reactions to succinylcholine is probably related to myoglobin excretion. Myoglobinuria from other causes is an established cause of acute oliguric renal failure where the characteristic histological feature is obstruction of the distal tubules by casts of myoglobin. In addition to the idiopathic paroxysmal type, myoglobinuria may result from trauma, McArdle's disease (deficiency of muscle glycogen phosphorylase) and anoxia from various causes, including carbon monoxide poisoning (Loughridge et al., 1958).

Abnormal reactions to succinylcholine have been described in two further primary muscle disorders, dystrophia myotonica and myotonia congenita. The effects of succinylcholine in thirteen patients with dystrophia myotonica and one patient with myotonia congenita were studied by Örndahl and Sternberg (1962) who showed that all the myotonic subjects exhibited a mechanical muscular response, more generalized in the dystrophia myotonica group. In dystrophia myotonica, myotonia may not appear clinically until the second or third decade but associated features of the disease may aid in its diagnosis at an earlier stage. These include a family history of either cataracts only or of the total syndrome in previous generations, and evidence of atrophy of the sternomastoid, facial and shoulder-girdle muscles, testicular or ovarian atrophy, cataracts and premature loss of scalp hair in the patient. In myotonia congenita, myotonia is present from early childhood and there are no associated clinical features. It is inherited as a Mendelian dominant. Muscle biopsies and electromyography may be helpful in diagnosis of the two conditions.

Patients who show prolonged muscle rigidity after succinylcholine should have their urine screened for the presence of myoglobin and if this is positive, prophylactic mannitol is indicated. Measurement of serum levels of creatine phosphokinase (Tammisto and Airaksinen, 1966) or creatine phosphokinase and aldolase (Genever, 1971) may give some indication of the extent of muscle damage in these patients. If renal failure does supervene, there is a particular hazard from a rapid rise in serum potassium in this as in other conditions where oliguria is associated with extensive skeletal muscle damage (Loughridge et al., 1958). The hazards of untoward hyperkalaemia occurring, in the absence of urinary suppression, after administration of succinylcholine to patients suffering from recent trauma, burns, tetanus and neuromuscular catastrophes such as

paraplegia have been emphasized (Mazze et al., 1969; Cooperman, 1970).

Of considerable current interest is the now well-established entity of nephrotoxicity due to the inhalational anaesthetic, methoxyflurane. Early reports of adverse renal effects of this agent (Artusio et al., 1960; Paddock et al., 1964) were soon followed by the emergence of a clear-cut clinical syndrome, that of nephrogenic, vasopressin-resistant diabetes insipidus, dehydration and azotaemia occurring usually within 24 hours of methoxyflurane anaesthesia. A significant mortality has been recorded and post-mortem examination of the kidneys has revealed a high incidence of oxalate crystals in large numbers within the lumina of renal tubules. In some patients, oliguria rather than polyuria has characterized the renal illness. Many reports have emphasized the factors of prolonged administration of methoxyflurane and obesity in the recipients, implying the probability of a dose-related phenomenon. Fever is not a characteristic feature of the illness, with the exception of a small number of patients in whom liver damage also occurred (Panner et al., 1970). In a prospective study of the problem of methoxyflurane toxicity Mazze et al. (1970) found a 50 per cent incidence of polyuria with increased serum sodium, serum osmolality, blood urea nitrogen, creatinine and uric acid in patients anaesthetized with methoxyflurane and oxygen. By contrast, Rosen et al. (1972), assessing the risks of self-administration of methoxyflurane during labour, found no evidence of renal complications at this relatively low dose.

While there remains no reasonable doubt that methoxyflurane in adequate amount can damage the kidneys, the precise mechanism of this reaction is less clear. Known metabolites of methoxyflurane include fluoride in both non-volatile organic and inorganic form, and probably oxalate. In relation to the latter, the demonstration of oxalate crystals in the renal tubules of fatal cases is of great interest but an unlikely explanation of the early polyuric phase of the renal illness. However, the amount of oxalate is far in excess of that not infrequently observed in other forms of renal failure, e.g. tubular necrosis (Macaluso and Berg, 1959; Aufderheide, 1971) and should, therefore, be considered an intrinsic part of methoxyflurane-mediated kidney damage. That fluoride may be responsible for vasopressin-resistant polyuria in these subjects is suggested by several observations. Mazze et al. (1970) found higher serum concentrations of fluoride in patients who developed polyuria following methoxyflurane administration than in those unaffected in this way. Taves et al. (1970) found increased inorganic fluoride levels in the blood 8 and 19 days after methoxyflurane anaesthesia in an obese patient who developed renal failure and in two others who had been exposed to the agent without consequence. Inorganic fluoride levels in the first patient were of a higher order than those reported by Goldemberg (1931) who produced a diabetes-insipidus like state in patients given repeated intravenous injections of 100 mg. sodium fluoride for the treatment of thyrotoxicosis. Kuzucu (1970) has suggested a synergistic role for tetracycline in methoxyflurane renal damage. A more probable explanation is that the degree of azotaemia is more severe in patients who have also received tetracycline as a result of its known depressive effect on protein anabolism. In summary, it seems likely that fluoride derived from metabolism of methoxyflurane may be toxic to the renal tubule cell resulting in polyuria resistant to vasopressin. The severity of *permanent* renal damage may well be related to the severity of intratubular oxalate deposition. From the practical point of view, methoxyflurane should be avoided in prolonged operative procedures, in the obese, and in patients with impaired renal function. Early haemodialysis in established cases may be of value as a means of removing both organic and inorganic fluoride, shown by Taves *et al.* (1970) to have comparable dialysance.

### Anaesthesia in Patients with Renal Disease

The problems of anaesthesia in the presence of renal disease are potentially greatest in patients with terminal chronic renal failure requiring a kidney graft. Renal reserve in such patients is negligible and they are dependent upon regular dialysis treatment to maintain life. The extent of the surgical programme is considerable and may involve bilateral nephrectomy and in some centres splenectomy before transplantation is undertaken. Two further clinical groups in which anaesthesia for therapeutic or diagnostic procedures may be necessary in the presence of impaired renal function are (1) patients with less advanced chronic disease undergoing surgery for calculous disease or enlargement of the prostate, and (2) patients with acute renal failure, particularly post-surgical or post-traumatic, where further emergency surgical procedures may become necessary. To some extent these last two groups present more acute problems to the anaesthetist for the patients are often less well prepared than are those on long-term regular dialysis awaiting kidney transplantation.

The particular hazards of anaesthesia in all these patients lie first in the general metabolic upset resulting from severe renal functional impairment and secondly in the failure of damaged kidneys to excrete anaesthetic drugs adequately. The main biochemical abnormalities to be considered are azotaemia, hyperkalaemia and metabolic acidosis, all of which are readily corrected by prior dialysis if time allows and facilities are available. Peritoneal dialysis, apart from its relative slowness, is adequate for this purpose in the absence of any local abdominal contraindication.

Uncontrolled *hyperkalaemia* predisposes to cardiac arrhythmias and cardiac arrest during anaesthesia particularly in the presence of associated metabolic acidosis, sodium or calcium deficiency. The harmful effects upon the heart of potassium retention correlate well with the serum level and the patient is at risk when this has risen above 6 milliequivalents per litre. While hyperkalaemia is most efficiently corrected by dialysis, in an emergency temporary lowering of the serum potassium may be achieved by the administration of intravenous glucose and insulin in the proportions of 50 G. glucose and 25 units of soluble insulin. The serum level falls as potassium

passes into cells, and the electrocardiographic changes of hyperkalaemia regress acutely. The risks of cardiotoxicity from a high potassium level in renal failure may be further lessened by the intravenous infusion of calcium, for example 20 ml. of a 20 per cent solution of calcium gluconate. Severe uncontrolled metabolic acidosis also predisposes to arrhythmias during anaesthesia. While this also is most safely corrected by dialysis, it may be necessary to give intravenous sodium bicarbonate to protect the heart in the presence of hyperkalaemia. Because of the considerable risk of overloading the uraemic subject with sodium and water, careful monitoring of the venous pressure is essential.

Other aspects of established *chronic* renal disease of importance for anaesthesia include anaemia and hypertension. *Anaemia*, due mainly to defective production by the damaged kidneys of the haemopoietic factor erythropoietin and in part to a haemolytic tendency, responds only to blood transfusion. Such replacement has two main dangers for these patients, namely fluid overload and excess potassium from stored blood, particularly in the presence of profound oliguria. These hazards may be overcome, however, if the blood is given during a preoperative dialysis. Further transfusion during surgery may be dictated by the very common abnormal bleeding tendency of uraemic subjects. It is widely accepted, however, that patients managed by chronic intermittent haemodialysis in preparation for kidney transplantation should receive the smallest possible number of blood units by transfusion. A particular hazard, to patients and staff alike, is that of transfer of the virus causing serum hepatitis; this risk can be minimized, however, by prior testing of all blood units for the presence of Australia (hepatitis-associated) antigen. A further argument for restriction of blood transfusion in prospective transplant recipients, is the risk of passive transfer of antibodies which may subsequently react with antigenic material in a grafted kidney. When transfusion becomes vital, this hazard can be minimized by administering only red blood cells, 'washed' to remove antibody-bearing leucocytes.

*Hypertension* due to excess renin release is an almost constant feature of advanced chronic renal disease. Not only may the actual level of blood pressure present problems to the anaesthetist but the precise nature of the antihypertensive drug chosen for its control may be of great relevance. Left ventricular hypertrophy and failure are the most significant complications of long-standing hypertension in relation to anaesthesia. Pulmonary oedema is readily corrected by prior dialysis against a hypertonic dialysate, though if this is too zealously pursued there is a risk of hypovolaemia threatening *hypotension* on induction of anaesthesia. These patients are usually also treated with digitalis which in the presence of renal failure may accumulate in the blood to levels which predispose to arrhythmias. Hypertension in renal disease usually responds to one of the oral anti-hypertensive drugs such as methyldopa, guanethidine or, if less severe, reserpine. In many instances it may be safe to discontinue treatment for a short period before surgery, but if not the anaesthetist must know which drug has been given so that any untoward change in the blood pressure during anaesthesia can be dealt with appropriately. For example, if a patient on reserpine develops undue hypotension during anaesthesia, nor-adrenaline may be required for its control. Other effects upon anaesthesia of the prior administration of anti-hypertensive drugs have been described (Miller *et al.*, 1968). Having observed that patients on methyldopa required lower halothane concentrations to maintain a given plane of anaesthesia they made a further study of the influence of this and other anti-hypertensive agents upon anaesthetic requirements in experimental animals. The prior administration of methyldopa or reserpine, both central nor-adrenaline depletors, was associated with reduced halothane requirement in dogs; halothane requirement was unaffected by guanethidine, known to have only a peripheral nor-adrenaline depleting effect. Rats given the anti-depressive amine-oxidase inhibitor iproniazid, known to *elevate* central nor-adrenaline content, showed an increase in cyclopropane requirement. These observations point to the importance of brain content of adrenaline and nor-adrenaline in determining individual requirement for general anaesthetic agents.

## Excretion of Anaesthetic Agents

Failure of damaged kidneys to excrete anaesthetic agents is of particular importance in the case of the non-depolarizing muscle relaxants. Abnormal post-operative prolongation of muscle paresis after gallamine triethiodide in patients with poor renal function has been reported. In the patient described by Feldman and Levi (1963) assisted respiration was required for 5 days and respiratory activity did not return to normal until a haemodialysis was performed. Prolonged muscle paresis after gallamine has been reported in three out of five patients undergoing bilateral nephrectomy prior to transplantation (Churchill–Davidson *et al.*, 1967). Insignificant prolongation of paralysis occurred in six nephrectomized subjects who received d-tubocurarine. Post-anaesthetic problems with d-tubocurarine in renal transplantation have been reported in two patients (Katz *et al.*, 1967). The clinical impression that gallamine is the more dangerous of the two drugs in the presence of renal failure is supported by experimental observations in the dog. It has been shown, using tritiated d-tubocurarine, that when the renal pedicles are tied biliary excretion of the drug is markedly increased, accounting for more than 38 per cent of the dose (Cohen *et al.*, 1967). Such an alternative pathway for excretion is apparently not available to gallamine triethiodide which in the dog is excreted in the bile in negligible quantities after renal pedicle ligation (Feldman *et al.*, 1969). It seems clear, therefore, that gallamine triethiodide should be avoided in patients with renal failure; where a muscle relaxant of this group is necessary, d-tubocurarine is permissible but the patients require careful post-operative supervision. There is no contra-indication to the use of succinylcholine since only 2 per cent of the drug is normally excreted in the urine, the remainder being metabolized.

Apart from avoidance of methoxyflurane, as already discussed, the choice of inhalational anaesthetic is little affected by renal dysfunction. Strunin (1966) advises halothane for transplantation surgery, using concentrations of 1–1·5 per cent to avoid undue hypotension. Arrhythmias are more likely to occur with cyclopropane anaesthesia, particularly in uraemia. Spinal anaesthesia for transplant recipients was used by Vandam *et al.* (1962) to avoid the need for relaxants, and hypotension was not a problem. The role of mannitol during transplantation surgery is not yet clearly established but it is likely to be of most value in diminishing the effects of ischaemia upon kidneys removed from cadaver donors.

The selection of drugs for pre-medication in uraemic subjects is influenced mainly by avoidance of undue hypotension. It should be remembered, moreover, that some patients with chronic renal failure are receiving anti-depressant drugs of amine-oxidase inhibitor type and are, therefore, at risk from abnormal reactions to either pethidine or morphine.

Prolongation of the anaesthetic effects of thiopentone in patients with azotaemia has been observed (Dundee and Richards, 1954). The role of the normal kidney in the excretion of *long* and *medium*-acting barbiturate drugs and the management of overdosage by forced diuresis are well reviewed by Linton *et al.* (1967) Mawer and Lee (1968). In the presence of renal failure, removal of the drugs by dialysis may become imperative.

## REFERENCES

Artusio, J. F., Jr., Van Posnak, A., Hunt, R. E., Tiers, F. M. and Alexander, M. (1960), "A Clinical Evaluation of Methoxyflurane in Man," *Anesthesiology*, **21**, 512.

Aufderheide, A. C. (1971), "Renal Tubular Calcium Oxalate Crystal Deposition; its Possible Relation to Methoxyflurane Anaesthesia," *Arch. Path.*, **92**, 162.

Barry, K. G., Cohen, A., Knochel, J. P., Whelan, T. J., Beisel, W. R., Vargas, C. A. and Leblanc, P. C. (1961), "Mannitol Infusion. II. The Prevention of Acute Functional Renal Failure During Resection of an Aneurysm of the Abdominal Aorta," *New Engl. J. Med.*, **264**, 967.

Barry, K. G. and Malloy, J. P. (1962), "Oliguric Renal Failure. Evaluation and Therapy by the Intravenous Infusion of Mannitol," *J. Amer. med. Ass.*, **179**, 510.

Bennike, K. and Jarnum, S. (1964), "Myoglobinuria with Acute Renal Failure Possibly Induced by Suxamethonium," *Brit. J. Anaesth.*, **36**, 730.

Boyce, F. J. and McFetridge, E. M. (1935), "So-called 'Liver Death'. A Clinical and Experimental Study," *Arch. Surg.*, **31**, 105.

Churchill-Davidson, H. C., Way, W. L. and de Jong, R. H. (1967), "The Muscle Relaxants and Renal Excretion," *Anesthesiology*, **28**, 540.

Cohen, E. N., Brewer, W. M. and Smith, D. (1967), "The Metabolism and Elimination of d-Tubocurarine H³," *Anesthesiology*, **28**, 309.

Cooperman, L. H. (1970), "Succinylcholine-induced Hyperkalaemia in Neuromuscular Disease," *J. Amer. med. Ass.*, **213**, 1867.

Dawson, J. L. (1964), "Jaundice and Anoxic Renal Damage: Protective Effect of Mannitol," *Brit. med. J.*, **1**, 810.

Dundee, J. W. and Richards, R. K. (1954), "Effect of Azotemia Upon the Action of Intravenous Barbiturate Anesthesia," *Anesthesiology*, **15**, 333.

Feldman, S. A., Cohen, E. N. and Golling, R. C. (1969), "The Excretion of Gallamine in the Dog," *Anesthesiology*, **30**, 593.

Feldman, S. A. and Levi, A. J. (1963), "Prolonged Paresis Following Gallamine," *Brit. J. Anaesth.*, **35**, 804.

Genever, E. E. (1971), "Suxamethonium-induced Cardiac Arrest in Unsuspected Pseudohypertrophic Muscular Dystrophy," *Brit. J. Anaesth.*, **43**, 984.

Goldemberg, L. (1931), "Tratamiento de la enfermedad de Basedow 'y del hipertiroidismo por fluor," *Rev. Soc. Med. Int. Soc. Tisiol.*, **6**, 217.

Habif, D. V., Papper, E. M., Fitzpatrick, H. F., Lowrance, P., Smythe, C. Mc. C. and Bradley, S. E. (1951), "The Renal and Hepatic Blood Flow, Glomerular Filtration Rate and Urinary Output of Electrolytes During Cyclopropane, Ether and Thiopental Anesthesia, Operation and the Immediate Post-operative Period," *Surgery*, **30**, 241.

Katz, J., Kountz, S. L. and Cohn, R. (1967), "Anesthetic Considerations for Renal Transplant," *Anesthesia and Analgesia Current Researches*, **46**, 609.

Kuzucu, E. Y. (1970), "Methoxyflurane, Tetracycline and Renal Failure," *J. Amer. med. Ass.*, **211**, 1162.

Linton, A. L., Luke, R. G. and Briggs, J. D. (1967), "Methods of Forced Diuresis and its Application in Barbiturate Poisoning," *Lancet*, **ii**, 377.

Loughridge, L. W., Leader, L. P. and Bowen, D. A. L. (1958), "Acute Renal Failure Due to Muscle Necrosis in Carbon-monoxide Poisoning," *Lancet*, **ii**, 349.

Macaluso, M. P. and Berg, N. O. (1959), "Calcium Oxalate Crystals in Kidneys in Acute Tubular Necrosis and Other Renal Diseases with Functional Failure," *Acta path. microbiol. scand.*, **46**, 197.

Mawer, G. E. and Lee, H. A. (1968), "Value of Forced Diuresis in Acute Barbiturate Poisoning," *Brit. med. J.*, **2**, 790.

Mazze, R. I., Escue, H. M. and Houston, J. B. (1969), "Hyperkalaemia and Cardiovascular Collapse Following Administration of Succinylcholine to the Traumatised Patient," *Anesthesiology*, **31**, 540.

Mazze, R. I., Schwartz, F. D., Slocum, H. C. and Barry, K. G. (1963), "Renal Function During Anaesthesia and Surgery. 1. The Effects of Halothane Anesthesia," *Anesthesiology*, **24**, 279.

Mazze, R. I., Shue, G. L. and Jackson, S. H. (1971), "Renal Dysfunction Associated with Methoxyflurane Anaesthesia," *J. Amer. med. Ass.*, **216**, 278.

Miles, B. E. and de Wardener, H. E. (1952), "Renal Vasoconstriction Produced by Ether and Cyclopropane," *J. Physiol.*, **118**, 140.

Miller, R. D., Way, W. L. and Eger, E. I. (1968), "The Effects of Alpha-methyldopa, Reserpine, Guanethidine, and Iproniazid on Minimum Alveolar Anaesthetic Requirement," *Anesthesiology*, **29**, 1153.

Örndahl, F. and Stenberg, K. (1962), "Myotonic Human Musculature: Stimulation with Depolarising Agents," *Acta med. scand.*, **172**, suppl. 389.

Paddock, R. B., Parker, J. W. and Guadagni, N. P. (1964), "The Effects of Methoxyflurane on Renal Function," *Anesthesiology*, **25**, 707.

Panner, B. J., Freeman, R. B., Roth-Moyo, L. A. and Markowitch, W. (1970), "Toxicity Following Methoxyflurane Anesthesia. I. Clinical and Pathological Observations in Two Fatal Cases," *J. Amer. med. Ass.*, **214**, 86.

Papper, E. M., Habif, D. V. and Bradley, S. E. (1950), "Studies of Renal and Hepatic Function in Normal Man During Thiopental, Cyclopropane and High Spinal Anesthesia," *J. clin. Invest.*, **29**, 838.

Parrish, A. E. and Levine, F. H. (1956), "Chlorpromazine-induced Diuresis," *J. Lab. clin. Med.*, **48**, 264.

Peters, G. and Brunner, H. (1963), "Mannitol Diuresis in Hemorrhagic Hypotension," *Amer. J. Physiol.*, **204**, 555.

Rosen, M., Latto, P. and Asscher, A. W. (1972), "Kidney Function After Methoxyflurane Analgesia During Labour," *Brit. med. J.*, **i**, 81.

Strunin, L. (1966), "Some Aspects of Anaesthesia for Renal Homotransplantation," *Brit. J. Anaesth.*, **38**, 812.

Tammisto, T. and Airaksinen, M. M. (1966), "Increase of Creatine Kinase Activity in Serum as Sign of Muscular Injury Caused by Intermittently Administered Suxamethonium During Halothane Anaesthesia," *Brit. J. Anaesth.*, **38**, 510.

Taves, D. R., Fry, B. W., Freeman, R. B. and Gillies, A. J. (1970), "Toxicity Following Methoxyflurane Anesthesia. II. Fluoride Concentrations in Nephrotoxicity," *J. Amer. med. Ass.*, **214**, 91.

Taves, D. R., Gillies, A. J., Freeman, R. B. and Fry, B. W. (1970), "Toxicity Following Methoxyflurane Anaesthesia. III. Haemodialysis of Metabolites," *J. Amer. med. Ass.*, **214**, 96.

Thurau, K. (1964), "Renal Hemodynamics," *Amer. J. Med.*, **36**, 698.

Vandam, L. D., Harrison, J. H., Murray, J. E. and Merrill, J. P. (1962), "Anesthetic Aspects of Renal Homotransplantation in Man—With Notes on the Anesthetic Care of the Uremic Patient," *Anesthesiology*, **23**, 783.

Walker, E. H., Parker, J. M. and Hunter, J. (1955), "The Effect of Atropine Sulphate on Blood and Urine Electrolytes in Man," *Canad. J. Biochem. and Physiol.*, **33**, 256.

# CHAPTER 2

# ANAESTHESIA AND THE LIVER

## LAVINIA LOUGHRIDGE

The incidence and severity of hepatic damage from anoxia during anaesthesia have almost certainly been underestimated. While clinical jaundice in the post-operative period is uncommon, more sensitive indices of acute hepatocellular damage such as serum enzyme levels are not routinely measured. The need for accuracy in assessing the normal pattern of post-operative, post-anaesthetic liver injury has been emphasized by the controversy which surrounds the role of halothane in the occasional incidence of severe liver necrosis. The vulnerability of the liver to anoxia during anaesthesia is in part explained by the fact that 80 per cent of its blood supply is accounted for by the portal vein and only 20 per cent by the hepatic artery.

It is proposed to discuss the effects of anaesthesia upon hepatic haemodynamics in the normal, hepatic toxicity of anaesthetic agents and the chemical, biochemical and pharmacological problems of anaesthesia in established parenchymal disease of the liver.

## Effects of Anaesthesia on the Normal Liver

Blood flow to the liver in normal man averages 1,000–1,200 millilitres per minute, of which less than one quarter is supplied by the hepatic artery. Methods used to measure hepatic blood flow during anaesthesia include bromsulphthalein (B.S.P.) clearance, tagged colloidal chromic phosphate clearance and clearance of the dye indocyanine green.

## Cyclopropane

Cyclopropane anaesthesia causes a profound fall in hepatic blood flow measured by either B.S.P. or colloidal chromic phosphate clearance. In order to eliminate other possible factors such as surgical manipulation, hypoxia or hypercapnia, the effects of anaesthesia with this agent without subsequent surgery were observed in 10 normal adult males, using indocyanine green clearance to measure hepatic flow (Price et al., 1965). Arterial blood $P_{CO_2}$ and $P_{O_2}$ were monitored and did not deviate significantly from their levels when the subjects were conscious. Increased splanchnic vascular resistance and diminished splanchnic blood flow were demonstrated despite an increase in systemic arterial pressure. The subsequent intravenous injection of 10-12 milligrammes of hexamethonium reversed the changes in splanchnic resistance and flow, indicating that cyclopropane anaesthesia is associated with increased sympathetic tone in the splanchnic area. Reduction in splanchnic oxygen uptake during cyclopropane anaesthesia, comparable in extent to the fall in hepatic blood flow was demonstrated by Shackman et al., 1953. This observation was not confirmed in normal adults subjected to cyclopropane anaesthesia without surgery (Price et al., 1966).

## Thiopentone

Observations on the effects of thiopentone anaesthesia on hepatic haemodynamics are conflicting. Patients anaesthetized with thiopentone plus nitrous oxide and succinylcholine showed no change in hepatic flow as measured by B.S.P. clearance. The same anaesthetic combination caused a significant reduction in liver blood flow measured by colloidal chromic phosphate though less in extent than with thiopentone alone (Levy et al., 1961).

## Halothane

Halothane anaesthesia in normal adults without subsequent surgery causes a fall in splanchnic blood flow without significant change in vascular resistance (Epstein et al., 1966). In these studies the expected fall in systemic arterial pressure associated with halothane anaesthesia occurred. Observations were repeated in five subjects during a period of induced hypercapnia which resulted in an increase in hepatic blood flow with reduction in splanchnic vascular resistance. It is concluded that halothane abolishes the customary splanchnic vasoconstriction induced by carbon dioxide. In contrast to cyclopropane, halothane depresses sympathetic activity in the splanchnic region. The fall in hepatic blood flow is comparable in degree to that caused by cyclopropane. No significant change in splanchnic oxygen utilization during halothane anaesthesia has been demonstrated. In summary, there is no evidence that halothane anaesthesia is potentially more dangerous than other agents in respect of changes in either hepatic blood flow or oxygen consumption.

## Ether

Ether anaesthesia causes no consistent change in hepatic haemodynamics (Levy et al., 1961).

## Spinal Anaesthesia

High spinal anaesthesia causes a reduction in hepatic blood flow. These changes in hepatic haemodynamics induced by anaesthetic agents are of little clinical significance in patients with healthy liver parenchymal cells and normal blood supply. They are almost certainly of the greatest importance in determining the profound deterioration in liver function which regularly follows anaesthesia and surgery in established liver disease, either chronic as in cirrhosis or acute as in viral hepatitis.

## Hepatotoxic Effects of Anaesthetic Drugs

The overall incidence of hepatic dysfunction after anaesthesia is low and with the exception of chloroform, which appears to damage the liver by a direct action accelerated by both anoxia and hypercarbia, anaesthetic drugs present remarkably little direct risk to the liver cell. In rare instances, however, liver damage of all grades of severity has been reported to follow administration of the majority of general anaesthetic agents, for example cyclopropane, ether, nitrous oxide, trichlorethylene, methoxyflurane and halothane. Before accepting that an anaesthetic agent is responsible, it is necessary first to exclude other possible contributory factors which include (1) latent chronic liver disease such as cirrhosis made clinically apparent by nonspecific hepatic haemodynamic changes of anaesthesia, (2) coincidental damage from other drugs such as tetracycline, phenothiazines and amine oxidase inhibitors, (3) effects of severe shock with hypotension during surgery and anaesthesia, (4) haemolysis due to transfusion incompatibility, and (5) the possibility that the patient was already harbouring a virus of infective or serum hepatitis.

These considerations have been involved in the controversy which surrounds the question of halothane liver damage. Because of its structural resemblance to a known hepatotoxin, carbon tetrachloride, halothane was subjected to the most stringent laboratory tests before its introduction to clinical anaesthesia. No evidence of liver toxicity was found. This fact and its proven value as an anaesthetic agent, otherwise free from significant side-effects, explain the reluctance to accept halothane as a serious risk to the liver. It is proposed to discuss the types of liver damage known to result from certain drugs and poisons and to present the evidence for and against halothane toxicity in a later section.

The types of hepatic injury caused by drugs, including anaesthetic agents, have been classified as follows (Sherlock, 1967).

1. Interference with the binding of serum bilirubin to albumin, e.g. sulphonamides given to premature infants with the risk of kernicterus occurring at relatively low serum bilirubin levels.

2. Interference with hepatocellular bilirubin metabolism,

e.g. novobiocin-induced jaundice in the neonate and increased serum bilirubin (usually not clinically evident) in many subjects given cholecystographic media. This latter may be of importance if such are operated upon immediately following these investigations, when the additional factor of hepatic circulatory impairment induced by anaesthesia may lead to clinical jaundice postoperatively.

3. Steroid-induced cholestasis, e.g. methyltestosterone liver damage. This reaction does not involve sensitivity and all subjects given the drug over a long period will show evidence of disturbed liver function such as abnormal retention of bromsulphthalein.

4. Sensitivity-type cholestasis—well represented by the phenothiazine group of drugs, particularly chlorpromazine. This reaction occurs only in susceptible individuals and is independent of dose. Jaundice appears 1–4 weeks after administration or at once if there has been previous exposure. Recovery is usually complete but may take several weeks or months. The incidence of chlorpromazine sensitivity is less than 0·5 per cent. The possibility of an underlying genetic basis is suggested by the observation that chlorpromazine-induced jaundice has occurred in 3 members of 2 generations of the same family. Other manifestations of hypersensitivity including rash, fever, eosinophilia, are sometimes present.

5. Sensitivity-type hepatic reaction, exemplified by liver damage caused by the amine-oxidase inhibitor iproniazid. The clinical and pathological features are indistinguishable from virus hepatitis. The liver shows diffuse rather than zonal necrosis (the same change as occurs with liver toxins such as chloroform). There is a high mortality in the region of 50 per cent. In the absence of precise methods of virological diagnosis, the possibility of virus hepatitis will enter into the differential diagnosis where a drug is suspected of causing liver damage of this type. It is into this clinical and histological group that the suspected cases of 'halothane jaundice' fall and the evidence is discussed below.

6. Direct liver injury, e.g. cytotoxic agents such as 6-mercaptopurine, intravenous tetracycline in high dosage, tannic acid (formerly used in the treatment of burns and formerly included in barium sulphate enemata), carbon tetrachloride and chloroform. The hepatic lesion from these agents is a zonal hepato-cellular necrosis, most severe at the centre of the hepatic lobule and, unlike 'hepatitis', showing little inflammatory reaction.

From the anaesthetist's point of view, the hepatotoxic risk of chloroform, and that of chlorpromazine in a very small susceptible percentage of the community are accepted. Despite many reports of severe, often fatal, hepatic damage following exposure to halothane, absolute proof of its involvement has been remarkably difficult to establish. While it remains possible that, on occasion, halothane has been implicated in error as the cause of post-operative, post-anaesthetic liver damage, the fact that halothane-induced liver damage *can* occur seems incontrovertible. The most frequent source of confusion concerning jaundice in the early post-operative period is almost certainly latent viral hepatitis. Sensitive methods for detecting hepatitis-associated (Australia) antigen will help to exclude serum hepatitis (virus B or long-incubation type hepatitis). A reliable test for infective (virus A or short-incubation type hepatitis) would be of considerable value in this and many other clinical situations. Search for a test diagnostic of hepatic damage induced by halothane continues. Detection of mitochondrial antibodies in the sera of individuals believed to be suffering from halothane-mediated liver damage may prove to be valuable. Studies of lymphocyte transformation used as evidence of a cell-mediated hypersensitivity response, such as might occur with drug sensitivity, have proved controversial in the case of halothane (Paronetto and Popper, 1970; Bruce and Raymon, 1972; Walton et al., 1972). Nor is there agreement upon the existence of diagnostic histological findings in the liver either on biopsy or at autopsy in fatal cases. Mitochondrial abnormalities not seen in viral hepatitis have been described on electron-microscopy of liver sections by Klion et al., 1969. However, even in the absence of a reliable diagnostic test, the weight of evidence is such as to render impractical any effort to achieve on behalf of halothane total exoneration from blame.

Amongst the most convincing *clinical* reports of halothane-mediated liver damage, have been those affecting anaesthetists repeatedly exposed to the agent in low dosage during the course of their work. Belfrage et al. (1966) gave details of a 33-year-old male anaesthetist who experienced a hepatitis-like illness with eosinophilia after 3½ months occupational exposure to halothane. All evidence of hepatic dysfunction subsided within 6–8 weeks but eosinophilia persisted. At this time, he was intentionally re-exposed to halothane and after 5 hours became ill with pyrexia, elevated serum transaminases, sub-clinical icterus, abnormal bromsulphthalein retention and a further increase in eosinophilia. Liver biopsy was unsuccessful; liver function tests returned to normal within 3 weeks. A further instance of professional exposure to halothane was that reported by Klatskin and Kimberg (1969) in which a 44-year-old male anaesthetist developed repeated hepatitis-like episodes during the course of his work. An identical episode followed within 4 hours of an intentional halothane challenge after a period away from all contact with the drug. Liver biopsy performed 4 years after the first illness was interpreted as showing early 'post-hepatitic' cirrhosis. Tygstrup (1963) had earlier described an impressive case history of a 54-year-old female patient who had had three separate exposures to halothane. The first was unremarkable but the second was followed by fever, abdominal pain and jaundice subsiding within a few weeks. Two years later the patient was given halothane for the third time and within 8 hours developed fever, diarrhoea, jaundice and hepatomegaly. Liver biopsies during both illnesses showed inflammatory changes indistinguishable from those of moderately severe virus hepatitis. The report of the National Halothane Study published in 1966 analysed retrospective clinical and pathological data from 82 patients who suffered post-operative fatal massive hepatic necrosis within 6 weeks out of a total of 856,500 anaesthetized subjects from 34 centres in the U.S.A. In nine of the 82 cases, hepatic necrosis could not be attributed to shock, previous liver disease or any other recognized cause. Seven of these nine patients had received halothane, and four had had more than one exposure. Liver histology in these cases resembled that of virus hepatitis, suggesting a drug-induced sensitivity-type of hepatitis if halothane was, in fact, the cause. If halothane was to blame, the incidence of the reaction was clearly very low, a finding in keeping with a drug reaction affecting susceptible individuals only.

The distinctive features of 'hepatitis' occurring in 41 patients after halothane anaesthesia and without other obvious cause have been summarized (Klatskin, 1968). In more than two-thirds of these cases, hepatic damage followed multiple exposures to halothane consistent with the development of sensitization. One third of these patients had experienced an unexplained bout of fever following an earlier exposure. All 7 patients who were re-exposed to halothane after recovery had a recurrence of hepatic illness. The average time interval between a single exposure and the subsequent onset of hepatitis was 6·5 days, much later than would be expected from either ischaemic damage or the effect of a direct liver poison. The longest time interval in these cases was 12 days, very much shorter than the incubation period of hepatitis virus acquired at the time of surgery. The possibility of a latent, previously acquired, viral hepatitis presenting within the narrow time interval after surgery is less likely. The average time interval for the onset of hepatitis after multiple exposures was halved, i.e. 3 days, an observation very much in favour of hepatic sensitization and closely resembling chlorpromazine jaundice in this respect. Clinical features atypical of viral hepatitis included high fever, rigors, rashes, leucocytosis and eosinophilia which was found in 40 per cent of those patients in whom a differential white cell count was made. The remarkably high mortality of 50 per cent is very unlike viral hepatitis but approximates very closely to the reported mortality from sensitivity-type hepatitis due to iproniazid.

Possible mechanisms of halothane-mediated liver damage have been widely discussed. There is general agreement that halothane is unlikely to be responsible for a direct hepatotoxic effect and that an idiosyncrasy, probably to a metabolite of the drug, must be involved. It has been suggested that trifluoroacetate, a chemically reactive compound to which a small proportion of inhaled halothane is normally metabolized by hepatic enzymes, may be responsible for the severe hepatic cell damage that can occur in susceptible individuals (Blake et al., 1972; Cohen, 1971).

In conclusion, there seems little doubt that acceptance of halothane as a *rare* cause of liver injury is inevitable. To abandon the use of halothane, a much valued anaesthetic, on these grounds would seem unreasonable. Certain restrictions upon its use have however been suggested. These include avoidance where possible for planned procedures involving short-interval anaesthesia. Halothane should of course be avoided where a previous episode of jaundice following administration has been observed. Assessment of fever following a previous exposure is more difficult, since this is a relatively common finding in the early post-operative period. Any other manifestation of sensitivity, such as rashes or eosinophilia after halothane should be regarded with suspicion. A reliable diagnostic or predictive test would be of the utmost importance. It has been observed that methoxyflurane, a closely related chemical compound, may provoke a serious reaction in individuals previously sensitized to halothane (Lindenbaum and Leifer, 1963). The example of halothane should prove valuable in future assessment of the significance of reported drug-induced liver damage. Methods used to treat patients with fulminant hepatic damage of this type have included haemodialysis and exchange transfusion, and of these exchange transfusion would appear to offer some chance of benefit in an otherwise desperate clinical situation.

**Anaesthesia in Patients with Liver Disease**

The problems of anaesthesia in the presence of liver disease are in some respects more complex than those of uraemia. In the first place, there is no equivalent of dialysis for the temporary pre-operative correction of the metabolic disturbance of hepato-cellular failure. Secondly, the customary haemodynamic effects of anaesthesia are more hazardous to the diseased liver parenchyma than to the damaged kidney. The greater vulnerability of the liver to anoxia may be due in part to the normally low oxygen content of its major blood supply, the portal vein. Portal cirrhosis, the most important form of chronic diffuse liver disease, leads to progressive failure of the numerous metabolic functions of the liver cells while the associated distortion of the intra-hepatic vasculature causes portal hypertension with all its complications. From the anaesthetist's point of view, failure of the damaged liver to synthesize prothrombin and other clotting factors leading to excessive bleeding during surgery, and defective metabolism of anaesthetic drugs are the most important aspects of advanced liver cell failure. It should be remembered that jaundice in cirrhosis, in contrast to biliary tract obstruction is a late clinical sign and a significant number of latent cirrhotics first come to light post-operatively as a result of temporary impairment of bilirubin metabolism, precipitated by anoxia during anaesthesia and surgery for unrelated conditions.

Defective coagulation due to liver cell failure is of particular importance during surgery for bleeding oesophageal varices. The precise mechanisms of impaired clotting in liver disease are more clearly defined than those of uraemia. They include failure of hepatic synthesis of prothrombin and factors V, VII, IX and X and inadequate vitamin K absorption from the intestine due to defective bile salt secretion. In addition, there may be thrombocytopenia associated with the enlarged spleen of portal hypertension. Where the prothrombin time is prolonged in liver disease, intramuscular vitamin $K_1$, 10 mg. daily, for several pre-operative days may correct it. In severe hepatocellular failure, prolongation of prothrombin time will persist and surgery is most hazardous. Prothrombin and factors VII, IX and X are well preserved in banked blood (Sherlock, 1968) while thrombocytopenia and factor V deficiency may be temporarily relieved by transfusion of fresh blood. Increased circulating fibrinolysins, causing reduction in the blood fibrinogen level, are an important factor in operative and post-operative haemorrhage in patients with liver disease. This defect can be corrected by fresh blood transfusion, by fibrinogen infusion or by intravenous epsilon-aminocaproic acid. Such treatment, however, may result in a converse tendency to excessive clotting which has been responsible for post-operative deaths from thrombosis, particularly in patients who have undergone liver transplantation.

The specific coagulation defects of liver disease make their contribution to the already massive blood transfusion requirements of patients undergoing surgery for bleeding varices. The many hazards of transfusing large volumes of stored blood have been reviewed (Bunker, 1966). These include citrate intoxication causing a fall in ionized calcium with potential hazards to the myocardium and to clotting efficiency, hypothermia from inadequate rewarming of large volumes of refrigerated blood and change in acid-base balance, initially a metabolic acidosis due to a dilutional fall in serum bicarbonate and ultimately, following metabolism of the citrate, a metabolic alkalosis.

The cirrhotic patient bleeding from oesophageal varices is already at grave risk of portal-systemic encephalopathy or actual coma and the effects of surgery and anaesthesia may be sufficient to tip the balance. Porto-caval anastomosis further reduces the blood supply to the damaged liver and permits potentially toxic nitrogenous compounds to pass directly into the systemic veins. If liver function is critically depressed, encephalopathy will develop acutely in the post-operative period and may persist in a chronic form. For this reason some evidence of hepato-cellular reserve is essential before porto-caval shunt can be contemplated. Reduction of serum albumin below a critical level of 2·5–3 G. per 100 ml. should be regarded as a contra-indication to such surgery. The mortality of porto-caval anastomosis undertaken as an emergency procedure is 40–60 per cent compared with 6–10 per cent for the same operation performed electively when the patient is not actively bleeding. If conservative measures to control haemorrhage including blood transfusion, direct compression by the Sengstaken gastro-oesophageal tube and intravenous vasopressin to constrict the splanchnic arteriolar bed, have failed, the operation of choice for the acute stage of bleeding is direct ligation of the varices via a trans-thoracic approach to the oesophagus.

The precise toxin or toxins involved in hepatic encephalopathy are uncertain but the most consistent abnormality to date is a raised blood ammonia level. Correlation between depression of consciousness and ammonia level is not invariably close, however, and some other product or products of protein metabolism normally transformed by the liver may be responsible. The acute management of post-operative portal-systemic encephalopathy includes total dietary protein restriction, provision of adequate calories by intravenous glucose, avoidance of hypokalaemia, control of intercurrent infection and suppression of the normal bowel flora by oral Neomycin to control the breakdown of protein products by intestinal bacteria, thus reducing absorption of ammonia and other potential toxins.

The problems of anaesthesia and surgery in obstructive jaundice include haemorrhage due to defective vitamin K absorption and such patients should receive routine pre-operative vitamin $K_1$. The risks of post-operative acute renal failure in the deeply jaundiced patient are described in the chapter on Anaesthesia and the Kidneys (p. 319), and the need for prophylactic mannitol during such surgery is emphasized. The problem of determining the site of obstruction, whether intra- or extra-hepatic, may lead to laparotomy in an occasional case of acute viral hepatitis of the so-called 'cholestatic' type with subsequent profound deterioration in liver cell function resulting from the effects of anaesthesia and surgery.

The technical, administrative and immunological problems of liver transplantation are vast. From the anaesthetist's point of view, coagulation defects causing undue blood loss and occasional hypercoagulability may be troublesome. In 'orthotopic' liver transplantation, the graft is placed in the normal hepatic bed requiring prior removal of the recipient's liver. For a period during surgery, such patients are totally without functioning liver tissue. 'Heterotopic' transplants present their own problems of adequate biliary drainage and suitable vascular anastomoses. The most suitable recipients of liver grafts are patients with biliary atresia or localized primary hepatic tumours rather than cirrhotics who have reached a terminal stage with long-standing complex metabolic disturbance.

The selection of anaesthetic drugs in patients with liver disease is important. The normal liver is responsible for the metabolism of morphine, pethidine, thiopentone, local anaesthetic agents and atropine. Hepatic transformation of morphine is largely dependent on conjugation with glucuronic acid, synthesis of which by the liver cell is impaired early in liver disease. Morphine is, therefore, strongly contra-indicated in the routine management and premedication of patients with liver disease. Pethidine is normally hydrolysed and also demethylated by the liver and its use is inadvisable in the presence of hepatic dysfunction. Atropine is largely hydrolysed by the liver, but in normal doses may be given for pre-medication in combination with a phenothiazine. Barbitone or phenobarbitone, normally excreted by the kidneys, are valuable in the clinical management of the restless cirrhotic patient. Chlordiazepoxide (Librium) may have a place in pre-medication for surgery in these patients. Paraldehyde should be avoided since it is partially transformed by the normal liver.

There is little evidence that thiopentone is unduly hazardous in patients with hepatic disease. The liver normally metabolizes thiopentone very slowly and its 'short action' is due to rapid redistribution throughout the body tissues, related to its high lipid solubility. Less than 1 per cent is excreted unchanged by the kidneys. It is advisable, however, to avoid excessive dosage particularly in the hypovolaemic cirrhotic who has recently bled.

Succinylcholine is normally hydrolysed by plasma pseudocholinesterases. In severe liver disease prolonged apnoea may occur due to impaired production by the liver cell of normal pseudocholinesterases. The hazards of succinylcholine in homozygotes for the production of abnormal pseudocholinesterases are well recognized; the heterozygote may also be at risk if hepatic production of normal pseudocholinesterases is impaired by coincidental chronic liver disease. The incidence of such heterozygotes in the population of Canada has been estimated at 3·8 per cent (Kalow and Gunn, 1959), the homozygous condition occurring in only 1 in 2,800 of the same population. The use of minimal doses and careful observation in the post-operative period are indicated when succinylcholine is used in patients with advanced liver disease. In the absence of associated renal dysfunction there is no contra-indication to the use of either d-tubocurarine or gallamine triethiodide.

The choice of inhalational anaesthetic for patients with liver disease is less critical, but efforts to avoid hypoxia and hypotension are of the greatest importance. There is no evidence that halothane is more dangerous in the presence of liver disease. Respiratory difficulty due to the mechanical factor of a raised diaphragm due to massive ascites may be encountered. Judicious pre-operative treatment by salt restriction and diuretics may be helpful.

## REFERENCES

Belfrage, S., Ahlgren, I. and Axelson, S. (1966), "Halothane Hepatitis in an Anaesthetist," *Lancet*, **ii,** 1466 (letter).

Blake, D. A., Barry, J. Q. and Cascorbi, H. F. (1972), "Qualitative Analysis of Halothane Metabolites in Man," *Anesthesiology*, **36,** 152.

Bruce, D. L. and Raymon, F. (1972), "Test for Halothane Sensitivity," *New Engl. J. Med.*, **286,** 1218.

Bunker, J. P. (1966), "Metabolic Effects of Blood Transfusion," *Anesthesiology*, **27,** 446.

Cohen, E. W. (1971), "Metabolism of the Volatile Anaesthetics," *Anesthesiology*, **35,** 193.

Epstein, R. M., Deutsch, S., Cooperman, L. H., Clement, A. J. and Price, H. L. (1966), "Splanchnic Circulation During Halothane Anesthesia and Hypercapnia in Normal Man," *Anesthesiology*, **27,** 654.

Kalow, W. and Gunn, D. R. (1959), "Some Statistical Data on Atypical Cholinesterase of Human Serum," *Ann. Hum. Genet.*, **23,** 239.

Klatskin, G. (1968), *Mechanisms of Hepatic Injury, in Toxicity of Anesthetics*, Ed. B. R. Fink, Williams and Wilkins Co., Baltimore.

Klatskin, G. and Kimberg, D. V. (1969), "Recurrent Hepatitis Attributable to Halothane Sensitization in an Anesthetist," *New Engl. J. Med.*, **280,** 515.

Klion, F. M., Schaffner, F. and Popper, H. (1969), "Hepatitis after Exposure to Halothane," *Ann. Intern. Med.*, **71,** 467.

Levy, M. L., Palazzi, H. M., Nardi, G. L. and Bunker, J. P. (1961), "Hepatic Blood Flow Variations During Surgical Anesthesia in Man Measured by Radioactive Colloid (Tagged Colloidal Chromic Phosphate)," *Surg. Gynec. Obstet.*, **112,** 289.

Lindenbaum, J. and Leifer, E. (1963), "Hepatic Necrosis Associated with Halothane Anesthesia," *New Engl. J. Med.*, **268,** 525.

Paronetto, F. and Popper, H. (1970), "Lymphocyte Stimulation Induced by Halothane in Patients with Hepatitis Following Exposure to Halothane," *New Engl. J. Med.*, **283,** 277.

Price, H. L., Deutsch, S., Cooperman, L. H., Clement, A. J. and Epstein, R. M. (1965), "Splanchnic Circulation During Cyclopropane Anesthesia in Normal Man," *Anesthesiology*, **26,** 312.

Price, H. L., Deutsch, S., Davidson, I. A., Clement, A. J., Behar, M. G. and Epstein, R. M. (1966), "Can General Anesthetics Produce Splanchnic Visceral Hypoxia by Reducing Regional Blood Flow?" *Anesthesiology*, **27,** 24.

Shackman, R., Graber, G. I. and Melrose, D. G. (1953), "Liver Blood Flow and General Anaesthesia," *Clin. Sci.*, **12,** 307.

Sherlock, S. (1967), "The Prediction of Hepatotoxicity Due to Therapeutic Agents in Man," *Drug Responses in Man*. Ciba Foundation, 138–154.

Sherlock, S. (1968), *Diseases of the Liver and Biliary System*, 4th Ed. Blackwell, Oxford and Edinburgh.

Summary of the National Halothane Study (1966), *J. Amer. med. Ass.*, **197,** 775.

Tygstrup, N. (1963), "Halothane Hepatitis," *Lancet*, **ii,** 466 (letter).

Walton, B., Dumonde, D. C., Williams, C., Jones, D., Strunin, J. M., Layton, J., Strunin, L. and Simpson, B. R. (1972), "Failure to Demonstrate Increased Lymphocyte Transformation in Patients with Post-operative Jaundice and Physicians with Alleged Halothane Hypersensitivity," *Brit. J. Anaesth.*, **44,** 904.

*CHAPTER* 3

# NUTRITION AND METABOLISM

## V. MARKS AND JACQUELINE STORDY

### Introduction

All vital processes require energy which is obtained from chemical reactions carried on in the living cells. In the animal kingdom the principal mechanism for the liberation of energy is the gradual oxidation of various metabolites. In some tissues, such as striated muscle, energy requirements may be met anaerobically by glycolysis—but only for short periods.

Ingested food is the fundamental source of all energy for vital processes. When food is consumed in excess of energy requirements the excess may be incorporated into the fabric of the body. When food intake is insufficient to meet energy requirements the deficit is made good by utilizing metabolic stores, e.g. glycogen and triglycerides, or—*in extremis*—tissue protein.

Metabolic processes causing breakdown of tissue are referred to as catabolic; those concerned either with construction or deposition of metabolic stores as anabolic. In the healthy adult subject of constant weight, anabolism and catabolism proceed simultaneously at approximately equal rates, so that there is neither net gain nor net loss in body tissues which are, nevertheless, in a state of constant flux.

After digestion and absorption, food is converted into a form in which it can be transported to the cells of the body where, through a complicated series of biochemical linkages it can be utilized for such energy requiring (i.e. endergonic) processes as the synthesis of proteins and other complicated structural elements of the cell, muscular contraction, nervous conduction, transport of substances across membranes and glandular secretion. The ability to 'capture' energy and divert it into physiologically 'useful' pathways is a function of intracellular transfer mechanisms which occur in conjunction with respiratory enzyme systems in the mitochondria which are distributed as small particles throughout the cytoplasm of the cells. The most important intracellular transfer systems are the NAD-NADH and NADP-NADPH nucleotides; the cytochromes and flavoproteins.

The precise means by which chemical energy is retained as such—and not immediately freed as heat—is one of the principal mysteries of life. Nevertheless many of the intermediate steps are known and discussed in detail in another chapter. (Tissue metabolism, p. 337).

Even under 'ideal' conditions only a small and variable proportion of the energy liberated by oxidation processes can be utilized by the cell for maintaining vital processes. Excess energy is lost as heat. It has been calculated that overall loss in this way accounts for 75 per cent of the energy released from ingested foodstuffs; only 25 per cent is available for use in functional systems. Ultimately, *all* of the energy produced in the body—with the exception of a very small amount that appears as mechanical work—will be dissipated as heat so that measurement of heat production can be used to estimate the expenditure of energy by the organism. Interference by physical or chemical agents with the coupling of energy liberating (exergonic) and energy requiring (endergonic) reactions, reduces the 'usefulness' of the energy liberated by oxidative processes. Thus drugs such as dinitrophenol, which break the link by uncoupling oxidative phosphorylation permit uncontrolled oxidation of energy yielding substrate. This leads to excessive catabolism with liberation of large amounts of heat and is the basis of one of the treatments for obesity. It is also the cause of hyperpyrexia in dinitrophenol and salicylate poisoning, and is of course damaging and even fatal to the cell's physical integrity.

### Milieu Interieur

The unicellular organism obtains its food either by engulfing it or by absorbing it from the environment (the milieu exterieur). In higher forms of life the constituent cells depend entirely upon the latter method for their vital requirements; foodstuffs and their digestive products being conveyed in the blood from the gut to the interstitial fluid which bathes each individual cell. In the fasting state energy-providing substrates, mainly in the form of nonesterified fatty acids (N.E.F.A. or F.F.A.) and to a much lesser extent glucose are added to the blood by adipose tissue and liver respectively for distribution to the tissues.

Blood and interstitial fluid are in a state of dynamic equilibrium with each other, together constituting what Claude Bernard termed the 'milieu interieur'. He was also the first to recognize its extraordinary constancy of composition.

The milieu interieur contains all the basic elements necessary to maintain vital functions as well as furnishing a medium in which they can take place. The rest of this chapter is concerned with the nature, source, homeostatic control and fate of energy-providing substrates and their biological utilization.

### METABOLISM

The term 'metabolism', in its broadest sense, includes all the chemical reactions involved in growth, development and maintenance of the nutritive state of an individual or animal. Basal metabolism, or basal metabolic rate, is used to describe the minimal amount of heat produced by the fasting individual, physically and mentally at rest in a room at 20°C. It represents the energy expended to maintain vegetative functions and is provided by oxidation of fats, carbohydrates, and to a lesser extent, proteins.

#### Respiratory Quotient

Carbohydrates and fats are the main fuels of the body and normally are completely oxidized to carbon dioxide and water so that the energy derived and the end products produced are identical to those produced by complete oxidation outside the body. In metabolic studies the ratio of the $CO_2$ liberated to the oxygen consumed is known as the respiratory quotient;

$$RQ = \frac{\text{volume } CO_2}{\text{volume } O_2}$$

With a knowledge of this figure it is possible to determine how large a contribution to energy metabolism is being made by fat and how much by carbohydrate. When carbohydrate serves as fuel the respiratory quotient is 1·0, and each litre of oxygen consumed corresponds to 5·05 Calories liberated as heat; with fat as fuel the respiratory quotient is 0·7 and each litre of oxygen consumed corresponds to 4·69 Calories liberated as heat.

#### Metabolic Rate

Under physiological conditions it is most unusual for either fuel to be used exclusively and the *RQ* tends to lie somewhere between the two extremes. For many purposes —including the approximate measurement of basal metabolic rate by the classical Benedict-Roth instrument—*RQ* is assumed to be 0·82 but for more accurate work it can be determined exactly by measuring total oxygen consumption and $CO_2$ production by any one of a variety of techniques. From a knowledge of the respiratory quotient and the total amount of oxygen consumed per unit time it is comparatively simple to calculate the amount of energy liberated by the individual. In the fasted resting individual this corresponds to the basal metabolic rate. This method of calculating metabolic rate is known as indirect calorimetry and has been extensively validated, in the past, by comparison with direct calorimetry in which total heat production by individuals was actually measured. Because direct calorimetry requires extremely complicated apparatus and is very exacting for the subject being tested, it is seldom if ever employed nowadays.

For very accurate measurement of metabolic rate (whether it be under basal conditions or not) it is necessary to measure urea excretion, as proteins in contrast to carbohydrates and fats, are only incompletely oxidized in the body. From a knowledge of the amount of urea produced per hour, the amount of oxygen consumed and the amount of $CO_2$ liberated, it is possible to assess, more or less accurately, the contribution made by each of the three major types of fuel to total energy metabolism.

Formerly, measurement of basal metabolic rate by indirect calorimetry, and its expression as a percentage of mean normal for individuals of similar age and size (expressed in terms of their surface area), was widely used as a test of thyroid and other endocrine gland function. For a variety of reasons, not the least of them being the inherent imprecision of the method, it is seldom used for this purpose nowadays. Nevertheless indirect calorimetry remains the only practicable method for measuring metabolic rate under experimental conditions and providing it is carried out with care it can yield important information that is not otherwise obtainable.

Basal metabolism, although a useful concept, does not correspond to the situation in everyday life where activity and the consumption of food increase the metabolic rate. Recently it has been observed that overfeeding does not necessarily result in an equivalent gain of adipose tissue. It is thought that the mechanism whereby these individuals increase their heat output, both at rest and during activity, may be involved in the aetiology of obesity. Conservation of food energy is observed during semistarvation and in these circumstances the resting metabolic rate and the energy costs of work are reduced.

## METABOLIC SUBSTRATES

The main constituents of diet that provide energy are fats, carbohydrates and—to a lesser extent—proteins. After complete oxidation these yield 9·3, 4·1 and 4·1 kilo-calories (C) per gram respectively.

The composition of diets varies enormously according to both cultural and individual preference. Consequently the contribution to the total metabolic energy pool made by each type of nutrient cannot be stated except in the most general terms. It has been suggested that in Western Society, where three meals a day constitute the dietary norm, carbohydrates contribute about 43 per cent, fats 44 per cent and protein about 13 per cent to the energy pool. In some individuals alcohol is an important additional source of energy: each gramme (1·25 ml.) of pure alcohol providing 7 calories after complete oxidation to $CO_2$ and water.

The metabolism and regulation of fats, carbohydrates and proteins are closely interrelated both inside and outside the cell. It is nevertheless convenient to consider each class of metabolite independently though it must be stressed that this is a device adopted so as to facilitate description.

## 1. CARBOHYDRATES

The main carbohydrates of the diet are starch and sucrose. In the adult roughly 50 per cent of the carbohydrate is ingested in the form of starch or dextrins which after hydrolysis yield glucose alone. Approximately 25 per cent is taken as sucrose which yields equal quantities of glucose and fructose, and 10 per cent as lactose which yields equal quantities of glucose and galactose. Other carbohydrates are generally present in only negligible amounts but may become significant in some situations.

Before they can be absorbed from the gut, complex carbohydrates must be completely degraded into their constituent monosaccharides, glucose, fructose and galactose, in which form they are transported across the intestinal mucosa and into the portal blood stream. Transmucosal transport is an active process which can take place against a concentration gradient. In the gut, glucose and galactose share the same energy requiring transport system while fructose utilizes an independent system. Though galactose is an essential constituent of many of the structural elements of the body such as mucopolysaccharides and glycolipids, dietary galactose takes little part in intracellular energy metabolism until it has been converted into glucose in the liver. The same is true of fructose. Normally neither sugar is demonstrably present in peripheral blood even after a large meal.

Glucose is the main carbohydrate of the body. It is, however, virtually confined in its native form to the extracellular fluid and the intracellular water of the liver and red blood cells. Together these compartments comprise a body pool of glucose to which new glucose molecules can be added or subtracted. At any one time it is quite small, seldom exceeding 20 grams. Its size is determined by the magnitude of the glucose space, i.e. the volume of distribution of glucose which corresponds more or less with the E.C.F. and the blood glucose concentration, i.e. Glucose pool = glucose space × glucose concentration in E.C.F. water.

Under normal physiological conditions the glucose pool is more or less constant in size though always in flux as glucose molecules leave it to enter the cells—where they are metabolized—and are replaced by new glucose molecules recently absorbed from the gut or liberated from the liver by glycolysis.

In the post-absorptive (fasting) state the outflow of glucose from the glucose pool into the tissues exactly balances the inflow of glucose from the liver. As the space is, for all practical purposes, of fixed size the net result is that the blood glucose concentration remains constant. This constancy is maintained—despite enormous fluctuations in supply and demand for glucose—by a number of homeostatic mechanisms the most important of which are autoregulatory and hormonally mediated.

Fructose is even more rapidly metabolized than glucose in the body. It is taken up exceedingly rapidly by the liver and somewhat more slowly by adipose tissue. Unlike glucose, fructose does not require insulin before it can enter adipose tissue cells and is also considerably more anti-ketogenic in liver. Because it is less irritant to veins when given intravenously fructose enjoys considerable popularity as a source of energy when intravenous feeding is indicated.

## 2. Fats and Fatty Acids

Fatty acids and their derivatives, the ketone bodies, are important metabolic fuels. The two main sources of fatty acids in the body are:

  (a) preformed fatty acids ingested in the diet;
  (b) fatty acids synthesised from carbohydrates in the liver and adipose tissue cells.

(a) Fats are generally ingested in the form of triglycerides and must be broken down in the gut into their constituent parts, i.e. fatty acids, mono- and di-glycerides and glycerol, before they can be absorbed. Inside the intestinal mucosa cells fatty acids are handled differently depending upon their chain length. Long chain fatty acids are resynthesised into triglycerides; attached to a special carrier protein ($\beta$ lipoprotein polypeptide or apoprotein) together with a small amount of cholesterol and phospholipid, and secreted into the lymphatic system as minute particles called chylomicrons. These little packages of fat, for that in effect is what they are, enter the general circulation via the thoracic duct whence they are distributed to the tissues. There they are acted upon by an enzyme called lipoprotein lipase which is present in especially high concentration in the walls of the capillaries of adipose tissue. The result of this enzymic breakdown is the liberation of triglyceride from lipoprotein and the further hydrolysis of the triglyceride into its constituent fatty acids. These in turn are rapidly taken up by the tissues locally to be used either as fuel or for making more triglycerides to be stored within the cell.

After absorption from the gut, medium chain triglycerides are secreted unchanged into the portal venous blood whence they are transported loosely bound to albumin to the liver. In the liver they can either be rapidly metabolized into keto-acids or converted into long chain fatty acids.

The distinction between the mode of absorption and metabolic fate of dietary fats, depending on whether they are composed of long chain or medium chain triglycerides, has found extensive clinical application, especially in the management of certain types of malabsorption syndrome and disorders of metabolism.

(b) Most fatty acids, apart from those with two or more double bonds (i.e. the poly-unsaturated fatty acids) can be synthesized in the body from simple precursors, by a complicated energy-requiring process. In mammals, enzymes capable of effecting fatty acid synthesis are concentrated mainly in adipose tissue and liver cells but in some species notably birds and fishes they occur exclusively in the liver. Though fatty acids can be synthesized from carbohydrates, there is not, as far as is known, any mechanism whereby the reverse process can occur.

Interest in adipose tissue as an important constituent of the overall energy economy of the body, is comparatively new. Formerly adipose tissue was looked upon largely as padding whose main function was to round off contours produced by other tissues, provide insulation against cold and serve as a fat store. This view of adipose tissue as a relatively inert supporting medium is no longer tenable following the demonstration in the mid-1950s that not only is adipose tissue in a constant state of flux but that fatty acids synthesized and stored in it are an important fuel in most tissues of the body, especially for the fasting subject.

Fatty acids occur in adipose tissue cells largely as triglycerides. Dynamic studies have shown that within individual adipose tissue cells triglycerides are constantly being broken down into their constituent parts, i.e. fatty acid and glycerol, and being resynthesized. Under basal conditions these two processes, called lipolysis and esterification respectively, occur at more or less equal rates with lipolysis preponderating slightly. As a result there is a slow net release of fatty acids from adipose tissue cells into the blood, where they are transported, loosely bound to albumin, to the liver and other tissues.

Triglycerides are produced in adipose tissue, as elsewhere, by esterification of glycerol-phosphate (formed by glycolysis from glucose) by fatty acids. These are themselves derived either from fat eaten in the diet or are produced locally in adipose tissue cells by total synthesis from glucose. For thermodynamic reasons the glycerol liberated during lipolysis cannot be re-used for re-esterification of fatty acids in adipose tissue cells.

## 3. Proteins

Even in affluent societies proteins make comparatively little contribution to energy metabolism. Their main function is to provide the basic elements from which the body's own tissue can be constructed and the raw materials from which hormones and enzymes can be synthesized. Before they can be absorbed ingested proteins must be hydrolysed in the lumen of the gut by gastric and intestinal proteases into smaller polypeptides and amino-acids. These are then transferred by active transmucosal transport mechanisms into the portal circulation whence they are distributed to the tissues of the body. Amino-acids are rapidly removed from the circulation. The liver, intestine and kidney are the most active tissues in this respect. Of the twenty or so amino-acids found in proteins, eight of them—namely tryptophane, phenylalanine, lysine, threonine, valine, methionine, leucine and isoleucine—are essential for maintaining nitrogen balance in human subjects. The remaining twelve or so amino-acids that occur naturally in proteins, and those that function as hormones or fulfil other special functions, are all capable of being synthesized in the body from essential amino-acids and other substrates.

Free amino-acids cannot be stored in the body as such. They are instead rapidly converted either into tissue proteins or, by a series of complicated steps involving transamination and other processes, into energy yielding substrates. A small reserve of protein is available however, in the liver (and possible the muscles) which, though actually a part of the architecture of the tissue, can be called upon when protein intake is temporarily inadequate for body requirements without producing gross structural damage.

Even in the adult, tissue proteins are in a constant state of flux. This is exemplified, in gross form by the constant synthesis of albumin in the liver, its secretion into the blood and eventual utilization by other tissues to meet their own protein requirements. In most tissues the production, destruction and replacement of proteins is more subtle but equally active. In the healthy subject overall protein anabolism and protein catabolism proceed at more or less the same rate. Though amino-acids derived from protein taken in the diet participate in the anabolic process there is neither net gain nor net loss in the total body protein. In such a subject the amount of nitrogen excreted in the urine (largely in the form of urea, and to a lesser extent as uric acid, ammonium and creatinine) exactly equals the amount of nitrogen taken as protein in the diet. During physical growth or when, for any reason, the total amount of tissue protein is increasing—as for example, during recovery from a debilitating illness—less nitrogen is excreted than is ingested and the subject is said to be in positive nitrogen balance.

As both protein anabolism and catabolism continue regardless of whether the subject is fed or fasting there is inevitably, in the completely fasted subject, an overall negative nitrogen balance. Nevertheless, except when other factors are operating, such as severe illness or tissue damage produced by trauma, actual wastage of amino-acids by conversion to urea is very small after the first few days of total starvation. During this interim period many metabolic re-adjustments take place, some of them at least partly under hormonal and autonomic nervous control. Likewise after refeeding, protein synthesis is carried out in an orderly and highly organized manner but the precise control mechanism is still poorly understood.

In the intact organism protein catabolism is reduced by the ready availability of energy providing substrates such as glucose, fructose and fats which are consequently sometimes referred to as protein sparers.

### Parenteral Feeding

In some diseases food, and thus nutrients, can no longer be taken by mouth. Two alternative procedures are available; the nasogastric tube and intravenous feeding. The aim of these procedures is not only to provide a maintenance diet but also to provide for any extra needs due to the disease condition. In burns, for example, the protein requirement may be doubled and in any trauma or sepsis the energy and nitrogen intake should be increased if a serious negative nitrogen balance is to be avoided. Parenteral feeding is indicated in pre-operative states where there is malnutrition secondary to disorders of the gastrointestinal tract such as cancer of the oesophagus or ulcerative colitis and post-operatively after gastrointestinal surgery. Parenteral feeding may also be valuable in the treatment of burns, chest and skull injuries, hypercatabolic acute renal failure and cachexia associated with many conditions.

An intravenous diet must provide an adequate supply of water, energy, amino acids, vitamins, electrolytes and minerals. Observations should be made on the patient's blood urea, serum proteins and electrolytes and their urine urea and electrolyte output which will give a rough guide to the metabolic balance. Energy is provided chiefly as emulsified fat because glucose solutions cannot be given in sufficient concentration to provide an adequate energy intake. The energy source and amino-acids should be given simultaneously to achieve maximum benefit on nitrogen balance and some carbohydrate (about 10 per cent) should also be included because of its specific action on protein metabolism. Fructose is often chosen as the carbohydrate for parenteral feeding because it is independent of insulin for its metabolism and is particularly valuable in liver disease.

Ethanol may also prove a useful energy substrate not only because of its high energy content (7 K.Cal./gm.) but also for its beneficial effects on protein anabolism and the patient's sense of well being.

Amino acids for intravenous feeding are available in two forms, protein hydrolysates and mixtures of crystalline amino-acids. Protein hydrolysates are preferable because all of the amino-acids are available for metabolism whereas synthetic amino-acid mixtures also contain dextro amino-acids which cannot be used for protein synthesis.

Sodium, potassium, calcium, magnesium and vitamins should be added in suitable quantities to the amino-acid solution. They must not be added to fat emulsions as they may destroy it.

Appropriate parenteral feeding will improve the rate of recovery of the patient and should be continued until the patient can take an adequate diet by mouth. For further details see p. 363).

### Hormonal and Neural Control of Energy Metabolism

The hormonal and neural control of energy metabolism is extremely complicated. It involves a large number of hormones of which insulin, glucagon, growth hormone, ACTH, cortisol, TSH, thyroxine, adrenaline and various unidentified intestinal factors are amongst the most important. Contrary to former belief the hormonal system does not function independently but is closely integrated with, and controlled by, the autonomic nervous system.

### Insulin

Insulin is currently believed to be the most important single hormone controlling metabolic processes. It not only profoundly affects glucose, but possibly even more important it controls lipid and amino-acid metabolism.

The best known but not necessarily the most important effect of insulin is its ability to lower the blood glucose concentration. It does this by a dual mechanism—on the one hand by increasing glucose uptake in the peripheral tissues, particularly by striated muscle and adipose tissue, and on the other by decreasing hepatic glucose release.

It has been shown that most mammalian cells do not permit free and rapid entry of glucose in an indiscriminate way. Instead there is an active transcellular transport mechanism which only acts on sugars of a particular chemical structure. The cells of the liver and seemingly the $\beta$-cells of the pancreas are unique among mammalian cells in that they appear not to have a specific transport system. The most highly differentiated cells of the body—namely the neurones—and the most lowly—namely the erythrocytes—share the distinction of having a specific sugar transport mechanism which is independent of insulin. Most other cells—including those of muscle, connective and adipose tissue—exhibit an extremely low rate of transcellular glucose transport in the absence of insulin; they are, in effect, insulin-dependent. When insulin is present glucose enters the cell readily from the E.C.F. and becomes available for intracellular metabolism.

There is now evidence that insulin has some action upon the metabolism of glucose by the brain though it appears to be relatively unimportant for normal function. The disastrous effects of insulin over-dosage are not due to insulin *per se* but to hypoglycaemia as the brain, unlike most other tissues of the body, has an absolute requirement for glucose for the provision of energy. Nervous tissue cannot utilise free fatty acids for this purpose although recently it has been shown that during prolonged starvation adaptation does occur and ketones may be utilized as well as, or instead of, glucose.

The biological half life of insulin in the blood is very short; in the region of 2–5 minutes but its biological actions may persist for longer. This explains the reactive hypoglycaemia that occasionally develops when glucose infusions are terminated abruptly. Under these conditions insulin released during the phase of hyperglycaemia continues to exert its effect even after the stimulus to further insulin secretion has ceased. Fortunately hypoglycaemia produced in this way is rarely sufficiently severe to cause symptoms as it would otherwise seriously limit the clinical usefulness of intravenous glucose infusions. A similar situation sometimes occurs spontaneously in mild diabetics who, three to five hours after eating a meal, may experience slight to moderate symptoms of spontaneous hypoglycaemia.

In the liver insulin decreases gluconeogenesis and glycogenolysis and encourages glycogen synthesis. In the absence of insulin, gluconeogenesis and glycogenolysis increase and glucose pours out of the liver into the E.C.F. Since the glucose so liberated is also inhibited from entering the peripheral tissues it can go nowhere except to increase the concentration in the glucose pool. This causes a rise in the blood glucose concentration and eventually leads to spillage into the urine. In itself this is not unduly harmful to the animal organism although it is extremely wasteful of protein which has to be broken down to provide the glucose precursors used by the liver for gluconeogenesis. What is far more harmful, however, is the steep rise in plasma ketones which causes the profound acid-base disturbance so characteristic of diabetic ketoacidosis.

The synthesis of fats and their release from adipose tissue is under hormonal control. Insulin promotes triglyceride synthesis not only by stimulating fatty acid synthesis but also by increasing the availability of glycerol-phosphate. It has already been pointed out that for thermodynamic reasons glycerol liberated by lipolysis cannot be utilized within adipose tissue cells for resynthesizing triglyceride.

Instead 'energy-rich' glycerol-phosphate formed during the metabolic conversion of glucose must be used. Because glucose cannot enter the adipose tissue cell except in the presence of insulin, one consequence of insulin deficiency is that lipolysis is unopposed by re-esterification. As a result there is a large net increase in fatty acid release from the adipose tissue cells. The liberation of free fatty acids from adipose tissue is hastened by any mechanism that increases intracellular lipolysis by activating the hormone-dependent lipase present in every adipose tissue cell. Enzyme dependent lipase activity is decreased by insulin and by prostaglandins but increased by most other hormones. It is still unknown which of these are important physiologically, but current evidence suggests that glucagon, adrenaline and nor-adrenaline released locally from sympathetic nerve terminals are probably the most important.

The main regulator of insulin secretion is currently believed to be the concentration of glucose in the blood perfusing the pancreatic islets; a high concentration of glucose in the blood stimulating insulin secretion; a low concentration inhibiting it. There are, however, many other factors such as fatty acids, amino-acids, gut hormones and the autonomic nervous system that affect insulin secretion. Sympathomimetic drugs, for example, adrenaline and nor-adrenaline and sympathetic nervous activity which activates $\alpha$-adrenergic receptors inhibit insulin secretion whilst those that activate $\beta$ adrenergic receptors stimulate insulin release. Consequently, any stress, whether physical or mental, that activates non-specifically the sympathetic nervous system inhibits insulin secretion unless an $\alpha$ receptor blockade is imposed artificially. Excessive sympathetic nervous activity is in fact one of the factors responsible for 'stress-induced diabetes'.

### Glucagon

If insulin is the main anabolic hormone of the body then its pancreatic bed fellow, glucagon, can lay claim to being the main catabolic hormone—at least under stressful conditions.

Glucagon is a polypeptide hormone produced by the $\alpha$-2 cells of the pancreas. It stimulates hepatic glycogenolysis and glucose release from the liver but does not directly increase peripheral glucose uptake. Advantage is taken of this fact therapeutically in the use of glucagon for raising the blood glucose concentration of patients with hypoglycaemia due to overtreatment with insulin or sulphonylureas, and in whom, for some reason, glucose itself cannot be given. Glucagon has no hyperglycaemic activity when the liver glycogen reserves are low as in patients with alcohol induced hypoglycaemia, hepatocellular necrosis or acute starvation.

Glucagon also stimulates insulin secretion by a direct action on the $\beta$-cells of the pancreas and it promotes lipolysis in adipose tissue. These actions are probably as important physiologically as its better known hyperglycaemic properties. Glucagon also promotes gluconeogenesis and accelerates amino-acid metabolism by the liver. One consequence of this is that urea production is increased. Indirectly therefore, glucagon increases protein breakdown in the body and increases nitrogen wastage.

When administered parenterally to the non-stressed, non-fasting individual the lipolytic effect of glucagon is masked by its insulinotropic effect. In other words, glucagon is so potent a stimulus to insulin secretion that under the conditions of pharmacological experimentation its ability to mobilize fatty acids from adipose tissue by increasing intracellular lipolysis is more than overcome by the increase in insulin secretion. If stimulation of insulin secretion is blocked by α-sympathetic nervous activity, however, glucagon can increase lipolysis and produce a rise in plasma free fatty acids, even in normal individuals.

There is growing evidence that glucagon secretion is enhanced by sympathetic nervous activity, largely through activation of adrenergic receptors on the surface of the α-2 cells of the pancreas.

Glucagon secretion is inhibited by high concentrations of free fatty acids in the blood, by hyperglycaemia and by hyperinsulinaemia. Indeed, insulin is essential for glucose to exert its glucagon inhibitory effect. In the absence of insulin, such as in the insulinoprivic diabetic, glucose does not suppress glucagon secretion even at very high blood concentration and plasma glucagon levels are grossly elevated.

There is some evidence that sulphonylureas inhibit glucagon secretion but it is still unknown how constant a phenomenon this is, or whether insulin is an essential intermediary.

### Effect of other Hormones on Energy Metabolism

Although many other hormones, apart from insulin and glucagon, are involved in control of energy metabolism in very few of them is the association as intimate or as acute as with the pancreatic hormones. The thyroid hormones, for example, play an important role in setting the general level of metabolic activity and sensitize cells to the metabolic effects of the catecholamines. Likewise cortisol and other glucocorticoids have profound but nevertheless sub-acute effects upon metabolic processes. In particular they inhibit protein synthesis and therefore indirectly favour protein catabolism and nitrogen wastage. The relative importance of cortisol compared with other catabolic agents in the genesis of the negative nitrogen balance produced by trauma and acute injury is still unknown. The role of growth hormone in the regulation of metabolic processes is also poorly understood, despite the enormous amount of work carried out on this hormone during the past decade. It may well be that like the other hormones mentioned in this section, growth hormone is more important in setting the stage against which insulin, glucagon and catecholamines can work than in producing rapid changes itself.

The catecholamines are, between them, amongst the most important of the lipolytic agents. They not only stimulate hormone-dependent lipase within the adipose tissue cells by direct action—but also increase fatty acid mobilization indirectly by inhibiting insulin and stimulating glucagon secretion.

In the past much importance was attached to the metabolic effects of adrenaline; comparatively less was given to those of nor-adrenaline, the neurohormone released at sympathetic nerve terminals. This was probably an error, even though, under pharmacological conditions, the metabolic effects of adrenaline are more easily demonstrated than those of nor-adrenaline. In intact animals nor-adrenaline is released in direct contact with the effector cell from which a metabolic response will be evoked, e.g. lipolysis by adipocytes. Consequently nor-adrenaline not only affects cellular metabolism but does so more selectively than adrenaline.

### Effect of Trauma on Metabolic Processes

Conditions which are associated with severe stress not only cause inhibition of insulin secretion by sympathetic nervous activity but also promote glucagon secretion. Between them these two effects lead to accelerated lipolysis in adipose tissue cells, especially when primed by sympathetic nervous activity locally. As a result free fatty acids are released into the blood in greatly increased amounts. They are transported, in the blood bound to albumin, to the liver where some are converted into triglycerides and others into ketoacids. Free fatty acids reaching peripheral tissue, such as muscle, inhibit, still further, glucose uptake and utilization which has already been grossly reduced as a result of insulin deficiency.

A further effect of an increased supply of free fatty acids in the liver is that it increases the rate of gluconeogenesis already near maximally stimulated by glucagon excess and insulin deficiency. As a result the release of glucose into the glucose pool is still further enhanced. A situation exists therefore, in which hepatic glucose is increased at the same time as glucose utilization is decreased. The main consequence of this is a rise in blood glucose concentration. Simultaneously plasma ketones and free fatty acids increase so that a clinical picture, not very dissimilar from that produced by insulin deficiency, is produced. The possibility that the well known metabolic consequences of surgery—namely obligatory protein loss; hyperglycaemia and impaired glucose tolerance, ketosis and hyperlipacidaemia—are wholly or largely a consequence of sympathetic nervous activity affecting insulin and glucagon secretion, is one of the most exciting concepts to emerge within recent years. If correct it can lead to therapeutically desirable action. It can be imagined, for example, that by using adrenergic blocking agents to prevent the inhibition of insulin secretion, or by using agents capable of overcoming glucagon secretion, the protein loss and body wasting provoked by trauma and hitherto considered an inevitable consequence of it, could at least be partially alleviated.

It was mentioned earlier that in normal subjects glucose has long been known to be a protein sparing agent. It now seems likely that this is achieved, in part at least, by its ability to inhibit glucagon secretion and stimulate insulin secretion. In the traumatized or otherwise stressed individual in whom these actions of glucose are prevented or counteracted by sympathetic nervous activity glucose cannot gain entrance to adipose tissue cells. It cannot prevent accelerated endogenous protein turn-over or prevent ketosis. This may explain why, to date, the only method of treatment found to be effective in reducing post-traumatic protein loss is the simultaneous administration of large doses of glucose and insulin intravenously.

## Vitamins

These important constituents of the diet play a vital role in metabolism. Their chemical and physiological actions vary. Some, for example, thiamine, nicotinic acid and riboflavin, act as essential co-factors for enzymes concerned with energy transformations within the cell, others such as folic acid and cyanocobalamin are involved in synthesis of nucleoproteins. Vitamin D (cholecalciferol) is important in calcium homeostasis and vitamin A (retinol) is necessary for the health and integrity of epithelial tissues as well as the formation of rhodopsin. By definition vitamins are substances that cannot be synthesized in the body at a rate consistent with the maintenance of good health. The fat soluble vitamins A and D can be stored in the liver and fatty tissues of the body respectively, so a daily dietary intake is not necessary, but if excessive amounts are taken the accumulation can cause toxic effects which may be fatal. Cholecalciferol is exceptional because 7-dehydrocholesterol can be converted to cholecalciferol by the action of ultra violet light on the skin thus the body is dependent upon a dietary supplement of the vitamin only if the ultraviolet radiation of the skin is inadequate. Recent research has shown that cholecalciferol, either from the skin or the diet, is converted by the liver to 25 hydroxy cholecalciferol which the kidneys subsequently convert to the active metabolites. This has led to the suggestion that Vitamin D should be re-classified as a hormone because the active metabolites are secreted by one tissue and carried by the blood to the target tissues, namely bone and the gastrointestinal mucosa.

## Mineral Elements

Mineral elements are also dietary essentials. Within the body they form the structural components of hard tissue and in soft tissues they act as co-factors in enzyme systems. In body fluids they have an important role in acid-base balance and maintenance of the irritability of nerves and the contractility of muscles. They may also form part of physiologically active compounds. Iron, for example, is an integral part of the haemoglobin molecule and iodine part of thyroxine.

## SUGGESTED FURTHER READING

Allen, P. C. and Lee, H. A. (1969), *A Clinical Guide to Intravenous Nutrition*. Oxford: Blackwell Scientific Publications.

Bondy, P. K. (Editor) (1969), *Diseases of Metabolism* (6th Edition). Philadelphia: Saunders and Co.

Lefebvre, P. J. and Unger, R. H. (Editors) (1972), *Glucagon; Molecular Physiology: Clinical and Therapeutic Implications*. Oxford: Pergamon.

Thompson, R. H. S. and Wootton, I. D. P. (Editors) (1970), *Biochemical Disorders in Human Disease* (3rd Edition). London: Churchill.

*CHAPTER* 4

# TISSUE RESPIRATION

### J. CHAMBERLAIN

Essentially tissue respiration is the means whereby the body liberates the chemical energy contained in the three basic food stuffs, carbohydrate, fat and protein and changes it into a readily usable form, adenosine triphosphate (ATP). For the most efficient conversion of this energy from the one form to the other, oxygen is necessary. This chapter will present the ways in which this can take place and the consequences of oxygen lack, and then discuss how this may be detected.

## Bio Energetics

Energy is fundamental to life. It is required for the production of complex substances such as nucleoproteins, for the maintenance of temperature, for the maintenance of electrical activity in the heart and brain, and for the mechanical work of muscles.

A number of questions arise before we can discuss the mechanism of energy utilization in the body. Firstly what exactly is energy? Secondly, where does the energy contained in food stuffs come from and thirdly what form does it take and how can we measure it?

Energy 'is the equivalent of, or the capacity to do, work'. It is best understood by thinking what it can do, rather than what it actually is. Thinking in this way we come across the various forms of energy, such as electrical energy, mechanical energy, thermal energy and chemical energy, each able to do work in different ways. Each form of energy is interconvertible, when one form is created, an exactly equal amount of another is lost (law of conservation of energy). This interconvertibility is basic to life, as the electromagnetic radiation of the sun, resulting from nuclear reactions, is converted to chemical energy by photosynthesis and then, by biological means, to chemical work (biosynthesis), osmotic work (transport and concentration) and mechanical work. The concept of inter-convertibility also helps the understanding of certain fundamental processes in tissue respiration, e.g. describing the energy conversion in the respiratory chain in terms of the redox potential change (*vide infra*).

## Intermediary Metabolism

A final common pathway is used to trap the potential energy in all three food stuffs. The starting point of this pathway is almost invariably the substance acetyl-Co.A.

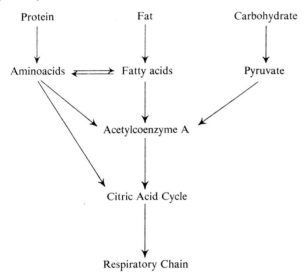

Fig. 1. Schema of relationship between fat, protein and carbohydrate metabolism and tissue respiration.

(During the course of protein metabolism certain substances such as α-ketoglutaric acid and succinic acid are formed which are members of the citric acid cycle and therefore gain entry at these points rather than through acetyl-Co.A.) Acetyl-Co.A. occupies a central position in

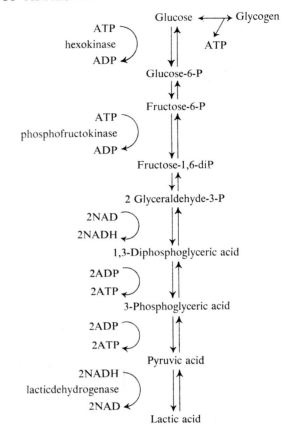

Fig. 2. Embden-Meyerhof pathway. Two molecules of 1,3-Diphosphoglyceric acid are formed from one molecule of fructose-1,6-diP.

adenosine triphosphate (ATP) are produced and two used up, and two molecules of nicotinamide adenine dinucleotide (NAD) are reduced to form reduced NAD (NADH)* which are then reoxidized during the conversion of pyruvate to lactate.

From glucose to pyruvic acid the process can be written:

$$\underset{\text{(glucose)}}{C_6H_{12}O_6} + 2ADP + 2P_1 + 2NAD^+ \rightarrow \underset{\text{(pyruvic acid)}}{2CH_3COCOOH} + 2ATP + 2NADH + 2H^+$$

From pyruvic acid to lactic acid:

$$\underset{\text{(pyruvic acid)}}{2CH_3COCOOH} + 2NADH + 2H^+ \rightarrow \underset{\text{(lactic acid)}}{2CH_3CHOHCOOH} + 2NAD$$

intermediary metabolism standing at the cross-roads of fat, carbohydrate and protein metabolism (Fig. 1). The exact mechanism whereby protein and fat produce acetyl-Co.A. is beyond the scope of this chapter. However their contribution to energy requirements is of paramount importance.

It will be necessary to look at carbohydrate metabolism in some detail as this is relevant to our later discussion on the means of detecting tissue hypoxia. In Figure 2 a simplified version of the Embden–Meyerhof pathway is seen. It is named in recognition of the two workers who contributed substantially to its formulation. The whole process involves the breakdown of glucose to lactic acid (glycolysis). During this process four molecules of

It should be noted that as fat and protein entry to the respiratory pool is primarily through acetyl-Co.A., the E-M pathway is not available to fat and protein and in the absence of oxygen their potential energy is unavailable for conversion to ATP.

In the presence of oxygen pyruvate is oxidized, and in the process, for each molecule of glucose originally

* Alternative nomenclature for NAD is Diphosphopyridine nucleotide (DPN). In the text the former terminology is used as recommended by the Commission on Enzymes of the International Union of Biochemistry.

If the reader comes across NAD⁺ in the literature this is recognition of the fact that its reduction involves the capture of two electrons, i.e. $NAD^+ + H^+ + 2\varepsilon = NADH$. If the state of ionization of the reactants and products is not known it is strictly correct to write NAD without the plus sign and to write out the term "reduced NAD" rather than use NADH.

supplied, 36 molecules of ATP are produced. As a result the conservation of energy is much more efficient in the presence of oxygen. This is why oxygen is so important to us. Those tissues such as the brain which derive almost all of their energy from oxidative phosphorylation die very quickly in the absence of oxygen. Certain evolutionary adaptations enable such animals as the diving turtle to remain submerged and active even when the oxygen tension in their blood is unrecordable. They survive because of the E–M pathway, but at the cost of a great loss of efficiency in energy conservation. Similarly the E–M pathway provides the means for supplying energy to actively contracting muscles when they outstrip their oxygen supply. It is also the mechanism which enables cells to survive when the arterial supply to the lower limbs is obstructed during reconstructive arterial surgery. Thus, while oxidative phosphorylation conserves most energy, the E–M pathway is very useful as a temporary stop-gap during hypoxia in certain tissues. (The terms *aerobic* and *anaerobic* glycolysis referring to glucose → pyruvate → Krebs cycle and to the E–M pathway respectively should be discarded. Glycolysis (glucose → pyruvate) is essentially an anaerobic process and oxidation occurs much later in the respiratory process.)

## Krebs Cycle and Oxidative Phosphorylation

The latent energy present in acetyl-CoA is incorporated into ATP as a result of two distinct but integrated processes, viz. the Krebs (citric acid or tricarboxylic acid) cycle and oxidative phosphorylation. The connecting links between the two systems are NAD and the flavoproteins. They are reduced (i.e. accept hydrogen) during the reactions of the citric acid cycle and are reoxidized during oxidative phosphorylation. Both systems are located on the mitochondrion and are thus intimately related to one another physically.

## Krebs Cycle (Fig. 3)

The cycle may be regarded as consisting of a series of carbon skeletons which act as vehicles for the delivery of hydrogen from the foodstuffs to the respiratory chain. During the process ATP and $CO_2$ are produced. NAD and flavoprotein are reduced and act as the connecting links between the citric acid cycle and the respiratory chain. In fact only 1 molecule of ATP is produced in the cycle, the bulk production occurring in the respiratory chain. Starting with pyruvate the overal reaction may be written:

$$CH_3COCOOH + 2\tfrac{1}{2}O_2 + ADP + P \rightarrow 3CO_2 + 2H_2O + ATP$$

The entry of one molecule of acetyl-Co.A. followed by a single turn of the cycle results in the following:

$$3NAD^+ + 6H \rightarrow 3NADH + 3H^+$$
$$Flavin + 2H \rightarrow Flavin\ H_2$$

Although most of the steps in the cycle are reversible

the α-ketoglutarate succinyl-Co.A step is not, so that the direction of the cycle is from citrate to oxaloacetate.

Control of the cycle is dependent on the availability of NAD which in turn depends on the rate of oxidation of

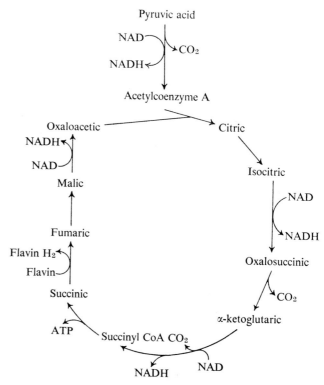

Fig. 3. Krebs cycle.

NADH in the respiratory chain. This rate is linked to the formation of high energy phosphate bonds during oxidative phosphorylation. Thus the rate of turnover of the citric acid cycle is dependent on the needs of the cell for high energy phosphate bonds.

## Oxidative Phosphorylation (Fig. 4)

It is possible to state what oxidative phosphorylation achieves if not exactly how it does so. What follows then

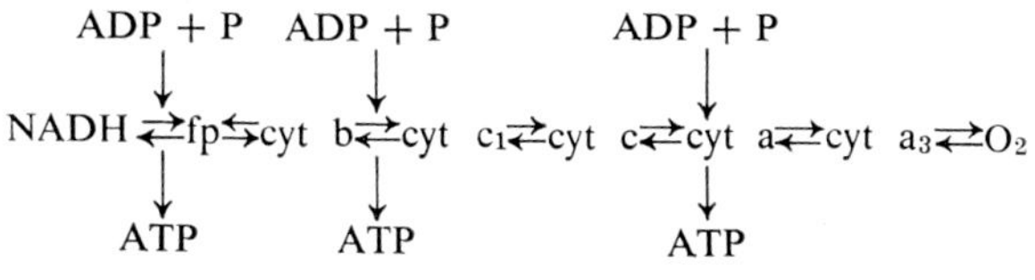

$$
\begin{array}{ccccc}
ADP + P & ADP + P & & ADP + P & \\
\downarrow & \downarrow & & \downarrow & \\
NADH \rightleftarrows fp \rightleftarrows cyt\ b \rightleftarrows cyt\ c_1 \rightleftarrows cyt\ c \rightleftarrows cyt\ a \rightleftarrows cyt\ a_3 \rightleftarrows O_2 \\
\downarrow & \downarrow & & \downarrow & \\
ATP & ATP & & ATP &
\end{array}
$$

Fig. 4. Oxidative phosphorylation and the respiratory chain. Shows the three positions of energy release.

is but a possible explanation of what occurs. Essentially oxidative phosphorylation consists of two distinct processes which have close links. It is firstly an oxidative process whereby the hydrogen produced during the citric acid cycle is oxidized to $H_2O$. Secondly it results in the phosphorylation of adenosine diphosphate (ADP) to ATP. The energy is trapped in ATP in the form of the 'high energy phosphate bond' ($\sim$P). The two processes are 'coupled' to one another, or in other words, phosphorylation will only happen in the presence of oxidation. This is because the

important observation as here we have a means of assessing tissue oxygenation *in vivo*.

The reactions of the respiratory chain may be summarized as follows:

$$3NADH + 3H^+ + 9ADP + 9P_1 + 1\tfrac{1}{2}O_2 \rightarrow 3NAD^+ + 9ATP + 3H_2O$$

$$\text{flavin } H_2 + 2ADP + 2P_1 + \tfrac{1}{2}O_2 \rightarrow \text{flavin} + 2ATP + H_2O$$

energy required for incorporation of the high energy phosphate bond into ATP is released as a result of the oxidative process. Occasionally uncoupling can occur, where the oxidative process continues in the absence of ATP production and the energy released is then dissipated as heat. A familiar example of an uncoupler is thyroxine which, in excess, results in the dissipation of the body's energy supply to heat with loss of weight and hyperpyrexia.

Oxidative phosphorylation is carried out by a series of enzymes linked to one another in the respiratory chain (Fig. 4). At one end of the chain is situated NAD and at the other cytochrome $a_3$. Essentially what happens is that NADH is presented at one end and has two electrons removed.

i.e. $$NADH \rightarrow NAD^+ + H^+ + 2e$$

These 2 electrons flow down the respiratory chain, rather like a current flowing down a wire, successively reducing the adjacent enzyme. The enzyme from which the electrons have been removed becomes reoxidized and receptive to further electrons. As when current flows through a wire, causing it to become hot (i.e. to give off energy), energy is released as electrons flow down the respiratory chain. The energy is picked up by ADP and P, and is incorporated into ATP as the $\sim$P.

In fact the reaction

$$ADP + P \leftrightarrow ATP$$

has an equilibrium far to the left and ATP would not form without energy to drive the reaction to the right.

As a result of the existence of several members in the respiratory chain it is possible to release small amounts of energy at a time. The energy difference between NADH and oxygen is more than three times that necessary to cause ATP formation from ADP and P. Therefore increasing the steps available enables energy release to occur in discrete steps with the formation of more ATP.

The last member of the chain, cytochrome $a_3$, reacts with molecular oxygen. It gives up its 2 electrons to oxygen to form $O^{--}$. This reacts with the $H^+$ ions produced earlier to form water.

$$2H^+ + O^{--} \rightarrow H_2O$$

We can see immediately that the supply of oxygen to the tissue will be reflected by the oxidation-reduction (redox) state of cytochrome $a_3$. Cytochrome $a_3$'s redox state will be reflected in cytochrome a's redox state and so on back down the chain. In other words the redox state of NAD:NADH will also reflect tissue oxygen availability. The ability to measure changes in the concentration of NADH *in vivo* by fluorometric methods makes this a most

Control of the rate of respiratory chain oxidation depends on the availability of several factors, viz. ADP and $P_1$, substrate supply of NADH, and oxygen. Thus the exact redox state of all the members of the chain will vary with the supply of these factors. Absence of oxygen will cause all members to be reduced. Abundance of all factors results in gradually increasing states of oxidation of the members with NADH 50 per cent oxidized at one end and cytochrome $a_3$ fully oxidized at the other. Under these circumstances the factor which limits the oxidation of NADH is the speed with which the respiratory chain can cope with oxidation. Reduction of ADP supply will give rise to a different redox state of the chain. In all, five such states have been described resulting from various combinations of factor supply.

## SUMMARY

Energy originating from the sun's radiation, trapped in the form of chemical energy in food, is converted into a form, ATP, which is readily available for the body's needs. The process involves breakdown of food to a common unit, acetyl-CoA, from which hydrogen is removed in the Krebs cycle, to produce reduced NAD and reduced flavoprotein. These being at a higher energetic level than oxygen, release energy in the process of being oxidized by the respiratory chain. This energy is partially trapped by the body as ATP which then uses this energy for mechanical, electrical and osmotic work. Lack of oxygen leads to a serious loss of efficiency in energy conservation.

### Abnormal Tissue Respiration resulting from Tissue Hypoxia

Most of the changes resulting from inadequate oxygen supplies to the tissues will be evident from the foregoing discussion. With complete cessation of oxygen supply, the oxygen remaining in the tissue will be used up until there is no more available to accept electrons from cytochrome $a_3$. The proportion of reduced cytochrome $a_3$ will increase, as electrons continue to be supplied along the respiratory chain, and it will in time become completely reduced. At the same time the relative proportion of reduced to oxidized form of all the other enzymes in the chain will increase until eventually they are all completely reduced, from cytochrome $a_3$ at one end to NADH at the other.

The requirement of the tissue for continued supplies of accessible energy (ATP) is met by the continued function of the E-M pathway. In this process, the conversion of pyruvate to lactate produces NAD to enable the glucose to pyruvate part of the pathway to function. The rate of glycolysis is also increased.

The end result of tissue hypoxia will be:

1. Reduced oxygen content with a fall in tissue $P_{O_2}$.

2. Reduction of the enzymes of the respiratory chain including NAD.

3. A decrease in creatine phosphate, with an increase in creatine. The creatine phosphate/creatine ratio will as a consequence decrease.

4. A decrease in ATP with an increase in ADP and P and a decrease of the ATP/ADP ratio. The increase in ADP stimulates glycolysis.

5. NADH rise: Normally cytoplasmic NADH is transferred to the mitochondria via 'shuttle' systems which depend for their operation on enzyme systems and Krebs cycle substrates. In hypoxia the shuttle system becomes inoperative and the NADH concentration builds up in the cytoplasm.

6. Lactate formation: Pyruvate will no longer be oxidized via the Krebs cycle but will be converted to lactate, with the result that tissue lactate increases as does the lactate/pyruvate ratio. In the process a certain amount of NADH is oxidized to NAD.

As lactate and pyruvate can diffuse out of the tissue, the increased lactate/pyruvate ratio may be reflected in the blood draining the tissue, and in any fluid which may be bathing it (e.g. CSF).

7. Tissue acidosis: As it is strictly speaking lactic acid which is produced, and as this is ionized at normal tissue pH, then $H^+$ ions are formed and tissue acidosis results. Diffusion causes the venous effluent and tissue fluid to become more acid.

8. $K^+$ ion release: The build up of the cellular $H^+$ ion concentration forces out $K^+$ ions which are also released into the blood.

9. Release of cellular enzymes (such as glutamic oxaloacetic acid, GOT) occurs when tissue hypoxia is severe. Cell death is probably not a pre-requisite for this to occur.

10. Cell death.

### Methods of Detecting Tissue Hypoxia

A simple method of detecting inadequate oxygen supply to the tissue in clinical practice would be of great value. Unfortunately no such method exists at the present time. The commonest approach is to measure the arterial oxygen tension ($Pa_{O_2}$). However, variations in blood flow and local tissue anatomy (e.g. in oedematous tissues) and in the $O_2$ carrying capacity of the blood make the relationship between the $Pa_{O_2}$ and tissue $P_{O_2}$ uncertain and as a result decrease the usefulness of this observation.

Experimentally various approaches have been used which all involve the measurement of some biochemical parameter. For the sake of our present discussion we will define tissue hypoxia as constituting a change in the redox state of the respiratory chain to a more reduced state from that which occurs when oxygen is in abundance. Adequate supplies of substrate (NADH) and ADP and $P_1$ are presumed. It should be remembered that this does not necessarily constitute a life threatening situation but means a less efficient conservation of the energy in foodstuffs.

Detecting changes in the redox state of the respiratory chain enzymes is the most direct approach of assessing adequate oxygen supplies. Analyses of lactate-pyruvate ratios and ATP and creatine phosphate levels are one step removed and thus are less certain methods owing to the influence of extraneous factors. The detection of enzymes released as a result of cell death is open to the same objection as well as being imprecise. Direct measurement of tissue $P_{O_2}$ although technically feasible relies on the detection of some biochemical change for the interpretation of its significance.

### 1. Changes in Redox State of the Respiratory Chain Enzymes

#### (a) Spectro-photometric Analysis

The individual respiratory chain enzymes when reduced may be identified by their characteristic light absorption. A knowledge of their specific extinction coefficients enables a calculation of their concentration from the absorption spectra. The first member of the chain to be affected by reduced oxygen supply is cytochrome $a_3$ and measurements of the redox state of this enzyme would be the most direct way of assessing tissue oxygenation. However, owing to the fact that the absorption spectra of the cytochromes are similar to haemoglobin, all blood must be removed from the preparation before measurements are made. Thus this technique is only suitable for excised tissues or preparations of mitochondria. Despite this, spectrophotometric analysis has proved to be a very effective method for determining the effect of various manoeuvres on the state of the respiratory chain enzymes *in vitro*.

#### (b) Fluorometric Analysis

Reduced NAD, but not the oxidized form, fluoresces strongly with a broad band around 470 m$\mu$ when excited with 366 m$\mu$ light from a mercury arc. Haemoglobin absorbs both the emitted and the excitation lights. However, both the oxidized and reduced forms of Hb absorb the light with equal intensity and so changes in the oxygenation of Hb do not alter the level of fluorescence. In consequence this technique may be used for *in vivo* analysis of the redox state of NAD. Blood vessels appear as black lines and their effect is to reduce the area from which the signal is produced. The degree of fluorescence is proportional to the degree of reduction of NAD. The NADH:NAD ratio is related to the oxygen available, providing adequate ADP and substrate NADH are present.

This method has been extensively used by one group in America and preliminary results are encouraging. However, it is technically quite difficult and at the moment is suitable only for experimental work.

### 2. Tissue $P_{O_2}$

Tissue $P_{O_2}$ is measured either by the insertion of a miniature oxygen electrode directly into the tissue, or by placing an electrode on the surface. The microelectrodes are usually made by the individual experimenter, although there is a commercially available electrode.

To avoid trauma to the tissue these electrodes have to be very small at their tip, usually only a few microns in diameter, and they are in consequence, quite difficult to make. Despite this several groups have been using them with considerable success.

As previously mentioned, tissue $P_{O_2}$, unrelated to any other measurement, is of limited value. It has been found that the rate of tissue respiration in the brain judged by the respiratory enzyme redox state, is unaffected down to local $P_{O_2}$ of 2 mm. Hg. In addition wide variation in tissue $P_{O_2}$ occurs depending on the relationship of electrode tip to the nearest arteriole. Put in another way there is a diffusion gradient through the tissue, the lowest $P_{O_2}$ being found at the point farthest from the arteriole.

Thus to place an $O_2$ electrode into a tissue at random, hoping to get some idea of the adequacy of tissue oxygenation is a useless exercise. Firstly, because one can never be sure whether one has struck the area with the lowest $P_{O_2}$, and second, even if one had it is impossible to obtain meaningful discrimination with these electrodes below a $P_{O_2}$ of 1 mm. Hg.

### 3. Tissue Biochemistry

Although limited in its clinical application a comprehensive review of all the parameters which change as a result of tissue hypoxia, is the most satisfactory approach at the present time to the study of tissue hypoxia. The techniques for the measurement of ATP, ADP, phosphate, creatine and creatine phosphate, lactate and pyruvate, are all well established and fairly easy to perform. More limited studies, such as the measurement of lactate and pyruvate, are, because of their more indirect nature, less certain to provide one with clear-cut facts.

### 4. Changes in Venous Blood

Here one relies on the measurements of substances which are diffusible, e.g. lactate, pyruvate, phosphate, oxygen, $K^+$, $H^+$. In addition when cell membrane function is disturbed certain substances may be released from the tissue in increased amounts e.g. enzymes.

For this approach to be useful certain prerequisites are necessary.

1. The blood sampled must be mainly from the organ or tissue under study. For example, there is no point in sampling from the internal jugular vein in the human, in the hope that this represents blood coming solely from the brain. There is considerable contamination from extracerebral structures. It is necessary to sample blood from the internal jugular bulb which is very little contaminated.

2. If the first condition is satisfied we must then inquire about the anatomy of the venous system within the organ itself. This point becomes clear if one considers a pathological situation. An area of ischaemia, receiving an inadequate blood supply, will in consequence provide only a small fraction of blood to the total venous drainage. Sampling downstream, and inquiring about such inadequately oxygenated areas, we might find that the abnormal values undoubtedly present in the blood draining that area, are obliterated by the vast excess of normal blood draining the adequately oxygenated areas.

Even in the normal situation certain anatomical peculiarities, such as a counter-current system, might occur. In the counter-current situation the vessels are arranged as a U loop, the tops of the U being quite close to one another. Blood entering one limb of the U has a high oxygen tension and blood leaving the other limb a lower tension. Because of this oxygen tends to diffuse directly through the adjacent tissue from inlet to outlet limb. This results in a much lower oxygen tension in the bottom of the U than would occur if no oxygen had escaped. This curious arrangement of blood vessels has been demonstrated in the normal brain.

One can see that the venous effluent under these circumstances could be unrepresentative of the tissue at the bottom of a U loop.

3. The rate at which a substance diffuses into the blood must be known. This is important both in relation to the timing of sampling and in drawing conclusions from ratios between different substrates. It is obvious that if the substrate under examination diffuses slowly from the cell then one must allow sufficient time to elapse before drawing conclusions about its concentration in the venous blood. Errors may occur due to failure to consider the implication of the timing of the measurement in the light of the clinical situation. If the cause of the tissue hypoxia is a reduced blood supply, little abnormality of the venous blood from the whole organ may be observed. If however the blood flow is restored, e.g. an aortic clamp is removed, then the ischaemic metabolites formed in the tissue will be washed out and the venous blood may then be quite abnormal. In this instance the venous blood may reflect pre-existing hypoxia.

If one wishes to draw meaningful conclusions from ratios in the venous blood, such as the lactate/pyruvate (L/P) ratio, then one must be certain that the rate at which both substances diffuse from the tissue is equal, otherwise changes of the ratio will be measured which are not representative of what is happening in the tissue.

4. A further possible cause of misinterpretation of venous values could be that the changes observed are the result of alterations in the arterial blood supply to the organ resulting from the method of the study. Arterial sampling and comparison of a-v differences will solve this problem.

5. Having satisfied oneself that there is a true change of venous values and that this blood is representative of the organ under study we need to inquire as to the exact interpretation of these changes. It is not sufficient to conclude that because one has the changes associated with tissue hypoxia that this is the only interpretation.

### (a) Venous $P_{O_2}$

Tissue hypoxia should cause a fall in the $P_{O_2}$ of the blood draining the hypoxic area. If the organ being studied is uniformly hypoxic, venous $P_{O_2}$ levels are likely to be of some use in detecting this. However, to judge whether a particular $P_{O_2}$ is critical, one must have some biochemical or other standard by which to assess it. If the $P_{O_2}$ in the venous blood from the brain falls to approximately 20 mm Hg it has been shown that other changes suggesting tissue hypoxia consistently occur. Thus a finding of this kind would be strong evidence that the brain was under-oxygenated. However, it would not be possible to argue the reverse and suggest that the presence of a $Pv_{O_2} > 20$ mm Hg meant that there was no tissue hypoxia (see Section 1). A striking example of this occurs in head injuries where the occurrence of 'red veins' has been noted. Arterio-venous shunts resulting from vasomotor paralysis, which is in turn due to tissue acidosis, cause highly oxygenated blood to drain into the venous system and this frequently causes a high venous $P_{O_2}$.

## (b) Biochemical Changes

All the biochemical parameters which are diffusible and thus appear in the venous blood as a result of increasing tissue levels, are non-specific for tissue hypoxia.

A detailed discussion of this fact is not appropriate here and the reader may consult the references for details. However, the facts relating to the measurement of lactate/pyruvate ratios (L/P ratios) and excess lactate may be stated as follows. (See Chamberlain and Lis (1968) and Cohen (1972).)

During hypoxia, lactate is produced by reduction of pyruvate by cytoplasmic NADH.

$$\text{Pyruvate} + \text{NADH} + \text{H}^+ \rightleftarrows \text{lactate} + \text{NAD}^+$$

If this equation is rearranged the influence on the L/P ratio of the redox state of NAD may be seen.

$$\frac{\text{Lactate}}{\text{Pyruvate}} = K \frac{\text{NADH} + \text{H}^+}{\text{NAD}^+}$$

If the ratio NADH/NAD increases as a result of tissue hypoxia then the L/P ratio will increase. However, tissue hypoxia results in an increase of NADH/NAD in the mitochondrion and will only be reflected by the ratio in the cytoplasm if the shuttle system between the mitochondria and the cytoplasm is functional. Hypoxia affects the efficiency of the system and so cytoplasmic ratio may not necessarily reflect mitochondrial ratios. If measurement of blood L/P ratios are made these will only reflect cytoplasmic L/P and NADH/NAD ratios, and therefore do not always accurately relate to mitochondrial values. It is evident from the equation that alterations in $\text{H}^+$ ion concentration will affect L/P ratios. An increased $\text{H}^+$ ion concentration should result in an increase in the L/P ratio, in the absence of changes in the NADH/NAD ratio. In fact abundant evidence exists which shows that *alkalosis* is associated with increased L/P ratio in arterial and venous blood. The reason for this discrepancy is not clear.

That changes in the venous blood of the kind outlined previously, do occur when a tissue is under oxygenated, is undisputed. The problem arises when one wishes to infer from observed biochemical changes the state of tissue oxygenation. At the moment insufficient evidence exists to enable one to interpret such changes precisely. However,

no better tool exists and the evaluation of these changes in the clinical field, requires more attention.

## 5. Cerebrospinal Fluid

Because of the difficulties associated with the interpretation of changes in the cerebral venous blood attention has recently been focused on the C.S.F. The existence of a barrier to easy diffusion of certain substrates from the brain to the blood suggested that the C.S.F. might be more representative of the biochemical state of the brain. It has been shown that the C.S.F. becomes more acid and has an increased L/P ratio after hypoxia. There is a lack of precise information however about the inter-relationships between lactate and pyruvate levels, the $\text{H}^+$ ion concentration, and the electrical potential difference that exists between the C.S.F. and the blood. At the moment, although it is true to say that brain hypoxia causes increased acidosis and L/P ratios in the C.S.F., the reverse argument may not be true.

A limitation to examining the C.S.F. in the clinical field is the demonstration of the slow equilibration of lumbar C.S.F. and ventricular C.S.F. in acutely varying conditions.

## 6. Arterial and Central Venous Blood

Various workers have studied arterial and venous blood for biochemical changes. Blood sampled from these sites is necessarily the resultant of whole body changes. Despite this it has become common clinical practice to measure $\text{H}^+$ ion concentration, $Pa_{O_2}$ and $Pv_{O_2}$ because useful information is obtained about adequacy of tissue oxygenation. The utility of such information is however probably confined to gross clinical conditions, such as cardiac arrest and low cardiac output states.

Looking for subtler inadequacies of tissue oxygenation is more difficult. It is possible that observing increases in the L/P ratio may be helpful although little change in the arterial ratio is found unless the arterial $P_{O_2}$ falls below 40 mm. Hg. A comparison of acid base changes and L/P changes would be useful.

Arterial $P_{O_2}$ measurements are popular but have limitations when considering the adequacy of tissue oxygenation. However, it is a simple technique to measure $P_{O_2}$ and it does at least ensure that one parameter, which the anaesthetist can control, is at a satisfactory level.

Central venous $P_{O_2}$ is not so easily measured and does not have the same specificity as, say, cerebral venous $P_{O_2}$. It will be even less likely to detect small areas of tissue hypoxia.

## Conclusion

Gross tissue hypoxia will usually be evident from clinical observation and certain simple measurements, e.g. $Pa_{O_2}$, the base deficit. It will also cause a number of biochemical changes some of which may be detected in the venous blood draining the hypoxic site. Less severe hypoxia is more difficult to detect at the moment and more work will be needed to establish whether changes in biochemical parameters such as increasing L/P ratios, are reliable indices of tissue hypoxia.

## FURTHER READING

Chamberlain, J. H. and Lis, M. (1968), "Measurement of Blood Lactate Levels and Excess Lactate as Indices of Hypoxia During Anaesthesia," *Anaesthesia*, **23**, 521.

Cohen, P. J. (1972), "The Metabolic Function of Oxygen and Biochemical Lesions of Hypoxia," *Anaesthesiology*, **37**, 148–177.

Jobsis, F. S. (1964), "Basic Processes in Cellular Respiration," in *Handbook of Physiology*, Chap. 2, p. 63.

Section 3, "Respiration," Vol. 2. American Physiological Society, Washington, D.C.

Nunn, J. F. (1969), "Oxygen," in *Applied Respiratory Physiology*, Chap. 12. Butterworth, London

*CHAPTER* 5

# HYPOTHERMIA

### D. BENAZON

If hypothermia is defined as the clinical state of subnormal body temperature, the terms 'normal temperature' and 'body temperature' demand closer definition.

### Normal Temperature

Normal temperature measured in the oropharynx usually varies between 36·0–37·5° (Wallace, 1968). Certain physiological variations are well recognized. These include diurnal variations of 1–2°C with the minima occurring at night and the maxima in the evening. These variations may show reversal following alterations in sleep rhythm.

Other physiological variations occur in association with menstruation and pregnancy. Thus the average daily temperature rises distinctly at ovulation and remains at this level until menstruation when it falls again. Should conception occur, the temperature may remain raised. These changes are only noticeable if the recordings are charted as each days measurement falls within the normal range of variations.

### Body Temperature and Gradients

John Hunter (1786) began the practice of measuring body temperature by means of a mercury thermometer placed beneath the tongue. This method is cheap and suffices when changes in body temperature are occurring very slowly and particularly when there is a rise of temperature above normal. It meets the needs of the commoner clinical situations.

However it was subsequently realized that oral temperature often differed from that measured elsewhere in the body and that large masses of body tissue, such as the skin, subcutaneous tissues and the extremities were often permitted to cool, although the temperature of deeper organs, such as brain and heart, was maintained. These tissues are known as the 'shell' and the 'core' respectively, and it is therefore apparent that the concept of

'average body temperature' is of limited use. Usually 'body temperature' will apply to the oropharyngeal temperature, but in writings concerned with hypothermia it more commonly applies to the oesophageal temperature.

Oesophageal temperature varies with the position of the sensing probe and Whitby and Deakin (1968) found that the lower quarter of the oesophagus gave the most reliable reading.

### Heat Balance

The temperature of the body core is determined by the balance between heat gain and heat loss.

In the natural state, exchange of heat occurs at the body surface, predominantly the skin, but some heat exchange occurs in the lungs.

The five factors involved are set out below and the symbols used in the equations are (Moore, 1972): $Q$—quantity of heat transferred (Joules or cal./sec./m.$^2$); $T$—temperature; $c$—core; $s$—surface; $w$—wall (of radiating surface); $a$—air; $\lambda$—thermal conductivity; $l$—depth of tissue.

1. Radiation $\quad Q_1 \propto T_s^4 - T_w^4$

2. Conduction $\quad Q_2 \propto (T_c - T_s)\dfrac{\lambda}{l}$

3. Convection $\quad Q_3 \propto (T_s - T_a)\sqrt{\text{air speed}}$

4. Evaporation $\quad Q_4 \propto 0.577(4.4 + 0.264\,V.)\Delta P_{H_2O}$

(i.e. latent heat of evaporation × air speed factor × change in water vapour pressure from surface to air).

5. Endogenous heat production $Q_5$.

The sum of these quantities should be zero if the body temperature is to remain constant.

These formulae have something to teach us, even though in use they need much modification due to the diversity of local conditions in the body. However, the possible importance of radiation losses is shown by the fourth power relationship in the equation. This can lead to cooling of exposed bodies even if the ambient air temperature is maintained. This can happen in ambulances or in incubators (Hey and Mount, 1957) when long wave radiations escape to adjacent cold wall surfaces, or to the sky.

In exposure situations, increased wind speed can produce severe chilling (Pugh, 1964) and it is apparent that effective protective measures must take into account all these paths for heat loss.

If heat loss continues, the body preserves the core temperature at the expense of the peripheral shell tissues, whose temperature is allowed to fall. At the same time the flow of blood in the surface and shell tissues is reduced by vascular constriction, thus increasing insulation and reducing heat loss. Metabolic heat production may also be increased from shivering and non-shivering sources.

The application of a calorimetry to the study of heat production in animals has led to the concept of a 'thermo-neutral' zone within which a homeothermic animal subjected to lowered environmental temperature compensates by alteration in peripheral blood flow and piloerection. If this environmental temperature falls below the 'critical temperature', then heat production rises due to increased activity, shivering and metabolic stimulation. The rate at which production of heat rises depends on the animal's size, insulation (e.g. fat layers), degree of acclimatization (see page 346) and species differences in the pattern of thermo-regulation.

Loss of heat due to evaporation may, in burned patients, lead to metabolic stimulation.

## The Control of Body Temperature

Heat regulation is a feed back system and is served by reflex mechanisms.

It includes receptors, afferent and efferent pathways, central nervous system connections and centres, and a battery of effector mechanisms (Hemingway and Price, 1968).

The essentials of this system are outlined in the scheme below.

**Receptors**—These are temperature sensitive receptors in the skin and also a temperature sensitive area in the rostral hypothalamus separate from the thermoregulation centre.

**Afferent Pathways**—via the dorsal roots and the spinal cord relays and via cranial nerves.

**Central Connections**—via reticular formation relays, and the main hypothalamic thermoregulation centre. Afferent input also passes to the cerebral cortex.

**Efferent Pathway**—(1) from the main hypothalamic centre, via brain stem tracts and the reticular integrating neurones to the rubrospinal and reticulospinal tracts of the spinal cord to the preganglionic neurones in the grey matter of the spinal cord and thence via the ventral roots to muscles.

(2) Other efferents descend in the sympathetic efferent pathways to sympathetic effectors.

**Cerebral Cortex**—this receives some of the afferent input and is responsible for the appreciation of cold and heat and for originating the various behavioural responses.

**Local Temperature Effects**—changes occur in cutaneous vasomotor tone produced by local temperature alterations, independent of central connections. This has been observed in patients with sympathectomized limbs and patients with cord transections (Johnson, 1965).

**Effectors**—(1) voluntary muscles concerned with increased activity during behavioural responses and shivering.

(2) Sympathetic effectors serving cutaneous vasoactivity, sweating, piloerection and release of catecholamines with increased metabolic thermogenesis.

## Significance of the Control Mechanisms

The skin receptors and the rostral hypothalamic temperature sensitive areas may produce opposing effects. Johnson showed that if the core temperature is below about 36·5°C, warming the trunk area of subjects failed to produce the usual reflex vasodilation in the hand. Thus presumably the central control centre is exerting an overriding influence.

He also showed that the sensation of cold is related to cortical appreciation of skin temperature and that shivering only occurs in muscles with intact central connections. Thus conscious quadriplegics who were rendered hypothermic but whose skin above the level of the transection was kept warm, did not feel cold and only shivered above the level of the lesion.

The local temperature effects are of considerable importance in patients with cord transections where central connections are interrupted.

The effector mechanisms vary in their practical significance.

1. Cutaneous vasoactivity: Blood flow in superficial tissues determines skin temperature, which in turn determines heat loss to the environment. This mechanism regulates heat balance in most ordinary situations, but represents a fine control only. It is mediated by sympathetic hormones released from adrenergic endings and the action on smooth muscle receptors is of the alpha type.

2. Shivering: This centrally mediated non-autonomic response consists of involuntary rhythmic contractions of voluntary muscle. Shivering leads to a large increase in heat production (up to five times the resting value). But it increases convective heat loss and is an inefficient and inconvenient long term response as it adversely affects co-ordination and fine movements.

3. Sweating: In man this response is mediated by the reflex connections already referred to and by cholinergic sympathetic fibres passing to the sweat glands. Those of greatest importance in thermal sweating are the eccrine glands which are widely distributed over the skin surface. The apocrine glands are different. They are localized in the more hairy regions of the body (axillae, areolae, perineum, etc.) and respond to catecholamine mediators. They do not become involved in thermal sweating unless the demand is extreme. Piloerection is of vestigial importance in man. It is an adrenergic mechanism mediated by a similar reflex mechanism.

4. Non-shivering thermogenesis and acclimatization:

Metabolism provides the energy for essential physiological processes and for heat production. Where hypothermic stress is applied, heat production may become the major metabolic activity. Thus in muscles that are shivering, 'useful work' may approach zero; yet there will be intense metabolic activity devoted to heat production.

In the short term, heat production from muscle shivering is the main source of extra heat. Johnson (1965) could find no evidence in his subjects who were curarized and cooled, of increased oxygen uptake, but more general metabolic stimulation might take time to develop, Figure 1.

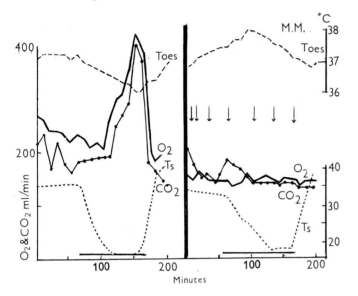

Fig. 1. The effect of muscle paralysis (induced by galla-mine 80 mgm. at each arrow) in abolishing the increase in oxygen consumption induced by cooling. Skin temperature ($T_s$). Oesophageal temperature ($T_{oes}$).

*By permission of the editors of the J. Physiol.*

In prolonged cooling and cold acclimatization, as well as in the reverse process of heat adaptation, there is evidence in animals and man of changes in metabolic activity independent of shivering or muscle hypertonus.

Cottle *et al.* (1956) investigated non-shivering thermogenesis and cold acclimatization in rats and found that animals placed in a cold environment at 5°C for several weeks first showed the usual reactions to cold such as muscle shivering, cutaneous vasoconstriction, piloerection and increased activity with increased metabolic rate. In time the piloerection subsided, skin temperature returned to normal, and shivering ceased. Metabolic activity however, remained high. Moreover they showed that cold acclimatized rats in an environment at 5°C were able to maintain their body temperature even when shivering was prevented by curarization.

In man it becomes more difficult to devise studies under standard conditions of temperature, humidity, activity, body size, diet, race, etc. However Simpson (personal communication) showed that in Jamaicans, in their own continuously hot environment, there was a marked fall in Basal Metabolic Rate (BMR), compared with Jamaicans in this country. Similarly Yoshimura *et al.* (1966) showed

that there were seasonal variations among Japanese with a rise of BMR in winter and fall in summer.

Wyndham *et al.* (1968) investigated differences between fat and normal men in their reactions to cold. They showed that the metabolic rate of fat men did not rise due to shivering until the air temperature had dropped to 10°C which was 10°C lower than the normal subjects, and that the latter then showed a higher skin temperature and lower rectal temperature than the fat subjects.

After a period in Antarctica, normal men showed a fall in metabolic rate and average skin temperature. They also put on weight and showed a similar delayed metabolic response to fall of air temperature to fat men. Skin temperature is influenced by the insulating effect of fatty layers and they found that the skin temperature of fat men dropped about 5°C lower than that of normal men before an increase in metabolism was evident.

### Neurohumoral and Cellular Responses to Cold

Let us consider where increased non-shivering thermogenesis arises and the mechanism of its control.

Even lower animals, including unicellular organisms and poikilotherms such as molluscs, fishes, amphibians and reptiles, show adaptations to thermal environmental changes. Many of these are at cellular and enzyme level and there is reason to believe that similar mechanisms underly the more complex adaptations that came later in the phylogenetic sequence. Having outlined the neural mechanisms it is necessary to discuss those neuro-humoral, hormonal and cellular mechanisms which are particularly concerned in non-shivering thermogenesis.

### Brown Adipose Tissue

Interest in hibernating animals focussed attention on the curious masses of brown fatty tissue found in various sites, especially the interscapular region in these animals. Brown fat cells are richer in protoplasm than those of white adipose tissue and are derived from a primitive adipose organ of reticuloendothelial origin. All mammalian species, including humans, have this tissue at birth, but usually it disappears with progress to maturity. In hibernating animals and rats it persists into adult life as an actively functioning organ, rich in steroids, enzymes and aminoacids and shows evidence of hypertrophy in cold stress conditions.

Smith (1964) suggested that a portion of the increase in non-shivering thermogenesis in such animals in cold environments is due to the activity of brown adipose tissue and that cold induced arousal from hibernation is caused by sympathetic stimulation of this gland, leading to increased metabolism and a rise of temperature and activity which spreads to the neighbouring thoracic organs and beyond.

There is evidence that this organ continues to function in the new born infant.

It is known from the work of Cross, Tizard and Trythall (1955) that mild hypoxia suppresses heat production in the human neonate. Animal experiments suggest that ganglion blocking agents have a similar effect and that noradrenaline infusion increased heat production. Whether these effects can be attributed entirely to Brown Adipose tissue responses is uncertain, particularly as in human neonates Brown fat deposits are less well developed than in some experimental animals. However, it is plain that anoxia, beta-blocking drugs and anaesthetics may be expected to depress non-shivering heat production, particularly in neonates.

### Other Trophic Changes

In cold adapted animals, the thyroid, adrenals, pituitary and gut show hypertrophy. The gut hypertrophy is presumably related to the need for increased caloric intake and the endocrine hypertrophy also suggests increased demands for their respective hormones.

Catecholamines have been shown to stimulate oxygen consumption in rats, particularly if they were cold adapted (Evonuk and Hannon, 1963). Leduc (1961) showed that during cold acclimatization in rats, urinary noradrenaline output increased initially and then fell to normal. He suggested that there developed increased sensitivity to the hormone and that this accounted for the increased non-shivering thermogenesis and the acclimatization process.

Both hexamethonium and piperoxan will reduce the raised oxygen consumption of cold adapted curarized rats (Hsei *et al.*, 1957) and noradrenaline has been shown to be a potent stimulator of oxygen consumption in rats, the non-shivering muscle taking a major part in this increased consumption (Depocas, 1960).

Thyroidectomy lowers non-shivering oxygen consumption in rats and possibly sensitizes muscle to noradrenaline induced thermogenesis. Adrenaline seems to be more a last line of defence in severe cold stress, particularly in the presence of thyroid deficiency, when it is released from chromaffin tissue and assists in thermogenesis. (Hsei *et al.*, 1957; Hsei and Carlson, 1957; Andersson *et al.*, 1967).

### Neurohumoral and Cellular Integration

The integration of these neurohumoral and hormonal actions into our understanding of cellular function is the next stage in enquiry.

Hormones are metabolically active substances, no different basically from other substrates. Their synthesis and degradation is integrated into the general body metabolism. Their production is controlled by the well known feedback mechanisms.

In the control of body temperature, balance is principally determined by the amount and oxidoreductive states of the pyridine nucleotides, NAD and NADH. NADH steps lie across almost every known synthetic pathway.

For instance, thyroxine treatment, or cold exposure, will diminish triglyceride synthesis and lead to diversion of NADH into the synthetic pathways for cholesterol and phospholipids. These are in turn substrates for the synthesis of steroids and for components of the mitochondrial electron transport chain.

Upon this complex system of interactions, the environmental cold stimulus imposes a directional pattern, possibly mediated as follows:

The activity of the hypothalamic heat regulatory centre, sympathetic motor discharge and catecholamine release could result in increased glycogenolysis with the production of glucose 1 phosphate. Hormonal influences will then determine the further course in the direction of classical glycolysis and other NADH and thyroid facilitated paths which lead to the diversion of substrates, such as α-glycerophosphate into the cytochrome-c dependent pathway of the mitochondrial electron chain. It is suggested that this may lead to the loss of chemical potential normally needed for further metabolic reactions and instead, the conversion of this energy to heat (Smith and Hoijer, 1962).

This is one possible way the presence of a cold environment could, in time, alter the direction of metabolic pathways and lead to the production of extra heat.

The significance of Serotonin in temperature regulation is suggested in the report of Vaidya and Levine (1971), who quoted a case of carcinoid syndrome treated with the Serotonin antagonist, parachlorophenylalanine, that responded to this drug by the development of hypothermia.

### Behavioural Responses

While there is good reason to believe that the autonomic and metabolic adaptations referred to above are important, it must be admitted that the most significant of man's responses to cold are probably behavioural. These include increased voluntary activity, the use of clothing to add insulation, etc. Thus it was shown by Norman (1965) that in polar conditions, only 9 per cent of the total time may be spent out of doors.

## Physiology of Hypothermia

We have considered thermoregulation in animals and man, and the extent of adaptation possible under the normal range of environmental conditions.

Let us now consider the implications if thermoregulation fails and the body temperature is allowed to fall.

### Antimetabolic Effect of Hypothermia

Many estimates of this effect have been made in the past, and these estimates can differ considerably depending on the conditions of the experiment.

Metabolic energy is derived from the oxidation of substrates to carbon dioxide and water. Estimations of carbon dioxide output as an index of metabolism have proved inaccurate owing to changes in the solubility of this gas, and the complex buffering mechanisms of the body. Oxygen uptake is more easily measured, and is the most commonly used index.

The body can derive energy on a temporary and limited basis via lactate without the immediate consumption of oxygen, although finally oxidation has to take place if energy transfer is to continue. If oxygen debt were to occur during hypothermia this should be indicated by the presence of acidosis and by a higher oxygen uptake during rewarming than during cooling. Tissue death would also result in diminished uptake, but the clinical effect should be apparent on rewarming. Bigelow *et al.* (1950) considered, but found no evidence for these possibilities.

Acidosis and oxygen debt can occur if perfusion and cooling of local blocks of tissue are inadequate. This may occur if perfusion techniques are inadequate or where circulatory arrest is employed.

Comparisons between different experiments are difficult if shivering is uncontrolled or if different reference temperatures are employed or steady state conditions are not present. Thus using rapid pervascular cooling, it has been shown that it is possible rapidly to reduce oesophageal temperature to 30°C and leave the total body oxygen consumption at 75 per cent normal value due to the very large temperature gradients produced by this technique (Clowes *et al.*, 1958).

The general trend shown by all investigations is approximately as follows:

| Body temperature | Metabolic rate (% of normal) |
|---|---|
| 30°C | 60–70 |
| 20°C | 25 |
| 15°C | 15 |
| 5°C | 5 |

McQuiston (1949) applied hypothermia in the management of severely cyanosed patients undergoing cardiac surgery with apparent benefit, on the assumption that the slowing of tissue metabolism with cooling would bring the tissue demands for oxygen more nearly within the limits of available supply.

Bigelow *et al.* (1950) carried investigations a stage further. They reasoned that at a sufficiently low level of metabolic oxygen demand, it should be possible to provide for all the tissue oxygen requirements, including that of the brain, from the available stores of oxygen in the tissues, and thus allow an extended period of circulatory arrest. The length of this period would depend on the degree to which cooling had depressed metabolism, but certainly periods of total circulatory arrest in excess of the 3–4 minutes permissible at normal temperature should be possible. They proved that dogs cooled to 30°C could survive 8–10 minutes circulatory arrest.

This opened up a vast new field of endeavour in cardiac surgery as it enabled the surgeon to gain access to the heart, and to operate in a field unobscured by blood and without undue haste.

Later work showed that this period of safe circulatory arrest could be extended to one hour at 10°C (nasopharyax) (Drew *et al.*, 1959).

With the advent of pump oxygenators, hypothermia gave additional safety and flexibility to the techniques of cardiopulmonary bypass by reducing the need for high flow rates because as the tissues cooled they required less oxygen. Also, short periods of circulatory arrest could be provided at key periods in the repair or when unexpected difficulties in perfusion technique were encountered.

## Central Nervous System in Hypothermia

Hypothermia leads to the slowing of all central nervous system activity. Narcosis supervenes at nasopharyngeal temperatures below 25°C, thus reducing the need for anaesthetic drugs at low temperature.

Electroencephelographic activity disappears at 15–20°C but is not completely reliable as an indicator of neuronal activity as it is affected by other variables including venous pressure, anaesthetics, and the presence of cerebral oedema.

Cerebrospinal fluid pressure and brain size both decrease with fall in temperature.

The degree of depression of cerebral metabolism with most methods of cooling is probably rather greater than for the rest of the body. This may be due to the very good blood supply, which encourages cooling.

However the cerebral vessels also become vasoconstricted and irritable with cooling at temperatures of 30°C, but at lower temperatures vasodilatation becomes more noticeable, so the total effect of hypothermia on the balance of oxygen provision and requirement in the brain is a little uncertain.

## Respiration

**Lungs.** Respiratory depression proceeds at about the same rate as the depression of oxygen demands and carbon dioxide production, and in subjects uninfluenced by drugs, such as some cases of accidental hypothermia, remains at a level sufficient to meet the body's needs. Most anaesthetic drugs tend to produce additional respiratory depression and for this reason anaesthetists prefer to control ventilation. This is in any case necessary if the chest is to be opened but where this is not to be the case, as in neurosurgical practice, it can be argued that control of respiration produces more problems than it solves. Certainly it is easy to overventilate a hypothermic patient and provided anoxia is avoided by means of high oxygen mixtures, a moderate rise of $P_{CO_2}$ is unlikely to produce much harm, and may even benefit the patient by the effect on the oxyhaemoglobin dissociation curve and cerebral vascular resistance.

Some increase in respiratory dead space due to bronchodilatation occurs in hypothermia and some areas of the lung may show reduced perfusion.

**Blood.** Gas transport is affected in three ways under hypothermic conditions.

1. There is increased solubility of oxygen and carbon dioxide in body fluids.

2. There is a shift of the oxyhaemoglobin dissociation curve to the left. Thus the tension of oxygen in the tissues must fall to a lower value than at normal temperature, before the haemoglobin will give up its oxygen.

3. There is increased activity of blood buffers, resulting in increased carbon dioxide carrying capacity.

How significant are these changes? Brewin (1964) estimates that there can be a highly significant increase in oxygen-carrying capacity.

| | Patient on air 38°C | Patient on $O_2$ (700 mm. Hg.) 38°C | Patient on $O_2$ (700 mm. Hg.) 10°C |
|---|---|---|---|
| $O_2$ ml. in solution per 100 ml. of Blood | 0·3 ml. | 2 ml. | 3·2 ml. |

As the normal arterio-venous oxygen difference is about 4–6 ml. per 100 ml. of blood, it can be seen that at 10°C most of the metabolic need for oxygen could be met from dissolved oxygen without utilizing the haemoglobin transport system.

Brewin estimates that fully oxygenated haemoglobin at 38°C loses 25 per cent of its oxygen when the $P_{O_2}$ falls to 40 mm. Hg., but only 10 per cent of its oxygen when there is the same fall of $P_{O_2}$ occurring at 10°C. Although tissues can function quite adequately at low oxygen tensions any tendency to anaerobic metabolism would result in acidosis, the resulting rise in hydrogen ion concentration would then shift the oxyhaemoglobin dissociation curve back to the right.

In practice there seems to have been little evidence that significant anoxia occurs during hypothermia, Provided tissue perfusion is adequate, neither acidosis nor tissue damage have been prominent. Despite this, many workers use 5 per cent carbon dioxide in oxygen mixtures in order to shift the oxyhaemoglobin dissociation curve back towards the right, Figure 2. There was support for this practice in dog experiments when survival from hypothermia was improved (Bigelow, 1950). It is possible that the carbon dioxide was also helpful in promoting vasodilatation in brain, muscle and elsewhere, thus improving tissue perfusion generally.

Hypothermic patients can easily be overventilated as they produce less carbon dioxide and because of the increased solubility of $CO_2$. It has been shown (Burton, 1954) that by maintaining the $Pa_{CO_2}$ at 40 mm. the EEG is improved and there is improved post-operative cerebral function and cardiac action. The heart may be more difficult to defibrillate in a grossly alkalotic subject.

The carriage of carbon dioxide is also influenced by temperature. Arterial blood at 38°C, and $Pa_{CO_2}$ 40 mm Hg., carries 2·7 ml. as physically dissolved $CO_2$ per 100 ml blood. This rises to 5·4 ml at 10°C, and influences the $H^+$ ion status of the blood.

However at low temperatures, the buffering power of haemoglobin in the cells is increased, allowing it to accept more hydrogen ions. This encourages the reaction below in the direction indicated. (i)

$$CO_2 + H_2O \rightarrow H_2CO_3 \rightarrow H^+ + HCO_3^- \qquad (i)$$

Thus, plasma $HCO_3^-$, the numerator in the pH equation, rises.

These remarks presuppose that the carbon dioxide tension is kept constant with change in temperature and that the buffer composition of the fluid, particularly the haemoglobin concentration, is unaltered. This may not be the case *in vivo*.

The change in intracellular buffers during cooling may result in a considerable fall in $[H]^+$ concentration with various undesirable effects on cellular function.

If hyperventilation is allowed and the $P_{CO_2}$ falls the tendency to alkalosis in plasma and cells will be accentuated and this further justifies the addition of carbon dioxide to the inspired air during cooling. This will result in the

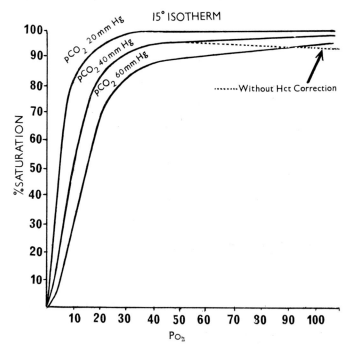

FIG. 2. Oxyhaemoglobin dissociation curve at 15°C, showing the influence of change in carbon dioxide tension.
*By permission of J. B. Lippincott Co., Philadelphia.*

absorption of large volumes of carbon dioxide which will then have to be eliminated during rewarming. Also the additional $HCO_3^-$ ions that have accumulated in the cells must pass out into the plasma again and this may not be a rapid process, particularly under hypothermic conditions, when the activity of carbonic anhydrase, which facilitates the reaction in equation (i), is depressed.

Uncertainty exists as to the optimum $P_{CO_2}$ at low temperature. Clinical evidence suggests that a $Pa_{CO_2}$ of about 40 mm. Hg. is favourable at both normal and low temperature.

### Measurements

The measurement of $[H]^+$ ion concentration with change of temperature presents further difficulties. In practice it is much more convenient to measure pH at a constant temperature of 38°C than at different body temperatures. 'Body temperature' is, as we have seen, impossible to define due to gradients, and thus pH and $P_{CO_2}$ may not be uniform. Also, it is necessary to stabilize electrodes at the various temperatures and allow for differences in the performance with change in temperature of the buffers used in determinations.

Thus it is usual to measure the pH of blood drawn from the circulation at low temperature after it has been warmed in the pH meter to 38°C and then apply the Rosenthal correction factor to produce an estimation of the actual pH at low temperature.

This correction factor is based on *in vitro* estimation of the change in pH with fall in temperature of blood in a closed container, i.e. a rise of 0·0147 pH units per 1°C fall in temperature (Rosenthal, 1948).

The direct measurement of blood $P_{CO_2}$ presents similar problems. If the $P_{CO_2}$ of blood taken at low temperature is measured after the temperature of that blood has been raised anaerobically to 38°C, the $P_{CO_2}$ will be very high due to [the altered solubility of the gas and hence the higher $P_{CO_2}$ at 38°C.

Alternatively, the pH may be determined as above, corrected with the Rosenthal factor and inserted in the Siggaard–Andersen equation to derive a $P_{CO_2}$. These results agree with experimental evidence from tonometer experiments. Siggaard–Andersen also give an equation for the conversion of $P_{CO_2}$ values measured at 38°C to the original blood temperature ($t$):

$$P_{CO_{2_t}} = \text{antilog} (\log P_{CO_{2_{38}}} - 0.021 (38 - t))$$

The non-respiratory component, base excess, does not change when the blood is rewarmed to 38°C and it can therefore be conveniently measured at this temperature.

### Acidosis

Metabolic acidosis can occur in hypothermia if perfusion techniques give uneven cooling and perfusion of tissues, or if circulatory arrest occurs. It is often most apparent during rewarming when lactate accumulated in peripheral areas that have been relatively anoxic, returns to the general circulation or when shivering occurs.

Acidosis may be harmful in a number of ways. The low pH may lead to depression of cellular activity and interfere with the ability of the tissues to take up oxygen. It also leads to an increase in serum potassium thus influencing the trans-membrane potential and cardiac activity. The ability of the liver and other tissues to deal with excess lactate is depressed by cold. The combined effects of acidosis and citrate from ACD blood have a particularly deleterious effect on the heart.

Treatment of the acidosis with buffer solutions ensures correction of $H^+$ ion balance. Either sodium bicarbonate or tris aminomethane buffer solution (THAM) may be used.

Bicarbonate is used most frequently and appears to be satisfactory. It may be given on the basis of this formula:

0·3 (Wt. in Kg. × base deficit in mEq./litre of blood)

but accurate titration of the patient's needs using repeated determinations of the acid base status is desirable.

THAM buffer has possible theoretical advantages and these are carefully considered, though largely rejected, by Bleich and Schwartz (1966).

### Blood Flow

Flow characteristics of blood alter with cooling particularly below 30°C. There is the usual increased viscosity that occurs with all fluids and in addition there is some haemoconcentration due to a loss of plasma volume and possibly sludging of red cells. For these reasons, low molecular weight dextran is often added to the priming volume of the extracorporeal circulation.

With improvement in the design of mechanical circulations and in the control of clotting, difficulties with coagulation defects have become uncommon. It is usual to heparinize patients treated with the extracorporeal circulation with heparin 1·5 mg./kg. and reverse this finally with protamine sulphate 3 mg./kg. approximately, the dose depending on *in vitro* determination of clotting time. Cooling itself does induce some reduced coagulability of the blood but this is insufficient to prevent clotting when use of the extracorporeal circulation is envisaged.

It has been possible to reduce the trauma to blood by careful design of machines, by the use of siliconized components, by avoiding excessive turbulence and excessive flow rates and by haemodilution techniques.

### The Peripheral Circulation

The peripheral resistance rises with cooling due to the viscosity effect noted previously. The behaviour of the vessels themselves varies with the temperature, but below 25°C there is a general vasodilatation. Above this temperature there may be vasoconstriction and increased irritability of vessels.

Circulatory reflexes are depressed progressively and are inactive below 20°C.

Arterial blood pressure falls with cooling, partly due to these factors, but also due to cardiac depression.

### The Heart

The heart rate falls with cooling due to a direct effect of cold on the pacemaker and on cardiac muscle.

Atropine and vagal section have no effect on this bradycardia, although this does not invalidate the use of atropine in hypothermia when the heart is relatively warm. Cold induced slowing leads to a prolonged systolic and isometric relaxation phase, whereas vagal slowing leads to a prolonged diastole.

It is possible to follow this bradycardia down to about 15–10°C when perhaps 1–2 beats/min are occurring, until, with further cooling, finally arrest occurs. During rewarming, normal rhythm may appear. In man, during cooling this orderly sequence may be broken at any temperature below about 30°C when ventricular arrhythmias may appear and may rapidly culminate in ventricular fibrillation and arrest of the circulation.

This instability and irritability of the heart muscle varies with the maturity of the subject and is much less prominent in young children. Other factors, such as pre-existing cardiac ischaemia, mechanical handling of the heart, biochemical disorders, anoxia, and overdistension of its chambers, may help to precipitate ventricular fibrillation.

Drugs have failed to prove reliable in the prevention of ventricular fibrillation.

At temperatures below 26°C, a mechanical pump is usually necessary to take over support of the circulation, although when the heart is not subject to direct interference, as in neurosurgical cases, temperatures as low as

26–25°C have been achieved routinely and in some cases of accidental hypothermia as low a temperature as 9·5°C has been recorded with recovery without the aid of a mechanical circulation (Niazi and Lewis, 1958).

A heart that is well oxygenated and undamaged by excessive dilatation or surgical trauma will usually restart readily if it can be rewarmed. Even if it is in ventricular fibrillation it may resume normal rhythm following the flick of a finger on to its surface, or it may need electrical defibrillation.

The electrocardiograph may show various arrhythmias and progressive prolongation of PR, QT, QRS and an elevated and markedly prolonged ST with depression of T wave, as cooling deepens. Most typical is the small positive wave on the downstroke of the R wave which appears about 30°C and is called the 'J' wave. This wave occurs in conditions other than hypothermia.

Cardiac output decreases with fall in temperature and heart rate, but stroke volume alters relatively little down to 25°C. Coronary blood flow continues to be well maintained and does not limit cardiac function.

## Hepatic Function

The cold liver is unable to metabolize glucose or citrate ions and may have difficulty in dealing with accumulated lactate during the rewarming period. For this reason infusions of dextrose, gluconates and excessive amounts of ACD blood are to be avoided during hypothermia. Many drugs depend on the liver for detoxification and this process is also depressed by cold. Function returns to normal on rewarming.

## Renal Function

There is a decrease in renal plasma flow with falling temperature and cardiac output. There is also some renal vasoconstriction and this leads to an additional fall in renal plasma flow. However selective reabsorption is also decreased because of depression of transport mechanisms for ions and water and only isosmotic reabsorption continues. Thus, at least above 20°C, urine flow is not greatly reduced and sodium excretion continues. Below this temperature, urinary output usually ceases.

## Pharmacology

Drugs may be used in hypothermic patients for the following reasons:
1. Sedation and analgesia.
2. To prevent shivering and vasoconstriction and thus facilitate cooling.
3. Control of respiration.
4. For circulatory effects.

The non-inhalational agents suffer from the disadvantage that there is a decreased ability by the liver, kidney, and other tissues to detoxify or eliminate these agents. Thus their action may be more prolonged.

Commonly used drugs in this group include chlorpromazine, pethidine and promethazine. They have other disadvantages including a tendency to produce hypotension.

Post-operative treatment with analgesics should take account of the fact that tissues may be incompletely rewarmed and circulatory stability uncertain. Thus reduced dosages should be used.

Inhalational agents have the advantage that their uptake and elimination is little affected by hypothermia and rewarming.

Relaxants have found a place in the prevention of shivering in hypothermia. There appears to be a diminished muscle sensitivity to non-depolarizing relaxants and an increased sensitivity to depolarizing agents (Cannard and Zaimis, 1959). Thus recurarization can be seen on rewarming if large doses of non-depolarizing agents have been given in the cold state. This has provided no practical limitation on their judicious use, and reversal with neostigmine and atropine in the usual doses is recommended.

Hypothermia does not contra-indicate the use of digitalis for the treatment of heart failure, although under hypothermic conditions, resistance to digitalis is often encountered.

Noradrenaline and methoxamine continue to produce vasoconstriction even below 10°C. The use of infusions of these drugs in an effort to maintain blood pressure during hypothermia using surface cooling has shown some success and appears to allow the heart to continue beating effectively without arrhythmia to about 26°C provided it is not subjected to mechanical disturbance.

## The Application of Hypothermia

Experience, guided by experiment on animals, has shown the limits of circulatory arrest tolerated at various temperatures (oesophageal) in man.

| | | |
|---|---|---|
| >32°C | . . | 3– 9 mins. |
| 32–28°C | . . | 9–15 mins. |
| 28–18°C | . . | 15–45 mins. |
| <18°C | . . | 45–60 mins. |

## Hypothermia in Cardiac and Vascular Surgery

Cooling the patient to approximately 30°C allows the correction of some cardiac defects such as secundum type atrial septal defects, and also a range of vascular operations, such as the treatment of carotid artery stenosis or aneurysm resections when a period of diminished circulation is necessary. More profound cooling is necessary however if longer arrest periods are required in order to correct more complex defects.

A moderate or deep level of hypothermia is sometimes employed together with cardiopulmonary bypass to reduce the perfusion rates needed.

Moderate hypothermia may be achieved by a surface cooling method, or by a simple blood stream cooling system employing a heat exchanger and pump. This pump system in no way assists the circulation of blood round the body. It merely circulates the blood from the patient, through the heat exchanger and back to the patient (Fig. 3. 1.).

With cooling to below 30°C ventricular fibrillation frequently occurs if the heart is disturbed, and then the vital organs are soon at risk from anoxia. Also the cessation of the circulation means that further cooling or rapid rewarming becomes impossible. Finally a cold fibrillating heart may be difficult to restart and so disaster may ensue. Thus cooling below 30°C is unsafe in cardiac surgery if reliance is to be placed on a spontaneously beating heart.

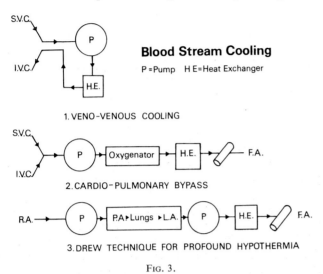

**Blood Stream Cooling**

P = Pump   H E = Heat Exchanger

1. VENO-VENOUS COOLING

2. CARDIO-PULMONARY BYPASS

3. DREW TECHNIQUE FOR PROFOUND HYPOTHERMIA

FIG. 3.

For these reasons if profound hypothermia is to be induced it becomes vital to maintain the circulation with pumps and thus take over from the heart and allow continued oxygenation, cooling and rewarming to occur in a controlled manner.

This may be achieved using either a system of pumps to take over the cardiac function, retaining the patient's own lungs in the circulation as in the Drew technique, or substituting complete cardiopulmonary bypass and an artificial oxygenator (Fig. 3 (2, 3.)).

## Surface Cooling and Rewarming

We have considered the necessity to avoid shivering and promote vasodilatation of the skin vessels if effective cooling is to occur.

Careful monitoring of blood pressure, pulse, electrocardiograph and oesophageal temperature is vital. An oesophageal temperature probe gives the most reliable indication of cardiac temperature and as it is vital that this should not drift too low, a chart of these measurements is essential in order that the trend of all variables may be readily assessed.

Cooling methods include the use of cold water immersion, ice bags, cold air, and refrigerated blankets. For cardiac surgery a collapsible plastic bath that can be erected on the operating table and then filled with cold or warm water as applicable, has found favour (Fig. 4). Cold water immersion helps to take some of the weight off the body (which partially floats) thus helping the circulation of blood through the subcutaneous tissues which lessens the risk of cold injury.

For adults, ice is continually added to the water, but for small children, the rate of cooling will be quite sufficient if the temperature of the coolant is kept at about 15°C.

It is advisable to remove the patient from the bath at about 33°C (oesophageal) as the temperature will continue to fall for some time as cold blood from the peripheral tissues continues to enter the main circulation. This is called the 'after drop' in temperature.

Once the curve of temperature change has started to flatten out, procedures involving the heart may commence. The circulation is stopped for the duration of the intracardiac repair by occlusion of the superior and inferior vena caval inflow of blood; subsequently removal of the occlusion allows resumption of an effective beat by the ventricles and thus restoration of the circulation.

Rewarming may then be commenced by means of warm water blankets placed in position under the patient at the start of the operation. Later the patient's wound may be dressed and covered with water-proof dressings and the rewarming process completed in the bath filled with warm water at 42°C. Ventricular fibrillation, if it occurs, may be treated with internal cardiac massage and electrical defibrillation. Warm saline (40°C) poured into the pericardial and pleural cavities may assist. If ventricular fibrillation commences during the course of the arrest period, reversion to normal rhythm should not be attempted until the intracardiac surgery is completed.

## Blood Stream Cooling

Venovenous cooling (Ross, 1954) is an alternative to surface cooling for moderate hypothermia. Following thoracotomy, the superior vena cava is cannulated and the blood is then pumped via a heat exchanger and a second cannula into the inferior vena cava. The pump may be hand operated and the procedure need not be instituted until the cardiac defect has been closely assessed upon opening the pericardium. This method demands extra cannulation procedures and returns cold blood straight to the heart thus favouring the development of arrhythmias. Peripheral 'shell' tissues are cooled less by this method, thus avoiding the 'after drop' but increasing the risk of acidosis.

Other types of bloodstream cooling that employ a femoral artery to femoral vein shunt or a left atrium to femoral artery shunt may be used. The latter procedure is sometimes employed in aortic surgery and may be used as a left ventricular bypass.

## Blood Stream Cooling with Assisted Circulation

The correction of some complex cardiac defects demands more time than can be provided by the surface or venovenous cooling methods already described. This can be provided in two ways, both demanding the use of an assisted circulation.

### Cardiopulmonary Bypass

This may be used with or without hypothermia. Blood is withdrawn from the venae cavae, oxygenated in the machine and returned via the femoral artery to perfuse the body. The blood and hence the body may be cooled. This reduces the body's metabolic demands and hence the need for the high flow rates necessary at 38°C. Also it allows the circulation to be stopped if this should prove

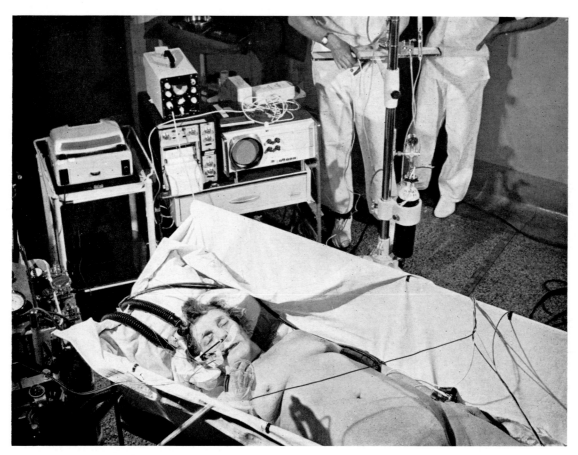

FIG. 4. Surface hypothermia, showing collapsible plastic bath and monitoring equipment for temperature, E.C.G., E.E.G. and blood pressure.

*Photograph: Dr. Keith Glennie Smith, Royal Victoria Hospital, Bournemouth.*

useful, the period of arrest permissible depending on the naso-pharyngeal temperature.

Another variation has been described by Subramanian *et al.* (1971) for use in babies up to 15 Kg. in weight. These infants are cooled by surface methods to 24°C oesophageal, and then the chest is opened and cardiopulmonary bypass used to lower the temperature further to 20°C, at which point surgery is carried out on the cardiac defect, with total arrest of the circulation for up to 60 min. Rewarming is carried out by means of the extra-corporeal circulation and surface rewarming, the bypass being discontinued at 34°C. The good results are attributed to slow, even cooling, rapid rewarming and the excellent operating conditions.

### Profound Hypothermia (Drew technique)

The aim of this method is to maintain the circulation by means of two pumps until a sufficiently low temperature (around 15°C nasopharyngeal) is reached to allow a long period of circulatory arrest covering the entire period of the repair. One pump passes blood from the right atrium into the pulmonary artery (and thus takes over from the right ventricle) and the other pumps blood from the left atrium into the femoral artery (and thus takes over from the left ventricle). A heat exchanger in the circuit provides for cooling or rewarming, and the system uses the patient's own lungs for oxygenation.

With both these methods, the ventricles often, but not inevitably, fibrillate at low temperature. It is seldom difficult to restore normal rhythm by a finger flick or electrical defibrillation, once rewarming has reached about 30°C. Then, with the heart beating well, the supporting circulation can be gradually withdrawn.

### Monitoring

Continuous measurement of the temperature in the naso-pharynx, oesophagus, muscles, etc., gives guidance to the gradients achieved and to the brain temperature, which approximates to the nasopharyngeal temperature. Excessive rates of cooling leave some tissues rather warm and hence increase the risk of acidosis during the circulatory arrest.

The electrocardiogram and the venous and arterial pressures are monitored, the latter by electromanometry. The electroencephalogram is of some value as an index of brain activity, particularly as a cross-check on the reliability of the pharyngeal temperature recording. Biochemical control, and the control of blood clotting, is essential, as is correct blood replacement using venous and arterial pressures as valuable guides.

### Post-operative Management

It is usual to continue the monitoring and observation of these patients in the intensive care unit post-operatively, until the circulation is safely stabilized. Respiratory support is sometimes necessary as is careful attention to analgesia and to the patient's comfort.

### Hypothermia for Neurosurgery

Surgical indications for hypothermia may include intra-cranial aneurysms, vascular anomalies, internal carotid artery stenosis and cerebral oedema of surgical or traumatic origin. Hypothermia reduces the risk of cerebral ischaemia caused by pressure on brain tissue or vascular occlusion.

Cerebral vessels tend to show vasoconstriction and increased irritability down to 30°C when vasodilatation becomes more apparent. Hence cooling below 30°C should provide the best results. Hypocapnia increases cerebral vasoconstriction. For this reason, some anaesthetists prefer to rely on spontaneous respiration in order to maintain an increased level of $P_{CO_2}$. Furthermore, Hewer (1964) believes that the pattern of spontaneous respiratory movements provides a vital indication of medullary ischaemia.

Hypotension and low cardiac output during hypothermia may cause cerebral ischaemia and should be controlled with careful blood replacement, vasopressors and avoidance of postural disturbances.

Moderate hypothermia, achieved by surface cooling methods, is used most frequently in neurosurgical cases. Cold air cooling has advantages over the iced water bath method in that less movement and hence cardiovascular disturbance, is produced and also cooling is more gradual and the after-drop in temperature less severe. More profound cooling has not been widely applied because of the need for an extracorporeal circulation and a major additional operation.

### Head Injury

The value of hypothermia in treatment is still open to doubt and has not achieved general application except in the treatment of hyperpyrexia when cooling to 35–32°C is employed.

### Cardiac Arrest

Hypothermia has been used in the management of patients after cardiac arrest, particularly if consciousness has not returned rapidly or if there has been pyrexia and signs of cerebral damage. Cooling is maintained for 2–3 days with the object of reducing cerebral oxygen demand and cerebral oedema.

### Eclampsia

Hypothermia has been used in an effort to reduce intra-cranial pressure and the metabolic load on kidneys and liver when heavy sedation has failed to control fits.

### Neonatal Asphyxia

Hypothermia has not been successful in management of these infants. There appears to be a real risk of severe cold injury (*see* section on the Newborn, p. 354) and many paediatricians believe that full-term infants that show no tendency to breathe have severe cerebral damage incompatible with complete recovery.

### Hyperpyrexia

Hyperpyrexia produced by virus encephalitis has been treated with apparent benefit by hypothermia. Damage to the hypothalamus following intracranial surgery may lead to hyperpyrexia which should be controlled by cooling to 35–32°C. It has also been recommended for the treatment of hyperpyrexia associated with thyrotoxic crisis and in the treatment of malignant hyperpyroxia.

## Other Conditions

Despite the saving in myocardial work and oxygen demands, there is little to be said for the use of hypothermia in the treatment of cardiac infarction due to the risk of hypotension and arrhythmias.

Many trials have been made of hypothermia in cancer therapy without any evidence of improvement.

### Accidental Hypothermia

#### Summary of Aetiological Groups

1. Naturally susceptible groups—newborn
   —the aged.
2. Secondary to Disease states.
   Endocrine disorders—Myxoedema
   —Hypopituitary states
   —Adrenal failure.

   Coma or confusional states—Diabetic hyper- or
   hypoglycaemic
   —Cerebrovascular
   accidents
   —Head injuries
   —Drug induced
   Chlorpromazine,
   Barbiturates
   Alcohol or
   Carbon-monoxide
   poisoning, etc.
   —Severe toxaemia
   —peritonitis
   —pancreatitis

   Conditions associated with immobility

   —Paraplegia, Parkinsonism, etc.
   —Severe arthritis
   —Inanition
   —Severe illness—Coronary thrombosis
   —Pulmonary embolism, etc.
3. Exposure—Immersion hypothermia and cold air exposure.
4. Chronic and episodic hypothermia.

## The Newborn

The ability of newborn animals to regulate their temperature differs with the species and with the age and maturity of the newborn. Babies in particular have poorly developed shivering responses.

Newborn kittens show a diminished ability to raise their metabolic rate in response to cold stress, although the response improves in the course of the first and second post-natal week (Hill, 1961).

Apart from possible defects of the thermoregulatory mechanism, premature infants are deficient in subcutaneous fat and therefore insulation.

There is convincing evidence that the survival rate among infants in the first few days of life is improved by maintaining them in a warm environment thus reducing the metabolic demands of thermoregulation. Silverman (1959) showed that survival rates in premature babies was significantly higher with an environmental temperature at 31·6°C compared with a control group at 28·9°C.

Furthermore it seems that neonates kept in an environment that allows the skin temperature to be maintained at 36·5°C grow faster than those whose skin temperature was 35°C (Glass, 1968). However, the 'warm' group were less resistant to cold and were less able to maintain body temperature if placed in a cool environment at 28°C.

It may be that short periods of exposure to cooler environments may 'train' the thermoregulatory mechanisms, although the increased energy requirements would need replacement. Brown adipose tissue is present in the interscapular region of infants and may have a part to play in non-shivering thermogenesis in cold adapted infants, similar to its function in lower animals.

## Cold Injury

This is an occasional complication of hypothermia in neonates and small children particularly, although it can occur in adults. It is due to small areas of subcutaneous fat necrosis. Duhn et al. (1968) reported an extensive case resulting in miliary calcified nodules in the subcutaneous tissues of an infant undergoing hypothermia treatment for asphyxia neonatorum. Although not in itself particularly dangerous, this finding has acted as a further discouragement to the use of hypothermia in this condition, where striking benefit has not been apparent.

## The Aged

A report published by the Royal College of Physicians of London (1966) showed that in a three month period in the Winter of 1966 about 9,000 hypothermic patients, mostly over 60 years of age, could have been admitted to hospitals in the U.K. Others must have been treated at home or passed unrecognized.

Aetiological factors included the very low temperature reached in the homes of many old people at night, often only a degree or two above the outside temperature, inadequate food intake and intercurrent diseases, some of which are listed above.

Macmillan et al. (1967) produced evidence that there was a defect of temperature regulation in the elderly survivors of accidental hypothermia. This defect included an inability to raise heat production and reduce heat loss by vasoconstriction and continued to be evident when responses were measured up to 3 years after recovery. Elderly control patients did not show this defect and thus it would seem that the elderly survivors of accidental hypothermia need extra supervision and protection in the winter season.

The clinical state and its dangers are well described by Rosin and Exton Smith (1964), and are summarized below.

With cooling there is a progressive disturbance of consciousness. The patients feel the cold but are apathetic. They have pale, sometimes cyanosed or 'puffy' skin and do not shiver. Their extremities have poor blood flow and may become gangrenous. Pulse rate is about 60/min and respiration depressed. Responses are slow and muscles may show marked rigidity. Neck stiffness may mimic meningism. Pancreatitis is a common complication.

Mortality is 30–80 per cent but partly reflects coexisting serious diseases.

Treatment presents difficulties. Rapid surface rewarming may result in vasodilatation, fall of blood pressure, and the return of large amounts of very cold surface blood to the main circulation. This may lead to cardiac arrest. Slow surface rewarming over 24 hours is the safest course.

Monitoring of temperature (oesophageal), ECG, venous and arterial pressures and biochemical variables, particularly $P_{CO_2}$, $P_{O_2}$, pH, etc., is helpful in management.

Intravenous fluids, including low molecular weight dextran, should be given to correct haemoconcentration and restore tissue perfusion, but care should be taken to avoid overtransfusion and pulmonary oedema. Head down tilt may help to maintain systemic blood pressure. Hydrocortisone hemisuccinate 100 mg 8 hourly and a broad spectrum antibiotic should be given intravenously.

Incipient gangrene in the legs has been treated successfully with epidural analgesia, although this may increase the risk of lowering the blood pressure.

Rewarming the patient by means of warm peritoneal dialysis has been described by Lash *et al.* (1967) and the use of the extracorporeal circulation in these patients has been described by Fell *et al.* (1968). There are possible advantages in this method in that the heart receives warm blood in the early and dangerous phase of rewarming, rather than cold blood as in surface rewarming.

## Hypothermia Associated with Disease States

The recognition of disease states may be difficult. Peritonitis can be missed rather easily, particularly as some muscle rigidity is common in the hypothermic patient.

Diabetic coma may present difficulties in diagnosis and treatment as a raised blood sugar is found in hypothermia. Also there is poor utilization of glucose and insulin in the cold state, and rewarming to 32°C is necessary if therapy is to be effective.

Myxoedema should be treated with triiododothyronine in small doses (10 μg. eight–twelve hourly). Overdosage may precipitate coronary insufficiency or adrenal failure.

Some of the other possible precipitating causes of accidental hypothermia are indicated above.

## Hypothermia Due to Exposure

Hypothermia continues to take a toll of otherwise healthy individuals. It is the primary cause of death in patients drowning in the waters around the UK.

Experiment has shown that survival in very cold water is aided by thick clothing and by keeping still, rather than active swimming. Even waterlogged clothing provides valuable insulation. It seems that muscle movement is undesirable as it results in reduced insulation in the body 'shell' due to vasodilatation in muscles, the massaging effect of movement on the blood in the tissues which is thereby squeezed into the general circulation, and also disturbance of the water layers trapped in clothing next to the skin.

Keatinge *et al.* (1969) have shown that a very marked hyperventilation may develop upon immersion in water at 4·7°C and that this may so incapacitate a swimmer that he may suddenly fail to swim after as little as $1\frac{1}{2}$ minutes

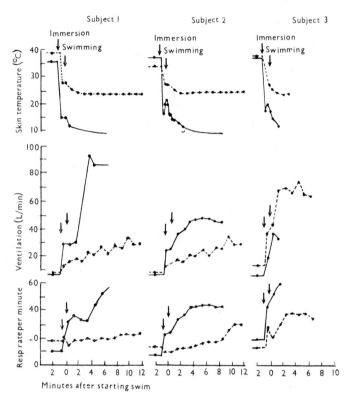

Fig. 5. Skin temperature, ventilation and ratio of breathing, before and during swims. • - - - • warm water (23.7°C) •———• cold water (4.7°C.)

(Fig. 5). This hyperventilation is reflex in origin. Fatter and more buoyant subjects may be able to swim through this period of reflex hyperventilation, which seems to subside as the skin receptors adapt to the cold stimulus. However, progressive hypothermia along with fatigue induced as a result of swimming fully clothed in water rendered more viscous by cold, caused even fat subjects to give up swimming within less than 12 minutes. Wooldridge (1969) suggests that this uncontrollable reflex hyperventilation is partly due to apprehension and may lose its danger if the person is given proper instruction.

There seems to be less risk in rewarming healthy young people, who have become hypothermic, as rapidly as possible, although the arterial pressure should be recorded every 10 minutes and the ECG monitored. Keatinge (1964) recommends rapid rewarming in a bath at 40°C, with the extremities held clear of the water.

Provided that the peripheral pulse is of good volume, rapid surface rewarming seems to be safe, but Hellman

(1971) favours slow rewarming where perfusion is poor, particularly if the blood is anoxic. In emergency situations, the administration of 95 per cent oxygen and 5 per cent carbon dioxide is recommended along with cardiac massage and possibly the centripetal injection of 0·5–1 litre of warm blood or balanced salt solution into the carotid artery. The carbon dioxide is given with the aim of avoiding any respiratory alkalosis due to hyperventilation of a hypothermic patient, and the intra-arterial infusion might assist coronary perfusion.

Lloyd (1971) makes the ingenious suggestion that warming could be achieved by ventilating the lungs with a mixture of carbon dioxide and oxygen, utilizing the heat produced when these gases are passed through a soda lime container.

## Inadvertent Hypothermia During Anaesthesia

Anaesthetic and premedicant drugs predispose the patient to hypothermia by reducing receptor sensitivity to cold, prevention of shivering, increased cutaneous vasodilatation and depression of the thermoregulatory centre and voluntary activity.

Violent shivering is often seen on emergence from halothane anaesthesia. It may be due to hypothermia produced during the preceding period of exposure on the operating table followed by early restoration of receptor and central nervous system activity due to the poor analgesic properties of halothane and its rapid elimination.

This shivering is undesirable as it may lead to large oxygen demands that the circulatory or respiratory system are unable to meet, and such patients do show cyanosis and decreased venous oxygen tension.

Newborn and premature infants are particularly at risk from hypothermia and central nervous system defects, such as hybrocephalus, in these infants, add to the hazard (Calvert, 1962). This can lead to fall of blood pressure, respiratory arrest, and prolonged post-operative recovery time (Hunter, 1964).

If large quantities of stored blood (at 4°C) are transfused, this should be prewarmed using a suitable blood warmer. (Ref. apparatus).

Cold blood given intravenously passes straight to the heart and if this organ is already cold, this blood with its low pH and high citrate ion concentration may lead to sudden hypotension or circulatory arrest.

Prevention should include proper control of ward, anaesthetic room and operating theatre temperatures, adequate blankets and clothing for patients on stretcher trolleys, etc. It is not easy to keep patients warm on operating tables. Electric blankets have possible dangers and water blankets with thermostatically controlled water flow, though cumbersome, seem the best solution for children.

A new approach has been the use of fibre optic radiant heat sources for the provision of warmth. This method is effective and avoids the inconvenience of radiant heat canopies or incubator walls, particularly on the operating table (Shaw, Franzel and Bordiuk, 1971).

## Chronic and Episodic Hypothermia

The condition of episodic hypothermia is discussed by Duff *et al.*, 1961, and chronic hypothermia by Hockaday *et al.*, 1962. These conditions appear to be due to some abnormality of the central control of tempearture leading either to complete loss of thermoregulation or to an abnormally low 'setting' of the patient's normal temperature.

## REFERENCES

Andersson, B., Eckerman, C., Hokfelt, B., Jobin, M. and Robertshaw, D. (1967), "Studies of the Importance of the Thyroid and Sympathetic System in Defence against Cold in the Goat," *Acta Physiol. Scand.*, **69**, 111.

Bigelow, W. G., Lindsay, W. K., Harrison, R. C., Gordon, R. A. and Greenwood, W. F. (1950), "Oxygen Transport and Utilization in Dogs at Low Body Temperature," *Amer. J. Physiol.*, **160**, 125.

Bleich, H. L. and Schwartz, W. B. (1966), "Tris Buffer (T.H.A.M.): An Appraisal of its Physiological Effects and Clinical Usefulness," *New Eng. J. Med.*, **274**, 782.

Brewin, E. G. (1964), "Physiology of Hypothermia," *Int. Anaesthesiol Clinics*, 803–827.

Burton, G. W. (1964), "Metabolic Acidosis during Profound Hypothermia," *Anaesthesia*, **19**, 118.

Calvert, D. A. (1962), "Inadvertent Hypothermia in Paediatric Surgery," *Anaesthesia*, **17**, 29.

Cannard, T. H. and Zaimis, E. (1959), "Effect of Lowered Muscle Temperature on the Action of Neuromuscular Blocking Drugs in Man," *J. Physiol. (Lond.)*, **149**, 112.

Clowes, G. H. A., Neville, W. E., Sabga, G. and Shibota, Y. (1958), "Relationship of Oxygen Consumption, Perfusion Rate, and Temperature to the Acidosis Associated with Cardiopulmonary Bypass," *Surgery*, **44**, 220.

Cottle, W. H. and Carlson, L. D. (1956), "Regulation of Heat Production in Cold Adapted Rats," *Proc. Soc. Exptl. Biol. Med.*, **92**, 845.

Cross, K. W., Tizard, J. P. M. and Trythall, D. A. H. (1955), "The Metabolism of New Born Infants Breathing 15% Oxygen," *J. Physiol. Lond.*, **129**, 69.

Drew, C. E., Keen, C. T. and Benazon, D. B. (1959), "Profound Hypothermia," *Lancet*, **1**, 745.

Duff, R. S., Farrant, P. C., Levaux, V. M. and Wray, S. M. (1961), "Spontaneous Periodic Hypothermia," *Quart. J. Med.*, **30**, 329.

Duhn, R., Schoen, E. J. and Siu, M. (1968), "Subcutaneous Fat Necrosis with Extensive Calcification after Hypothermia in Two Newborn Infants," *Paediatrics*, **41**, 3, 661.

Evonuk, E. and Hannon, J. P. (1963), "Cardiovascular and Pulmonary Effects of Noradrenaline in the Cold Acclimated Rat," *Fed. Proc.*, **22**, 411.

Fell, R. H., Gunning, A. J. and Bardken, K. D. (1968), "Severe Hypothermia as a Result of Barbiturate Overdose Complicated by Cardiac Arrest," *Lancet*, **I**, 392, Feb.

Glass, L., Silverman, W. A. and Sinclair, J. C. (1968), "Effect of the Thermal Environment on Cold Resistance and Growth of Small Infants after the First Week of Life," *Paediatrics*, **41**, 6, 1033.

Hellman, H. (1971), *Lancet*, **ii**, 1257.

Hemingway, A. and Price, W. M. (1968), "The Autonomic Nervous System and Regulation of Body Temperature," *Anaesthesiol.*, **29**, **4**, 693.

Hewer, A. J. H. (1964), "Hypothermia for Neurosurgery," *Int. Anaesthesiol Clinics*. Vol. II. No. 4. p. 919.

Hey, E. N. and Mount, L. E. (1967), "Heat Losses from Babies in Incubators," *Arch. Dis. Childh.*, **42**, 75.

Hill, J. R. (1961), *British Medical Bull.*, **17**, 2, 164–167, May.

Hockaday, T. D. R., Cranston, W. I., Cooper, K. E. and Mottram, R. F. (1962), "Temperature Regulation in Chronic Hypothermia," *Lancet*, **2**, 428.

Hsei, A. C. L. and Carlson, L. (1953), "Role of the Thyroid in the Metabolic Response to Low Temperature," *Amer. J. Physiol.*, **188**, 40.

Hsei, A. C. L., Carlson, L. D. and Gray, G. (1957), "Role of the Sympathetic Nervous System in the Control and Chemical Regulation of Heat Production," *Amer. J. Physiol.*, **190**, 247, 157.

Hunter, A. R. (1964), "Inadvertent Hypothermia during Anaesthesia," *Internat. Anaesthesiol Clins.* Vol. II. No. 4, pp. 1003–8.

Hunter, J. (1786), "Animal Oeconomy."

Johnson, R. H. (1965), "Neurological Studies in Temperature Regulation," *Ann. Roy. Coll. Surg. Engl.*, **36**, 6, 339.

Keatinge, W. R. (1964), "Hypothermia in Healthy People," *Internat. Anaesthesiol Clin.* Vol. II. No. 4, p. 1008.

Keatinge, W. R., Prys-Roberts, C., Cooper, K. E., Honour, A. J. and Haight, J. (1969), "Sudden Failure of Swimming in Cold Water," *Brit. Med. J.*, **1**, 480.

Lash, R. F., Burdette, J. A. and Ozdil, T. (1967), "Accidental Profound Hypothermia and Barbiturate Intoxication. A Report of Rapid 'Cool' Rewarming by Peritoneal Dialysis," *J. Amer. Med. Ass.*, **201**, 269.

Leduc, J. (1961), "Catecholamine Production and Release in Exposure and Acclimation to Cold," *Acta. Physiol. Scand.*, **53**, Suppl., 183.

Lloyd, E. L. (1971), "Treatment After Exposure to Cold," *Lancet*, **ii**, 1376.

Macmillan, A. L., Corbett, J. L., Johnson, R. H., Crampton Smith, A., Spalding, J. M. K. and Wolner, L. (1967), "Temperature Regulation in Survivors of Accidental Hypothermia in the Elderly," *Lancet*, **II**, 165. 22nd July.

McQuiston, W. O. (1949), "Anaesthetic Problems in Cardiac Surgery in Children," *Anaesthesiol*, **10**, 590.

Moore, R. E. (1972), *Modern Trends in Physiology*, pp. 112–126, Butterworth.

Niazi, S. A. and Lewis, F. J. (1958), "Profound Hypothermia in Man," *Ann. Surg.*, **147**, 264.

Norman, J. N. (1965), *Brit. Antarctic Survey Bull.*, **6**, 1.

Pugh, L. G. G. (1964), "Deaths from Exposure on Four Inns Walking Competition, March 14/15, 1964," *Lancet*, **i**, 1210.

Report of Committee on Accidental Hypothermia (1966). *Royal College of Physicians* (*London*).

Rosenthal, T. B. (1948), "The Effect of Temperature on pH of Blood and Plasma *in vitro*," *J. Biol. Chem.*, **173**: 25.

Rosin, A. J. and Exton-Smith, A. N. (1964), "Clinical Features of Accidental Hypothermia, with some Observations on Thyroid Function," *Brit. Med. J.*, **5374**, 16–9, Jan.

Ross, D. N. (1954), "Venous Cooling. A New Method of Cooling the Blood Stream," *Lancet*, **1**: **1108**.

Shaw, A., Franzel, I. and Bordiuk, J. (1971), "Prevention of Neonatal Hypothermia by a Fiber-Optic 'Hot Pipe' System: A New Concept," *J. Paediatric Surg.*, **6**, No. 3, 354–358.

Silverman, W. A. (1959), "The Physical Environment and the Premature Infant," *Paediatrics*, **23**, 166.

Simpson, M. (1969). Personal communication and in press.

Smith, R. E. and Heijer, D. J. (1962), "Metabolism and Cellular Function in Cold Acclimation," *Physiol. Reviews*, **42:1**, 60–142.

Smith, R. E. (1964), "The Physiological Role of Brown Adipose Tissue," *Ann. Acad. Scient. Fennicae.*, Series A.N., **71/28**, 391–397.

Subramanian, S., Wagner, H., Vled, P. and Lambert, E. (1971), "Surface Induced Deep Hypothermia in Cardiac Surgery," *J. Paediatric Surg.*, **6**, 612–617.

Vaidya, A. B. and Levine, R. J. (1971), *New Engl. J. Med.*, **284**, 255–257.

Wallace, W. F. W. (1968). *Brit. Med. Journal*, **2**, 174.

Whitby, J. D. and Deakin, L. J. (1968), "Temperature Differences in the Oesophagus," *Brit. J. Anaesth.*, **40**, 991.

Wooldridge, M. J. (1969). *Brit. Med. J.*, **1**, 711.

Yoshimura, M., Yukihoshi, T., Yoshioka, T. and Takeda, H. (1966), "Climatic Adaptation of Basal Metabolism," *Fed. Proc.*, **25**, 1169–1176.

Wyndham, C. H., Williams, C. A. and Loot, S. H. (1968), "Reactions to Cold," *J. Applied Physiol.*, **24**, 3, 282.

*Apparatus*

*Blood Warmer.* Grant Instruments Ltd., Barrington, Cambridge, England.

*Water Blankets.* Infant Warming Blanket, Pump, Thermostat. Aquamatic K. Blanket. Gormann Rupp, Belville, Ohio, U.S.A.

*CHAPTER* 6

# NEONATAL PHYSIOLOGY

### W. J. GLOVER

Many physiological differences exist between the newborn infant and the adult. This chapter deals with those differences which are most relevant to the anaesthetist who may be involved in the care of the infant in the delivery-room, in the operating theatre, or in the intensive care area.

## THE SIGNIFICANCE OF BIRTH WEIGHT

The mean birth weight in the United Kingdom is about 3,300 g. In the past the term 'premature' was applied to all infants weighing less than 2,500 g. but it is now realized that many of these infants are born after a pregnancy of normal duration.

Infants weighing less than 2,500 g. are therefore described as *low birth weight* babies and those infants who are under-weight in relation to the duration of pregnancy are described as *small-for-dates* babies. *Preterm* infants are those born before the 37th week of pregnancy.

Compared with infants of normal weight, infants of low birth weight are more likely to suffer from congenital malformations, hypoglycaemia, respiratory distress syndrome or asphyxia. They also have greater difficulty in maintaining body temperature.

## THE CONTROL OF BODY TEMPERATURE

There have now been several controlled trials which show that the mortality rises considerably if small babies are nursed in surroundings more than a degree or so below the optimum range. The cause of the increased mortality is uncertain. Additional facts have led to acceptance of the view that the newborn infant is a true homeotherm. Maintenance of body temperature is therefore of prime importance in the delivery-room, the operating theatre, the intensive care area and the nursery.

### Basal Heat Production

The basal metabolic rate of the newborn baby is higher than that of the adult per unit body weight but it is considerably less per unit surface area (Hey, 1971). Resting heat production per unit surface area is particularly low in preterm babies of low birth weight during the first month of life.

### Heat Loss

The average newborn has about twice the surface for heat loss for each kilogram of tissue compared with the average adult (Cross, 1965). Although thermoregulatory control over skin blood flow is well developed even in very small babies, heat is readily lost because tissue insulation in the newborn babies is so much less than in adults. Tissue insulation is even less in babies of low birth weight (Hey, Katz and O'Connell, 1970). Under ideal environmental conditions for the newborn about one quarter of basal heat production is lost by evaporation of water from the skin and respiratory tract. The remainder is lost by radiation and convection. In warm surroundings the evaporative heat loss may increase considerably due to sweating and in cold surroundings the heat loss by radiation and convection will increase.

### Response to Cold

Most newborn mammals respond to cold exposure by a large increase in oxygen consumption and heat production. In several species and in the human infant this is largely achieved without shivering. Within the past few years it has been shown that the main source of this additional heat production is the oxidation of fat within the brown adipose tissue (Hull, 1966). Brown adipose tissue is widely distributed in the neonate, between the muscles of the neck and back, in the axillae and groins and especially around the kidney and adrenal glands.

Oxygen is required for oxidation of the fat in brown adipose tissue and the infant's increased oxygen consumption as a result of cold stress may be of the order of 60 per cent. Consequently, an infant who is already in respiratory distress will deteriorate further if nursed in a cool environment. As anaesthesia will suppress this metabolic response to cold (Hey, 1971), the temperature of an infant will fall considerably in the operating theatre if steps are not taken to minimize heat loss.

A baby's ability to respond to cold stress is impaired by severe hypoxia. This is of particular importance in respiratory distress syndrome.

### Response to Warmth

As already stated, thermoregulatory control over skin blood flow is well developed and skin blood flow increases sufficiently in warm surroundings to reduce tissue insulation to one-third its amount in the cold (Hey and Katz, 1970).

Unfortunately infants have a limited ability to sweat and the reasons for this are not clear as there are more sweat glands per unit area than in the adult. Preterm infants are even less capable of sweating and those born more than 8 weeks before term seem unable to sweat at all, possibly because of glandular immaturity. Consequently the average newborn baby cannot maintain thermal equilibrium if the environmental temperature is as high as body temperature.

### Neutral Thermal Environment

Between the extremes of environment which cause either the metabolic response to cold or sweating there is a narrow neutral zone. In this zone body temperature can be controlled by changes in posture and blood flow alone and oxygen consumption is minimal. This neutral zone can not be defined in terms of temperature alone because heat loss is determined by many factors, e.g. radiation, ambient humidity, presence or absence of draughts and, most important, whether the infant is clothed or naked.

Under standard conditions, free from thermal stress, the main factors determining the neutral environmental temperature are age and weight. The low basal heat production (per unit surface area) and low tissue insulation make it necessary to maintain a high environmental temperature (32–35°C) to provide neutral conditions for a *naked* infant in the neonatal period. An adult under the same conditions would require an environmental temperature of only 29°C (Hey, 1972).

### Optimum Warmth

As the infant's rectal temperature may be maintained by increased heat production, it is difficult to detect that the environmental temperature is too low. One must also guard against too warm an environment because the neutral range is small and the infant has great difficulty in maintaining body temperature when the environmental temperature is above the upper limit of the neutral zone. In practice therefore it is advisable to maintain the environmental temperature at the lower limit of the neutral range, rather than the upper limit.

If an infant is *clothed* and *well wrapped*, in a cot in a draught-free room of moderate humidity, then a room temperature of 24°C is required for a full-term baby more than 2 days old and 31°C for a 1 Kg. baby in the first few days of life (Hey and O'Connell, 1970).

In recent years it has become common practice to keep babies who require constant observation naked in incubators. In this situation it is necessary to control the environment within narrow and precise limits. Under these circumstances a temperature of 32°C provides neutral conditions for a full-term baby of more than 2 days old and a temperature of 35°C is required for a 1 Kg. infant in the first few days of life (Hey, 1972).

It is important to realize that if the room temperature outside the incubator is low then the perspex walls of the incubator will be relatively cold and the infant will lose heat by radiation to them. It is estimated that the incubator air temperature should be raised by 1°C (above the temperatures quoted above) for every 7°C by which the incubator air temperature exceeds room temperature. As 35°C is the highest incubator temperature allowable under British Standards it is suggested that all incubators should be kept in a room with a temperature of 27–30°C (Hey, 1972). Incubators should not be subjected to direct sunlight as this will change the radiant environment.

In order to make access to the baby easier, radiant heat canopies have recently been introduced as an alternative to incubators. Great care is still necessary to maintain a neutral environment. If a sensing thermistor is strapped to the baby's abdomen it may become detached resulting in hyperthermia. In addition, the thermistor must be extremely accurate. For example, an abdominal skin temperature of 36·1°C is appropriate for a 3 Kg. baby whereas a temperature of 36·4°C is more appropriate for a baby of 1·5 Kg. or less (Hey, 1972).

In the operating theatre the infant can be placed on a thermostatically controlled heating pad or water blanket and the limbs wrapped in foil or cotton wool. If these precautions are taken the temperature of the operating theatre need not be raised to a level that is uncomfortable for the operating team as that would impair their efficiency. The theatre ventilation should not be set at a high level of air changes as this would increase convective heat loss. Humidification of the inspired gases will reduce evaporative heat loss from the respiratory tract but the patient's temperature can usually be maintained without taking this step.

It is important to remember that a non-anaesthetised baby can be suffering from the cold even if the rectal temperature is normal, i.e. one must remember the distinction between *being* cold (hypothermia) and *feeling* cold (subject to a cold environment) (Hey, 1972).

## RESPIRATORY SYSTEM

### Transition from Foetal to Neonatal State

The lungs are filled with fluid before birth. This fluid differs in composition from amniotic fluid and plasma and it appears to be an ultrafiltrate of plasma with selective reabsorption or secretion. A variable amount of this fluid is squeezed out from the air passages in the final stages of delivery and as the compressed chest emerges some air is drawn in to replace the fluid previously present. Most of the fluid still remains in the lungs at this stage. This residual fluid is absorbed mainly by the lymphatics and to a lesser extent by the capillaries during the first 24 hours after birth.

The reasons for the onset of the first breath and the maintenance of regular respiration are complex and require further study. During the first breath considerable force is required to overcome the viscosity of the fluid in the lungs, the surface tension at the air/fluid interface and the tissue resistive forces. Pressures measured in the oesophagus during the first breath are of the order of −10 to −70 cm. $H_2O$ on inspiration maintained for 0·5–1·0 sec. and 20–30 cm. $H_2O$ on expiration. Much of the inspired air remains in the lungs as residual volume. After the first few breaths the lungs are almost completely and evenly expanded and the functional residual capacity reaches about 75 per cent of its ultimate volume within a few minutes. Once respiration is established infants maintain an arterial $P_{CO_2}$ greater than in foetal life, a $P_{CO_2}$ which is reduced and a pH not greatly altered.

The lungs must be mature before they are capable of sustaining life. The alveoli must form by flattening of the cuboidal epithelium at the terminal air sacs and the pulmonary vasculature must develop until the pulmonary capillaries are sufficient for gaseous exchange. In the human this stage is reached at about 28 weeks gestation. In parallel with this anatomical development biochemical development of the lungs must also occur. The normal alveolar lining layer produces surface active phospholipids and adequate amounts of these substances are required to maintain lung stability and avoid atelectasis. In the normal infant this degree of biochemical development is also reached at about 28 weeks gestation.

These phospholipids (also known collectively as pulmonary surfactant) have been identified as a number of saturated lecithins and are synthesized in the lung tissue by the type II alveolar cells and excreted into the air space to form surface active lining layers.

Until recently it was not known why the lung remained expanded. The relationship between the pressure ($P$), surface tension ($T$) and radius ($r$) of a sphere is expressed by the La Place equation $P = \dfrac{2T}{r}$. This means that the smaller the sphere the higher the pressure within that sphere. One would therefore expect the pressure in the smaller alveoli of the lung to be relatively high with a tendency for them to empty into adjacent larger alveoli at lower pressure. This would cause an unstable situation with extensive atelectasis. It does not happen because, as Clements first demonstrated, extracts of normal lungs have the remarkable property of altering surface tension; the smaller the surface area, the lower the surface tension (Clements, Brown and Johnson, 1958). This explained the phenomenon that the smaller air spaces in the lung remained expanded instead of becoming atelectatic. These surface active lecithins are very much reduced or absent in infants dying from respiratory distress syndrome and this may account for the generalized atelectasis in this condition. This disease occurs almost entirely in preterm infants.

### The Neonatal Lung

A fairly stable functional residual capacity is established by 8–10 min. after birth. Continuing ventilation is associated with decreasing pulmonary vascular resistance leading to a great increase in pulmonary blood flow (*see below*). The absorptive process of the fluid in the lungs by the lymphatics and pulmonary capillaries takes several hours and therefore the increase in the specific compliance of the lung does not reach its maximum for 24 hours (Nelson, 1966). Airway resistance is high for the same period possibly due to bronchospasm and clearance of some fluid from the airways. At birth the infant is in a state of relative asphyxia but this is rapidly corrected. By one hour of age the pH is normal and the alveolar ventilation stable.

After a few hours two important differences exist between

the blood gases of the normal neonate and those of the older child or adult:

1. The arterial oxygen tension in the neonate is about 80 mm. Hg. whereas that in the adult is about 95 mm. Hg. Nelson attributes this mainly to veno-arterial shunting through the foramen ovale (Nelson, 1966). However, Cook and Motoyama believe that it is due to pulmonary ventilation not being properly matched with increased pulmonary perfusion (Cook and Motoyama, 1968). Total shunting in the normal neonate is at least 20 per cent of cardiac output compared with less than 5 per cent in the adult.

2. The alveolar and the arterial carbon dioxide tensions are approximately 35 mm. Hg. compared with the adult level of 40 mm. Hg. Alveolar ventilation is considerably higher per unit of lung volume and per unit of body weight than in the adult. This in turn is due to the higher oxygen consumption per unit of lung volume or body weight (Cook and Motoyama, 1968).

The resting oxygen consumption per unit of body weight is twice that of the adult, 7 ml./Kg./min. compared with 3·5 ml./Kg./min. As already stated earlier the minimum oxygen requirements exist when the neonate is nursed in a neutral thermal environment. Exposure to cold, causing the metabolic response to cold, or to heat, causing hyperthermia, will increase the oxygen consumption considerably. Therefore there is a much greater demand placed on the lung of the infant, even under optimum conditions, than in older patients. Consequently there is less respiratory reserve in the infant than in older individuals.

The exact basis for the higher respiratory rates which occur at rest in infants and young children is not known. It has been suggested that individuals adjust their respiratory rate and tidal volumes so that ventilation is accomplished with minimum work. Dead space, like most lung volumes, correlates well with height throughout childhood. Most workers agree that the ratio of dead space to tidal volume is the same in infants as in adults, i.e. 30 per cent.

The infant's respiratory system is well developed to deal with normal demands. However, any respiratory disease which increases excessively the mechanical work of breathing can cause very great physical energy expenditure in a baby. In extreme cases the work of breathing may cost more in consumed oxygen than can be delivered through the failing lungs (Polgar and Promadhat, 1971). The factors which contribute to this situation are the 'soft' rib-cage, the recumbent body position and the preference for nose breathing.

The preference for nose breathing is a very serious factor in infants with bilateral choanal atresia as the infant will not breathe through its mouth and asphyxia may ensue. The situation is immediately relieved by inserting an oropharyngeal airway.

### The Use of Oxygen

The administration of oxygen can cause blindness due to retrolental fibroplasia in babies of short gestation and the more immature the infant the greater is the risk of retinal damage. High retinal arterial oxygen tensions (above 150 mm. Hg.) cause retinal artery vasoconstriction in immature babies and this seems to initiate the process leading to retrolental fibroplasia.

If the oxygen tension is monitored from the umbilical artery in the immediate newborn period lower values will be obtained than exist in the vessels perfusing the eye and brain. This is due to the normal right-to-left shunting already described. When large shunts exist, as in respiratory distress syndrome, an arterial oxygen tension of 60–90 mm. Hg. in the umbilical artery blood sample may be acceptable (Baum and Tizard, 1970). Monitoring from a small indwelling needle in the radial artery will give a much more reliable indication of the arterial oxygen tension in the vessels perfusing the eye. The danger of pulmonary damage from prolonged administration of high inspired oxygen mixtures must also be remembered but this complication is not limited to the young.

In caring for ill infants there should be no hesitation in raising the inspired oxygen concentration as much as is necessary to maintain acceptable arterial oxygen tensions. Retrolental fibroplasia will not occur unless the arterial oxygen tension is abnormally high and the danger of pulmonary damage from high inspired oxygen concentrations is not acute enough to outweigh the serious and immediate consequences of severe oxygen desaturation.

When additional oxygen is given the inspired oxygen mixture should be checked regularly with an oxygen analyser and the infant's arterial oxygen tension should also be monitored, especially in immature infants.

## CARDIOVASCULAR SYSTEM

### Foetal Circulation

*In utero* the placenta provides a means of gaseous exchange and nutrition for the foetus. Most of the blood in the descending aorta passes via the hypogastric arteries and their continuation the umbilical arteries to the placenta and returns to the foetus via the umbilical vein. From the umbilical vein the blood passes via the ductus venosus, thereby by-passing the liver, to the right atrium. From the right atrium the blood goes through the foramen ovale to the left atrium and thus to the left ventricle and ascending aorta. The superior vena caval blood returning to the right atrium enters the right ventricle and then the pulmonary artery from which it passes through the ductus arteriosus to enter the descending aorta.

### Circulatory Changes at Birth

After birth the lungs and liver must serve the functions of the placenta and therefore the circulation must adjust accordingly. The circulation via the umbilical arteries ceases and the ductus venosus should close. The patent ductus arteriosus and foramen ovale should close so that the blood flows through the pulmonary circulation before reaching the left heart and aorta.

The main mechanism which causes an increase in blood flow through the pulmonary circulation is ventilation of the lungs with air thereby exposing the pulmonary vessels to a higher oxygen tension. This causes a decrease in the pulmonary vascular resistance probably by a direct local effect rather than by a reflex via the aortic and carotid chemo-receptors. The first breath therefore causes an increase in pulmonary blood flow which raises the left atrial pressure above that of the inferior vena cava and right atrium. Consequently the foramen ovale closes functionally by a valve-like action the membrane which is on the left atrial side.

The blood from both inferior vena cava and superior vena cava now enters the pulmonary artery from the right side of the heart. As the resistance in the pulmonary vessels falls so the blood flow through the pulmonary vascular bed increases rapidly with a consequent diminution in the flow through the ductus arteriosus. In the first hour after birth there may be left-to-right and right-to-left shunts via the ductus in normal infants. The right-to-left shunt decreases rapidly within the first hour and after this time is unusual in the resting normal infant (Rudolf, 1968). If the ductus remains open a left-to-right shunt will develop. The pulmonary vascular resistance does not fall to adult levels immediately otherwise a large shunt would develop from left-to-right through the still patent ductus leading to an overwhelming pulmonary blood flow. As the left ventricular output is increased after birth and the systemic vascular resistance rises, a large left-to-right shunt causing an additional output from the left ventricle might precipitate failure.

Oxygenation of the systemic arterial blood causes constriction of the ductus and functional closure occurs within a few hours but histological closure may take 2–3 weeks (Rudolph, 1968). A significant reduction in arterial oxygen tension may reopen a constricted ductus in the first few days. This is of considerable importance to the anaesthetist because the lowered oxygen tension will cause an increase in pulmonary vascular resistance leading to a right-to-left shunt through the ductus. This could cause a considerable degree of desaturation in the systemic circulation. Patency of the ductus persists for several months after birth in several preterm infants. A possible cause may be inadequate ventilation and hypoxia.

At birth the walls of the ventricles are of equal thickness. After birth the left ventricular wall increases in thickness because of the greater resistance it must overcome. The pulmonary artery and right ventricular pressures in the human infant drop to near adult levels by 7–14 days and then there is a further slow fall for 5–7 weeks.

## Cardiac Output

The average cardiac output of the human infant is about 180 ml./Kg./min. and is double the adult value per Kg. The heart rate and cardiac output in both the foetus and the newborn are so high that there is not much room for further increase (Dawes, 1971).

## Systemic Pressure and Peripheral Resistance

In the newborn baby the mean arterial pressure is about 40 mm. Hg. below the mean of the adult and once the readjustments immediately following birth are complete there is a low peripheral resistance. The blood flow to the extremities is about double that of the adult and the cerebral blood flow is high (Young, 1963). The physiological activity of the vasomotor sympathetic mechanism to skin

blood vessels is well developed, and comparable with the adult. Therefore they act well in attempting to conserve heat in the non-anaesthetized baby as already mentioned under 'Heat loss'.

## BODY FLUIDS

### Total Body Water

Approximately 80 per cent of the total body weight in the newborn is fluid. This proportion drops to 75 per cent in the young child and 55–60 per cent in the adult. There are wide variations in body composition between individual newborn infants due to differences in the size of the skeleton and thus in the proportions of bone and soft tissue as well as in fat content (Wilkinson, 1969).

### Distribution of Water

The extracellular volume (plasma plus interstitial fluid) in the neonate is relatively increased and constitutes about 40 per cent of the body weight at birth. It falls to 32–35 per cent at weights of 5–20 Kg. and 25 per cent in adults.

The intracellular fluid in the newborn amounts to only 30 per cent body weight compared with over 40 per cent in adults.

The blood volume represents about 10 per cent of the total fluid volume throughout life. Consequently, because of the high proportion of fluid in the newborn the blood volume is about 80 ml./Kg. body weight whereas in adult males it is about 65–70 ml./Kg. and in females about 55–65 ml./Kg. varying inversely with the amount of body fat present.

### Water Balance

In the first few days of life there is normally a large loss of weight, approximately 10 per cent. This is related to the duration of the restriction of water intake and can be reduced by starting a water intake soon after birth. Of this 10 per cent loss less than one-third can be accounted for by the urine passed. Apart from some of the remainder which is used for metabolic processes, most of the weight loss is due to insensible loss via the expired air and skin. Once feeding begins, fluid metabolism rapidly increases reaching a peak at 2 years of age. At 2 years of age the daily turnover of total body water content is 15 per cent compared with 9 per cent in the adult. This reflects a higher metabolic rate in proportion to weight and results in a higher insensible loss (via the skin and lungs) and higher renal water loss (Smith, 1968). Consequently, the infant and young child will become depleted much more rapidly than the adult.

### Water Requirements

For parenteral replacement (provided there are no abnormal losses) it is suggested that no fluid is required for the first 36–48 hours after birth. Then 45–65 ml./Kg./24 hours should be given if oral feeding has not commenced (Smith, 1968). Larger amounts (100 ml./Kg./24 hours) are required in older infants and young children after which the requirement drops gradually to the adult level.

## Renal Function

The neonatal kidney has a remarkable capacity to conserve sodium and potassium in the first week of life. If given a water load, infants excrete it well but they can not excrete a given water load within 4 hours. Adults can achieve this.

The urine of infants is hypotonic compared with that of older children and their renal clearances of urea, sodium, potassium and chloride are always low even when the plasma concentrations are raised. However the range of function of infantile kidneys is adequate for the infant's needs in neonatal life. If large quantities of glucose solution or saline are given, especially intravenously, the limited capacity to excrete a water load and the low renal clearances of sodium and potassium may lead to retention of large quantities of fluids.

It is always difficult to decide exactly how much water, minerals and calories to give each child in the neonatal period because the margin between enough and too much is so small (Wilkinson, 1969).

## Metabolic Aspects

One week after birth the normal neonate taking breast milk will retain in the body 65 per cent of its intake of protein, sodium and potassium and incorporate it in new tissue. The neonate consumes and retains on a body weight basis much more than the adult. Of the large intake only about 20 per cent has to be excreted in the urine so the neonate needs only about 10 per cent of the adult renal capacity. Therefore on a diet of breast milk under normal circumstances the neonate kidney is amply fitted for the functions it has to perform. It is not surprising that the capacity to excrete large quantities of additional water and mineral salts is limited. Consequently when fluid is administered to the neonate it should resemble as closely as possible, in quality and quantity, the losses sustained (Wilkinson, 1969).

The kidney of the neonate is capable of reducing the concentration of sodium from 140 m.Eq./litre in glomerular filtrate to less than 10 m.Eq./litre in the urine from the fourth to the seventh to tenth days after birth. The neonatal kidney is therefore highly efficient at reabsorbing sodium. Although normally little potassium is passed, excess potassium can be excreted if administered.

If an excess of sodium chloride and water is given intravenously infant kidneys cope less well than adult kidneys.

An infant weighing 3·5 Kg. with an insensible water loss of 90 ml. and a urinary output of 30–100 ml./24 hours is losing 120–190 ml. water/day. In the absence of abnormal losses it is suggested that the total intake of fluid in a neonate should not exceed 66 ml./Kg./24 hours.

## RESPONSE TO RELAXANTS

There is a great deal of controversy concerning the effects of muscle relaxants in the newborn. This is partly due to the conflicting reports concerning the response of the youn infant to relaxants.

The earliest report of a difference in response to relaxants in neonates was by Stead (1955). He reported that infants aged less than one month with intestinal obstruction showed a myasthenic-like sensitivity to d-tubocurarine and an increased tolerance to succinylcholine compared with older patients. Telford and Keats (1957) found that the newborn required 5 times as much succinylcholine per unit body weight as the adult and that there was a fall in the amount required from birth to the age of 10 years.

Using electromyographic techniques, Churchill-Davidson and Wise found that the neonate's response to the depolarizing relaxant decamethonium was like that of a myasthenic and that the infant required 3 times the equivalent adult dose of decamethonium (Churchill-Davidson and Wise, 1964). Nightingale, Glass and Bachman (1966), also using electromyographic techniques, found a shorter duration of action of succinylcholine in infants and young children. They suggested that this was due to a higher rate of metabolism of the drug and they found a progressive increase in the duration of action up to $12\frac{1}{2}$ years of age.

Bush and Stead (1962) showed that, clinically, the infant at birth requires only half the normal dose by weight of d-tubocurarine. This sensitivity decreases and disappears at about one month of age. Churchill-Davidson and Wise (1963) again using electromyographic techniques found that the average dose of d-tubocurarine required for paralysis of the hand muscles was the same, on a weight basis, in the infant and the adult. However they found the tidal volume of the infant reduced whereas the tidal volume of the adult was unchanged. Reversal by neostigmine was prompt.

The reasons for the responses of the newborn to relaxants are not understood. It seems that there is an increased tolerance to succinylcholine throughout childhood whereas the decreased requirements of d-tubocurarine exist only in the first month or so of life. Consequently no single factor is likely to explain both responses.

The many physiological differences which exist between the neonate and the adult such as the high extracellular fluid volume, the high resting minute volume, the high metabolic rate and the liability to hypothermia in the operating theatre may all contribute to the differences reported.

## REFERENCES

Baum, J. D. and Tizard, J. P. M. (1970), "Retrolental Fibroplasia: Management of Oxygen Therapy," *British med. Bull.*, **26**, 171.

Bush, G. H. and Stead, A. L. (1962), "The Use of d-Tubocurarine in Neonatal Anaesthesia," *Brit. J. Anaesth.*, **34**, 721.

Churchill-Davidson, H. C. and Wise, R. P. (1963), "Neuromuscular Transmission in the Newborn Infant," *Anesthesiology*, **24**, 271.

Churchill-Davidson, H. C. and Wise, R. P. (1964), "The Response of the Newborn Infant to Muscle Relaxants," *Canad. Anaesth. Soc. J.*, **11**, 1.

Clements, J. A., Brown, E. S. and Johnson, R. P. (1958), "Pulmonary Surface Tension and Mucus Lining of the Lungs: Some Theoretical Considerations," *J. appl. Physiol.*, **12**, 262.

Cook, C. D. and Motoyama, E. K. (1968), "Respiratory Physiology in Infants and Children," in *Anesthesia for Infants and Children*, 3rd Edition, Chap. 3, p. 32 (R. M. Smith, Ed.). St. Louis: Mosby.

Cross, K. W. (1965), "Respiration and Oxygen Supplies in the Newborn," in *Handbook of Physiology*, Section 3, "Respiration", Vol. II, Chap. 52, p. 1329. Washington, D.C.: American Physiological Society.

Dawes, G. S. (1971), "Fetal and Neonatal Respiration," in *Recent Advances in Paediatrics*, 4th Edition, Chap. I, p. 1 (D. Gairdner and D. Hull, Eds.). London: Churchill.

Hey, E. N. (1971), "The Care of Babies in Incubators," in *Recent Advances in Paediatrics*, 4th Edition, Chap. 6, p. 171 (D. Gairdner and D. Hull, Eds.). London: Churchill.

Hey, E. N. (1972), "Thermal Regulation in the Newborn," *Brit. J. Hosp. Med.*, **8**, 51.

Hey, E. N. and Katz, G. (1970), "The Range of Thermal Insulation in the Tissues of the New-born Baby," *J. Physiol.*, **207**, 667.

Hey, E. N., Katz, G. and O'Connell, B. (1970), "The Total Thermal Insulation of the New-born Baby," *J. Physiol.*, **207**, 683.

Hey, E. N. and O'Connell, B. (1970), "Oxygen Consumption and Heat Balance in the Cot-nursed Baby," *Archs. Dis. Childh.*, **45**, 335.

Hull, D. (1966), "The Structure and Function of Brown Adipose Tissue," *Brit. med. Bull.*, **22**, 92.

Nelson, N. M. (1966), "Neonatal Pulmonary Function," *Pediat. Clin. N. Amer.*, **13**, 769.

Nightingale, D. A., Glass, A. G. and Bachman, L. (1966), "Neuromuscular Blockade by Succinylcholine in Children," *Anesthesiology*, **27**, 736.

Polgar, G. and Promadhat, V. (1971), "Specific Tests and Procedures in Children," in *Pulmonary Function Testing in Children*, Chap. 4, p. 42 (G. Polgar and V. Promadhat, Eds.). Philadelphia: Saunders.

Rudolph, A. M. (1968), "The Foetal Circulation, Circulatory Adjustments After Birth and the Influence of Congenital Heart Lesions on Pulmonary Haemodynamics," in *Paediatric Cardiology*, Chap. 3, p. 48 (H. Watson, Ed.). London: Lloyd-Luke.

Smith, R. M. (1968), "Fluid Therapy and Blood Replacement," in *Anesthesia for Infants and Children*, Chap. 26, p. 406 (R. M. Smith, Ed.). St. Louis: Mosby.

Stead, A. L. (1955), "The Response of the Newborn Infant to Muscle Relaxants," *Brit. J. Anaesth.*, **27**, 124.

Telford, J. and Keats, A. S. (1957), "Succinylcholine in Cardiovascular Surgery of Infants and Children," *Anesthesiology*, **18**, 841.

Wilkinson, A. W. (1969), "Disturbances During Infancy and Childhood," in *Body Fluids in Surgery*, 3rd Edition, Chap. 12, p. 245 (A. W. Wilkinson, Ed.). Edinburgh and London: Livingstone.

Young, M. (1963), "The Fetal and Neonatal Circulation," Chap. 46, p. 1619 in *Handbook of Physiology*, Section 2, *Circulation*, Vol. II. Washington, D.C.: American Physiological Society.

*CHAPTER 7*

# PARENTERAL NUTRITION

## STEWART FARQUHARSON

It is still widely accepted that major medical or surgical illness will inevitably be associated with severe wasting of the body tissues. All too often, nutritional requirements are considered to be of secondary importance to other therapeutic procedures. In fact convalescence will be shortened and the incidence of many surgical complications reduced by correct nutrition. Indeed, survival may depend on supplying the correct metabolic substrate, which, in many circumstances, can only be given parenterally.

### History

Historically the concept of parenteral nutrition is by no means new. Alcohol (as ale and wine) was given intravenously by Sir Christopher Wren in 1656 to dogs, using a pig's bladder and silver cannula; in 1831 the place of intravenous infusions in general was firmly established by Latta when he resuscitated moribund cholera patients with salt solutions. Hodder administered intravenous milk to cholera victims in 1873, but the first notable success with parenteral nutrition was that of Henriques and Anderson, who in 1913, maintained a goat in good health for 16 days with a continuous infusion of glucose, sodium and potassium salts and amino acids obtained by hydrolysis of goat muscle.

Fat emulsion was first given by Yamakawa in 1920, but the first such infusion for prolonged daily usage was the soya bean preparation, Intralipid, introduced by Wretlind in 1957. Routine administration of amino acids became possible with the introduction of Aminosol (casein hydro-lysate) by Wretlind in 1944, and the recent advance in this field is the introduction of pure synthetic preparations of laevo amino acids.

### The Catabolic Response

Basic to the understanding of the patient's nutritional needs is a knowledge of some aspects of protein and carbohydrate metabolism not only during starvation but also when stress and/or trauma are superimposed.

The carbohydrate reserves in the body are of the order of 100–300 g. of glycogen. Thus, during starvation carbohydrate alone can supply no more than 1,200 calories.* Once this carbohydrate is metabolized (in a maximum of around 12 hours) the body will proceed to metabolize proteins and fats. It is widely accepted that the reason for the protein catabolism is to provide carbohydrate metabolic intermediates, the process of gluconeogenesis.

Fat cannot provide carbohydrates. Indeed fat metabolism demands a steady supply of carbohydrates if ketoacidosis is to be prevented. Glucose is also an essential substrate for the brain. With the onset of acute starvation catabolism occurs at a rate of 10–15 g. of nitrogen daily. The administration of only 100 g. of glucose reduces this to 3–4 g. of nitrogen. Insulin is almost certainly the stimulus inhibiting the gluconeogenesis (Cahill, 1970). During

---

* 1 calorie is the popularly accepted abbreviation for 1 kilocalorie. With the introduction of S.I. units, 1 kilocalorie would become 4,184 joules.

prolonged starvation the body appears to adapt to the metabolism of ketoacids, as the negative nitrogen balances fall to about 3–4 g.

Even so nearly all calories are produced from fat, since 1 g. of fat provides about 7 times as many calories as 1 g. of lean tissue, and they tend to be catabolised in approximately equal quantities (Moore, 1959; Kinney, 1970).

The protein catabolism is a somewhat wasteful process since some amino acids are not easily converted to the carbohydrate metabolic intermediates. It is imperative to realise that the fat patient shows an identical protein catabolism. Many clinicians withhold nutrition from the obese, failing to appreciate this point.

Body proteins are by no means static. They are continually being broken down (catabolism) and rebuilt (anabolism), and these processes are in dynamic equilibrium in health. It is generally accepted that there is no location of any actual protein reserves in the body, but there are very significant differences in the rate of protein turnover in different areas. After starvation and refeeding experiments in rats, 3 broad groups may be identified (Waterlow, 1962; Jin Soon Ju, 1959), where:

1. Protein is very static, such as brain or collagen.
2. Protein is rapidly depleted during early starvation. This involves the protein notably of the liver, serum albumen, intestinal mucosa and pancreas. The protein is said to be labile.
3. Protein is depleted slowly initially, but the process is accelerated once the liver in particular is depleted. This applies notably to the body musculature.

It has been clearly demonstrated that the lysosomes are an important site of catabolic enzymes (Sawant *et al.*, 1964) and normally they are highly stable intracellular organelles. It has been shown that starvation alone increases the levels of lysosomal enzymes (Desai, 1969). The association between lysosomes and catabolism has been considered in great detail (Carlo, 1971).

Further important work by Waterlow (1968) demonstrated that during periods of reduced protein intake, albeit just sufficient for the maintenance of growth, the organism still shows the same overall rate of catabolism and anabolism but now a far smaller amount of nitrogen is excreted. This adaptation seems to explain the frequently observed fact that the malnourished show a reduced catabolic response to trauma, whereas the well nourished show the greatest degree of early catabolism.

Catabolism has important undesirable secondary effects. Protein breakdown will inevitably release potassium ions and fixed acids in the form of sulphates and phosphates. If catabolism is reduced by nutrition the postoperative loss of potassium ions is largely prevented. It is said that for each gramme of nitrogen lost there is the liberation of 16–18 mEq. of potassium and about 3·3 mEq. of fixed acid (Carlo, 1971). In all probability depletion of hepatic protein has secondary effects on enzyme and antibody levels. Furthermore, substrates are known to stabilize their enzyme systems (Munro, 1968) and so withdrawal of food can be expected to reduce the level of anabolic systems, including RNA.

The patient undergoing surgery is usually starved for a period of 12 hours or more and this is sufficient to deplete the carbohydrate reserves and initiate gluconeogenesis. The surgical patient now exposed to stress and surgical trauma shows enhanced catabolism: there are many factors known to be involved and there must surely be others yet undiscovered:

1. Starvation usually persists in the postoperative period since most patients undergoing major surgery receive only 400–600 calories in the form of isotonic dextrose solutions.

2. Any fit well nourished adult who goes to bed and rests will inevitably go into negative $N_2$ balance to the extent of around 2 g. a day (Dietrich, 1948). The mechanism is presumed to be a result of tissue atrophy.

3. There is an increased metabolic rate following surgery, usually of the order of 25–30 per cent (Kinney, 1967). This figure is greatly exceeded where complications such as sepsis occur.

4. Insulin antagonism: the high level of glucocorticoids to be found after stress and injury is well known to promote further the conversion of proteins to carbohydrates. The extent and duration of the high cortisol level have been fully investigated (Plumpton, Besser and Cole, 1969). Growth hormone has a similar action and is present in increased amounts (Johnston, 1967), and this probably applies to glucagon. Nonetheless, although the greatest importance has been attached to the high level of cortisol, adrenalectomized animals on a constant replacement regime show an identical catabolic response (Selye, 1954), which suggests that hydrocortisone is unlikely to be a major factor in postoperative catabolism and that catecholamines may be involved.

5. It has been suggested that at the sites of reparative processes, perfusion and therefore oxygen supplies, must be limited, at least initially, and so energy is provided by the very uneconomic anaerobic metabolism of glucose to lactate (Cahill, 1970).

6. The mobilization of amino acids is necessary to make proteins for repair processes.

7. In some cases there will be excessive protein losses as in burns or ulcerative colitis. (In burns there may also be considerable heat loss associated with evaporation of large quantities of water, thereby demanding even greater catabolism).

8. The lysosomal enzyme levels are raised far higher than by starvation alone, by metabolic acidosis (Schummer, 1968) and shock states or by the action of adrenaline (Glenn, 1970). Surgical trauma causes adrenaline release: this may prove to be of greater relevance than cortisol release.

9. Age and sex effect the catabolic response. The young, with a higher rate of protein turnover show the greater catabolism and males incur a greater degree than females.

Some authorities regard catabolism as a physiological process and an invariable accompaniment of severe trauma or illness (Davidson and Passmore, 1966), but, as has been so pertinently pointed out (Peaston, 1967) the catabolic response cannot be considered physiological when stress and trauma are in themselves pathological. A number of factors have been found to reduce catabolism:

1. Feeding. Numerous investigations have shown that post-operative feeding can reduce or even abolish the catabolic response. Pre-operative feeding presumably merely by abolishing the gluconeogenesis of starvation may be especially effective (Rush, 1970). Rush started parenteral nutrition with carbohydrate and amino acids two days pre-operatively and was able to achieve a positive $N_2$ balance in 13 out of 19 patients subjected to major upper abdominal surgery. This compares with average losses of 10–15 g. of $N_2$ a day in such patients treated with the usual regimes. Furthermore, Rush using a high electrolyte intake was able to achieve slightly positive potassium balance as compared to average losses of 50–100 mEq. daily, in the postoperative patient.

2. Environmental temperature. Both Caldwell (1962) and Cuthbertson et al. (1968) have demonstrated a marked reduction of catabolism in a warmer environment. Cuthbertson's study, involved nursing the patient at a temperature of 30°C and a humidity of 35 per cent (any higher becomes uncomfortable). A remarkable feature of this investigation was that postoperative oliguria was almost abolished.

3. Control of the stress factor. In a very interesting investigation by Setbon (1970) postoperative patients were heavily sedated with neuroleptanalgesic drugs, and given trophysan and sorbitol in only moderate amounts. Using this technique he was able to achieve a positive $N_2$ balance within 24 hours of the operation in most patients. This study is highly suggestive that adrenaline release is closely related to postoperative catabolism, as droperidol and allied drugs induce a degree of adrenergic blockade.

4. Avoidance of acidosis. The importance of prevention and treatment of postoperative metabolic acidosis must never be underestimated. A vicious circle can be induced where the acidosis promotes catabolism and the catabolism enhances the acidosis.

The degree of catabolic response to be found after some surgical procedures have been measured on many occasions. A broad generalization would be that uncomplicated major upper abdominal or thoracic surgery without feeding regimes induces negative nitrogen balances of the order of 10–15 g. daily for around 5 days, and major surgery where complications occur will lead to losses of 15–25 g. daily. The following table shows the generally accepted equivalents:

$$1 \text{ gm. } N_2 = \begin{cases} 25\text{–}30 \text{ g. lean tissue} \\ 6\cdot25 \text{ g. protein} \\ 5\text{–}6 \text{ g. amino acids} \end{cases}$$

Simple arithmetic explains how dramatic weight loss can occur with surgical complications. In peritonitis with paralytic ileus for example, daily nitrogen losses of at least 15 g. can be anticipated, equivalent to lean tissue losses of 400–500 g. Such complications would be expected to last for many days.

The advantages of adequate nutrition during the operative period can now be suitably summarized:

Maintenance of body weight and reduction or abolition of the catabolic response which may deplete the patient of proteins. Protein deficiency is associated with prolonged convalescence and greater susceptibility to post operative complications such as infection, slow healing, wound deshiscence, and the breakdown of anastomoses (Hadfield, 1965). Maintenance of body proteins can only help in the maintenance of antibodies, enzymes and almost certainly RNA. Metabolic effects are minimized. Acidosis and potassium loss are reduced. The liver is protected against anaesthetics and/or shock (Brit. J. Anaesth., 1972). Where major operative complications occur, survival is often impossible without full nutrition.

## Catabolism and Insulin

The effect of the stress situation on carbohydrate metabolism has already been mentioned. The insulin antagonism is attributable to the presence of raised levels of circulating cortisol, glucagon, growth hormone and adrenaline. The result is hyperglycaemia with poor utilization of glucose. Insulin is necessary for the entry of glucose into most body cells such as striated muscle, cardiac muscle and adipose tissue (as opposed to brain and erythrocytes where it does not appear to be necessary). Interestingly, the insulin level is also raised post-operatively (Johnston, 1967). Although the effects of insulin on carbohydrate metabolism are well known, the highly anabolic actions are not so widely appreciated. It promotes the uptake of amino acids by cells and consequently the synthesis of muscle protein (Waterlow, 1968). Conversely, amino acids have actually been shown to stimulate insulin secretion. Finally, insulin stimulates triglyceride formation and is therefore strongly antiketotic. (See chapter 3, p. 330).

## THE CONSTITUENTS OF PARENTERAL NUTRITION

For anabolism to occur, nitrogenous sources must be given with adequate calories. It is usually stated that the optimal ratio is 150–250 calories for each g. of $N_2$. Carbohydrates must be given all the time as they are necessary for all aspects of metabolism of which the anabolism of amino acids and utilization of fats are but two examples. Amino acids given without carbohydrate will be deaminated to a major extent. Carbohydrates also play an important role as structural units in other molecules. It is apparent that all solutions other than fats will have to be hypertonic if sufficient calories are to be given by infusion, without overloading the patient with fluid.

## CALORIE SOURCES

### Glucose

Physiologically glucose is the most common carbohydrate received by man. It should not be forgotten that glucose is an essential substrate for the brain. The rate of intake should not exceed 0·5 g./Kg./hour.

When glucose is given in the postoperative or stress situation it does have some drawbacks although these can be managed with strict attention to detail.

1. Insulin antagonism at this time means that the blood glucose must be carefully monitored and insulin will be required, if osmotic diuresis is to be prevented. Isotope studies show that glucose is diluted by approximately 25 per cent of the body mass, but that this approaches 100 per cent when given with adequate insulin (Thoren, 1964).

2. Hypoglycaemia may occur when a glucose infusion is stopped, especially in small children. Therefore infusions should be given at an even pace and slowly tailed off.

3. Thrombophlebitis rapidly occurs when glucose is infused into peripheral veins, and so central venous catheterization is usually necessary. It is sometimes maintained that the anabolic effect of insulin necessarily given concurrently with the glucose outweighs the disadvantages, and there is some evidence to support this (Allison, 1971). Glucose is now regaining its popularity since it has been shown that fructose, albeit in high dosage, can provoke acidosis (Sahebjami and Scarlettar, 1971).

### Fructose

Fructose does have some important advantages over glucose, especially in the situations of stress. Fructose enters the metabolic pathways by phosphorylation and there appear to be two routes, via fructokinase to fructose-1-phosphate (insulin independent) and by hexokinase to fructose-6-phosphate which is insulin dependent. Renal losses of fructose are less than those of glucose when given without insulin in spite of the fact that the renal threshold is far lower (around 10 mg. per cent). This is due to the fact that it is very rapidly diluted in the whole body water and that metabolism is much faster as evidenced by:

1. A rapid conversion to pyruvate with a concommitant rise in the RQ and a fall in plasma phosphate.
2. A more rapid conversion to glycogen. Other advantages of fructose over glucose are a greater antiketogenic effect, enhancement of the metabolism of alcohol, a more stable blood glucose and a lower incidence of thrombophlebitis in peripheral veins.

Both glucose and fructose are reducing sugars and they can denature amino acids if sterilized by heat together; the so-called Maillard reaction. Dudrick *et al.* (1970a) makes up fresh solutions of sterile glucose and amino acids using a 0·22μ membrane filter and so avoids this important problem.

### Sorbitol

Sorbitol is a sugar which occurs naturally in fruits. Metabolism takes place in the liver where the enzyme sorbitol dehydrogenase converts it to fructose, and there is a subsidiary pathway by the enzyme aldose reductase, to glucose, the former being more important quantitatively.

Its antiketogenic effect is even greater than that of fructose. This may be attributed to the fact that during oxidation to fructose an additional molecule of NADH is produced. It has been found that a higher ratio of NADH to NAD reduces the oxidation of fatty acids to acetate (Murisasco *et al.*, 1966).

Sorbitol causes less thrombolophlebitis than fructose and it may be given into peripheral veins during short term parenteral nutrition. This may be related to a pH of the solution of 6–7, as opposed to glucose and fructose with a pH range of 3–4·5. Although sorbitol was originally introduced as a diuretic, metabolic utilization of the agents when used at recommended infusion rates is around 90–95 per cent (Bye, 1969; Lee *et al.*, 1971).

### Ethanol

Historically ethanol was the first nutritious substance to be given parenterally. It has a high calorific value at 7·1 cal./g. The metabolic pathway is via acetaldehyde to pyruvate to enter the citric acid cycle. The rate of metabolism in man is of the order of 8–10 ml./hour and is a little less in women; this limits the concentration that may be given to about 5 per cent.

It can therefore only be described as an adjuvant to parenteral nutrition. Its pharmacological action on the CNS may be of benefit in sedation to the intensive care patient. In addition it promotes peripheral blood flow.

There are some important drawbacks to its use insofar as metabolism is very dependent on good liver function and this precludes its use in the very small infant. Its diuretic effect is well known. Signs of intolerance have sometimes been observed when, as would frequently be required, it is given with antibiotics. (Wenzel, 1970).

### Xylitol

Xylitol is a normal metabolic intermediate in the pentose shunt. Particular interest in its use in parenteral nutrition has arisen after the discovery that the production of ribose from glucose (or other hexoses) is slowed in the stress situation. This is due to the fact that the enzyme glucose-6-phosphate dehydrogenase, which catalyses the production of 6 phosphogluconic acid, the main metabolic route for ribose formation, appears to be somewhat inhibited, although the mechanism is not understood. Ribose is an intrinsic component, not only of nucleic acids, but also of mucopolysaccharides, glycoproteins and glycolipids, and of great importance to the clinician is the fact that nucleic acids affect all further protein synthesis. Of further interest is the fact that metabolism of xylitol is independent of insulin (Lang, 1967) and proceeds well in liver disease (Wenzel, 1970) it is strongly antiketogenic, it is very well tolerated in peripheral veins and metabolic rates are increased by continued exposure to the drug (Bassler, 1967).

At present, however, its use is prohibited in the U.K. at least, following deaths associated with its administration, although these may well have been due to impurities. It is undergoing further clinical trials at the time of writing.

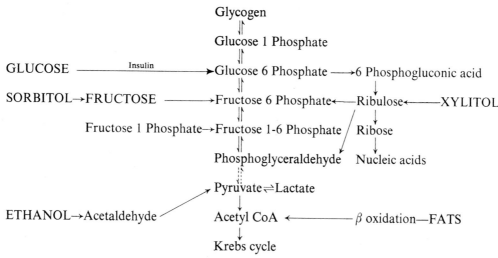

Principal metabolic pathways for intravenous calorie sources.

## Fats

Complete parenteral nutrition is impossible without intravenous fats. Intravenous preparation of fat has the great advantage of supplying large quantities of calories in small volumes of fluid which are not hypertonic and extremely well tolerated by veins. The calorific value of fat is 9·3 cal./g.

Although fat therapy is a safe routine procedure, today, historically the administration of fat emulsion was associated with a high incidence of complications: there were two kinds of reaction. Firstly, an acute situation characterized by chest pain, dyspnoea, hypotension, cyanosis and rigors, and secondly, a chronic toxicity, called the overloading syndrome, which tended to occur after around two weeks administration, which was manifested by fever, nausea, hepatosplenomegaly, jaundice and gastro-intestinal bleeding. This reaction has been attributed to impurities rather than the fat itself. In one preparation a highly toxic agent, gossypol, was identified (Leveen et al., 1961).

Further aspects of the history and method of preparation have been extensively reviewed (Shuttleworth, 1962; Hallberg et al., 1967). In essence, an attempt has been made to manufacture artificial chylomicrons. The very high interfacial tension between the vegetable oil and water is reduced by emulsifying agents and isotonicity is achieved with sugar solution or glycerol. Particle size should not exceed 2 μ (embolism occurs at 4 μ). Metabolism proceeds by two methods, hydrolysis by the enzyme lipoprotein lipase and by the removal of whole particles by the reticulo endothelial system.

There are only two fat preparations available in the U.K.: one derived from soya beans (Intralipid) and the other from cotton seeds (Lipiphysan). Undoubtedly, the most satisfactory preparation especially where long term therapy is likely to be necessary is the soya bean preparation. The incidence of side effects with this preparation is very low (Hallberg et al., 1967). The cotton seed oil preparation may have a place for short term therapy. The recommended rate of administration is 1–3 g. fat/kg./day, although far higher doses have been given (Hadfield, 1966). For long termt herapy 2 gm./kg. should be considered the maximum. One should be prepared to use large doses when hyper-

alimentation is indicated. It is recommended that heparin be added to fat emulsions at a rate of 5 units/ml. for two reasons: to enhance the clearing of the fat emulsion by lipoprotein lipase (Geyer, 1960) and to prevent a possible hypercoagulability state (Amris et al., 1964). The utilization is in fact remarkably rapid, approximately 70 per cent being metabolized in 5 hours (Geyer et al., 1948).

Contraindications to I.V. fat therapy are liver damage, coagulation disorders and pathological hyperlipaemia as occurs in diabetics and the nephrotic syndrome. Fat therapy must be considered to be relatively contraindicated in pregnancy as it has been incriminated in promoting the onset of labour (Heller, 1971). Fats should not be given in the first 24 hours postoperatively as there is always some impairment of liver function at this time.

## Amino Acids

The daily requirement of amino acids is about 0·8–1·0 g./kg./day. This equates with the commonly quoted figure of 14 g. of $N_2$/day as meeting the daily requirements for an adult. This estimate should be raised where hypermetabolic states may be expected.

Blood, plasma and serum albumen contain proteins. None of these agents is useful in parenteral nutrition as a source of nitrogen because the breakdown to individual amino acids is far too slow. Albumen, however, is largely responsible for the very important colloid osmotic effect of plasma proteins, holding water in the circulation. In some conditions where parenteral nutrition is indicated, albumen (or plasma) should be given because profuse exudative processes can be expected to occur (as in peritonitis) and the liver may well be incapable of maintaining the serum albumen.

## Amino Acid Preparations

The composition of an amino acid preparation is of the utmost importance. It is well known that there are eight essential amino acids and it is important that the ratio of these essential amino acids is balanced, otherwise a reduction in anabolic activity must occur. Furthermore, there are some semi-essential amino acids. These are amino acids that cannot be synthesized fast enough from simple units such as glycine. Into this group comes histidine and possibly proline and alanine (Fekl, 1969). Arginine is of the greatest importance in an amino acid mixture, occupying as it does, a central position in the urea cycle. Its absence leads to a potentially dangerous rise in the blood ammonia level.

**Casein hydrolysates** such as the preparations Aminosol and Amigen have been the basis of British practice in intravenous amino acid therapy after a series of reports by Peaston and his colleagues. There are important limitations on the routine use of Aminosol:

1. A high sodium content of approximately 160 mEq./l.

2. It is an impure preparation pharmacologically. In fact as much as 30 per cent of the preparation is in the form of peptides which cannot be utilized and which may become allergenic.

3. Doubts have been expressed as to whether the preparation contains sufficient tryptophan.

### Crystalline Amino Acid Mixtures

Body tissues are built from laevo-amino acids. During manufacture both optical isomers will be produced. Racemic mixtures are available (e.g. Trophysan). However, apart from methionine and phenylalanine, the dextro isomers cannot be used for tissue synthesis. The other dextro isomers are largely excreted in the urine and can promote an osmotic diuresis. A certain proportion is deaminated and used as a carbohydrate source.

Pure laevo-amino acids are available as two different kinds of preparation. Those, such as Vamin, which contain all the amino acids and others which contain the essential and semi-essential amino acids (Aminoplex, Aminofusin) with glycine as an inexpensive non-specific source of nitrogen. Theoretically, metabolic work must be saved by supplying all the amino acids. Undoubtedly, the pure laevoamino acid preparations show the best results on $N_2$ balance studies, but they are the most expensive; economics apart, they would seem to be the preparation of choice.

### The Indications for Parenteral Nutrition

1. **Preoperative.** Patients with long standing inadequate oral intake, severe diarrhoea or malabsorption can greatly benefit from preoperative parenteral nutrition. Iatrogenic malnutrition may well be added in hospital while such a patient undergoes recurrent radiological investigation. The patient with upper intestinal malignancy or ulcerative colitis could be expected to show far better anastomotic and wound healing with adequate intravenous feeding which ideally should start preoperatively.

2. **Postoperative.** Patients who cannot be expected to take food orally for many days due to peritonitis or trauma for example, should start parenteral nutrition immediately. Abdominal fistulae are now treated very successfully in some centres in the U.S.A. using parenteral nutrition alone (Dudrick, 1970b). Malignancy of the head and neck involving major surgical procedures is an indication for full intravenous feeding (Littlewood and Peaston, 1965). If feeding by mouth or through a nasogastric tube were

employed, regurgitation over the anastomoses could jeopardize healing of anastomoses. Furthermore pulmonary aspiration is far more likely when the pharyngeal anatomy has been altered by operation.

3. **Increased Catabolism.** There is a group of conditions where oral feeding may in fact be possible, but intake cannot be expected to approach the metabolic needs of the patient. Such conditions are severe burns, postoperative patients with complications, major traumatic cases, cranial trauma especially where there is increased muscle tone or frank rigidity. Parenteral nutrition is strongly indicated in cases of hypercatabolic renal failure.

4. **Prolonged vomiting or diarrhoea.** Included in this group would be conditions such as hyperemesis gravidarum or diarrhoea which not infrequently follows tube feeding (although this has been reduced by the addition of methyl cellulose).

5. **Paediatrics.** Neonates with major gastrointestinal anomalies such as tracheoesophageal fistula or gut atresia may need parenteral nutrition. 8 cm. of small bowel seems to be the critical length necessary for suitable adaptation and survival (Dudrick, 1970b). Respiratory distress syndrome and major debilitation is another indication.

6. **Other medical conditions.** Patients with respiratory failure or acute polyneuritis, for example, often have transitory paralytic ileus. In most major medical illnesses appetite is usually reduced while energy requirements are increased, although supplementation can usually be given via the gastrointestinal tract. This is clearly not a complete list. The overriding principle is that parenteral nutrition should be given when oral feeding sufficient to meet the metabolic needs cannot be given in the immediately foreseeable future. A major consideration too is the danger of pulmonary aspiration, associated with oral or tube feeding, in the patient who is dyspnoeic or who has a reduced level of consciousness.

### PRACTICAL CONSIDERATIONS AND DESIGN OF A DIET

There is no intravenous diet available which can be expected to be satisfactory in every situation. In order to design a suitable regime certain basic information is essential, including the patient's weight, the renal and hepatic functions, serum electrolytes, proteins, haematological and acid/base status. An assessment must be made as to whether nutritional demands would be expected to be normal or increased. It is emphasized that the patient with major trauma, infection or burns can be expected to have requirements at least double those of the resting state. The following table gives an indication of a patient's needs per kg./day.

|  | *Basal* | *Increased* |
|---|---|---|
| Water | 30–40 m. | 50–60 ml. |
| Calories | 30 | 50–60 |
| Protein | 0·8–1·0 g. | 1·5–2·5 g. |
| Carbohydrate | 2–3 g. | 4–8 g. |
| Fat | 1–2 g. | 3 g. |

(Adapted from Allen and Lee, 1969.)

In calculating the fluid requirement, the patient's clinical condition, existing fluid balance status and any abnormal losses are taken into account; similarly, the electrolyte requirements are greatly affected by pre-existing conditions such as renal failure or abdominal fistulae. During parenteral nutrition there is an enhanced potassium requirement, since anabolism involves the incorporation of the intracellular ions, and for optimal utilization, at least 5–10 mEq. should be given for each g. of nitrogen (assuming normal renal function).

Carbohydrate in the diet should be given at an even rate throughout the whole 24-hour period. This not only reduces the possibility of osmotic diuresis but also ensures a steady supply of calories to anabolize amino acids and metabolize the fats. This necessitates the use of a single 'complete' solution or a system utilizing one or more Y connections.

Vitamins must not be omitted. B vitamins being vitally concerned with carbohydrate metabolism and vitamins A and C essential for healing processes. Full vitamin replacement and the administration of trace elements becomes increasingly important with time, and this aspect will be considered in greater detail in relation to long term therapy.

Clinicians working the U.K. are well advised to use the intravenous diets suggested by Irving and Rushman (1971). At the time of writing all proprietary amino acid solutions in the U.K. contain electrolytes in varying amounts. Dudrick's solution or a system which uses amino acid and sugar solutions to which ions may be added allows greater flexibility in practice.

## SOME EXAMPLES OF PARENTERAL REGIMES

### Maintenance

|  | Contents |
|---|---|
| Sorbitol 30 per cent 1,500 ml. + (KCl as required) | Vol. 2,000 ml. Cal. 2,000 |
| 10 per cent amino acid solution 500 ml. | $N_2$ 8·5 g. |

### High Calorie

| | Contents |
|---|---|
| 40 per cent glucose or fructose 1,500 ml. | Vol. 4,000 ml. |
| 20 per cent fat emulsion 1,000 ml. + 5,000 units heparin/l | Cal. 5,000 |
| 10 per cent L-amino acids 1,500 ml. | $N_2$ 25 g. |

It is appreciated that there is considerable difference in the availability of preparations to clinicians in different countries; having understood the principles, he must choose a regime from those available to him and relevant to the patient's clinical condition.

### The Addition of Insulin

The carbohydrate intake in the second regime is still well below traditional upper limit of 0·5 g./kg./hour. If glucose is the carbohydrate of choice and the patient is in a postoperative or stress situation, insulin will be required. There is no general agreement on the amount of insulin required. Furthermore, the requirement will fall as the postoperative phase is passed and/or the islet cells respond by increasing the endogenous insulin secretion. The anticipated insulin requirement is of the order of 10–25 units/100 g. of glucose and this can either be given subcutaneously in divided doses or intravenously with the sugar solution. The blood glucose should be kept below 180 mg./100 ml.* It should be remembered that there is often a reduced insulin requirement when fructose is used.

### The Effect of Other Conditions

In many patients requiring parenteral nutrition there will be pre-existing diseases which necessitate variation in the I.V. diet:

1. **Liver Disease.** Fat and ethanol are contraindicated. Glucose is certainly the carbohydrate of choice. The intake of protein should be stopped where there is any risk of acute hepatic failure. An intake of L-amino acids does not seem to be contraindicated in infective hepatitis (Long et al., 1970).

2. **Diabetes.** Fat is contraindicated and fructose is the carbohydrate of choice.

3. **Renal Failure.** The Giordano-Giovannetti diet is a compromise between a protein free intake which promotes catabolic wasting and the normal diet which causes an unacceptable accumulation of nitrogenous waste products. Many patients however are unable to take it either because of an associated uraemic gastroenteropathy or because of accidental or surgical trauma to the gastrointestinal tract.

An intravenous modification of the Giordano-Giovannetti diet using 50–70 per cent glucose and laevo amino acids has been used at the University of Pennsylvania Medical Centre with considerable success. The patient's condition as judged by a sense of well being, abolition of nausea and vomiting, and biochemical parameters such as blood urea, serum phosphate and standard bicarbonate have been greatly improved. There was a reduction too in the need for dialysis (Long et al., 1970).

Protein requirement in such patients is of the order of 0·4 g. protein/kg./day (Fekl, 1969). Amino acids given during dialysis are wasted since they are easily lost into the dialysate. Where a patient is undergoing peritoneal dialysis there is a considerable loss of amino acids and albumen and a high intake of these agents is actually indicated.

4. **Paediatrics.** The problems of parenteral nutrition in paediatrics have been well reviewed by Harries (1971). The methods used have been meticulously described. He recommends using peripheral veins relying on a high intake of Intralipid to minimize the thrombophlebitis. He maintains that three weeks parenteral nutrition is possible by this method. Dudrick, in the U.S.A. (where I.V. fats are still unavailable) uses a superior vena caval catheter, inserted via an external jugular vein, which is tunnelled subcutaneously to emerge from the scalp, thereby leaving a maximal distance between the skin wound and vein, an important point for the prevention of septicaemia (Dudrick, 1968).

---

* When the blood glucose is very unstable management will be made easier by starting with a lower glucose intake.

## Long Term Therapy

When 'maintenance' regimes are given and the duration of feeding is not expected to be more than about 4 or 5 days, the use of peripheral veins is suitable, although the vein should be changed daily to reduce the incidence of thrombophlebitis.

Success with long term therapy depends on obsessional attention to detail with regard to catheter care, and the administration of vitamins for example. Central venous catheterization is essential. Inferior vena caval catheterization is not suitable as it is associated with a high incidence of thromboembolism which is frequently septic. This is attributable to the short distance between the skin and vein at the femoral insertion and the likelihood of soiling the puncture site with urine or faeces.

Superior vena caval catheterization may be achieved via the basilic vein, the subclavian vein, either via the infraclavicular (Aubaniac, 1952; Dudrick, 1969), or supraclavicular approach, or via the external or internal jugular vein (English et al., 1969). When very long therapy is likely to be required, infraclavicular puncture should be chosen. It should not be lightly undertaken as there is a significant incidence of complications such as pneumothorax, hydrothorax and air embolism. An excellent review of caval catheterization and its complications has recently been published (Burri and Henkemeyer, 1971).

After insertion, the catheter must be firmly secured, preferably by a stitch very near the puncture site to prevent it slipping to and fro and introducing pathogenic organisms. The giving set must be very securely attached and a free reflux of blood obtained on lowering the infusion bottle. An occlusive dressing is applied to the puncture site and finally a chest X-ray taken to check the position of the catheter. Clearly a shorter length of cannula is less likely to act as a focus for infection. Where a cutdown is used the vein should not be ligated. Infusion sets must be changed daily and the occlusive dressing taken down daily so that the puncture site may be inspected, cleaned and then sprayed with an antibiotic or antiseptic preparation, preferably incorporating an antifungal agent. With this degree of care drips may run for many weeks, although Dudrick recommends changing subclavian infusions every 30 days. Obvious infection of the puncture site is an indication for removal of the central venous catheter, as is otherwise unexplained fever, when blood cultures should be taken and the catheter tip cultured after removal.

## Vitamins and Trace Elements

At present, one can only speculate on the vitamin requirements of patients undergoing long term parenteral nutrition. As already explained, metabolic demands are often greatly increased and this will mean greater requirements. A further complicating fact is that in the absence of gastrointestinal feeding the vitamins produced by the intestinal flora must be greatly curtailed. The only safeguard is greatly to exceed the normal daily requirements which are as follows:

| | |
|---|---|
| Vitamin A | 3,000–5,000 I.V. |
| Vitamin D | 500 I.V. |
| Vitamin C | 100 mg. |
| Thiamine (B$_1$) | 2 mg. |
| Riboflavine (B$_2$) | 2 mg. |
| Nicotinamide (B$_3$) | 20 mg. |
| Pantothenic Acid (B$_5$) | 10 mg. |
| Pyridoxine (B$_6$) | 2 mg. |
| Cyanocobalamin (B$_{12}$) | 1–5 $\mu$gm. |
| Vitamin K | 1–2 mg. |
| Folic Acid | 0·4 mg. |

(Largely compiled from *Documenta Geigy*, Scientific Tables, 7th Edition.)

Sometimes included in the B group of vitamins are biotin and choline, the latter can be made in the body when there is an adequate tryptophan intake. Vitamin E is an antioxidant, its importance is still debated.

From the clinical point of view, it is safe to say that a patient would be kept in good health using preparations such as 'Pabrinex' or 'Parentrovite' for two weeks, after which the need for a more complete vitamin preparation becomes necessary (when 10 ml. of multivitamin infusion, SAS Scientific Chemicals, London, for example, should be given at least every other day.) From this time the patient should have weekly injections of Vitamin K (Menadiol) 10–20 mg. and Folic acid 5–10 mg. Vitamin B12 100 $\mu$gm. should be given monthly.

Magnesium can scarcely be considered to be a trace element. Symptoms of magnesium deficiency are very similar to those of hypocalcaemia (twitching and tetany) and in addition bizarre psychiatric disturbances may occur. It has been clearly demonstrated that with a reduced or absent intake the serum level rapidly falls (Coats and Maynard, 1968). Six to ten mEq. of this ion are necessary daily. Calcium is vital in small children but is scarcely necessary in adults for some months so long as vitamin D is given because of the enormous reserves in the body skeleton. An intake of 235 mg. of phosphorus is provided by 500 ml. 20 per cent Intralipid (Lee, 1972) and this should be sufficient; the serum phosphate should however be monitored. Phosphates are also present in protein hydrolysate solutions (e.g. 10 per cent Aminosol, 555 mg./L.). Fat emulsions also provide essential fatty acids. Iron can be given as weekly injections of Iron Dextran Complex 1 ml. (providing 50 mg. of elemental iron). Finally trace elements such as zinc, copper, manganese, molybdenum, chromium and iodine are found as contaminants of protein hydrolysate solutions, but are provided also by twice weekly infusions of plasma.

## Acute Gastric Erosion

It is widely appreciated that food to a large degree protects the stomach from the corrosive action of pepsin and gastric acid. Where parenteral methods of nutrition are employed this is no longer the case, and it is strongly recommended that where there is no surgical contraindication regular antacid be given to reduce the incidence of this serious potential hazard to the intensive care patient.

## Nitrogen Balance

The efficacy of the intravenous regime can be measured by nitrogen balance studies. During parenteral nutrition the input is known precisely. Urinary losses of nitrogen can be measured by the Kjeldahl technique. The method however is beyond the capacity of most laboratories and a suitable alternative is based on the measurement of 24-hour urine samples for the losses of urinary urea, which can be assumed to represent 80 per cent of the nitrogen loss. 28/60 of the result in grams gives the measurement of the daily nitrogen loss. Corrections must be applied for changes in the blood urea (Peaston, 1967) and any amino-aciduria which is easily estimated colorimetrically by the ninhydrin reaction (Matthews *et al.*, 1964).

Today malnutrition should not be allowed to occur in our surgical or medical patients. Relative or complete failure of the gastro-intestinal tract can be overcome by giving all known nutrients intravenously. With scrupulous attention to detail, excellent overall health may be maintained for many months, as can normal growth and development: 400 days total parenteral nutrition has been achieved (Dudrick, 1969).

## REFERENCES

Allen, P. C. and Lee, H. A. (1969), *A Clinical Guide to Intravenous Nutrition*, p. 143. Blackwell Scientific Publications.

Allison, S. P. (1971), "Insulin and Carbohydrate in Parenteral Feeding," in *Parenteral Nutrition*, An International Symposium in London, April 30th–May 1st, 1971. (A. W. Wilkinson, Ed.). London: Churchill Livingstone, 1972.

Amris, C. J., Brøckner, J. and Larsen, V. (1964), "Changes in the Coagulability of Blood During the Infusion of Intralipid," *Acta chir. scand.*, suppl. 325, p. 70.

Aubaniac, R. (1952), "L'injection intraveineuse sousclaviculaire," *Presse méd.*, **60**, 1456.

Bassler, K. H. (1967), "Adaptive Processes Concerned with Absorption and Metabolism of Xylitol," *International Symposium on Metabolism, Physiological and Clinical Use of Pentoses and Pentitols*, p. 190. Hakone, Japan, Aug. 27–29, 1967.

*Brit. J. Anaesth.* (1972), **44**, 123. Editorial, "Anaesthesia and the Liver."

Burri, C. and Henkemeyer, H. (1971), "Review of the Use of 3241 Caval Catheters," in *Parenteral Nutrition*, An International Symposium in London, April 30th, May 1st, 1971, p. 234. (A. W. Wilkinson, Ed.). London: Churchill Livingstone, 1972.

Bye, P. A. (1969), "The Utilization and Metabolism of Intravenous Sorbitol," *Brit. J. Surg.*, **56**, 653.

Cahill, G. F. and Aoki, T. T. (1970), "The Starvation State and Requirements of the Deficit Economy," in *Intravenous Hyperalimentation*, p. 20 (G. Cowan and W. Scheetz, Eds.). Philadelphia: Lea and Febiger, 1972.

Caldwell, F. T. (1962), "Metabolic Response to Trauma II. Nutritional Studies with Rats at Two Environmental Temperatures," *Ann. Surg.*, **155**, 119.

Carlo, P. E. (1971), "Therapeutique nutritionelle en chirurgie et traumatologie. Consequences metaboliques de la restriction calorique et de l'agression," *Agressologie*, **12**, 303.

Coats, D. A. and Maynard, A. T. (1968), "Long-term Parenteral Nutrition," *Proc. of an International Symposium*, p. 478. Nashville, Tenn., April 4–6, 1968.

Cuthbertson, D. P., Smith, C. M. and Tilstone, W. J. (1968), "The Effect of Transfer to a Warm Environment (30°C) on the Metabolic Response to Injury," *Brit. J. Surg.*, **55**, 513.

Davidson, Sir S. and Passmore, R. (1966), *Human Nutrition and Dietetics*. London: Livingstone.

Desai, I. D. (1969), "Regulation of Lysosomal Enzymes. I. Adaptive Changes in Enzyme Activities During Starvation and Refeeding," *Canad. J. Biochem.*, **47**, 785.

Dietrich, J. E. (1948), *Bull. N.Y. Acad. Med.*, **24**, 364.

Dudrick, S. J. (1968), "Discussion: Growth, Weight Gain and Positive Nitrogen Balance with Long Term, Total Parenteral Nutrition," *International Symposium on Parenteral Nutrition*. Nashville Tenn., April 4–6, 1968.

Dudrick, S. J., Wilmore, D. W., Vars, H. M. and Rhoads, J. E. (1969), "Can Intravenous Feeding as the Sole Means of Nutrition Support Growth in the Child and Restore Weight Loss in an Adult?" *Ann. Surg.*, **169**, 974.

Dudrick, S. J., Steiger, E., Long, J. M., Ruberg, R. L., Allen, T. R., Vars, H. M. and Rhoads, J. E. (1970a), "General Principles and Techniques of Intravenous Hyperalimentation," in *Intravenous Hyperalimentation* (G. Cowan and W. Scheetz, Eds.). Philadelphia: Lea and Febiger, 1972.

Dudrick, S. J., Ruberg, R. L., Long, J. M., Allen, T. R. and Steiger, E. (1970b), "Uses, Non-uses and Abuses of Intravenous Hyperalimentation," in *Intravenous Hyperalimentation* (G. Cowan and W. Scheetz, Eds.). Philadelphia: Lea and Febiger, 1972.

English, I. C. W., Frew, R. M., Piggott, J. F. and Zaki, M. (1969), "Percutaneous Catheterization of the Internal Jugular Vein," *Anaesthesia*, **24**, 4, 521.

Fekl, W. (1969), "Some Principles of Modern Parenteral Nutrition," *Scand. J. Gastro-Enterology*, **4**, suppl. 3, 17.

Geyer, R. P., Chapman, J. and Stare, F. J. (1948), "Oxidation *In Vivo* of Emulsified Radioactive Trilaurin Administered Intravenously," *J. biol. Chem.*, **176**, 1469.

Geyer, R. P. (1960), "Parenteral Nutrition," *Physiol. Rev.*, **40**, 150.

Glenn, T. M. and Lefer, A. M. (1970), "Role of Lysosomes in the Pathogenesis of Splanchnic Ischaemia Shock in Cats," *Circulation Res.*, **27**, 5, 783.

Hadfield, J. I. H. (1965), "Preoperative and Postoperative Intravenous Fat Therapy," *Brit. J. Surg.*, **52**, 291.

Hadfield, J. I. H. (1966), "High Calorie Intravenous Feeding in Surgical Patients," *Clin. Med.*, **73**, 25.

Hallberg, D., Holm, I., Obel, A. L., Schuberth, O. and Wretlind, A. (1967), "Fat Emulsions for Complete Parenteral Intravenous Nutrition," *Postgrad. med. J.*, **43**, 307.

Harries, J. T. (1971), "Intravenous Feeding in Infants," *Arch. Dis. Child.*, **46**, 855.

Heller, L. (1971), "Problems of Parenteral Nutrition in Pregnancy," in *Parenteral Nutrition*, An International Symposium in London, April 30th–1st May, 1971, p. 180 (A. W. Wilkinson, Ed.). London: Churchill Livingstone, 1972.

Irving, M. H. and Rushman, G. B. (1971), "Parenteral Nutrition for the Surgical Patient," *Anaesthesia*, **26**, 4, 450.

Jin, Soon Ju and Nasset, E. S. (1959), "Changes in Total Nitrogen Content of Some Abdominal Viscera in Fasting and Realimentation," *J. Nutr.*, **68**, 633.

Johnson, I. D. A. (1967), "The Role of the Endocrine Glands in the Metabolic Response to Operation," *Brit. J. Surg.*, **54**, 438.

Kinney, J. M. (1967), "The Effect of Injury on Metabolism," *Brit. J. Surg.*, **54**, 435.

Kinney, J. M. (1970), "Energy Significance of Weight Loss," in *Intravenous Hyperalimentation*, p. 85. (G. Cowan and W. Scheetz, Eds.). Philadelphia: Lea and Febiger, 1972.

Lang, K. (1967), "Utilization of Xylitol in Animals and Man," *International Symposium on Metabolism, Physiological and Clinical Use of Pentoses and Pentitols*, p. 151. Hakone, Japan, Aug. 27–29, 1967.

Lee, H. A., Morgan, A. G., Waldram, R. and Bennett, J. (1971), "Sorbitol: Some Aspects of its Metabolism and Role as an Intravenous Nutrient," in *Parenteral Nutrition*, An International Symposium in London, April 30th–May 1st, 1971. London: Churchill Livingstone, 1972.

Lee, P. J. (1972), Personal communication. Paines and Byrne Ltd., Greenford, Middlesex.

Leveen, H. H., Giordano, P., Spletzer, J. (1961), "The Mechanism of Removal of Intravenously Injected Fat," *Arch. Surg.*, **83**, 311.

Littlewood, A. H. M. and Peaston, M. J. T. (1965), "Nutritional Problems in Radical Cancer Surgery and the Metabolic Response to Intravenous Feeding," *Symposium on Parenteral Nutrition*. London: Wembley Press Ltd., 1967.

Long, J. M., Dudrick, S. J., Steiger, E., Ruberg, R. L. and Allen,

T. R. (1970), "Use of Intravenous Hyperalimentation in Patients with Renal or Liver Failure," in *Intravenous Hyperalimentation*, p. 147. (G. Cowan and W. Scheetz, Eds.). Philadelphia: Lea and Febiger, 1972.

Matthews, D. M., Muir, G. G. and Baron, D. N. (1964), "Estimation of α-amino Nitrogen in Plasma and Urine by the Colorimetric Ninhydrin Reaction," *J. clin. Path.*, **17**, 150.

Moore, F. D. (1959), *Metabolic Care of the Surgical Patient*. Philadelphia: Saunders.

Munro, H. N. (1968), "Role of Amino Acid Supply in Regulating Ribosome Function," *Fed. Proc.*, **27**, 1231.

Murisasco, A., Unal, D., Jauffret, P. and de Belsunec, M. (1966), "The Clinical Use of Sorbitol 30 per cent Solution for Intravenous Infusion," *Aggressologie*, VII, **3**, 253.

Peaston, M. J. T. (1967), "Maintenance of Metabolism During Intensive Patient Care," *Postgrad. med. J.*, **43**, 317.

Plumpton, F. S., Besser, G. M. and Cole, P. V. (1969), "Corticosteroid Treatment and Surgery," *Anaesthesia*, **24**, 3.

Rush, B. F., Richardson, J. D. and Griffen, W. O. (1970), "Positive Nitrogen Balance Immediately After Abdominal Operations," *Amer. J. Surg.*, **119**, 70.

Sahebjami, H. and Scarlettar, R. (1971), "Effects of Fructose Infusion on Lactate and Uric Acid Metabolism," *Lancet*, **i**, 366.

Sawant, P. L., Desai, I. D. and Tappel, A. L. (1964), "Digestive Capacity of Purified Lysosomes," *Biochem. Biophys. Acta*, **85**, 93.

Schummer, W. and Sperling, R. (1968), "Shock and its Effect on the Cell," *J. Amer. med. Ass.*, **205**, 4, 215.

Selye, H. (1954), "Conditioning Versus Permissive Actions of Hormones," *J. Clin. Endocrinol.*, **14**, 122.

Setbon, L. (1970), "Le metabolisme azoté sous neuroleptanalgesique postoperatoire," *Cahiers d'anesthesio*, **18**, 981.

Shuttleworth, K. E. D. (1962), "Intravenous Fat Therapy (Hunterian Lecture R. C. S.)," *Annals R.C.S.* 1963, **32**, 164.

Thoren, L. (1964), "Parenteral Nutrition with Carbohydrate and Alcohol," *Acta chir. scand.*, suppl. **325**, 75.

Waterlow, J. C. (1962), "Factors Influencing Protein Metabolism in the Organism," *CIBA Foundation Symposium*, 1962, p. 90. London: J. and A. Churchill.

Waterlow, J. C. (1968), "Observations on the Mechanism of Adaptation to Low Protein Intakes," *Lancet*, **ii**, 1091.

Wenzel, M. (1970), "Carbohydrates in Parenteral Nutrition," *Deutsches med. J.*, 339.

# BLOOD TRANSFUSION AND NOTES ON RELATED ASPECTS OF BLOOD CLOTTING AND HAEMOGLOBINOPATHIES

D. C. O. JAMES

## Historical Introduction

References in ancient Egyptian texts, Greek writings and medieval European records reflect the importance attached through the ages to the life giving properties of blood.

Initial attempts in the 17th century (e.g. by Lower in England and Denys in France) to effect transfusion of blood from one animal to another led eventually to transfusions from animals to humans, with disastrous consequences resulting in legal sanctions against the practice for about two centuries. Eventually, Blundell (1818) and others obtained occasional, though unpredictable successes using humans for both donors and recipients and thereby restored interest in the possibilities of blood transfusion therapy.

The key event in further progress was the work of Karl Landsteiner, whose researches into the differences between individuals of the same species led to the discovery of human blood groups. He described the blood groups A, B and O (1900) and two of his co-workers described the fourth and rarest group (AB) of this system. Using animals immunized with human red cells, Landsteiner and Levine discovered the M, N and P groups and again using rabbits and guinea pigs immunized with erythrocytes of the monkey, Macacus rhesus, Landsteiner and Wiener discovered the Rhesus groups in 1939, a finding of paramount clinical importance.

In spite of the discovery of the ABO blood group system in the early 1900's, another major transfusion problem remained, namely the lack of a safe anticoagulant. In 1914–15 it was shown that non-toxic amounts of citrate could be used for this purpose and this led eventually to the development in 1943 by Loutit and Mollison of an acid-dextrose solution which has been in use in Britain since that time as ACD solution. This has the following composition:

| | |
|---|---|
| Disodium citrate (monohydric) | 2 g. |
| Dextrose (anhydrous) | 3 g. |
| Water | 120 ml. |

to be mixed with 420 ml. of blood.

Blood stored in this way cannot be used after 21 days and numerous attempts have been made to extend its expiry date, e.g. by adding adenine, etc., or by modification of the anticoagulant, e.g. use of citrate phosphate-dextrose (CPD). Some promising advances have been made.

More recent developments and successes have followed the finding that red cells, suitably treated, could be frozen and thus preserved apparently indefinitely with little loss of cell viability. There is little doubt that this principle will be used on an increasing scale in the future. The advent of 'artificial blood' although not yet in sight may be nearer than is thought generally. The advantages of a simple temporary oxygen carrier devoid of a multitude of potentially dangerous biological antigens, as found in human blood, are obvious and worthy of a more concentrated research programme than so far employed.

## Blood Groups

Human blood groups are important clinically since they are systems of antigens which may react with corresponding antibodies *in vivo* to produce harmful or even fatal results—(*see* Hazards of Blood Transfusion). Antigenic characteristics (or determinants) which represent the immunological differences between the red cells, etc. are under genetic control (*see* Inheritance of Blood Groups).

To date, a total of about eleven distinct blood group systems have been demonstrated, one of which ($Xg^a$) is unique in being sex linked. However, of the many blood group systems known, ABO and Rhesus are by far the most important in routine clinical work although from time to time transfusion reactions and Haemolytic disease of the Newborn (HDN) occur due to less common blood group antigens.

White cells and platelets carry some of the antigens found on red cells, e.g. those of ABO, MN and P systems but apparently not others, e.g. the Rhesus system. Until recently, both white cells and platelets were thought to carry other (HL-A) antigens not found on mature red cells and which were of particular importance in organ transplantation and rejection phenomena. Using automated techniques with increased sensitivity it has been shown, however, that some red cell antigens, e.g. $Bg^a$ do have partial if not complete identity with certain HL-A antigens (Morton *et al.*, 1969, 1971). These leucocyte antigens are the subject of the rapidly developing field of 'tissue' or more correctly lymphocyte typing in relation to organ transplantation, etc. and will be considered later (*see* Hazards of Blood Transfusion).

*Antigen* is taken to mean any substance that has the ability to evoke an *in vivo* immune response upon parenteral injection into an immunologically competent animal. A most important requirement, especially for its detection, is that the antigen can react with the products of such a response, i.e. the corresponding antibody, both *in vivo* and *in vitro*.

*Antibodies* are specific serum proteins produced in the lymphoid tissue as a result of stimulation with an antigen and can react with the latter *in vivo* and *in vitro*.

*Alleles* in this context are taken to mean alternative forms of the genes (and hence the blood group antigens) concerned at a single locus on a chromosome.

## Inheritance of Blood Group Antigens

A set of 23 chromosomes inherited from each parent resulting in a total of 46 chromosomes is found in the human somatic cell. The male is distinguished by the replacement of one of the two x chromosomes of the female by the smaller y chromosome.

The genes controlling antigenic structure of a particular blood group system occupy specific loci on corresponding chromosomes. Such genes may be identical (homozygous, e.g. *BB*) or different (heterozygous, e.g. *BO*). Unless the gene is modified or suppressed then it can be demonstrated *in vitro* as a particular blood group antigen, e.g. A or B; however, some genes do not produce demonstrable effects, e.g. the gene for group O. Hence an individual's genotype (i.e. the sum of the genetic blood group characteristics obtained from both parents) may not be the same as his phenotype (the demonstrable genes present), thus a phenotype of B may be of genotype *BB* or *BO* (*see* Table 1).

### TABLE 1

ABO GROUPS AND CORRESPONDING GENOTYPES

| Blood group (phenotype) | Possible genotypes |
|---|---|
| A | *AA* |
| | *AO* |
| B | *BB* |
| | *BO* |
| O | *OO* |
| AB | *AB* |

The fact that gene inheritance is Mendelian allows the prediction of the possible blood group of an unborn child. In practice this often permits the selection of blood of suitable group for exchange transfusion prior to its delivery. Legally it may play an essential part in medico-legal cases involving paternity issues. An example is shown in Fig. 1.

To illustrate the mode of inheritance—a particular

type of mating, as that in which a group A male mates with a group O female can be considered. The group A male may be of genotype *AA* or *AO* and the female will be of genotype *OO*, therefore within this mating subdivisions exist, namely (a) *AA* with *OO* and (b) *AO* with *OO*. The outcome of the two matings is shown in Fig. 1, namely, that the children of such a mating would be group (phenotype) A or O. Blood of group A and group O would be selected in advance for this case, should an exchange transfusion be under consideration.

## Chemistry of the Blood Group Antigens

The studies of Morgan and Watkins, Kabat and others have shown that A, B, H and Lewis substances are glycoproteins combined with carbohydrates and appear to be closely related in structure and composition. They are thought to consist of a number of relatively short oligosaccharide chains attached at intervals to a peptide basis. The same five sugars and fifteen amino acids are found in pure A, B, H and Le$^a$ substance. Differences in specificity depend partly on which sugar occupies the terminal position or side chains of the molecule and partly on the nature of the linkages between one sugar and the next.

Recent work has shown that the I antigen is a very complex system of antigens derived from a precursor glycoprotein devoid of A, B, H Le$^a$ and Le$^b$ activity. Similarly, the M and N antigens are now yielding to biochemical analysis. Strangely enough, the important Rhesus antigen has so far defied efforts to unravel its structure.

## Blood Group antibodies

Antibody activity is mostly confined to the gamma globulin fraction of plasma, forming the general group known as Immunoglobulins (Ig) which consists of five

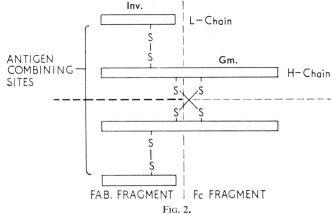

FIG. 2.

distinct classes called IgM, IgG, IgA, IgD and IgE based on physicochemical and serological properties. The blood group antibodies are associated with the IgM, IgG and IgA classes. The chemistry of IgG but not IgM and IgA has been fairly well worked out and the structure of a typical IgG molecule is shown in Fig. 2.

In general, IgG represents the immune 'warm' acquired 7S antibodies with molecular weight of about 160,000 and which can cross the placenta, e.g. immune anti-D. IgM

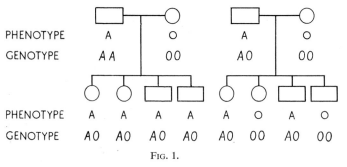

FIG. 1.

represents mainly naturally-occurring cold antibodies having a high molecular weight of about 900,000 which cannot cross the placenta, e.g. anti-A and anti-B. IgA antibodies form an intermediate group which also cannot cross the placenta.

## The ABO Blood Group System

Following Landsteiner's discovery of the ABO blood group system, von Dungern and Hirszfield (1911) not only first described subgroups of A but also showed that ABO genes were inherited. However, the exact mode of inheritance was determined by Bernstein (1924). The relationship of the gene O (recognized as Blood Group O) to the antigens H, A and B, has been explained by Morgan

TABLE 2

GENERAL COMPARISON OF BLOOD GROUP ANTIBODY
TERMINOLOGIES AND PROPERTIES

|  | *'Naturally occurring'* antibodies | *'Immune'* antibodies |
|---|---|---|
| Synonyms | Complete Saline agglutinating | Incomplete* Albumin agglutinating |
|  | 'Cold' (20°C and below) | 37°C |
| Recent term | $\gamma M$, $\beta_2 M$ | $\gamma G$ |
| Present name | IgM | IgG* |
| Molecular weight | 900,000 | c.160,000 |
| Sedimentation | 19S | 7S |
| Placental transmission | No | Yes |

\* Occasionally IgG antibodies occur as incomplete and/or complete antibodies.

and Watkins. Thus beginning with a precursor mucopolysaccharide substance which is moulded by the gene *H* into H substance, the H in turn is partly converted by the independent genes *A* or *B* into A or B antigens. *O* is an amorphous gene which effects no conversion hence group O cells contain only H substance. The H antigen is of considerable importance then since it appears to be the basic ground substance from which the A and B antigens are derived. Occasionally anti-H, a 'cold' antibody, may achieve clinical significance if of high titre and if the individual has to undergo operation under hypothermic conditions.

## Secretors

The antigens of the ABO system are found as glycolipid, alcohol—soluble components of all body tissue except perhaps brain and spinal cord. However, approximately 78 per cent of individuals have the same antigens (corresponding to their ABO group) in a water-soluble form in their body secretions, e.g. saliva, urine, sweat, but not in C.S.F. Such individuals are termed "secretors" and this hereditary characteristic has been used in genetic studies.

## The Subgroups of A

Von Dungern *et al.*, showed that there were two types of group A antigen $A_1$ and $A_2$, also that serum from group B individuals contains two types of anti-A antibodies. One reacted with all group A and group AB red cells, the other is an anti-$A_1$ which only reacts with $A_1$ or $A_1B$ cells. The difference between $A_1$ and $A_2$ appears to be qualitative since a number of $A_2$ individuals and almost 26 per cent of $A_2B$ individuals have anti-$A_1$ in their serum, i.e. $A_1$ has some component which is missing in $A_2$. $A_1$ can also be identified using an anti-$A_1$ lectin prepared from the seeds of Dolichos biflorus. Other subgroups of A exist all of which are weaker than $A_2$ (which is weaker than $A_1$) and have been designated $A_3$, $A_4$, $A_5$, $A_x$, etc. The A subgroups are sometimes clinically significant because:

(1) Anti-$A_1$, although usually an unimportant cold antibody not active over 30°C occasionally has a higher thermal range and can then cause a transfusion reaction.

(2) Weak subgroups of A including $A_2$ can only be detected with high potency testing sera and failure to detect them may result in grouping the individual incorrectly as group O instead of $A_2$ or group B instead of $A_2B$. Subsequent transfusion with group O blood may lead to a reaction or accelerated destruction of the patient's A cells.

Weak subgroups of the B antigen exist but are extremely rare.

## The ABO Isoantibodies

Anti-A and Anti-B occur with such precise regularity that Landsteiner formulated his "Rule" that their presence or absence must be ascertained for the definitive establishment of the groups (*see* Table 3). In addition 2 per cent of

TABLE 3

ANTIGEN AND ANTIBODY CONTENT OF THE RED CELLS AND
SERUM OF THE ABO BLOOD GROUP SYSTEM

| Group | Antigen on red cells | Antibodies in serum | Frequency in English population (%) |
|---|---|---|---|
| O | NONE | anti-A, anti-B | 47 |
| A | A | anti-B | 42 |
| B | B | anti-A | 8 |
| AB | A and B | NONE | 3 |

$A_2$ individuals and 26 per cent of $A_2B$ contain anti-$A_1$. Because of this predictable occurrence of these antibodies in all individuals without apparent antigenic stimulation they are referred to as 'naturally occurring'. They appear in the serum three to six months after birth—remaining throughout life. Their absence in infants of less than three months demands care in determination of the blood group, especially since at that age the A antigen is immature and may be only weakly reactive. The mechanism by which anti-A and anti-B are produced is still disputed. Experimental evidence supports the theory that A and B antigens are ubiquitous in nature, e.g. in the bacterial flora of the intestinal canal, hence while a group A individual would not produce anti-A against a bacterial A antigen he would produce an anti-B and vice versa.

Immune anti-A and anti-B may be found in individuals lacking the antigen and who have received it via transfusions, pregnancies or various vaccines such as tetanus and diphtheria toxoids (all of which may contain traces of A or B antigens). These immune antibodies differ in important respects from their naturally occurring counterparts thus they bind complement and are haemolytic both *in vivo* and *in vitro*, further they are most active at 37°C. Their possible and unsuspected presence in group O donor blood, the so called 'universal donor' should be noted since on many occasions the transfusion of group O blood to group A or B recipients has produced a brisk haemolytic reaction. Since the immune antibody is in the donor plasma, its potential danger will not be demonstrated on the major crossmatch which tests only donor cells against recipient serum. Its presence must be suspected and excluded if, during the blood grouping of the donor, haemolysis is noticed in the tube containing incubated donor serum and control group A cells. A haemolytic titre of one in four or less is within normal limits; higher titres may make the donor a 'dangerous universal donor' and the blood should only be given to a group O recipient.

Basic blood grouping techniques have continued almost unchanged since the Landsteiner era, but more recently automation has been used in this field and most Blood Transfusion Centres as well as larger hospitals, now use automatic equipment for carrying out this exacting but monotonous routine work.

### The Rhesus (Rh) Blood Group System

When the Rhesus blood group system was discovered in 1940 by Landsteiner and Wiener it was thought that only one antigen was involved—tests having shown that 85 per

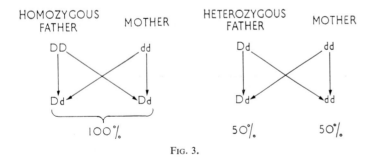

Fig. 3.

cent of white individuals reacted with sera from rabbits immunized against Rhesus macacus red cells. Such individuals were termed Rhesus Positive and the remaining 15 per cent Rhesus Negative. This anti-rhesus antibody appeared to be identical with that described by Levine and Stetson (1939) as the cause of Haemolytic disease of the Newborn in their patient and thus the human antibody was also named anti-Rh. Later work showed that these antibodies were, in fact, not identical.

With more refined techniques the Rhesus system was shown to contain at least five important antigens (of

which the D antigen remains by far the most important from the clinical viewpoint) and two main terminologies are in current use, that of Fisher and Race (used in this review) and that of Wiener (U.S.A.). Fisher (1943) postulated the existence of three pairs of allelomorphic genes occupying three separate but closely linked loci on each of a pair of chromosomes. The genes and the antigens they controlled were called C and its allele c, E and e and D and d. Rhesus 'Negative' is taken to imply the absence of the D antigen (D negative) when applied to recipients but blood donors *must* be cde/cde. It should be noted that the genes for C and c and E and e are co-dominant and that the antigen c is, after D, the most potent and common cause of Haemolytic disease of the Newborn. Anti-d has not yet been found and this fact not only has theoretical implications but it means that the presence or absence of that antigen cannot be verified *in vitro*. Thus the decision whether an individual is homozygous or heterozygous for the D antigen can only be a statistical one, based on the frequency with which D occurs in relation to the antigens C, c, E and e, all of which can be demonstrated *in vitro* using the corresponding antibody. The genotype report therefore always refers to the 'probable genotype' except in the case of cde/cde. A knowledge of the father's genotype (especially in respect of D) is of paramount importance in families where severe Haemolytic disease of the Newborn has been encountered (see Figure 3). An individual who is homozygous for D would pass on the D antigen to all his offspring while in the heterozygous case there would be a 50% chance of one half of the offspring being D negative.

### Antigenic Variants

The D antigen is thought to be a mosaic composed of many factors called $Rh^A$ $Rh^B$ $Rh^C$ $Rh^D$, etc. Where one or more components is missing the antigen is called a $D^u$. $D^u$ individuals are usually detected because their cells will react with some anti-D sera but not with others. One variety of $D^u$ is hereditary and here the D antigen may react so weakly *in vitro* that an antiglobulin test must be used to detect it. Another variety (non-hereditary) is due to the transposition of the C antigen in relation to the D. It can depress the D expression and is an example of 'gene interaction'. Rare individuals occur who are lacking in some Rh antigens, e.g. the variety—D—has the D antigen but not C or E while the Rh null variety or – – –/– – – has no Rhesus antigen at all.

### Rh Antibodies

Anti-Rh antibodies are most commonly found as incomplete agglutinins and require the addition of colloids such as albumin to the suspending media or the use of the antiglobulin technique of Coombs or enzymes for their detection. Naturally-occurring Rh antibodies are uncommon and in general D negative individuals never have anti-D antibodies unless they have received an antigenic stimulus through blood transfusion or pregnancy. Antibody production is dependent upon antigenicity and the frequency of occurrence of Rh antibodies suggests that the order of potency is D > c > C > E > e.

Rh antibodies do not bind complement and are therefore not haemolytic.

## Rh Groups and Haemolytic Disease of the Newborn (HDN)

Haemolytic disease of the Newborn may be considered as an acquired haemolytic anaemia of the newborn of varying degree. The anaemia may be severe or very mild and it can cause intrauterine death. After delivery and without adequate treatment the associated hyperbilirubinaemia may cause bilirubin encephalopathy (kernicterus) and result in permanent brain damage.

Haemolytic disease of the Newborn occurs when the mother lacks some blood group antigen and is immunized by foetal red blood cells, especially at delivery. In the event of subsequent pregnancies the resulting isoantibodies cross the placental barrier and react with the foetal erythrocytes leading to their destruction. Anti-D is by far the most important antibody in this respect. Paradoxically, the same immune anti-D given prophylactically after delivery of the first D-positive child to a D-negative mother has been shown conclusively to inhibit the sensitizing effect of the foetal cells on the mother. This treatment promises to end Haemolytic disease of the Newborn, due to the D antigen (which causes about 92 to 95 per cent of all cases). The remainder of cases of Haemolytic disease of the Newborn due to anti-A or anti-B which are severe enough to require treatment are rare (about one in 3,000 or less of all newborn infants): other blood group antibodies concerned include anti-c, anti-K, anti-k, anti-E and anti-Fy$^a$.

## Other blood group systems

Since the discovery of the ABO groups in 1900 many other blood group factors have been discovered. The discovery has usually resulted from the finding of an atypical antibody in the serum of a recipient of several transfusions or in that of a pregnant woman. In view of their lesser clinical significance only a very brief outline of them is considered here.

In the main the M, N, S and P groups are 'cold' agglutinins, i.e. giving strong reactions at about 20°C with little or no reactivity at 37°. The significance of the corresponding antibodies in patients subjected to operation under hypothermic conditions remains unanswered but they are otherwise of little clinical importance unless their thermal range exceeds 30° above which they may be able to effect a reduced red cell survival time. Some have been known to cause transfusion reactions, others have been associated with Haemolytic disease of the Newborn. It is doubtful if the P$_1$ antigen has a role in histocompatibility and graft survival, as was originally thought.

Kell (K), Cellano (k), Duffy (Fy$^a$ and Fy$^b$), Kidd (Jk$^a$) and their related antigens are usually only detected by the antiglobulin (Coombs) reaction. They are often associated with transfusion reactions and occasionally cause Haemolytic disease of the Newborn, especially K and k which are exceptionally potent antigens, being second in strength only to D of the Rh system.

The I blood group system differs from others in many respects especially with regard to its slow maturation, its almost universal occurrence and the quantitative difference only existing between I Positives and Negatives. Anti-I and anti-i are cold agglutinins and may be found especially in the sera of patients suffering from primary atypical pneumonia and in autoimmune acquired haemolytic anaemia of the 'cold' antibody type. There is also a suspected inter-relationship between the I-i, ABO and P blood group systems.

Until the early 1960's all known red cell antigens were thought to be controlled by autosomal genes. The discovery of Xg as a sex linked blood group, i.e. occurring on the x chromosome may assist considerably in chromosome mapping.

## The Antiglobulin (Coombs) Test

The antiglobulin test, since its rediscovery and application by Coombs et al. (1945), resulted in the discovery of the Kell blood group system and has proved to be the outstanding serological finding in recent years.

The principle of the test was relatively simple and depended on the reasoning that since antibodies are globulins, then the injection of human sera or purified globulin into a susceptible animal would produce anti-human globulin antibodies. This reagent, suitably diluted, could be used to detect antibodies (globulins) on human red cells by allowing it to react with the antibody on the cell surface under controlled conditions, resulting in agglutination of the cells. The red cell itself simply becomes an indicator for the reaction.

Coombs and co-workers outlined two applications of the test—one to be performed on serum, referred to as the INDIRECT test, and one to be used on red cells, known as the DIRECT test. The INDIRECT test is most frequently used to detect antibodies in the sera of pregnant women, or to learn whether antibodies are present in the recipient of a transfusion, as for example, in the crossmatch or compatibility test. The DIRECT test is used to detect antibodies already adsorbed or coated on the red cell surface. This may occur in Haemolytic disease of the Newborn in which case coating takes place in utero so that testing of cord blood will indicate whether the infant will be affected. Also, in cases of auto-immunization, e.g. acquired haemolytic anaemia, the test may be positive.

## Leucocyte (Lymphocyte) Agglutinins

The advent of 'tissue typing' for organ transplantation has accelerated the growth of knowledge regarding leucocyte antigens and antibodies. An extensive literature on white cell histocompatibility (HL-A) antigens is now available. The significance of leucocyte (lymphocyte) antigens and antibodies in blood transfusion is referred to later under Hazards of Blood Transfusion.

## Blood Transfusion

A basic knowledge of human blood groups and antibodies is essential for those concerned with requesting or supervising blood transfusion procedures since otherwise they may be unaware of the many advantages and important hazards of this life saving procedure. The emphasis of this section is on the practical aspects of blood transfusion. For more detailed discussions the reader should refer to Mollison's textbook *Blood Transfusion in Clinical Medicine*, 1972.

## Blood Donors

Blood for transfusion is obtained in the UK from volunteer donors: in most other countries either all donors are paid or both systems operate. Donor protection includes restricting the frequency of donation to two or three times per year, the use of plasmapheresis wherever possible and insistence on a minimum haemoglobin level of 12·5 g. per cent for females and 13·5 g. per cent for males. Recipient protection depends mainly on accurate history taking from the donor to exclude maladies thought or known to be undesirable. Venereal diseases are excluded serologically. Patients who give a history of malaria or brucellosis should be excluded since these diseases are known to be transmissible by blood transfusion.

Very important advances have been made in the last five years in detecting carriers of the serum hepatitis virus. All blood donations issued from Blood Transfusion Centres in the United Kingdom are tested for Australia Antigen (Au-SH), which appears to have a strong association with the serum hepatitis virus. All blood donors retained on the British National Donor Panel must be Australia Antigen negative. The impact of these precautions on the incidence of serum hepatitis following blood transfusion remains to be evaluated but there are no grounds for complacency as yet.

## Care of Blood

Blood should not be issued for transfusion if it shows any evidence of haemolysis or is time expired (21 days).

The correct temperature for storage is 4° to 6°C (38°–42°F) and the refrigerator should have an automatic temperature recording device and a battery operated alarm system. The temperature limits must be rigidly observed to preserve the red cells and minimize the multiplication of chance bacterial contaminants. Blood must never be allowed to freeze unless in a suitable medium such as glycerol, as used in long term preservation processes, since transfusion of blood which has been frozen and thawed may cause death. Food and pathological specimens must never be stored in the blood refrigerator. Blood for transfusion should not be out of the refrigerator for more than 30 minutes before transfusion, otherwise it should be discarded. Similarly, packed red cells, unless concentrated in a sterile closed system, e.g. plastic transfer pack, must be used within twelve hours and reconstituted plasma, fibrinogen or albumin within three hours. Bottles of blood which have been partly used should always be discarded. No medicaments should be introduced into a blood bottle prior to use.

## Volume and Rate of Transfusion

The following factors must be considered:

1. The age of the patient.
2. The general condition.
3. The state of the circulation.
4. The indication for the transfusion.

The young adult with a normal myocardium will tolerate the rapid infusion of large volumes of colloid. On the other hand the chronically anaemic patient with an enfeebled myocardium or patients with respiratory or cardiac disorders or infective and toxic conditions should be transfused cautiously. The availability of potent diuretics, if correctly used, has significantly reduced the risk of circulatory overloading from over transfusion. Severe injury with blood loss exceeding 20 per cent of the circulating blood volume requires rapid and adequate restoration of the volume as the immediate aim.

In the treatment of anaemia it may be assumed that one bottle of whole blood will raise the haemoglobin level about 1·0 g. per cent. If, in the absence of continuing blood loss the volume of whole blood required to raise the haemoglobin to the required level exceeds one third of the calculated blood volume, the transfusion should be given in two parts, separated by two days and the use of packed red cells should be considered.

The rate of administration should not normally exceed 20–40 drops per minute. In chronic anaemia with haemoglobin below 3·7 g. per cent, cachexia, cardiac or respiratory disease, this rate may be halved and the venous pressure should be monitored for indication of overtransfusion. Patients with a septic condition or toxaemia should be treated with similar caution. Large volumes of fluid even if administered slowly over a long period should not be given as a single continuous transfusion in such conditions: it should be divided and given slowly as a number of small transfusions. It is usually recommended that no major surgical procedure should be carried out unless the haemoglobin is at least 10·4 g. per cent. Where pre-operative transfusions are necessary these should be completed at least twenty-four hours prior to the operation, partly to avoid the possibility of a reaction occurring at a time when the subjective signs would be masked by anaesthesia, but also because the oxygen dissociation curve of red cells stored in citrate is shifted to the left (storage lesion of red blood cells). For about twenty-four hours after transfusion such cells are incapable of releasing as much oxygen to the tissue as normal red cells, hence by diluting the patient's own blood in this way, there exists a temporary phase when the net effect is a decrease of oxygen availability for the tissues (Valtis and Kennedy, 1954).

## Choice of Replacement Fluids

Transfusion should only be undertaken after careful assessment of the patient's clinical condition to determine the nature and volume of fluid to be transfused and the rate of administration. The patient may require whole blood, packed red cells, washed red cells, whole plasma or a specific blood component.

A transfusion should never be given without a definite indication in view of the element of risk involved (*see* Hazards of Blood Transfusion). It should never be used to correct moderate or slight degrees of anaemia. Emergency transfusions carry greater risks than well planned elective transfusions. Likewise the risk involved in giving single unit transfusions to adults often exceeds the possible benefits therefrom and these should be actively discouraged.

With continuing experience of blood transfusion therapy and important changes in emphasis in the mode of its application—the use of the standard product, i.e. stored whole blood, is rapidly giving way to a more sophisticated usage and range of blood products. Replacement fluids may be classified under:

A. Blood
B. Plasma and specific plasma components.
C. Plasma substitutes.
D. Electrolyte solutions (*see* Chapter 2).

## A. Blood

Blood is still the most important therapeutic substitute for the treatment of severe blood losses. The various ways in which it may be obtained are shown in Table 4.

## B. Plasma and Specific Plasma Components

Since the shelf life of stored blood is only three weeks, it is not surprising that there has been a ceaseless search for methods of producing long term stable blood fractions. Table 5 shows some current stable plasma preparations and plasma components.

## C. Plasma Substitutes (otherwise called plasma expanders, blood substitutes, etc.)

Natural plasma products or derivatives still form the best replacement fluids and some, e.g. Plasma Protein

TABLE 4

A. BLOOD. SOME FORMS IN WHICH BLOOD MAY BE OBTAINED FOR TRANSFUSION

| Form | Indication | Expiry | Comments |
|---|---|---|---|
| 1. Stored whole blood: <br>(a) Blood 420 ml. ACD 120 ml. <br><br>(b) Blood 500 ml. Heparin (1500 IU) | 1. Haemorrhage—acute or chronic <br>2. Anaemia—acute or chronic <br>3. Oligaemic shock <br>4. Blood dyscrasias, e.g. aplastic anaemia <br>Where dilution of transfused blood not desirable use (b) | 21 days <br><br><br>24 hours | ACD is the anticoagulant of choice for routine purposes <br><br>Heparinized blood deteriorates rapidly |
| 2. Concentrated red cells | Anaemias in which increased haemoglobin level but not blood volume required | 12 hours (glass bottles) <br><br>21 days (plastic transfer packs) | Especially advised for patients with heart disease, chronic and severe anaemia, severe sepsis and toxaemia, also for the very young and the very old |
| 3. Fresh whole blood | 1. Specifically for bleeding due to thrombocytopenia <br>2. Immediately pre-op where platelet count less than 40,000 mm³ | 12 hours* | Give as whole blood if increased haemoglobin level desired, otherwise as platelet-rich plasma or platelet concentrate |
| 4. 'Almost fresh' whole blood | Exchange transfusion in neonates | 2 days | Use when minimal plasma potassium content and maximal survival of transfused red cells required |
| 5. 'Washed' red cells (leucocyte poor) | 1. Paroxysmal nocturnal haemoglobinuria <br>2. Patients with known leucocyte or platelet antibodies <br>3. Transfusion reaction unrelated to red cell antigen systems (plasma reactors) <br>4. Ideally, all patients selected for and post organ transplantation <br>5. Patients with known immune deficiencies, on massive irradiation or heavy immuno-suppression therapy. | 6 hours when manual techniques employed | Complete removal of leucocytes, has not yet been achieved |
| 6. Frozen red blood cells | As for 1 and 5 above | 6 hours after reconstitution | More expensive to produce than 1 but always available when required |

* The expiry time of 12 hours, previously thought essential for satisfactory platelet survival and activity has recently been extended to 2–3 days at 4°C.

TABLE 5

**B. PLASMA.** SOME FORMS IN WHICH HUMAN PLASMA OR ITS COMPONENTS MAY BE OBTAINED

| Form | Indication | Expiry | Comments |
|---|---|---|---|
| 1. Dried pooled plasma, issued with sterile pyrogen free distilled water for preparation | 1. To increase fluid volume when red cells not necessary or available<br>2. Burns | 3 hours after preparation (8 years in dry form) | Prepared from ten donor pool hence slightly increased risk of serum hepatitis |
| 2. Fresh frozen plasma | Treatment of clotting factor deficiencies such as occur in:<br>  Haemophilia<br>  Massive transfusions<br>  Over dosage with coumarin and indandione anticoagulants | To be used immediately after thawing | Risk of serum hepatitis as for blood |
| 3. Plasma Protein Fraction (PPF) concentrate (18 g. protein per bottle) | As for 1 above | Two years | Does not contain fibrinogen or gamma globulin. Hepatitis virus inactivated by 6 hour pasteurization |
| 4. Albumin (25 g. per bottle) | Hypoalbuminaemia | 3 hours after preparation | Heat treated hence no risk of serum hepatitis |
| 5. Fibrinogen (3–4 g. per bottle) | Afibrinogenaemia following massive bleeding, fibrinolytic therapy, defibrination | 3 hours after preparation | Risk of serum hepatitis (as for blood) |
| 6. Cryoprecipitate | Factor VIII deficiency | 3 months | Risk of serum hepatitis as for blood |
| 7. Factor VIII (dried) | 1. Haemophilia A<br>2. Factor VIII deficiency following massive transfusions | 3 hours after preparation | Porcine and bovine concentrate used for patients with Factor VIII inhibitors |
| 8. Factor IX concentrate often presented as<br>9. 2, 7, 9, 10 concentrate | Haemophilia B (Christmas disease)<br>1. Congenital deficiencies with bleeding<br>2. Over dosage with coumarin drugs<br>3. Haemorrhagic disease of the newborn | One year (three hours after preparation) | Still on clinical trial in U.K. |
| 10. Platelet-rich plasma or platelet concentrate | 1. Bleeding associated with thrombocytopenia<br>2. Initial low platelet count (below 40,000 c. mm.) prior to major surgery<br>3. Often required during massive transfusions | 2–3 days at 4°C | Expiry date recently extended |
| 11. Leucocyte transfusions | 1. Myelo-suppression and leukopenia in patients on cytotoxic therapy<br>2. Primary granulocytopenia<br>3. Severe overwhelming infection | Direct transfusion using NCI-IBM cell separator on donor | Ideally HL-A typed blood given but danger of graft v. host reaction |

TABLE 6

C. PLASMA. SUBSTITUTES

| Form | Indication | Expiry | Comments |
|---|---|---|---|
| 1. Dextran | 1. Initial treatment of haemorrhagic shock until compatible blood available<br><br>2. Shock conditions in burns, crash injuries, sepsis<br><br>3. Conditions where capillary circulation impaired (thrombosis, vascular insufficiency) | 10 years | 6% Dextran 70 (Macrodex) and 10% dextran 40 (Rheomacrodex) are most often used today. An extensive literature exists as to their respective merits. Blood for grouping and cross-matching should be taken before dextran is infused |
| 2 Gelatin preparations:<br>(a) Oxypolygelatin<br>(b) Modified fluid gelatin<br>(c) Crosslinked gelatin | Shock due to haemorrhage, burns, etc. | | Crosslinked gelatin (Haemacel) is the best documented but in general there is insufficient data at present to recommend the use of gelatin preparations |
| 3. Polyvinyl pyrolidone (PVP) | Use discontinued | | PVP cannot be metabolized in the body |
| 4. Hydroxyethyl starch (HES) 6% | Volume expander | | Undergoing clinical trials—insufficient data for evaluation |

Fraction and Albumin have been heat treated during processing and therefore should be free from the hepatitis virus. However, the supply of these products is unlikely ever to meet the demand for them—hence the need for infusion solutions containing artificial colloids. The requirements for a satisfactory artificial colloidal infusion solution include:

1. Should be capable of being administered at such a concentration that its colloidal osmotic pressure is equivalent to that of normal blood plasma.

2. When employed to increase plasma volume after blood loss, there should be at least 50 per cent retention for at least six and preferably for 12 hours.

3. The viscosity should not cause added work to the heart.

4. It should not interfere with haemostasis or blood coagulation at levels normally employed.

5. It should not interfere seriously with blood grouping.

6. It should be metabolized or eliminated from the body without causing delayed interference with the function of any organ, even after repeated administration.

The advantage of a satisfactory artificial colloidal solution would be:

1. It would help to save blood.

2. The risk of virus and other infections would be eliminated.

3. Such solutions could be kept available at places where emergency administration may be necessary, e.g. in ambulances.

4. Blood serology could be ignored and the solutions could be given irrespective of blood group.

5. Incidence of pyrogenic reactions, etc. would be reduced.

6. Long term storage would not present a problem.

7. The product would be available in unlimited quantities.

The plasma substitutes which are available are shown in Table 6.

**Changes in Stored Blood**

Certain changes occurring in stored blood are shown in Table 7.

**Effects of Storage on Blood and Plasma Clotting Factors**

**(a) Red cells.** In general, red cells in stored blood die at the rate of 1 per cent for each day of storage and when stored under optimal conditions at 4° to 6°C for 21 days should have a survival rate of not less than 70 per cent for

TABLE 7

CHANGES IN STORED CITRATED BLOOD (4 to 6°C)

*According to Strumia and others*

| Days | 0 | 7 | 14 | 21 | 28 |
|---|---|---|---|---|---|
| pH | 7·1 | 6·85 | 6·75 | 6·68 | 6·65 |
| Glucose mg% | 350 | 300 | 245 | 210 | 190 |
| Plasma | | | | | |
| Haemoglobin mg% | 0–10 | 25 | 50 | 100 | 150 |
| Potassium mEq./l. | 3–4 | 12 | 24 | 32 | 40 |
| Ammonia μg% | 50 | 260 | 470 | 680 | — |
| Lactic acid mg% | 20 | 70 | 120 | 140 | 150 |

the first 24 hours after transfusion. The changes *in vitro* leading to loss of viability are still poorly understood.

## Influence of Storage Medium

Red cells stored with trisodium citrate alone deteriorate rapidly. Likewise storage with heparin results in clotting after 24 hours and the red cells deteriorate rapidly with an increased loss of potassium compared with red cells stored in ACD.

Dextrose has a very favourable effect on preservation, probably by providing energy for the synthesis of organic phosphate compounds particularly diphosphoglycerate and adenosine triphosphate (ATP) (Maizels, 1941).

Acidification is beneficial hence the superiority of ACD over trisodium citrate alone. The ATP content of red cells falls more slowly in ACD solution with trisodium-citrate-dextrose and there is good correlation between the ATP content of stored red cells and their post transfusion survival.

## Influence of Storage Temperatures

The accepted range of 4° to 6°C represents a temperature giving good preservation and one which is safely above the freezing point of blood. Red cell survival is significantly reduced if blood is stored at 25°C and deterioration is rapid at 37°C. Low temperatures also inhibit chance bacterial contaminants although certain gram negative bacilli can proliferate at blood bank temperatures.

**(b) Plasma clotting factors.** Factor I (Fibrinogen) is stable in 'fresh' bank blood and fresh frozen plasma and can be successfully concentrated, permitting the administration of large amounts of fibrinogen in relatively small volumes of liquid. It carries the same risk of serum hepatitis as blood.

Factor II (Prothrombin) is stable in Bank blood under normal conditions of storage.

Factor V (Labile factor, Ac globulin) deteriorates during storage but the data are conflicting regarding its rate of disappearance *in vitro*.

Factor VII (Stable factor) is stable in bank blood under the usual conditions of storage.

Factor VIII (Antihaemophilic Factor) deteriorates rapidly during storage of bank blood—as much as 50 per cent may be lost after one to two weeks. It is best stored as fresh frozen plasma at −20° to −30° or as cryoprecipitate or Factor VIII concentrate also kept at the same temperature range.

Factor IX is stable in bank blood.

Factor XI storage properties are not well documented.

**(c) Platelets.** Therapeutic benefit from platelet transfusion is short-lived because platelets have a relatively short life span of about ten days, this is immaterial where the platelets are only required to effect haemostasis. Platelet preparations should be given as soon as possible after collection. There is a significant loss in viability after storage but there is now evidence suggesting that platelets may be given up to 2 days and some think up to 3 days after collection.

**(d) Leucocytes.** Certain conditions, e.g. agranulocytosis and profound neuropenia due to massive chemotherapy, etc. represent conditions where leucocyte transfusions might properly be indicated. Early attempts have been made in the United Kingdom at least to effect this, using a continuous cell separating technique. Ideally both donor and recipient should have the similar red cell and white cell typing.

## Hazards of Blood Transfusion

Avoidance of transfusion hazards is the responsibility of the clinician and again it is stressed that every transfusion carries an element of risk and should never be given without a definite indication.

It is often forgotten that the donor also has to be protected against certain hazards. Thus a donor should not be bled (1) more often than 2–3 times yearly or (2) if pregnant and for one year following pregnancy or (3) if the haemoglobin in a female is less than 12·5 g. per cent, in a male less than 13·5 g. per cent—thus avoiding adverse effects on the iron balance. Additionally the donor is always at risk of vasovagal attacks, tetany due to hyperventilation, air embolism especially when blood is taken into glass bottles and sepsis at the point of insertion of the taking needle. A brief review of the main hazards to the patient is listed below:

1. **Mortality.** Mortality as a result of transfusion is about 0·1–1 per cent and is thought to be comparable with that of appendicitis or any simple procedure carried out under general anaesthesia. 3,000 persons die annually in the U.S.A. due to transfusion, comparable figures are not available in the U.K.

2. **Transmission of disease.** The most important of the transmitted diseases are viral hepatitis, syphilis, malaria and brucellosis. Of these syphilis is excluded by serological tests and malaria and brucellosis by donor history as far as possible. The greatest problem is still serum hepatitis although it is possible that recent work on the Australia antigen (thought to be related to the hepatitis virus) and screening of all donors for that antigen may eventually assist in overcoming this particular hazard. Until recently the importance of non-icteric hepatitis was not properly recognized.

Icteric form—frequency lies between 0–25 per cent. In UK it may lie between 2–5 per cent, in Sweden about 10 per cent, USA 10–20 per cent and Japan 25 per cent (paid donors having the highest frequency). The risk to the recipient increases with each transfusion.

Mortality of the icteric form is 1–12 per cent.

No absolute measure for the prevention of transfusion hepatitis yet exists. Thus only extremely strict selection of blood donors and absolute restriction to blood transfusion deemed urgent can be advocated at present.

3. **Bacterial contamination.** Probably 2 per cent of stored blood is bacterially contaminated from either the skin or air even with strict control. The optimal storage conditions (4° to 6°C) are thus essential and blood left out of the refrigerator for more than 30 minutes at any one time should be discarded. The greatest danger is caused by gram negative bacteria, cryophilic organisms, some of which grow at refrigeration temperature.

4. **Pyrogenic reactions.** These may be due to pyrogens—polysaccharide products of bacterial metabolism—in

the container or anticoagulant fluid. Tests for pyrogens on equipment and anticoagulant solutions are therefore essential before use. The incidence of pyrogenic reactions has decreased significantly following the use of disposable transfusion giving sets.

5. **Incompatibility.** A compatible blood transfusion is one in which transfused cells survive as long as the host red cells as well as vice versa. Incompatibility is where the survival time of transfused cells is reduced; this is not identical with haemolytic reactions which occur less frequently. Although the half-life of transfused cells is about 32 days, it has been shown that in 30 per cent of all transfusions especially in multi-transfused patients, the red cells only survive 14–16 days and then disappear from the vascular system, suggesting that the routine crossmatch by no means detects all patient-donor incompatibilities. The risk of iso-immunization is additive and is about 1 per cent per blood transfusion.

6. **Haemolytic reactions.** The majority are usually due to blood group incompatibility—and may have a frequency of 0·2–0·3 per cent or higher. Mortality variously estimated at 1 in 10,000 or more transfusions has been decreased recently with improved expertise in renal dialysis. A haemolytic type of reaction may also be caused by blood improperly stored or stored for too long or already haemolysed, e.g. by overheating or freezing.

7. **Allergic reactions.** Urticarial and asthmatic reactions are rarely of clinical importance and are usually controlled with antihistamines, having an incidence of 1–1·5 per cent of all transfusions.

8. **Citrate toxicity.** Stored blood contains 120 ml. ACD solution and rapid transfusion of large volumes may cause tremors and cardiac arrhythmias due to metabolic acidosis. This is most likely to occur in severe shock, liver disease, in neonates or under hypothermic conditions. Plasma potassium elevation accompanies the decrease in pH. Normally the sodium citrate is rapidly metabolized to sodium bicarbonate in the liver and two litres of citrated blood can be transfused in about 20 minutes without danger of citrate intoxication. While 1 g. of calcium gluconate is usually given per litre of citrated blood, Boyan and Howland (1969) suggest that calcium is not necessary and can sometimes be dangerous.

9. **Acidity of preserved blood.** ACD blood has a pH of about 7·1 decreasing to 6·6 with storage. Massive transfusion may cause a metabolic acidosis unless the blood is warmed under controlled conditions and 3·75 g. sodium bicarbonate given intravenously per 5 litres of blood is recommended by some workers to neutralize the acidosis.

10. **Dangers of cold blood.** Anaesthetized patients have a diminished temperature regulation and if transfused rapidly with large volumes of cold blood suffer a fall in heart and body temperature. Oxygen consumption also increases. Children in particular are unable to compensate quickly for the fall in temperature and are prone to ventricular fibrillation and cardiac arrest (as in exchange transfusions). The value of using warm blood exclusively for massive transfusion, i.e. over 5 litres or so has been amply demonstrated. However, the blood must never be warmed over 40°C and warming devices must be thermostatically controlled whenever possible.

11. **Potassium intoxication.** Fresh stored blood contains about 4–5 mEq./l. of plasma potassium—this may rise to 30 mEq./l. or more by the expiry date. Blood over 10 days old should not be given in large volumes to patients with impaired renal function, e.g. in shock or to neonates.

12. **Circulatory overloading.** At one time this was the commonest cause of death following transfusion but has now greatly diminished with the advent of potent diuretics. However, lengthy operations involving both continuous blood loss and transfusions often result in an over-transfused patient. Knowledge of the central venous pressure and use of dyes or isotopes for measuring plasma volume (PV) and hence total blood volume (TBV) has reduced the hazards but the haemodynamic fluid shifts due to shock, etc. must always be allowed for when interpreting haematocrit and PV results in such patients. It is also good practice to auscultate the lung bases periodically when giving large volumes of blood or when transfusing the elderly patient.

13. **Effects of anaesthetics and drugs.** In patients under the influence of anaesthetics or drugs during transfusion the only two signs suggesting that incompatible blood may have been transfused are (1) hypotension despite apparently adequate blood replacement and (2) abnormal bleeding.

14. **Graft versus Host (GVH) reactions.** These reactions are now recognized in increasing frequency in human patients; in all known cases they have been caused by administration of blood containing histo-incompatible immuno-competent lymphocytes to patients with severe disorders of the thymus-dependent immune system (e.g. lymphopenic hypogammaglobulinemia) or those previously exposed to massive irradiation or heavy immunosuppression and therefore unable to reject foreign cells. GVH disease in man is fatal unless the recipient has some remaining immuno-competence or the donor cells are compatible (Meuwissen et al., 1969).

To prevent this fatal complication of blood transfusion in patients susceptible to GVH diseases, special precautions should be taken to remove lymphocytes before administration.

15. **Rhesus (D) Positive blood.** Apart from the random immunization dangers of blood transfusion—a specific risk is attached to the transfusion of Rhesus (D) Positive blood to D Negative individuals. Thus, except as a life saving procedure, Rhesus (D) Positive blood should never be given to a female below menopausal age since it could be the cause of Haemolytic disease of the Newborn. Younger D negative males should also not be transfused with D Positive blood since they are more likely to produce anti-D than older males.

**The Transfusion Reaction**

The hazards of blood transfusion have already been discussed and it is again emphasized that the greatest of these is a *clerical* error. Technical mistakes account for a very small proportion of all reactions.

Allergic or febrile reactions unless very severe are treated with antihistamines but the transfusion is continued cautiously.

Where a haemolytic or severe febrile reaction is suspected or detected, the transfusion is stopped and the remainder of the transfused blood and the giving set are returned to the Blood Transfusion laboratory accompanied by a fresh blood specimen from the patient.

The basic scheme of investigating a blood transfusion reaction is shown in Fig. 4. Should a positive result be obtained, more detailed tests, e.g. antibody titres, cell survival studies, etc. will normally be carried out at the discretion of the Pathologist.

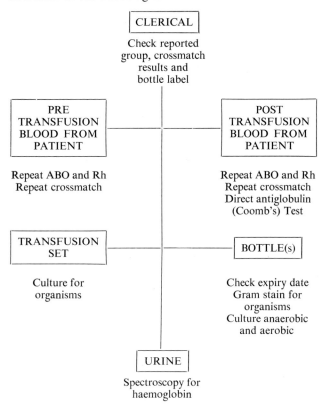

Fig. 4. Basic scheme of investigation of a blood transfusion reaction

## COAGULATION PROBLEMS IN RELATION TO BLOOD TRANSFUSION

### The Coagulation Mechanism

The importance of blood coagulation has been recognized since earliest recorded history and eventually led up to the Morowitz classical theory of coagulation (1905) which may be shown as:

$$
\begin{array}{ccc}
\text{BLOOD} & & \text{TISSUE} \\
& \searrow \quad \swarrow & \\
& \text{THROMBOKINASE} & \\
& \downarrow & \\
& \text{Ca} & \\
& \downarrow & \\
\text{PROTHROMBIN} & \longrightarrow & \text{THROMBIN} \\
& \downarrow & \\
\text{FIBRINOGEN} & \text{———} & \text{FIBRIN}
\end{array}
$$

He thus appears to have recognized the importance of the extrinsic and intrinsic systems even at this early date.

In the 1930's the one stage prothrombin determination of Quick and the two stage prothrombin procedure of Warner and co-workers brought coagulation studies into the routine clinical laboratory. Using these techniques, the cause of sweet clover disease of cattle as a bleeding disorder, was traced to decreased prothrombin after consumption of spoiled sweet clover. This led to the isolation of a dicoumarin derivative from spoiled clover and to the eventual inclusion of this and allied drugs in the modern range of conventional anticoagulants.

The rapid increase in knowledge of the coagulation mechanism led to several often unrelated names for each factor recognized. An International Committee now designates a number to each new factor which it recognizes (Table 8).

### TABLE 8

INTERNATIONAL NOMENCLATURE FOR BLOOD COAGULATION

| Factor | Synonym |
|---|---|
| I | Fibrinogen |
| II | Prothrombin |
| III | Tissue factor, tissue thromboplastin |
| IV | Calcium |
| V | Pro-accelerin, labile factor |
| VI | — |
| VII | Proconvertin, stable factor |
| VIII | Antihaemophilic globulin (AGH) or factor (AHF) |
| IX | Christmas factor, plasma thromboplastin component (PTC) |
| X | Stuart-Prower factor |
| XI | Plasma Thromboplastic Antecedent (PTA) |
| XII | Hageman factor |
| XIII | Fibrin Stabilizing Factor |

Although certain reactions in blood coagulation have long been considered to be enzymatic, recently there has developed a concept which holds that nearly all plasma coagulation factors circulate as pro-enzymes and are converted to enzymes during the process of clotting. The function of each enzyme derived from the pro-enzyme appears to be the activator of the pro-enzyme which succeeds it in the coagulation sequence. Thus blood coagulation may be considered as the result of a series of reactions in which the product of reaction 1 is the enzyme which catalyzes reaction 2 and the product of 2 is the enzyme which catalyzes reaction 3 and so on to the formation of fibrin. This concept (1964) has been called the 'enzyme cascade' (Macfarlane) of blood coagulation which is outlined in Fig. 5.

The 'intrinsic system' represents reactions leading to coagulation of blood without addition of exogenous substances. 'Extrinsic system' involves the participation of exogenous tissue factor. Reference to the figure shows that in the intrinsic system activated factor VIII (i.e. factor VIIIa) activates factor X while in the extrinsic

## THE 'CASCADE' THEORY OF COAGULATION

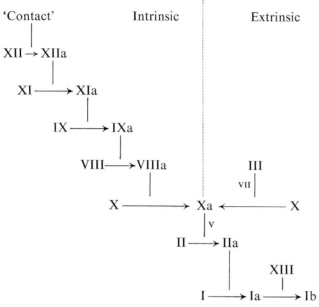

FIG. 5. After Macfarlane, R. G. (1964), *Nature*, **202**, 498 and Macfarlane, R. G. (1965), *Thromb. et diath. haem.*, Suppl. **17**, 45.

system tissue factor, factor VII and calcium are all involved in this reaction. The cascade concept has not displaced the much older notion of intrinsic and extrinsic systems since these differ in their speed of reaction, thus via the intrinsic system thrombin formation may take as long as 4–5 min. to completion compared with 10–15 sec. when the extrinsic system (i.e. including tissue factor) is operative. It is not intended to study each step in detail but some points need special emphasis.

Factor XII. The intrinsic system begins with the activation of factor XII to XIIa by contact with any foreign surface, e.g. collagen, fibre, skin, etc.

The mechanism of activation is not understood and may involve removal of an inhibitor. The activated factor XII (XIIa) then appears to act as an enzyme in activating factor XI.

Factor X appears to be the beginning of the final common pathway of blood coagulation since it is the first factor involved in both intrinsic and extrinsic systems.

The 'extrinsic' system describes coagulation resulting from the addition of tissue extracts to whole blood. Tissue factor activity may be extracted from many organs including fresh lung, placenta and brain tissue. The role of this system in haemostasis and in inflammatory processes is not clear but is likely to be more important in the latter. Only extremely small amounts of tissue factor are necessary and the clotting reactions occur very rapidly. It may be that every wound causes the release of some tissue factor into the damaged vessels where it may induce rapid fibrin formation although this does not explain the mechanism of bleeding, e.g. in haemophilia. It is however clear that the extrinsic system does play an important part in pathological processes such as disseminated intravascular coagulation.

### Implications of the Enzyme Cascade Concept

Macfarlane stresses the potential of the system for amplification since the enzymes are catalysts and a small quantity of enzyme would be expected to convert a large quantity of substrate to product. Since the product is also an enzyme each step leads to rapidly increasing enzymatic activity. The concept is a very acceptable one although it does not fully explain all known facts about coagulation and especially the function of platelets in the coagulation mechanism.

### Blood Coagulation Disturbances after Massive Blood Transfusion

The most important disturbances in the coagulation mechanism of patients who require massive transfusions during surgery are (1) a marked reduction in the number of platelets, (2) a decrease in factors V and VIII, both effects being due to dilution. Such disturbances are often seen when the patient receives more than 5 litres of blood in 24 hours. Fresh blood is indicated for (1) while fresh blood or fresh frozen plasma can be used for (2).

### Investigation of Abnormal Bleeding at Operation

The possible causes of abnormal bleeding at operation have been very adequately reviewed elsewhere (Ulin, 1964). However, in such an event, and especially where previous haematological investigations have not been carried out— a routine screening for possible haematological causes of bleeding should include:

1. Kaolin Cephalin Clotting Time and/or Hicks and Pitney screen test.
2. A total platelet count.
3. A plasma fibrinogen estimation measuring clottable protein.
4. A test for abnormal blood fibrinolytic activity.

The above are adequate as initial tests to exclude significant clotting abnormalities. It should be noted that the list does not include bleeding and clotting times since these are insensitive and reveal only gross abnormalities. Of the two alternatives in 1 above the Kaolin Cephalin Clotting Time is quicker and easier to perform.

The plasma fibrinogen *must* be estimated using a clotting technique. Chemical and immunological methods measure both fibrinogen and fibrin degradation products (formed during abnormal fibrinolysis and Arvin therapy) and may sometimes give grossly misleading high results.

Abnormal fibrinolysis is demonstrated by incubating a clotted blood sample in a water bath at 37°C for one hour with inspection at quarter hourly intervals—if present, the clot will have become smaller or totally disappeared. A more sensitive method involves the measurement of the euglobulin lysis time which provides a quantitative assessment of fibrinolytic activity.

Finally, it is important that blood samples for clotting

tests be taken by a clean venepuncture and placed in containers with the correct anticoagulant. Thus:

| Test | Anticoagulant to be used |
|------|--------------------------|
| Kaolin Cephalin test | — Disodium citrate |
| Hicks and Pitney | — Disodium citrate |
| Platelet count | — EDTA |
| Fibrinogen | — Disodium citrate |
| Fibrinolytic activity | — Disodium citrate *and* a clotted blood specimen |

## The Significance of Disseminated Intravascular Coagulation in Blood Transfusion Reactions and in the Shocked Patient

Disseminated intravascular coagulation (DIC) is a relatively new concept in the detection of disease. It is defined as acute, transient coagulation occurring in the blood flowing throughout the vascular tree and which may obstruct the microcirculation. It may or may not result in an accumulation of fibrin but does involve the transformation of fibrinogen into fibrin (Hardaway, 1966).

Briefly it is postulated that coagulation and fibrinolytic activity are two processes which go on continuously and normally in the vascular tree. They are in fact thought to be in dynamic equilibrium, with constant removal of this fibrin mainly by the body's fibrinolytic system. Thus:

$$\text{COAGULATION} \rightleftharpoons \text{FIBRINOLYSIS}$$

However, certain factors may accelerate intravascular clotting so that fibrin accumulates. Such shifts in the equilibrium result in disseminated intravascular coagulation (DIC).

Typical findings in an episode of DIC are:

1. Sudden appearance of unexplained hypotensive shock with possible cyanosis and death.
2. Appearance of a clinical bleeding tendency which may be dramatic and can cause death.

The bleeding tendency may be due to:

(a) Partial or complete afibrinogenaemia and often deficiency of other clotting factors.
(b) Platelet deficiency.
(c) Presence of fibrin degradation products which act as circulating anticoagulants.
(d) Activation of the fibrinolytic system.

It is often difficult to decide whether intravascular coagulation or fibrinolysis have occurred either singly, together or in sequence. Although each case must be considered as a separate entity, it is a general finding that when fibrinolytic activation is *secondary* to intravascular coagulation then the number of circulating platelets is characteristically decreased whereas in *primary* fibrinolytic activation (hyperplasminaemia) the plasminogen level is low but the platelet count is seldom decreased.

Plasminogen levels do not fall in uncomplicated fibrin formation and hence may serve to exclude intravascular clotting.

3. Finding of capillary thrombi at autopsy (particularly if epsilon amino caproic acid (EACA) has been given).
4. Focal haemorrhagic necrosis in the liver, kidneys, etc., due to capillary obstruction by fibrin. The necrosis may cause death in renal failure.

### Some Syndromes of Disseminated Intravascular Coagulation (DIC)

Many clinical syndromes are undoubtedly episodes of DIC. Of immediate interest are the following:

1. Shock (inadequate capillary perfusion) due to:

(a) Haemorrhage.
(b) Trauma.
(c) Burns.

2. Haemolytic syndromes including haemolytic blood transfusion reactions.

3. Obstetric syndromes:

(a) Concealed accidental ante-partum haemorrhage with premature separation of the placenta.
(b) Abortion.
(c) Amniotic fluid embolism.
(d) Retained dead foetus.

4. Extracorporeal circulation.

It is essential to note that the two immediate effects of DIC are inadequate capillary perfusion (shock) and an acute clotting defect. Although all shock (inadequate capillary perfusion) does not result from DIC, DIC invariably results in shock. Likewise all clotting defects do not result from DIC but DIC always results in a clotting defect.

### Shock Following Incompatible Blood Transfusion

An incompatible blood transfusion may result in a haemolytic transfusion reaction with release of thromboplastin-like substance from the red cells. The syndrome that often results is without doubt due to DIC—the shock being caused by widespread obstruction of the microcirculation by micro-fibrin clots formed from the circulating fibrinogen. Chest pain, although partly due to bronchiolar constriction due to histamine, like substances, may also be due to the blocking of pulmonary blood vessels by agglutinates; likewise renal failure (and pain) may well be due to the obstruction of the renal microcirculation by fibrin, which undoubtedly occurs.

### Principles of Treatment

If DIC is assumed to be the cause of abnormal bleeding (as indicated by laboratory tests), here a low platelet count and afibrinogenaemia are sensitive indicators, then immediate treatment is essential. If the afibrinogenaemia is associated with fibrinolytic activation then an acute life-threatening haemorrhagic state may develop.

Treatment must therefore include administration of fibrinogen until plasma level exceeds 100 mg. per cent, with fresh whole blood to replace the platelets and additional fresh frozen plasma, if necessary, to supply other clotting factors.

Where DIC is thought to be still occurring then immediate *heparin* therapy is indicated to inhibit the clotting process and prevent further fibrin formation. The use of epsilon amino caproic acid (EACA) to inhibit secondary fibrinolytic activity should only be considered as a last resort since the fibrinolysis is protecting the patient from the complications of intravascular coagulation. Further, any fibrin formed in the presence of EACA is incapable of being lysed later by the body's fibrinolytic system and so can only organize with resultant complications of fibrous tissue formation. EACA should never be used unless (a) violent fibrinolytic activation can be demonstrated, (b) life threatening bleeding is present, (c) blood clot formed after the drug becomes effective can be removed.

Occasionaly DIC may result from transfusion, in which case anticoagulation with heparin should precede replacement therapy.

## HAEMOGLOBINOPATHIES

Von Korber (1866) made the original observation that placental (foetal) blood was less easily denatured (decolourized) by alkali than adult blood and concluded that there were two human haemoglobins, adult and foetal. The subsequent work of Herrick (1910) on sickle-cell anaemia and of Cooley and Lee (1925) on thalassaemia laid the foundations of our knowledge of the haemoglobinopathies. Pauling *et al.* (1949) used electrophoresis to demonstrate the abnormal sickle cell haemoglobin (Hb-S) while Brunori *et al.* (1970) and Perutz (1970) using X-ray analysis have made outstanding contributions to our present understanding of the chemical structure and function of human haemoglobins.

Lehmann and Huntsman (1966) and others have demonstrated the genetic nature of these diseases, that they have a geographical distribution, have an association with malaria, give rise to bone changes and have genetical variants capable of producing phenotypes with a wide range of clinical expressions. The bone changes in particular have enabled research workers to study the migration of ancient populations and spread of disease in earlier times.

### Normal Haemoglobins

Oxygen transport is carried out by the haemoglobin molecule. In the adult (Hb-A) this molecule consists of two pairs of polypeptide chains termed alpha ($\alpha$) and beta ($\beta$), consisting of 141 and 146 amino acid residues respectively. A haem group is associated with each individual globin chain in such a way as to protect its iron atom from oxidation while leaving it free to combine reversibly with oxygen. Lehmann (1964) showed that three normal human haemoglobins exist, namely adult (Hb-A), foetal (Hb-F) and Hb-A$_2$. Each consists of 4 chains, of which two are alpha ($\alpha$) chains but the other two differ. Hb-A ($\alpha_2\beta_2$) makes up 98 per cent of total adult haemoglobin, the remainder consisting of Hb-A$_2$ ($\alpha_2\delta_2$) and Hb-F. Hb-F ($\alpha_2\gamma_2$) which makes up 50–70 per cent of total haemoglobin in neonates decreases to less than 2 per cent in early childhood. Thus the three haemoglobins may be represented as:

$$\begin{array}{ccc}
\alpha\alpha \text{ (alpha)} & \alpha\alpha \text{ (alpha)} & \alpha\alpha \text{ (alpha)} \\
\times & \times & \times \\
\beta\beta \text{ (beta)} & \delta\delta \text{ (delta)} & \gamma\gamma \text{ (gamma)} \\
\text{Hb-A} & \text{Hb-A}_2 & \text{Hb-F}
\end{array}$$

### Haemoglobinopathies

**Definition:** These are diseases caused by inherited abnormalities of the globin part of the haemoglobin molecule. Those so far encountered are due to either:

(1) a defect in the synthesis of a specific polypeptide chain (thalassaemia including sickle cell anaemia); or
(2) a biochemical alteration in polypeptide structure abnormal haemoglobin); or
(3) a combination of (1) and (2).

In thalassaemia the result is underproduction of haemoglobin and a shortened red cell survival, due to unbalanced synthesis of globin chains. In the case of abnormal haemoglobins, the deletion or substitution of amino acids at important points in the haemoglobin molecule may cause both inefficient oxygenation and reduced red cell survival. Figure 6 explains the basic problem in the development of certain thalassaemias. While alpha ($\alpha$) chain production becomes almost maximal by about the third month of intrauterine life and remains at this level, gamma ($\gamma$) chain production begins to fall off by the sixth month and reaches 2–3 per cent by the sixth month of postnatal development. Conversely, beta ($\beta$) chain production is low during intrauterine life but takes over from the gamma chain sequence during the early postnatal phase, becoming maximal by the 5th–6th month. Delta ($\delta$) chain production normally remains at 1–2 per cent of the $\beta$ chains present.

Thalassaemias are classified mainly according to the globin chain of which there is deficient production. Of these, the beta chain (or $\beta$-thalassaemia) is the most widespread inherited abnormality, being found in almost every population studied but $\alpha$-thalassaemia is not so prevalent. In homozygous $\beta$-thalassaemia (thalassaemia major) the synthesis of chains is almost completely inhibited and a severe anaemia begins at 3–6 months (*see* Fig. 1) i.e. the time when $\beta$ chain synthesis first exceeds $\gamma$ chain in production. Hb-F production continues at a rate far below that necessary to maintain an acceptable haemoglobin level. The Hb-A$_2$ level also increases. On the other hand, $\alpha$-thalassaemia involves defective alpha ($\alpha$) chain production, which is reflected in the under-production of all three normal haemoglobins, A ($\alpha_2\beta_2$), A$_2$ ($\alpha_2\delta_2$) and F ($\alpha_2\gamma_2$). The gamma ($\gamma$) chains, in fact, now unite to form an abnormal ($\gamma_4$) haemoglobin known as Hb-Bart's. In the homozygote the result is perinatal death from hydrops foetalis.

Figure 7 shows the chain sequence of amino acids characterizing Hb's A, S and C. Those in italics show the substitutions. Hb-A is normal adult haemoglobin having glutamic acid in position 6 of the beta chain. In the abnormal sickle cell haemoglobin (Hb-S) this amino acid has been replaced by valine while in the abnormal Hb-C molecule position 6 is occupied by lysine. Hb-S is the most severe of the haemolytic anaemias arising from common

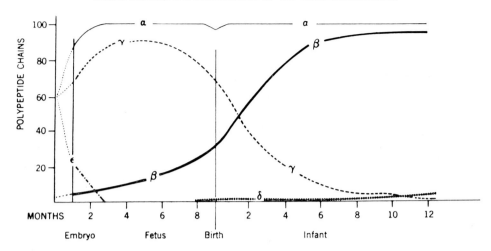

FIG. 6. Course of various human haemoglobin polypeptide chain formation during early life. (After Wintrobe.)

variants of Hb-A and is important since its solubility in the reduced state is about a hundredth of that of Hb-A. Consequently, the red cell Hb-S remains in solution as long as the environment is rich in oxygen but when the latter is reduced either artificially, e.g. by exposure to high altitudes or in the tissues, the haemoglobin crystallizes out and distorts the red cell to the sickle cell shape (Fig. 9). The cells are lysed, being sequestered excessively in the R.E. system and can occlude the microcirculation in many parts of the body, hence the sickle cell crises commonly found in this disease.

For fuller details on the subject, the reader should consult the references at the end of this article. However, certain aspects of these disorders are of especial interest and importance to anaesthetists.

Patients with β-thalassaemia major are fairly easily diagnosed from the medical history and physical signs, and thus management can be considered prior to anaesthesia. Of greater importance because of its higher frequency is β-thalassaemia minor (sickle cell trait) and also haemoglobin S-C disease (in which the individual carries two abnormal alleles, haemoglobin S and haemoglobin C): these are sometimes only detected after operation when the patient may develop 'sickle cell crisis'.

As a general rule, all patients of negro origin should be tested for sickle cell disease prior to operation under general anaesthetic, in view of the higher incidence (20 per cent of West Africans and 10 per cent of West Indians and American negroes) compared with white individuals. In many hospitals, it is customary for blood from such patients to be sent to the laboratory prior to operation for a sickling test (*details below*). Should the test be positive, the blood

is then electrophoresed, partly to confirm the previous result and partly to identify the actual abnormal haemoglobin concerned, since although it is the commonest, Hb-S is not the only one to produce a sickling effect (Fig. 8).

**Preparation of Sickle Cells**

The sickling phenomenon may be demonstrated by sealing a thin fluid film of the blood under test between slide and cover-glass using a mixture of paraffin-wax and petroleum jelly, and incubating the preparation at 37°C. Since the test depends on exhausting the available oxygen under the coverslip, it is more usual to include also a reducing agent, e.g. sodium metabisulphite or sodium dithionite to accelerate the process. In sickle-cell anaemia well marked sickling may be obvious after incubation for an hour (*see* Fig. 9).

It is particularly important to remember that the sickle carrier is generally fit and that sickling occurs only under conditions of severe hypoxia. Patients with sickle-cell haemoglobin-C disease are often completely unaware that they suffer from this disorder. Hypoxia sufficient to cause an infarctive sickling crisis may occur during infections or anaesthetic accidents, as well as by flying or residing at high altitudes. However, although it seems agreed that patients with more severe sickle-cell disorders should not be allowed to fly as aircrew, the position of sickle-cell carriers is by no means agreed.

It is generally accepted that general anaesthesia may be hazardous in patients with sickle-cell conditions, especially those with genotype S-S and S-C and in S-beta thalassaemia. The anaesthetic management of such patients has been summarized (Oduro and Searle, 1972) as simple techniques,

| Sequence peptide | 1 | 2 | 3 | 4 | 5 | 6 | 7 |
|---|---|---|---|---|---|---|---|
| Hb-A (adult) | Valine | Histidine | Leucine | Threonine | Proline | Glutamic acid | Glutamic acid |
| Hb-S (sickle) | Valine | Histidine | Leucine | Threonine | Proline | *Valine* | Glutamic acid |
| Hb-C | Valine | Histidine | Leucine | Threonine | Proline | *Lysine* | Glutamic acid |

FIG. 7. The β chain sequence of amino acids characterizing haemoglobins -A, -S and -C.

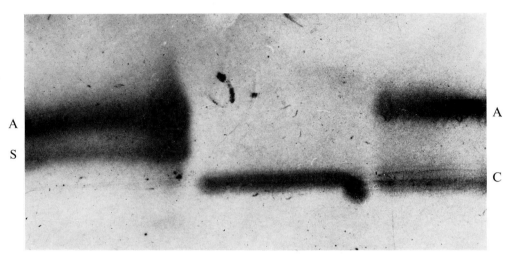

A
S

A
C

FIG. 8. Electrophoretic strip showing Hb-A, Hb-S and Hb-C.

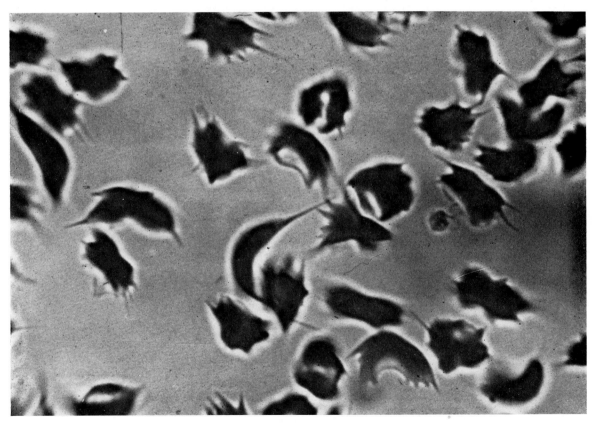

FIG. 9. Photograph of sickled cells.

with adequate oxygenation, ventilation, maintenance of the circulating volume and efficient postoperative care.

Many methods and regimes have been tried for the prevention and treatment of sickle-cell crisis—none has received universal acceptance. Reports of metabolic acidosis occurring in patients with 'painful crises' and thus providing a rationale for an alkalinization therapy during anaesthesia are not supported by other workers: the value of urea for the same purpose remains to be proven: the use of exchange transfusion has merit but may not be practicable in areas where blood availability is low. Lehmann and Huntsman advise keeping the patient warm, alleviating pain, dealing with secondary infections and attempting to prevent further formation of thrombi in the circulatory system. For this purpose they refer to the use of injections of magnesium sulphate, used as a calcium antagonist and to the value of plasma expanders such as Rheomacrodex. They also seem to favour alkaline therapy. A more recent and perhaps effective treatment is available in some hospitals, namely, hyperbaric oxygen.

Blood transfusions and iron therapy are best avoided but the former, if required, should be given as packed cells to avoid the risk of cardiac failure (*see* Hazards of Blood Transfusion). Attempts to remove the excess iron using desferrioxamine do not seem to have been particularly successful.

Finally, the methods outlined above do not cure the inherited abnormality and at this molecular level, the value of marrow transplantation should be seriously considered in the homozygous disease, if the necessary expertise and facilities are available. Earlier failures in this field do not provide sufficient reason for ignoring recent developments in tissue typing techniques etc. which are such that the outlook for successful marrow transplantation now appears to be much more optimistic (Cordon *et al.*, 1973).

## REFERENCES

Bernstein, F. (1924), "Ergebnisse einer biostatischen zusammenfassenden Betrachtung über die erblichen Blutstrukturen des Menschen," *Klin. Wschr.*, **3**, 1495–1497.

Boyan, C. P. and Howland, W. S. (1969), "Immediate and Delayed Mortality Associated with Massive Blood Transfusions," *Surg. Clin. N. Amer.*, **49**, 217–222.

Coombs, R. R. A., Mourant, A. E. and Race, R. R. (1945), "Detection of Weak and 'Incomplete' Rh Agglutinins: A New Test," *Lancet*, **ii**, 15.

Cordon, A. *et al.* (1973), "Three Unfractionated Bone Marrow Grafts," January Meeting of British Transplantation Society at Birmingham.

Cossart, Y. E. and Vahrman, J. (1970), "Studies of Australia-SH Antigen in Sporadic Viral Hepatitis in London," *Brit. Med. J.*, **1**, 403.

Dungern, E.v. and Hirszfeld, L. (1911), "Über gruppenspezifische Strukturen des Blutes III," *Z. Immun. Forsch.*, **8**, 526–562.

Fisher, R. A., cited by Race, R. R. (1944), "An 'Incomplete' Antibody in Human Serum," *Nature, Lond.*, **153**, 771–772.

Gruber, U. F. (1969), *Blood Replacement*. Berlin: Springer-Verlag.

Hardaway, R. M. (1966), *Syndromes of Disseminated Intravascular Coagulation*. U.S.A.: Charles C. Thomas.

Lehmann, H. and Huntsman, R. G. (1966), *Man's Haemoglobins*. Amsterdam: North-Holland.

Loutit, J. F. and Mollison, P. L. (1943), "Advantages of a Disodium-citrate-glucose Mixture as a Blood Preservative," *Brit. Med. J.*, **ii**, 744.

Maizels, M. (1941), "Preservation of Organic Phosphorus Compounds in Stored Blood by Glucose," *Lancet*, **i**, 722.

Marengo-Rowe, A. J. (1971), "Haemoglobinopathies," *Brit. J. Hosp. Med.*, **6**, 617.

Mewissen, H. J., Stutman, O. and Good, R. A. (1969), "Functions of the Lymphocytes," *Seminars in Haem*, **6**, 28–66.

Mollison, P. L. (1972), *Blood Transfusion in Clinical Medicine*. Blackwell Scientific Publications.

Morton, J. A., Pickles, M. M. and Sutton, L. (1969), "The Correlation of the Bg$^a$ Blood Group with the HL-A7 Leucocyte Group: Demonstration of Antigenic Sites on Red Cells and Leucocytes," *Vox Sang.*, **17**, 536.

Morton, J. A., Pickles, M. M., Sutton, L. and Skov, F. (1971), "Identification of Further Antigens on Red Cells and Lymphocytes," *Vox Sang.*, **21**, 141–153.

Oduro, K. A. and Searle, J. F. (1972), "Anaesthesia in Sickle-Cell States: A Plea for Simplicity," *Brit. Med. J.*, **4**, 596–598.

Satinoff, M. I. (1972), "Origins and Geographical Spread of the Thalassaemias and Abnormal Haemoglobins," *J. Hum. Evol.*, **1**, 79.

Strumia, M. M. (1963), "General Principles of Blood Transfusion," *Transfusion*, **3**, 303.

Ulin, A. W. *et al.* (1964), "Bleeding in the Surgical Patient," *Ann. N.Y. Acad. Sci.*, **115**, Art. 1.

Valtis, D. J. and Kennedy, A. C. (1954), "Defective Gas-transport Function of Stored Red Blood Cells," *Lancet*, **i**, 119.

Weatherall, J. D. (1967), "The Thalassaemias," *Seminars Haem.*, **4**, 72.

# CHAPTER 2

# APPLIED PHYSIOLOGY OF THE BODY FLUIDS

P. J. HORSEY

## Measurement of the Body Spaces

The use of radioactive isotopes for the measurement of water distribution has reached a stage which necessitates revision of earlier concepts. Total body water can be measured with either Deuterium or Tritium with an accuracy of the order of $\pm 2$ per cent. A precisely measured dose of the isotope is taken by mouth or injected intravenously and equilibration samples are taken after 4 hours in normal subjects, longer equilibration times being allowed in patients with oedema or ascites. The method depends upon atomic exchange of hydrogen into the water molecules, and it is believed that the entire body water is accessible.

Total body water expressed as a percentage of body weight is highest at birth when it constitutes 75 per cent, falling to 65 per cent at one month and about 60 per cent at one year. In men there is a progressive fall from 60 to 50 per cent as age increases and in women from 50 to 45 per cent at corresponding ages—figures much lower than those deduced from earlier methods (Edelman and Leibman, 1959).

Once total body water is known, either of its two compartments can be calculated if the other is measured. As there is no known method by which cell water can be measured directly, intracellular water is computed by subtracting the extracellular volume from the total. Again, recent developments require a revision of former beliefs about the relative volumes.

Every worker who sets out to measure extra-cellular fluid does so by injecting a substance which he assumes will equilibrate throughout the interstitial fluid and be halted at the cell membranes of every tissue of the body. If it is metabolized or excreted during the time allowed for equilibration allowances have to be made for this. The substances used in these measurements are either crystalloids or ions. Mannitol, inulin and sucrose are examples of crystalloids; bromide, sulphate, sodium and chloride are the ions most commonly used. The crystalloids are larger molecules which require longer equilibration times and unlike the ions, cannot be injected in the form of radioactive isotopes. Strictly speaking measurements made with these substances should be referred to as the '24 hr. mannitol space' or the '1 hr. sulphate space' but they seldom are. To designate them as extracellular fluid volume, particularly when disease or injury may have interfered with normal tissue perfusion, is to introduce unwarranted assumptions. Current textbooks usually give the ratio of intracellular to extracellular fluid as $2\frac{1}{2} - 3:1$. The most accurate data available from methods employing isotopes assign almost equal proportions to the two

compartments. Edelman and Leibman (1959) in their masterly review give the ratio of cell water to extracellular water as $55:45$ and this has been confirmed by subsequent work. With rare exceptions, chronic disease is characteristically associated with a fall in intracellular volume and expansion of the extracellular space so that extracellular water may be equal to or even exceed the volume of water within the cells.

## The Extracellular Space

That part of the extracellular fluid outside the vascular tree used to be referred to as interstitial fluid. It was thought of as a single homogeneous pool of fluid which was in close functional association with plasma. The development of isotope dilution studies has shown that this was an oversimplification and at the same time has explained the discrepancies between former and present views on the volume and composition of the intracellular fluid. The extracellular fluid which is readily permeated by both crystalloids and ions is called 'interstitial lymph' fluid by Edelman and Leibman. It forms 20 per cent of the total body water and is that part of the body fluid which is in dynamic equilibrium with the capacitance side of the vascular compartment—it acts as a reservoir from which water and sodium can be mobilized into the circulation, or which will accept large amounts of water and sodium when circumstances favour extravascular filtration. In view of recent developments in parenteral fluid therapy, the interstitial lymph fluid may appropriately be designated as "functional" extracellular fluid. This implies that there are other components of extracellular fluid which are less closely concerned with homeostasis of plasma volume. The various components of the extracellular space are shown in Table 1.

TABLE 1

THE EXTRACELLULAR FLUID

Total extracellular water 45 per cent
(After Edelman and Liebman, 1959)

| | % Total body water |
|---|---|
| 1. Plasma water | 7·5 |
| 2. Interstitial lymph water | 20·0 'Functional ECF' |
| 3. Dense connective tissue water | 7·5 |
| 4. Bone water | 7·5 |
| 5. Transcellular water | 2·5 |

Note that there are two 'pools' of extracellular fluid, one in dense connective tissue (cartilage, ligaments, tendons) and the other in bone each of which is equal in volume to the plasma. Water in these tissues plays little part in losses or dislocations of fluid as they affect surgical patients. Its main interest is that earlier determinations of extracellular fluid volume did not take it into account and assigned both its water and its sodium content to the intracellular compartment.

## The Transcellular Fluid

The transcellular fluid is extracellular fluid but has had to pass through cells in order to become so. It is of more direct interest because it includes water within the lumen of the gastro-intestinal tract which may expand and be lost in large amounts at the expense of the functional extracellular fluid.

## The Nature and Dynamics of the Functional ECF

Guyton et al. (1966) describe the interstitial fluid in this compartment as consisting of a gelatinous ground substance traversed by collagen fibres. These workers have produced evidence that the normal interstitial fluid pressure is negative and varies between −8 and −4 mm Hg. As long as this negative pressure is maintained large volumes of water can be accumulated in a relatively immobile state in the gelatinous matrix of the ground substance which fills the interstitial spaces. The space itself behaves like an elastic chamber with non-linear characteristics (Gauer and Henry, 1963). As fluid accumulates within it there is a gradual increase in pressure towards zero when a precipitous increase in compliance occurs and oedema forms. The transient rise in central venous pressure with rapid saline infusion was recognized long ago by Bayliss and Starling (1894). These workers attributed this to accommodation of the extra fluid within the capacitance side of the circulation but it is now held to be due to very rapid filtration into the interstitial fluid which becomes progressively less rapid as the filtered volume increases. In this way a change in behaviour of venous pressure to non-colloidal volume expansion indicates that interstitial fluid volume is increased to the point of saturation. This has obvious implications in the interpretation of the response of central venous pressure to such volume expansion.

## Guides to the Adequacy of Circulating Volume

During the decade of the 1960's there was a great improvement in the management of the 'shocked' surgical patient. Much of this was attributable to the development of more aggressive fluid therapy which was justified by monitoring of the central venous pressure and the hourly urine volume. Both measurements have their place, but both must be used critically if they are not to lead to overtransfusion.

## The Central Venous Pressure

The sternal angle is commonly taken as the zero reference point for measurement of the central venous pressure (CVP). Robson (1968) showed that the average right atrial pressure was 6·2 + 1·5 cm. of saline; as the sternal angle is about 5 cm. above the level of the atrium in the supine position, a normal pressure will be below 3 cm. of saline and may even be negative if the sternal angle is taken as zero. For this reason either the mid-axillary line should be used or 5 cm. added to the observed level if the sternal angle is used.

The earlier attitude to CVP measurements was well summarized by Artz (1966) who stated that fluids could be given to patients in shock without fear of overload as long as the CVP did not exceed 15 cm. of water. Since then it has been increasingly apparent that CVP may be a very unreliable guide to blood volume in hypotensive states (Wilson et al., 1971) and a much more cautious attitude has arisen. Frank (1969) and Berman and Spencer (1972) warn that neither clinical examination of the lungs nor measurement of the CVP will provide any evidence of the development of interstitial pulmonary oedema and they advocate frequent chest radiography for its detection. James and Myers (1972) draw attention to the lag between the infusion of fluid and its reflection in raised CVP and Cohn et al. (1970) stress that the CVP is an unreliable guide to end-diastolic left ventricular pressure—which is what it is tacitly assumed to indicate—when either of the ventricles is functioning abnormally. Thus after myocardial infarction the CVP is usually lower than the end-diastolic left ventricular pressure and in pulmonary embolism it is likely to be higher.

The present position is that measurement of the CVP should be done whenever the usual indices of adequate circulation provide insufficient guides to management. It is of particular help in so-called endotoxic shock in which the very high mortality can be reduced by bold infusion of fluids, the amount and rate being guided principally by the behaviour of the venous pressure. It is the response of the CVP to rapid infusions of small volumes of fluid which is the best guide to therapy. Wilson and his colleagues (1971) describe an acute venous pressure response as a rise in CVP of 2 cm. of water or more in response to 200 ml. of fluid given in ten minutes and persisting for more than ten minutes. If this is seen, no more fluid should be given for the time being.

## Monitoring the Urine Volume

During surgery the kidney is subjected to very high levels of antidiuretic hormone; in spite of this the urine volume can be increased by any osmotically active solute. Sodium as saline or Ringer-lactate solution is the commonest solute given for this purpose and it must be appreciated that the resulting increase in urine volume is quite variable from one subject to another. If a preconceived hourly urine volume is sought it is very likely that it will only be attained at the expense of a strongly positive water and sodium balance (Mackenzie and Donald, 1969). The figure to aim for is often quoted as 50 ml./hour but Doty et al. (1970) stated that in many cases such an output could only be achieved by over-expansion of the extracellular fluid. Such an accumulation is usually tolerated in the young without necessarily being beneficial; in the elderly it may be harmful. If the urine volume is being measured, minute volumes of 0·4–0·6 ml. (approximately 30 ml./hour) should be accepted as being compatible with normal renal function.

## Changes in Volume of Extracellular Fluid

There are two important general principles to grasp before going on to consider their application.

1. 'Although this important volume of body water can both contract and expand, it much more commonly expands than contracts.' (Moore, 1959.)

2. The concentration of sodium in the extracellular fluid is an extremely fallible guide to the stores of exchangeable sodium in the body. 'The advent of the flame photometer has shown that a low serum sodium concentration ($Na_s$) may occur in any seriously ill patient.' (Edelman, 1956.)

Starling (1909) recognized that the kidney exhibited a high degree of what he termed 'sensibility'—the power of reacting to various stimuli in a manner appropriate to the survival of the organism. For many years it has been tacitly assumed that maintenance of normal osmolarity and pH of the body fluids was of such obvious importance to survival that all else would be subordinated to these ends. There is now clear evidence that maintenance of extracellular fluid volume often takes precedence over normal osmolar relationships and occasionally distortions of $H^+$ ion excretion will be perpetuated in order that sodium shall be conserved. Teleologically, as Gauer and Henry point out, dilutional hyponatraemia is apparently a lesser evil than circulatory collapse. One can therefore accept as a generalization that the post-operative period is likely to be associated with expansion of this space and dilution of the extracellular fluid.

## The Serum Sodium Concentration—$Na_s$

The serum sodium concentration, though less capricious in its fluctuations than that of potassium, is a very poor guide to the need to give or to withhold sodium. Before deciding that a particular level of $Na_s$ requires 'correcting' the sequence of events which preceded its development must be taken into account: in addition, the variables known to influence $Na_s$ must all be considered (Edelman et al., 1958).

These variables are

1. The exchangeable sodium stores of the body $Na_e$.
2. The exchangeable potassium stores of the body $K_e$.
3. The total body water, TBW.

They are related in the following way

$$Na_s \propto \frac{Na_e + K_e}{TBW}$$

## Total Exchangeable Sodium

With the single exception of Addison's disease, patients with normal kidneys who are chronically ill tend to have raised body sodium stores. Trauma, by a variety of mechanisms, causes the body to retain sodium and is therefore similarly associated with an increase in exchangeable sodium if sodium intake is continued.

## Total Exchangeable Potassium

There is no known disease in which body potassium content is raised: in sharp contrast to sodium, both acute and chronic illness and trauma are associated with progressive loss of body potassium. Surgical patients may lose as much as 100 mEq. of potassium in the first 36 to 48 hours after a major operation. Thereafter the loss diminishes to what Moore calls a 'potassium constant' for the starving patient of about 25 mEq. a day (Moore and Ball, 1952). This loss is due to renal excretion of potassium.

## Total Body Water

One of the least appreciated but most predictable results of surgery is that it causes the body to retain water avidly, provided that the water is administered as 'osmotically free' water which in practice generally means as 5 per cent dextrose with no sodium.

Whatever the external water intake it must also be remembered that a major operation results in a catabolism of what Moore calls mixed tissue, high in fat content. Such tissue in its combustion will release as much as 600 to 1,000 ml. of sodium-free water a day which becomes extracellular in the process (Moore, 1959). The denominator of the equation which determines $Na_s$ is therefore very likely to become greater after trauma and there is now little doubt that the characteristic hyponatraemia is due chiefly to dilution of the normal or increased exchangeable sodium with excess water. If potassium balance is also negative (which is very likely) this will accentuate the tendency for $Na_s$ to fall.

When confronted with a patient known to have an abnormally low $Na_s$ it is important to try and deduce what the probable sodium stores of the body are likely to be and also to determine if cardiovascular function supports a diagnosis of sodium deficiency. If capillary refill is rapid, the periphery is warm and the blood pressure is maintained when the patient is sat up, it is unlikely that extracellular fluid volume is depleted or that attempts to raise $Na_s$ will be beneficial. If very low levels are encountered e.g. below 120 to 125 mEq./l. in patients free from cardiovascular disease it is reasonable to use hypertonic (1·8%) saline when there are signs of E.C.F. depletion, but once levels above 125 mEq./l. are restored isotonic saline should be substituted.

Normal levels of $Na_s$ are all too often accepted as indications that significant sodium depletion has not occurred: it can be just as misguided to withhold isotonic saline (or Ringer-lactate) from a patient because he has a normal serum sodium level as it may be to give it solely because he has a low level. As in hyponatraemia, the decision to give sodium should be determined by clinical evidence that extracellular fluid volume is depleted. There are often clear biochemical signs of this and the serum sodium concentration is by no means necessarily one of them. Wallace et al. (1966) described 47 cholera victims with severe depletions of the extracellular fluid (Table 2). Note the high average $Na_s$ in both groups: all were rapidly infused with a fluid resembling Ringer-lactate with a sodium concentration of 140 mEq./l. One may summarize the matter by saying that whenever there is good evidence of loss of extracellular fluid, the fluid given to make good the loss should contain sodium in at least isotonic concentration.

TABLE 2

PATIENTS WITH CLASSICAL AND EL TOR CHOLERA

| | Classical (14) | | El Tor (33) | |
|---|---|---|---|---|
| | Mean | Range | Mean | Range |
| Serum Na | 148 | 130–157 | 151 | 142–161 |

## Loss of Functional Extracellular Fluid at Operation

By repeated measurements of the 18 or 20 minute radiosulphate space during surgery, Shires and his colleagues (1961) demonstrated large contractions of the volume of the space so measured. The amounts of fluid 'lost' were considerable—as much as 3 or 4 litres—and it was claimed that they varied with the degree of trauma involved.

Any such contraction of a volume of dilution may be due to one of two quite different causes—either there has been a major shift in the components of the volume of dilution or there has been a failure of the isotope to gain access to some of the 'space'. The clinical implications of these two mechanisms are quite different and the first came to be accepted somewhat uncritically and the second to be overlooked.

There have been several reports by subsequent investigators, of which that by Gutelius and Shizgal (1968) is a good example, which failed to substantiate the large falls in functional extracellular fluid volume previously described. Reports such as these have modified the early enthusiasm for infusions of very large volumes of sodium and water during surgery. The position has been reached whereby most agree that there is a pool of traumatic oedema at the operative site but there is by no means general agreement that any benefit is to be obtained by expanding the functional extracellular fluid to compensate for this. Against doing so is the knowledge that patients undergoing major surgery do not manifest the signs of sudden large losses of extracellular fluid. There is no haemoconcentration and if blood volume is maintained cardiovascular function is not obviously disordered. On the other hand the profound oliguria which accompanies such surgery can often be prevented by infusions of saline or Ringer-lactate and this is generally conceded to indicate that renal perfusion is better and renal oxygen requirements are reduced. The choice now lies between giving no sodium-containing fluids during surgery and giving moderate amounts such as 5 ml./kg./hour up to a maximum of 1 to 1½ litres. Authorities such as Moore (1967) and Hayes (1968) have come down in favour of the proponents of giving moderate amounts of Ringer-lactate during major surgery: provided that the 24 hour fluid intake (excluding blood loss and replacement) does not excede 2½ litres and the amounts given during operation are included, such a schedule does seem to offer advantages over the 'no sodium' one.

## High Serum Sodium Concentrations

Anaesthetists are now very likely to be confronted with hypernatraemic patients in intensive care units. There are two common causes of this disorder—relative water depletion and the use of hypertonic sodium bicarbonate.

## Hypernatraemia Due to Water Depletion

Just as low levels of $Na_s$ should direct attention to the possibility of excess body water, so should the finding of abnormally high levels immediately arouse suspicion of water depletion. In such cases the water depletion is usually a relative one in that water has been lost in excess of an osmotically equivalent sodium load. In other words patients with hypernatraemia may be sodium depleted.

In this condition serum sodium levels of 160 to 180 mEq./l. may be found, and levels above 200 mEq./l are reported. Unconscious patients, particularly if they receive high protein feeds by intragastric tubes, are at risk. The repeated use of osmotic diuretics such as mannitol will have the same result, often accelerated by increased water loss due to hyperpnoea and fever. All these factors may operate in patients after head injuries whose daily water intake may need to be increased to 3½ or 4 litres and who go into increasing negative water balance if restricted to a 2 litre daily intake.

The chief risk such a patient runs if hypernatraemia is discovered is that he will receive a rapid and large infusion of 5 per cent dextrose. There is evidence, particularly in children, that the transition from hypernatraemic water depletion to water intoxication can readily be caused (Hughes Davies, 1966), and sodium should be included in the initial repleting fluid. Concentrations of 30–75 mEq./l. are suitable for infants and young children, and adults should receive at least 75 mEq./l. The use of formulae for calculating the fluid deficit from $Na_s$ is often misleading in hyponatraemia, but when high levels due to predominant water depletion are found, the approximate deficit can be calculated as follows:

Observed $Na_s$ × Observed body water

= Normal $Na_s$ × Normal body water.

If observed $Na_s$ is 160 mEq./l. and normal body water is assessed as 40 litres
Then

$$160 \times TBW = 140 \times 40$$

$$TBW = \frac{140 \times 40}{160} = 35 \text{ litres}$$

Water deficit is 40 − 35 = 5 litres.

About a third of the deficit should be given in the first four hours, using fluids with sodium concentrations of between 30 and 75 mEq./l. The remainder is given as 5 per cent dextrose or 'fifth normal' saline more slowly over the next 36–48 hours and is added to the normal water requirements for this time.

## Hypernatraemia Due to Sodium Bicarbonate

Most anaesthetists have seen serum sodium concentrations in the range 160–180 due to uncontrolled infusion of molar (8·4%) sodium bicarbonate. This is usually the result of putting up a half litre flask of the very hypertonic solution without a careful prescription of the exact volume to be given. Provided that signs of overloading the circulation are not present—which they seldom are—this osmotic trespass is surprisingly well tolerated. The natural inclination to reduce the high sodium concentration with rapid infusion of 5 per cent dextrose should be resisted.

### The Intracellular Fluid

For many years it was believed that the cells were hypertonic with respect to their interstitial fluid environment. Cell water is not easy to define in terms of osmolarity because the osmotic activity of many cell proteins is not known: 'bound' water, which is water which cannot be transported across cell membranes in response to osmotic gradients, is governed by the concentration of cell proteins and probably accounts for 16–40 per cent of intracellular water (Olmstead, 1966).

During the last decade there has been general acceptance that the body cells in health behave as perfect osmometers —that is to say they will imbibe or eject water in response to the osmotic forces acting across the cell membranes. There are obvious exceptions to this; the cells of the distal renal tubule, for example, will maintain a gradient between interstitial fluid (290 m.Osmol./l.) and urine at four times this concentration, but the non-secretory cells do not allow sustained osmotic gradients to persist.

Studies of mammalian response to water deprivation all point to the relative expendibility of cell water which is in sharp contrast to the rigorous conservation of extracellular water. Water within the cells can only become extracellular if the osmotically active potassium holding it there is excreted. It is therefore not unexpected that water depletion is associated with renal conservation of sodium and excretion of potassium.

### Water Balance in Surgical Patients

A clinical belief which is deeply entrenched is that a patient totally deprived of water for 12–18 hours becomes significantly 'dehydrated':* there is abundant evidence that the body tolerates water deficits of at least two litres without measurable effect on cardiovascular function (Henschel, 1963). In very hot conditions men do not drink enough to replenish evaporative water loss but undergo a voluntary dehydration often amounting to between 2 and 4 per cent of body weight (Schmidt-Nielsen, 1964). In the clinical setting, Wilkinson (1956) has reported a number of patients subjected to gastrectomy with total fluid deprivation for 48 hours. Although not obviously deleterious, such constraint is at best disagreeable and is likely to reduce ciliary activity on the mucosal surface of the tracheo-bronchial tree. It is therefore reasonable to give parenteral water (as 5 per cent dextrose) to any patient who is unable to drink for more than 12 hours after operation.

Before prescribing a daily fluid schedule one must be aware that setting up an intravenous infusion of 5 per cent

---

* Throughout this chapter it is assumed that the patients under discussion are afebrile, under resting conditions and in temperate ambient temperatures.

dextrose reduces the capacity of the kidneys to excrete water to about 25 per cent of that possible on a normal diet (Kerrigan et al., 1955). The antidiuretic hormone activity provoked by major surgery approximately halves this capacity during the first 36–72 hours so that some patients will go into a strongly positive water balance on an intake of 3 litres a day. Zimmermann and Wangensteen (1952) reported three cases of water intoxication whose average water intake was less than 3 litres a day, and they drew attention to the vulnerability of the elderly undergoing major surgery. Many rather complex methods based on surface area have been suggested to calculate the water requirements of surgical patients, but the total volume of 5 per cent dextrose given can reasonably be covered by:

> 1 litre on the day of operation;
> 1½ litres on day 1;
> 2 litres on day 2 and subsequent days.

In addition to this intake, saline or Ringer-lactate may be given during operation as described above, and an additional half litre of isotonic saline is given on each post-operative day.

## REFERENCES

Artz, C. P. (1966), Editorial, "Volume Replacement in Shock," *Surg. Gynec. Obstet.*, **122**, 112.

Bayliss, W. M. and Starling, E. H. (1894), "Observations on Venous Pressures and their Relationship to Capillary Pressures," *J. Physiol.*, **16**, 159.

Berman, I. R. and Spencer, F. C. (1972), Editorial, "The Wet Lung: Diagnostic Considerations," *Ann. Surg.*, **175**, 458.

Cohn, J. N., Khatri, I. M. and Hamosh, P. (1970), "Bedside Catheterization of the Left Ventricle," *Amer. J. Cardiol.*, **25**, 66.

Doty, D. B., Hufnagel, H. V. and Moseley, R. V. (1970), "The Distribution of Body Fluids following Hemorrhage and Resuscitation in Combat Casualties," *Surg. Gynec. Obstet.*, **130**, 453.

Edelman, I. S. (1956), "The Pathogenesis of Hyponatremia: Physiologic and Therapeutic Implications," *Metabolism*, **5**, 500.

Edelman, I. S., Leibman, J., O'Meara, M. P. and Birkenfeld, L. W. (1958), "Interrelationships between Serum Sodium Concentration, Serum Osmolarity and Total Exchangeable Sodium, Total Exchangeable Potassium and Total Body Water," *J. Clin. Invest.*, **37**, 1236.

Edelman, I. S. and Leibman, J. (1959), "The Anatomy of Body Water and Electrolytes," *Amer. J. Med.*, **27**, 256.

Frank, E. D. (1969), Editorial, "The Hazard of Interstitial Pulmonary Edema," *Ann. Surg.*, **169**, 641.

Gauer, O. H. and Henry, J. P. (1963), "The Circulatory Basis of Fluid Volume Control," *Physiol. Rev.*, **43**, 424.

Gutelius, J. R. and Shizgal, H. M. (1968), "The Effect of Trauma on Extracellular Water Volume," *Arch. Surg.*, **97**, 206.

Guyton, A. C., Scheel, K. and Murphree, D. (1966), "Interstitial Fluid Pressure. Its Effect on Resistance to Tissue Fluid Mobility," *Circ. Res.*, **19**, 412.

Hayes, M. A. (1968), "Water and Electrolyte Therapy after Operation," *New Eng. J. Med.*, **278**, 1054.

Henschel, A. (1963). In: *Thirst—First International Symposium on Thirst in the Regulation of the Body Water*. Editor: Wayner, M. J. Oxford: Pergamon Press.

Hughes-Davies, T. H. (1966). Letter: "Treatment of Hyperosmolar States in Children," *Lancet*, **1**, 822.

James, P. M. and Myers, R. T. (1972), "Central Venous Pressure Monitoring," *Ann. Surg.*, **175**, 693.

Kerrigan, G. A., Talbot, N. B. and Crawford, J. D. (1955), "Role of the Neurohypophyseal-Antidiuretic-Renal System in Everyday Clinical Medicine," *J. Clin. Endocrin.*, **15**, 265.

Mackenzie, A. I. and Donald, J. R. (1969), "Urine Output and Fluid Therapy during Anaesthesia and Surgery," *Brit. med. J.*, **3**, 619.

Moore, F. D. (1959). In: *Metabolic Care of the Surgical Patient.* Philadelphia: W. B. Saunders.

Moore, F. D. and Ball, M. R. (1952). In: *The Metabolic Response to Surgery.* Springfield, Illinois: Charles C. Thomas.

Moore, F. D. and Shires, G. T. (1967). Editorial *Moderation, Surgery*, **166**, 300.

Olmstead, E. G. (1966). In: *Mammalian Cell Water.* London: Henry Kimpton.

Schmidt-Nielsen, K. (1964). In: *Desert Animals.* Oxford: Clarendon Press.

Shires, G. T., Williams, J. and Brown, F. T. (1961), "Acute Changes in Extracellular Fluid Associated with Major Surgical Procedures," *Ann. Surg.*, **154**, 803.

Starling, E. H. (1909), *Herter Lectures*, p. 109. Chicago: W. T. Keener.

Wallace, C. K., Carpenter, C. C. J., Sack, R. B., Khanra, 6. R., Werner, A. S., Duffy, T. P., Oleinick, A. and Lewis, G. W. (1966), "Classical and El Tor Cholera: A Clinical Comparison," *Brit. med. J.*, **2**, 447.

Wilkinson, A. W. (1956), "Restriction of Fluid Intake after Partial Gastrectomy," *Lancet*, **2**, 428.

Zimmermann, B. and Wangensteen, O. H. (1952), "Observations on Water Intoxication in Surgical Patients," *Surgery*, **31**, S54.

*CHAPTER* 3

# THE SIGNIFICANCE OF ACID-BASE BALANCE

## S. A. FELDMAN

Claude Bernard postulated that in order for an animal to be independent of his environment he must be able to control his 'milieu interieur'. He was particularly concerned with the maintenance of temperature, electrolyte concentration and the tonicity of the body fluids. In recent years we have come to realize that not only is it necessary to control these physiological variables of the internal environment but it is also essential to maintain the $H^+$ ion concentration within certain very narrow limits. Failure to do so results in acidaemia or alkalaemia with serious effects on bodily function.

### Why is H⁺ Ion Important?

Undoubtedly, the most important effect of derangement of the $H^+$ ion concentration is due to its effect upon the enzyme activity in the body. Enzymatic reactions have an optimum pH at which the speed of reaction is maximum. This is strictly analogous to the optimum temperature for enzyme reactions. The speed of reaction is decreased as the $H^+$ ion concentration is altered, moving it away from the optimum pH. Thus the enzyme catalase has an optimum pH of 7·2 whilst the series of enzymes that constitute plasma pseudo-cholinesterase have an optimum pH of 8·2. As a result of the wide variation in the optimum pH of the enzyme systems in the body, an increase in the $H^+$ ion concentration will speed up some reactions whilst slowing down others. All metabolically active processes are involved and the result is metabolic chaos. Whilst cooling a patient tends to result in a fairly uniform decrease in metabolic activity, a change in pH has a more random and unpredictable effect. For this reason pH changes produce widespread effects in every active organ in the body.

pH changes will also affect the degree of ionization of partially ionized molecules. This effect will vary according to pK of the compound considered. One well documented example of this is the effect of hyperventilation on the 'free' or 'unbound' serum calcium. The lowering of the 'free' serum calcium that occurs during hyperventilation may result in spontaneous tetany. The effect on ionization will alter the degree of plasma binding of drugs. Lowering of the $H^+$ ion concentration decreases the ionization of thiopentone resulting in less being bound to plasma protein and therefore a relatively greater effective plasma concentration.

The effect of acidaemia upon the action of *d*-tubocurare has been attributed to an alteration in ionization of the phenolic hydroxyl groups with a consequent increase in receptor affinity. This explanation, based on the classical formulation of *d*-tubocurare has been challenged by Katz *et al.* (1963) on the basis that the change in charge density consequent upon an alteration in ionization would be insufficient to account for the increased potency of the drug at an increased $H^+$ ion concentration.

The activities of certain drugs are affected by changes in $H^+$ ion other than by virtue of the effect on protein binding. Some years ago Stuzman and Allen (1941) showed that adrenaline was less active in acidaemia. In a very acidaemic animal adrenaline can be administered intravenously without any change in blood pressure or pulse. If the acidaemia is rapidly corrected, as may occur when such an animal is hyperventilated, then the effect of circulating adrenaline may be revealed and cardiac arrhythmias, tachycardia and hypertension will result.

Other drugs that are directly antagonized by acidaemia, include the digitalis glycosides, the amphetamines and insulin. The antagonistic effect of excess $H^+$ ion to insulin is magnified by the depressant effect of acidaemia upon the phosphorylation enzyme system which in part accounts for the resistance that develops to insulin in diabetic acidaemia.

Acidaemia is associated with a shift of ions across the cell membrane resulting in a loss of potassium from within the cell into the extracellular fluid. This exchange will normally be reversed upon correction of the acidaemia, but may cause an excessive potassium loss in the urine. As a result of the shift of potassium, from the intracellular fluid into the extracellular fluid, the transmembrane potential will be decreased. This may produce the ECG changes typical of hyperkalaemia and an effect on the neuromuscular end plate that will be antagonistic to nondepolarizing muscle relaxants.

Acidaemia produced by the administration of $CO_2$ will produce a discharge of catechol amines from the adrenal medulla (although this effect may be reduced by certain anaesthetics). There will be an initial positive inotropic and chronotropic effect upon the heart and an increase in peripheral vascular resistance. Cardiac output, stroke volume, cardiac rate and myocardial contractility will be increased. If the acidaemia increases it ultimately reaches a point when the direct metabolic depressant effect becomes apparent and cardiac output and peripheral resistance will fall.

In addition to these general effects, changes in pH also have localized effects on the cerebral and pulmonary circulation, on smooth muscle, cardiac muscle, nervous conduction and upon renal function. The cerebral vascular resistance falls whilst the resistance to blood flow in the pulmonary circulation increases.

## Where is the 'Internal Environment?'

When one estimates pH it is usually the $H^+$ ion concentration of the plasma that is measured. Depending as it does upon the ratio of $HCO_3^-$ to $CO_2$, it is reasonable to expect the plasma $H^+$ ion concentration to reflect changes that have occurred in the pH of the extracellular fluid. It is also unlikely that it will respond rapidly and accurately to changes occurring inside the cell if these involve a change in $HCO_3^-$ ions, which are principally extracellular ions, as these ions diffuse slowly across the cell membrane. It is necessary therefore to consider whether it is the E.C.F. or the I.C.F. that constitutes the 'internal environment'. Robin (1963) considered this and concluded that as most metabolic enzyme systems reside inside the cell, adjacent to the mitochondria, the true internal environment was probably inside the phospholipid membrane of the mitochondria themselves. It is, therefore, essential when assessing the significance of any derangement of the $H^+$ ion, measured in the plasma, that it is considered how accurately this reflects the changes inside the cell. It cannot be over-emphasized that measurements of plasma pH are indirect estimations of the acid-base state of the cells themselves, which contain over one half of the total body water. One must also bear in mind the great variation in buffering capacities found in different cells; generally the most metabolically active cells, those of the liver and kidneys, have the greatest buffering capacity whilst the

more inert cells of connective tissue have less buffering potential.

## The Clinical Effects of Acidaemia

As might be predicted from a consideration of the widespread effects of $H^+$ ion derangement, acidaemia effects virtually all physiological function. It is a hazard to life by virtue of its effect upon the central nervous system, the respiratory system, the circulation and endocrine function (Brooks and Feldman, 1962).

## Control of Acid-Base Balance by the Body

As a result of ingesting a diet containing protein, the end product of metabolism will be fixed or metabolic acids. These metabolic acids are ultimately excreted by kidney and contribute to the acidity of the urine.

The major buffer systems of the body are intracellular, however, it is the less efficient extracellular bicarbonate/carbonic acid buffer, that makes the largest contribution to body $H^+$ ion homeostasis. This is the result of the rapid and usually effective physiological control exercised over this system by virtue of the body's ability to adjust its excretion of $CO_2$ by altering ventilatory exchange. The nature of the respiratory centre's response has been the subject of recent investigations. In 1961, Lambertsen *et al.*, demonstrated that when $CO_2$ was administered, 45 per cent of the ventilatory response could be accounted for by alteration in blood $H^+$ ion content. It has been demonstrated that the site of the remaining 55 per cent of the increase in ventilation is due principally to the influence of the $CO_2$ upon the pH of the csf. It follows therefore that any alteration in the buffering capacity of this fluid will profoundly affect the ventilatory $CO_2$ response. The csf bicarbonate level only changes very slowly in response to alterations in plasma levels.

Any increase in carbonic acid is rapidly diluted by its passage into the total body water. The buffering transients of the various components of this pool vary. Thus there exists the very rapid acceptance of $CO_2$ by haemoglobin to form carbamino haemoglobin—the rapidity of this reaction is such that up to one-fifth of the resting $CO_2$ production is carried in this form. Due to the presence of carbonic anhydrase within the RBC, the haemoglobin buffer system acts rapidly. Other systems especially the buffering potential of collogen and bone may not be fully equilibrated in 24 hours. As few body tissues have the buffering capacity of the RBCs *in vitro* observations made of the acid-base status of whole blood, using a $CO_2$ equilibration technique, may not reflect the actual true state of the total body fluid (Shwartz and Relman, 1965).

The body's ability to control the bicarbonate concentration is rather more limited and less rapid than its control of $CO_2$, as this ion is principally restricted to the extracellular fluid from which it can be excreted by the kidney. This is the result of limited conductance across cell membranes (with the exception of the membrane of the RBC, where its conductance equals that of chloride). Excretion of this ion by the kidney depends upon the presence of carbonic anhydrase in the cells of the renal tubules and is hindered by $Na^+$ and fluid depletion.

## Central Nervous System

Alteration of H$^+$ ion concentration from the normal $40 \times 10^{-9}$ m.mol. (pH 7·4) causes depression of cerebral function. The greater the deviation from normal the greater the effect. This is especially noticeable with increasing degrees of acidaemia. The greater the H$^+$ ion concentration the more confused and unresponsive the patient; eventually unconsciousness is produced. The effects of acidaemia on cerebral function will summate with the effects of any hypnotic or narcotic drug that the patient may have received.

In addition to the effects on higher cerebral function, there is also depression of the vasomotor and respiratory centres. The depression of respiration is clinically similar to that seen after a large overdose of morphine, slow and gasping in nature with tracheal and jaw tug during inspiration. In later stages of acidaemia respiratory arrest will occur, although there is some evidence, from experiments on dogs, to suggest that if artificial ventilation is instituted a form of spontaneous respiration will recommence at even higher H$^+$ ion levels.

## The Circulation

Acidaemia causes depression of contractility in the isolated heart, and a fall in stroke volume. In the intact animal, especially if the excess H$^+$ ion is due to hypercarbia, the depressant effect of acidaemia is initially masked by the release of endogenous catechol amines which offset the depressant effects of the H$^+$ ion and cause tachycardia, increased minute output and frequently cardiac arrhythmias. If the hypercarbia is progressive the depressant effect of the acidaemia will eventually be revealed. Although there is some experimental evidence to suggest that metabolic acidaemia also causes the release of catechol amines, its usual clinical effect is a fall in cardiac output, bradycardia and occasionally, arrhythmias.

The peripheral circulation is sluggish in acidaemia. This is due in part to the depression of the vasomotor centre but also to a direct effect upon the smooth muscle of the arteriolar walls. These actions, together with the fall in cardiac output, cause hypotension with dilated vessels and warm extremities with peripheral and central cyanosis. The hypotension responds poorly, if at all, to infusions of catechol amines.

Blood coagulation is affected by the acidaemia and it is common to observe a constant bloody ooze from cut surfaces.

## Respiration

The initial effect of acidaemia upon ventilation is to stimulate the respiratory centre and to increase gaseous exchange in the lung. This effect is largely due to a direct effect upon brain itself and is little affected by denervating the peripheral chemoreceptors. If the acidaemia is progressive, then it has been demonstrated by the administration of high inspired $CO_2$ to animals, that gasping respiration develops, followed by apnoea. These experimental observations are in keeping with clinical experience that profound acidaemia will produce central depression of

ventilation both by a direct effect on the brain and secondary to the diminished cardiac output and progressive cerebral hypoxia.

The clinical presentation of a patient with acidaemia is of an unconscious or semi-conscious person, with hypotension, warm cyanosed and commonly sweaty extremities, with full veins. Respiration is slow, gasping and associated with tracheal tug. Cardiac arrhythmias are frequent. If untreated, it is a progressive condition leading to the patient's death.

## Alkalaemia

The occurrence of temporary acute acidaemia during strenuous exercise is a common physiological occurrence whereas acute alkalaemia does not occur under normal circumstances except in the rapid ascent to heights where hyperventilation occurs as the response to the low partial pressure of oxygen. In these circumstances most people feel some discomfort, such as dizziness, nausea, blurring of vision, breathlessness and excessive fatigue. The effects of acute alkalaemia upon the bodily processes not in man have not been subject to as much attention as the effects of acidaemia. It is reasonable to assume that it will affect enzyme systems and so cause widespread disturbances of metabolic function.

## Central Nervous System

The effects of alkalaemia on cerebral function are complicated by the increase in cerebral vascular resistance that occurs when the $P_{CO_2}$ is lowered (Kety and Schmidt, 1948). As a result an effect on consciousness or cerebral function may be interpreted as either an effect of the alkalaemia or the consequence of cerebral hypoxia resulting from the diminished perfusion and the shift in the oxygen dissociation curve (Bohr effect).

## Circulation

The effect of alkalaemia is most marked upon the peripheral circulation where it produces cutaneous vasoconstriction. The sluggish blood flow through the skin may cause peripheral cyanosis associated with the stagnant hypoxia.

## Blood

Hyperventilation causes a shift of the dissociation curve to the left (Bohr effect) (Fig. 1). As a result less oxygen is available to the tissues at a given partial pressure. The result of this shift is minimal except in tissues of high metabolic activity where a relative hypoxia could be produced.

## Hyperventilation and Buffer Base

It has been shown that the long term effect of hyperventilation is to cause a loss of bicarbonate from the plasma and cerebro-spinal fluid. This is principally achieved by excreting base in the urine. As a result of this an acclimatized individual living at high altitudes has a normal $CO_2$/bicarbonate ratio and normal pH, although both the values for $P_{CO_2}$ and bicarbonate may be lower than normal.

Elkinton *et al.* (1955) demonstrated a fall in buffer base as a result of respiratory alkalaemia. This was confirmed, using artificial hyperventilation, by Papadopoulus and Keats (1959) and Bunker (1964). Some of this loss is due to a reversal of the chloride shift and a reversion of haemoglobin to a basic form, although the total loss of base is

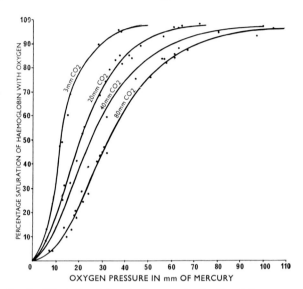

FIG. 1. Effect of variations in $P_{CO_2}$ on the $O_2$ dissociation curve.

so great that it necessitates postulating an absolute deficiency of bicarbonate. The extent of the reduction of bicarbonate depends upon the degree of hyperventilation. Explanations that have been suggested to explain this phenomenon include the existence of an intracellular compensating mechanism; the possibility that it is the result of tissue hypoxia caused by vasoconstriction and the shift in the oxygen dissociation curve, or that it is the result of disordered metabolism caused by derangement of the enzyme systems $[H]^+$ ion change.

### The Clinical Causes of $H^+$ Ion Disturbances

The $H^+$ ion concentration depends upon the ratio of $CO_2/HCO_3^-$. Acidosis exists when there is either an absolute excess of $CO_2$ or a deficit of $HCO_3^-$, alkalosis being the reverse state. If conditions are not compensated for by an adjustment of the other component of the ratio, a change in the $H^+$ ion concentration occurs and acidaemia or alkalaemia is produced.

### Respiratory Acidaemia

Acidaemia can be caused by an excess of $CO_2$ (respiratory) or a deficit of bicarbonate (metabolic). Alkalaemia can be the result of hyperventilation (respiratory) or the administration of base (metabolic). *Respiratory Acidaemia* is the result of an excess production of $CO_2$ in relation to the effective rate of removal. As alveolar ventilation is normally controlled by the respiratory centre, with exquisite sensitivity to maintain a $Pa_{CO_2}$ of 40 mm. Hg.,

respiratory acidaemia represents either a failure of respiratory control or of alveolar ventilation.

Anaesthesia inevitably causes some depression of the respiratory centre's responsiveness and a rise in $Pa_{CO_2}$. This can be demonstrated by the shift that occurs in the $CO_2$ response curve indicating that it requires a higher partial pressure of $CO_2$ to cause the same increase in alveolar ventilation. It has been shown that normal sleep is associated with a dicreased responsiveness of the respiratory centre and a rise in $Pa_{CO_2}$ to 42–44 mm. Hg. Premedication with narcotic drugs, barbiturates, volatile anaesthetics, hypoxia and acidaemia itself all cause respiratory depression, leading to respiratory acidaemia.

Depression of alveolar ventilation may be secondary to loss of sensitivity of the respiratory centre, or it may be due to inability to effect adequate alveolar exchange of $CO_2$. This may be due to many causes—such as airway obstruction, increased airway resistance, pulmonary pathology or inadequate movement of the chest wall and diaphragm; which may be the result of residual muscle paralysis.

### Metabolic Acidaemia

Metabolic acidaemia is due to a loss of base, producing a relative excess of $CO_2$ and therefore $H^+$ ion. Often there is partial respiratory compensation for a base deficit (metabolic acidosis). If this is to be effected ventilation has to be increased. The encroachment upon respiratory reserve produced by such a compensating mechanism produces a condition analogous to the limitation of respiratory reserve caused by pulmonary disease. It is for this reason that metabolic acidosis is of significance in anaesthesia as it produces the same physiological defect in the patient as pulmonary disease. For this reason any base deficit should be corrected before anaesthesia and surgery.

The usual replacement formula based upon the suggestion made by Astrup is that the number of millimols of bicarbonate administered should equal

$$\frac{\text{base deficit} \times \text{body weight kg}}{0 \cdot 3}$$

A more rational way of calculating the number of millimols of bicarbonate to be given would be

$$\text{base deficit} \times \text{distribution volume}$$

As replacement is given in the form of sodium bicarbonate the initial distribution is approximately equal to the sodium space, or about 15–18 l. for a 70 kg. man.

Base deficit is due to one of two mechanisms:

(a) Loss of base from the body,
(b) Excessive production of fixed acids.

### (a) *Loss of Base*

Bicarbonate can be lost from the body in intestinal secretions, in mucus and in urine. The commonest clinical situation producing a metabolic acidosis is chronic intestinal obstruction but it also occurs following pancreatic fistulae, mucous secreting tumours of the large bowel, chronic renal disease and as a late effect of ureteric transplantation. In these circumstances the primary loss is from E.C.F.

The administration of sodium chloride solution will, if renal function is good, result in the conservation of base and the excretion of $Cl^-$ ions. Similarly, sodium lactate infusion will provide base once the lactate has been metabolized. Both these compensatory mechanisms take time, renal compensation may take many hours or days to be complete. For this reason sodium bicarbonate should be used to prepare a patient, with metabolic acidosis, for urgent surgery.

Failure to correct the base deficit preoperatively will result in the patient developing a much wider range of alterations in the $H^+$ ion content of his blood as a result of a given change of $Pa_{CO_2}$. If his base deficit was 12 mEq./l. he would suffer a greater change in $H^+$ ion concentration than a normal patient after a given alteration of $Pa_{CO_2}$. This follows from the hydrogen ion formula (1). If the denominator ($HCO_3^-$) is reduced, the same increase in the numerator ($CO_2$) will produce a greater change in the $[H^+]$.

$$[H^+] = K^1 \frac{CO_2}{[HCO_3^-]} \times 10^{-9} \text{ m.mols.} \qquad (1)$$

### (b) Excessive Production of Fixed Acids

This usually is the result of tissue anoxia either due to too little perfusion (cardiac arrest, tourniquets, emboli, aortic clamps, hypotension, catechol amine infusions, etc.), or perfusion with blood containing too little oxygen to meet the metabolic demands (respiratory depression, apnoea or breathing hypoxic mixtures). As a result of incomplete metabolism, lactic and pyruvic acid is produced in the I.C.F. which is buffered by the bicarbonate and protein system causing a loss of base. It is important to realize that the measured plasma bicarbonate may not completely reflect the extent of the intracellular acidaemia in these patients and a total replacement of base deficit on the basis of number of mEq./l. deficit $\times$ 0·3 $\times$ body wt kg may be insufficient to correct the total base depletion. When bicarbonate is given to neutralize a fixed acid, 1 millimol of $CO_2$ will be released for every mEq. bicarbonate used. It is therefore to be expected that the $Pa_{CO_2}$ will rise during the infusion of bicarbonate and this should be corrected by hyperventilation.

Other causes of a metabolic acidosis include the rapid administration of acid citrate in the form of ACD blood, the production of keto acids in diabetic ketosis and the ingestion of excessive amounts of salicylates.

### Alkalaemia

This is usually iatrogenic and follows imposed hyperventilation (respiratory alkalaemia) or the excessive administration of alkaline solutions such as bicarbonate (metabolic alkalaemia).

Prolonged hyperventilation producing compensated respiratory alkalosis, occurs after acclimatization to high altitudes and after prolonged artificial hyperventilation. This will result in a reduction of the buffer base content of both plasma and csf. As a result of this compensatory depletion of buffer base the $H^+$ content of the blood remains normal at a lower $Pa_{CO_2}$. This will result in an excessive increase in $H^+$ ion content after quite moderate increases in $Pa_{CO_2}$ when normal ventilation is resumed, as in metabolic acidosis (vide supra). This is the probable explanation of the observation that patients in whom prolonged hyperventilation has been carried out, start breathing spontaneously at low $Pa_{CO_2}$ levels.

Metabolic alkalosis is occasionally seen as a late occurrence after massive infusions of ACD blood. The citrate having been partially metabolized in the liver produces an excess of bicarbonate and alkalamia.

### Conclusion

Some of the widespread effects of derangement of $H^+$ ion concentration have been considered. It can be seen that not only are the effects of these changes widespread but that as a result of these effects the life of the patient is endangered. Unless the stability of the $H^+$ ion concentration in the internal environment, is maintained metabolic function will be grossly deranged and the life of the patient imperilled.

### REFERENCES

Bernard, C. (1833), Lecons sur les Effets des Substances Toxiques et Medicamenteuses. Bailliere et fils, Paris.

Brackett, N. C., Cohen, J. J. and Schwartz, W. B. (1965), New Engl. J. Med., 272, 6.

Brooks, D. K. and Feldman, S. A. (1962), "Metabolic Acidosis—A New Approach to Neostigmine Resistant Curarisation," Anaesthesia, 17, 161.

Bunker, J. P. (1964), "Neuroendocrine and Other Effects of Carbohydrate Metabolism During Anesthesia," Anesthesiology, 24, 575.

Elkinton, J. R., Singer, R. B., Barker, E. S. and Clark, J. K. (1955), "Effects in Man of Respiratory Alkalosis," J. clin. Invest., 34, 1671.

Katz, R. L., Ngai, S. H. and Papper, E. M. (1963), "The Effect of Alkalosis on the Neuromuscular Blocking Agents," Anesthesiol., 24, 18.

Kety, S. S. and Schmidt, C. F. (1948), "Effect of Altered Arterial Tensions of Carbon Dioxide and Oxygen on Cerebral Blood Flow and Cerebral Oxygen Consumption of Normal Young Men," J. Clin. Invest., 27, 584.

Lambertson, C. J., Gelford, R. and Kemp, R. A. (1965), "Dynamic Response Characteristics of Several $CO_2$-reactive Components of Respiratory Control System," Cerebrospinal Fluid and the Regulation of Ventilation (Brooks, Kao and Lloyd, Eds.). Oxford: Blackwell.

Papadopoulas, C. N. and Keats, A. S. (1959), "Metabolic Acidosis of Hyperventilation Produced by Controlled Respiration," Anesthesiol., 20, 156.

Robin, E. D. (1963), "Intracellular pH. The Regulation of Human Respiration," Ed. Cunningham, D. J. and Lloyd, B. B. Blackwell.

Schwartz, W. B. and Relman, A. S. (1965), New Engl. J. Med., 272, 318.

Stutzman, J. W. and Allen, C. R. (1941), "Adrenolytic Action of Cyclopropane," Proc. Soc. Exper. Med. and Biol., 47, 218.

### FURTHER READING

Davenport, H. W. (1958), The ABC of Acid Base Chemistry. Chicago.

Nunn, J. F. (1969), Applied Respiratory Physiology. London: Butterworth.

# CHAPTER 1

# FACTORS AFFECTING THE ACTION OF DRUGS

ARIEL. F. LANT

## Introduction

With the increased complexity and sophistication of modern drug therapy, it is becoming virtually impossible for any one individual to acquire complete knowledge of the actions and potential hazards of all available therapeutic agents. This poses a particularly difficult problem for the anaesthetist, since the drugs employed in anaesthetic practice cover an unusually wide spectrum of compounds of diverse structure, physical and pharmacological properties. Although the mechanisms of action of few are explicable in molecular terms, advances made in the sphere of biochemical pharmacology in the past decade have shown that the pharmacodynamics of drug action in general are governed and often determined by certain common physicochemical principles. In this chapter, attention has been focussed on some of these fundamental principles with the aim of providing the requisite background for understanding the actions of drugs and the basis for their rational use in clinical practice.

## Drug Disposition

The ultimate purpose in administering any drug is to achieve an adequate concentration at its site or locus of action sufficient to trigger the desired pharmacological effect. After administration by whichever route, the medium of drug transfer is the plasma water, and it is through this medium that the drug arrives at its site of action or tissue receptor. Only a small proportion of the total number of drug molecules in the circulation reaches and reacts with the receptor, the absolute number depending on the relative activities of various processes which influence the concentration of free drug in the plasma.

After a drug enters the circulation, a number of fates await it. A variable proportion becomes bound to *plasma protein* and is no longer diffusible. Part is bound to *tissue structures* which have nothing to do with the specific drug effect. A small fraction reaches the site of action and reacts with the *specific receptors* (*see* p. 415). Circulating free drug is in a state of dynamic equilibrium with these three processes. The equilibrium state is, however, constantly being disturbed by loss of free drug either by excretion of the unchanged molecule or as metabolites formed by processes of metabolic transformation and conjugation.

It is clear that from the time of administration till its ultimate elimination from the body the state of distribution of a drug at any given time is dependent on the relative activities of the processes of plasma and tissue binding, metabolism and excretion depicted in Fig. 1.

Furthermore, participation in these various processes involves either directly or indirectly the crossing of a succession of membrane barriers. These barriers range from rather simple membranes like the blood capillary and red cell to the complex multicellular barriers of the gastric mucosa, intestinal and renal tubular epithelia. It is, therefore, important to consider the mechanisms whereby drugs traverse body membranes and the physico-chemical properties of molecules and membranes that characterize these transport processes.

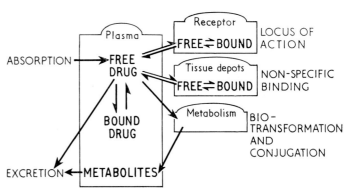

Fig. 1. Schematic representation of the factors which influence the plasma concentration of a drug.

## Passage of Drugs across Cell Membranes

**Membrane Structure** (Conference on Biological Membranes, 1966; Whittaker, 1968; Korn, 1969)

Natural membranes can be broadly classified into two groups: those which surround individual cells (plasma membranes) and those which surround subcellular structures (cytoplasmic membranes such as the endoplasmic reticulum and the envelopes enclosing intracellular organelles). Although there may be considerable individual variations in structural detail, the general picture which has emerged from chemical, X-ray diffraction and electron microscopic studies is of a basically similar architecture for all cell membranes. This consists of a bimolecular layer of lipid molecules covered with an adsorbed monolayer of protein on both sides, the long axes of the lipids being perpendicularly orientated in relation to the membrane surface. The thickness of the membrane is of the order of 75–100Å. The question of whether body membranes consist of a continuous lipid barrier or a discontinuous lipid mosaic interspersed with aqueous channels or 'pores' remains a controversial issue. The presence of 'pores' seems necessary to account for the ready passage of water and small lipid insoluble molecules and ions across the membrane. This is particularly so for the blood capillary membrane which behaves as a typical 'lipoid-pore' barrier; lipid-soluble substances penetrate readily at a rate determined by their lipid/water partition coefficients, whilst water-soluble substances penetrate less readily at rates determined by molecular size and electrical charge. However, whereas lipid-soluble substances appear to traverse the entire capillary surface, even the smallest hydrophilic molecules (including water) behave as though only a small fraction (about 0·2 per cent) of the total cross-sectional area of the capillary surface was available for transfer. Such behaviour is consistent with the belief that membrane structure incorporates a system of pores, and studies of comparative permeability to various substances have allowed measurements to be derived of equivalent pore radii of different natural membranes. However, thus far it has not proved possible to visualize pores with certainty even with the high resolving power of the electron microscope.

**Transport Mechanisms** (Schanker, 1962; 1964; Whittam, 1964; Curran and Schultz, 1968)

There are two general mechanisms whereby drugs cross membranes: (a) passive transfer, in which the membrane behaves as an inert system through which the drug passes; (b) specialized transport, in which the membrane plays an active role in the process of transferring the drug through it.

**Passive Transfer**

**Simple diffusion and filtration.** Most drugs cross membranes by *simple diffusion* where the rate of transfer is proportional to the concentration gradient across the membrane, and the driving force is thermal agitation of the molecules in accordance with Fick's law. As well as being related to surface area and thickness of the membrane, the speed of transfer is also determined by inherent properties of the drug such as its molecular size, spatial configuration, degree of ionization if it is an electrolyte and lipid solubility. In general, substances of low molecular weight diffuse readily, but as size increases, the lipid solubility of the molecule becomes more important. The significance of lipid solubility was first emphasized by the work of Overton (1899) who showed that the permeability of membranes to lipid-soluble molecules increased as the molecule became more soluble in non-polar solvents. The subsequent finding that the potency of various inhalational anaesthetics correlated with their oil/water partition coefficients formed the basis of the 'lipid solubility' theory of anaesthesia (Meyer-Overton). However, correspondence between lipid solubility and anaesthetic potency does not necessarily imply a cause and effect relationship and may represent a phenomenon quite distinct from the fundamental mechanism of action of general anaesthetics at a cellular or molecular level. There is no doubt, however, that in the case of most drugs, lipid solubility is a major determinant in the ability to penetrate the cell membrane. It is of particular importance in relation to those drugs which undergo partial ionization at body pH, for membrane permeability to the non-

ionized form of a weak electrolyte is very much greater than to the ionic form. Indeed the membrane can be regarded as virtually impermeable to the latter. The amount of drug present in the lipid-soluble unionized form is a function of the dissociation constant of the native molecule and the pH of the fluid in which it is dissolved (*vide infra*).

On the other hand, a number of lipid insoluble substances cross a membrane as if it were a fine sieve, smaller molecules and ions crossing faster than larger ones to an extent not affected by pH. Presence of a system of 'pores' or polar discontinuities in the lipoprotein barrier offers a means whereby such hydrophilic substances can cross the membrane. Although "pores" have not been visualized with certainty even with the electron microscope, their presence has been inferred from studies of comparative membrane permeability to various substances and their average size can be expressed mathematically in the form of an "equivalent pore radius." Small lipid-insoluble molecules may diffuse directly through aqueous-filled pores, or when a hydrostatic or osmotic pressure difference exists across the membrane, the flow of water in bulk through the "pores" may drag with it any solute molecules whose dimensions are small enough to penetrate the 'pores.' This process has been called 'solvent drag.' A figure of about 4Å is representative of the equivalent pore radius of the plasma membrane of most cells and thus penetration by pore filtration is restricted to substances, whose molecular radius in at least one dimension is less than 4Å. Thus urea (MW 60), with an equivalent radius of 1·6Å, passes readily across cell membranes. Most drug molecules have radii considerably larger than this and filtration by pores is, therefore, of minor importance as a route of cell entry for drugs. Attempts to correlate molecular and pore sizes may be misleading, for example in the case of penetration of membranes by ions. The volume of an ion may be much larger than indicated by molecular weight on account of hydration. Furthermore, with some ions transfer may be more dependent on charge than size. For example, although the size of the hydrated ions of $K^+$ and $Cl^-$ is about the same, the permeability of the red cell membrane to $Cl^-$ is very much greater than to $K^+$.

The situation is different in the case of certain body membranes such as the sheet-like structures formed by the epithelial cells of blood and glomerular capillaries. Although these membranes possess the lipoidal characteristics of the membranes of their constituent cells, the sheets of cells do not fit together tightly with the result that the effective pore size may be as high as 30Å in radius. The result is that these membranes are highly 'porous' and most drugs pass from one side to the other with relative ease. Plasma albumin (MW 69,000) is borderline in size and tends to be restrained by the normal capillary and glomerular membranes as are molecules of drug which are albumin-bound.

**Diffusion and drug ionization** (Albert, 1952; Brodie and Hogben, 1957; Schanker, 1963; Brodie, 1964a). The majority of drugs are weak electrolytes capable of undergoing ionization in aqueous solution. The cell membrane is preferentially permeable to the lipid-soluble non-ionized form but resists penetration of the water-soluble ionized form. The extent of ionization of a drug is a function of its dissociation constant and the pH of the surrounding solution. By international convention, the dissociation constants for both acids and bases are expressed on the same scale in the form of $K_a$. Because these constants are small, it is more convenient to use the expression $pK_a$, which represents the negative logarithm of the dissociation constant. The $pK_a$ scale is analogous to pH notation and provides a useful way of comparing the strengths of acids and bases. The stronger an acid, the lower its $pK_a$, the stronger a base, the higher its $pK_a$ (Fig. 2).

The relationship between $pK_a$ and the proportion of total drug which has undergone ionization can be represented by the Henderson–Hasselbalch equation which results from application of the law of mass action.

$$\text{For a weak acid, } pH - pK_a = \log \frac{\text{(ionized form)}}{\text{(unionized form)}}$$

$$\text{For a weak base, } pH - pK_a = \log \frac{\text{(unionized form)}}{\text{(ionized form)}}$$

At 50 per cent ionization, the logarithmic fraction equals unity and $pH = pK_a$. If $C_I$ and $C_{II}$ are the concentrations of total drug on sides I and II of a biomembrane, the ratio $R = C_I/C_{II}$, can be expressed in the following form:

$$\text{For a weak acid, } R = \frac{1 + \text{antilog } (pH_I - pK_a)}{1 + \text{antilog } (pH_{II} - pK_a)}$$

$$\text{For a weak base, } R = \frac{1 + \text{antilog } (pK_a - pH_I)}{1 + \text{antilog } (pK_a - pH_{II})}$$

From these relationships, it is clear that a small change in pH can make a large change in the extent of ionization, particularly if the values of $pK_a$ and pH lie close together. The pH partition hypothesis can be employed to calculate the theoretical distribution of drugs across various body membranes where distinct pH differences are known to exist in the media bathing either side of the membrane. Thus there is an unequal distribution of weak acids and bases between the highly acid gastric juice and plasma with its pH close to neutral. In the stomach, strong acids with $pK_a$ less than 1 are largely in ionized form and are not absorbed. Drugs of weaker acidity such as salicylates ($pK_a$ 3·0–3·5) or barbiturates ($pK_a$ 7·5–7·9)

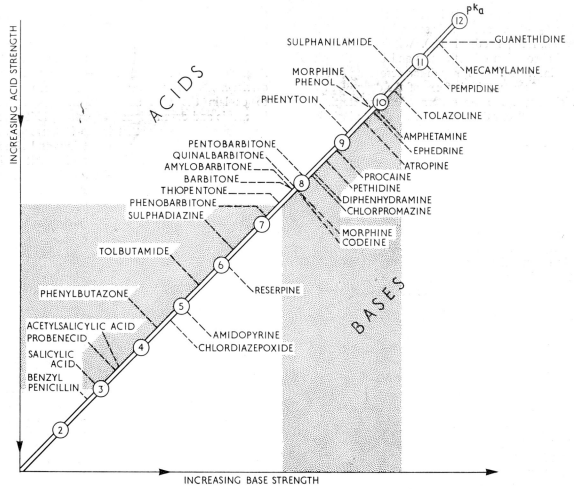

Fig. 2. $pK_a$ values of some commonly used drugs. The shaded areas represent the ranges of $pK_a$ for weak acids (3·0–7·5) and weak bases (7·5–10·5) whose urinary excretion displays the phenomenon of pH-dependence. Values have been obtained from Brodie and Hogben (1957); Schanker et al. (1957); Anton (1961); Brodie (1964a); Gosselin and Smith (1966); Hart, Guarino and Schanker (1969).

exist as unionized molecules which, being lipid soluble, are readily absorbed. Alkalinization of the stomach contents by addition of $NaHCO_3$, decreases the absorption of salicylate through conversion of a large part of the drug to the ionized form whereas a drug like thiopentone ($pK_a$ 7·6) is but little affected by increase in pH since even at pH 8 it is largely in nonionized form. On the other hand absorption of weak bases can be markedly increased when stomach contents are neutralized (Brodie, 1964a). Absorption from the intestine resembles that from the stomach in that there is rapid penetration by lipid-soluble non-ionized molecules. Passage of drugs across the mucosa is dictated to a considerable extent by the $pK_a$ and the differential pH gradient. It is the gradient between the pH at the absorbing (membrane) surface and plasma rather than that existing between plasma and the bulk contents within the lumen which determines the degree to which ionization affects absorption. Experimental work has shown that the pH in the immediate environment of the intestinal mucosa is about 5·3, a value somewhat more acidic than that usually associated with intestinal contents. Strong acids and bases are present in both intestine and plasma mainly in ionized form and are poorly absorbed.

In general, there is negligible intestinal absorption of acids with $pK_a < 2·5$ and of bases with $pK_a > 8·5$ (Schanker et al., 1958; Brodie, 1964a). Within these limits there is good absorption of both acids and bases though the extent in individual cases may differ according to the lipid solubility of the non-ionic form of the drug. Other factors which may make the pattern of gastrointestinal absorption deviate from that predicted by theory include variations in blood supply and motility of the gut, viscosity and pH of secretions as well as drug formulation.

Degree of ionization and the lipid-solubility of the unionized drug moiety play a major role in determining the rate at which many drugs penetrate into the C.S.F. and brain. The blood-brain and blood-C.S.F. boundaries which comprise the 'blood brain barrier' behave basically like other lipid biomembranes. Drugs with very high lipid solubility such as the anaesthetic gases diffuse across freely to an extent limited not by lipid solubility but almost entirely by rates of blood flow. In the case of more polar compounds, however, the role of ionization becomes increasingly important. Because there is only a very small pH gradient between plasma and C.S.F. (the pH of the latter normally being 0·1 unit less than plasma), distribution of drugs between the two compartments is largely a function of $pK_a$ and the lipid solubility of the undissociated molecules present. The degree of binding of drug to plasma protein is also critical because the rate of diffusion across a membrane is proportional to the *unbound* and not *total* concentration of drug in the plasma (*see* p. 412).

Realization of the important roles of lipid solubility and extent of ionization which underlie the pH-partition hypothesis have provided much insight into the mechanisms whereby drugs penetrate cell boundaries. It has become clear that alterations in extracellular pH, whether of respiratory or metabolic origin, can have far-reaching consequences on the biological efficacy of any drug which undergoes ionization in body fluids, for distribution of drug, ability to attain equilibrium at the tissue site of action, metabolism and elimination may all be profoundly affected.

The special role of the renal tubular epithelium in relation to drug elimination will be considered later.

**Specialized Transport** (Hoffman, 1964; Skou, 1965; Csáky, 1965; Heinz, 1967; Neame and Richards, 1972).

A number of naturally-occurring non-electrolytes are readily transported across cell membranes under physiological conditions although they are too large to traverse 'pores' and too polar to dissolve in the lipid biophase. In some cases, a remarkable degree of stereospecificity of the membrane exists as for example in the selective intestinal absorption of l-amino acids as compared to their d-enantiomorphs (Wiseman, 1968). Such lipid-insoluble materials are believed to traverse the membrane by a specialized transport system which involves the formation of a complex with a 'carrier' in the membrane. 'Carriers' are pictured as membrane components which combine with substrate at one surface of the membrane, the complex then moves across the membrane under its own diffusion gradient, substrate is released and the carrier returns to the original surface for another trip. Ussing (1952) has suggested the analogy of the ferry boat. A considerable literature has developed on the subject of carrier-mediated transport which has been extended also to explain the transmembrane movements of certain inorganic and organic ions (Robertson, 1968). It must be emphasized, however, that in no instance has a carrier substance been isolated with certainty and although it is likely to be lipoprotein in composition, its existence is still speculative (*see* Wilbrandt and Rosenberg, 1961; Pardee, 1968; Wasserman, Corradino and Taylor, 1969).

At least three types of carrier-mediated transport are recognized:

(a) **Active transport.** If the substrate molecule is moved against a concentration gradient or, in the case of an ion, against an electrochemical gradient, chemical energy is needed and the process is called 'active transport'. The maximum rate of carrier-mediated transport is limited by the concentration of carrier molecules in the membrane. The transport system can become saturated with substrate if the concentration of substrate molecules is high enough, formation and breakdown of the carrier-substrate complex within the membrane following Michaelis-Menten kinetics (*see* p. 416). In many cases, the system displays a high degree of structural- and stereo-specificity for chemical configuration. If two substances of similar chemical structure are transported, one will competitively inhibit the other. Because active transport is 'uphill transport', and requires the expenditure of cellular energy, it can be blocked by metabolic inhibitors. The details of how the chemical reactions of cellular metabolism are coupled to the transport mechanism are not fully understood. Active transport systems are widely distributed in living tissues. An example of an active transport system of considerable significance is the 'sodium pump' found within cell membranes. It uses energy from the hydrolysis of adenosine triphosphate (ATP) to expel Na and accumulate K and is responsible for maintaining the low concentration of Na and high concentration of K found in most body cells (see Fig. 3). At least two separate transport systems

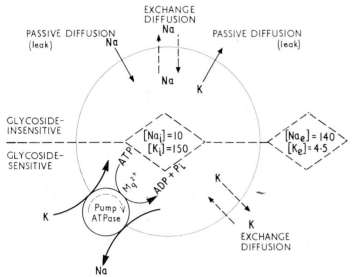

Fig. 3. Diagrammatic representation of the interrelationships between active and passive cation movements in cells and the sensitivity of ion fluxes to the inhibitory effects of cardiac glycosides. Cell volume and cation content are kept constant by the balance which normally exists between the downhill movements of passive diffusion (leak) and the active transport of Na and K via the sodium pump in the membrane. The curved arrows connected by the circle represent the active ion fluxes which oppose the attainment of diffusion equilibrium. The outward pumping of Na is linked to the inward pumping of K. The glycoside-sensitive, $Mg^{2+}$, $Na^+$, $K^+$—ATPase, located in the cell membrane either constitutes the pump or is a major component of its mechanism (see Skou, 1965; Glynn, 1968; Lant, Priestland and Whittam, 1970). ATP = adenosine triphosphate; ADP = adenosine diphosphate; $P_i$ = inorganic phosphate; $[Na_i]$, $[K_i]$ = intracellular Na and K concentrations (mmol/kg. intracellular water); $[Na_e]$, $[K_e]$ = extracellular Na and K concentrations (mmol/l.).

have been discovered in renal tubular epithelium which are energy-dependent and fulfil the criteria for processes of active transport. However, judging from the wide heterogeneity of chemical substances which can be handled, these systems appear to lack any clear structural requirements as to substrate configuration (Weiner and Mudge, 1964).

A few synthetic drugs are absorbed from the intestine by an active transport mechanism because they closely resemble natural substrates. An example is the antihypertensive agent, α-methyldopa, which is structurally related to phenylalanine (Young and Edwards, 1966).

(b) **Facilitated diffusion.** This term is applied to carrier-mediated transport in which the substrate moves down a concentration gradient just as in the case of simple diffusion but considerably faster than by the latter process alone. Thus, for example, glucose readily traverses the red cell membrane attaining the same concentration inside as on the outside, by a process which displays specificity,

saturability and sensitivity to certain metabolic inhibitors (LeFevre, 1961). A number of volatile anaesthetics compete with monosaccharides for the carrier within the red cell membrane and it is possible that these agents may therefore traverse the membrane both by simple and facilitated diffusion (Greene and Webb, 1969).

(c) **Exchange diffusion.** This term describes the transport system in which the carrier complex moves the substrate from one surface of the membrane to the opposite and, after releasing the substrate, reacts with another molecule of substrate which it then returns to the original surface (Ussing, 1949). No net movements of substrate occur by this route. An example would be the rapid exchange between substrate and its isotope placed on either side of a membrane (see also Ussing, 1960; Glynn, Hoffman and Lew, 1971).

### Pinocytosis and Phagocytosis

This is the process by which cells engulf small drops of the external medium and occurs classically in amoebae and mammalian macrophages (Holter, 1962; Gosselin, 1967). The mammalian intestinal mucosa may engulf fat droplets and perhaps other large molecules in this way (Palay and Karlin, 1959). The absorption of cyanocobalamin-intrinsic factor complex in the ileum may involve pinocytosis (Mackenzie and Donaldson, 1969) but whether such a process affects drug absorption in general to any significant extent is unknown.

### Drug Transfer across Specialized Membranes

**Blood-brain Barrier** (Davson, 1960; Rall et al., 1961; Bradbury and Davson, 1964; Schanker, 1965; Davson, 1967; Lajtha and Ford, 1968)

The resistance of the brain and C.S.F. to penetration by various substances led to the formulation of the concept of a 'blood-brain barrier'. In recent years, it has become clear that the boundaries between blood and brain and blood and C.S.F., though differing anatomically, behave in an analogous manner to other lipoidal plasma membranes with regard to their permeability to drugs. The blood-brain barrier consists essentially of the blood capillary wall and a surrounding layer of glial cells closely applied to the basement membrane of capillary endothelium. Because of this investment of the brain capillaries by a cellular sheath, their permeability characteristics are closer to those of the plasma membranes of cells rather than the more porous structure of capillary endothelium. The blood-C.S.F. boundary consists mainly of the epithelium of the choroid plexus. The blood-brain and blood-C.S.F. boundaries resist the entrance of highly ionized compounds such as quaternary ammonium derivatives like d-tubocurarine or gallamine. With drugs that undergo only partial ionization at plasma pH, penetration rates are proportional to the lipid/water partition coefficient of the unionized molecules, allowing for variations in the individual degrees of binding to plasma protein (Brodie, Kurz and Schanker, 1960). Highly lipid soluble drugs such as the inhalation anaesthetics enter the brain so rapidly that barriers to diffusion are not demonstrable and blood flow becomes the main rate-limiting factor. A less obvious example of high lipid solubility affecting the onset and duration of drug action is the behaviour of thiopentone as an intravenous anaesthetic agent. Thiopentone is largely non-ionic at plasma pH and has a very high partition coefficient. Its oxygen homologue, pentobarbitone, is even less ionized at pH 7·4 and is much less protein-bound, but because of the low partition coefficient of the non-ionized form, its penetration is very slow. The low lipid solubility of barbitone is also responsible for its slow penetration despite a negligible degree of protein binding and similar degree of ionization

possible routes whereby lipid-insoluble compounds may leave the C.S.F. First, they may be swept out via the valve-like structures of the arachnoid villi as C.S.F. drains in bulk from the subarachnoid space to the dural blood sinuses. The porosity of these villi is so great that a small molecule like mannitol and a large molecule like albumin flow out at similar rates (Prockop, Schanker and Brodie, 1961). Second, the epithelium of the choroid plexuses offers an alternative exit route. Available evidence indicates the presence in the choroidal cells of two distinct active transport mechanisms, one pumping out organic anions and the other cations. These specialized transport

## TABLE 1

COMPARISON OF THE STRUCTURES AND PHYSICOCHEMICAL PROPERTIES OF THREE BARBITURATE DERIVATIVES

| Drug | X | Y | Z | $pK_a$ | Fraction non-ionized at pH 7·4 | Fraction bound to plasma protein at pH 7·4 | Partition coefficient (n-heptane/water) of non-ionized form |
|---|---|---|---|---|---|---|---|
| Thiopentone | $-CH_2-CH_3$ | $-CH-(CH_2)_2-CH_3$ with $CH_3$ | $=S$ | 7·6 | 0·61 | 0·75 | 3·30 |
| Pentobarbitone | $-CH_2-CH_3$ | $-CH-(CH_2)_2-CH_3$ with $CH_3$ | $=O$ | 8·1 | 0·83 | 0·40 | 0·05 |
| Barbitone | $-CH_2-CH_3$ | $-CH_2-CH_3$ | $=O$ | 7·5 | 0·56 | <0·02 | <0·002 |

Data from Hogben et al. (1959) and Brodie, Kurz and Schanker (1960).

to thiopentone (Table 1). Thus, for any weak electrolyte to act upon the central nervous system, it should have a suitable combination of the following properties which will allow ready penetration of the blood-brain barrier: low ionization at plasma pH; low binding to plasma protein and a fairly high lipid-water partition coefficient. Increase in the degree of ionization by deliberate molecular modification may hinder passage of drugs across the blood-brain barrier. (For example, atropine and physostigmine (eserine) are tertiary amines which penetrate brain tissue readily whilst their quaternarized derivatives, atropine methyl sulphate and neostigmine are more highly ionized and are effectively excluded from the central nervous sytem. The latter drugs have the advantages of evoking the same autonomic effects in the periphery as the parent molecules from which they are derived, but their parenteral use is free from the complications of central effects. The boundary, consisting of ependyma and pia which separates brain and C.S.F., has a high degree of permeability so that diffusion of most molecules, including lipid insoluble compounds, is essentially unrestricted (Lanman and Schanker, 1965).

Unlike entry of drugs into the central nervous system, passage of drugs out of the C.S.F. is less dependent on lipid solubility and extent of ionization. There are two

mechanisms appear to function separately, a situation analogous to that occurring in the renal tubular epithelium (see later).

**Placenta** (Ginsburg and Jeacock, 1964; Moya, 1965; Moya and Smith, 1965; Villee, 1965; Smithells and Morgan, 1970; Burt, 1971; Ginsburg, 1971).

Although there has been a considerable interest in recent years in the potential teratogenicity of drug therapy in pregnancy, surprisingly little is known of the mechanisms governing transplacental passage of drugs. It has become clear that it is an over-simplification to regard the placenta as a homogeneous semi-permeable barrier although the features of drug transfer do, in many cases, parallel those of other lipid biomembranes. The situation is, however, complicated by the extensive anatomical and physiological changes which the placenta undergoes in the course of development. The mature placenta is a remarkably active organ which is not only capable of transporting many substances of physiological importance, but also possesses organized enzyme systems capable of synthesizing hormones such as gonadotrophin, oestrogens and progesterone. Because of the understandable technical difficulties involved, there is extremely little quantitative information on the kinetics of drug penetration of the placenta at different stages of pregnancy. Nevertheless, the concept of the blood-placenta barrier as a modified lipid membrane has gained ground from the behaviour of drugs with differing degrees of ionization and lipid solubility. Drugs with high degrees of ionization and low lipid solubility such as the quaternary ammonium neuromuscular blocking drugs, apparently penetrate poorly, whilst drugs that are fat soluble at physiological pH penetrate almost instantaneously (Moya and Thorndike, 1962, 1963). Thus, for example, thiopentone attains rapid equilibrium with foetal blood as do the inhalational anaesthetics. Other drugs known to traverse the placental barrier include narcotic analgesics of the opiate group (Beckett and Taylor, 1972), phenothiazine derivatives, sulphonamides. Local anaesthetics such as lignocaine, bupivacaine or mepivacaine, whether given in labour by the epidural, caudal or paracervical routes, cross the placenta without difficulty and may cause dose-related bradycardia in the foetus (Rosefsky and Petersiel, 1968; Shnider and Way, 1968; Reynolds and Taylor, 1971). Various antibiotics including penicillins, cephalosporins tetracyclines, the aminoglycoside and macrolide derivatives, cross the placenta, but rather slowly and at varying rates. The gradient of drug achieved across the placenta is primarily a function of the amount administered to the mother. However, other factors such as distribution in the maternal and foetal extracellular spaces, metabolism and excretion in the mother, infant and placenta and also maternal and foetal blood flow rates are of importance. The speed of maternal-foetal equilibration is also influenced by the degree of binding to plasma proteins because binding can clearly occur on either side of the placenta. The foetal plasma proteins act as a reservoir for drug molecules after they cross the placenta in free form and the speed of equilibration can be retarded particularly in cases where the process of diffusion is rate-limiting. The inhalational anaesthetics diffuse and equilibrate very rapidly, the rate of equilibration being limited more by variations in placental blood flow than by protein-binding.

Pathological changes in the placenta secondary to hypoxia, hypertension, dehydration, etc., can all affect the selectivity of the membrane barriers and alter the efficacy of the protective mechanism which nature has provided for the foetus (see also Sect. 5, Ch. IIA—Placental Circulation). This is specially important in the newborn since it is placed in a vulnerable state by having immature and inefficient drug-metabolizing and detoxifying systems (see later). More systematic studies of drug transfer kinetics across the placenta are needed before firm conclusions can be drawn and predictions made as to the safety of drugs administered during various stages of gestation, during labour and at delivery.

## Binding of Drugs and Molecular Mechanisms of Drug Action

### Plasma-protein Binding

Within the vascular compartment, a variable proportion of the drug is reversibly bound to plasma proteins. Only the free or unbound drug is diffusible and pharmacologically active. For this reason, to speak of the 'plasma level' of a drug has only limited meaning. The value of functional significance is the *unbound* component. The protein most generally involved in drug-binding is albumin, a single chain peptide structure with a non-specific reactivity for binding a variety of drugs. The muscle relaxant *d*-tubocurarine is somewhat of an exception in that it appears to bind predominantly to gamma globulin (Stovner, Theodorsen and Bjelke, 1971a).

### Nature of Binding Forces

Although the subject of much study, the detailed mechanisms reponsible for holding drugs in combination with protein remain obscure. The major physicochemical forces which may be involved in binding are as follows:

**1. Attractive forces. (a) Covalent bonding.** This is the familiar strong bond which holds together the carbon atoms of organic molecules (Pauling, 1960). It is formed by sharing of a pair of electrons by two atoms and has a bond energy of about 40 to 200 kcals/mole. Such bonding is usually irreversible at ordinary temperatures unless enzymatic cleavage is involved. Because of its high stability, the covalent bond plays little part in the readily reversible binding of drugs to protein. It may have an important role in reaction mechanisms which involve the formation of unusually stable complexes such as, for example, the inactivation of cholinesterase by organophosphate insecticides (Hobbiger, 1968).

**(b) Electrostatic or ionic binding.** This arises from electrostatic attraction between oppositely charged particles. Electrons of one atom are transferred to a different atom. The bond strength is of the order of 4 to 6 kcals/mole. Combination of acidic or basic drugs which undergo ionization at plasma pH may bind in this way to oppositely charged sites on the protein molecule.

**(c) Hydrogen bonding.** The hydrogen nucleus, a proton, has a strong electropositive nature. It is able to accept readily an electron pair in part from each of two electron donor atoms such as oxygen, nitrogen or fluorine and forms a bridge approximately 3 Å long between them. The bond strength ranges between 2 and 7 kcals/mole. Water, by its chemical nature, can readily form hydrogen bonds both by its constituent H and O atoms.

**(d) Hydrophobic bonding.** This type of bonding represents an interaction between non-polar molecules or groups and the aqueous environment. Formation of hydrophobic bonds is associated with a decrease in entropy implying that some more ordered structure has been formed. It is believed that a layer of 'structured' or 'icelike' water forms either round the drug molecule or in the immediate proximity of the binding protein. Dissolution of this 'iceberg' when drug and binding-protein meet may contribute to the free energy of hydrophobic binding. A characteristic of this type of binding is its lack of high structural specificity on the part of the involved molecules. There has been considerable interest in the role which changes in water structure in the vicinity of nonpolar binding-sites in protein or other tissue macromolecules may play in the molecular mechanism of anaesthesia.

**(e) Van der Waals forces.** These represent short-range attractive forces which develop whenever two atoms approach each other closely. They are in essence the result of slight distortions in the electron clouds surrounding each nucleus. The bond energy is only 0·5–2·0 kcals/mole but in the case of close-fitting groups of atoms or molecules, such forces may become sizeable and cause the groups to cling together. At least three different types, named Keesom, Debye and London forces respectively, have been distinguished as components of this group (Featherstone, 1968).

**2. Repulsive forces. (a) Ionic and dipole repulsions.** Clearly, where similarly charged chemical groups come close together, a decrease in drug-protein binding interaction is to be expected. The repulsive Born force comes into this category.

**(b) Steric hindrance.** This refers to certain three-dimensional characteristics of chemical structure such as the orientation of certain radicals or the inflexibility of certain bonds to distortion, which influence the overall reactivity of a drug molecule. Certain variations in molecular architecture may thus hinder the ability of substances to bind with protein or other macromolecules.

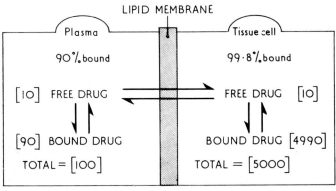

Fig. 4. Theoretical steady-state distribution between a tissue cell and plasma of a drug such as chlorpromazine which has a higher binding affinity for intracellular protein than for plasma albumin. Only the unbound moiety equilibrates across the membrane.

### Extent of protein-binding

It is evident that for binding to be reversible, the tertiary structure of the binding protein must remain intact. The overall extent of drug-protein binding depends on the concentration of drug, the capacity and number of sites for interaction and the affinity of the drug for them (Fig. 4). Although the detailed mechanisms involved in binding are not fully understood, it is probable that several of the binding forces considered above are involved together in the process. In some cases, the degree of binding is considerable as, for example, has been found with iodinated derivatives of β-phenylpropionic acid ($C_6H_5 \cdot CH_2 \cdot CH_2 \cdot COOH$); the compound hydroxy-triiodo-ethyl-cinnamic acid was used at one time as a contrast medium in diagnostic cholecystography. The half-life of the albumin complex of this drug is about 2·5 years (Astwood, 1957). In other instances, hardly any protein-binding occurs as, for example, in the case of the pyrazolone analgesic,

antipyrine (Brodie, Kurz and Schanker, 1960) or the nondepolarizing muscle relaxant, pancuronium (Stovner, Theodorsen and Bjelke, 1971b). Protein-binding of drugs may be impaired in certain disease states; thus, for example, the binding of phenytoin to plasma albumin is decreased in uraemia (Reidenberg et al., 1971).

### Protein-binding and Volatile Anaesthetics

Volatile anaesthetics have a greater solubility in plasma and whole blood than can be accounted for by their lipid or water solubility alone. This has directed attention to possible interactions with circulating proteins such as albumin and haemoglobin (Featherstone, 1963; Featherstone and Schoenborn, 1964). Binding to fixed protein or other macromolecular components of tissue cells may also play an important role in the mechanisms of anaesthesia at a molecular level (Featherstone and Muehlbaecher, 1963). Experimental work on the association of volatile anaesthetics with various protein molecules including haemoglobin and myoglobin has shown that this interaction occurs without the anaesthetic undergoing any chemical change and that under physiological conditions, ionic or covalent bonds are not involved. Available evidence points to this being a triple association involving anaesthetic, water and protein molecules. These appear to be held together by the concerted effects of hydrogen bonding, hydrophobic bonding and Van der Waals forces, though the precise details of the binding mechanism have not been worked out yet (Keyes and Lumry, 1968; Schoenborn, 1968).

**Kinetics of binding** (Goldstein, 1949; Martin, 1965; Meyer and Guttman, 1968).

The interaction of a drug $D$ with the unoccupied binding sites of a protein $P$ can be considered as a reversible reaction obeying the law of mass action:

$$[D] + [P] \underset{k_2}{\overset{k_1}{\rightleftharpoons}} [DP]$$

drug     protein     drug-protein complex

where $k_1$ and $k_2$ are the rates of forward and reverse reactions respectively and $DP$ is the drug-protein complex.

At equilibrium, the forward and reverse reactions are equal and

$$\frac{[D] \cdot [P]}{[DP]} = K_D \qquad (1)$$

where $K_D$ equals the dissociation constant.

If the drug is able to combine with a certain number of binding sites, $n$, on each protein molecule, the total number of these sites equals $n[P_T]$ where $[P_T]$ equals the total concentration of protein.

It follows that $n[P_T] = [P] + [DP]$

$$\therefore \quad \frac{[D]\{n[P_T] - [DP]\}}{[DP]} = K_D$$

$$[D] \cdot n[P_T] - [D] \cdot [DP] = K_D \cdot [DP]$$

and

$$\frac{[DP]}{n[P_T]} = \frac{[D]}{[D] + K_D} \qquad (2)$$

If $F$ equals the fraction, ratio of bound drug to total number of drug molecules, then by definition

$$F = \frac{[DP]}{[DP] + [D]} = \frac{1}{1 + \frac{[D]}{[DP]}}$$

However, it has been shown above that

$$[DP] = \frac{n[P_T] \cdot [D]}{[D] + K_D}$$

$$\therefore \quad F = \frac{1}{1 + \frac{K_D}{n[P_T]} + \frac{[D]}{n[P_T]}} = \frac{[P_T]}{[P_T] + \frac{K_D}{n} + \frac{[D]}{n}} \quad (3)$$

From this equation, it is evident that since in plasma, $P_T$ is fixed, and $n$ and $K_D$ are determined by the particular drug under consideration, the fraction of bound drug becomes inversely related to the concentration of drug $[D]$, the terms $K_D/n[P_T]$ and $n[PT]$ being invariant. At sufficiently high concentrations, all drugs saturate the binding sites; if the concentration is increased further, additional drug is free, and $F$ decreases toward zero. Although at such concentration levels the maximum amount of drug is bound, this still represents only a very small fraction of total drug. As the drug concentration $[D]$ declines, for example through processes of elimination from the body, $F$ tends to increase. If the binding affinity is very high ($K_D$ very low) and provided the number of binding sites is high enough, practically all the drug present will be bound and $F$ approaches unity.

## Structural Requirements for Binding

There appears to be no correlation between chemical structure and the extent and stability of binding to plasma protein such as albumin. Binding occurs with a diversity of drugs ranging from single anions and cations to complex aromatic and heterocyclic compounds. It also occurs with hydrophilic as well as lipid-soluble substances. Increase in lipid solubility, however, is associated with increase in degree of protein binding, and this suggests that hydrophobic forces may be of importance. Thus, thiopentone is more lipid soluble than its oxygen analogue pentobarbitone and is also more highly bound to plasma albumin (see Table 1).

The lowered polarity resulting from ethyl and allyl quaternarization of the nitrogen atoms in the molecules of gallamine and alcuronium may account for the higher binding affinity of these muscle relaxants for plasma albumin as compared with $d$-tubocurarine. The latter compound binds preferentially to globulin and this behaviour has been ascribed to greater hydrophilic nature associated with presence in the molecule of $d$-tubocurarine of two free phenolic hydroxyl groups (Stovner, Theodorsen and Bjelke, 1971b).

## Significance of Binding

Except for the very small fraction of drug bound to specific receptors in the tissues, protein-bound drug molecules are pharmacologically inert and are hindered

from gaining access to the sites of metabolism and excretion. Yet, binding to protein is not as disadvantageous as it might seem at first sight. Provision of a 'reservoir' from which free drug is liberated slowly prolongs biological activity and tends to prevent the wide fluctuations in plasma concentration of unbound drug which might otherwise occur. The reversibility of the drug-plasma protein interaction may be likened to the stabilizing behaviour of a buffer system. (Although at true equilibrium, the rate at which $DP$ would be formed ($k_1$) and the rate at which it is dissociated ($k_2$) equal one another, this is rarely the situation in vivo.) The plasma levels of unbound drug tend naturally to decline through occurrence of processes of metabolism and elimination. Because of the ready reversibility of the drug protein complex, there is a continuous dissociation of bound to unbound drug and provided the total amount of bound drug, $DP$, is sufficient, this buffering effect tends to replenish and maintain the circulating level of unbound drug. If the processes of excretion and metabolic inactivation occur at sufficiently rapid rates at, for example, active transport sites in the kidney or enzymatic sites in hepatic tissue, the concentration of free drug molecules may be lowered locally to infinitesimal levels. As a result, the equilibrium of the plasma protein-drug interaction is shifted to the left with rapid conversion of bound to unbound drug to an extent dependent on the rate constant for dissociation, $k_2$. This explains why drugs such as penicillins which are highly bound to plasma protein may nevertheless be virtually cleared from plasma in a single passage through the kidney.

## Drug Displacement from Binding Sites

Analysis of the binding characteristics of various drugs to plasma albumin has shown that whereas, at physiological pH, several binding sites exist for basic compounds, acidic drugs attach to no more than two primary binding sites and often to only one (Thorp, 1964). Where only a single binding site is available as, for example, with sulphonamides, the carrying capacity of plasma is limited to one molar equivalent of its albumin content. This is about $7 \times 10^{-4}M$, which at an average molecular weight for sulphonamides of 300, is equivalent to a plasma concentration of drug of about 20 mg/100 ml. Beyond this concentration, the fraction of unbound drug increases rapidly and it becomes available for diffusion to tissue sites of metabolism and excretion. A maximum plasma concentration of drug may eventually be reached regardless of dosage, because the processes of metabolism and elimination have kept pace with the increased availability of unbound drug. A number of acidic drugs with high affinity for binding may compete for and may displace each other from the same protein binding sites. Thus, for example, phenylbutazone, coumarin anticoagulants, sulphinpyrazole and salicylic acid are all capable of displacing 'long-acting' sulphonamides from plasma albumin (Anton, 1960; 1961). Since these sulphonamides are not rapidly metabolized, the displaced molecules diffuse from the plasma to the tissues where their antibacterial action is continued despite the fact that the total plasma concentration of sulphonamide is decreased. Similar competitive displacement from plasma albumin may increase the effective antibacterial activity of acidic antibiotics such as the semi-synthetic penicillins (Kunin, 1966). Thus a reduction of only 5 per cent in the plasma protein-binding of oxacillin by administration of sulpha-methoxy-pyridazine almost doubles the plasma concentrations of unbound oxacillin in the circulation (Kunin, 1966). Displacement of plasma bound drug by another chemical may have dangerous results, especially where the binding to plasma albumin is extensive and the free drug normally represents only a very small fraction of the total. Thus, the potentiating effect of certain sulphonamides on the hypoglycaemic action of tolbutamide (Christensen, Hansen and Kristensen, 1963) or the increase in anticoagulant efficacy of coumarin and indanediane compounds by co-administration of clofibrate (Oliver et al., 1963), phenylbutazone (Eisen, 1964; Aggeler et al., 1967; O'Reilly and Aggeler, 1970) or tolbutamide (Welch, et al., 1969) can be explained on the basis of this same mechanism (see also Hussar, 1967; Prescott, 1969). The non-diuretic benzothiadiazine derivative, diazoxide, binds firmly to one major site on plasma albumin (Sellers and Koch-Weser, 1969). As well as being markedly diabetogenic, diazoxide is an effective antihypertensive agent when administered by rapid intravenous injection. It is not metabolized to any significant extent and hence any appreciable displacement from its binding site by other more strongly bound drugs such as, for example, warfarin, could result in sustained and serious hypotension.

Drugs may displace endogenous substances such as bilirubin that are bound to plasma albumin (Schmid et al., 1965). Premature infants have relatively low levels of albumin and the acidic binding sites are readily saturated with bilirubin (Odell, Cohen and Kelly, 1969). After administration of certain sulphonamides to such infants, bilirubin may be displaced from its albumin complex (Odell, 1959a and b) and the resultant increase in circulating unbound bilirubin may lead to the development of kernicterus. The premature infant is in a particularly vulnerable position because the glucuronyl transferase system in the liver is not properly developed and hence elimination of bilirubin as its glucuronide is retarded (Done, 1964). It follows that neonates should not be given acidic drugs such as sulphonamides, salicylates, phenylbutazone or indomethacin which are highly bound to albumin and can readily uncouple bilirubin from its binding site (Done, 1966). The reverse situation may also occur in that a number of naturally occurring substances may compete with exogenous drugs for the same limited number of protein-binding sites. Thus, for example, fatty acids are transported in plasma bound to albumin. Release of free fatty acids into the blood as a result of physiological stimuli may serve to displace drug bound to albumin.

Few drugs have a primary affinity for plasma globulins, but a number of endogenous hormones including thyroxine and cortisol bind to α-globulins and d-tubocurarine binds to γ-globulins. It has been suggested that the mechanism of action of certain antirheumatic drugs such as phenyl-

butazone and indomethacin may be linked to their ability to displace endogenous corticosteroids from their binding to the globulin, transcortin, thereby increasing the tissue concentrations of free corticosteroid (Maickel, Miller and Brodie, 1965). Subsequent work has not supported this hypothesis (Stenlake et al., 1968).

### Cellular Binding

**Non-specific Storage Depots** (Brodie and Hogben, 1957; Brodie, 1964b, 1965)

A number of molecular structures besides the plasma proteins may bind drugs. Many tissues serve as storage depots because drugs combine with cellular constituents and as a result accumulate in higher concentrations than in extracellular fluid. The major part of this tissue binding is 'non-specific' in the sense that it is not involved in the process whereby the drug interacts with a cell component or receptor to evoke a specific pharmacological effect. Such secondary binding is nevertheless of considerable importance in providing extensive pools for drug storage in the body. Without these, many drugs would be metabolically inactivated and excreted so quickly that their effects would be too transient to be of therapeutic value. Non-specific binding is generally a reversible process. The stored drug remains in dynamic equilibrium with unbound drug which is then free to diffuse into the circulation and replenish drug eliminated by processes of metabolism and excretion (Fig. 4). Some drugs are stored in connective tissue because they are bound to the strongly anionic radicals of mucopolysaccharides. Gallamine has a strong affinity for mucopolysaccharide which is shared by suxamethonium but not by other muscle relaxants (Fig. 5). Bones, teeth and nails may serve as reservoirs for drugs such as heavy metals and tetracyclines (Segal, 1963; Stewart, 1968). Other drugs such as the antimalarials, mepacrine and chloroquine, have a special affinity for binding to tissue nucleoprotein (Shannon et al., 1944; Rubin, Bernstein and Zvaifler, 1963); in the case of chloroquine, significant amounts have been detected in blood and urine of patients for as long as five years after the last administration of the drug.

By contrast, there are a few drugs which have no significant binding affinities for tissue constituents, and for them body water may serve as a storage reservoir. Thus barbitone and amidopyrine are examples of drugs which remain confined to body water as unbound molecules until they are excreted from the body.

**Adipose tissue.** Drugs with high lipid/plasma partition ratios tend, understandably, to accumulate in adipose tissue. The significance of fat as a storage depot for lipid-soluble drugs is emphasized by the fact that in obesity, fat content may amount to over 35 per cent of the body weight whilst even in starvation, the level does not fall much below 10 per cent. Body fat behaves as a relatively homogeneous substance attracting lipophilic drugs in quite an indiscriminate manner. Binding is mainly by the close-range intermolecular attraction of Van der Waal forces. A good illustration of the role of lipid storage in determining drug pharmacodynamics is

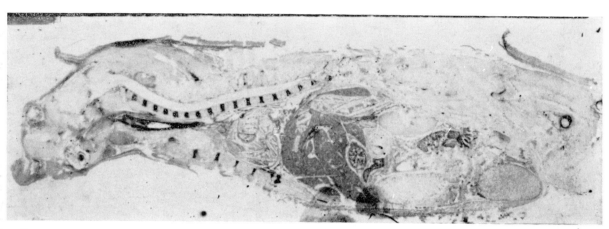

FIG. 5. Autoradiograph showing the localization of $^3$H-gallamine in cartilagenous tissues of the rat. (*Reproduced by courtesy of Dr. S. A. Feldman*)

the behaviour of thiobarbiturates. At one time, the ultra-short action of thiopentone was attributed to rapid metabolic inactivation. This view is now known to be incorrect since the barbiturate is metabolized and excreted slowly (Brodie et al., 1950; Brodie, 1952). After a single dose, most tissues well supplied with blood, including brain and muscle, rapidly take up considerable amounts of thiopentone in proportion to their bulk and the plasma levels fall abruptly; thereafter the tissue levels decline slowly in parallel with plasma levels (Mark, 1963). On the other hand, the level of drug in fat is low at first and then rises rapidly to a peak level of about ten times that in plasma in about 3 hours. At this time, about 70 per cent of the drug remaining in the body is localized to adipose tissue. The main clinical implication of this high lipid localization coupled with a slow rate of metabolism is that the duration of anaesthesia after a large dose of thio-barbitone may be prolonged out of all proportion to the dosage needed for induction of anaesthesia. Although not thiobarbiturates, hexobarbitone and other N-methylated derivatives of barbituric acid are also localized extensively in fat. There are two main reasons for this: First, presence of the N-methyl group at position 3 renders them such weak acids that they are essentially unionized at pH 7·4. Second, the methyl group also increases lipid solubility by eliminating the hydrogen bonding between the adjacent nitrogen and oxygen atoms at positions 3 and 4 of the barbiturate ring. The compound N-methyl thiopentone is both a thiobarbiturate *and* possesses a methyl sub-stituent at position 3. It is characterized by a very high degree of lipid solubility coupled with a relatively slow rate of metabolism (Papper et al., 1955).

Further examples of lipid-soluble drugs which accumu-late preferentially in body fat are the α-receptor blocking drugs, phenoxybenzamine and dibenamine (Brodie, Aronow and Axelrod, 1954).

### Specific Tissue Binding

**Concept of Drug Receptors.** It is self-evident that any drug must achieve adequate concentrations at its site of action if it is to produce its desired effects. Although obviously a function of the amount given, the amount ultimately reaching the site of action is necessarily de-pendent on the relative avidities of other processes such as non-specific binding, metabolism and excretion, which are all competing for disposal of the active form of the drug (Fig. 1). Most drugs display a degree of specificity of action and correlation of pharmacological activity with chemical structure which leads us to presume that the biological response is the consequence of an interaction with a specific tissue element called the *drug receptor*. The theory that drugs produce their effects through discrete cellular sites had its origins in the pioneer work of Ehrlich and Langley in the late nineteenth century. However, identification and characterization of drug receptors has proved extremely difficult. With the vast majority of drugs, the nature of the receptor is still unknown and has to be discussed in the abstract. Although this vagueness is but a reflection of ignorance, the *concept* of the receptor has nevertheless proved most valuable since it has allowed

the application of thermodynamic principles in seeking to explain the fundamental action of drugs at a molecular level. Such theoretical analyses of the mechanisms of drug-receptor interaction have been undertaken by many pharmacologists following on the classical studies of Clark (1926). The interested reader is referred to reviews by Paton (1961); Ariëns (1964); Furchgott (1964); Burgen (1966) and Van Rossum (1968).

A receptor can be considered as the functional compon-ent of a cell with which a drug combines reversibly to initiate a response. There has been considerable lack of agreement between biochemists, physiologists and pharma-cologists as to what exactly is meant by the term 'receptor' (Schild, 1962; Albert, 1971). In the present state of knowledge, it seems best to avoid the confusion of semantic arguments and equate 'drug receptor' with 'site of action'. Two of the most important mediators of molecular speci-ficity in biological systems—enzymes and antibodies—are proteins, and it has therefore been reasonable to assume that the receptor, too, is a specialized section of a protein or related macromolecule. When a specific macromolecule affected by a drug 'does something' which is readily measurable, attempts to isolate and purify the receptor substance may be fruitful. Thus, for example, the elucida-tion of the molecular mechanisms of action of drugs which inhibit specific enzymes, e.g. anticholinesterases or folic acid reductase inhibitors (see later), has been possible because the sophisticated techniques of enzymology could be utilized and readily applied. However, when it comes to investigating possible receptor proteins without enzymic or other readily measured activity, the problem is much more difficult, the approaches become indirect and results often highly speculative.

If a working hypothesis is accepted that a receptor is part of a protein molecule, drug-receptor interaction can be looked upon as a special case of reversible protein-binding involving the combined operation of the various binding forces considered above (p. 411). The essential difference between this type of binding and non-specific binding is that only drug-receptor interaction is followed by the drug response.

The secondary and tertiary structures of protein are unstable systems held together by interaction of a con-siderable number of these same relatively weak binding forces. The structure of the whole depends on the struc-tural integrity of the constituent subunits. When a foreign molecule interacts with a part of chemical grouping of a cellular macromolecule, the development of new forces at the binding site or sites may lead to a general alteration in tertiary structure and influence the stability of the protein as a whole (Koshland, 1963). Many of the ideas on mech-anisms of drug-receptor interaction have developed directly from knowledge of substrate-enzyme combination. Thus, the receptor for drug molecules may be looked upon as analogous to the active site or centre of an enzyme. Since changes in enzyme conformation have been shown to accompany formation of enzyme-substrate complexes, it may be inferred that similar conformational changes occur secondary to drug-receptor interaction. One important difference lies in the consequences. In the case of the enzyme, the induced structural change in the protein leads to a change in the substrate. In the case of the receptor, molecular disturbances occur in the matrix of the protein of which the receptor is a constituent part; these changes of conformational perturbation then initiate a chain of biochemical and physiological events which characterize the pharmacological response to the drug.

**Consequences of drug-receptor interaction** (Gill, 1965; Mautner, 1967; Waud, 1968).

The major part of an administered dose of drug is either directed to non-specific binding sites, metabolized or excreted, without ever reaching the select receptor. Interaction of the minute fraction of drug which does combine with its receptor can manifest itself in a number of ways.

Drugs which combine with the receptor and generate a response are called *agonists*. They must posses two important properties. First, they must have *affinity* for the receptor and second, *intrinsic activity* (Ariëns, van Rossum and Simonis, 1957) or *efficacy* (Stephenson, 1956) —the power to initiate the subsequent response.

The quantitative analyses of drug-receptor interaction developed by Clark (1926) and Gaddum (1937) have emphasized that pharmacological response is proportional to the number of receptors occupied (*occupation theory of drug action*). Paton (1961) has suggested a different interpretation based on the proposal that the response to a drug is not a function of the number of receptors occupied but of the rate of drug-receptor combination (*rate theory of drug action*). These two theories may not be mutually exclusive and it is conceivable that the occupation theory may be valid for certain receptors whilst the rate theory is valid for others (Furchgott, 1964).

Agonists that produce a smaller maximal effect than other agonists reacting with the same receptor are said to have intermediate efficacy and are called *partial agonists*. If a partial agonist and full agonist act on the same receptor simultaneously, the effects may be additive or the partial agonist may competitively antagonize the full agonist, depending on the relative concentrations of the two drugs. In certain situations, a substance may react with the same receptor as a full agonist but, because it lacks intrinsic activity, its action becomes that of a *competitive antagonist*.

**Kinetics of drug-receptor interaction**

The reaction between a drug and its receptor is a reversible process governed by the law of mass action. It can be expressed mathematically in a manner analogous to the reaction of non-specific protein-binding considered on p. 412. Thus, if an agonist $D$ reacts with a receptor $R$:

$$[D] + [R] \underset{k_2}{\overset{k_1}{\rightleftharpoons}} [DR]$$

Drug   Receptor        Drug-receptor
                        complex.

However, unlike non-specific binding, drug-receptor interaction is characterized by a second event in which the

drug-receptor complex acts further to evoke a pharmacological effect, $Q_D$. The complex mechanisms involved in this second event are largely obscure at the present time. The reasonable assumption may, however, be made that during this phase of response the receptor reappears, otherwise drug action would imply destruction of the receptor which is in general known not to be the case. The complete scheme of events may be described as follows:

$$[D] + [R] \underset{k_2}{\overset{k_1}{\rightleftharpoons}} [DR] \overset{k_3}{\longrightarrow} Q_D + [R]$$

where $k_1$, $k_2$ and $k_3$ = the rate constants for each partial reaction.

At equilibrium $K_D = \dfrac{k_2}{k_1} = \dfrac{[D][R]}{[DR]}$ (cf. equation 1, p. 412), where $K_D$ = the dissociation constant of the drug-receptor complex.

If the total receptor concentration equals $[R_T]$, it follows that $[R_T] = [R] + [DR]$. On substituting in the above equation we obtain

$$K_D = \frac{[D]\{[R_T] - [DR]\}}{[DR]} \quad \text{or} \quad \frac{[DR]}{[R_T]} = \frac{[D]}{K_D + [D]}$$

Now, $Q_D = k_3[DR]$ indicating that the response is proportional to the concentration of $DR$.

If $Q_{max}$ equals the maximal response which the system is capable of, then, $Q_{max} = k_3[R_T]$.

$$\frac{Q_D}{Q_{max}} = \frac{[DR]}{[R_T]} = \frac{[D]}{K_D + [D]} \tag{4a}$$

$$\therefore \quad Q_D = \frac{Q_{max} \cdot [D]}{K_D + [D]} = \frac{Q_{max}}{\dfrac{K_D}{[D]} + 1} \tag{4b}$$

The derivation of these last equations is identical to that of the well-known *Michaelis-Menten equation* which expresses the velocity $V$ of an enzyme reaction as a function of the concentration of substrate, $S$, the enzyme-substrate dissociation constant, $K_s$ and the maximal velocity when the enzyme is saturated with substrate, $V_{max}$:

$$v = \frac{V_{max}}{\dfrac{K_s}{S} + 1} \tag{5}$$

When $v = V_{max}/2$, $S$ is equal to $K_s$. The value of $S$ which is experimentally found to give half the maximum velocity is written as $Km$, *the Michaelis constant*, so that under these conditions $Km = K_s$. With the drug-receptor interaction, the parallel situation arises when $Q_D = Q_{max}/2$, whereupon $[D]$ becomes equal to $K_D$.

If the pharmacological activity of a drug is assumed to be proportional to the magnitude of the response, $Q_D$, then the ratio $Q_D/Q_{max}$ of equation (4a) will be a constant for each particular drug. This ratio of maximum effect is given the symbol $\alpha^E$, and expresses the *efficacy* or *intrinsic activity*. $\alpha^E$ is usually expressed as a constant relative to a standard drug which evokes maximum effect in the particular biological system under consideration. The reciprocal of the dissociation constant, $K_D$, gives a measure of the *affinity* of a drug for its receptor. It may conveniently be expressed as $pK_D$, by analogy with pH, where $pK_D = -\log_{10}K_D$; thus the higher the value of $pK_D$, the greater the affinity of a drug.

Equation (4b) may be transformed to its reciprocal form just as Lineweaver and Burk transformed the Michaelis-Menten equation.

$$\frac{1}{Q_D} = \frac{K_D}{Q_{max}} \cdot \frac{1}{[D]} + \frac{1}{Q_{max}} \qquad (6)$$

The advantage of this manœuvre is that when the variables $1/Q_D$ and $1/[D]$ are plotted against one another, a straight line is obtained whose slope equals $K_D/Q_{max}$, whilst the intercept of the $1/[D]$ axis, i.e. when $1/Q_D = 0$, equals $-1/K_D$ and thus gives a direct measure of affinity. This double-reciprocal plot has been widely applied to the analysis of the kinetics of enzyme inhibition (Dixon and Webb, 1964); it has also provided considerable theoretical insight into the mechanisms of drug antagonism. For further details, the reader is referred to the articles by Stephenson (1956), Ariëns, van Rossum and Simonis (1957), Ariëns (1964), van Rossum (1964; 1968) and Waud (1968).

**Chemical identity of receptors** (Belleau, 1967; Ehrenpreis, Fleisch and Mittag, 1969; Albert, 1971). The best way to gain information about the chemical nature of a receptor would be to identify and isolate it. Unfortunately, this direct approach is beset with pitfalls and difficulties, and despite considerable progress in recent years in this direction, no true receptor substance has yet been isolated with certainty. The study of structure-activity relationships (SAR) has offered a most valuable way of gaining indirect data on receptor structure. This approach is based on the fundamental premise that the interaction of an agonist molecule with its receptor involves the mutual attraction of chemically reactive groups which are spatially orientated in a pattern complimentary to one another. Many of the inferences regarding the chemical structure of receptors have been drawn from SAR studies undertaken particularly amongst autonomic neurotransmitters and narcotic analgesics (Burger and Parulkar, 1966).

Study of SAR data on members of the polymethylene bis-methonium compounds has indicated that the receptors for the cholinergic transmitter at autonomic ganglia and the skeletal neuromuscular junction have different structures. The prototype structure for this series is a symmetrical molecule containing two cationic groups separated by a simple aliphatic chain:

$$_3(CH_3)\overset{+}{N} - (CH_2)_n - \overset{+}{N}(CH_3)_3.$$

When the biological activity of derivatives with differing chain length was investigated, the ganglionic site was found to interact most strongly with $C_5$ (pentamethonium) or $C_6$ (hexamethonium) compounds. These drugs cause ganglion blockade by preventing the receptor from responding to acetyl choline. On the other hand, compounds with longer chain length such as $C_{10}$ (deca-

methonium) and succinylcholine show greatest selectivity for the neuromuscular end plate, suggesting that the anionic sites on the latter receptor are spaced further apart.

On the basis of detailed SAR studies of sympathomimetic drugs, it appears that the grouping

$$C_6H_5 - \overset{\mid}{\underset{\mid}{C}} - \overset{\mid}{\underset{\mid}{C}} - N \diagup$$

is the one that fits the essential sites of attachment of the adrenergic or adrenoceptive receptor (Belleau, 1966; Bloom and Goldman, 1966; Ehrenpreis, Fleisch and Mittag, 1969). A model can be constructed which defines the relationship between catechol amine structure and the hypothetical $\alpha$ and $\beta$ sites of a single adrenergic or 'adrenoceptive' receptor. Three essential chemical features

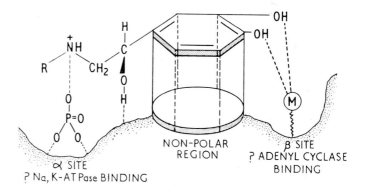

Fig. 6. Diagram of a catecholamine and the concept of its fit with a receptor model containing an $\alpha$ site which forms an ionic bond and a $\beta$ site at which chelation with a metal, M, (possibly magnesium) occurs. At the $\alpha$ site, binding may occur to membrane-bound ATPase with catalysis of ATP hydrolysis; the $\beta$ site may be located on the enzyme adenylcyclase and thus binding may involve formation of cyclic AMP.

appear to be (1) a flat surface to which the benzene ring can be applied closely, (2) a cationic site where ion pairing can occur, (3) a chelation site which may involve a metallic ion like $Mg^{2+}$ or formation of hydrophobic bonding with aqueous layers in the vicinity of the receptor surface. These are depicted diagrammatically in Fig. 6. Substitution on the N atom especially of bulky alkyl groups like isopropyl (as in isoprenaline or propranolol) increases the affinity of a compound for the $\beta$ site, probably by steric hindrance of the ion-pairing necessary to $\alpha$ site attachment. The phenolic-OH groups attached to the benzene nucleus contribute to intrinsic activity at the $\beta$ site. The alcoholic-OH at the $\beta$ carbon atom on the side-chain appears to serve mainly to strengthen attachment to the $\alpha$ site of the receptor (i.e. causing an increase in affinity); its presence gives rise to an asymmetrical carbon in the molecule and optically active stereoisomers. For both agonists and antagonists pharmacological activity is much greater in the (−)isomer.

SAR amongst stereoisomers has been particularly valuable in allowing certain inferences to be drawn about the three-dimensional structure of receptor surfaces. This has been done extensively with narcotic analgesics and has allowed the construction of a model of a hypothetical receptor surface for morphine and its congeners. In this case only the D (−)-isomers can fit the surface features of the receptor and in both the natural and synthetic compounds, only D (−)-molecules have analgesic activity (Beckett and Casey, 1954, 1965; *see also* Lewis, Bentley and Cowan, 1971).

Although construction of models of receptor structure is a highly speculative undertaking it has the particular merit of seeking to explain the molecular action of drugs in physicochemical terms. Further work in this direction should not only provide an answer to the fundamental

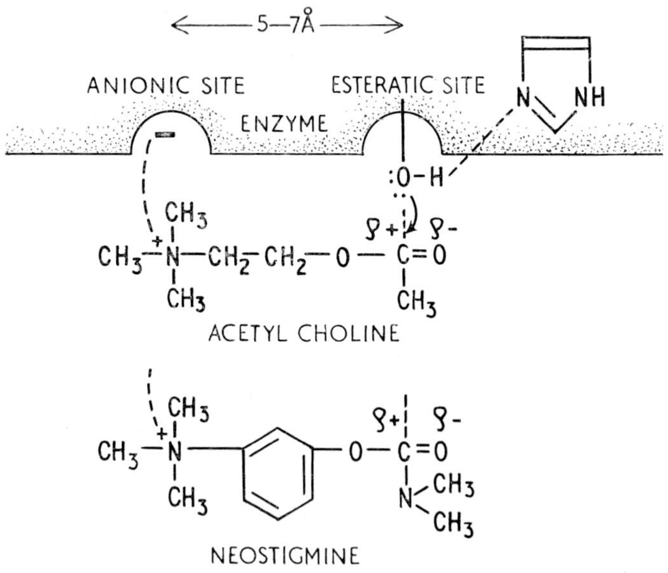

Fig. 7. Substrate and inhibitor interactions with the active centre of AChE. :O—H represents the essential electron-rich group at the esteratic site which makes a nucleophilic attack on the substrate by donating electrons to the electrophilic $\rangle$C = O radical of the ester. The nucleophilic group to the enzyme is made more nucleophilic by formation of H-bonding with the imidazole N atom of a neighbouring histidine residue. Attachment of the carbon atom to the serine oxygen leads to formation of the acyl-enzyme complex (acetylated enzyme, if the substrate is acetyl choline). [Based on Wilson, 1967]

problem of how drug interaction with the cell receptor is translated into pharmacological response but should make it feasible to design new drugs with even greater specificity of action.

**Enzyme receptor sites.** A number of drugs appear to act through known specific enzymatic mechanisms. The mechanism of action may involve direct inhibition of an enzyme. Alternatively, the inhibition may be indirect; if the drug has close chemical similarities with the normal substrate, it may serve as a substrate substitute for the enzyme and thereby block a key reaction in a vital metabolic sequence. In either event, the subunit of the enzyme macromolecule which contains the functional three-dimensional region for binding the specific substrate, i.e. the active or catalytic centre, may be regarded as the drug receptor. An important difference between binding of drugs to receptor sites of macromolecules in general

and the active sites of enzymes in particular is that in the former case, initiation of the pharmacological response does not usually involve making or breaking of covalent bonds in the agonist, whereas this can readily occur in reactions of enzymatic catalysts.

**Inhibition of cholinesterase.** Anticholinesterases are classic examples of drugs whose pharmacological effects are mediated by inhibition of a specific enzyme. There are two types of mammalian cholinesterase with different specificities and affinities for both substrates and inhibitors (Lehmann and Lidell, 1962). These are true- or acetyl-cholinesterase (AChE) and butyryl cholinesterase (BuChE) or pseudocholinesterase; the latter enzyme is considered in detail on p. 440. The clinical effects of anticholinesterase drugs are almost entirely due to inhibition of AChE whose physiological substrate is acetylcholine.

Acetylcholine has in its molecule only two functional groups, an ester and quaternary ammonium group, which it can offer for attachment to an enzyme receptor site. The active centre of cholinesterase is believed to consist of two sites approximately 7 Å apart, an *anionic site* that forms an ionic bond with the cationic "onium" head of acetylcholine and an *esteratic site* at which the ester bond is actually split (Fig. 7). The anionic site is composed of ionized carboxyl groups whose main function is to anchor the cationic head of the substrate and keep it there for the few microseconds needed for hydrolysis to occur. The esteratic site represents an electron-rich centre which includes an essential serine residue. The initial interaction at the esteratic site is thought to be electron donation to the electrophilic carboxyl C atom. This carbon is then linked to a serine OH group and choline is split off, leaving an acetylated esteratic site. The acetylated enzyme has only a very transient existence and is rapidly hydrolysed in about 100 microseconds to yield acetic acid and the regenerated free enzyme. This may be represented as follows:

$$\text{(E)-H} + S \underset{k_{-1}}{\overset{k_1}{\rightleftharpoons}} [\text{(E)-H} \cdots S] \overset{k_2}{\longrightarrow} \text{(E)-acyl} + \text{choline}$$
$$\downarrow k_3$$
$$\text{(E)-H} + \text{acetic acid}$$

where (E)-H represents AChE and $S$ equals substrate, acetyl choline in this case; (E)-acyl is the unstable acylated enzyme which rapidly decomposes to regenerate the original enzyme.

Anticholinesterases may compete with acetyl choline for the active sites of the enzyme and interfere with hydrolysis of the natural substrate. They may do this in two ways:

**(a) Rapidly reversible inhibitions** by combining only with the anionic site, e.g. edrophonium, which is a *bis*-quaternary ammonium compound not containing an ester radical.

**(b) Acylation,** namely formation of an acylated enzyme which is considerably more stable than the acetylated enzyme formed by reaction with acetylcholine. Anticholinesterases acting via an acylation mechanism are the carbamates and organophosphates. The carbamates, e.g. the quaternary amine, neostigmine, form a carbamylated

AChE which reacts with water at less than one millionth the rate of the corresponding acetylated form (Fig. 7). The organophosphates react at the esteratic site to form a phosphorylated AChE which is extremely stable. If the alkyl groups attached to the organophosphate are $-CH_3$ or $-C_2H_5$, significant regeneration of the enzyme occurs spontaneously in several hours. With isopropyl groups as in DFP, however, the phosphoryl-enzyme bond undergoes negligible spontaneous hydrolysis; recovery of AChE activity depends on synthesis of new enzyme protein, a process that may take months (Aldridge, 1969). Reactivation of the phosphorylated enzyme can be achieved much more rapidly by employing certain nucleophilic agents such as hydroxylamine (Fig. 8). Unfortunately, high doses of hydroxylamine are needed and these are not tolerated *in vivo*. It was reasoned that if a hydroxylamine derivative could be synthesized which also possessed a cationic head that would fit simultaneously into the anionic site of the enzyme (i.e. at a distance of approximately 7 Å from the N-OH radical) reactivation potency might be enhanced further (Wilson, 1959). A number of quaternary pyridine aldoximes, such as pralidoxime and TMB-4, fulfil this requirement and are rapid and less toxic reactivators.

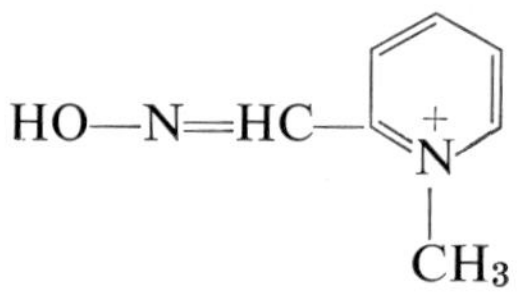

pralidoxime

They are of considerable value as antidotes in the treatment of poisoning by organophosphate insecticides.

Evidence gleaned from a number of experimental approaches including thermodynamic studies and investigation of structure-activity relationships, raises the possibility that, rather than there being several different cholinergic receptors, the active centre of AChE may represent the fundamental cholinergic or cholinoceptive receptor. It is conceivable, though not proven, that the so-called muscarinic and nicotinic 'receptors' may merely represent altered conformations of the same enzyme protein bearing a standard active centre as receptor site for the neurotransmitter (for further details, *see* Conference on Cholinergic Mechanisms, 1967).

**Inhibition of other enzymes.** Examples of other drugs whose pharmacological activity is a direct expression of enzyme inhibition include inhibitors of carbonic anhydrase (e.g. acetazolamide); of xanthine oxidase (e.g. allopurinol); of aldehyde oxidase (e.g. disulfiram, *see* p. 329).

**Antimetabolites.** The antibacterial sulphonamides are representative of a class of drugs which exert their biological effects by acting as antimetabolites. There is a close chemical similarity between sulphonamides and p-aminobenzoic acid (PABA), an essential growth factor and biosynthetic intermediate in the metabolism of many bacteria. PABA is normally condensed enzymatically with a glutamylpteridine compound to form dihydropteroic acid, a precursor of folic acid. Sulphonamides, because of their close structural likeness to PABA can also act as substrate for the condensing enzyme and thereby

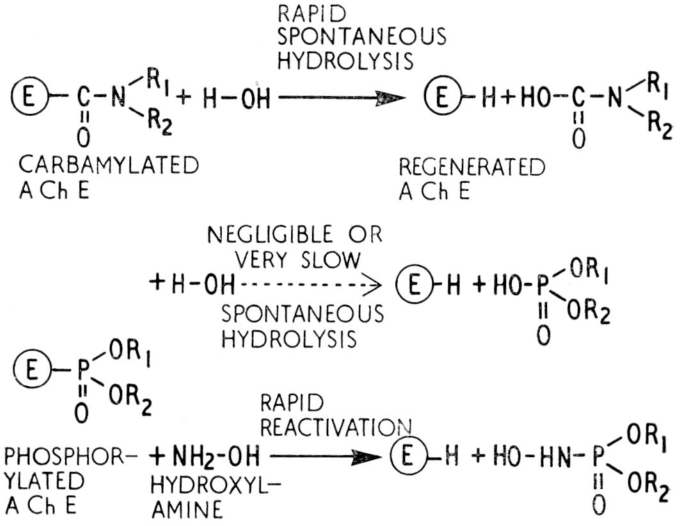

FIG. 8. Spontaneous and stimulated reactivation of carbamylated (a) and phosphorylated (b) forms of AChE. The native enzyme is represented as Ⓔ— H.

inhibit competitively the normal entry of PABA into the folic acid pathway (Brown, 1962). The ultimate consequence is bacterial folic acid deficiency manifested as a reversible inhibition of bacterial growth.

Antimetabolites have also been developed for use in cancer chemotherapy. Some of these act by the mechanism of counterfeit incorporation into biosynthetic pathways. The pyrimidine antagonist, 5-fluorouracil, differs from uracil merely by substitution of F for H at position 5 in the ring. Fluorouracil is handled metabolically like uracil forming a riboside and riboside phosphate.

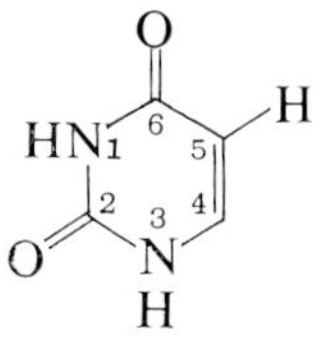

uracil 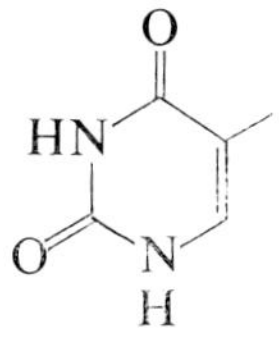                5-fluorouracil

The enzyme thymidine synthetase which normally methylates uracil to thymidine is inhibited. In addition fluorouracil is converted to the corresponding nucleoside triphosphate and then incorporated into messenger-RNA in place of uracil (Heidelberger, 1967). Miscoding may result through misinterpretation of codons containing fluorouracil during the assembly of aminoacids into polypeptide chains.

## Drug Action not Mediated by Receptor Interaction

The pharmacological effects of a variety of drugs do not appear to involve attachment to receptors possessing a high degree of structural specificity. Substances as unrelated chemically as diethyl ether, nitrous oxide, halothane or xenon all produce very similar effects of depression of the central nervous system. As a group, the volatile anaesthetics are remarkable for the lack of any obvious correlation between chemical structure and pharmacological activity. The term 'chemically inert' which has frequently been applied to this class of drugs is somewhat misleading. First, there is now good evidence that many of these compounds undergo significant metabolism in the body (see p. 460). Second, under certain conditions, hydrophobic associations may develop with other substances including water as in clathrate formation or bonding to tissue or circulating macromolecules. However, because the volatile anaesthetics do not enter into a reaction of distinct chemical specificity with the organism, most approaches aimed at defining the molecular environment in which these drugs act have focussed attention on correlations between potency and certain physical properties. Many such correlations have been noted as for example with vapour pressure, polarizability, molecular size and shape, free energy of drug-membrane adsorption (Mullins, 1954; Featherstone and Muehlbacher, 1963; Symposium on The Molecular Pharmacology of Anaesthesia, 1968; Seeman, Roth and Schneider, 1971). The well-known correlation with oil/gas partition coefficients formed the basis for the Meyer-Overton hypothesis. The 'microcrystal' theory of Pauling (1961) and 'iceberg' concept of Miller (1961) emphasize the critical role of the aqueous rather than the lipid phase of nervous tissue in the molecular mechanism of anaesthesia. Both of these theories are based on a close correlation noted between narcotizing partial pressures of anaesthetics and the partial pressures necessary to form hydrates at $0°C$. Subsequent work on fluorinated anaesthetics has revealed gross deviations from the correlation with hydrate dissociation pressure and has swung the emphasis once more on the property of lipid solubility (Miller, Paton and Smith, 1965; Eger et al., 1969).

However, it is certainly not valid to assume that because of a correlation between potency and a particular physicochemical property, this necessarily explains the cellular mechanism of drug action. The major difficulty with non-specific drug action such as characterizes the volatile anaesthetics is that we are still quite ignorant as to what precisely these drugs are acting upon, and controversy still exists between possible primary effects on the plasma membrane of cells as opposed to effects on intracellular organelles (Allison and Nunn, 1968; Saubermann and Gallagher, 1973). In such a situation, it may be helpful to consider anaesthetic-induced narcosis in terms of thermodynamic activity.

Use of the concept of thermodynamic activity in describing non-specific drug action was developed by Ferguson (1939). According to the tenets of thermodynamics, the chemical activity of a substance is the same in all phases of an equilibrium system, so that by determining the activity in one phase, we have automatically determined the activity of all others even if the identity and location of these other places is not known. Thermodynamic activity represents a measure of those molecules which are free to exert their biological effect, and in the case of volatile anaesthetics can be estimated from the ratio of partial pressure at a particular temperature ($P_t$)

to saturation pressure at the same temperature ($P_s$). It is thus much more meaningful to speak of the comparative potencies of different anaesthetics in terms of 'activities' rather than in conventional terms of 'moles per litre'. The problem of standardizing comparative potency of different anaesthetics has been tackled in another way by Eger and his co-workers who have developed a common measure of potency in the form of the minimal anaesthetic concentration (MAC). MAC is defined as the minimal alveolar concentration which prevents muscular movement in the dog in response to a painful stimulus such as tail clamping or stimulation of mucous membranes with an electric current. Using MAC as an index of potency of different gaseous anaesthetic agents, including fluorinated derivatives, a closer correlation has been found between potency and lipid solubility than with other physicochemical properties such as vapour pressure (Eger et al., 1965) or dissociated pressure of hydrate crystals (Eger et al., 1969). In general, although the thermodynamic approach has proved of much value in providing a theoretical background to the study of nonspecific drug action, it has not provided an explanation for the mechanism of action of such drugs.

Experimental work with isolated membranes particularly of erythrocytes has emphasized the consequences of interaction of anaesthetic agents with the plasma membrane. Anaesthetics penetrate and expand biomembranes (Seeman and Roth, 1972). If this expansion is critical to the mechanism of anaesthetic action, occupation of the cell membrane by anaesthetic agents may be expected not only to cause electrostabilization but also to disorganize membrane architecture and induce conformational changes in membrane—associated proteins (Seeman, 1973). Such changes may account for the secondary disturbances in carrier-mediated transfer of ions and neutral solutes across the membrane.

Unfortunately, there is insufficient experimental evidence at the present time to decide upon a definitive theory of non-specific drug action which can fully explain the molecular mechanisms of action of volatile anaesthetics (see Chapter 2, Section IIc).

### Excretion of Drugs

The unbound diffusible fraction of a drug may be eliminated from the body either unchanged or in forms modified by metabolism or as a mixture of both native drug and biotransformed products. The processes involved in a drug metabolism are considered later (ch. 2). The basic mechanisms operating in excretion are applicable to both the unaltered or metabolized drug molecule.

Drugs may be excreted through the lung, kidneys, biliary system, intestine, salivary and sweat glands. By far the major route for most drugs is the kidney with the exception of the inhalation anaesthetics which are eliminated predominantly via the lungs.

**Renal Excretion** (Milne, Scribner and Crawford, 1958; Orloff and Berliner, 1961; Weiner and Mudge, 1964; Milne, 1966; Weiner, 1967; Lant, 1972).

Excretion of drugs by the kidney involves the triple

processes of glomerular filtration (passive), proximal tubular secretion (active), tubular diffusion (passive).

Plasma is filtered at the glomerular capillaries whose porous membranes permit the passage of most solutes. Unbound drug diffuses into the glomerulus in an amount proportional to the transfer of plasma water and hence filtration does not disturb the plasma equilibrium between bound and unbound drug. Meaningful values for clearance of drug from the plasma are only obtainable if the degree of protein-binding is known at the relevant drug concentration. Factors such as hypertension or dehydration which reduce glomerular filtration rate (GFR) reduce the filtered load, whilst correction of such abnormalities or infusion of mannitol may increase GFR and filtered load. The plasma ultrafiltrate then flows down the nephron, the subsequent fate of filtered drug molecules depends on their physicochemical properties. The lining of the tubules consists of a continuum of closely-packed epithelial cells with characteristics similar to other biomembranes. The principles which govern passage of drug back from the filtrate across the tubular epithelium are the familiar ones relating to transfer of solute across other lipid boundaries. Polar compounds including ions are not lipid-soluble and do not diffuse back, unless they are of small enough size to traverse the pores or are undergoing reabsorption by a carrier-mediated transport system. Drugs with high lipid/water partition coefficients will undergo ready tubular reabsorption.

**Active secretion in the proximal tubule.** The tubular epithelium closely resembles that in the biliary tract and choroid plexus in having a dual character with regard to transfer of drugs. It functions as a lipid boundary in permitting ready passage of unionized lipid-soluble molecules, and in addition also possesses two carrier-mediated mechanisms for transporting many organic acids and bases from plasma to urine. Unlike glomerular filtration, both the protein-bound and free drug forms are available for active tubular secretion. As free drug is removed by the tubular cells, there is rapid dissociation of the drug-protein complex to maintain the equilibrium with plasma water. Very strong protein-binding may, however, limit the rate of tubular secretion because uptake of drug by the cells, the first step of active transport, is dependent on the initial content of free drug in plasma water.

Results of competitive experiments have shown that the secretory pathways for organic acids and bases are quite separate. Although the characteristics of secretion by both pathways fulfil the criteria for active transport, neither mechanism is as selective as those for naturally occurring substances. The tubules are able to secrete a large number of acids and bases of diverse chemical structures, molecular sizes and ionic strengths (Weiner and Mudge, 1964). The acid-secreting mechanism transports the ionized forms of a variety of acidic drugs ranging from sulphonic acids to amino acid conjugates, ester and ether glucuronides, ethereal sulphates, acetylated sulphonamides, benzothiadiazines, heterocyclic carboxylic acids such as the penicillins and cephalosporins, aliphatic organic acids such as acylglycine and oxalic acid, enolic compounds such as phenylbutazone. The competition

displayed between these various anionic compounds for the secretory mechanisms has been taken advantage of in the clinical use of probenecid. Probenecid blocks the rapid renal secretion of penicillin and prolongs the duration of action of the antibiotic. This is of particular value in septicaemic infections and also where use of a particularly expensive derivative, such as carbenicillin, is indicated and dosage can be thereby kept to a minimum without decreasing clinical efficacy.

Secreted organic bases vary from the weakly basic primary (e.g. histamine), secondary (e.g. mecamylamine) and tertiary (e.g. N-methyl nicotinamide) amines to the highly ionized quaternary ammonium compounds such as choline and hexamethonium.

An interesting parallelism can be drawn between the non-specific functions of the renal secretory mechanisms which handle organic acids and bases and the microsomal enzyme systems which metabolize drugs in the liver. In discussing the evolutionary significance of the hepatic enzyme system which functions essentially to convert non-polar to polar substances, Brodie and Hogben (1957) speculate that this development was necessary for the 'emancipation of life from the sea'. It is conceivable that the proximal tubule system has evolved in an attempt to enhance the elimination of polar and non-polar compounds and thereby keep the plasma content of potential toxins at lower levels than would otherwise obtain by glomerular filtration alone.

**Diffusion and pH-dependent excretion.** In addition to the non-specific transport systems considered above, elimination of drugs occurs also by passive diffusion across the tubular epithelium. Drugs which are water soluble and of moderate molecular size as, for example, the polymeric carbohydrate, inulin (MW 5500) or cyanocobalamin (MW 1355) do not diffuse across the tubular cells. Such substances are filtered at the glomerulus and are neither reabsorbed nor secreted by the tubules. They can, therefore, be used for measuring GFR. Other water-soluble compounds of small molecular size such as urea may diffuse readily across the tubular epithelium. The clearance of such substances is less than the glomerular filtration rate, is unaffected by pH but is sensitive to changes in urine flow. Thus renal clearance is increased when high flow rates are induced with an osmotic diuretic like mannitol, for with high urinary flow rate, there is insufficient time for significant back-diffusion to occur. Processes of diffusion are potentially bidirectional, but as water is progressively abstracted from the tubular fluid on its passage down the nephron, intraluminal concentrations of dissolved drug increase and back-diffusion occurs.

The majority of non-volatile drugs are weak electrolytes and the relative proportions of unionized and ionized components on either side of the tubular epithelium will conform to the tenets of the pH-partition hypothesis and therefore depend on pH and $pK_a$ as shown by the Henderson–Hasselbalch equation. Weak acids tend to be excreted more rapidly in alkaline urine, weak bases in acid urine. The quantitative aspects of non-ionic diffusion and its influence upon the urinary excretion of weak electrolytes are considered in detail by Milne, Scribner and Crawford (1958). Variations in drug clearance with altered urinary pH which are achieved in practice are usually lower than the theoretical maxima for a number of reasons. These include the following factors: the tubular epithelium does not usually display an absolute impermeability to the ionized forms of weak acids or bases; when urine flow rate is high, there may be incomplete equilibration in the time available; back-diffusion in the distal nephron may be restricted on account of the relatively low rate of blood flow in the renal medulla.

Although atypical in a number of respects, output of ammonia by the kidney is probably one of the most

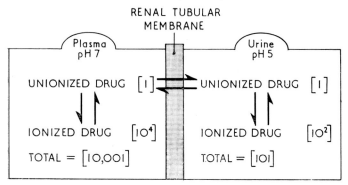

FIG. 9. Theoretical steady-state distribution of salicylate ($pK_a = 3 \cdot 0$) between urine and plasma. The concentrations of unionized and ionized forms of the drug in the two compartments have been calculated from the Henderson-Hasselbach equation. pH values have been rounded off for simplicity. Only the unionized moiety equilibrates across the tubular epithelium. At physiological pH, most of plasma salicylate is in the ionized form and is reversibly bound to albumin. Increase in urinary pH from 5 to 8 increases the fraction of drug in unionized form from $[10^2]$ to $[10^5]$ and thereby aids elimination from the body.

important examples of pH-dependent excretion. In this instance, the main direction of diffusion is from its site of production in the tubular cells into the lumen. Diffusion of ammonia into highly acid urine and its combination with secreted $H^+$ to form $NH_4^+$ constitutes a major mechanism for eliminating acidic products of metabolism and thereby maintaining acid-base homeostasis. In general, excretion of acidic or basic drugs is pH-dependent if the unionized fraction is lipid soluble and if the $pK_a$ is within the range of $3 \cdot 0$–$7 \cdot 5$ for weak acids and $7 \cdot 5$–$10 \cdot 5$ for weak bases (Milne, 1965) (see Fig. 2). This, therefore, includes the weak acids, salicylic, phenobarbitone, nitrofurantoin, certain sulphonamides, nalidixic acid and phenylbutazone; the weak bases, mepacrine, procaine, amphetamine, pethidine, imipramine and amitriptyline. A full list of compounds displaying pH-dependent excretion is given in Milne (1966).

The phenomenon of pH-dependent excretion has found an important application in the clinical management of acute poisoning. Appropriate manipulation of urinary pH may expedite the elimination of a drug present in the plasma in toxic concentrations. Rapid alkalinization of the urine by intravenous administration of sodium bicarbonate or lactate has been found useful in treating

aspirin ($pK_a$ 3·5) and phenobarbitone ($pK_a$ 7·2) overdosage (see Fig. 9). Most other barbiturates have higher $pK_a$ values and their urinary excretion is virtually unaffected by changes in urinary pH. Rapid acidification of the urine is more difficult to attain in practice. There is a slow drop in urinary pH after oral administration of ammonium chloride, and intravenous use of this salt may be hazardous. Intravenous administration of the hydrochlorides of arginine or lysine is safer and usually efficacious. Urinary acidification may be valuable in treating overdosages, with pethidine, amphetamine or its analogue fenfluramine, especially where there is impairment of hepatic function and the normal metabolism of these compounds is disturbed.

### Clinical Role of Renal Excretion

Removal of unchanged drug by the kidney is a less common means of terminating drug action *in vivo* than metabolic degradation. However, for those drugs whose elimination is primarily renal, the state of renal function is

TABLE 2

ELIMINATION RATE CONSTANT FOR VARIOUS ANTIMICROBIAL AGENTS

| Drug | Rate constant of elimination | |
| --- | --- | --- |
| | Normal renal function | Anuria |
| Penicillins | | |
| Benzylpenicillin | 1·40 | 0·03 |
| Ampicillin | 0·60 | 0·11 |
| Cephalosporins | | |
| Cephaloridine | 0·40 | 0·03 |
| Cephalexin | 0·70 | 0·03 |
| Tetracyclines | | |
| Chlortetracycline | 0·12 | 0·08 |
| Doxycycline | 0·03 | 0·03 |
| Macrolides and related agents | | |
| Erythromycin | 0·50 | 0·13 |
| Lincomycin | 0·15 | 0·06 |
| Polymyxins | | |
| Colistin | 0·31 | 0·08 |
| Aminoglycosides | | |
| Streptomycin | 0·27 | 0·01 |
| Kanamycin | 0·25 | 0·01 |
| Gentamicin | 0·30 | 0·02 |

[Data from Dettli, Spring and Ryter (1971).]

very important in relation to possible cumulation and toxic effects (Reidenberg, 1971) (see Sect. IID, Ch. 1). From the anaesthetists' point of view, the main drugs to be borne in mind in this respect are the nondepolarizing muscle relaxants (Churchill-Davidson, Way and de Jong, 1967; Gibaldi, Levy and Hayton, 1972), ganglion blockers, various antibacterial agents and cardiac glycosides (Bennett, Singer and Coggins, 1970; O'Grady, 1971; Doherty *et al.*, 1971; Prescott, 1972). Table 2 lists the elimination rate constants for a number of antibiotics whose main route of elimination is the kidney. The aminoglycosides poly-myxins and oxytetracycline potentiate the actions of non-depolarizing muscle relaxants in man and are particularly liable to do so when there is cumulation in the presence of renal insufficiency (Feldman and Levi, 1963; Weinstein and Dalton, 1968; Riordan and Gilbertson, 1971; Pittinger and Adamson, 1972).

### Pulmonary Excretion (Papper and Kitz, 1963; Eger, 1964)

Inhalation anaesthetics are metabolized to a small extent in the body (see later); they are, however, mainly eliminated in unchanged form at the lungs, their site of absorption. The healthy alveo-capillary membrane allows free diffusion of anaesthetic gases in both directions and poses no significant barrier to their transfer. The factors which govern the elimination of volatile anaesthetics are in effect the same ones that are concerned in the uptake of these agents. In essence, three factors are of special importance. First, the *solubility of the agent in blood* expressed as the blood/gas partition coefficient ($\lambda$) representing the ratio of anaesthetic concentration in blood to anaesthetic concentration in the gas phase when the two are in equilibrium. The coefficient varies from as high as 12·10 in the case of diethyl ether to 2·30 for halo-thane and 0·14 for insoluble anaesthetics like ethylene. Second, *cardiac output* as reflected in pulmonary blood flow, since this will influence the rate at which efficient elimination of gases can occur from the blood traversing the alveoli. Third, the *tension gradient* of anaesthetic existing between the mixed venous blood and alveoli.

Elimination of the anaesthetic takes place as a reversed image of the uptake phase. When a low-solubility agent such as nitrous oxide or cyclopropane ($\lambda = 0.47$) is discontinued, the arterial blood concentration falls very quickly as venous blood is almost cleared completely of anaesthetic in the lungs. A steep concentration gradient is thus provided which, with the high blood flow/mass ratio of brain tissue (a vessel rich group-VRG body tissue), favours rapid transfer of anaesthetic from brain to cerebral capillary blood and consciousness is rapidly regained. Conversely, after discontinuing a high-solubility agent, once equilibration of body water has occurred, the arterial tension falls slowly and desaturation of brain tissue tends to be limited by the rate of elimination of anaesthetic from the whole of body water. Recovery is therefore slow.

The factors influencing uptake distribution and elimination of inhalational anaesthetics are considered in detail in Chapter 3.

### Biliary Excretion (Schanker, 1962; Williams, Millburn and Smith, 1965; Williams 1967; Stowe and Plaa, 1968; Smith, 1973)

The excretion of drugs via the liver cells into bile has not been studied extensively. Available evidence indicates that the endothelium of the hepatic sinusoids behaves as an extremely porous barrier which allows ready equilibra-tion between plasma and bile of virtually all compounds whose molecular size is less than that of albumin. The membrane of the hepatic parenchymal cell has a porosity which is less than that of the sinusoidal epithelium but greater than that of many other cells. Quite a number of relatively hydrophilic compounds are thus able to traverse the liver cells. Although many drugs diffuse in small quantity into bile in the unchanged state, the majority undergo metabolic transformation in the liver and appear in bile as conjugates such as glucuronides, glycine or gluta-mine conjugates, ethereal sulphates, etc. Experimental studies in animals have shown that drugs of low molecular weight ($<200$) only appear in bile to the extent of less than 5 per cent of the dose, including the conjugates. Their main route of excretion is via the kidney. Compounds of higher molecular weight, particularly if they contain a suitably placed polar group such as $^-OH$ or $^-OCH_3$ in the molecule, are more likely to be excreted in bile provided they can be metabolized and conjugated. Thus, for example, excretion in bile is the major route of elimination of the drug carbenoxolone following glucuronide conjuga-tion in the liver (Parke, 1968). Many conjugates are polar acidic compounds which, being high ionized, are not readily reabsorbed from the intestine. They may be excreted unchanged in the faeces or may be split by enzyme activity emanating from intestinal cells or the bacterial microflora to yield other compounds which can be absorbed. An enterohepatic circulation of the compound and its metabolites may therefore arise which rather than assist in drug elimination, has the opposite effect of pro-longing drug action (Williams, Millburn and Smith, 1965). Such continuous recirculation of foreign compounds and metabolites could have toxicological significance.

In addition, there is evidence for at least two carrier-mediated systems for transporting organic acids and bases from blood to bile analogous to the secretory mechanisms of the renal tubule. Like the kidney, the biliary systems have the features of active transport mechanisms of low structural specificity.

### Kinetics of Drug Elimination (Butler, 1958; Nelson, 1961; Wagner, 1967; Levy, 1971)

After a dose of any drug is administered by whatever route, its ultimate fate will be its elimination from the body. The term 'elimination' is used here to include all the processes which operate to reduce the effective drug concentration in body fluids. Most elimination mechan-isms are approximately *first order*, that is, the rate of elimination is proportional to the concentration of drug in the body at any given time. Thus, a plot of concentration of drug in plasma versus time gives a typical exponential curve. If $D$ equals the total drug in the body at time $t$, $D_0$ is the drug present at zero time and $K$ equals the rate constant for elimination (in this case the sum of rate constants for metabolism, urinary excretion or other process disposing of drug), then

$$D = D_0 \, e^{-Kt}$$

and

$$\log D = \log D_0 - \frac{K}{2 \cdot 303} \cdot t$$

If $t_{\frac{1}{2}}$ equals the time for $D_0$ to decrease to one half the initial concentration, i.e. $D = D_0/2$, it follows that

$$t_{\frac{1}{2}} = \frac{2 \cdot 303 \log 2}{K} = 0 \cdot 693/K$$

$t_{\frac{1}{2}}$, the half time for elimination is often termed the *biological half-life*; from this equation, it is clearly independent of $D_0$.

When a drug is mainly excreted via the kidney, the plasma half-life is determined by the volume of distribution ($V_d$) and by the renal clearance of the drug ($C_D$) (Butler, 1958). Thus

$$t_{\frac{1}{2}} = 2 \cdot 303 \cdot \log 2 \cdot \frac{V_d}{C_D}$$

The volume of distribution and renal clearance tend to be inversely related because a major influence on their respective magnitudes is the inherent diffusibility of drugs across lipid biomembranes. Thus, for example, a highly lipid-soluble drug might possess an apparent $V_d$ much greater than total body water; its renal clearance would be low because of substantial back diffusion from the tubular fluid, possibly by a pH-dependent mechanism. The biological half-life would be long provided rapid metabolic inactivation in the liver was not occurring at the same time. The formula for $t_{\frac{1}{2}}$ is not affected by protein-binding of the drug provided the same measurement of drug concentration (i.e. either total concentration or protein-free component) is used for calculating $V_d$ and $C_D$. In practice, $t_{\frac{1}{2}}$ values vary widely. For example, the half-life of a drug like PAH will be very short because $V_d$ is small (localization of drug to the extracellular fluid) and $C_D$ is at the level of renal blood flow. In the case of the antimalarial mepacrine, because of its high affinity for intracellular binding sites and low excretion rate, $t_{\frac{1}{2}}$ is unusually long and significant amounts of drug may be found in the body for as long as two months after a single dose.

If the major elimination mechanisms of a drug can become saturated, and the concentration of drug rises above saturation level, then elimination will follow *zero order kinetics* (constant rate). Examples of this are the renal and biliary transport systems for drug secretion for which there is always a maximum transport capacity or *Tm*. If the plasma level of a drug is so high that *Tm* is exceeded, zero order kinetics will be obeyed until the concentration falls below the saturation level; subsequent elimination will be exponential and follow first order kinetics. The elimination of ethanol is an example where zero order kinetics apply. Ethanol is very slowly excreted through the kidneys and lungs, its chief route of elimination being oxidation by liver alcohol dehydrogenase via a NAD-coupled reaction:

$$C_2H_5OH + NAD^+ \rightleftharpoons CH_3CHO + NADH + H^+ \rightarrow$$
$$CH_3CO \cdot CoA$$
acetyl coenzyme A

The rate of metabolism in man is essentially constant at about 10 ml./hr. regardless of the concentration of alcohol,

and zero order kinetics arise mainly because $NAD^+$ cannot be made available at a sufficient rate (Mendelson, 1970; Hawkins and Kalant, 1972). Using the same notation as for first order kinetics, a zero order reaction obeys the following equation:

$$D = D_0 - Kt$$

If $t_{\frac{1}{2}}$ equals the time taken for $D$ to decrease to a value of $D_0/2$, then by substitution, $t_{\frac{1}{2}} = D_0/2K$, indicating that in this instance, the half-life is directly related to the initial concentration of drug. It is only as the circulating concentration of ethanol falls to low levels at which $NAD^+$ supply is no longer the limiting factor, that elimination kinetics become exponential.

## REFERENCES

Aggeler, P. M., O'Reilly, R. A., Leong, L. and Kowitz, P. E. (1967), "Potentiation of Anticoagulant Effect of Warfarin by Phenylbutazone," *New Engl. J. Med.*, **276**, 496–501.

Albert, A. (1952), "Ionization, pH and Biological Activity," *Pharcam. Rev.*, **4**, 136–168.

Albert, A. (1971), "Relations between Molecular Structure and Biological Activity: Stages in the Evolution of Current Concepts," *A. Rev. Pharmac.*, **11**, 13–36.

Aldridge, W. N. (1969), "Organophosphorus Compounds and Carbamates, and Their Reaction with Esterases," *Br. med. Bull.*, **25**, 236–240.

Allison, A. C. and Nunn, J. F. (1968), "Effects of General Anaesthetics on Microtubules: A possible Mechanism of Anaesthesia," *Lancet*, **2**, 1326–1329.

Anton, A. H. (1960), "The Relation Between the Binding of Sulfonamides to Albumin and Their Antibacterial Efficacy," *J. Pharmac. exp. Ther.*, **129**, 282–290.

Anton, A. H. (1961), "A Drug-induced Change in the Distribution and Renal Excretion of Sulfonamides," *J. Pharmac. exp. Ther.*, **134**, 291–303.

Ariëns, E. J. (1964), *Molecular Pharmacology. The Mode of Action of Biologically Active Compounds.* Volume One. New York and London: Academic Press.

Ariëns, E. J., Van Rossum, J. M. and Simonis, A. M. (1957), "Affinity, Intrinsic Activity and Drug Interactions," *Pharmac. Rev.*, **9**, 218–236.

Astwood, E. B. (1957), "Occurrence in the Sera of Certain Patients of Large Amounts of a Newly Isolated Iodine Compound," *Trans. Ass. Am. Physns*, **70**, 183–191.

Beckett, A. H. and Casy, A. F. (1954), "Synthetic Analgesics: Stereochemical Considerations," *J. Pharm. Pharmac.*, **6**, 986–1001.

Beckett, A. H. and Casy, A. F. (1965), "Analgesics and their Antagonists: Biochemical Aspects and Structure-activity Relationships," *Progr. mednl. Chem.*, **4**, 171–218.

Belleau, B. (1966), "Steric Effects in Catecholamine Interactions with Enzymes and Receptors," *Pharmac. Rev.*, **18**, 131–140.

Belleau, B. (1967), "Stereochemistry of Adrenergic Receptors. Newer Concepts on the Molecular Mechanism of Action of Catecholamines and Antiadrenergic Drugs at the Receptor Level," *Ann. N.Y. Acad. Sci.*, **139**, 580–605.

Bennett, W. M., Singer, I. and Coggins, C. H. (1970), "A practical Guide to Drug Usage in Adult Patients with Impaired Renal Function," *J. Am. med. Ass.*, **214**, 1468–1475.

Bloom, B. M. and Goldman, I. M. (1966), "The Nature of Catecholamine-adenine Mononucleotide Interactions in Adrenergic Mechanisms," *Adv. Drug Res.*, **3**, 121–169.

Bradbury, M. W. and Davson, H. (1964), "The Blood-brain Barrier," in *Absorption and Distribution of Drugs*, ed. Binns, T. B., pp. 77–85. Edinburgh: E. and S. Livingstone Ltd.

Brodie, B. B. (1952), Physiological Disposition and Chemical Fate of Thiobarbiturates in the Body," *Fedn. Proc.*, **11**, 632–639.

Brodie, B. B. (1964a), "Physico-chemical Factors in Drug

Absorption," in *Absorption and Distribution of Drugs*, ed. Binns, T. B., pp. 16–48. Edinburgh: E. and S. Livingstone Ltd.

Brodie, B. B. (1964b), "Distribution and Fate of Drugs: Therapeutic Implications," in *Absorption and Distribution of Drugs*, ed. Binns, T. B., pp. 199–251. Edinburgh: E. and S. Livingstone Ltd.

Brodie, B. B. (1965), "Displacement of One Drug by Another from Carrier or Receptor Sites," *Proc. R. Soc. Med.*, **58**, 946–955.

Brodie, B. B., Aronow, L. and Axelrod, J. (1954), "The Fate of Dibenzyline in the Body and the Role of Fat in its Duration of Action," *J. Pharmac. exp. Ther.*, **111**, 21–29.

Brodie, B. B. and Hogben, A. M. (1957), "Some Physico-chemical Factors in Drug Action," *J. Pharm. Pharmac.*, **9**, 345–380.

Brodie, B. B., Kurz, H. and Schanker, L. S. (1960), "The Importance of Dissociation Constant and Lipid-solubility in Influencing the Passage of Drugs into the Cerebrospinal Fluid," *J. Pharmac. exp. Ther.*, **130**, 20–25.

Brodie, B. B., Mark, L. C., Papper, E. M., Lief, P. A., Bernstein, E. and Rovenstine, E. A. (1950), "The Fate of Thiopental in Man and a Method for its Estimation in Biological Material," *J. Pharmac. exp. Ther.*, **98**, 85–96.

Brown, G. M. (1962), "The Biosynthesis of Folic Acid. II. Inhibition by Sulfonamides," *J. biol. Chem.*, **237**, 536–540.

Burgen, A. S. V. (1966), "The Drug-receptor Complex," *J. Pharm. Pharmac.*, **18**, 137–149.

Burger, A. and Parulkar, A. P. (1966), "Relationships Between Chemical Structure and Biological Activity," *A. Rev. Pharmac.*, **6**, 19–48.

Burt, R. A. P. (1971), "The Foetal and Maternal Pharmacology of some of the Drugs used for the Relief of Pain in Labour," *Br. J. Anaesth.*, **43**, 824–836.

Butler, T. C. (1958), "Termination of Drug Action by Elimination of Unchanged Drug," *Fedn. Proc.*, **17**, 1158–1162.

Christensen, L. K., Hansen, J. M. and Kristensen, M. (1963), "Sulphaphenazole-induced Hypoglycaemic Attacks in Tolbutamide-treated Diabetics," *Lancet*, **2**, 1298–1301.

Churchill-Davidson, H. C., Way, W. L. and de Jong, R. H. (1967), "The Muscle Relaxants and Renal Excretion," *Br. J. Anaesth.*, **28**, 540–546.

Clark, A. J. (1926), "The Reaction Between Acetyl Choline and Muscle Cells," *J. Physiol., Lond.* **61**, 530–546.

Conference on Biological Membranes: Recent Progress. (1966), *Ann. N.Y. Acad. Sci.*, **137**, Art. 2. pp. 403–1048.

Conference on Cholinergic Mechanisms (1967). *Ann. N.Y. Acad. Sci.*, **144**, Art. 2, pp. 383–936.

Csáky, T. Z. (1965), "Transport Through Biological Membranes," *A. Rev. Physiol.*, **27**, 415–450.

Curran, P. F. and Schultz, S. G. (1968), "Transport Across Membranes: General Principles," in *Handbook of Physiology*. Section 6. *Alimentary Canal.* Vol. III. *Intestinal Absorption*, ed. Code, C. F. pp. 1217–1243. Washington, D. C.: American Physiological Society.

Davson, H. (1967), *The Physiology of the Cerebrospinal Fluid*. London: J. and A. Churchill Ltd.

Dettli, L., Spring, P. and Ryter, S. (1971), "Multiple Dose Kinetics and Drug Dosage in Patients with Kidney Disease," *Acta Pharmac. Tox.*, **29**, suppl. 3, 211–244.

Dixon, M. and Webb, E. C. (1964), "Enzyme Kinetics," in *Enzymes*, pp. 54–166. London: Longmans, Green and Co. Ltd.

Doherty, J. E., Hall, W. H., Murphy, M. L. and Beard, O. W. (1971), "New Information regarding Digitalis Metabolism," *Chest*, **59**, 433–437.

Done, A. K. (1964), "Developmental Pharmacology," *Clin. Pharmac. Ther.*, **5**, 432–479.

Done, A. K. (1966), "Perinatal Pharmacology," *A. Rev. Pharmac.*, **6**, 189–208.

Eger, E. I. (1964), "Respiratory and Circulatory Factors in Uptake and Distribution of Volatile Anaesthetic Agents," *Br. J. Anaesth.* **36**, 155–171.

Eger, E.I., Brandstater, B., Saidman, L.J., Regan, M.J., Severinghaus, J. W. and Munson, E. S. (1965), "Equipotent Alveolar Concentrations of Methoxyflurane, Halothane, Diethyl Ether, Fluroxene, Cyclopropane, Xenon and Nitrous Oxide in the Dog," *Anesthesiology*, **26**, 771–777.

Eger, E. I., Lundgren, C., Miller, S. L. and Stevens, W. C. (1969), "Anesthetic Potencies of Sulfur Hexafluoride, Carbon Tetrafluoride, Chloroform and Ethrane in Dogs," *Anesthesiology*, **30**, 129–135.

Ehrenpreis, S., Fleisch, J. H. and Mittag, T. W. (1969), "Approaches to the Molecular Nature of Pharmacological Receptors," *Pharmac. Rev.*, **21**, 131–181.

Eisen, N. G. (1964), "Combined Effect of Sodium Warfarin and Phenylbutazone," *J. Am. med. Ass.*, **189**, 64–65.

Featherstone, R. M. (1963), "Binding on Proteins and Fat," in *Uptake and Distribution of Anesthetic Agents*, ed. Papper, E. M. and Kitz, R. J., pp. 42–50. New York: McGraw-Hill Book Co. Inc.

Featherstone, R. M. (1968), "Introduction to Symposium on the Molecular Pharmacology of Anesthesia," *Fedn. Proc.*, **27**, 870–871.

Featherstone, R. M. and Muehlbaecher, C. A. (1963), "The Current Role of Inert gases in the Search for Anesthesia Mechanisms," *Pharmac. Rev.*, **15**, 97–121.

Featherstone, R. M. and Schoenborn, B. P. (1964), "Protein and Lipid Binding of Volatile Anesthetic Agents," *Br. J. Anaesth.*, **36**, 150–154.

Feldman, S. A. and Levi, J. A. (1963), "Prolonged Paresis following Gallamine: A Case Report," *Br. J. Anaesth.*, **35**, 804–806.

Ferguson, J. (1939), "The Use of Chemical Potentials as Indices of Toxicity," *Proc. R. Soc., B.*, **127**, 387–404.

Furchgott, R. F. (1964), "Receptor mechanisms," *A. Rev. Pharmac*, **4**, 21–50.

Gaddum, J. H. (1937), "Discussion on the Chemical and Physical Bases of Pharmacological Action," *Proc. R. Soc., B.*, **121**, 598–601.

Gibaldi, M., Levy, G. and Hayton, W. L. (1972), "Tubocurarine and Renal Failure," *Br. J. Anaesth.*, **44**, 163–165.

Gill, E. W. (1965), "Drug Receptor Interactions," *Prog. mednl. Chem.*, **4**, 39–85.

Ginsburg, J. (1971), "Placental Drug Transfer," *A. Rev. Pharmac.*, **11**, 387–408.

Ginsburg, J. and Jeacock, M. K. (1964), "The Placental Barrier," in *Absorption and Distribution of Drugs*, ed. Binns, T. B., pp. 86–102. Edinburgh: E. and S. Livingstone Ltd.

Glynn, I. M. (1968), "Membrane Adenosine Triphosphatase and Cation Transport," *Br. med. Bull.*, **24**, 165–169.

Glynn, I. M., Hoffman, J. F. and Lew, V. L. (1971), "Some 'Partial Reactions' of the Sodium Pump," *Phil. Trans. R. Soc. Lond. B.*, **262**, 91–102.

Goldstein, A. (1949), "The Interactions of Drugs and Plasma Proteins," *Pharmac. Rev.* **1**, 102–165.

Gosselin, R. E. (1967), "Kinetics of Pinocytosis," *Fedn. Proc.*, **26**, 987–993.

Gosselin, R. E. and Smith, R. P. (1966), "Trends in the Therapy of Acute Poisonings," *Clin. Pharmac. Ther.*, **7**, 279–299.

Greene, N. M. and Webb, S. R. (1969), "Facilitated Transfer of Halothane in Human Erythrocytes," *Anesthesiology*, **31**, 548–552.

Hart, L. G., Guarino, A. M. and Schanker, L. S. (1969), "Gastric Dialysis as a Possible Antidotal Procedure for Removal of Absorbed Drugs," *J. Lab. clin. Med.* **73**, 853–860.

Hawkins, R. D. and Kalant, H. (1972), "The Metabolism of Ethanol and its Metabolic Effects," *Pharmac. Rev.*, **24**, 67–157.

Heidelberger, C. (1967), "Cancer Chemotherapy with Purine and Pyrimidine Analogues," *A. Rev. Pharmac.*, **7**, 101–124.

Heinz, E. (1967), "Transport Through Biological Membranes," *A. Rev. Physiol.*, **29**, 21–58.

Hobbiger, F. (1968), "Anticholinesterases," in *Recent Advances in Pharmacology*, 4th edition, ed. Robson, J. M. and Stacey, R. S., pp. 281–310. London: J. and A. Churchill Ltd.

Hoffman, J. F. (1964) (editor), *The Cellular Functions of Membrane Transport*. Englewood Cliffs: Prentice-Hall, Inc.

Hogben, C. A. M., Tocco, D. J., Brodie, B. B. and Schanker, L. S. (1959), "On the Mechanism of Intestinal Absorption of Drugs," *J. Pharmac. exp. Ther.*, **125**, 275–282.

Holter, H. (1962), "Pinocytosis," in *Enzymes and Drug Action*, ed. Mongar, J. L. and de Reuck, A. V. S., pp. 30–42. London: J. and A. Churchill Ltd.

Hussar, D. A. (1967), "Therapeutic Incompatibilities: Drug Interactions," *Am. J. Pharm.*, **139**, 215–233.

Kalow, W. and Genest, K. (1957), "A Method for the Detection of

Atypical Forms of Human Serum Cholinesterase. Determination of Dibucaine Numbers," *Can. J. Biochem. Physiol.*, **35**, 339–346.

Kattamis, Ch., Davies, D. and Lehmann, H. (1967), "The Silent Serum Cholinesterase Gene," *Acta Genet.*, **17**, 299–303.

Keyes, M. and Lumry, R. (1968), "Binding of Anesthetics to Proteins: Linkage Between the Sixth-ligand Site of Heme Iron Ion and the Nonpolar Binding Sites of Myoglobin," *Fed. Proc*, **27**, 895–897.

Korn, E. D. (1969), "Cell Membranes: Structure and Synthesis," *A. Rev. Biochem.*, **38**, 263–288.

Koshland, D. E. (1963), "Correlation of Structure and Function in Enzyme Action," *Science*, **142**, 1533–1541.

Kunin, C. M. (1966), "Clinical Pharmacology of the New Penicillins. II. Effect of Drugs which Interfere with Binding to Serum Proteins," *Clin. Pharmac. Ther*, **7**, 180–188.

Lajtha, A. and Ford, D. H. (1968) (editors), *Brain Barrier Systems*. Progress in Brain Research. Volume 29. Amsterdam: Elsevier Publishing Company.

Lanman, R. C. and Schanker, L. S. (1965), "Passage of Lipid-insoluble Substances from Cerebrospinal Fluid (CSF) to Brain," *Pharmacologist*, **7**, 161.

Lant, A. F. (1972), "Renal Excretion and Nephrotoxicity of Drugs," in *Renal Disease*, 3rd ed. Black, D. A. K., pp. 591–613. Oxford: Blackwell Scientific Publications.

Lant, A. F., Priestland, R. N. and Whittam, R. (1970), "The Coupling of Downhill Ion Movements Associated with Reversal of the Sodium Pump in Human Red Cells," *J. Physiol., Lond.*, **207**, 291–301.

LeFevre, P. G. (1961), "Sugar Transport in the Red Blood Cell: Structure–activity Relationships in Substrates and Antagonists," *Pharmac. Rev.*, **13**, 39–70.

Lehmann, H. and Liddell, J. (1962), "The Cholinesterases," in *Modern Trends in Anaesthesia*, 2, ed. Evans, F. T. and Gray, T. C., pp. 164–205. London: Butterworths.

Levy, G. (1971), "Kinetics of Drug Action in Man," *Acta Pharm. Tox.*, **29**, suppl. 3, 203–210.

Lewis, J. W., Bentley, K. W. and Cowan, A. (1971), "Narcotic Analgesics and Antagonists," *A. Rev. Pharmac.*, **11**, 241–270.

Mackenzie, I. L. and Donaldson, R. M. (1969), "Vitamin $B_{12}$ Absorption and the Intestinal Cell Surface," *Fedn. Proc.*, **28**, 41–45.

Maickel, R. P., Miller, F. P. and Brodie, B. B. (1965), "Interaction of Non-steroidal Anti-inflammatory Agents with Corticosteroid Binding to Plasma Proteins," *Pharmacologist*, **7**, 182.

Mark, L. C. (1963), "Thiobarbiturates," in *Uptake and Distribution of Anesthetic Agents*, ed. Papper, E. M. and Kitz, R. J., pp. 289–297. New York: McGraw-Hill Book Company, Inc.

Martin, B. K. (1965), "Potential Effect of the Plasma Proteins on Drug Distribution," *Nature, Lond.*, **207**, 274–276.

Mautner, H. G. (1967), "The Molecular Basis of Drug Action," *Pharmac. Rev.*, **19**, 107–144.

Mayer, S., Maickel, R. P. and Brodie, B. B. (1959), "Kinetics of Penetration of Drugs and Other Foreign Compounds into Cerebrospinal Fluid and Brain," *J. Pharmac. exp. Ther.*, **127**, 205–211.

Mendelson, J. H. (1970), "Biological Concomitants of Alcoholism," *New Engl. J. Med.*, **283**, 24–32; 71–81.

Meyer, M. C. and Guttman, D. E. (1968), "The Binding of Drugs by Plasma Proteins," *J. pharm. Sci.*, **57**, 895–918.

Miller, K. W., Paton, W. D. M. and Smith, E. B. (1965), "Site of Action of General Anaesthetics," *Nature, Lond.*, **206**, 574–577.

Miller, S. L. (1961), "A Theory of Gaseous Anesthetics," *Proc. natn. Acad. Sci. U.S.A.*, **47**, 1515–1524.

Milne, M. D. (1965), "Influence of Acid-base Balance on Efficacy and Toxicity of Drugs," *Proc. R. Soc. Med.*, **58**, 961–963.

Milne, M. D. (1966), "Drugs, Poisons, and the Kidney," in *Renal Disease*, 2nd edition, ed. Black, D. A. K., pp. 546–560. Oxford: Blackwell Scientific Publications.

Milne, M. D., Scribner, B. H. and Crawford, M. A. (1958). "Non-ionic Diffusion and the Excretion of Weak Acids and Bases," *Am. J. Med.*, **24**, 709–729.

Moya, F. (1965), "Mechanisms of Drug Transfer Across the Placenta with Particular Reference to Chemotherapeutic Agents," in *Antimicrobial Agents and Chemotherapy—1965*, ed. Hobby, G. L., pp. 1051–1057. American Society for Microbiology.

Moya, F. and Smith, B. E. (1965), "Uptake, Distribution and Placental Transport of Drugs and Anesthetics," *Anesthesiology*, **26**, 465–476.

Moya, F. and Thorndike, V. (1962), "Passage of Drugs Across the Placenta," *Am. J. Obstet. Gynecol.* **84**, 1778–1798.

Moya, F. and Thorndike, V. (1963), "The Effects of Drugs Used in Labour on the Fetus and Newborn," *Clin. Pharmac. Ther.* **4**, 628–653.

Mullins, L. J. (1954), "Some Physical Mechanisms in Narcosis," *Chem. Rev.*, **54**, 289–323.

Neame, K. D. and Richards, T. G. (1972), *Elementary Kinetics of Membrane Carrier Transport*. Oxford: Blackwell Scientific Publications.

Nelson, E. (1961), "Kinetics of Drug Absorption, Distribution, Metabolism, and Excretion," *J. pharm. Sci.*, **50**, 181–192.

Odell, G. B. (1959a), "Studies in Kernicterus. I. The Protein Binding of Bilirubin," *J. clin. Invest.*, **38**, 823–833.

Odell, G. B. (1959b), "The Dissociation of Bilirubin from Albumin and Its Clinical Implications," *J. Pediat*, **55**, 268–279.

Odell, G. B., Cohen, S. N. and Kelly, P. C. (1969), "Studies in Kernicterus. II. The Determination of the Saturation of Serum Albumin with Bilirubin," *J. Pediat.*, **74**, 214–230.

O'Grady, F. (1971), "Antibiotics in Renal Failure," *Br. med. Bull.*, **27**, 142–147.

Oliver, M. F., Roberts, S. D., Hayes, D., Pantridge, J. F., Suzman, M. M. and Bersohn, I. (1963), "Effect of Atromid and Ethyl Chlorophenoxy-isobutyrate on Anticoagulant Requirements," *Lancet*, **1**, 143–144.

O'Reilly, R. A. and Aggeler, P. M. (1970), "Determinants of the Response to Oral Anticoagulant Drugs in Man," *Pharmac. Rev.* **22**, 35–96.

Orloff, J. and Berliner, R. W. (1961), "Renal Pharmacology," *A. Rev. Pharmac.*, **1**, 287–314.

Overton, E. (1899), "Ueber die allgemeinen osmotischen Eigenschaften der Zelle, ihre vermutlichen Ursachen und ihre Bedeutung für die Physiologie," *Vertljschr. naturforsch. Ges. Zurich*, **44**, 88–135.

Palay, S. L. and Karlin, L. J. (1959), "An Electron Microscopic Study of the Intestinal Villus. II. The Pathway of Fat Absorption," *J. biophys. biochem. Cytol.* **5**, 373–384.

Papper, E. M. and Kitz, R. J. (1963) (editors), *Uptake and Distribution of Anesthetic Agents*. New York: McGraw-Hill Book Company Inc.

Papper, E. M., Peterson, R. C., Burns, J. J., Bernstein, E., Lief, P. and Brodie, B. B. (1955), "Physiological Disposition of Certain N-alkyl Thiobarbiturates," *Anesthesiology*, **16**, 544–550.

Pardee, A. B. (1968), "Biochemical studies on active transport," *J. gen. Physiol.*, **52**, 279–295 S.

Parke, D. V. (1968), "Metabolic Studies with Carbenoxolone in Man and Animals," in *A Symposium on Carbenoxolone Sodium*, ed. Robson, J. M. and Sullivan, F. M., pp. 15–25. London: Butterworths.

Paton, W. D. M. (1961), "A Theory of Drug Action Based on the Rate of Drug-receptor Combination," *Proc. R. Soc., B*, **154**, 21–69.

Pauling, L. (1960), *The Nature of the Chemical Bond*, 3rd edition. New York: Cornell University Press.

Pauling, L. (1961), "A Molecular Theory of Anesthesia," *Science*, **134**, 15–21.

Pittinger, C. and Adamson, R. (1972), "Antibiotic Blockade of Neuromuscular Function," *A. Rev. Pharmac.*, **12**, 169–184.

Prescott, L. F. (1969), "Pharmacokinetic Drug Interactions," *Lancet*, **2**, 1239–1243.

Prescott, L. F. (1972), "Mechanisms of Renal Excretion of Drugs (with Special Reference to Drugs used by Anaesthetists)," *Br. J. Anaesth.*, **44**, 246–251.

Prockop, L. D., Schanker, L. S. and Brodie, B. B. (1962), "Passage of Lipid-insoluble Substances from Cerebrospinal Fluid to Blood," *J. Pharmac. exp. Ther.*, **135**, 266–270.

Rall, D. P., Moore, E., Taylor, N. and Zubrod, C. G. (1961), "The Blood-cerebrospinal Fluid Barrier in Man," *Archs Neurol., Chicago*, **4**, 318–322.

Reidenberg, M. M. (1971), *Renal Function and Drug Action*. Philadelphia: W. B. Saunders Co.

Reidenberg, M. M., Odar-Cederlof, I., Von Bahr, C., Borga, O. and Sjoqvist, F. (1971), "Protein Binding of Diphenylhydantoin and Desmethylimipramine in Plasma from Patients with Poor Renal Function," *New Engl. J. Med.*, **285**, 264–267.

Reynolds, F. and Taylor, G. (1971), "Plasma Concentrations of Bupivacaine during Continuous Epidural Analgesia in Labour: The Effect of Adrenaline," *Br. J. Anaesth.*, **43**, 436–440.

Riordan, D. D. and Gilbertson, A. A. (1971), "Prolonged Curarization in a Patient with Renal Failure," *Br. J. Anaesth.*, **43**, 506–508.

Robertson, R. N. (1968), *Protons, Electrons, Phosphorylation and Active Transport*. Cambridge: University Press.

Rosefsky, J. B. and Petersiel, M. E. (1968), "Perinatal Deaths associated with Mepivacaine Paracervical-Block Anesthesia in Labor," *New. Engl. J. Med.*, **278**, 530–533.

Rubin, M., Bernstein, H. N. and Zvaifler, N. J. (1963), Studies on the Pharmacology of Chloroquine," *Archs Ophthal., N.Y.*, **70**, 474–481.

Saubermann, A. J. and Gallagher, M. L. (1973), "Mechanisms of General Anesthesia: Failure of Pentobarbital and Halothane to Depolymerize Microtubules in Mouse Optic Nerve," *Anesthesiology*, **38**, 25–29.

Schanker, L. S. (1962), "Passage of Drugs Across Body Membranes," *Pharmac. Rev.*, **14**, 501–530.

Schanker, L. S. (1963), "Pharmacologic Implications of Drug Ionization," in *Uptake and Distribution of Anesthetic Agents*, ed. Papper, E. M. and Kitz, R. J., pp. 52–56. New York: McGraw-Hill Book Company Inc.

Schanker, L. S. (1965), "Passage of Drugs into and out of the Central Nervous System," in *Antimicrobial Agents and Chemotherapy—1965*, ed. Hobby, G. L., pp. 1044–1050. American Society for Microbiology.

Schanker, L. S., Shore, P. A., Brodie, B. B. and Hogben, C. A. M. (1957), "Absorption of Drugs from the Stomach. I. The Rat," *J. Pharmac. exp. Ther.*, **120**, 528–539.

Schanker, L. S., Tocco, D. J., Brodie, B. B. and Hogben, C. A. M. (1958), "Absorption of Drugs from the Rat Small Intestine," *J. Pharmac. exp. Ther.*, **123**, 81–88.

Schild, H. O. (1962), "Receptors," in *Enzymes and Drug Action*, ed. Mongar, J. L. and de Reuck, A. V. S., pp. 435–443. London: J. and A. Churchill Ltd.

Schmid, R., Diamond, I., Hammaker, L. and Gundersen, C. B. (1965), "Interaction of Bilirubin with Albumin," *Nature, Lond.*, **206**, 1041–1043.

Schoenborn, B. P. (1968), "Binding of Anesthetics to Protein: an X-ray Crystallographic Investigation," *Fedn. Proc.*, **27**, 888–894.

Seeman, P. (1973), "The Membrane Actions of Anesthetics and Tranquilizers," *Pharmac. Rev.*, **24**, 583–655.

Seeman, P. and Roth, S. (1972), "General Anesthetics Expand Cell Membranes at Surgical Concentrations," *Biochim. Biophys. Acta*, **255**, 171–177.

Seeman, P., Roth, S. and Schneider, H. (1971), "The Membrane Concentrations of Alcohol Anesthetics," *Biochem. Biophys. Acta*, **225**, 171–184.

Segal, B. M. (1963), Photosensitivity, Nail Discoloration and Onycholysis," *Archs intern, Med.*, **112**, 165–167.

Sellers, E. M. and Koch-Weser, J. (1969), "Protein Binding and Vascular Activity of Diazoxide," *New Engl. J. Med.*, **281**, 1141–1145.

Shannon, J. A., Earle, D. P., Brodie, B. B., Taggart, J. V. and Berliner, R. W. (1944), "The Pharmacological Basis for the Rational Use of Atabrine in the Treatment of Malaria," *J. Pharmac. exp. Ther.*, **81**, 307–330.

Shnider, S. M. and Way, E. L. (1968), "The Kinetics of Transfer of Lidocaine (Xylocaine^R) across Human Placenta," *Anesthesiology*, **29**, 944–950.

Skou, J. C. (1965), "Enzymatic Basis for Active Transport of $Na^+$ and $K^+$ Across Cell Membrane," *Physiol. Rev.*, **45**, 596–617.

Smithells, R. W. and Morgan, D. M. (1970), "Transmission of Drugs by the Placenta and the Breasts," *Practitioner*, **204**, 14–19.

Stenlake, J. B., Davidson, A. G., Jasani, M. K. and Williams, W. D.

(1968), "The Effect of Acetylsalicylic Acid, Phenylbutazone and Indomethacin on the Binding of 11-hydroxysteroids to Plasma Proteins in Patients with Rheumatoid Arthritis," *J. Pharm. Pharmac.*, **20**, Suppl. 248–253 S.

Stephenson, R. P. (1956), "A Modification of Receptor 'Theory,'" *Br. J. Pharmac. Chemother.*, **11**, 379–393.

Stewart, D. J. (1968), "Tetracyclines: Their Prevalence in Children's Teeth," *Br. dent. J.*, **124**, 318–320.

Stovner, J., Theodorsen, L. and Bjelke, E. (1971a), "Sensitivity to Tubocurarine and Alcuronium with Special Reference to Plasma Protein Pattern," *Br. J. Anaesth.*, **43**, 385–391.

Stovner, J., Theodorsen, L. and Bjelke, E. (1971b), "Sensitivity to Gallamine and Pancuronium with Special Reference to Serum Proteins," *Br. J. Anaesth.*, **43**, 953–958.

Stowe, C. M. and Plaa, G. L. (1968), "Extrarenal Excretion of Drugs and Chemicals," *A. Rev. Pharmac.*, **8**, 337–356.

Symposium on The Molecular Pharmacology of Anesthesia (1968), *Fedn. Proc.*, **27**, 870–913.

Thorp, J. M. (1964), "The Influence of Plasma Proteins on the Action of Drugs," in *Absorption and Distribution of Drugs*, ed. Binns, T. B., pp. 64–76. Edinburgh: E. and S. Livingstone Ltd.

Ussing, H. H. (1949), "Transport of Ions Across Cellular Membranes," *Physiol. Rev.*, **29**, 127–155.

Ussing, H. H. (1952), "Some Aspects of the Application of Tracers in Permeability Studies," *Adv. Enzymol.*, **13**, 21–65.

Ussing, H. H. (1960), "The Alkali Metal Ions in Isolated Systems and Tissues," in *Handbuch der experimentellen Pharmakologie*, ed. Eichler, O. and Farah, A., volume 13, pp. 1–195. Berlin: Springer-Verlag.

Van Rossum, J. M. (1964), "Receptor Theory in Enzymology," in *Molecular Pharmacology. The Mode of Action of Biologically Active Compounds*, ed. Ariëns, E. J., volume II, pp. 199–255.

Van Rossum, J. M. (1968), "Drug-receptor Theories," in *Recent Advances in Pharmacology*, 4th edition, ed. Robson, J. M. and Stacey, R. S., pp. 99–133. London: J. and A. Churchill Ltd.

Villee, C. A. (1965), "Placental Transfer of Drugs," *Ann. N.Y. Acad. Sci.*, **123**, 237–242.

Wagner, J. G. (1967), "Equations for Excretion Rate and Renal Clearances of Exogenous Substances not Actively Reabsorbed," *J. clin. Pharmac.*, **7**, 89–92.

Wasserman, R. H., Corradino, R. A. and Taylor, A. N. (1969), "Binding Proteins from Animals with Possible Transport Function," *J. gen. Physiol.* **54**, 114–137 S.

Waud, D. R. (1968), "Pharmacological Receptors," *Pharmac. Rev.*, **20**, 49–88.

Weiner, I. M. (1967), "Mechanisms of Drug Absorption and Excretion. The Renal Excretion of Drugs and Related Compounds," *A. Rev. Pharmac.*, **7**, 39–56.

Weiner, I. M. and Mudge, G. H. (1964), "Renal Tubular Mechanisms for Excretion of Organic Acids and Bases," *Am. J. Med.*, **36**, 743–762.

Weinstein, L. and Dalton, A. C. (1968), "Host Determinants of Responses to Antimicrobial Agents," (second and third parts of article), *New Engl. J. Med.*, **279**, 524–531; 580–588.

Welch, R. M., Harrison, Y. E., Conney, A. H. and Burns, J. J. (1969), "An Experimental Model in Dogs for Studying Interactions of Drugs with Bishydroxycoumarin," *Clin. Pharmac. Ther.*, **10**, 817–825.

Whittaker, V. P. (1968), "Structure and Function of Animal-cell Membranes," *Br. med. Bull.*, **24**, 101–106.

Whittam, R. (1964), *Transport and Diffusion in Red Blood Cells*. London: Edward Arnold (Publishers) Ltd.

Wilbrandt, W. and Rosenberg, T. (1961), "The Concept of Carrier Transport and its Corollaries in Pharmacology," *Pharmac. Rev.*, **13**, 109–183.

Williams, R. T. (1967), "Patterns of Excretion of Drugs in Man and other Species," in *Drug Responses in Man*, ed. Wostenholme, G. and Porter, R., pp. 71–82. London: J. and A. Churchill Ltd.

Williams, R. T., Millburn, P. and Smith, R. L. (1965), "The Influence of Enterohepatic Circulation on Toxicity of Drugs," *Ann. N.Y. Acad. Sci.*, **123**, 110–122.

Wilson, I. B. (1959), "Molecular Complemenatrity and Antidotes for Alkylphosphate Poisoning," *Fedn. Proc.*, **18**, 752–758.

Wilson, I. B. (1967), "Conformation Changes in Acetylcholinesterase," *Ann. N.Y. Acad. Sci.*, **144**, 664–674.

Wiseman, G. (1968), "Absorption of Amino Acids," in *Handbook of Physiology*. Section 6. *Alimentary Canal*. Volume III. *Intestinal Absorption*, ed. Code, C. F., pp. 1277–1307. Washington, D.C.: American Physiological Society.

Young, J. A. and Edwards, K. D. G. (1966), "Competition for Transport Between Methyldopa and Other Amino Acids in Rat Gut Loops," *Am. J. Physiol.* **210**, 1130–1136.

## SUGGESTIONS FOR FURTHER READING

Adriani, J. (1963), "General Anesthetics. 1. Absorption, Distribution and Elimination," in *Physiological Pharmacology*, ed. Root, W. S. and Hofmann, F. G., pp. 3–42. New York: Academic Press.

Binns, T. B. (1964) (editor), *Absorption and Distribution of Drugs*. Edinburgh: E. and S. Livingstone Ltd.

Bunker, J. P. and Vandam, L. D. (1965) (chairmen), "Effects of Anesthesia on Metabolism and Cellular Functions," *Pharmac. Rev.* **17**, 183–263.

Burger, A. (1967) (editor), *Drugs Affecting the Peripheral Nervous System*. Medicinal Research Series. Volume 1. New York: Marcel Dekker, Inc.

Csáky, T. Z. (1969), *Introduction to General Pharmacology*. London: Butterworths.

Fingl, E. and Woodbury, D. M. (1965), "General Principles," in *The Pharmacological Basis of Therapeutics*, ed. Goodman, L. S. and Gilman, A., 3rd edition, pp. 1–36. New York: The Macmillan Company.

Goldstein, A., Aronow, L. and Kalman, S. M. (1968), *Principles of Drug Action. The Basis of Pharmacology*. New York: Hoeber Medical Division.

Gourley, D. R. H. (1967), "Factors Modifying Drug Action in the Body," in *Modern Trends in Pharmacology and Therapeutics*, ed. Fulton, W. F. M., pp. 1–40. London: Butterworths.

Mongar, J. L. and deReuck, A. V. S. (1962) (editors), *Enzymes and Drug Action*. Ciba Foundation Symposium. London: J. and A. Churchill Ltd.

Smith, R. L. (1973), *The Excretory Function of Bile. The Elimination of Drugs and Toxic Substances in Bile*. London: Chapman and Hall.

Symposium on Clinical Effects of Interaction Between Drugs (1965), *Proc. R. Soc. Med.*, **58**, No. 11. Part 2.

Whittam, R. and Wheeler, K. P. (1970), "Transport Across Cell Membranes," *A. Rev. Physiol.*, **32**, 21–60.

*CHAPTER 2*

# METABOLISM OF DRUGS

ARIEL F. LANT

The majority of drugs employed in anaesthetic practice, whether volatile or non-volatile, are metabolized to some extent in the body. The duration of action of a drug, its pharmacological properties and often its freedom from side effects may be considerably influenced by rate and patterns of metabolism. The biochemical reactions involved in drug metabolism are of considerable number and diversity. A feature common to nearly all is the increased polarity and water solubility of the metabolic products when compared with the parent drug. This progressive polarization is of considerable importance in facilitating drug elimination. Decreased lipid solubility makes the compound both less able to traverse cell membranes and less likely to be stored in fat depots. More polar metabolites undergo less back-diffusion via the renal tubular epithelium into the plasma. Their renal clearance tends, therefore, to be higher. The carrier-mediated secretory mechanisms for anions and cations in both the proximal tubular cells and hepatic parenchymal cells operate readily upon polar substances to reduce their biological half-lives.

The fact that the body has developed mechanisms for metabolizing drugs and other foreign materials may be looked upon as an evolutionary adaptation to terrestial life, permitting the disposal of lipid soluble substances ingested in food (Brodie, 1962). The disposal is brought about by transforming, with the aid of certain enzyme systems, the lipid-soluble materials into polar compounds. Fish and other marine organisms lack these enzyme systems but they are able to excrete lipid-soluble materials directly by diffusion through the gill membranes into the surrounding water.

The metabolism of volatile anaesthetics is considered in detail in Chapter 5.

### Pathways of Drug Metabolism

The metabolism of drugs in general may be viewed as occurring in two phases. First, *metabolic transformation or biotransformation*—a series of non-synthetic reactions including oxidations, reductions and hydrolyses, whereby functional chemical groups are either unmasked or introduced. As a result, the activity of the parent drug may be activated, inactivated or altered. Second, *conjugation*—representing a series of biosynthetic reactions in which the parent drug or its metabolites are coupled to endogenous substrates often of carbohydrate or amino acid structure. The synthetic reactions almost invariably result in converting drugs into polar excretory products which are pharmacologically inactive. Although some drugs are metabolized by one phase processes only, e.g. the progressive oxidation reactions of ethanol (*see* p. 424), most undergo two-phase metabolism, that is, metabolic transformation followed by conjugation. A typical example:

Phenobarbitone (active) → [aromatic hydroxylation] → p-hydroxyphenobarbitone (inactive) → [conjugation] → p-hydroxy phenobarbitone glucuronide or ethereal sulphate (inactive)

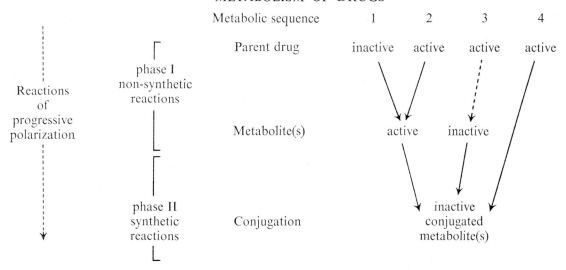

FIG. 1. Summary of the various patterns of drug metabolism involving non-synthetic and synthetic reactions. Interrupted lines indicate the possible occurrence of a series of intermediate reactions.

Although much of the information on drug metabolism has been obtained from studies in experimental animals, available clinical studies indicate that similar mechanisms operate also in man. However, there may be considerable species differences in the rates at which various reactions proceed. For example, a drug may undergo rapid metabolic inactivation and have a short duration of action in animals yet be more slowly inactivated and have longer duration of action in man (see later). The general pathways of drug metabolism are shown in schematic form in Fig. 1. The parent drug may be pharmacologically inactive or active. If inactive, it requires to be converted to an active metabolite as depicted in *sequence 1*. An example of this is given by the following reaction, which is of considerable historical importance:

In this case, an inactive parent drug in converted by azo-reduction to the active chemotherapeutic agent, sulphanilamide, and the active drug is subsequently inactivated by a synthetic acetylation reaction.

If the parent drug is pharmacologically active, three metabolic routes are open to it.

(a) *Sequence 2.* Conversion may occur to a metabolite which is pharmacologically active, but may differ in qualitative or quantitative characteristics from the parent drug.

Thus, for example:

Both these compounds are hydrazine derivatives of isonicotinic acid and both are effective antituberculous agents. However, the isopropyl compound, iproniazid, has marked antidepressant qualities which are probably linked to its ability to inhibit monoamine oxidase, and in addition it may produce a sensitivity-type hepatitis indistinguishable from viral hepatitis.

The principal metabolite of phenacetin is *p*-acetamidophenol or N-acetyl-*p*-aminophenol (paracetamol), both compounds possessing analgesic-antipyretic activity (Conney *et al.*, 1966). Paracetamol is subsequently inactivated largely by conjugation with glucuronic acid by typical conjugation reactions yielding a glucuronide and small amount of sulphate ester:

Occasionally metabolism leads to the formation of harmful substances including carcinogens (Miller and Miller, 1965). The process whereby an inactive compound is changed by metabolism into a toxic substance has been called *lethal synthesis* (Peters, 1969). A classic example is the conversion of the relatively inactive fluoroacetic acid into fluorocitric acid. The latter compound is an analogue of citric acid and acts as a metabolic inhibitor of the vital Krebs cycle enzyme, aconitate hydratase.

(b) *Sequence 3.* Conversion may occur through one or more steps to inactive metabolites, which may or may not undergo subsequent conjugation. This sequence of metabolism is a very common mode of drug inactivation. Hydroxylation of the phenyl group at C5 in the phenobarbitone molecule is a typical example (*see* p. 428).

(c) *Sequence 4.* Sometimes a drug follows a pattern of metabolism involving the synthetic reaction only. Thus an active drug may undergo direct conjugation by addition of glucuronic acid, methyl sulphate or other radicles to the molecule.

For example, the major route of metabolism of chloramphenicol in man is by formation of the monoglucuronide:

$NO_2$          $NO_2$

HO·CH    Cl     HO·CH    Cl

CH—NH·CO·CH    CH—NH·CO·CH

CH$_2$OH    Cl    CH$_2$O—C$_6$H$_9$O$_6$    Cl

chloramphenicol (active)        chloramphenicol glucuronide (inactive)

### Nature of Drug-Metabolizing Enzymes
(Brodie, 1962; Gillette, 1966; Gillette, Davis and Sasome, 1972)

Like other metabolic processes, the metabolism of drugs is catalysed by enzymes. Drugs are sometimes metabolized by the same enzymes which handle endogenous substrates. Thus certain steroid hormones are metabolized in the liver by the same microsomal enzymes which metabolize foreign drugs (Conney *et al.*, 1965). However, the vast majority of drugs are metabolized by special hepatic enzymes which do not appear to participate in the processes of intermediary metabolism.

**Microsomal Enzymes** (Mason, North and Vanneste, 1965; Holtzman *et al.*, 1968).

A series of drug metabolizing enzymes is located in the microsomes obtained when liver cell homogenates are subjected to differential centrifugation. The microsomal fraction consists mostly of fragmented elements of the plasma membrane and endoplasmic reticulum. In the intact cell the latter constitutes a network of lipoprotein channels extending throughout the cytoplasm and is continuous with the plasma- and nuclear-membranes. Under electron microscopy, some of the reticulum membranes are smooth (SER) whilst others are studded with ribosomes, making their appearance rough.

The rough microsomes are concerned with protein synthesis whilst drug-metabolizing enzymes are associated with the SER.

Drug metabolizing enzymes are unusual in a number of respects. They lack specificity and undertake biological oxidation of substances of widely differing nature provided they are lipid soluble; the products are more hydrophilic than the parent drug molecules. The drug metabolizing enzymes differ from the usual dehydrogenases of intermediary metabolism in having a requirement for the coenzyme, reduced nicotinamide adenine dinucleotide phosphate (NADPH) and also oxygen.

The mechanism of microsomal oxidation processes has been the subject of much study. It is believed that NADPH is part of a coupled redox system involving a flavoprotein, probably *cytochrome c reductase*. The electron transfer system incorporates as the terminal electron acceptor, a haem compound, cytochrome P-450, so-called because the

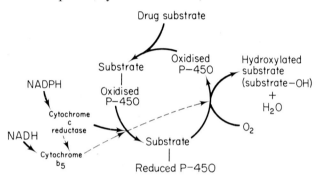

Fig. 2. Diagrammatic scheme of reactions involved in hydroxylations of drugs by cytochrome P-450 system.

spectral absorption peak of the carbon monoxide-reduced cytochrome ligand occurs at 450 nm. (Omura *et al.*, 1965; Alvares *et al.*, 1969). Oxidized P-450 combines with drug substrates and then the cytochrome moiety is reduced via the NADPH-cytochrome c reductase chain. The reduced P-450 drug complex then combines with molecular oxygen to result in hydroxylated drug products with the regeneration of oxidized P-450 so that the cycle can be repeated (Fig. 2). Participation of a second cytochrome, $b_5$, has been suggested, possibly involved in transfer of an electron into the system at the stage when reduced P-450—drug complex combines with molecular oxygen (Estabrook *et al.*, 1971). It is still uncertain whether the terminal transferase reaction represents the activity of a single non-specific hydroxylating enzyme or whether a plurality of enzymes is involved.

Two classes of drugs can be delineated on the basis of spectral changes caused on combination with the oxidized form of P-450. Type I substances are those which cause an absorption trough at about 420 nm. and peak at about 385 nm.; included in this category are hexobarbitone, pentobarbitone, ethylmorphine and aminopyrine. Type II substances produce an absorption trough at 390 nm. and peak at 430 nm.; this group includes aniline and nicotinamide. Other compounds such as acetanilid are intermediate in spectral studies and appear to cause both type I and type II changes (Schenkman, Remmer and Estabrook, 1967). It is of interest that halothane exerts a biphasic effect on NADPH-dependent oxidative reactions in rat liver microsomes, depressing the metabolism of type I substrates whilst stimulating the metabolism of the type II compound, aniline (Brown, 1971).

The finding that various compounds cause two types of spectral change in liver microsomes has raised hopes that this phenomenon may help to explain the inhibitory effects which some drugs have on each other's metabolism (*see* p. 437). However, anomalies exist in individual rates of inhibition and in the patterns of inhibitory response in different species indicating that the process of inhibition of microsomal metabolism is complex and may not be explicable on the basis of a single, universally applicable, mechanism (Gillette, 1971).

The endoplasmic reticulum of liver cells also contains other enzymes (capable of metabolizing drugs) such as reductases, esterases and also the transferases which are

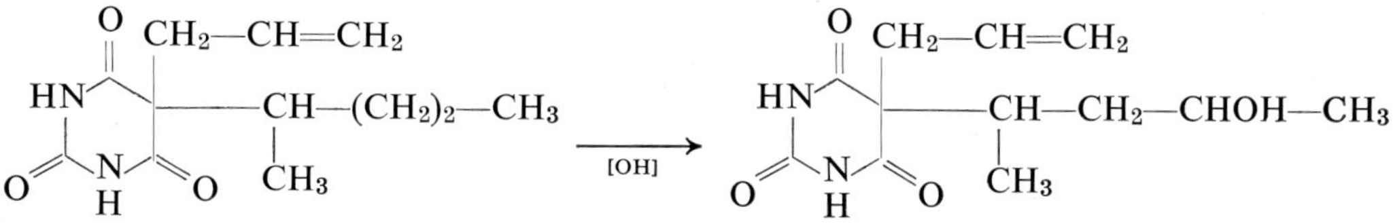

quinalbarbitone

hydroxyquinalbarbitone

involved in glucuronide formation. Some of these microsomal systems are also NADPH-dependent and involve participation of cytochrome P-450.

### Non-microsomal Enzymes

Drugs may, however, also be metabolized by enzymes present in mammalian cells but not in the microsomal fraction. Some of these enzymes are in the cell cytoplasm, as for example, aldehyde dehydrogenases or the enzymes concerned with sulphate and peptide conjugation as well as acetylation of various drugs (*see* p. 432). Other non-microsomal enzymes such as amine oxidases and various esterases are present in plasma.

A further source of drug-metabolizing enzymes is the bacterial flora of the intestinal tract. Because of the partially anaerobic environment in which they function, most of the metabolic transformations undertaken by these bacterial enzymes are reductions or hydrolyses. Such reactions may be of particular importance in the metabolism of incompletely absorbed drugs or compounds which on absorption are then excreted in bile and undergo a significant enterohepatic circulation.

### Types of Chemical Reaction (Brodie, Gillette and La Du, 1958; Williams, 1963; Williams and Parke, 1964; Greene, 1968; Parke, 1968a)

### I. Metabolic Transformation (Non-Synthetic Reactions)

Drugs undergo three main types of non-synthetic reaction:

1. Oxidations.
2. Reductions.
3. Hydrolyses.

### (1) Oxidations

#### A. Microsomal Oxidations

Most oxidative transformations involving drugs are mediated by enzymes located in the microsomal fraction of mammalian liver. The wide range of oxidations can all be ascribed to one common mechanism—*hydroxylation*.

In the following examples, the use of [OH] refers to oxidative reactions carried out through the activity of microsomal enzyme in presence of the coenzyme NADPH, and $O_2$. Unstable intermediates are enclosed in square brackets.

**(a) Aromatic hydroxylation** $R - C_6H_5 \rightarrow R - C_6H_4OH$. An example already considered is the conversion of phenobarbitone to p-hydroxyphenobarbitone (p. 428).

**(b) Aliphatic or side-chain hydroxylation.** Example:

**(c) Oxidative dealkylation**

$$R{-}NH{-}CH_3 \rightarrow [R{-}NH{-}CH_2OH]$$
$$\rightarrow R{-}NH_2 + HCHO$$

$$R{-}O{-}CH_3 \rightarrow [R{-}O{-}CH_2OH]$$
$$\rightarrow R{-}OH + HCHO$$

There may be oxidative removal of alkyl groups from nitrogen or oxygen moieties:

*N-dealkylation*, e.g.:

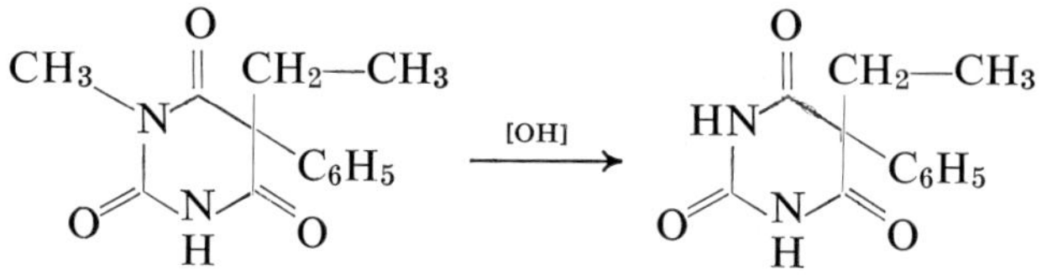

methylphenobarbitone

phenobarbitone

*O-dealkylation*, e.g.

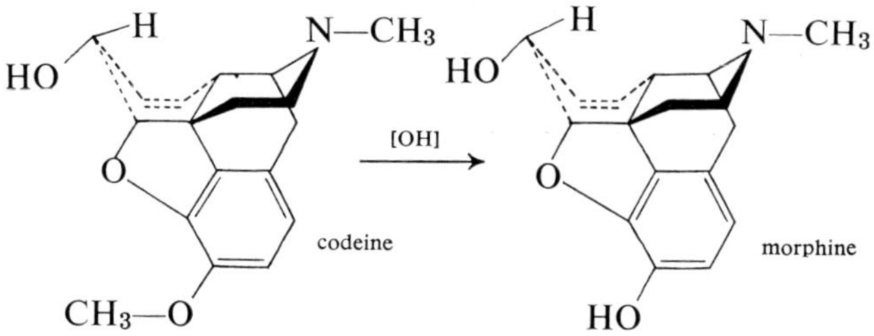

codeine

morphine

**(d) N-oxidation and N-hydroxylation** $R - NH_2 \rightarrow [R - NOH]^+ \rightarrow R - N = O + H^+$

Aromatic primary amines undergo hydroxylation of the amino group to form hydroxylamino compounds:

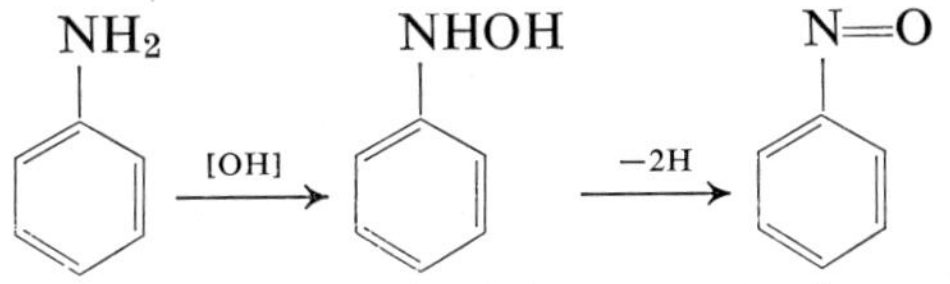

NH₂ → [OH] → NHOH → −2H → N=O

aniline     phenylhydroxylamine     nitrosobenzene

Secondary and tertiary amines may be metabolized to their corresponding N-oxides; the N-oxide may not only be the terminal metabolite but in some cases also an intermediate in the oxidative N-dealkylation of the parent drug. A number of commonly used tertiary amines such as chlorpromazine, chlorcyclizine, guanethidine and imipramine form N-oxides (Bickel, 1969).

**(e) S-oxidation**

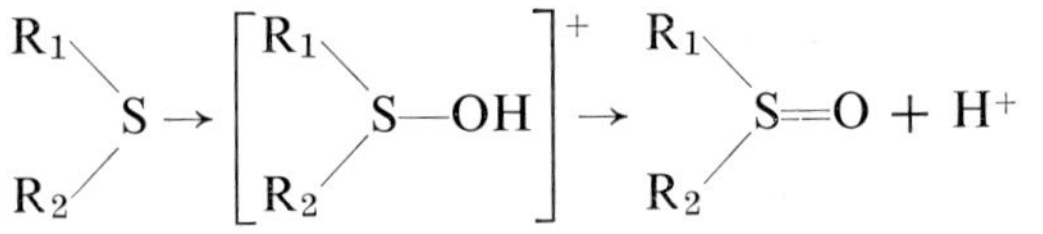

$$\frac{R_1}{R_2}S \rightarrow \left[\frac{R_1}{R_2}S-OH\right]^+ \rightarrow \frac{R_1}{R_2}S=O + H^+$$

The heterocyclic sulphur atoms of phenothiazine derivatives are oxidized to sulphoxides, e.g.:

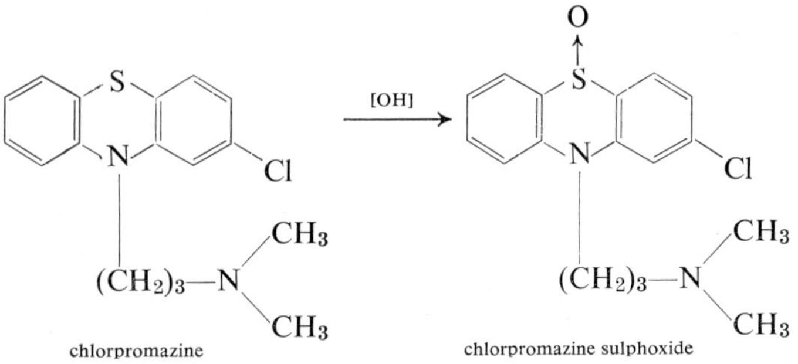

chlorpromazine → [OH] → chlorpromazine sulphoxide

(structures with (CH₂)₃—N(CH₃)₂ side chains and Cl)

**(f) Desulphurization.** Replacement of a sulphur atom by oxygen, e.g.:

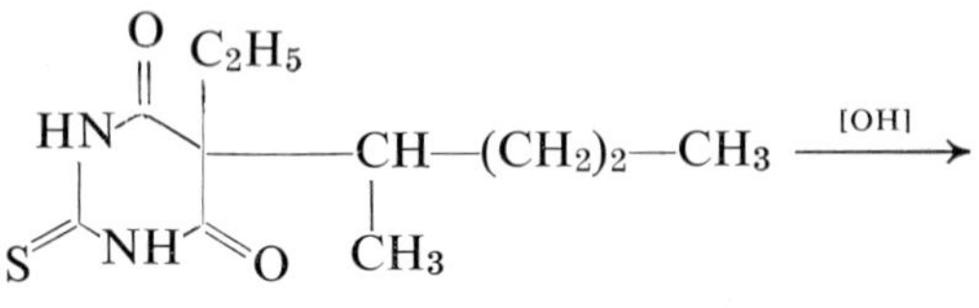

thiopentone → [OH] → pentobarbitone

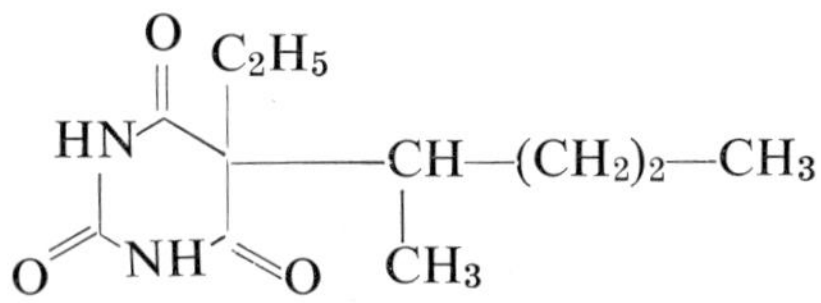

**(g) Oxidative deamination**

$$\frac{R_1}{R_2}CH-NH_2 \rightarrow \left[\frac{R_1}{R_2}C\frac{OH}{NH_2}\right] \rightarrow \frac{R_1}{R_2}C=O + NH_3$$

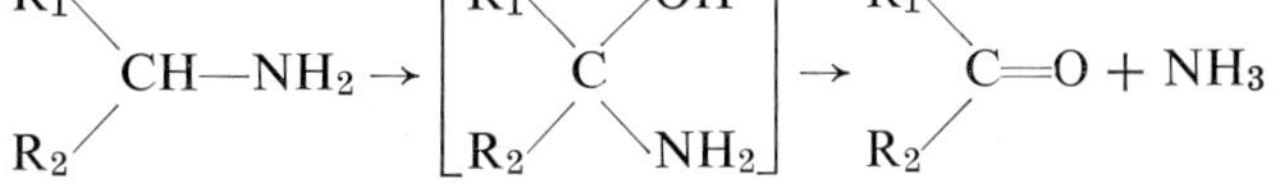

In addition to the well-known monoamine oxidase (MAO) which is a mitochondrial enzyme (see below), there is also microsomal deaminase activity in the liver which deaminates α methyl-substituted amines such as amphetamine.

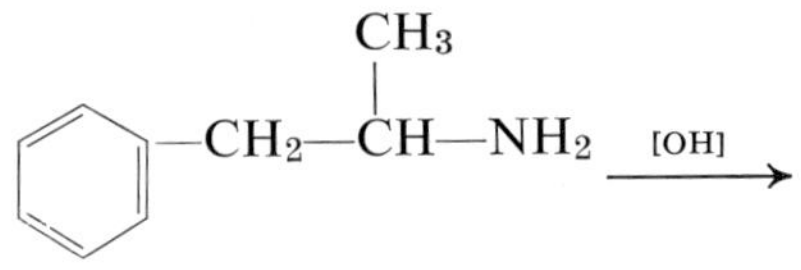

amphetamine → [OH] → phenylacetone + NH₃

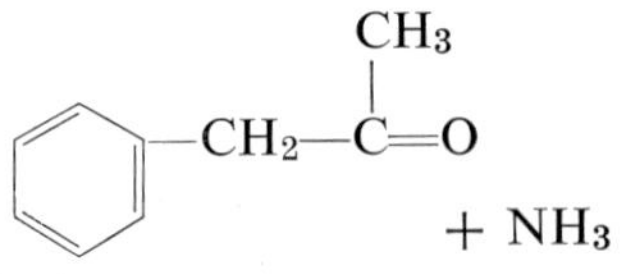

## B. Non-microsomal oxidations

Drugs may also undergo oxidative metabolism by mammalian enzymes which are not part of the hepatic microsomal system. Some of these enzymes are *mitochondrial*, such as the mono- and di-amine oxidases, others are cytoplasmic as for example alcohol and aldehyde dehydrogenase and xanthine oxidase. The metabolic transformations undertaken include aromatization of cyclohexane derivatives, oxidation of alcohols and aldehydes and oxidative deamination of aliphatic and aryl-substituted aliphatic amines.

**(a) Alcohol and aldehyde oxidation.** A variety of primary alcohols are metabolized by the relatively non-specific enzyme alcohol dehydrogenase found in the soluble fraction of hepatic cells. The substrates may be primary alcohols such as ethanol (see p. 424) or alcohols formed as intermediates during microsomal oxidation of other drugs, e.g. side-chain hydroxylation of barbiturates at C5 of the ring (see p. 428).

Aliphatic and aromatic aldehydes, including several purine derivatives, may be oxidized to their corresponding carboxylic acids by the soluble enzymes, aldehyde oxidase, xanthine oxidase and a NAD⁺-dependent aldehyde dehydrogenase. The latter enzyme appears to be responsible for the oxidation of chloral hydrate:

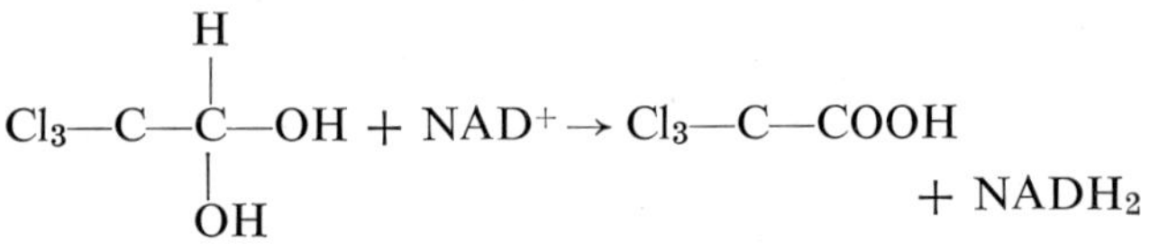

$$Cl_3-C\underset{OH}{\overset{H}{|}}-OH + NAD^+ \rightarrow Cl_3-C-COOH + NADH_2$$

chloral hydrate     trichloracetic acid

As with the alcohols, aldehyde formation may occur during microsomal metabolism and be followed by oxidation via cytoplasmic oxidative enzymes.

**(b) Deamination.** Several non-microsomal deaminating enzymes are known. These include tissue mono- and di-amine oxidases and amine oxidases circulating in plasma. Although the term monoamine oxidase (MAO) is widely used, it does not necessarily refer to a single enzyme; the enzyme probably exists in a number of forms. It is a mitochondrial enzyme found particularly at sites of formation and storage of bioamines. It metabolizes the catecholamines (dopamine, noradrenaline and adrenaline) and their *o*-methyl derivates as well as tyramine and the tryptophan derivatives, tryptamine and 5-hydrotryptamine. It does not, however, metabolize phenyl-ethylamines carrying an α methyl group, such as amphetamine or ephedrine. One of the functions of amine oxidases is to detoxify potentially toxic amines either ingested in food or produced in the body. The sympathomimetic amine, tyramine, together with other amines such as phenylethylamine and histamine, is present in considerable quantity in cheeses and various yeast extracts such as Marmite. These amines are normally inactivated by mono- and di-amine oxidase in intestinal

$$C_2H_5 \quad \overset{S}{\underset{\parallel}{} } \quad \overset{S}{\underset{\parallel}{} } \quad C_2H_5$$
$$\underset{C_2H_5}{\overset{}{\diagdown}} N-C-S-S-C-N \underset{C_2H_5}{\overset{}{\diagup}}$$
disulfiram

mucosa and liver. In patients treated with MAO inhibitors, the enzymes are inhibited to a variable extent. As a result, dietary amines are not metabolized efficiently and may in quantity trigger the release of catecholamines accumulated in tissue storage granules. A hypertensive crisis may thus be evoked.

## 2. Reductions

### A. Microsomal Reductions

The hepatic endoplasmic reticulum contains enzymes which reduce drugs. Both azo- and nitro-compounds are reduced by flavoprotein systems, azo-reductase being $NADPH_2$-dependent whilst nitro-reductase requires either $NADPH_2$ or $NADH_2$. Both enzymes function best anaerobically.

**(a) Azo- and nitro-reductase.** Azo reduction is illustrated by the classic reaction in which the dye Prontosil is reduced to yield the active antibacterial agent, sulphanilamide (*see* p. 325). Various aromatic nitro compounds such as nitrophenols and chloramphenicol are reduced to their corresponding amines by microsomal nitro-reductase.

**(b) Reductive dehalogenation.** This reaction involves the removal of chlorine, bromine or iodine atoms from halogenated organic molecules. Most susceptible to removal is chloride whilst the carbon-fluorine bond appears to be metabolically more stable. Reactive dehalogenation is of importance in the metabolism of halogenated hydrocarbons used as inhalational anaesthetics (Van Dyke and Chenoweth, 1965; Cohen, 1971). In the case of halothane, both dehalogenation and subsequent oxidation are processes probably undertaken by the hepatic microsomal system. Thus, for example:

$$F_3-C-CH\underset{Cl}{\overset{Br}{\diagup}} \rightarrow F_3-C-CH_3 \rightarrow F_3-C-COOH$$
halothane            trifluoroethane        trifluoracetic acid

On the basis of urinary excretion of trifluoracetic acid and bromide in two patients, it has been calculated that about 18 per cent of halothane absorbed undergoes metabolic transformation in man (Rehder *et al.*, 1967).

### B. Non-microsomal Reductions

**Mammalian enzymes.** The reduction of disulphide and sulphoxide compounds proceeds through the action of cytoplasmic enzymes which are distinct from the hepatic microsomal system. Disulphides are reduced to mercaptans and sulphoxides to sulphides by this mechanism. For example, the drug disulfiram, used in the treatment of alcoholism, is reduced to its corresponding thiol.:

$$\longrightarrow 2 \left[ \underset{C_2H_5}{\overset{C_2H_5}{\diagup}} N-C-SH \right]$$
diethyl-dithio-carbamic acid

**Bacterial Enzymes.** Reduction of drugs may occur through action of enzymes of the gastrointestinal flora. The native drug may be reduced before absorption or the products of host enzymic metabolism excreted into bile may be acted upon further within the intestinal lumen. Reduction of N-oxides and azo-benzene compounds may occur by this mechanism.

## 3. Hydrolyses

Drug metabolism by hydrolysis is largely restricted to esters and amides. The responsible esterases and amidases isolated from different mammalian and bacterial sources have different substrate specificities.

### A. Microsomal hydrolyses

Esterase and amidase activity may be associated with the microsomal enzyme system of the liver. For example, pethidine is hydrolysed in man by microsomal esterase and not by plasma esterase:

$$CH_3-N\underset{}{\overset{C_6H_5}{}}COO\cdot C_2H_5 \longrightarrow$$
pethidine

$$CH_3-N\underset{}{\overset{C_6H_5}{}}COOH + C_2H_5OH$$
meperidinic acid            ethanol

### B. Non-microsomal Hydrolyses

**Mammalian enzymes.** *Hydrolysis of esters and amides.* There are a number of esterases such as acetylcholinesterase and pseudocholinesterase which differ from the hepatic microsomal enzymes. These enzymes are found in various mammalian tissues such as plasma, red cells and nervous tissue. A wide variety of ester drugs are hydrolysed to their

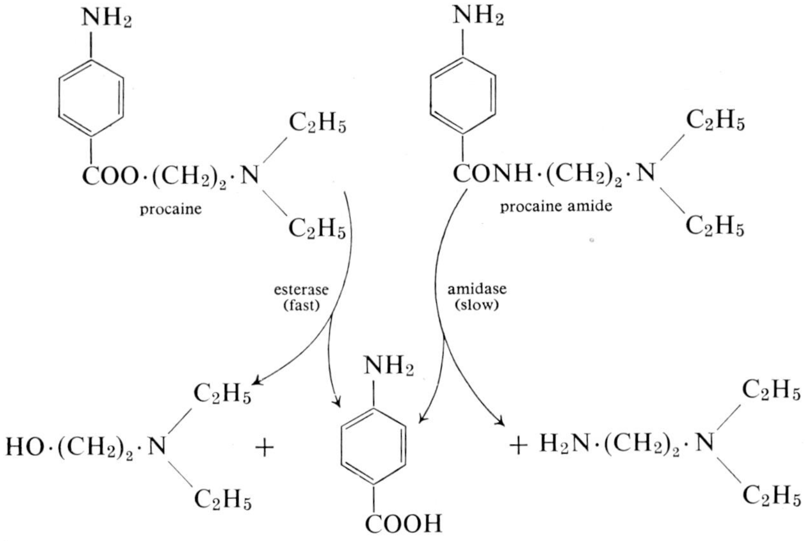

FIG. 3.

constituent acids and alcohols by this mechanism. There are a number of interesting species differences. Thus, for example, atropine does not undergo significant hydrolysis in man but is rapidly hydrolysed by certain rabbits who have a genetically determined high level of atropine esterase in the plasma (Gosselin, Gabourel and Wills, 1960; Margolis and Feigelson, 1964).

Amides are generally more stable than the corresponding esters and undergo slower hydrolysis to form acid and amine. This has been taken advantage of in development of new drugs. For example, procaine is rapidly hydrolysed and inactivated by plasma esterases. Its amide analogue is hardly hydrolysed at all in the plasma and only undergoes slow hydrolysis in the tissues. The pharmacological activity of procaine amide is therefore more prolonged (Mark *et al.*, 1951). (*See* Fig. 3.)

*Hydrolytic scission of heterocycles.* Hydrolysis of heterocyclic compounds may take the form of cleavage of the ring structure. For example, the hydrogenated benzothiadiazine diuretics may undergo scission by hydrolysis of the thiadiazine ring (Pinson *et al.*, 1962).

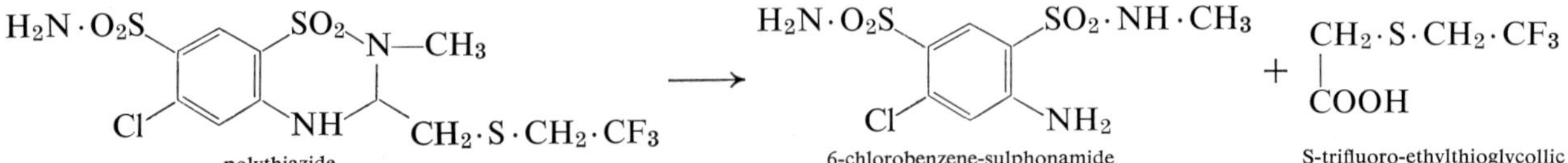

**Bacterial enzymes.** A number of esters and glycosides may be hydrolysed by enzymes of the intestinal flora (Scheline, 1968; Williams, 1971). For example, coumarin anticoagulants may undergo scission of the heterocyclic ring to yield substituted phenolic compounds.

## II. Conjugation of Drugs (Synthetic Reactions)

A conjugation reaction is a biochemical synthesis which occurs between drugs and their metabolites and a substance of endogenous origin. The endogenous substrate is often called the *conjugating* or *donor agent* and is usually a derivative of carbohydrate or aminoacid metabolism. Conjugation is not confined to foreign compounds. It plays a major role in the metabolism of a number of substances of physiological importance. Thus detoxication and transport of bile pigments (as glucuronides), bile salts (as taurine and glycine conjugates), synthesis and inactivation of catechol amines (N-methylation of noradrenaline; inactivation by *o*-methylation) are examples of conjugation reactions.

The following conjugation reactions have been shown to occur in man:

1. Glucuronide formation.
2. Peptide formation—conjugates with glycine, glutamine and other amino acids.
3. Ethereal sulphate formation.
4. Methylation.
5. Acetylation.
6. Glutathione conjugation.
7. Thiocyanate formation.

### 1. Glucuronide Formation (Dutton, 1966; Smith and Williams, 1966)

This is probably the most important of all the types of conjugation. Whereas other conjugating reactions are limited to certain chemical structures, a remarkably wide range of different chemical structures can participate in glucuronide formation. Compounds possessing phenolic, alcoholic, carboxylic amino or thiol radicals can form

O-, N- or S-glucuronides according to the chemical nature of the functional group undergoing conjugation. Formation of glucuronides involves the transfer of the glucuronyl residue from its active form where it is attached to the coenzyme, uridine diphosphate-glucuronic acid (UDPGA) to the acceptor drug molecule. The reaction is catalysed by a group of microsomal enzymes known as UDP-transglucuronylases or glucuronyl transferases. Thus:

$$R—OH + UDPGA \rightarrow R—O—C_6H_9O_6 + UDP$$

acceptor drug    "activated" glucuronic acid    glucuronide    uridine diphosphate

In general, glucuronide conjugates are $\beta$-pyranoside structures:

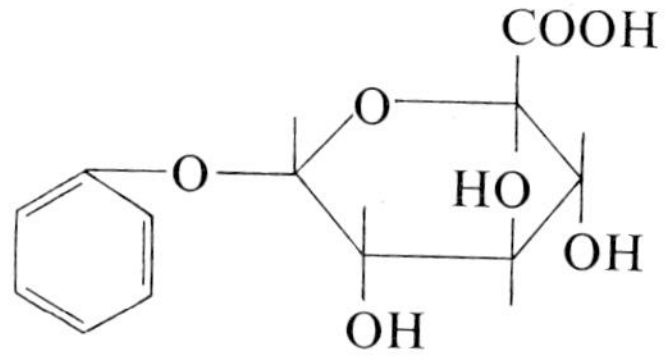

phenyl $\beta$-D-glucuronide
(ether-glucuronide)

The UDP-glucuronic acid is synthesized in the soluble fraction of liver cells from glucose 1-phosphate through oxidation of the coenzyme uridine diphosphate-glucose. The transferase system is in the microsomal fraction.

The wide range of compounds which form glucuronides is illustrated in Table 1. Drugs which do not possess one of the listed reactive groups may undergo preliminary metabolic transformation by non-synthetic reactions and their metabolites may then have an available radical for linkage with glucuronic acid. Glucuronide synthesis and UDP-glucuronic acid are at a low level in the foetus and new-born as is also glucuronyl transferase activity. Inactivation of drugs normally eliminated as glucuronides may therefore be defective in this situation (see pp. 414 and 439). Based on the finding that D-glucaric acid is a product of D-glucuronic acid metabolism (Marsh, 1963) urinary glucaric acid excretion has been employed as an indirect measure of the in vivo activity of drug-conjugating enzymes in the liver (Hunter et al., 1971).

TABLE 1

EXAMPLES OF DRUGS POSSESSING DIFFERENT FUNCTIONAL GROUPS WHICH UNDERGO CONJUGATION WITH GLUCURONIC ACID IN MAN. The italicized hydrogen (H) is replaced by the glucuronyl residue $C_6H_9O_6$, to form the glucuronide conjugate. Glucuronides may give a positive reducing test for sugar (e.g. clinitest) and a check should therefore be made on ingestion of drugs whenever urine is found to give a negative specific reaction for glucose but positive reaction for reducing sugar.

(Data from Smith and Williams (1966).)

| Functional group | Structure | Drug example |
|---|---|---|
| *Hydroxyl* | | |
| phenol | R—O*H* | morphine; paracetamol |
| primary alcohol | —CH₂—O*H* | chloramphenicol |
| *Carboxyl* | | |
| aromatic | R—COO*H* | salicylic acid |
| primary aliphatic | —CH₂—COO*H* | indomethacin |
| *Amino and Imino* | | |
| carbamate | —O—CON*H*₂ | meprobamate |
| sulphamoyl | —SO₂—N*H*— | sulphonamide N¹-conjugation |
| *Sulphydryl* | —S*H* | diethyl thiocarbamic acid (p. 433) |

Among the drugs which form peptide conjugates in man are salicylic and nicotinic acids. Thus PAS is excreted as a mixture of glycine and glutamine conjugates. Isoniazid, like iproniazid (see p. 429), is first hydrolysed to isonicotinic acid; this acid then conjugates with glycine to form isonicotinuric acid.

### 3. Ethereal Sulphate (Sulphate Ester) Formation

Formation of organic sulphate esters occurs through conjugation of aromatic, aliphatic and steroid hydroxyl groupings, and aromatic amines with an activated form of sulphate. The sulphate is transferred from the coenzyme PAPS (3′phosphoadenosine-5′-phosphosulphate) by sulphate-transferring enzymes such as the sulphokinases. There are a number of different sulphokinases for different acceptor molecules. The general reaction may be expressed as follows:

$$R—OH + PAPS \rightarrow R—O—SO_2OH + 3′phosphoadenosine-5′-phosphate$$

"activated" sulphate     sulphate ester

### 2. Peptide Formation

Formation of peptide conjugates of glycine and glutamine is a characteristic synthetic reaction of aromatic and certain steroidal acids. The reaction involves the 'activation' of the acceptor acid molecule by formation of its acetyl coenzyme A derivative which then interacts with the amino acid:

### 4. Methylation

Methylation reactions are of considerable importance since they play a major role in a number of physiological pathways of metabolism, notably, for example, in the case of bioamines (Sandler and Ruthven, 1969). Methylation is a reaction in which a methyl group is transferred from its attachment to the coenzyme S-adenosyl methionine to

$$R—COOH \xrightarrow{ATP + CoA—SH} R·CO—S·CoA \xrightarrow{NH_2·CH_2·COOH} R·CO·NH·CH_2·COOH$$

aromatic acid     aroyl-coenzyme A     glycine conjugate

phenols, amines and certain thiol compounds. The reaction is catalysed by several different methyl transferase enzymes. Catechol *o*-methyl transferases methylate catechols and catechol amines, and are involved in the inactivation of endogenous and exogenous catechol amines:

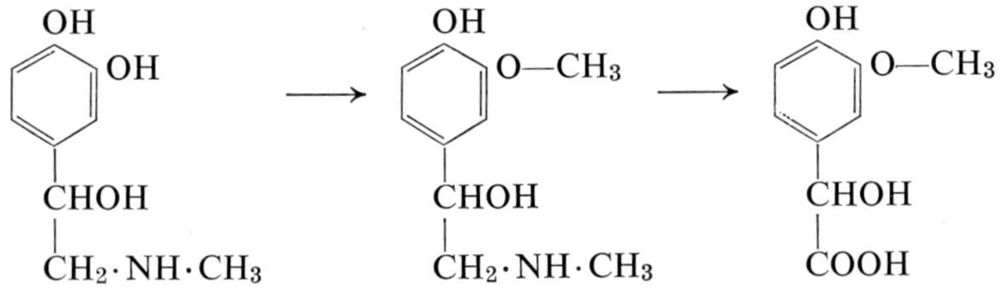

Adrenaline      metadrenaline      3-methoxy, 4 hydroxy-mandelic acid (VMA)

## 5. Acetylation

The functional groups on the acceptor molecules involved in this conjugation reaction are primary amino, sulphonamido and hydrazino radicals. The acetyl group is transferred from acetyl coenzyme A by acetyl transferases found mainly in the soluble fraction of liver cells. The important acetylation of sulphonamides to yield $N^1$- and $N^4$-acetyl derivates (*see* p. 429) occurs by this route. The general reaction may be depicted as follows:

$$R-NH_2 + CH_3CO \cdot S \cdot CoA \xrightarrow{acetyl\ transferase}$$
$$R-NH \cdot CO \cdot CH_3 + CoA \cdot SH$$

## 6. Glutathione Conjugation

A number of aromatic hydrocarbons (e.g. naphthalene), halogenated benzene derivates (e.g. nitrobenzene), aniline and sulphonamide derivatives form conjugates with glutathione, the latter probably existing in an activated form. The native drugs are often metabolized first to epoxides by microsomal oxidation. These intermediates then conjugate with glutathione, the final excretory products being derivatives of N-acetyl cysteine, known as mercapturic acids. For example:

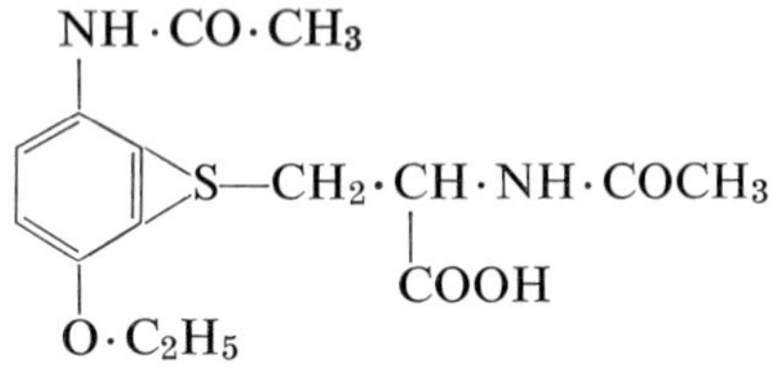

phenacetin mercapturic acid

## 7. Thiocyanate Formation

Cyanide may be formed *in vivo* as a by-product of metabolism of naturally-occurring glycosides ingested in food such as, for example, amygdalin. Detoxification occurs by conjugation with sulphur to form thiocyanate, the reaction being catalysed by the mitochondrial enzyme, sulphur transferase (or rhodanese):

$$CN^- + S_2O_3^{2-} \rightarrow CNS^- + SO_3^{2-}$$
cyanide   thiosulphate   thiocyanate   sulphite

### Patterns of Drug Metabolism

The overall pattern of metabolism of even a relatively simple drug molecule may involve a number of metabolic transformations and conjugations. For example, the analgesic phenacetin may undergo aromatic hydroxylation, dealkylation (*see* p. 429) and deacetylation. The metabolites of the first two reactions form glucuronide and sulphate conjugates; phenacetin itself may form a mercapturic acid (6 above). More complex drugs may be subjected to multiple metabolic attacks on the molecule, leading to a host of metabolites and conjugates. The possible metabolic transformations which may be undergone by barbiturates (Bush and Sanders, 1967) include:

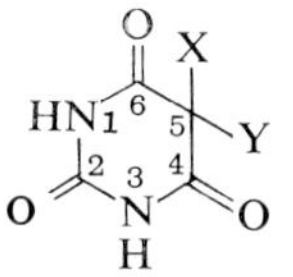

Oxidation of substituent chains X and Y at C5
N-dealkylation at $N^1$ and $N^3$
Desulphuration of thiobarbiturates at C2
Hydrolytic cleavage of ring structure

In the case of the organic inhalation anaesthetics, besides dehalogenation (*see* p. 433), metabolism may proceed by cleavage of ether linkages or removal of carbon atoms from the molecule. (Van Dyke and Chenoweth, 1965; Greene, 1968; Brown and Vandam, 1971; Cohen, 1971). The metabolic degradation of methoxyflurane can be summarized as follows:

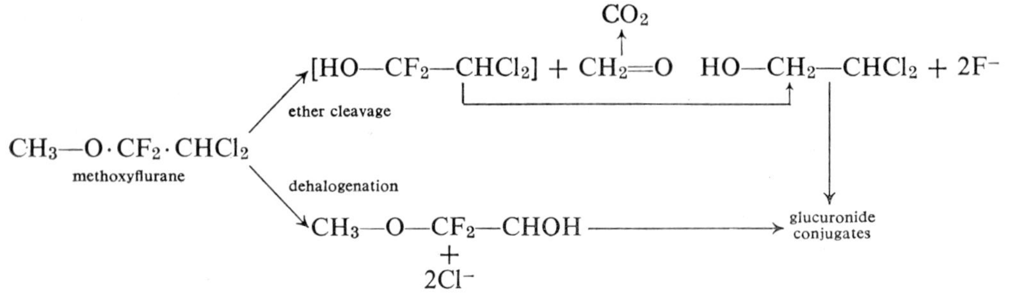

The fact that volatile anaesthetics possess a distinct degree of metabolic reactivity and display varying patterns of bio-transformation raises a number of interesting points. Although the extent of metabolism may not be enough to alter significantly the clinical depth of anaesthesia, the rate of elimination of the more polar metabolites is likely to be slower than that of the unchanged parent molecule. This may result in the metabolites persisting well beyond the anaesthetic period. The question has been raised as to whether some of the intermediate products of metabolism may not be potentially toxic. This appears to be the case for example with methoxyflurane where nephrotoxicity occasionally associated with its use is attributable to metabolic release of inorganic fluoride which blocks the concentrating capacity of the distal nephron (Mazze et al., 1971; Frascino et al., 1972). Because of the high lipid solubility of the parent molecule, there is significant storage in body fat with the result that fluoride may continue to be released slowly for some time after anaesthetic exposure has ceased (Corbett and Ball, 1971; Fry, Taves and Merin, 1973). Also, free radicals may acquire significant antigenicity on combining with suitable protein macromolecules. Furthermore, repeated occupational exposure in anaesthetists and surgical personnel may lead to increased rates of drug metabolism by processes of self-induction (Cohen, 1969, 1971; Corbett and Ball, 1971; Cascorbi et al., 1971) (see p. 462).

## Effects of Drugs on Drug Metabolism

(Burns and Conney, 1965; Conney, 1967; Prescott, 1969; Cooksley and Powell, 1971)

The activity of the enzymes involved in drug metabolism may be either inhibited or stimulated by drugs. With the increasing multiplicity and complexity of modern drug therapy, interactions resulting from the effects of one drug upon its own metabolism or that of another drug may have far-reaching pharmacological and toxicological consequences.

### Inhibition

Interference with metabolic processes occurring in hepatic microsomes may intensify and prolong the biological activity of a drug.

SKF 525-A ($\beta$-diethylaminoethyl diphenylpropylacetate hydrochloride) is one of the most potent drugs which inhibit microsomal enzymes concerned in drug metabolism. SFK 525-A has no appreciable pharmacological activity of its own but in animals it interferes with oxidative hydroxylation of barbiturates, N-dealkylation of morphine, hydrolysis of procaine and glucuronide formation. Its mode of action is obscure.

**Disulfiram.** Metabolism of drugs occurring at sites other than the endoplasmic reticulum may be inhibited by other drugs. For example, the cytoplasmic enzyme, aldehyde dehydrogenase, is competitively inhibited by the drug disulfiram. Disulfiram has no pharmacological effects on its own but if ethyl alcohol is ingested in its presence, an unpleasant syndrome of flushing, hypotension and dyspnoea develops; this is attributable to the accumulation of acetaldehyde secondary to inhibition of the next oxidative step of alcohol metabolism.

**Monoamine oxidase inhibitors (MAOI).** These drugs have complex pharmacological actions which are not well understood. They undoubtedly cause an elevation in the levels of free monoamines such as noradrenaline and 5-hydroxytryptamine in the central nervous system, but how this is related to their mood-elevating action is uncertain. MAOI have little or no potentiating effect on the cardiovascular effects of natural catechol amines, probably because o-methylation and tissue uptake rather than oxidative deamination are the main processes of physiological inactivation (Sandler and Ruthven, 1969; see also pp. 433 and 436). However, MAOI do potentiate the cardiovascular effects of exogenous and indirectly-acting sympathomimetic amines. Dangerous interactions in the form of hypertensive crises may occur between MAOI and substances which release (e.g. reserpine) or replete (amine precursors such as l-dopa in broad beans) mono-amines either centrally or peripherally (Sjöqvist, 1965). As well as their obvious actions on mitochondrial amine oxidases, certain MAOI also appear to inhibit the drug-metabolizing enzymes of hepatic microsomes. This may explain the prolonged but otherwise normal pharmacological response seen in man when drugs such as pethidine, barbiturates or phenothiazines, which undergo microsomal metabolism, are given to patients on chronic MAOI therapy.

**Other drugs.** In man, the metabolism of tolbutamide and phenytoin may be slowed by co-administration of coumarin anticoagulants (Solomon and Schrogie, 1967), phenylbutazone or chloramphenicol (Christensen and Skovsted, 1969). A number of other drugs have been found to inhibit microsomal drug-metabolizing enzymes in animals. These include chlorcyclizine, glutethamide, opiates, and also DPEA (2, 4 dichloro-6, phenylphenoxyethylamine). In some cases, after initial inhibition, compounds may then stimulate these enzymes. This biphasic behaviour has been noted particularly with potent inhibitors like chlorcyclizine and SKF 525-A.

### Stimulation (Enzyme Induction)

Administration of one drug can reduce the duration and intensity of pharmacological activity of another drug by stimulating its metabolic inactivation. Drugs exert this action by increasing the amount of drug-metabolizing enzymes in liver microsomes. This is referred to as enzyme induction and experimental evidence indicates that the mechanism of this effect involves synthesis of more microsomal drug-metabolizing enzymes including cytochrome P-450. After administration of certain drugs in animals for a number of days, there is a significant increase in the incorporation of labelled amino acids and in total protein concentration. By correlating biochemical data with the electron microscopic observations, it has been shown that increase in enzyme activity is accompanied by a marked proliferation of smooth-surfaced membranes of the endoplasmic reticulum of the liver (Ernster and Orrenius, 1965; Remmer and Merker, 1965). Agents which block protein synthesis in different ways, such as ethionine, puromycin and actinomycin D, prevent the induction of microsomal enzyme activity (Orrenius and Ericsson, 1966). Stimulation of metabolism secondary to microsomal enzyme induction occurs only when drugs are administered *in vivo*; addition of drugs to *in vitro* microsomal preparations has no stimulating effect. Increased enzyme activity may take several days to reach a maximum. Although the phenomenon is reversible it may take some time for enzyme activity to return to pre-treatment levels. For example, about ten weeks are required before the extent of microsomal hydrolysis of phenylbutazone returns to normal on discontinuing the drug in dogs.

Several hundred drugs are now known to stimulate the activity of drug-metabolizing enzymes (Conney, 1967). The pharmacological actions of these compounds are remarkably diverse and there is no apparent relationship between their actions or molecular structure and their ability to induce enzymes. The only feature common to most is that they are lipid soluble at physiological pH. The term "xenobiotic"* compounds has been coined (Mason, North and Vanneste, 1965) to describe this large group of chemical substances (including environmental agents) which, though foreign to the normal metabolic network of the organism, influence the function of, or are themselves altered by, essential enzymatic reactions. Amongst commonly used drugs which are active enzyme inducers in animals may be listed barbiturates and other hypnotics, inhalational anaesthetics, anticonvulsants, phenothiazines, benzodiazepines, tricyclic antidepressants, oral hypoglycaemic agents, analgesics including phenylbutazone, antihistamines and uricosurics. Since steroid hormones are normal body substrates for the oxidative microsomal enzymes in the liver (*see* p. 433), drugs that are effective stimulators of drug-metabolizing enzymes also stimulate microsomal hydroxylation of steroids.

In addition to therapeutic agents, certain foreign substances present in the environment also act as enzyme inducers. The accidental finding that spraying of animal rooms with halogenated hydrocarbon insecticides shortened the biological activity of hexobarbitone in rats led to the discovery that pesticides such as chlordane and dicophane (DDT) also act as enzyme inducers. Certain carcinogenic polycyclic hydrocarbons such as 3,4-benzpyrene and 1,2,5,6-dibenzanthracene are also potent enzyme inducers (Conney *et al.*, 1971).

The mechanism of induction may not be the same for all the different chemical types of enzyme stimulator. Phenobarbitone and many other compounds including the halogenated pesticides give rise to a relatively general induction of microsomal enzyme activity which involves hydrolytic, reductive and glucuronyl transferase activities; the inductive effect is accompanied by marked proliferation of the SER. By contrast, the carcinogenic polycyclic hydrocarbons stimulate a more limited group of reactions and have little or no effect on the proliferation of the smooth membraned endoplasmic reticulum (Fouts and Rogers, 1965).

Repeated administration of a drug may result in induction of the enzymes responsible for its biotransforma-

* "stranger to life" (ξένος, strange; βίος, life).

tion. Thus chronic therapy with certain drugs may by the process of 'self-induction' speed up their own metabolism, lower the effective plasma levels and decrease biological efficacy. Thus, for example, chronic exposure of animals to methoxyflurane increases the activity of the microsomal enzyme system responsible for dechlorinating this volatile anaesthetic (*see* p. 437) (Van Dyke, 1966). Development of *tolerance* to barbiturates may be related to self-induced acceleration of their own hepatic microsomal metabolism. In most cases, the phenomenon of tolerance to drugs as, for example, in the case of opiates is not an expression of enhanced metabolism but of adaptive changes at the drug receptor sites (Remmer, 1962).

Although most of the stimulatory effects of drugs and other foreign chemicals on drug and steroid metabolism have been demonstrated in animals, the phenomenon of enzyme induction may have important implications in relation to therapy in clinical practice. Differences between species make it impossible to predict that all the compounds shown in animals to induce hepatic microsomal enzymes will necessarily also act as inducers in man (Welch *et al.*, 1969). Nevertheless, a number of important examples of interactions caused by stimulation of metabolism of one drug on another have been documented in man. Phenobarbitone stimulates the metabolism of a number of clinically useful drugs and may thereby decrease their pharmacological activity. Phenytoin metabolism is accelerated in epileptics who are given phenobarbitone therapy at the same time. Phenobarbitone also enhances the hydroxylation of coumarin derivatives with diminution in anticoagulant efficacy (Cucinell *et al.*, 1965). There may be serious consequences if, for example, stabilization of a patient on a coumarin anticoagulant is undertaken during a period of regular barbiturate administration. If administration of the enzyme inducer is then stopped and coumarin therapy continued without an appropriate reduction in dosage, there may be a substantial rise in plasma levels of the anticoagulant and danger of haemorrhage. Such sequence of events has been reported after withdrawal of chloral hydrate and phenobarbitone in patients maintained on oral anticoagulant therapy (Cucinell *et al.*, 1966). Other examples of interactions explicable on the similar basis of enzyme induction are the lowered plasma levels of amidopyrine and its derivative dipyrone when regular treatment with phenylbutazone, phenobarbitone or glutethamide is given at the same time (Burns *et al.*, 1965). These selected instances of metabolic interaction emphasize one aspect of the potential risks of multiple drug therapy. Many of the effects of drugs on their own metabolism and that of other substances—both exogenous and endogenous—have been insignificantly investigated as yet in man. Much more research is needed, for example, to appreciate fully the long-term effects of chronic human exposure to environmental pesticides on the enzymatic mechanisms for metabolizing drugs (Conney *et al.*, 1967). Occurrence of enzyme induction may complicate the interpretation of chronic toxicity tests since by stimulation of their own metabolism drugs may become less toxic as a state of tolerance develops. Furthermore, the familiar use of crossover studies may be influenced by modification of the pharmacological effects of the second dose of drug by the first, as a result of stimulation of drug-metabolizing enzymes in the liver.

Enzyme induction has, however, been exploited to clinical advantage in one instance. Drug-metabolizing enzymes are either absent or present in negligible amounts in premature infants and the newborn (Fouts and Hart, 1965). This deficiency applies not only to oxidative but also to conjugative enzyme systems. Inadequate glucuronide formation makes the neonate particularly vulnerable to kernicterus since bilirubin cannot be conjugated and excreted properly. The hazard may be increased if neonatal hyperbilirubinaemia is further aggravated by displacement of bilirubin from plasma albumin through administration of other drugs such as salicylates, sulphonamides, etc., competing for protein binding sites (see p. 413). By administering a powerful and relatively harmless enzyme inducer in late pregnancy, the foetal microsomal enzyme system may be induced, conjugation stimulated and serum bilirubin levels lowered. Both phenobarbitone (Maurer et al., 1968) and alcohol (Waltman et al., 1969) have been used prophylactically for this purpose with success.

### Influence of Genetic Factors

**Species Differences** (Brodie and Reid, 1967; Williams, 1967; Burns, 1968)

Species differences of both qualitative and quantitative type occur in the metabolic transformation of drugs. The drug metabolizing microsomal enzymes found in mammals are not present in fish and amphibians. The teleological basis for this interesting difference has been considered on p. 428. However, even amongst mammals, wide differences exist in drug metabolism amongst the different species and no obvious rationale is apparent to account for the differences. Furthermore, even when pathways for metabolism are the same, rates vary, and different species may deal with the same drug by quite separate routes.

The marked species differences in duration of action of hexobarbitone have been shown to be due to genetic and environmental differences in its in vivo metabolism (Vessell, 1968). For example, the biological half-life of the drug in mice is only 19 min., whereas in dogs it is over 4 hr. This correlates inversely with the activity of the hepatic microsomal enzymes in the two species; microsomal activity in the mouse is about seventeen times that in the dog liver (Quinn, Axelrod and Brodie, 1958). Species differences exist in the capacity to conjugate drugs. Dogs are unable to acetylate aromatic primary amines ($R-NH_2$), yet they can acetylate the N-sulphamoyl radicle of sulphonamides ($R-SO_2NH_2$). Cats form glucuronides with difficulty due to low tissue activity of glucuronyl transferase. With the exception of the cat, most laboratory animals metabolize drugs more rapidly than man.

Differences in pathways of metabolism may have toxicological significance. For example, phenacetin is predominantly metabolized in man by de-ethylation to form paracetamol (p. 433); in the dog, the parent drug undergoes de-acetylation yielding the compounds p-phenetidine and p-aminophenol which lack analgesic activity and may cause methaemoglobinaemia (Kiese, 1965).

Sex differences in drug metabolism have been noted in the rat, possibly related to more rapid drug turnover by the hepatic microsomal enzymes in the male than the female. Thus, for example, hydroxylation of barbiturates and N-demethylation of morphine is more rapid in male rats (Kato and Gillette, 1965). Most other laboratory animals do not show a sex difference in metabolism and, fortunately for the clinician, neither does man.

Considerations such as these show that species differences undoubtedly complicate the projection of experimental data from animal to man. Sometimes this can be a serious obstacle in the development and screening of new drugs. A drug may be active in one or more animal species yet be relatively ineffective or overtly toxic when used clinically. The difficulties which face the extrapolation of information obtained in animals to problems of human therapy make it all the more important to expand knowledge of the comparative aspects of drug metabolism. As fundamental information accumulates from studies in various species including man, it will be possible to undertake the molecular manipulation of old drugs and synthesis of new drugs on a truly rational basis.

### Strain Differences (Pharmacogenetics)

As well as the differences in responses to drugs which occur between species, there may be variations amongst individual strains within one species. In recent years, there has been an increasing awareness of the wide individual differences which exist in man in his response to drugs and in his ability to metabolize drugs. *Pharmacogenetics* is a relatively new branch of pharmacology which deals with study of the genetic factors and mechanisms which account for these variations (Evans and Clarke, 1961; Kalow, 1962, 1967; Porter, 1964; Conference on Evaluation and Mechanisms of Drug Toxicity, 1965; Symposium on Experimental and Clinical Aspects of Pharmacogenetics, 1965; Clarke et al., 1968).

As we have seen, drug metabolism is mediated by a series of enzymatic reactions. The activity of each enzyme is determined by at least one gene. Hereditary difference in genetic material may alter the structure or amount of a key enzyme involved in drug metabolism. The result may be disturbed drug inactivation or an inability to maintain critical cellular metabolites in the presence of the drug.

Inherited characteristics may be controlled either by many genes—multifactorial inheritance—or by a single gene or gene pair. In the former case, the distribution of the given characteristic shows a continuous variation and follows a unimodal or Gaussian (normal) curve. Inheritance of characteristics of multifactorial origin shows no obvious Mendelian pattern and because of the dependence on many genes, it may be extremely difficult to detect any single biochemical correlate of the characteristic. On the other hand, with characteristics that depend on single genes, the distribution of the trait in the population will be discontinuous. A bimodal or trimodal distribution may be obtained in which the population is seen to consist of two or three distinct groups. In this situation, it may be possible to recognize an individual biochemical correlate such as lack or critical alteration in structure of a single protein, e.g. a key enzyme in drug metabolism (Motulsky, 1965). When a drug is given to a large number of persons under controlled conditions, the collective response may be either continuous or discontinuous. Each step of a discontinuous system may represent a genetically-determined phenotype. The term *polymorphism* is used to describe the existence of two or more phenotypes within the same population in the environment at the same time. It thus implies the occurrence of a genetic trait determined by a single gene (monogenic) which is occurring at a frequency which cannot be accounted for by mutation alone (Kalow, 1962; 1965). Polymorphic systems revealed by drugs can be divided into two groups:

(1) polymorphism of the metabolic transformation and conjugation reactions undergone by the drug molecule;
(2) polymorphism of the effects of drugs upon altered enzyme systems or physiological mechanisms.

An important criterion fulfilled by both types of polymorphism is that because the enzymes involved do not occupy key positions in the mechanisms of intermediary metabolism, the consequences of genetically determined alterations in their structure and function do not become clinically apparent unless the appropriate drug stimuli are given. Two illustrative examples from each group will be discussed: In group I, the polymorphisms involving (a) plasma pseudo-cholinesterase and (b) liver acetyltransferase; in group 2, the polymorphisms involving (a) glucose 6 phosphate dehydrogenase (G6PD) and (b) unstable haemoglobins (H and Zurich).

### Group 1 Polymorphisms

**(a) Suxamethonium and pseudocholinesterase.** Plasma pseudocholinesterase hydrolyses a number of drugs including procaine (*see* Fig. 3, p. 434) and suxamethonium:

of suxamethonium-sensitivity. About 1 in 2,500 to 3,000 individuals is homozygous for this 'atypical' esterase. Other less common variants which have been discovered include a 'fluoride-resistant' esterase (Harris and Whittaker, 1962) and enzymatic deficiency due to presence of the so-called 'silent or amorphic' allele (Kattamis, Davies and Lehmann, 1967). It appears, therefore, that formation of pseudocholinesterase is controlled by at least four allelic genes: that controlling normal esterase ($E^u$ or $Ch^u$), 'atypical' esterase (dibucaine-resistant enzyme ($E^a$ or $Ch^D$), fluoride-resistant esterase ($E^f$ or $Ch^F$) and a silent gene ($E^s$ or $Ch^s$) which in the homozygous state results in complete absence of esterase activity. (Lehmann and Liddell, 1969; Rubinstein *et al.*, 1970). Other rarer genetic variants of serum cholinesterase have also been described (La Du, 1971; 1972).

**(b) Isoniazid and liver acetyl transferase.** Isoniazid is deactivated by acetylation in the liver. The enzyme N-acetyl transferase catalyses the transfer of the acetyl group from acetyl coenzyme A to isoniazid as well as to other drugs (p. 436). The human enzyme is in the soluble fraction of hepatic cells and is 'non-inducible'. When plasma concentrations of isoniazid were measured 6 hr. after oral administration of the drug in a group of 267 individuals, a histogram of the frequency distribution showed bimodality (Evans, Manley and McKusick, 1960). Some people metabolized the drug slowly, some rapidly. This allowed the population to be divided into two groups which were designated 'slow inactivators' and 'rapid inactivators'. Family studies showed that the trait, slow inactivator, was recessive. Over half of all Caucasians are homozygous for the recessive gene and are slow inactivators. Slow inactivators are more susceptible to developing peripheral neuropathy which may be attributable to a greater tendency to form isoniazid hydrazones with essential endogenous metabolites such as pyruvate and pyridoxal (Peters, Miller and Brown, 1965). This complication can be prevented by administration of pyridoxine. Development of antinuclear antibodies and LE-like syndrome is commoner in slow inactivator hypertensives treated with hydrallazine than in rapid acetylators.

$$CH_3)_3\overset{+}{N}—(CH_2)_2—O—\overset{\overset{O}{\|}}{C}—(CH_2)_2—\overset{\overset{O}{\|}}{C}—O—(CH_2)_2—\overset{+}{N}(CH_3)_3$$

choline                                                        succinyl monocholine

↓ Hydrolysis

Soon after suxamethonium was introduced into anaesthetic practice, occasional patients were noted to respond with an atypical apnoea. Studies by Kalow and Genest (1957) showed that the plasma esterase from suxamethonium-sensitive persons differed from the usual esterase not in quantity but in its qualitative properties. The 'atypical' esterase was less susceptible to inhibition by dibucaine (cinchocaine) and a number of other esterase inhibitors. The 'atypical' esterase (dibucaine-resistant) variant accounts for most of the genetically determined instances

Sulphadimidine and the substituted hydrazine drugs, hydrallazine and phenelzine, are also acetylated by the same hepatic acetyl transferase and display the same genetic variation in metabolism. Sulphanilamide, *p*-amino benzoic (PAB) and *p*-aminosalicylic (PAS) acids, however, undergo monomorphic acetylation and there is, therefore, no phenotype specially susceptible to develop toxicity to these drugs. This suggests the existence in man of two acetylating systems, one polymorphic and the other monomorphic (Evans, 1965).

$$CO \cdot NH—NH_2$$

isoniazid

major route →

$$CO \cdot NH—NH \cdot COCH_3$$

acetylated isoniazid

hydrolysis · hydrazone formation

COOH

isonicotinic acid

$$CONH—N{=}\overset{\overset{\displaystyle CH_3}{|}}{C}—COOH$$

pyruvic acid isonicotinoyl hydrazone

## Group 2 Polymorphisms

**(a) Glucose-6-phosphate dehydrogenase.** The link between drug-induced haemolysis and deficiency of glucose 6-phosphate dehydrogenase (G6PD) in red cells is an example of a polymorphism where unusual drug effects arise because of genetically-mediated differences in cell metabolism.

It has been estimated that the trait is present in more than 100 million people in the world. Particular ethnic and geographical groups have a high incidence, e.g. American negroes (15–20 per cent), Sephardic Jews and Kurds (50 per cent) and Sardinians (10–30 per cent). The defect appears to be due to a gene of intermediate dominance which is linked to the X-chromosome. The normal function of G6PD, a key enzyme in the hexose monophosphate shunt pathway, is to provide a ready source of NADPH; this acts as cofactor of the enzyme glutathione reductase, and maintains glutathione in its reduced state (GSH). Deficiency in G6PD leads to impairment of glutathione reduction through lack of NADPH. This is associated with a decreased ability of the red cell to protect itself against various substances capable of causing oxidative denaturation of haemoglobin and haemolysis. A large number of drugs are known to be potentially haemolytic in subjects with G6PD deficiency, ranging from the 8-amino-quinoline antimalarials to sulphonamides, nitrofurantoin, naphthalene derivatives, salicylates (Beutler, 1969). Some subjects have an associated chronic non-spherocytic haemolytic anaemia whilst in others, haemolysis may be precipitated by ingestion of the broad bean, *Vicia fava*. The precise sequence of events leading to haemolysis when drugs interact with G6PD-deficient red cells is still poorly understood (Fraser and Vesell, 1968). High incidences of G6PD deficiency are found in areas where malaria is endemic and the geographical distribution suggests that G6PD deficiency, like the sickle cell trait, is protective against *P. falciparum* malaria.

Detailed studies have shown that G6PD deficiency displays a number of polymorphisms. Different qualitative variants of G6PD have been discovered using electrophoretic techniques, some of these differing only in one amino acid substitution from the normal enzyme (Kirkman, 1968; Motulsky, Yoshida and Stamatoyannopoulos, 1971). The type of G6PD deficiency observed in Mediterraneans ($Gd^{Mediterranean}$) differs from that commonly found in the American Negro ($Gd^{A-}$) in that in the former, the abnormal enzyme is particularly unstable *in vivo*. The rate of inactivation is so rapid that it barely exceeds the rate of synthesis. The result is that G6PD activity may only be detectable in reticulocytes and not at all in mature red cells (Marks and Banks, 1965; Piomelli *et al.*, 1968).

**(b) Unstable haemoglobins.** Inherited variations in the structure of haemoglobin may also confer abnormal sensitivity to certain drugs capable of producing methaemoglobin, even though the reductive processes in the red cell are operating normally. Several different unstable haemoglobins have been described involving both $\alpha$ and $\beta$ chains of haemoglobin (Beutler, 1969). Two particular examples are first, haemoglobin Zurich in which the histidine residue in position 63 of the $\beta$ chain is replaced by arginine; second, haemoglobin H, which is a tetramer of four $\beta$ chains ($\beta_4$). Unstable haemoglobins readily become denatured into insoluble aggregates, a process which is hastened by drugs that catalyze the oxidation of haemoglobin. The role of methaemoglobin formation is not clear. In most cases, the mode of inheritance is dominant. Individuals possessing such unstable haemoglobins may develop unusually severe haemolytic anaemia after administration of sulphonamide drugs.

Haemoglobin S, which differs from normal adult haemoglobin A ($\alpha_2\beta_2$) in replacement of glutamic acid by valine at position 6 of both $\beta$-chains, characteristically forms molecular aggregates in the absence of oxygen. Anaesthesia may be a potential hazard in patients with sickle haemoglobin since hypoxia may produce intravascular sickling with either massive intravascular haemolysis or blockage of blood vessels by red cell conglomerates and resultant infarction (Motulsky and Stamatoyannopoulos, 1968). With careful attention to maintaining adequate ventilation and oxygenation, and avoiding hypovolaemia and hypotension, the risks of producing a sickling crisis by general anaesthesia can be minimized (Howells *et al.*, 1972; Searle, 1973).

For more detailed accounts of the ways in which genetic

factors influence individual responses to drugs and examples of other drug-induced polymorphisms associated with clinical disorders, the reader is referred to reviews by Kalow (1964); Parke (1968b); Evans (1968); Beutler (1969); La Du (1971), the Conference on Pharmacogenetics (1968), and the Section on "Genetic Aspects of Drug Metabolism in Man" in Vesell (1971).

## REFERENCES

Alvares, A. P., Schilling, G., Levin, W., Kuntzman, R., Brand, L. and Mark, L. C. (1969), "Cytochromes P-450 and b5 in Human Liver Cytochromes," Clin. Pharmac. Ther., 10, 655–659.

Beutler, E. (1969), "Drug-induced Hemolytic Anemia," Pharmac. Rev., 21, 73–103.

Bickel, M. H. (1969), "The Pharmacology and Biochemistry of N-oxides," Pharmac. Rev., 21, 325–355.

Brodie, B. B. (1962), "Drug Metabolism—Subcellular Mechanisms," in Enzymes and Drug Action, ed. Mongar, J. L. and de Reuck, A. V. S., pp. 317–343. London: J. and A. Churchill Ltd.

Brodie, B. B., Gillette, J. R. and La Du, B. N. (1958), "Enzymatic Metabolism of Drugs and Other Foreign Compounds," A. Rev. Biochem., 27, 427–454.

Brodie, B. B. and Reid, W. D. (1967), "Some Pharmacological Consequences of Species Variation in Rates of Metabolism," Fedn. Proc. 26, 1062–1070.

Brown, B. R. (1971), "The Diphasic Action of Halothane on the Oxidative Metabolism of Drugs by the Liver: An in-vitro Study in the Rat," Anesthesiology, 35, 241–246.

Brown, B. R. and Vandam, L. D. (1971), "A Review of Current Advances in Metabolism of Inhalation Anesthetics," Ann. N.Y. Acad. Sci., 179, 235–243.

Burns, J. J. (1968), "Variation of Drug Metabolism in Animals and the Prediction of Drug Action in Man," Ann. N.Y. Acad. Sci., 151, 959–967.

Burns, J. J. and Conney, A. H. (1965), "Enzyme Stimulation and Inhibition in the Metabolism of Drugs," Proc. R. Soc. Med., 58, 955–960.

Burns, J. J., Cucinell, S. A., Koster, R. and Conney, A. H. (1965), "Application of Drug Metabolism to Drug Toxicity Studies," Ann. N.Y. Acad. Sci. 123, 273–286.

Bush, M. T. and Sanders, E. (1967), "Metabolic Fate of Drugs: Barbiturates and Closely Related Compounds," A. Rev. Pharmac., 7, 57–76.

Cascorbi, H. F., Vesell, E. S., Blake, D. A. and Helrich, M. (1971), "Halothane Biotransformation in Man," Ann. N.Y. Acad. Sci., 179, 244–248.

Christensen, L. K. and Skovsted, L. (1969), "Inhibition of Drug Metabolism by Chloramphenicol," Lancet, 2, 1397–1399.

Clarke, C. A., Evans, D. A. P., Harris, R., McConnell, R. B. and Woodrow, J. C. (1968), "Genetics in Medicine: A Review. Part II. Pharmacogenetics," Q. Jl. Med., 37, 183–219.

Cohen, E. N. (1969), "Metabolism of Halothane-2¹⁴C-2 in the Mouse," Anesthesiology, 31, 560–565.

Cohen, E. N. (1971), "Metabolism of the Volatile Anesthetics," Anesthesiology, 35, 193–202.

Conference on Evaluation and Mechanisms of Drug Toxicity (1965), "Part III. Genetic factors in drug toxicity," Ann. N.Y. Acad. Sci., 123, 167–218.

Conference on Pharmacogenetics (1968), Ann. N.Y. Acad. Sci., 151, Art. 2, 691–1001.

Conney, A. H. (1967), "Pharmacological Implications of Microsomal Enzyme Induction," Pharmac. Rev., 19, 317–366.

Conney, A. H., Schneidman, K., Jacobson, M. and Kuntzman, R. (1965), "Drug-induced Changes in Steroid Metabolism," Ann. N.Y. Acad. Sci., 123, 98–109.

Conney, A. H., Sansur, M., Soroko, F., Koster, R. and Burns, J. J. (1966), "Enzyme Induction and Inhibition in Studies on the Pharmacological Actions of Acetophenetidin," J. Pharmac. exp. Ther., 151, 133–138.

Conney, A. H., Welch, R. M., Kuntzman, R. and Burns, J. J. (1967), "Effects of Pesticides on Drug and Steroid Metabolism," Clin. Pharmac. Ther., 8, 2–10.

Conney, A. H., Welch, R., Kuntzman, R., Chang, R., Jacobson, M., Munro-Faure, A. D., Peck, A. W., Bye, A., Poland, A., Poppers, P. J., Finster, M. and Wolff, J. A. (1971), "Effects of Environmental Chemicals on the Metabolism of Drugs, Carcinogens, and Normal Body Constituents in Man," Ann. N.Y. Acad. Sci., 179, 155–172.

Cooksley, W. G. E. and Powell, L. W. (1971), "Drug Metabolism and Interaction with Particular Reference to the Liver," Drugs, 2, 177–189.

Corbett, T. H. and Ball, G. L. (1971), "Chronic Exposure to Methoxyflurane: A Possible Occupational Hazard to Anesthesiologists," Anesthesiology, 34, 532–537.

Cucinell, S. A., Conney, A. H., Sansur, M. and Burns, J. J. (1965), "Drug Interactions in Man. I. Lowering Effect of Phenobarbital on Plasma Levels of Bishydroxycoumarin (Dicoumarol) and Diphenylhydantoin (Dilantin)," Clin. Pharmac, Ther., 6, 420–429.

Cucinell, S. A., Odessky, L., Weiss, M. and Dayton, P. G. (1966), "The Effect of Chloral Hydrate on Bishydroxycoumarin Metabolism. A Fatal Outcome," J. Am. med. Ass., 197, 366–368.

Dutton, G. J. (1966), "The Biosynthesis of Glucuronides," in Glucuronic Acid. Free and Combined, Chapter 3, pp. 185–299. New York: Academic Press.

Ernster, L. and Orrenius, S. (1965), "Substrate-induced Synthesis of the Hydroxylating Enzyme System of Liver Microsomes," Fedn. Proc., 24, 1190–1199.

Estabrook, R. W., Franklin, M. R., Cohen, B., Shigamatzu, A. and Hildebrandt, A. G. (1971), "Influence of Hepatic Microsomal Mixed Function Oxidation Reactions on Cellular Metabolic Control," Metabolism, 20, 187–199.

Evans, D. A. P. and Clarke, C. A. (1961), "Pharmacogenetics," Br. med. Bull., 17, 234–240.

Evans, D. A. P. (1965), "Individual Variations of Drug Metabolism as a Factor in Drug Toxicity," Ann. N.Y. Acad. Sci., 123, 178–187.

Evans, D. A. P. (1968), "Clinical Pharmacogenetics," in Recent Advances in Medicine, ed. Baron, D. N., Compston, N. and Dawson, A. M., 15th edition, pp. 203–242. London: J. and A. Churchill Ltd.

Evans, D. A. P., Manley, K. A. and McKusick, V. A. (1960), "Genetic Control of Isoniazid Metabolism in Man," Br. med. J., 2, 485–491.

Fouts, J. R. and Hart, L. G. (1965), "Hepatic Metabolism During the Perinatal Period," Ann. N.Y. Acad. Sci., 123, 245–251.

Fouts, J. R. and Rogers, L. A. (1965), "Morphological Changes in the Liver Accompanying Stimulation of the Microsomal Drug Metabolizing Enzyme Activity by Phenobarbital, Chlordane, Benzpyrene or Methylcholanthrene in Rats," J. Pharmac. exp. Ther., 147, 112–119.

Frascino, J. A., O'Flaherty, J., Olmo, C. and Rivera, S. (1972), "Effect of Inorganic Fluoride on the Renal Concentrating Mechanism. Possible Nephrotoxicity in Man," J. Lab. clin. Med., 79, 192.

Fraser, I. M. and Vesell, E. S. (1968), "Effects of Drugs and Drug Metabolites on Erythrocytes from Normal and Glucose-6-phosphate Dehydrogenase-deficient Individuals," Ann. N.Y. Acad. Sci., 151, 777–794.

Fry, B. W., Taves, D. R. and Merin, R. G. (1973), "Fluorometabolites of Methoxyflurane: Serum Concentrations and Renal Clearances," Anesthesiology, 38, 38–44.

Gillette, J. R. (1966), "Biochemistry of Drug Oxidation and Reduction by Enzymes in Hepatic Endoplasmic Reticulum," in Advances in Pharmacology, ed. Shore, P. and Garattini, S., vol. 4, pp. 219–261. New York: Academic Press.

Gillette, J. R. (1971), "Factors Affecting Drug Metabolism," Ann. N.Y. Acad. Sci., 179, 43–66.

Gosselin, R. E., Gabourel, J. D. and Wills, J. H. (1960), "The Fate of Atropine in Man," Clin. Pharmac. Ther., 1, 597–603.

Greene, N. M. (1968), "The Metabolism of Drugs Employed in Anesthesia," Anesthesiology, 29, 127–144; 327–360.

Harris, H. and Whittaker, M. (1962), "The Genetics of Drug Sensitivity with Special Reference to Suxamethonium," in Enzymes and

*Drug Action*, ed. Mongar, J. L. and de Reuck, A. V. S., pp. 301–313. London: J. and A. Churchill Ltd.

Holtzman, J. L., Gram, T. E., Gigon, P. L. and Gillette, J. R. (1968), "The Distribution of the Components of Mixed-Function Oxidase Between the Rough and Smooth Endoplasmic Reticulum of Liver Cells," *Biochem. J.*, **110**, 407–412.

Howells, T. H., Huntsman, R. G., Boys, J. E. and Mahmood, A. (1972), "Anaesthesia and Sickle-Cell Haemoglobin," *Br. J. Anaesth.*, **44**, 975–987.

Hunter, J., Maxwell, J. D., Carrella, M., Stewart, D. A. and Williams, R. (1971), "Urinary D-glucaric Acid Excretion as a Test of Hepatic Enzyme Induction in Man," *Lancet*, **1**, 572–575.

Kalow, W. (1962), *Pharmacogenetics; Heredity and the Response to Drugs*. Philadelphia: W. B. Saunders Co.

Kalow, W. (1964), "Pharmacogenetics and Anesthesia," *Anesthesiology*, **25**, 377–387.

Kalow, W. (1965), "Dose-response Relationships and Genetic Variation," *Ann. N.Y. Acad. Sci.*, **123**, 212–218.

Kalow, W. (1967), "Pharmacogenetics and the Predictability of Drug Responses," in *Drug Responses in Man*, ed. Wostenholme, G. and Porter, R., pp. 220–239. London: J. and A. Churchill Ltd.

Kalow, W. and Genest, K. (1957), "A Method for the Detection of Atypical Forms of Human Serum Cholinesterase. Determination of Dibucaine Numbers," *Can. J. Biochem. Physiol.*, **35**, 339–346.

Kato, R. and Gillette, J. R. (1965), "Sex Differences in the Effects of Abnormal Physiological States on the Metabolism of Drugs by Rat Liver Microsomes," *J. Pharmac. exp. Ther.*, **150**, 285–291.

Kattamis, C., Davies, D. and Lehmann, H. (1967), "The Silent Serum Cholinesterase Gene," *Acta Genet.*, **17**, 299–303.

Kiese, M. (1965), "Relationship of Drug Metabolism to Methemoglobin Formation," *Ann. N.Y. Acad. Sci.*, **123**, 141–155.

Kirkman, H. N. (1968), "Glucose-6-phosphate Dehydrogenase Variants and Drug-induced Hemolysis," *Ann. N.Y. Acad. Sci.*, **151**, 753–764.

La Du, B. (1971), "Plasma Esterase Activity and the Metabolism of Drugs with Ester Groups," *Ann. N.Y. Acad. Sci.*, **179**, 684–693.

La Du, B. (1972), "Pharmacogenetics: Defective Enzymes in Relation to Reactions to Drugs," *A. Rev. Med.*, **23**, 453–468.

Lehmann, H. and Liddell, J. (1969), "Human Cholinesterase (Pseudocholinesterase): Genetic Variants and their Recognition," *Br. J. Anaesth.*, **41**, 235–244.

Margolis, F. and Feigelson, P. (1964), "Genetic Expression and Developmental Studies with Rabbit Serum Atropinesterase," *Biochem. biophys. Acta*, **90**, 117–125.

Mark, L. C., Kayden, H. J., Steele, J. M., Cooper, J. R., Berlin, I., Rovenstine, E. A. and Brodie, B. B. (1951), "The Physiological Disposition and Cardiac Effects of Procaine Amide," *J. Pharmac. exp. Ther.*, **102**, 5–15.

Marks, P. A. and Banks, J. (1965), "Drug-induced Hemolytic Anemias Associated with Glucose-6-phosphate Dehydrogenase Deficiency: a Genetically Heterogenous Trait," *Ann. N.Y. Acad. Sci.*, **123**, 198–206.

Marsh, C. A. (1963), "Metabolism of D-glucuronolactone in Mammalian Systems. Identification of D-glucaric acid as a normal Constituent of Urine," *Biochem. J.*, **86**, 77–86.

Mason, H. S., North, J. C. and Vanneste, M. (1965), "Microsomal Mixed-function Oxidations: The Metabolism of Xenobiotics," *Fedn. Proc.*, **24**, 1172–1180.

Maurer, H. M., Wolff, J. A., Poppers, P. J., Finster, M., Pantuck, E., Kuntzman, R. and Conney, A. H. (1968), "Reduction in Concentration of Total Serum-bilirubin in Offspring of Women Treated with Phenobarbitone During Pregnancy," *Lancet*, **2**, 122–124.

Mazze, R. I., Trudell, J. R. and Cousins, M. J. (1971), "Methoxyflurane Metabolism and Renal Dysfunction: Clinical Correlation in Man," *Anesthesiology*, **35**, 247–252.

Miller, J. A. and Miller, E. C. (1965), "Metabolism of Drugs in Relation to Carcinogenicity," *Ann. N.Y. Acad. Sci.*, **123**, 125–140.

Motulsky, A. G. (1965), "The Genetics of Abnormal Drug Responses," *Ann. N.Y. Acad. Sci.*, **123**, 167–177.

Motulsky, A. G. and Stamatoyannopoulos, G. (1968), "Drugs, Anesthesia and Abnormal Hemoglobins," *Ann. N.Y. Acad. Sci.*, **151**, 807–821.

Motulsky, A. G., Yoshida, A. and Stamatoyannopoulos, G. (1971), "Variants of Glucose-6-phosphate Dehydrogenase," *Ann. N.Y. Acad. Sci.*, **179**, 636–643.

Omura, T., Sato, R., Cooper, D. Y., Rosenthal, O. and Estabrook, R. W. (1965), "Function of Cytochrome P-450 of Microsomes," *Fedn. Proc.*, **24**, 1181–1189.

Orrenius, S. and Ericsson, J. L. E. (1966), "Enzyme-membrane Relationship in Phenobarbital Induction of Synthesis of Drug-metabolizing Enzyme System and Proliferation of Endoplasmic Membranes," *J. Cell Biol.*, **28**, 181–198.

Parke, D. V. (1968a), "The Metabolism of Drugs," in *Recent Advances in Pharmacology*, ed. Robson, J. M. and Stacey, R. S., 4th edition, pp. 29–74. London: J. and A. Churchill Ltd.

Parke, D. V. (1968b), "Factors which Affect the Metabolism of Drugs," in *Recent Advances in Pharmacology*, ed. Robson, J. M. and Stacey, R. S., 4th edition, pp. 75–98. London: J. and A. Churchill Ltd.

Peters, J. H., Miller, K. S. and Brown, P. (1965), "Studies on the Metabolic Basis for the Genetically Determined Capacities for Isoniazid Inactivation in Man," *J. Pharmac. exp. Ther.*, **150**, 298–304.

Peters, R. A. (1969), "The Biochemical Lesion and its Historical Development," *Br. med. Bull.*, **25**, 223–225.

Pinson, R., Schreiber, E. C., Wiseman, E. N., Chiaini, J. and Baumgartner, D. (1962), "The Fate and Excretion of Polythiazide in the Dog," *J. med. pharm. Chem.*, **5**, 491–503.

Piomelli, S., Corash, L. M., Davenport, D. D., Miraglia, J. and Amorosi, E. L. (1968), "In Vivo Lability of Glucose-6-Phosphate dehydrogenase in $Gd^{A-}$ and $Gd^{Mediterranean}$ Deficiency," *J. clin. Invest.*, **47**, 940–948.

Porter, I. H. (1964), "Genetic Basis of Drug Metabolism in Man," *Toxic. appl. Pharmac.*, **6**, 499–511.

Prescott, L. F. (1969), "Pharmacokinetic Drug Interactions," *Lancet*, **2**, 1239–1243.

Quinn, G. P., Axelrod, J. Brodie, B. B. (1958), "Species, Strain and Sex Differences in Metabolism of Hexobarbitone, Amidopyrine, Antipyrine and Aniline," *Biochem. Pharmac.*, **1**, 152–159.

Rehder, K., Forbes, J., Alter, H., Hessler, O. and Stier, A. (1967), "Halothane Biotransformation in Man: a Quantitative Study," *Anesthesiology*, **28**, 711–715.

Remmer, H. (1962), "Drug Tolerance," in *Enzymes and Drug Action*, ed. Mongar, J. L. and de Reuck, A. V. S., pp. 276–300. London: J. and A. Churchill Ltd.

Remmer, H. and Merker, H. J. (1965), "Effect of Drugs on the Formation of Smooth Endoplasmic Reticulum and Drug-metabolizing Enzymes," *Ann. N.Y. Acad. Sci.*, **123**, 79–97.

Rubinstein, H. M., Dietz, A. A., Hodges, L. K., Lubrano, T. and Czebotar, V. (1970), "Silent Cholinesterase Gene: Variations in the Properties of Serum Enzyme in Apparent Homozygotes," *J. clin. Invest.*, **49**, 479–486.

Sandler, M. and Ruthven, C. R. J. (1969), "The Biosynthesis and Metabolism of the Catecholamines," *Progr. mednl. Chem.*, **6**, 200–265.

Scheline, R. R. (1968), "Drug Metabolism by Intestinal Microorganisms," *J. pharm. Sci.*, **57**, 2021–2037.

Schenkman, J. B., Remmer, H. and Estabrook, R. W. (1967), "Spectral Studies of Drug Interaction with Hepatic Microsomal Cytochrome," *Molec. Pharmac.*, **3**, 113–123.

Searle, J. F. (1973), "Anaesthesia in Sickle Cell States. A Review," *Anaesthesia*, **28**, 48–58.

Sjöqvist, F. (1965), "Psychotropic Drugs (2). Interaction Between Monoamine Oxidase (MAO) Inhibitors and Other Substances," *Proc. R. Soc. Med.*, **58**, 967–978.

Solomon, H. M. and Schrogie, J. J. (1967), "Effect of Phenyramidol and Bishydroxycoumarin on the Metabolism of Tolbutamide in Human Subjects," *Metabolism*, **16**, 1029–1033.

Smith, R. L. and Williams, R. T. (1966). "Implications of the Conjugation of Drugs and Other Exogenous Compounds," in *Glucuronic Acid. Free and Combined*, Chapter 7, pp. 457–491. New York: Academic Press.

Symposium on Experimental and Clinical Aspects of Pharmaco-genetics (1965), *Fedn. Proc.*, **24**, 1259–1292.

Van Dyke, R. A. (1966), "Metabolism of Volatile Anesthetics. III. Induction of Microsomal Dechlorinating and Ether-cleaving Enzymes," *J. Pharmac. exp. Ther.*, **154**, 364–369.

Van Dyke, R. A. and Chenoweth, M. B. (1965), "Metabolism of Volatile Anesthetics," *Anesthesiology*, **26**, 348–357.

Vesell, E. S. (1968), "Genetic and Environmental Factors Affecting Hexobarbital Metabolism in Mice," *Ann. N.Y. Acad. Sci.*, **151**, 900–912.

Waltman, R., Bonura, F., Nigrin, G. and Pipat, C. (1969), "Ethanol in Prevention of Hyperbilirubinaemia in the Newborn. A Controlled Trial," *Lancet*, **2**, 1265–1267.

Welch, R. M., Harrison, Y. E., Conney, A. H. and Burns, J. J. (1969), "An Experimental Model in Dogs for Studying Interactions of Drugs with Bishydroxycoumarin," *Clin. Pharmac. Ther.*, **10**, 817–825.

Williams, R. T. (1963), "Detoxication Mechanisms in Man," *Clin. Pharmac. Ther.* **4**, 234–254.

Williams, R. T. (1967), "Comparative Patterns of Drug Metabolism," *Fedn. Proc.*, **26**, 1029–1039.

Williams, R. T. (1971), "The Metabolism of Certain Drugs and Food Chemicals in Man," *Ann. N.Y. Acad. Sci.*, **179**, 141–154.

Williams, R. T. and Parke, D. V. (1964), "Metabolic Fate of Drugs," *A. Rev. Pharmac.*, **4**, 85–114.

## SUGGESTIONS FOR FURTHER READING

Brodie, B. B. (1967), "Physicochemical and Biochemical Aspects of Pharmacology," *J. Am. med. Ass.*, **202**, 600–609.

Gillette, J. R., Davis, D. C. and Sasome, H. A. (1972), "Cytochrome P-450 and its Role in Drug Metabolism," *A. Rev. Pharmac.*, **12**, 57–84.

Goldstein, A., Aronow, L. and Kalman S. M. (1968), *Principles of Drug Action. The Basis of Pharmacology*. New York: Hoeber Medical Division.

Mongar, J. L. and de Reuck, A. V. S. (1962) (editors), *Enzymes and Drug Action*. Ciba Foundation Symposium. London: J. and A. Churchill Ltd.

Parke, D. V. (1968), *The Biochemistry of Foreign Compounds*. International Series of Monographs in Pure and Applied Biology. Oxford: Pergamon Press.

Spirtes, M. A. (1965), "Fate of Drugs in the Body," in *Pharmacology in Medicine* (Drill), ed. DiPalma J. R., 3rd edition, pp. 26–46. New York: McGraw-Hill Book Company, Inc.

Vesell, E. S. (1971) (editor), *Drug Metabolism in Man. Ann. N.Y. Acad. Sci.*, **179**, 773 pp.

Williams, R. T. (1959), *Detoxication Mechanisms, The Metabolism and Detoxication of Drugs, Toxic Substances and Other Organic Compounds*, 2nd edition. London: Chapman & Hall Ltd.

Wolstenholme, G. and Porter, R. (1967) (editors), *Drug Responses in Man*. A Ciba Foundation Symposium. London: J. and A. Churchill Ltd.

*CHAPTER* 3

# UPTAKE, DISTRIBUTION, AND ELIMINATION OF INHALED ANAESTHETICS

## EDMOND I. EGER

The anaesthetist controls the course of an inhalation anaesthetic by indirect manipulation of anaesthetic tension in the brain. Inhaled anaesthetics cannot be directly presented to the brain. Instead they must be administered through the lungs to arterial blood and thence to brain and other tissues. At each step (inspired gas to alveoli, alveoli to blood, and blood to brain), a decrease in anaesthetic tension gradient is present until equilibration is complete.

What causes the difference in tension between inspired and alveolar gas? Three factors are involved: ventilation (Eger and Larson, 1964), uptake (Eger, 1963a) and concentration (Eger, 1963b). If unimpeded, ventilation would cause the alveolar tension rapidly to reach that inspired. With a 'normal' alveolar minute volume of 4 l./min. and a functional residual capacity of 2 l., the alveolar concentration would equal 98 per cent of that inspired within 2 minutes. However, the effect of ventilation is countered by uptake into blood. Just as ventilation raises alveolar concentration by bringing anaesthetic into the lungs, uptake decreases alveolar concentration by removing agent. Ignoring for the moment the concentration effect, the alveolar anaesthetic tension is determined principally by the balance between anaesthetic input (ventilation) and anaesthetic loss (uptake).

There are three things which determine how much agent is taken up by blood. First, solubility of the agent:

the higher the solubility in blood the greater the uptake. Solubility is expressed as a ratio of the concentration distribution (i.e. the ratio of the concentrations in each phase) of an agent in equilibrium between two phases (Eger and Larson, 1964). This is a partition coefficient and numerically is equal to the Ostwald solubility coefficient. For example if alveolar nitrous oxide concentration were 80 volumes per cent and if this were in equilibrium with 37·6 volumes per cent in pulmonary blood, the nitrous oxide blood/gas partition coefficient would be $37·6/80 = 0·47$. Another way of saying this is for every 100 molecules/ml. of nitrous oxide in air there are 47 molecules per ml. of blood. Nitrous oxide has a relatively low blood solubility compared to halothane (blood/gas coefficient = 2·3). In turn, halothane is much less soluble than diethyl ether (blood/gas coefficient = 12·1). Thus, for a given alveolar concentration, ether is taken up in greatest quantity, halothane less so and nitrous oxide least. This means that the greatest difference between alveolar and inspired concentration occurs with ether, a lesser but still sizeable difference is found with halothane, while only a small difference is seen with nitrous oxide (Fig. 1). A list of some partition coefficients is given in Table 1.

The second factor determining uptake is cardiac output; as it increases, uptake increases. This is simply a function of the larger volume of blood exposed to anaesthetic in the

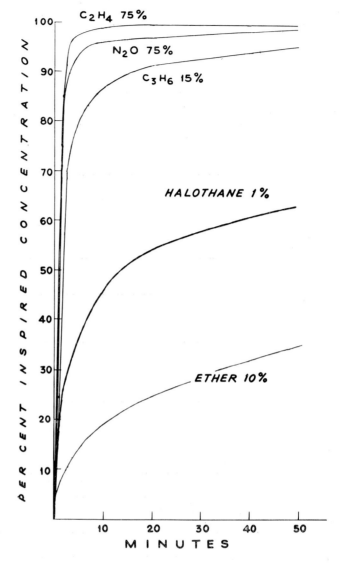

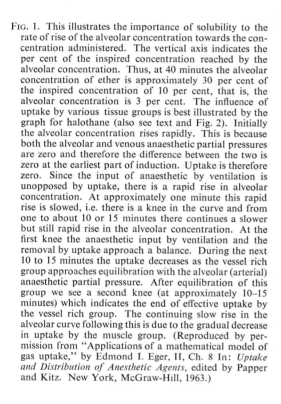

FIG. 1. This illustrates the importance of solubility to the rate of rise of the alveolar concentration towards the concentration administered. The vertical axis indicates the per cent of the inspired concentration reached by the alveolar concentration. Thus, at 40 minutes the alveolar concentration of ether is approximately 30 per cent of the inspired concentration of 10 per cent, that is, the alveolar concentration is 3 per cent. The influence of uptake by various tissue groups is best illustrated by the graph for halothane (also see text and Fig. 2). Initially the alveolar concentration rises rapidly. This is because both the alveolar and venous anaesthetic partial pressures are zero and therefore the difference between the two is zero at the earliest part of induction. Uptake is therefore zero. Since the input of anaesthetic by ventilation is unopposed by uptake, there is a rapid rise in alveolar concentration. At approximately one minute this rapid rise is slowed, i.e. there is a knee in the curve and from one to about 10 or 15 minutes there continues a slower but still rapid rise in the alveolar concentration. At the first knee the anaesthetic input by ventilation and the removal by uptake approach a balance. During the next 10 to 15 minutes the uptake decreases as the vessel rich group approaches equilibration with the alveolar (arterial) anaesthetic partial pressure. After equilibration of this group we see a second knee (at approximately 10–15 minutes) which indicates the end of effective uptake by the vessel rich group. The continuing slow rise in the alveolar curve following this is due to the gradual decrease in uptake by the muscle group. (Reproduced by permission from "Applications of a mathematical model of gas uptake," by Edmond I. Eger, II, Ch. 8 In: *Uptake and Distribution of Anesthetic Agents*, edited by Papper and Kitz. New York, McGraw-Hill, 1963.)

alveoli. In excitement uptake may be much increased by this factor. In shock the reverse occurs and the unusually rapid rise in alveolar tension that results may lead to anaesthetic overdosage, especially with the more soluble agents.

The third factor is the anaesthetic tension gradient from alveoli to venous blood. Uptake increases in proportion to the size of the gradient. This gradient (and hence uptake) equals zero after equilibration with all parts of the body. The gradient is greatest at the time of least saturation, i.e. during induction. To understand what determines the changes in this gradient during and following induction one must understand the relative distribution of blood within the body (Eger, 1963b). Between 70–80 per cent of the cardiac output is directed to roughly 6 per cent of the body tissues. This group of tissues (brain, kidney, hepatoportal system, heart, endocrine glands) is a vessel rich group (VRG) which, because of the high blood flow/mass ratio, rapidly attains equilibrium with the anaesthetic tension in arterial blood. As equilibrium is approached, the agent's tension in the venous blood

leaving these tissues also rises until, at equilibrium, it equals the arterial (and tissue) tension. This process is complete within 10 to 15 minutes if no concomitant rise in arterial tension occurs, and thus after this time, 70–80 per cent of the blood returning to the lungs is at the same tension as that found in the alveoli and arterial blood. The alveolar-venous blood gradient is, therefore, rapidly reduced to 20–30 per cent of its initial size and uptake must be similarly reduced (Fig. 2). Three other tissue groups continue to remove anaesthetic from arterial blood long after saturation of the VRG. Skin and muscle (MG) form 50 per cent of the body bulk and at rest receive about 18 per cent of the cardiac output. Saturation of this group proceeds slowly and is not complete for at least an hour and a half even when arterial tension is held constant. Fat (FG) comprises roughly 19 per cent of the body volume and has a blood flow per unit volume slightly less than resting muscle. Perhaps 5–6 per cent of the cardiac output flows through fat. However, saturation of the FG proceeds much more slowly than that of the MG since all anaesthetics are considerably more soluble in fat. The last

TABLE 1

PARTITION COEFFICIENTS OF SOME ANAESTHETIC GASES AT $37°C \pm 0.5°C$

| Anaesthetic Gas | Blood/Gas | Tissue/Blood | Oil/Gas |
|---|---|---|---|
| Ethylene | 0·140 | 1·0 (Heart)<br>1·2 (Brain) | 1·28 |
| Xenon | 0·17 | 1·20 (Brain-White)<br>0·74 (Brain-Grey)<br>0·73 (Muscle)<br>0·74 (Liver)<br>0·72 (Heart)<br>7·94 (Fat) | 1·9 |
| Cyclopropane | 0·45 to 0·6 | 0·91 (Muscle)<br>1·36 (Liver) | 11·8 |
| Nitrous Oxide | 0·47 | 1·13 (Heart)<br>1·06 (Brain)<br>1·0 (Lung) | 1·4 |
| Fluroxene | 1·37 | 1·43 (Brain-White)<br>1·43 (Brain-Grey)<br>2·27 (Muscle)<br>1·37 (Liver) | 47·7 |
| Halothane | 2·3 | 2·6 (Brain)<br>2·6 (Liver)<br>1·6 (Kidney)<br>3·5 (Muscle)<br>60 (Fat) | 224 |
| Divinyl Ether | 2·8 | | 58 |
| Chloroform | 8·4 | 1·0 (Heart)<br>1·0 (Brain) | 265 |
| Trichloroethylene | 9·15 | | 960 |
| Diethyl Ether | 12·1 | 1·14 (Brain)<br>1·2 (Lung) | 65 |
| Methoxyflurane | 13·0 | 2·34 (Brain-White)<br>1·70 (Brain-Grey)<br>1·34 (Muscle) | 970 |

Table 1 lists the partition coefficients of the common and some uncommon anaesthetic gases in order of their blood/gas partition coefficients. Those at the top of the table have the lowest and those at the bottom have the highest coefficients. This parallels the rate at which induction and recovery may be achieved with these agents. The tissue/blood partition coefficients are, with the exception of fat, all close to one. The greatest deviation is found with halothane in muscle. The oil/gas partition coefficients may be used to indicate potency. For man, the oil/gas coefficient times the minimum alveolar concentration (MAC) required to eliminate movement in response to a painful stimulus equals a constant of approximately 140. Many of the sources for these partition coefficients are given in Eger and Saidman, 1964. Other sources include Conn, H. L., Jr., 1961, Gregory and Eger, 1968, and Regan and Eger, 1967.

tissue group, the vessel poor group (VPG), is so poorly perfused that it has little or no effect on uptake and distribution although it makes up a significant fraction of the body (22 per cent). Bone, cartilage, tendons, ligaments and other relatively avascular tissues are in this group.

From the above, the alveolar-venous blood anaesthetic gradient may be seen to go through at least three stages.

rate at which the alveolar concentration rises (concentration effect) (Eger, 1963a and c). A higher inspired concentration results in a relatively more rapid approach of alveolar concentration to that inspired. At 100 per cent inspired concentration, the alveolar tension rise is equally rapid for all anaesthetics regardless of differences in solubility. That is, uptake (which is directly related to

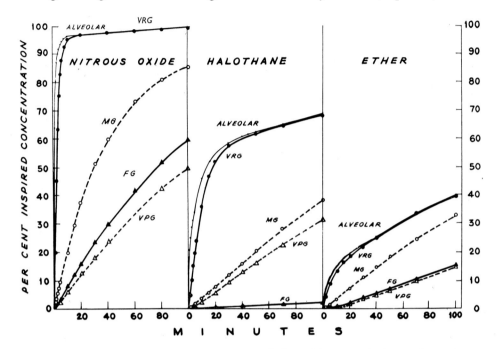

FIG. 2. The figure illustrates the concomitant anaesthetic partial pressure rise in alveoli, vessel rich group (VRG), muscle group (MG), fat group (FG) and vessel poor group (VPG) for the anaesthetics nitrous oxide, halothane and ether. The rates of rise of alveolar concentration (uppermost curve for each anaesthetic) towards the concentration being inspired are identical with those in Figure 1. Underlying the alveolar curve and rapidly rising towards it is the partial pressure rise in the vessel rich group. A significant separation between partial pressures in alveoli and vessel rich group exists only early in anaesthesia; for the first five minutes for nitrous oxide and for ten minutes for halothane. This is the period of sizeable uptake by the vessel rich group. Following this time, uptake by the vessel rich group is inconsequential. The rate of rise of partial pressure in the muscle group is significantly less than that in the vessel rich group. The difference between the anaesthetic partial pressure in the muscle group and the alveoli is large for approximately one hour in the case of nitrous oxide and for several hours in the case of halothane. The partial pressure rate of rise in the fat group is inversely related to the fat/blood partition coefficient. It is fairly rapid in the case of nitrous oxide but extremely slow in the case of halothane. Equilibration of halothane with the fat group probably requires several weeks. The vessel poor group is too poorly perfused to be of significance in uptake. (Reproduced with permission from "Applications of a mathematical model of gas uptake" by Edmond I. Eger, II, Ch. 8 In: *Uptake and Distribution of Anesthetic Agents.* Edited by Papper and Kitz. New York, McGraw-Hill, 1963.)

Initially all tissue groups are unsaturated and remove most of the anaesthetic from the blood passing through them. The anaesthetic tension in venous blood leaving all tissues is low. As induction progresses, the VRG rapidly becomes saturated; and the venous tension may rise thereafter to 70–80 per cent of arterial. The remaining 20–30 per cent alveolar-venous gradient is slowly reduced over a period of hours as equilibration is reached in the MG. During this entire period and beyond, the FG remains unsaturated and thus prevents venous and arterial (alveolar) tension from reaching equality during the course of 3–30 hours of anaesthesia.

Although it has been ignored thus far, the inspired concentration of agent may exert a profound influence on the

solubility) no longer counteracts the ventilatory input of anaesthetic. The rate of alveolar tension rise toward that inspired is determined solely by ventilation when the inspired concentration is 100 per cent. The lower the concentration the greater the effect of solubility.

This can be explained in a crude fashion. Imagine what happens when we fill a mythical lung with 1 per cent of a new gas. The solubility of the new gas is such that half of the gas is removed and the concentration thereby decreases by half. If, however, we fill the mythical lung with 100 per cent of this gas and half is removed, the resulting concentration is not 50 per cent, but remains 100 per cent. That is, uptake does not affect the alveolar concentration. Between these extremes, the effect of uptake is decreased but still present. This is illustrated in Figure 3 for nitrous oxide (Stoelting and Eger). Initially the lung (as indicated by a rectangular box) is filled with 80 per cent nitrous oxide. If half of the nitrous oxide is removed as indicated in Section A of that figure, the concentration does not fall to 40 per cent nitrous oxide, but rather to 66·7 per cent. Furthermore, if the mythical lung, instead of decreasing in size, maintains its initial size by drawing in more gas having the same composition as that originally placed in the lung, the alveolar concentration of nitrous oxide would be further raised as indicated in the right hand portion of Figure 3. Addition of the two nitrous oxide boxes containing 40 and 32 per cent indicates that the final nitrous oxide percentage would be 72 per cent, far higher than the 40 per cent which would

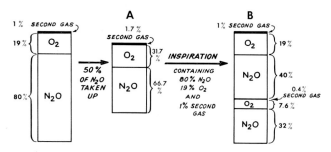

FIG. 3. This is an example of both the concentration effect and the second gas effect (see text for details). (Reproduced with permission from "Additional explanation for the second gas effect: A concentrating effect," by Robert K. Stoelting and Edmond I. Eger, II, *Anesthesiology*, **30**, 273, 1969.)

be reached if the reduction were proportional to the amount removed.

The concentration effect is of clinical importance for those gases that have an appreciable solubility and may be administered at high inspired concentrations—nitrous oxide, cyclopropane, fluroxene, and ether. This explains the more rapid rate of rise of alveolar nitrous oxide compared to cyclopropane in Figure 1: although the two have similar partition coefficients (except for fat) nitrous oxide is administered at a far higher inspired concentration.

The uptake of large volumes of anaesthetic as indicated in Figure 3 for nitrous oxide may appreciably increase the total volume of gas inspired. Epstein (1964) has shown that this increased inspiratory volume carries with it any other gas given concomitantly and hence accelerates the rise in alveolar concentration of the second gas (Fig. 4). He has called this the 'second gas effect'. Stoelting *et al.* have shown that there is an additional explanation for the second gas effect which might be called a 'concentrating effect'. Both explanations are illustrated in Figure 3. Initially there is 1 per cent of some second gas present in the lungs. As half of the nitrous oxide is removed, the concentration of this second gas increases to 1·7 per cent although the absolute volume does not change (middle panel). The relative concentration increases because of the reduction in total volume. This is the concentrating portion of the second gas effect. If the lung is not allowed to collapse, but is replenished with gas containing the same concentration

as initially filled the lung, then more of the second gas is brought into the lung as indicated in the panel on the right in Figure 3. This is the increased inspiratory ventilation suggested by Epstein as the cause for the second gas effect (Epstein *et al.*, 1964). In this case the increase

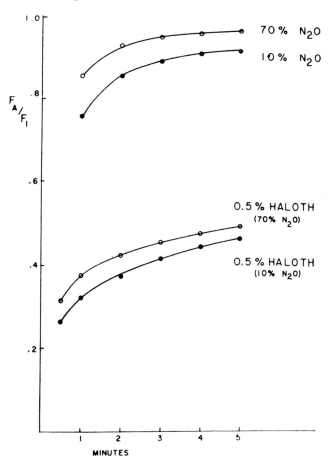

FIG. 4. This illustrates both the concentration effect and the second gas effect. In this experiment, performed by Epstein, two anaesthetics were administered. One was 70 per cent nitrous oxide and 0·5 per cent halothane, the other was 10 per cent nitrous oxide with 0·5 per cent halothane. Ventilation was the same in both cases. $F_A/F_I$ is the ratio of alveolar to inspired anaesthetic concentrations. The administration of the higher concentration of nitrous oxide (70 per cent vs. 10 per cent) resulted in a more rapid rise of the alveolar concentration toward the concentration being inspired. This is the concentration effect. Although the inspired concentration of halothane was the same in both experiments the alveolar rate of rise was greater when the halothane was given with 70 per cent nitrous oxide. This is the second gas effect. (Reproduced with permission from "Influence of the concentration effect on the uptake of anesthetic mixtures: the second gas effect," by R. M. Epstein, H. Rackow, E. Salanitre and G. L. Wolf, *Anesthesiology*, **25**, 364, 1964.)

in inspired ventilation actually reduces the concentration of the second gas from 1·7 to 1·4 per cent. The importance of concentration versus increased inspired ventilation to the second gas effect depends upon the solubility of the second gas. If the solubility is great in blood (methoxyflurane, ether) then the main explanation of the second gas effect lies in the increased inspired ventilation. If solubility is small (nitrous oxide, cyclopropane), then the concentrating effect will be most important. The second gas effect is dependent upon the uptake of large volumes of the first gas, or anaesthetic. Uptake of large volumes of anaesthetic may occur upon induction with nitrous oxide or with diethyl ether. The second gas effect is therefore limited to these anaesthetics. The rate of induction with any gas given simultaneously with these anaesthetics will be accelerated.

Each of the above factors (ventilation, cardiac output, alveolar-blood gradient and inspired concentration) may interact with the other. For example by bringing more anaesthetic into the lungs per unit time, an increase in ventilation reduces the difference between inspired and alveolar tensions (Fig. 5). However, the relative effect of an increase in ventilation is different for gases of different solubilities. Changes in ventilation have a small effect on the least soluble anaesthetics such as ethylene, nitrous oxide, and cyclopropane, but have a profound effect on the very soluble anaesthetics such as methoxyflurane, ether, and chloroform. A doubling of ventilation during induction may result in a near doubling of alveolar concentration with the soluble agents (Eger, 1963a). This is seen in the right hand portion of Figure 5 where ventilation is varied from 2 to 8 litres per minute. After 10 minutes of administration at a 2 litre per minute alveolar ventilation, the alveolar ether concentration has risen by only 10 per cent. Whereas at 8 litres per minute it has risen by about 35 per cent, that is, a 3·5 fold difference. Compare this with the moderately soluble halothane where, at the same point in time, the same change in ventilation produces a rise in alveolar concentration from 30 per cent to approximately 65 per cent. That is, a little more than 2 fold increase. The increase with nitrous oxide is negligible both because of the low solubility and because of the concentration effect which, as noted previously, diminishes the impact of uptake. Similarly, an increase in cardiac output results in an increased inspired-alveolar anaesthetic gradient; but this change in gradient is small for the less soluble agents and large for the very soluble agents (Fig. 5).

The anaesthetic partial pressure in the brain closely follows the anaesthetic partial pressure in the alveoli. The lag is short because of the high brain blood flow. However, changes in ventilation and circulation may alter the flow of blood to brain and thereby alter the rate at which anaesthesia may be induced. For example an increase in ventilation causes the alveolar concentration to rise more rapidly, but the reduction in $P_{CO_2}$ which accompanies hyperventilation decreases cerebral blood flow and thereby delays induction. The impact of this alteration in cerebral blood flow on the rate of induction is related to solubility (Munson and Bowers, 1967). With the poorly soluble anaesthetics there is an appreciable delay. With the very soluble anaesthetics the more rapid rise in alveolar concentration more than compensates for the reduction in cerebral blood flow and hyperventilation therefore still produces a more rapid induction of anaesthesia with soluble anaesthetics. Similar observations may be made on the effect of the reduction in cardiac output associated with shock (Munson et al., 1968). This results in a more rapid rise in the alveolar concentration. However, if cerebral blood flow is concomitantly reduced then the higher alveolar anaesthetic partial pressures obtained are not reflected as rapidly in the brain and it will appear that the induction of anaesthesia is proceeding at a normal rate, except for poorly soluble anaesthetics where there is a delay. If, however, the perfusion to the brain is spared in shock, then the rate of rise of anaesthetic partial pressure in the brain, and consequently induction, is more rapid than usual. The changes in cerebral blood flow relative to cardiac output that occur during shock in man are not known, but animal work suggests that both are lowered

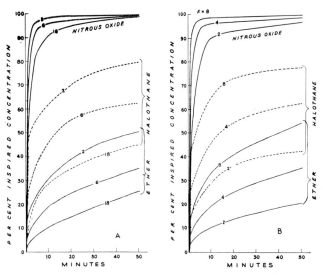

Fig. 5. This illustrates the effect of changes in circulation or ventilation on the rate of rise of the alveolar concentrations of three anaesthetics: ether, halothane and nitrous oxide. The left portion of the figure gives the effect of changing cardiac output from 2 to 6 to 18 litres per minute. The right illustrates the effect of changing ventilation from 2 to 4 to 8 litres per minute. The relative effect is most pronounced with the most soluble agent, ether, both for changes in ventilation and circulation. The least effect is seen with the least soluble agent, nitrous oxide. (Reproduced with permission from "Applications of a mathematical model of gas uptake," by Edmond I. Eger, II, Ch. 8 In: *Uptake and Distribution of Anesthetic Agents.* Edited by Papper and Kitz, New York, McGraw-Hill, 1963.)

with, however, some sparing of cerebral flow (Rittman and Smith, 1966).

Thus far we have assumed that ventilation/perfusion ratios were equal throughout the lung. Abnormalities of this sort, including the presence of arteriovenous shunts across the lung, result in an alveolar-arterial gradient which is proportional to the degree of abnormality. Comparing the arterial tensions attained with and without a ventilation/perfusion abnormality, the greatest difference occurs with the least soluble agents. Thus rate of induction of anaesthesia is least affected with the most soluble agents in the presence of such an abnormality (Eger and Severinghaus, 1964; Saidman and Eger, 1967). The reason for the greater impact of ventilation/perfusion abnormalities on the less soluble anaesthetics is illustrated in Figure 6. A in this figure illustrates the relationships that might be obtained when ventilation/perfusion ratios are equal throughout the lungs. In this case, the end-tidal anaesthetic concentration of 10 mm.Hg. accurately reflects the alveolar and arterial partial pressure. In Figure B and C, Figure 6, one lung is obstructed and the remaining lung assumes the ventilation normally entering the obstructed side; that is, the ventilation to the unobstructed side is doubled. If the gas is very soluble, then doubling the ventilation essentially doubles the alveolar concentration (*see* Figure 5, ether) and the anaesthetic partial pressure in the unobstructed side is nearly twice normal as illustrated in Figure B. Although the anaesthetic partial

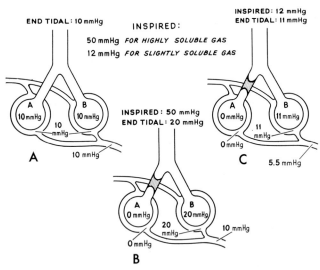

Fig. 6. This illustrates the effect of obstruction of ventilation to one lung on the arterial anaesthetic partial pressure of a highly soluble (B) and poorly soluble (C) gas. (A) represents the normal lung with a normal end-tidal anaesthetic partial pressure equal in both lungs and in the arterial blood. See text for further description. (Reproduced with permission from "The influence of ventilation/perfusion abnormalities upon the uptake of inhalation anaesthetics," by L. J. Saidman and E. I. Eger, II, *Clinical Anesthesia*, Vol. 1, Ch. 5, p. 79, 1967.)

pressure from the obstructed lung is zero until recirculation occurs, the mean arterial pressure is 10 mm. Hg., or the same as in the absence of the ventilation/perfusion abnormality. If, however, we are speaking of a slightly soluble gas, then the increase in ventilation to the unobstructed lung scarcely elevates the alveolar partial pressure (again see Figure 5, nitrous oxide). Since the anaesthetic partial pressure in the ventilated lung is only slightly elevated, and the anaesthetic partial pressure initially returning from the unventilated lung is zero, the mean arterial pressure is little more than half normal.

Insertion of an anaesthetic system between anaesthetic source and patient introduces three new factors to be considered. First, the volume of such a system acts as a buffer to changes in anaesthetic tension (Eger, 1963). The larger the system the more slowly do changes occur. Second, the rubber of the system may take up appreciable quantities of agent and thus act to buffer both the rise and the fall of tension within the system (Eger and Larson, 1962; Eger and Brandstater, 1963). The rubber/gas partition coefficients for methoxyflurane and halothane

are 742 and 121, respectively, values sufficiently high to remove significant amounts of each agent during induction. Such removal is illustrated in Figure 7. A three litre per minute inflow is led into the rubber portions of an anaesthetic circuit which are connected in a circle. The

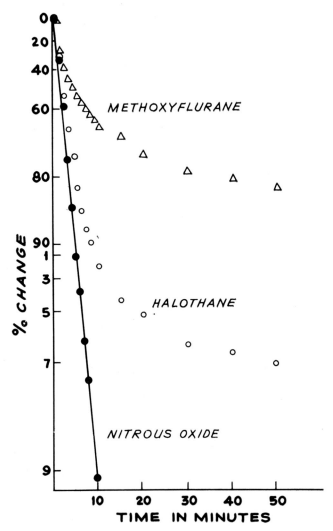

Fig. 7. This illustrates the effect of uptake by the rubber in an anaesthetic system on the concentration of anaesthetic which a patient might inspire. The vertical axis indicates the per cent of the inflowing concentration of anaesthetic existing within the system (i.e. the concentration in the system divided by the inflowing concentration). Inflow rate into the system is 3 litres per minute and the system volume is approximately 6·25 litres. (Reproduced with permission from "Solubility of methoxyflurane in rubber," by Edmond I. Eger, II and B. Brandstater, *Anesthesiology*, **24**, 679, 1963).

rise in concentration within the circle toward the concentration being introduced is depicted as a downward trend, 100 per cent change existing when the two concentrations are equal. The predicted rate of change is indicated by the continuous line. The experimental points for nitrous oxide, a gas not taken up in appreciable quantities by rubber, overlies this line. Both halothane and methoxyflurane deviate from this line and deviate in proportion to the difference in their solubilities. The removal of halothane is relatively small but the removal of methoxyflurane is large. Even after 50 minutes 20 per cent of the methoxyflurane introduced into the system is removed by the rubber. This, of course, is a significant hindrance to the development of an adequate inspired anaesthetic tension. Third, the amount of anaesthetic that reaches the lungs is not only dependent on ventilation, but is also limited by the inflow rate into the system (Eger, 1960; Severinghaus, 1966). Since inflow and ventilation act on successive points, whichever is least gives the uppermost limit to the rate of rise of alveolar anaesthetic partial

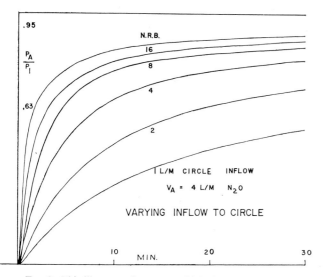

FIG. 8. This illustrates the rate at which the alveolar concentration of nitrous oxide approaches the concentration inflowing into the anaesthetic system. The inspired concentration (not shown) lies between these two concentrations. The vertical coordinate is the ratio of alveolar to inflowing anaesthetic partial pressures ($P_A/P_I$). Alveolar ventilation ($V_A$) is constant at 4 litres per minute. The inflow rate varies from 1 to 16 litres per minute. The uppermost curve indicates that which would be found with a non-rebreathing system. That is, at infinite inflow. This also shows that a high inflow rate (greater than 4 litres per minute) is necessary to assure a rapid rise in alveolar concentration during induction. (Reproduced with permission from unpublished work of John W. Severinghaus.)

pressure. For example, during apnoea the alveolar concentration will not rise regardless of inflow rate. Conversely, regardless of the degree of hyperventilation, the alveolar concentration will not rise if inflow is zero. Usually, of course, alveolar ventilation and inflow are finite rather than these extremes. Figure 8 shows the effect of varying inflow while ventilation remains constant and Figure 9 shows the effect of varying alveolar ventilation with inflow constant. In both cases, the fixed factor limits the alveolar rate of rise toward the inflowing concentration regardless of how much the other factor varies.

Uptake may occur not only by a tissue but by an enclosed gas space within the body. Uptake by such a space presents certain problems of volume or pressure change which are not present in the case of uptake by a tissue. If an air (nitrogen) filled space exists within the body and an anaesthetic such as nitrous oxide is administered

via the lungs, then one of two things may happen to the space. If the walls of the space are compliant then the space expands (Eger and Saidman, 1965). Nitrous oxide enters the gas phase, but nitrogen cannot leave because of its low solubility. The amount of expansion depends on the nitrous oxide concentration in the lungs. At a 50 per cent concentration the maximum expansion doubles the size of the space, while at 75 per cent it quadruples the size. If the gas space is a pneumothorax, such expansion might seriously embarrass respiration or circulation (Hunter, 1955). Other compliant spaces in the body

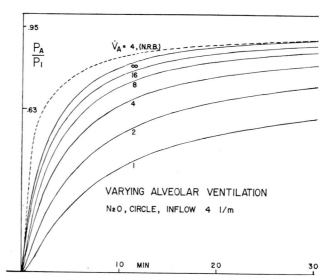

FIG. 9. This figure also illustrates the approach of alveolar to inflowing concentration. However, as opposed to the previous figure, the inflow rate is constant at 4 litres per minute and the alveolar ventilation is allowed to vary from 1 litre per minute to infinity. The uppermost curve indicates the rate of rise with a non-rebreathing system when alveolar ventilation is 4 litres per minute. Notice that at infinite ventilation the inflow rate still imposes a limit on the alveolar rate of rise. The difference between the curve resulting from infinite ventilation and that obtained with a non-rebreathing system is due to the difference in system volume. (Reproduced with permission from unpublished work of John W. Severinghaus.)

include bowel gas (Eger and Saidman, 1965) and air emboli (Munson and Merrick, 1966). If the walls of the space are not compliant then entrance of the anaesthetic without concomitant loss of nitrogen produces a rise in pressure. Such a rise, if it impairs local circulation, might prove hazardous during a procedure such as pneumoencephalography (Saidman and Eger, 1965). Other noncompliant (or low compliance) spaces include the sinus and middle ear (Waun et al., 1967; Matz et al., 1967).

Uptake of anaesthetic agents varies with the manner of presentation to the patient. The inspired, or inflowing concentration may be kept constant and in this case the alveolar concentration rises until at equilibrium it reaches that inspired or inflowing. The former is the situation we have described above. However, this would represent a constantly changing depth of anaesthesia with continual deepening until equilibrium is reached. This is contrary to common practice which is rapidly to obtain a certain depth of anaesthesia which is maintained thereafter at roughly the same level. A constant alveolar anaesthetic concentration more closely approximates this technique. The inflowing and inspired concentration, then, must be constantly changing (decreasing) until equilibrium is attained (Eger and Saidman, 1964).

Uptake at constant inspired concentrations may be considerably different from uptake at constant alveolar concentrations. With the former, uptake is subject to less change with time as the solubility of the anaesthetic increases. At constant alveolar concentration the pattern is always qualitatively the same regardless of solubility. A

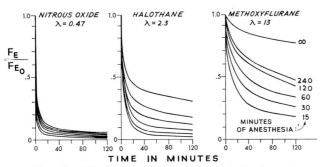

FIG. 10. This illustrates the importance of duration of anaesthesia on the rate at which the alveolar concentration falls. The minutes of anaesthesia indicate the minutes of constant alveolar concentration of the respective anaesthetics. The times in each case are (from lowest to highest curves) 15, 30, 60, 120, 240 minutes and an infinite period. λ is the blood/gas partition coefficient. The vertical axis is the expired concentration ($F_E$) divided by the expired concentration immediately prior to the cessation of anaesthesia ($F_{E_0}$). (Reproduced by permission from "Influence of ventilation and solubility on recovery from anaesthesia: an *in vivo* and analog analysis before and after equilibrium," by R. K. Stoelting and E. I. Eger, II, *Anesthesiology*, **30**, 290, 1969.)

high initial uptake is followed by a rapid reduction to a lower level. This rapid reduction occurs in five to fifteen minutes and represents a saturation of the vessel rich group. Uptake continues to decrease thereafter but at a much slower rate. This decrease is related to saturation of the muscle group and fat group.

After total body equilibration, elimination of anaesthetics occurs nearly as an inverted reproduction of uptake (Eger, 1963; Mapleson, 1963). The output of less soluble anaesthetics is high at first but rapidly declines to a lower level. The output level continues to fall thereafter at a slow and ever decreasing rate. The output of soluble agents is high initially but only gradually decreases with time. The decrease in alveolar concentrations during recovery parallels the decrease in output of agent; recovery is, therefore, rapid with nitrous oxide and slow with ether.

Total body equilibration is of course never achieved in clinical practice. The impact of incomplete equilibration is illustrated in Figure 10. As the duration of anaesthesia increases, the rate at which the alveolar concentration falls on recovery is progressively slower (Mapleson, 1963; Stoelting and Eger, 1969). However, for any given period of anaesthesia the rate of fall is always most rapid with the least soluble anaesthetic. Even with total body equilibra-

tion, the rate of fall is rapid with a poorly soluble anaesthetic, nitrous oxide. As solubility increases, so does the importance of duration of anaesthesia on the rate at which the alveolar concentration falls during recovery. Clinically then, we may anticipate that prolonged anaesthesia with methoxyflurane considerably lengthens the time required for recovery. This is not the case with the poorly soluble anaesthetic, nitrous oxide.

Differences in ventilation during recovery have the same effect (but in an opposite direction) as during induction. An increase in ventilation accelerates recovery; a decrease in ventilation proiongs recovery. The greater

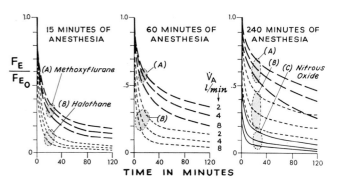

FIG. 11. This illustrates the effect of ventilation following anaesthesia of various durations. In each case, as ventilation is increased from 2 to 4 to 8 litres per minute alveolar ventilation, the fall in the alveolar anaesthetic concentration is accelerated. The impact of these changes in ventilation is increased with increasing anaesthetic solubility and with increasing duration of anaesthesia. (Reproduced with permission from "Influence of ventilation and solubility on recovery from anaesthesia: an *in vivo* and analog analysis before and after equilibrium," by R. K. Stoelting and E. I. Eger, II, *Anesthesiology*, **30**, 290, 1969.)

effect is on the more soluble anaesthetic (Fig. 11). The effect of variations in ventilation also depends on the duration of anaesthesia. If anaesthesia is short, then variations in ventilation have little impact on recovery. That is, the shorter the anaesthetic, the more an anaesthetic acts like a poorly soluble gas (Stoelting and Eger).

During recovery from nitrous oxide anaesthesia, the outpouring of the agent far exceeds the uptake of inspired gas (air) because nitrous oxide is 30 times more soluble than nitrogen. The result of this may be (1) to displace or dilute the inspired oxygen concentration (Fink, 1955) and (2) to decrease the inspired volume required to maintain alveolar carbon dioxide tension constant (Rackow *et al.*, 1961). The reduction in alveolar oxygen concentration that results is called diffusion anoxia. Figure 12 illustrates the reduction in haemoglobin saturation that might be expected when the patient breathes air following a nitrous oxide-oxygen anaesthetic.

In summary, inhalation anaesthesia may be viewed as the development of a series of tension gradients. We begin with a high anaesthetic tension in the cylinder or vaporizer which progressively decreases as we pass from the cylinder to anaesthetic circuit, from circuit to alveoli, and from alveoli to brain or other tissues. The development of these gradients determines the course of anaesthesia.

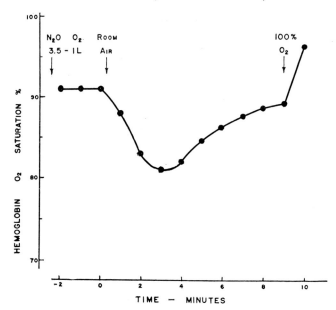

FIG. 12. This depicts the reduction in haemoglobin saturation that occurs on cessation of nitrous oxide-oxygen anaesthesia and initiation of ventilation with 80 per cent nitrogen. A 10 per cent reduction in saturation is seen at approximately 2 to 3 minutes, the time of greatest outpouring of nitrous oxide. As the output of nitrous oxide is reduced, the oxygen saturation returns towards control values. (Reproduced with permission from "Diffusion anoxia," by B. R. Fink, *Anesthesiology*, **16**, 511, 1955.)

Some of these gradients are subject to manipulation by the anaesthetist while others are partially or completely beyond his control. In any case the rational administration of inhalation anaesthesia requires an understanding of the factors governing these gradients so that they may be best controlled or accounted for.

## REFERENCES

Conn, H. L., Jr. (1961), "Equilibrium Distribution of Radioxenon in Tissue: Xenon-hemoglobin Association Curve," *J. Appl. Physiol.* **16**, 1065.

Eger, E. I., II (1960), "Factors Affecting the Rapidity of Alteration of Nitrous Oxide Concentration in a Circle System," *Anesthesiology*, **21**, 348.

Eger, E. I., II, Larson, C. P., Jr. and Severinghaus, J. W. (1962), "The Solubility of Halothane in Rubber, Soda Lime and Various Plastics," *Anesthesiology*, **23**, 356.

Eger, E. I., II (1963), "Applications of a Mathematical Model of Gas Uptake," Ch. 8 in *Uptake and Distribution of Anesthetic Agents*. Edited by Papper and Kitz. New York: McGraw-Hill.

Eger, E. I., II (1963), "A Mathematical Model of Uptake and Distribution," Ch. 7 in *Uptake and Distribution of Anesthetic Agents*. Edited by Papper and Kitz. New York: McGraw-Hill.

Eger, E. I., II (1963), "Effect of Inspired Anesthetic Concentration on the Rate of Rise of Alveolar Concentration," *Anesthesiology*, **24**, 153.

Eger, E. I., II and Brandstater, B. (1963), "Solubility of Methoxyflurane in Rubber," *Anesthesiology*, **24**, 679.

Eger, E. L., II and Larson, C. P., Jr. (1964), "Anaesthetic Solubility in Blood and Tissues: Values and Significance," *Brit. J. Anaesth.*, **36**, 140.

Eger, E. I., II and Saidman, L. J. (1964), "Anesthetic Uptake at a Constant Alveolar Concentration," Ch. 2 in *Clinical Anesthesia*. Vol. 3. Philadephia: F. A. Davis Co.

Eger, E. I., II and Saidman, L. J. (1965), "Hazards of Nitrous Oxide Anesthesia in Bowel Obstruction and Pneumothorax," *Anesthesiology*, **26**, 61.

Eger, E. I., II and Severinghaus, J. W. (1964), "Effect of Uneven Pulmonary Distribution of Blood and Gas on Induction with Inhalation Anesthetics," *Anesthesiology*, **25**, 620.

Epstein, R. M., Rackow, H., Salanitre, E. and Wolf, G. L. (1964), "Influence of the Concentration Effect on the Uptake of Anesthetic Mixtures: the Second Gas Effect," *Anesthesiology*, **25**, 364.

Fink, B. R. (1955), "Diffusion Anoxia," *Anesthesiology*, **16**, 511.

Gregory, G. A. and Eger, E. I., II (1968), "Partition Coefficients in Blood and Blood Fractions at Various Concentrations of Cyclopropane," *Fed. Proc.*, **27**, 705.

Hunter, A. R. (1955), "Problems of Anaesthesia in Artificial Pneumothorax," *Proc. Soc. Med.*, **48**, 765.

Mapleson, W. W. (1963), "Quantitative Prediction of Anesthetic Concentrations," Ch. 9 in *Uptake and Distribution of Anesthetic Agents*. Edited by Papper and Kitz. New York: McGraw-Hill.

Matz, G. J., Rattenborg, C. G. and Holaday, D. A. (1967), "Effects of Nitrous Oxide on Middle Ear Pressure," *Anesthesiology*, **28**, 948.

Munson, E. S. and Bowers, D. L. (1967), "Effects of Hyperventilation on the Rate of Cerebral Anesthetic Equilibration," *Anesthesiology*, **28**, 377.

Munson, E. S. and Merrick, H. C. (1966), "Effect of Nitrous Oxide on Venous Air Embolism," *Anesthesiology*, **27**, 783.

Munson, E. S., Eger, E. I., II and Bowers, D. L. (1968), "The Effects of Changes in Cardiac Output and Distribution on the Rate of Cerebral Anesthetic Equilibration. Calculations Using a Mathematical Model," *Anesthesiology*, **29**, 533.

Rackow, H., Salanitre, E. and Frumin, M. J. (1961), "Dilution of, Alveolar Gases During Nitrous Oxide Excretion in Man," *J. Appl. Physiol.*, **16**, 723.

Regan, M. J. and Eger, E. I., II (1967), "Effect of Hypothermia in Dogs on Anesthetizing and Apneic Doses of Inhalation Agents," *Anesthesiology*, **28**, 689.

Rittman, W. W. and Smith, L. L. (1966), "Cerebral Blood Flow Following Severe Hemorrhage," *Surg. Gynec. Obstet.*, **123**, 67.

Saidman, L. J. and Eger, E. I., II (1965), "Change in Cerebrospinal Fluid Pressure During Pneumoencephalography Under Nitrous Oxide Anesthesia," *Anesthesiology*, **26**, 67.

Saidman, L. J. and Eger, E. I., II (1967), "The Influence of Ventilation/Perfusion Abnormalities Upon the Uptake of Inhalation Anesthetics," *Clinical Anesthesia*, Vol. 1, Ch. 5, p. 79.

Severinghaus, J. W., "Role of Lung Factors," Ch. 6 in *Uptake and Distribution of Anesthetic Agents*, edited by Papper and Kitz, p. 59. New York: McGraw-Hill.

Stoelting, R. K. and Eger, E. L., II (1969), "Additional Explanation for the Second Gas Effect: A Concentrating Effect," *Anesthesiology*, **30**, 273.

Stoelting, R. K. and Eger, E. I., II (1969), "Influence of Ventilation and Solubility on Recovery from Anesthesia: An *in vivo* and Analog-Analysis Before and After Equilibrium," *Anesthesiology*, **30**, 290.

Waun, J. E., Sweitzer, R. S. and Hamilton, W. K. (1967), "Effect of Nitrous Oxide on Middle Ear Mechanics and Hearing Acuity," *Anesthesiology*, **28**, 846.

# CHAPTER 4

# UPTAKE, DISTRIBUTION, AND ELIMINATION OF THE MUSCLE RELAXANTS

## ELLIS N. COHEN

Pharmacologic response following administration of a drug depends upon the effective concentration which is reached at its site of action. The rate at which such a concentration is attained, and the time course over which it remains effective are influenced by many factors. In the intact organism the situation is dynamic and only rarely does the steady state obtain.

A number of considerations interrelate in the uptake and distribution of all foreign compounds. These include the route of administration, transport to the site of action, transfer across cell membranes, redistribution to various depots, protein binding, biotransformation, and elimination of the drug from the body (Fig. 1). A factor of major significance concerns the ability of the drug to penetrate cell membrane barriers. The determining factors here depend upon the physical–chemical characteristics of the molecule, including water solubility, lipid solubility, ionization constant, molecular size, spatial relationships, etc.

Although the individual muscle relaxants vary considerably in their mechanism of action, duration of response, side effects, etc., most relaxants have certain characteristics in common. These compounds are usually quaternary amines of large molecular weight, highly ionized, and possess high water, but only limited lipid solubility. Most do not undergo significant destruction in the body (exception succinylcholine; pancuronium), and are excreted unchanged in the urine or in the bile. It follows that the duration of action of the muscle relaxants depends primarily upon redistribution, and the further possibility of cumulative effects must be considered.

but only slightly soluble in olive oil (0·44 per cent) or in a typical organic solvent such as heptane (0·01 per cent). Its pK approaches 14, so that the drug must be considered highly ionized at all pH ranges.

In translating the above information to the *in vivo*

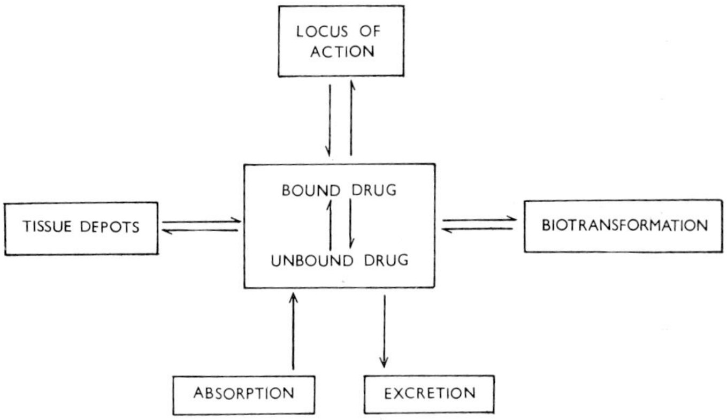

FIG. 1. Inter-relating factors affecting drug distribution. (Absorption and Distribution of Drugs, Binns, T. B., Williams and Wilkins Co., Baltimore, 1964, p. 17.)

situation, one would expect d-tubocurarine to distribute rapidly throughout the water compartments of the body and very slowly penetrate the lipid membrane barriers existing in the stomach, gut, placenta, brain, or renal tubules. By the same token, one would anticipate its efficient renal elimination. In essence, this is what occurs. d-Tubocurarine taken orally or rectally is without significant effect. This fact was well known to the Peruvian Indians

*d-Tubocurarine*

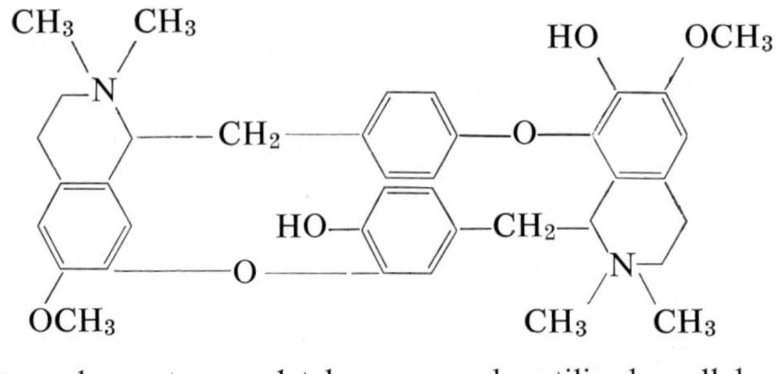

d-Tubocurarine is the oldest and most completely studied of the muscle relaxants. Although its history goes back well over 400 years, introduction of the drug into clinical anaesthesia took place scarcely 30 years ago. d-Tubocurarine is a naturally occurring alkaloid derived from the plant, Chondodendron Tomentosum. Chemically, it is an isoquinoline derivative, possessing two quaternary amines located 14Å units apart; the latter being characteristic of many, but not all muscle relaxants. It is water soluble to the extent of 5·0 gm./100 ml. (5·0 per cent),

who utilized small doses of the crude drug (Wourari) for its gastric action. On the other hand, the danger in handling crude concentrates of the drug in the presence of an open cut was well recognized. Both a blood-brain and a placental barrier to d-tubocurarine have been shown to exist, and the kidney provides the major route of elimination from the body.

Following the intravenous injection of a paralysing dose of d-tubocurarine (0·3 mg./kg.), one can study the dynamics of its vascular and extravascular distribution (Fig. 2).

During the first phase of distribution (half life of 7–10 minutes) there is a rapid redistribution of drug within the vascular and extravascular water compartments, and equilibrium develops between the amount of drug in solution and that bound to plasma protein. During the second phase (half life of 30–45 minutes) the drug disappears from the extracellular fluid due to urinary elimination and diffusion into the various tissue compartments. The final phase of vascular redistribution depends upon the slower processes of continued renal or biliary elimination.

The initial distribution of *d*-tubocurarine within the vascular system is confined to plasma, and the drug does not enter the red blood cells. Binding to various plasma

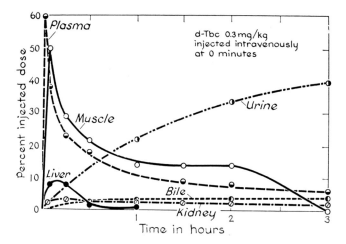

FIG. 2. Experimental data for the distribution of *d*-tubocurarine within six known compartments. (*Anesthesiology*, **27**, 64, 1966, Fig. 4.)

proteins takes place, and equilibrium dialysis indicates that approximately one-third of the drug is protein bound (Fig. 3). The unbound drug rapidly redistributes throughout the extravascular water compartment, and the process is essentially completed within 15 to 20 minutes. By the end of the first hour, the plasma contains slightly more than 10 per cent of the originally injected dose. During the later phases of vascular redistribution the plasma concentration slowly decays, and by the sixth hour only traces of *d*-tubocurarine are to be found.

The concentration of *d*-tubocurarine within the muscle compartment closely parallels that present in the plasma, although the proportionate amount of drug in the muscle tissue is considerably less. Muscle mass represents 40–45 per cent of body weight of which only 10–15 per cent is extracellular fluid. Equilibration of the *d*-tubocurarine between the plasma and muscle compartments takes place within these extracellular spaces. A localized concentration of *d*-tubocurarine is present at the muscle receptor areas. Autoradiographic studies indicate that high concentrations of *d*-tubocurarine are localized at the synaptic clefts of the motor endplate. There is also anatomical and physiological evidence for a high concentration present at the motor nerve terminal. The rapid muscle paralysis which follows

the intravenous injection of *d*-tubocurarine relates to this localized concentration of drug in the motor endplate area. This in turn may be the result of specific tissue affinities at the receptor site, plus the unusually close spatial relationship existing between capillaries and the muscle endplate.

The renal elimination of *d*-tubocurarine is evidenced by the localization of drug in the kidney parenchyma (4–6 times the plasma concentration), and by the rapid accumulation of drug in the urine. By the end of the third hour, 35 per cent of the injected dose is present in the urine. Within 24 hours, 75 per cent of the drug can be recovered in an unchanged state. Studies of renal plasma clearance in the dog indicate the mean plasma clearance is 2·74 ml./min./kg. which is comparable to that of urea. The renal elimination of *d*-tubocurarine may thus be accounted

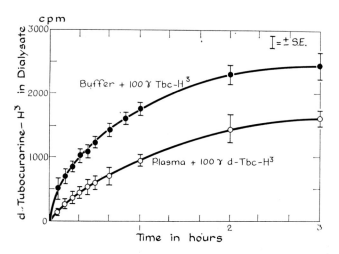

FIG. 3. Protein binding of *d*-tubocurarine-H³. (*Anesthesiology*, **28**, 309, 1967, Fig. 2.)

for in terms of glomerular filtration without evoking the additional mechanism of tubular secretion. The absence of tubular reabsorption of *d*-tubocurarine, which is the result of its lipid insolubility and high ionization, ensures rapid elimination of the drug.

The significant role of the kidney in the elimination of *d*-tubocurarine is emphasized in the patient with altered renal function. Loss of fluids or a reduction in intake leading to moderate dehydration is sufficient to prolong the time course for the renal elimination of *d*-tubocurarine and results in a sustained plasma level of drug. The importance of severe alteration in renal function may be evaluated by experiments in the nephrectomized animal. If we compare the normal versus the nephrectomized animal, it may be seen that bilateral nephrectomy produces little change in the initial plasma *d*-tubocurarine levels (first 20 minutes) since these are primarily related to factors of redistribution (Fig. 4). Subsequently, in the absence of renal function, we find sustained plasma levels of the drug. However, despite the total lack of renal function, plasma levels continue to fall slowly. By 3 hours, the plasma level of *d*-tubocurarine in these nephrectomized animals is actually below paralysing concentration. As noted later, this decline reflects the availability of an alternative (hepatic) route of elimination.

The liver possesses a rapid circulation and *d*-tubocurarine attains its peak concentration within 5 minutes of intravenous injection. This peak concentration, however, rapidly drops and approaches trace levels by one hour. Biliary elimination of the *d*-tubocurarine proceeds at a steady rate, dependent upon plasma drug concentration. Under normal circumstances the biliary route accounts for elimination of 10–20 per cent of the *d*-tubocurarine within 24 hours. Since plasma levels are primarily dependent upon renal elimination of the drug, we find higher plasma levels in the nephrectomized animal (*see above*). Under these

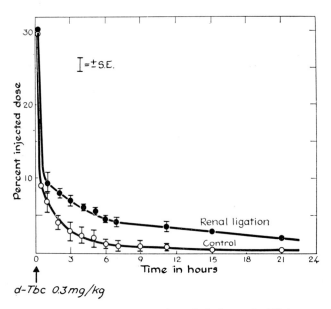

Fig. 4. Plasma concentration of *d*-tubocurarine-H³ in control dogs and in those with bilateral renal ligation. (*Anesthesiology*, **28**, 309, 1967, Fig. 4.)

circumstances, biliary elimination increases, and in animal experiments a fourfold increase occurs with over 40 per cent of the drug eliminated via the bile in a 24 hour period. This increased biliary elimination of *d*-tubocurarine accounts for the fall in plasma levels observed in the nephrectomized animal. In a similar fashion, following administration of very large doses of *d*-tubocurarine (1 mg./kg.), the liver increases its normal rate of elimination and also acts as a drug reservoir until further elimination is effected via the kidneys. Since the ratio of d-tubocurarine in bile to that in plasma exceeds 40 to 1, an active transport system presumably is involved. It has been shown that this transport system for *d*-tubocurarine may be saturated by high concentrations of this drug or other quaternary ammonium compounds. As with the urine, *d*-tubocurarine is recovered from the bile largely in an unchanged state, indicating that metabolism does not play a significant role in the elimination of this drug.

As discussed earlier, the *d*-tubocurarine molecule is highly ionized and lipid insoluble. These characteristics create a barrier to its transfer across membranes possessing

lipid properties. The importance of this lipid barrier in preventing the tubular reabsorption of *d*-tubocurarine in the kidney has already been mentioned. In addition, it has been shown that both a blood-brain and a placental barrier exist to *d*-tubocurarine. The former barrier is very efficient, excluding *d*-tubocurarine from the cerebrospinal fluid following its intravenous injection. The latter barrier, while effective in the physiological dose range, becomes relatively less efficient when massive doses of *d*-tubocurarine are administered, and under these extreme circumstances some drug may thus reach the foetus.

The use of the analog computer to develop model systems which can simulate drug distribution is an established procedure. Not only does this approach serve to provide insight into the processes involved, but under

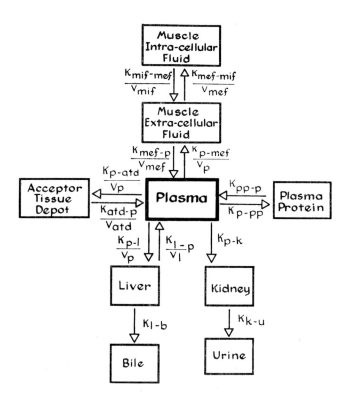

Fig. 5. A nine compartment representation for the distribution of *d*-tubocurarine. Initially *d*-tubocurarine is present in the plasma compartment and arrows indicate further transport between compartments. (*Anesthesiology*, **27**, 64, 1966, Fig. 1.)

certain circumstances it may be used to postulate distributions in experimentally inaccessible compartments. The value of such a tool is seen in Figures 5 and 6 where nine compartments have been utilized to develop simulated distribution curves for *d*-tubocurarine. A close similarity is seen between these curves and those illustrated in Figure 2 which were developed from direct animal experimental data. It is to be noted that an additional depot is required for the model system shown in Figure 6 in order to coincide with the experimental curves in Figure 2. This depot is needed to temporarily hold or indiscriminately bind the *d*-tubocurarine. Such a possibility has been suggested by Cavallito and termed an "acceptor tissue depot". This depot represents an area in which the drug

## DISTRIBUTION OF *D*-TUBOCURARINE

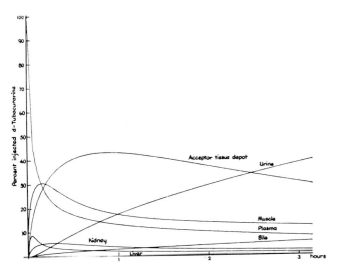

FIG. 6. Simulated distribution of *d*-tubocurarine as recorded on a X-Y plotter. (*Anesthesiology*, 27, 64, 1966, Fig. 3.)

is held and from which it exerts no local pharmacologic response. Recent whole body autoradiographic studies in the rat validate the presence of such a depot. In these studies, it was shown that organs such as the spleen and lungs temporarily filter drug out of the blood stream and retain it. Finally, these same autoradiographic studies indicate that the heart muscle has a special affinity for *d*-tubocurarine, and that concentrations are in excess of those in circulating blood. Concentrations in the heart are

5–8 fold greater than those of muscle tissue elsewhere in the body. The importance of this observation is yet to be evaluated, although very high concentrations of *d*-tubocurarine ($2 \times 10^{-4}$ M) have been shown to exert negative inotropic effects.

*Dimethyl d-tubocurarine*

Dimethyl *d*-tubocurarine is prepared by the methylation of *d*-tubocurarine. The resultant compound is interesting in that replacement of the phenolic hydroxyls by the less reactive methyl groups leads to a pronounced increase in potency. The drug is soluble in water to the extent of 0·3 gm./100 ml. (0·8 per cent), but practically insoluble in organic solvents such as ether, benzene, or chloroform. In most respects dimethyl *d*-tubocurarine behaves in a similar fashion to its parent compound.

Following the intravenous injection of dimethyl *d*-tubocurarine in the cat, there is a rapid decrease in plasma concentration related to transfer of the drug into the interstitial fluid compartment. By 30 minutes, only 10 per cent of the drug remains in the plasma. (Similar to *d*-tubocurarine, the dimethyl ether is initially confined to the plasma and does not enter the red blood cells.) The drug then slowly disappears from the plasma compartment related to its urinary elimination. By 7 hours, 80 per cent of the drug is recovered in the urine in its unchanged state, and by 15 hours, the plasma level represents only 0·8 per cent of the originally injected dose.

In the experimental animal, bilateral renal ligation produces sustained plasma levels of dimethyl *d*-tubocurarine as compared to the control. Unlike *d*-tubocurarine, elevated plasma levels persist for at least 5 hours. No information is available as to its biliary elimination, but this route must be considered unlikely in view of the sustained plasma levels. Experimental evidence has also been presented for a blood-brain barrier to dimethyl *d*-tubocurarine. This becomes less efficient under severe stress conditions such as hypotension, hypothermia, or hypoxia.

The plasma protein binding of dimethyl *d*-tubocurarine has been studied in an ultrafiltrate of human plasma, and 70 per cent of the labelled drug was shown to be bound to plasma protein after 48 hours.

*Gallamine*

$$O—CH_2—H_2—N—(C_2H_5)_3$$
$$(C_2H_5)_3—N—CH_2—CH_2—O—\underset{}{\bigcirc}—O—CH_2—CH_2—N—(C_2H_5)_3$$

Gallamine is a synthetic ether of pyrogallol and differs from most muscle relaxants in that it contains three quarternary ammonium groups. Two of these onium groups are 14 Å units apart, satisfying the thesis for optimum activity. There is evidence that the third onium group contributes less to the potency of the compound. Gallamine is highly soluble in water (166 gm./100 ml.), and comparatively insoluble in ether, benzene, or chloroform. On the other hand, its solubility in olive oil on a mg. basis is 10·9 per cent.

Following the intravenous injection of a paralysing dose of gallamine (2·0 mg./kg.) in the dog, the blood concentration drops rapidly. Within 5 minutes, only 25 per cent of the drug remains in the circulation, by 30 minutes the blood contains 12·2 per cent of the injected dose, and at the end of the first hour 7·4 per cent of the drug is present. Six hours after intravenous injection, only 1·6 per cent of the

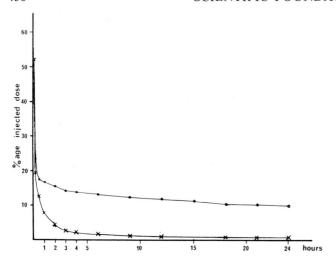

FIG. 7. Effect of bilateral renal ligation on the distribution of gallamine in the blood—(X are control animals and dots represent no renal blood flow). (*Anesthesiology*, **30**, 593, 1969, Fig. 3.)

Whole body autoradiography studies in the rat validate these observations and also indicate an increased accumulation of drug in the foetus with time. These same studies, however, suggest that the blood-brain barrier remains intact. These studies also indicate that substantial amounts of gallamine are present in the lung, liver, spleen, and kidneys.

In the intact animal a high proportion (81 per cent) of the injected gallamine leaves the blood within the first ten minutes. Although further equilibration between blood and tissues continues, urinary elimination quickly becomes the principal means for lowering the blood level and terminating its clinical action. This is attested by the difference in rates of reduction of blood gallamine levels in dogs with intact kidneys and those with ligated renal pedicles. As stated earlier, the difference in response to *d*-tubocurarine versus gallamine reflects the alternative biliary route of elimination available to the former, but denied the latter. One must, of course, keep in mind the importance of the size of the initially administered dose in relation to the dynamics of distribution. With larger doses, efficient function of the kidneys is more important than with smaller doses where the effects may rapidly be terminated by redistribution alone.

original material remains in the blood. Unlike *d*-tubocurarine, gallamine appears to equilibrate between red blood cells and the plasma. In man approximately 42 per cent of the drug is present in red blood cell fraction at 3 hours.

Decamethonium possesses the simplest structure of the commonly used neuro-muscular blocking agents, and was designed as a compound providing 14 Å distance between

## Decamethonium

$$(CH_3)_3—N—CH_2—CH_2—CH_2—CH_2—CH_2—CH_2—CH_2—CH_2—CH_2—CH_2—N—(CH_3)_3$$

The urinary elimination of gallamine proceeds rapidly with 65 per cent of the drug present in the urine at the end of the third hour. 84 per cent of the injected drug is recovered in the urine within 24 hours and is unchanged from the original molecule. The biliary elimination of gallamine is of minor significance with only 3·5 per cent of the drug excreted via this channel.

The effect of bilateral renal ligation on the blood levels of gallamine is most dramatic (Fig. 7). Although there is little change in the initial rapid decrease in gallamine concentration (first 10–15 minutes), high sustained blood levels of drug soon result. By 30 minutes, 17·5 per cent of the injected drug is still circulating, and from this point on there is a slow decline in blood concentration with 9·8 per cent of the injected dose still present at 24 hours. This 24 hour blood level in the renally ligated dogs corresponds to that present between 30 and 60 minutes in animals with intact renal function. Unlike *d*-tubocurarine, there does not appear to be an alternative biliary route to handle the increased drug concentrations, and biliary elimination in these dogs does not vary from the control. The importance of these observations is to contra-indicate the use of gallamine in the renally damaged or nephrectomized patient.

Clinically, it has been observed that the placental barrier to gallamine is incomplete, and that foetal depression may follow intravenous injection of the drug to the mother.

two quaternary ammonium groups separated by the interposition of 10 carbon atoms. Under these conditions, maximal myoneural blocking action is present. Decamethonium is highly soluble in water to the extent of 10 gm./100 ml. (10 per cent), although it is very slightly soluble in chloroform and insoluble in ether. Decamethonium is only 0·06 per cent soluble in olive oil and 0·01 per cent soluble in heptane. Thus it possesses the least lipid solubility characteristics of the commonly used muscle relaxants.

Following its intravenous injection in the cat, decamethonium rapidly leaves the blood stream, and within 10 minutes only 28 per cent of the drug remains in the circulating blood. By 20 minutes, the blood contains 18 per cent of the injected dose, and at the end of the first hour only 8 per cent. Although the drug is mainly confined to the plasma, about 3–10 per cent of the decamethonium may be found in the red cell fraction.

The urinary excretion of decamethonium in the cat indicates that 50 per cent of the drug is present in the urine within the first hour, and in man up to 90 per cent can be recovered in 24 hours. There is little evidence for the metabolism of decamethonium (less than 1 per cent), and the drug appears in the urine in its unchanged state. The liver plays only a minor role in the elimination of the drug, and biliary concentrations are less than that in blood.

Whole body autoradiographic studies in the rat support other studies indicating a blood-brain barrier and a placental barrier for decamethonium. The placental barrier is more efficient for decamethonium than for any of the other muscle relaxants. Autoradiographic studies also demonstrate that the lung and spleen extract decamethonium from the blood stream in a similar fashion to that which occurs with *d*-tubocurarine. The concentration of drug in heart muscle, however, does not reach the high levels attained with the latter drug.

This drug may be considered as composed of two molecules of acetylcholine. It contains 2 quarternary nitrogen

the injected drug is present in the urine. It is of interest to note that the hydrolysis of succinylcholine occurs only when the drug is present in the serum.

In view of its rapid hydrolysis, it is very difficult to obtain precise information on the uptake and fate of this drug. Studies with radioactively labelled materials injected in cats indicate that only 20 per cent of the total radioactivity remains in the plasma at 5 minutes. By the second hour this concentration has been reduced to 1·5 per cent (Fig. 8). Conversely, the cumulative urinary elimination of radioactivity (largely succinylmonocholine) accounts for approximately 50 per cent of the injected dose within the first hour.

*Succinylcholine*

$$(CH_3)_3\!-\!N\!-\!CH_2\!-\!CH_2\!-\!O\!-\!\overset{\overset{\textstyle O}{\|}}{C}\!-\!CH_2\!-\!CH_2\!-\!\overset{\overset{\textstyle O}{\|}}{C}\!-\!O\!-\!CH_2\!-\!CH_2\!-\!N\!-\!(CH_3)_3$$

atoms spaced 15 Å units apart. It differs in a significant fashion from the other muscle relaxants in its susceptibility to hydrolysis. The two ester groups are readily split by warm alkali or enzymatically by pseudocholinesterase.

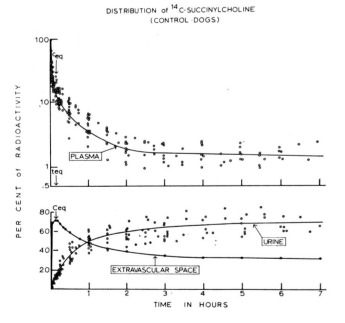

DISTRIBUTION of $^{14}$C-SUCCINYLCHOLINE
(CONTROL DOGS)

FIG. 8. Disappearance from plasma, cumulative urinary elimination and passage into the extra-vascular space of radiocarbon ($^{14}$C) following intravenous administration of a trace dose of $^{14}$C-succinyldicholine to control dogs. (*Anesthesiology*, **29**, 435, 1968, Fig. 1.)

By 7 hours, 70 per cent of the injected radioactivity has been recovered in the urine, with 1·4 per cent still present in the plasma, and leaving 28·6 per cent untraced.

The first stage hydrolysis of succinylcholine is very rapid, and the average adult has sufficient enzyme to convert 80 mg. of succinylcholine per minute. Unlike enzymatic destruction, alkaline hydrolysis of succinylcholine is a first order reaction with the amount of hydrolysis proportional to drug concentration. Under usual circumstances, less than 5 per cent of the succinylcholine is destroyed by this route. It follows that most of the injected succinylcholine is metabolized within the first minute. On the other hand, that drug which leaves the plasma intact and enters the region of the endplate is no longer exposed to enzymatic activity. It is the further diffusion of these unaltered molecules away from the endplate region into the interstitial fluid that actually terminates the action of the drug.

Lack of entry of radioactivity into the cerebrospinal fluid indicates the presence of a blood-brain barrier. The placental barrier is far less efficient, and clinical experiments show that with high doses of drug administered to the mother it succeeds in penetrating the foetal circulation.

Subsequent to its administration, a fraction of the succinylcholine is bound to plasma protein. The degree of binding is not entirely clear. *In vivo* studies in cats suggest that binding is negligible for the first 45 minutes, although equilibrium dialysis studies indicate that 30 per cent of the radioactivity is bound to plasma protein. It was further shown in these studies that gamma globulin was more effective than serum albumin in binding succinylcholine.

*Pancuronium*

Succinylcholine is highly water soluble (100 gm./100 ml.), but only sparingly soluble in benzene or chloroform.

The enzymatic hydrolysis of succinylcholine takes place in two steps, the first step leading to the formation of succinylmonocholine and choline. In the second stage, succinylmonocholine is further broken down to choline and succinic acid. Normally, pseudocholinesterase activity in man is rapid and efficient so that less than 2 per cent of

This bis-quaternary ammonium steroid demonstrates strong neuromuscular blocking effects in animal and man, but is essentially devoid of steroid activity. It is approximately five times as potent as *d*-tubocurarine, and exhibits a similar time of onset and duration of action. It is freely soluble in water, poorly fat soluble, and the aqueous buffer to octanol coefficient has been determined as less than 99 to 1. No precise protein binding data are available, although it has been suggested on the basis of structural and clinical experiments that the binding of pancuronium to plasma proteins does not occur.

Following its intravenous administration in the dog, rat, cat, and mouse, there is rapid disappearance of radioactivity from the plasma. In the cat the plasma half life is 4 minutes, while in the mouse only 6·1 per cent of the radioactivity remains at this time. Disappearance from the plasma can be shown to occur in two phases; the first phase related to a rapid distribution to the interstitial fluid, and the second phase (half life 32 minutes in the cat) combining the effects of excretion, metabolism and movement to other compartments.

Following an intravenous injection of 0·8 mg./kg. in the cat, 30 per cent of the injected dose is eliminated in the urine within 8 hours, and an additional 24 per cent is excreted in the bile. Although most of the drug eliminated by these routes is in unaltered form, some 30 per cent is present as hydroxylated derivatives. Large amounts of the injected drug and its metabolites are retained in the liver (24 per cent at 8 hours). In the mouse, trace concentrations persist at 28 days.

Placental transfer of pancuronium does occur in the human (defined in terms of urinary excretion of pancuronium by the neonate), but the amount of drug reaching the foetus is apparently small and not of clinical importance. Studies in several animals species substantiate this observation. Little or no drug appears to enter the central nervous system.

## Summary

The muscle relaxants possess certain physical and chemical characteristics in common, which determine their myoneural blocking action and influence their uptake and distribution in the body. As highly ionized, water soluble, lipid insoluble compounds, their distribution is essentially limited to the extracellular water compartments. Renal elimination, on the other hand, is enhanced by a lack of tubular reabsorption. With the exception of succinylcholine, metabolism of the muscle relaxants does not play a significant role in their immediate distribution or elimination.

## FURTHER READING

Agoston, S., Kersten, U. W. and Meijer, D. K. F. (1973), "The Fate of Pancuronium Bromide in the Cat," *Acta Anaesth. Scand.*, **17**, 129.

Cohen, E. N., Brewer, H. W. and Smith, D. (1967), "The Metabolism and Elimination of *d*-tubocurarine-H³," *Anesthesiology*, **28**, 309.

Cohen, E. N., Corbascio, A. and Fleischli, G. (1965), "The Distribution and Fate of *d*-tubocurarine," *Jour. Pharm. and Exper. Therap.*, **147**, 120.

Cohen, E. N., Hood, N. and Golling, R. (1969), "Uptake and Distribution of Labelled Muscle Relaxants in the Rat Using Whole Body Autoradiography," *Anesthesiology*, **29**, 987.

Dal Santo, G. (1964), "Kinetics of Distribution of Radioactive Labelled Muscle Relaxants. I. Investigations with ¹⁴C Dimethy-*d*-tubocurarine," *Anesthesiology*, **25**, 788.

Dal Santo, G. (1968), "Kinetics of Distribution of Radioactive Labelled Muscle Relaxants. III. Investigations with ¹⁴C Succinyldicholine and ¹⁴C Succinylmonocholine During Controlled Conditions," *Anesthesiology*, **29**, 435.

Eckenhoff, J. E., Editor (1959), "A Symposium on Muscle Relaxants," *Anesthesiology*, **20**, 407.

Feldman, S. A., Cohen, E. N. and Golling, R. (1969), "The Excretion of Gallamine in the Dog," *Anesthesiology*, **30**, 593.

Fleischli, G. and Cohen, E. N. (1966), "An Analog Computer Simulation for the Distribution of *d*-tubocurarine," *Anesthesiology*, **27**, 64.

Luthi, U. and Waser, P. G. (1965), "Vertilung and Metabolismus von ¹⁴C—Decamethonium in Katzen," *Arch. Int. Pharmacodyn.*, **156**, 319.

Papper, E. M. and Kitz, R. J. (1963), "Uptake and Distribution of Anesthetic Agents." New York: McGraw-Hill Co.

*CHAPTER 5*

# METABOLISM OF VOLATILE ANAESTHETIC AGENTS

MALCOLM F. TYRRELL

Until recently it was generally accepted that, with the exception of trichlorethylene, all volatile anaesthetic agents were excreted unchanged via the lungs. This statement is no longer tenable today; over the last few years it has been shown that most, if not all, inhalational agents undergo biotransformation within the body. When one looks at the molecular structure of these agents it is perhaps surprising that their inert behaviour in the body was accepted for so long. Many have a plentiful supply of ether and vinyl

linkages and halogen radicles; all eminently vulnerable to the action of the enzyme systems. There are probably three reasons why the immutability of volatile anaesthetics was accepted for so long.

Firstly, it is all too easy to accept a dogmatic statement uncritically. It has been suggested, probably correctly, that much of the most fruitful research comes from a close examination of such statements! Secondly, most theories of anaesthesia are based upon physical properties and do

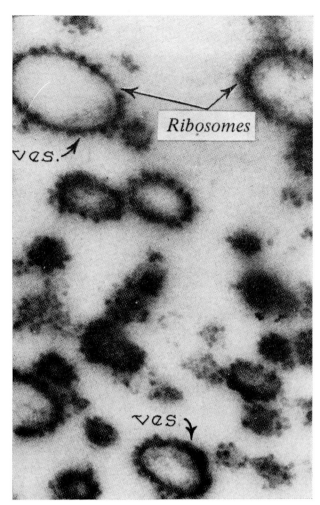

Fig. 1

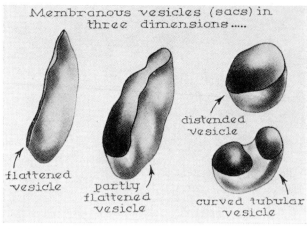

Fig. 2

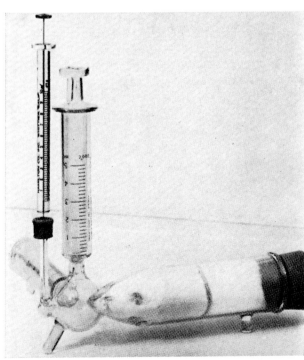

Fig. 3

Fig. 1. Electron micrograph ($\times$ 80,000) of microsome fragment of homogenized cells of the pancreas. The microsome fraction consists of vesicles and tubules which have granular surfaces (due to ribosomes) or agranular surfaces. The agranular fraction is thought to be concerned with drug metabolism. (From *Histology* by Ham (1969), 6th Edn. J. B. Lippincott Co., Philadelphia, modified from Palade, G. E. and Siekevitz, P. (1956), *J. Biophys. Biochem. Cytol.*, **2**, 271.)

Fig. 2. Diagrammatic illustration of the various forms assumed by cytoplasmic membranous vesicles. The cut surface of each vesicle shows how it would appear in a section. (From *Histology* by Ham (1969), 6th Edn. J. B. Lippincott Co., Philadelphia.)

Fig. 3. Apparatus for the administration of volatile anaesthetics to the mouse. Liquid anaesthetic is introduced into chamber from micro-syringe. (Cohen, E. N. and Hood, N. (1969a), *Anesthesiology*, **30**, 306.)

not depend upon the chemical reactivity of the agent. This has tended to direct attention away from a possible intracellular role for the volatile agents. Finally, the real advances in this field have followed the application of sophisticated isotope technology, which has only been available during the last decade. Such is the extent of interest in the metabolism of volatile anaesthetics that in America a commercial isotope organization is able to provide $^{14}$C-labelled samples of most volatile agents as stock items.

## SITE OF METABOLISM

Within the cell there is a network of strands and vesicles throughout the cell sap, namely the endoplasmic reticulum. This fraction of the cell contents may be separated by use of the ultracentrifuge. One constituent of the endoplasmic reticulum is the microsome fragment, which consists of a series of vesicles of varying shapes and sizes, but considerably smaller than the mitochondria (Figs. 1 and 2). Most drug metabolism, including that of the volatile anaesthetics, is brought about by enzymes found in the microsome fragment. The most important organ in this metabolism is the liver, but of course such microsomal enzyme systems exist elsewhere, notably in the brain and kidneys.

Parenthetically, another constituent of the endoplasmic reticulum is the microtubular system. This system forms the supporting framework of the cell and is clearly demarcated in many plant cells and some mammalian cells including neurones. Allison and Nunn (1968) have demonstrated that clinical concentrations of some anaesthetic agents produce depolymerization and dispersal of labile microtubules in certain organisms, consistent with an interaction between the anaesthetic and microtubule protein.

The enzymes of the microsome fragment do not appear to be substrate specific, but may be categorized in terms of the chemical transformation produced; they may produce ether cleavage or dehalogenation, for example. These enzyme systems may be stimulated or inhibited by exposure to drugs—this causes 'enzyme induction' or 'inhibition'.

### Enzyme Stimulation (Induction)

It has been demonstrated that repeated administration of a drug often produces an altered response to subsequent exposure to that drug and to other drugs. This has been shown to occur both in animals and man. It has been found that pre-treatment of an animal with such drugs as phenobarbital or methylcholanthrene, both enzyme inducers, leads to a subsequent increase in the metabolism of volatile anaesthetics (Van Dyke, 1966). It has also been shown that the volatile agents may influence the biotransformation of other drugs.

Particular interest to anaesthetists is the finding that anaesthetists metabolize halothane more efficiently than non-anaesthetists (Cascorbi et al., 1970). This provides some evidence, albeit circumstantial, that chronic exposure to sub-anaesthetic concentrations of anaesthetic agents produces enzyme induction and an increase in its metabolism. Several studies have confirmed that trace amounts of anaesthetic gases are present in the operating theatre during and after their administration (Linde and Bruce 1969, Whitcher et al., 1971). Also measurable quantities of anaesthetics have been found both in the expired gas and blood of operating theatre personnel (Hallen et al., 1970). Unfortunately the consequences of the possible increase in metabolism in these circumstances is not yet known and therefore the importance of these observations cannot be assessed. However, it is known that some of the metabolites of the volatile agents may be toxic to such organs as the liver and kidney (q.v.). It has also been alleged that sensitization of individuals to these agents may occur. Other reports suggest that the volatile agents may have a teratogenic effect; there is evidence that they increase the spontaneous abortion rate in pregnant nurses and doctors exposed to such trace concentrations (Cohen et al., 1970). Until there is some clarification of the role played by metabolites in these reported toxic effects, it would seem reasonable to ensure that the working environment of medical personnel in operating theatres contains as low a concentration of anaesthetic as possible, if necessary by the use of scavenging or diversion techniques.

### Enzyme Inhibition

Enzyme inhibition may occur following the pre-treatment of an animal with anti-metabolites, such as disulphuram. In rats this prevents the hepatotoxicity of chloroform. More interestingly, it has been shown by Sawyer and his co-workers and others, that the metabolism of volatile agents is influenced by the inhaled concentration (Sawyer et al., 1971). High concentrations inhibit metabolism while trace amounts are actively and extensively metabolized, this suggests that enzyme saturation has occurred, as high concentrations of anaesthetics also inhibit metabolism of other drugs in a dose dependent fashion.

## EXPERIMENTAL METHODS

This area of research has expanded with the availability of isotope techniques, which allows sufficient sensitivity for the study of biotransformation. It also follows that all isotopes used in such work must be of high purity; any impurities would lead eventually to false positive results. Gas radiochromatography is usually used to establish the radioactive and chemical purity of labelled samples prior to their use (Trudell et al., 1972).

In reviewing experimental work done in this field, two facts must be borne in mind. Firstly, the majority of research has been performed in animals and the results obtained are not necessarily applicable to man, however, information in humans is now accumulating. Secondly, the isotopes are often administered by highly unusual routes, for instance the volatile agents have been administered intraperitoneally to animals and intravenously to animals and man. Although the results of such experiments are of value in the context of the individual trial, they are not qualitatively comparable to the inhalation of the agent under clinical conditions.

One of the most useful techniques developed in the study of the volatile agents is that of low-temperature, whole-body autoradiography. Cohen and Hood modified the technique introduced by Ullberg (1958) to study the volatile agents including chloroform, diethyl ether and halothane (Cohen and Hood, 1969a, b and c). Mice were allowed to inhale the labelled anaesthetic for 10 minutes (Fig. 3), and then sacrificed at 0, 15 and 120 minutes after being returned to room air. The animals were immediately frozen in liquid nitrogen, mounted in carboxymethylcellulose, refrozen and hemisectioned. The hemisections were mounted against a photographic emulsion and exposed for periods up to 10 days under solid $CO_2$ or liquid nitrogen, in view of the volatility of the agents. The radioisotopes emit $\beta$-radiation which reduces the silver halide of the emulsion, in much the same way as light, so leaving an exact record of the distribution and intensity of radioactivity (Fig. 4). Further, thin sections of the original hemisections were cut, allowed to warm and were re-exposed. In this way the distribution of non-volatile metabolites was identified (Fig. 5). Finally, each organ was biopsied and the amount of radioactivity present quantified using a scintillation counter. Thus, this technique has allowed detection and distribution of the volatile agents and volatile and non-volatile metabolites in all organs of the body at varying time intervals after administration.

In other studies mentioned in this chapter, detection and quantification of radioactive metabolites rely on such techniques as gas-liquid, thin layer and column chromatography and radioactive counting techniques, the most useful being scintillation counting.

## METABOLISM OF INDIVIDUAL AGENTS

The second half of this chapter is devoted to a review of the current knowledge of the metabolism of the individual anaesthetic agents. Although the chapter heading limits the subject to a discussion of the volatile agents, for completeness the section is extended to include anaesthetic gases and inorganic anaesthetics.

## HYDROCARBONS

*Ethylene* ($H_2C{=}CH_2$). This simple compound may be produced by liver mitochondria under normal conditions. $^{14}C$-labelled ethylene administered to rats is converted to $^{14}CO_2$ and non-volatile urinary metabolites (Van Dyke and Chenoweth, 1965a). Using low temperature, whole-body autoradiography high concentrations of non-volatile metabolites have been found in the liver (Cohen, 1971).

*Cyclopropane* ($C_3H_6$). Work by Van Dyke and Chenoweth (1965a) suggest that in rats $^{14}C$-cyclopropane is converted to $^{14}CO_2$.

## HALOGENATED HYDROCARBONS

*Chloroform* ($CHCl_3$). It has been shown that chloroform undergoes biodegradation to $^{14}CO_2$ and $^{36}Cl$-labelled non-volatile urinary metabolites (Van Dyke *et al.*, 1964). Using low-temperature autoradiography in mice it has been shown that 4 per cent of administered radioactivity is present in the liver as non-volatile metabolites two hours after administration (Cohen and Hood, 1969a). The identity

of these metabolites has not yet been established. Chloroform has a high fat/blood solubility coefficient and is retained in fat depots for extended periods; this probably accounts for the continued steady production of $^{14}CO_2$ for some twelve hours after its administration (Van Dyke *et al.*, 1964).

It has been mentioned that anti-metabolites reduce the hepatotoxicity of chloroform, suggesting that metabolites of chloroform may be responsible for hepatic damage. Not surprisingly, enzyme induces increase the incidence of hepatotoxic effects (Scholler, 1970).

*Trichloroethylene* ($CCl_2{=}CHCl$). The metabolism of trichloroethylene was established as early as 1933 (Bruning and Schretka, 1933). Following administration of $^{36}Cl$-trichloroethylene some 20 per cent is metabolized, 10 per cent to trichloroacetic acid and 10 per cent to trichloroethanol. Both metabolites have been identified in the urine, excretion being very slow and reaching a maximum some two days after administration.

*Halothane* ($CF_3CHClBr$). Halothane has been the most extensively studied volatile agent from the point of view of biotransformation. Early work by Duncan and Raventos (1959) failed to demonstrate any appreciable metabolism of halothane; however, with the introduction of sophisticated isotope methods it has been shown that up to 20 per cent of an inhaled dose of halothane may be accounted for in terms of non-volatile urinary metabolites (Rehder *et al.*, 1967) and many trials attest to the biodegradation of the agent (Van Dyke *et al.*, 1964; Stier, 1964, 1967; Rehder *et al.*, 1967).

The biotransformation of halothane is probably extremely complex and certainly shows considerable variation from species to species. However, several general comments can be made. The $CF_3$ bonding is disrupted only with difficulty and consequently very little $CO_2$ is produced and the fluorine appearing in the urine is organically bound, only trace quantities (less than 0·5 per cent) being present as inorganic or free fluorine. This is in marked contrast to methoxyflurane. The chloride and bromide bonds are readily broken by microsomal enzymes. The main urinary metabolites of halothane are probably bromide ion (Rehder *et al.*, 1967) and trifluoroacetic acid (Stien, 1964, 1967).

Employing low-temperature whole-body autoradiography Cohen and Hood (1969c) have demonstrated an accumulation of non-volatile metabolites in the liver of mice following the administration of $^{14}C$-halothane (Fig. 5.) The metabolites, which are detectable up to twelve days after exposure, are fluorine containing and retain the $CF_3$ configuration.

In animals enzyme induction occurs following pretreatment with enzyme inducers such as phenobarbital or by the repeated administration of halothane itself, leading to increased metabolism of halothane. A 423 per cent increase in liver non-volatile metabolites occurred in mice given five weekly intravenous administrations of $^{14}C$-halothane (Cohen and Hood, 1969c). The fact that a group of anaesthetists metabolized halothane more efficiently than non-anaesthetists has received previous comment.

It has proved extremely difficult to identify the non-volatile metabolites occurring in the liver and urine.

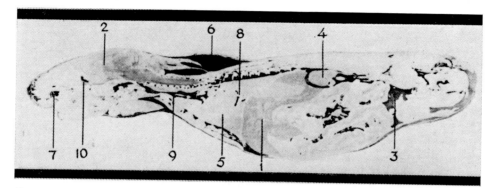

FIG. 4. Autoradiograph prepared from hemisection of mouse sacrificed immediately following inhalation of C¹⁴-halothane. 1, liver; 2, brain; 3, fat; 4, kidney; 5, heart; 6, brown fat; 7, nasal mucous membrane; 8, lung; 9, blood; 10, Hardner's gland. (Cohen, E. N. and Hood, N. (1969c), *Anesthesiology*, **31**, 553.)

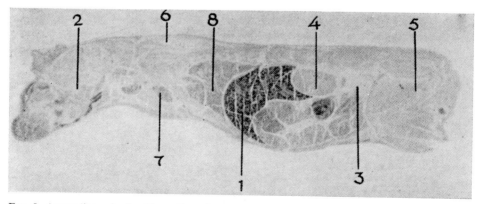

FIG. 5. Autoradiograph of a 40μ-section of mouse sacrificed 120 minutes following inhalation of C¹⁴-halothane. Section dried for 48 hours at −15°C then heated to 80°C for 4 hours. 1, liver; 2, brain; 3, fat; 4, kidney; 5, muscle; 6, brown fat; 7, blood; 8, lung. (Cohen, E. N. and Hood, N. (1969c), *Anesthesiology*, **31**, 553.)

$$CF_3CHBrCl \xrightarrow[O_2]{TPNH} [CF_3CHOHCl] \rightarrow [CF_3CHO] \xrightarrow{?} CF_3COOH \rightarrow CO_2$$

(Diagram: $CF_3CH_2OH$ Glucuroride above $CF_3CHO$ and $CF_3COOH$ with $?$ marks)

$$\begin{bmatrix} & O \\ & \| \\ CF_3-C\cdot \end{bmatrix}$$

$$CF_3COO^-$$

$$CF_3-CO-NH-CH_2-CH_2-OH$$

Proteins
Polypeptides
Amino acids
Lipids

Suggested Metabolism of Halothane
(from Cohen, E. N. (1971), *Anesthesiology*, **35**, 193)

Animal studies suggest that in the urine many metabolites may be present and must have molecular weights over 700, suggesting an association with polypeptides. Thus far only low molecular weight metabolites, including trifluoroacetic acid, have been particularly identified in man. Metabolites present in the liver also seem to be of a high molecular weight and on a subcellular basis appear to be associated with the cell membrane, mitochondria and microsomes (Cohen, 1971).

labelled $CO_2$ and urinary non-volatile metabolites presumably following ether cleavage (Van Dyke *et al.*, 1963). Certainly liver microsomal enzymes are capable of ether cleavage. Low temperature autoradiography has confirmed the presence of non-volatile metabolites in the body of the mouse with accumulation in the liver (Cohen and Hood, 1969b). These *in vivo* metabolites were studied by radiochromatography and mass spectrometry and found to be labelled fatty acids, cholesterol and glycerides. It would

$$CH_3CH_2-O-CH_2CH_3 \rightarrow CH_3-CHO + CH_3CH_2OH \rightarrow Glucuronide$$

$$CH_3CH_2OH \longrightarrow CH_3COOH \rightarrow CO_2$$

Acetyl Co A
Fatty acids
Glycerides
Cholesterol

Suggested Metabolism of Diethyl ether
(from Cohen, E. N. (1971), *Anesthesiology*, **35**, 193)

The possible toxicity of halothane to the liver is a difficult and controversial subject (Bunker, J. P. *et al.*, 1969). The role played by metabolites in the very rare hepatotoxic reactions to halothane is conjectural. In fact there are two ways in which these metabolites might be implicated, it has been suggested that there is an increase in hepatotoxic reactions following repeated exposure to halothane (Belfrage *et al.*, 1966; Bunker *et al.*, 1969; Klatskin and Kimberg, 1969) and in several instances this has been attributed to be a sensitization response. If such a response occurs the presence of a haptene has to be postulated although it is unlikely to be a small molecule such as halothane. However, halothane metabolites linked with protein could form a high molecular weight structure with potential antigenic properties. Alternatively, the metabolites of halothane could be hepatotoxic themselves; certainly several, including trifluoroacetic acid and trifluoroethanol, have been shown to be toxic in animals. A sequence of repeated exposure to halothane, enzyme induction and increase in metabolism might allow toxic levels of metabolites to accumulate.

## ETHERS

*Diethyl Ether* ($C_2H_5-O-C_2H_5$). Following intraperitoneal injection in rats $^{14}C$-labelled ether produces

follow that diethyl ether is transformed to $^{14}C$-acetate and thus enters the common metabolic pool, producing metabolites found in the body under normal conditions. Unlike halogenated anaesthetics, rats exposed chronically to ether show no abnormalities. Rats similarly exposed to methoxyflurane and halothane demonstrate failure to thrive with weight loss and hepatomegaly (Leong *et al.*, 1970).

## HALOGENATED ETHERS

*Fluroxene* ($CF_3CH_2-O-CH=CH_2$). $^{14}C$-labelled fluroxene undergoes metabolism to trifluoroethanol, trifluoroacetic acid and $^{14}CO_2$ in the mouse (Blake *et al.*, 1967), $^{14}CO_2$ being obtained from the vinyl carbon only. Recent studies suggest that mice die within 5 to 24 hours following fluroxene anaesthesia, the death rate being related to dose and pre-treatment with an enzyme inducer; this would indicate that a metabolite might be responsible (Cascorbi and Singh-Amaranath, 1972). Using low-temperature whole-body autoradiography non-volatile metabolites are found to accumulate in the liver of the mouse after two hours (Tyrrell, 1970), as yet these metabolites have not been identified.

In man, $^{14}C$-labelled fluroxene was administered to two volunteers and 12·1 per cent and 15·4 per cent of the administered dose of radioactivity was recovered from the

$$CF_3CH_2-O-CH=CH_2 \rightarrow CF_3CH_2OH + HOCH=CH_2$$

$$\begin{bmatrix} & OH & OH \\ & | & | \\ CF_3CH_2-O-CH-CH_2 \end{bmatrix} \text{Glucuronide}$$

$$CO_2 + C\!F_3CH_2OH \longrightarrow CF_3COOH \rightarrow CO_2$$

Suggested Metabolism of Fluroxene
(from Cohen, E. N. (1971), *Anesthesiology*, **35**, 193)

urine in 24 hours. Interestingly these two individuals showed widely disparate efficiency in metabolizing halothane (Blake and Cascorbi, 1970).

**Methoxyflurane** ($CH_3-O-CF_2CHCl_2$). Animal experiments using $^{14}C$ and $^{36}Cl$-labelled methoxyflurane have shown the presence of $^{14}CO_2$ and labelled non-volatile metabolites in the urine (Van Dyke and Chenoweth, 1965b). Induction of microsomal enzyme systems producing ether cleavage and dechlorination has been demonstrated *in vivo* following pre-treatment with phenobarbital and methoxyflurane itself. Pentobarbital increases the rate of deposition of fluorine in bones following the administration of methoxyflurane, the supposition being that increased metabolism has occurred.

Recently, these animal studies have been substantiated in man using $^{14}C$-methoxyflurane. Holaday and his co-workers (1970) showed that 7 to 21 per cent of the drug underwent ether cleavage and in one subject a further 40 per cent was dechlorinated. The same workers went on to identify dichloroacetic acid, methoxydifluroacetic acid and fluorine ion as metabolites. It will be noted that the $CF_2$ bonding in this agent is readily attacked by biological enzyme systems contrasting with the $CF_3$ group in halothane where little free fluorine is found.

Free fluorine is a very significant metabolite of methoxyflurane. Since 1966 sporadic case reports of a toxic nephropathy following the use of this agent have appeared; this nephropathy is characterized by polyuria and weight loss, hypernatraemia, increased serum osmolarity and elevated blood urea (Crandell *et al.*, 1966). A recent randomized prospective clinical trial has confirmed the occurence of this syndrome in man (Mazze *et al.*, 1971). Further research has indicated that the nephropathy is dose dependent and that free fluorine is the responsible metabolite (Mazze *et al.*, 1972). In rats a histological picture of mitochondrial swelling and rupture was seen in the cells of the proximal tubule of the kidney following methoxyflurane anaesthesia. An identical picture was seen following injection of free fluorine. The severity of the changes correlated directly with the concentration of the agent. In man an additional study has shown a dose dependent nephrotoxity also correlating with serum inorganic fluorine following methoxyflurane anaesthesia (Cousins and Mazze, 1972).

Obviously the advisability of using methoxyflurane is in question in patients with renal disease and in operations showing a high incidence of renal complications. However, the doses of the agent used in the above studies and producing clinical nephropathy were high, and there has been

Suggested Metabolism of Methoxyflurane
(from Mazze *et al.* (1971), *Anesthesiology*, **35**, 247)

no evidence of renal dysfunction in obstetric analgesia, for instance, where low concentrations are used.

**Ēthrane** ($CHF_2$—O—$CF_2$.CHClF) and **Forane** ($CHF_2$—O—$CHCl.CF_3$). Although work in this field is not completed, the recently introduced and closely related ethers would seem to undergo only limited biodegradation. With Ēthrane there is evidence of deposition of fluorine in bone and recovery of inorganic and organic fluorine in the urine in man (Case, 1970). Liver perfusion studies in miniature swine have not demonstrated any metabolites of Forane recoverable in the portal drainage (Halsey et al., 1971).

## INORGANIC ANAESTHETICS

Under this heading are included the rare gases, xenon and krypton and nitrogen, nitrous oxide and carbon dioxide; all are weak anaesthetics requiring high partial pressures to produce anaesthesia. Interestingly there is evidence that even the rare gases are capable of association with metals and that xenon is chemically reactive.

Nitrous oxide is, of course, quite a reactive chemical but there is no definite evidence of biotransformation. Unfortunately there is no stable radioactive isotope of nitrous oxide which will allow its study (although stable isotopes have been prepared). However, there is circumstantial evidence that biotransformation may occur, as it is not biologically inert. Depression of the bone marrow and reticuloendothelial system have been described and a teratogenic effect suggested (Shepard and Fink, 1968). It has been shown to produce enzyme induction suggesting some metabolic activity (Van Dyke, 1971).

## CONCLUSIONS

From the standpoint adopted only a few years ago that inhalational agents were inert and excreted unchanged, it can now be seen that we are faced with an entirely different situation. Not only do the volatile agents undergo extensive biotransformation, but metabolites are produced which are potentially toxic to such organs as the liver and kidney. These dangers exist not only for the patient but also for his close attendants in the operating theatre environment. Obviously this is a field requiring much further study. However, the problems involved in handling trace quantities of radioactive material and the separation and identification of metabolites, particularly in man, are enormous. Significantly, much current work in this area at present is being directed at cellular and sub-cellular function, an ever expanding field in many branches of medical research.

## REFERENCES

Allison, A. C., Nunn, J. F. (1968), "Effects of Anaesthetics on Microtubules," *Lancet*, **2**, 1326.

Belfrage, S., Ahlgren, L. and Axelson, S. (1966), "Halothane Hepatitis in Anaesthetists, *Lancet*, **2**, 1466.

Blake, D. A. and Cascorbi, H. F. (1970), "A Note on the Biotransformation of Fluroxene in Two Volunteers," *Anesthesiology*, **32**, 560.

Blake, D. A., Rozman, R. S., Cascorbi, H. F. and Krantz, J. C. (1967), "Biotransformation of Fluroxene. 1. Metabolism in Mice and Dogs *in vivo*," *Biochem. Pharmacol.*, **16**, 1237.

Bruning, A. and Schnetka, M. (1933), "Über den Nachweis von Trichloräthylen und Anderen Halogenhaltigen Organischen Lösungsmitteln," *Arch. Gewerbepathol Gewerbehyg*, **4**, 840.

Bunker, J. P., Forrest, W., Mosteller, F. *et al.* (1969), *National Halothane Study*. U.S. Gvt. Printing Office. Bethesda.

Cascorbi, H. F., Blake, D. A. and Helrich, M. (1970), "Differences in the Biotransformation of Halothane in Man," *Anesthesiology*, **32**, 119.

Cascorbi, H. F. and Singh-Amaranath, A. V. (1972), "Fluroxene Toxicity in Mice," *Anesthesiology*, **37**, 480.

Chase, R. E. (1970), "Biotransformation of Ethrane in Man, 24th." Postgrad, Assembly, New York, p. 61.

Cohen, E. N. (1971), "Metabolism of Volatile Anesthetics," *Anesthesiology*, **35**, 193.

Cohen, E. N. and Hood, N. (1969a), "Application of Low Temperature Autoradiography to the Study of the Uptake and Metabolism of Volatile Anesthetics in the Mouse. 1. Chloroform," *Anesthesiology*, **30**, 306.

Cohen, E. N. and Hood, N. (1969b), "Application of Low Temperature Autoradiography to the Study of the Uptake and Metabolism of Volatile Anesthetics in the Mouse. II. Diethyl Ether," *Anesthesiology*, **31**, 61.

Cohen, E. N. and Hood, N. (1969c), "Application of Low Temperature Autoradiography to the Study of the Uptake and Metabolism of Volatile Anesthetics in the Mouse. III. Halothane," *Anesthesiology*, **31**, 553.

Cohen, E. N., Belville, J. W. and Brown, B. W. (1971), "Pregnancy, Anesthesia and Miscarriage. A Study of Operating Room Nurses and Anesthetists," *Anesthesiology*, **35**, 343.

Cousins, M. J. and Mazze, R. I. (1972), "Dose-response Study of Methoxyflurane Nephrotoxicity in Man," *Abstracts Proceedings 5th World Congress, Anaesthesiology*, p. 115. Excerpta Medica. Amsterdam.

Crandell, W. B., Pappass, S. G. and Macdonald, A. (1966), "Nephrotoxicity Associated with Methoxyflurane Anesthesia," *Anesthesiology*, **27**, 591.

Hallen, B., Ehrner-Samuel, H. and Thomason, M. (1970), "Measurements of Halothane in the Atmosphere of the Operating Theatre and in Expired Air and Blood of the Personnel during Routine Anaesthetic Work," *Acta Anaesth. Scand.*, **14**, 17.

Halsey, M. J., Sawyer, D. C., Eger, E. I., Bahlman, S. H. and Impelman, D. M. K. (1971), "Hepatic Metabolism of Halothane, Methoxyflurane, Cyclopropane Ethane and Forane in Miniature Swine," *Anesthesiology*, **35**, 43.

Holaday, D. A., Rudofsky, S. and Trenhaft, P. S. (1970), "Metabolic Degradation of Methoxyflurane in Man," *Anesthesiology*, **33**, 579.

Klatskin, G. and Kimberg, D. V. (1969), "Recurrent Hepatitis Attributable to Halothane Sensitization in an Anesthetist," *New Eng. J. Med.*, **280**, 515.

Linde, H. W. and Bruce, D. L. (1969), "Occupational Exposure of Anesthetists to Halothane, Nitrous Oxide and Radiation," *Anesthesiology*, **30**, 363.

Leong, B. K. J., Sparschu, G. L., Torkelson, T. R. *et al.* (1970), "Chronic Toxicity of Anesthetics," *Abstr. Proceedings Conference on Cellular Toxicity of Anaesthetics*, Seattle.

Mazze, R. I., Shue, G. L. and Jackson, S. H. (1971), "Renal Dysfunction Associated with Methoxyflurane Anesthesia. A Randomized Prospective Clinical Evaluation," *J.A.M.A.*, **216**, 278.

Mazze, R. I., Cousins, M. J. and Kozek, J. C. (1972), "Dose Related Methoxyflurane Nephrotoxicity in Rats," *Anesthesiology*, **36**, 571.

Rehder, K., Forbes, J., Aller, H., Hessler, O. and Stier, A. (1967), "Halothane Biotransformation in Man, a Quantitative Study," *Anesthesiology*, **28**, 711.

Sawyer, D. C., Eger, E. I. II and Bahlman, S. H. (1971), "Concentration Dependence of Hepatic Halothane Metabolism," *Anesthesiology*, **34**, 230.

Scholler, K. L. (1970), "Modification of the Effects of Chloroform on the Rat Liver," *Brit. J. Anaesth.*, **42**, 603.

Shepard, R. H. and Fink, B. R. (1968), "Teratogenic Activity of Nitrous Oxide in Rats," in *Toxicity of Anesthetics* (Ed. B. R. Fink), p. 308. Baltimore: Williams and Wilkins.

Stier, A. (1964), "Trifluoroacetic Acid as Metabolite of Halothane," *Biochem. Pharmacol.*, **13**, 544.

Stier, A. (1967), "The Biotransformation of Halothane," *Anesthesiology*, **29**, 388.

Trudell, J. R., Watson, E. and Cohen, E. N. (1972), "Impurities in $^{14}$C-labelled Halothane," *Anesthesiology*, **37**, 93.

Tyrrell, M. F. (1970), Unpublished observations.

Ullberg, S. (1958), "Autoradiographic Studies on the Distribution of Labelled Drugs in the Body," *Proceedings 2nd U.N. International Conference on Peaceful Uses of Atomic Energy*, **24**, 248.

Van Dyke, R. A. (1966), "Metabolism of Volatile Anesthetics III. Induction of Microsomal Dechlorinating and Ether Cleavage Enzymes," *J. Pharmacol. Exp. ther.*, **154**, 364.

Van Dyke, R. A. quoted in Cohen, E. N. (1971), "Metabolism of Volatile Anesthetics," *Anesthesiology*, **35**, 193.

Van Dyke, R. A. and Chenoweth, M. B. (1965a), "Metabolism of Volatile Anesthetics," *Anesthesiology*, **26**, 348.

Van Dyke, R. A. and Chenoweth, M. B. (1965b), "The Metabolism of Volatile Anesthetics. II. *In vitro* Metabolism of Methoxyflurane and Halothane in Rat Liver Slices and Cell Fractions," *Biochem. Pharmacol.*, **14**, 603.

Van Dyke, R. A., Chenoweth, M. B. and Van Poznak, A. (1964), "Metabolism of Volatile Anesthetics. I. Conversion *in vivo* of several Anesthetics to $^{14}CO_2$ and Chloride," *Biochem. Pharmacol.*, **13**, 1239.

Whitcher, C. E., Cohen, E. N. and Trudell, J. R. (1971), "Chronic Exposure to Anesthetic Gases in the Operating Room," *Anesthesiology*, **35**, 343.

# ANAESTHETIC APPARATUS

# CHAPTER 1

# AUTOMATIC LUNG VENTILATORS

JOHN S. ROBINSON

## Basic Principles

The function of ventilators is to move gases in and out of the lungs, and the power for this movement can either come from the pressure of the gases themselves or from an external source of energy such as an electric motor. Apart from inflating the lung with gas, energy is also necessary to cycle the ventilator, that is to terminate the inspiratory phase and to re-cycle the expiratory phase to bring it back to the inspiratory phase. The cycling of the ventilator can be accomplished by the same energy source as that used to move the gases, but sometimes a totally independent source of energy, such as an electronic timing circuit is used. The principle of operation of any lung ventilator is therefore divisible into 4 phases: (1) the inspiratory phase; (2) the inspiratory to expiratory cycling; (3) the expiratory phase; and (4) the expiratory to inspiratory cycling.

### 1. The Inspiratory Phase

The flow of gases into the lungs during inspiration can be accomplished in two ways only; (1) The machine may generate a pattern of pressure in the gases delivered to the airways that will be reflected by the flow pattern into the lungs. This will produce an alveolar pressure wave and a flow pattern that will result from the pressure pattern applied by the machine, the compliance of the patient's lungs and of his airways resistance. (2) In the other method, the instrument produces a set pattern of flow of gases into the lungs so that the airway presssure, alveolar pressure and volume patterns are dependent upon the compliance and airway resistance of the patient acting against this flow. What we are really saying is that, either the *pressure pattern* applied to the airway by the instrument is set by the machine and is unaltered by the patient's characteristics, or alternatively the *flow pattern* applied, by the machine, to the airways is unaltered by the patient's characteristics. Thus, there are two basic methods of producing the inspiratory phase: (1) a pressure generator; and (2) a flow generator.

There are functional differences in the various methods of getting gas volumes into the lungs during inspiration and it seems to be widely believed that the distribution of inspired gas in the lungs is determined by the inspiratory flow and pressure patterns. Otis and his colleagues (1956) gave a theoretical basis for these views. Some manufacturers have claimed that their particular device, by controlling the flow pattern, promotes more uniform intrapulmonary gas mixing, but such views have not been upheld by objective measurement of gas mixing in the lung. Thus, Watson (1963) showed that gas distribution during artificial ventilation, as measured by physiological dead space, was uninfluenced by the pattern of flow or pressure applied to the airway. Using a nitrogen wash-out technique, Bergman (1969) also showed that gas mixing was uninfluenced by the patterns of flow and pressure applied to the airway. Of real importance, however, is the length of the inspiratory period, if this falls below one second then the physiological dead space increases and the lung compliances falls; on the other hand if the inspiratory period is prolonged beyond 1·5 seconds then there is no improvement in gas distribution. It has been shown that these results are the same irrespective of whether flow into the lung decreases during inspiration, as it would if a constant pressure was applied to the airway, or whether it remains constant, as it would if a constant flow was applied to the airway.

It is pointless, therefore, to discuss the various patterns of inspiratory flow, pressure and volume generated unless the method of cycling from inspiration to expiration is also included in the appraisal because we need to determine the total timing of the inspiratory flow and the integral of this flow with time—*the tidal volume*. Similar considerations preclude the examination of the expiratory phase without consideration of the expiratory to inspiratory cycling. The appraisal of the clinical importance of the functional characteristics of various ventilators will therefore be considered after the basic mechanisms of all the phases have been described.

### 2. Inspiratory to Expiratory Cycling

**Time Cycling.** When the change to expiration is produced by a timing mechanism which is uninfluenced by any changes in the patient's lungs, then the ventilator is *time cycled*. This mechanism may be electro-mechanical, as in the East Radcliffe, Cape or Engström instruments, or it may be effected by an electronic timing circuit as in the Barnet or Loosco Infant Ventilator. As the mechanism is uninfluenced by any changes in the patient's lungs, it follows that the pressure developed in the lungs and the flow and the volume delivered at the termination of inspiration can all vary. The actual values reached are determined by the characteristics of the patient's lungs acting on either the flow or pressure generating mechanisms of the instrument. Certain ventilators, though essentially time cycled, may deliver a pre-set volume during the inspiratory period because the power of the machine is so great. Thus the Cape and Engström can be described as time cycled volume pre-set.

**Volume cycling.** When the inspiratory to expiratory change occurs because a volume delivered by the ventilator has passed from some point in the machine, then the machine is volume cycled, thus the duration of the inspiratory phase and the flow and pressure developed at the end of the phase can all vary. This method of cycling has in the past been uncommon. It usually takes the form of a piston or concertina bag emptying its contents into the patient. The volume delivered is set by means of a mechanical or electrical trip device on the piston or concertina bag. The Bourne paediatric ventilator and the Barnet Mark III ventilator, in its volume cycling mode, can act in this way.

Now that reliable and cheap electronic flow meters are available, true volume cycling of flow generators has become possible. This means that the flow pattern during inspiration can be altered to the three basis patterns, constant, accelerating and decelerating flows. The machine monitors the inspired flow and integrates it with time to give the inspired tidal volume. The expired flow is similarly integrated to give expired tidal volume. Any discrepancy between inspired $V_T$ and expired $V_T$ can thus be sensed to ring an alarm. Such machines therefore do not need respiratory monitor alarms and the inspired respiratory flow pattern can be altered so that the theoretical optimal ventilation can be obtained for different pathophysiological changes in the lungs. Two types of these machines are on the market, the Servo Ventilator 900 (Elema-Schönander) and the Pneumotron (British Oxygen Co. Ltd.).

**Pressure Cycling.** If the machine cycles when a predetermined pressure has been reached in the upper airway or in some part of the gas circuit, then the machine is pressure cycled. Although this form of cycling cannot alter the airway pressure at the end of the inspiratory phase, it is more sensitive than any other form of cycling and the length of the inspiratory phase, the volume delivered and the flow occurring at the end of inspiration can all alter. This can create many difficulties in use and will be considered later. This type of pressure cycling occurs in the Harlow ventilator, the Bird series of ventilators and with the Blease Pulmoflator.

**Flow cycling.** When the change from inspiration to expiration occurs because the flow from the machine reaches a pre-determined minimal value, flow cycling occurs. This uncommon type of cycling is to be found on the Bennett ventilator.

### 3. The Expiratory Phase

This is analagous to inspiration and can only occur as the result of either flow or pressure generated. The most obvious method of allowing exhalation is by venting the airway directly to the atmosphere. The flow of gas from the lungs can be retarded by various means so that a small constant pressure above that of atmosphere is held during the expiratory phase. Conversely, if the patient's expiratory gas flow is directed to the entrainment orifice of a venturi, during expiration, then a constant sub-atmospheric pressure will be applied. This is the mechanism by which the Bird Mark 8, the Bennett PR 11 and the Loosco Infant Ventilator produce their 'negative' expiratory phases. Other forms of 'negative' expiratory phases can be obtained by directing the patient's expiration to bellows which are actively expanded during the expiratory phase so that a sub-atmospheric pressure is created in the patient's airway.

### 4. Expiratory to Inspiratory Cycling

The change from the expiratory phase to the inspiratory phase can be cycled by the same mechanisms as the inspiratory to the expiratory phase, but in practice only two forms are in common use:

1. Time cycled, in which the change over occurs after a pre-set period of time, and
2. Pressure cycled, in which the change over occurs when the airway pressure falls to a pre-set level.

There are a number of machines in which more than one type of cycling is operative, these will be discussed where appropriate.

**Time Cycling.** When the expiratory phase terminates from a timing mechanism which is uninfluenced by any characteristics which exist in the patient's lungs at the moment of cycling then the instrument is *time cycled*. This is the normal expiratory/inspiratory cycling which is found on most ventilators. The pressure and the volume of gas in the lungs at the time of cycling and the presence or absence of flow in the airway will, therefore, depend upon the length of the expiratory phase and the airways resistance.

**Pressure cycling.** The type of cycling depends upon the time taken to reach a given pressure in the mouth or some closely related pressure in the machine, and this occurs irrespective of the volume that may have been expired and the flow that may be existing at the time. This is a very uncommon type of cycling, but another type of pressure cycling is quite common, that of patient cycling or patient triggering. The patient produces a sub-atmospheric pressure at the end of expiration by an inspiratory effort and this sub-atmospheric pressure is transmitted to a diaphragm somewhere in the ventilator where it is sensed by an electrical or pneumatic switch which terminates expiration. This type of mechanism is to be found in the Bird, Harlow, Bennett and Barnet series of ventilators.

**The bellows or bag in bottle.** A number of anaesthetic ventilators use their pressure or flow generation and cycling mechanisms to empty an anaesthetic bag or bellows suspended in a bottle and compressed by the gases delivered by the ventilator. The reason for this is so that the patient may breathe a different gas mixture from that used to drive the ventilator, which is usually compressed air. During expiration the patient may exhale directly to the atmosphere or via a carbon dioxide absorption circuit back into the bellows. The functional effects of this arrangement are very little different to the effects of the gas from the ventilator entering the patient's lungs directly, the only difference being that due to the effect of compression upon the volume of air in the bottle. This is negligible if the volume of the bottle is small.

**Inspiratory pressure generators.** The most basic form

of pressure generator is the constant pressure generator, which comprises a concertina bellows compressed by a weight or a spring; the mechanism of the East Radcliffe, the Manley and the Barnet ventilators. Almost without exception the most successful constant inspiratory pressure generators are time cycled from inspiration to expiration.

Let us consider the pressure, flow and volume patterns which would result when a constant airway pressure is applied to a patient with normal compliance and airways resistance (Fig. 1). The applied airway pressure causes a high initial gas flow into the lungs, because the pressure difference between the alveoli and the airways is greatest at the beginning of inspiration. Then, there is a gradual increase in the oesophageal pressure (which can with certain reservations be equated with alveolar pressure). This increase in the alveolar pressure decreases the pressure gradient within the lungs so that at the end of the inspiratory period the alveoli and airway pressures are almost equal and flow ceases. Now if the airway pressure is applied for just sufficiently long enough for the flow into the lungs to cease and inspiratory to expiratory cycling to start, then the patterns in Fig. 1 are produced. If, however, the inspiratory phase was prolonged longer than that required for equilibration between the oesophageal and airway pressures then a plateau of oesophageal pressure would occur, but there would be no further flow into the lungs because the pressure difference between the oesophagus and the airway has reached equilibrium. If the compliance of the patient being ventilated by a constant pressure time cycled ventilator is low then the rate of rise of oesophageal pressure would be greatly increased because there is a decreased flow and volume entering the lungs with the same applied airway pressure. The equilibrium with the airway pressure is reached early in the inspiratory phase giving an oesophageal pressure pattern similar to that caused by extending the length of the inspiratory phase. The final alveolar pressure reached will be insufficient to overcome the decrease in compliance and therefore the tidal volume falls (Fig. 2). The applied airway pressure must therefore be raised to overcome the effects of a low compliance.

If the airways resistance is increased then the pressure and flow patterns that would occur with a constant pressure time cycled device are shown in Fig. 3. The applied square wave of airway pressure will remain the same, but because the airways resistance is high the oesophageal pressure will not rise at the same rate as it does with a normal airway resistance. The flow into the lungs therefore starts more slowly and the rate of flow out of the lungs is also reduced —because the rate of rise and fall in the oesophageal pressure has diminished. If the total inspiratory time is kept the same as that of Figs. 1 and 2, then the tidal volume must decrease because a lower flow is occurring for the same period of time. However, if the inspiratory time is sufficiently prolonged then the tidal volume will not decrease because the lower flow into the lungs is allowed to continue for a longer period of time.

Three conclusions can be drawn about the behaviour of these time-cycled constant pressure generators:

1. If the compliance is low then the flow will decline much more rapidly because the rate of rise of the oesophageal pressure is more rapid. The tidal volume will be reached much sooner and will be reduced in

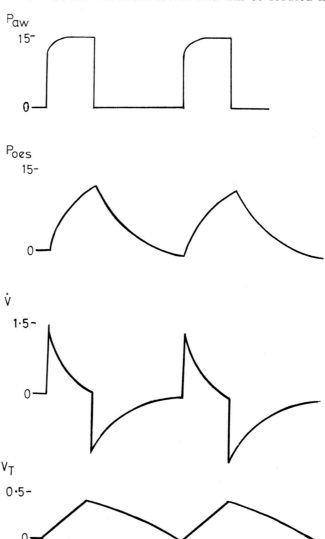

FIG. 1. Pressure flow and volume patterns produced against 'normal' lungs by a constant pressure generator (East Radcliffe) which was time cycled at both from inspiration to expiration and expiration to inspiration. The expiratory phase is due to venting the lungs to atmosphere.

$Paw$ = airway pressure (cm $H_2O$)
$P_{oes}$ = oesophageal pressure (cm $H_2O$)
$\dot{V}$ = gas flow (litres/sec)
$V_T$ = tidal volume (litres)

The units are the same for all the figures in this chapter.

size unless the applied airway pressure is raised to compensate for the low compliance.

2. When the airways resistance is increased the initial flow is decreased and the decay of flow becomes much slower, therefore unless the inspiratory phase is lengthened, the low flow acting for a normal inspiratory period will decrease the tidal volume.

3. If patients have a normal compliance and the inspiratory period is lengthened unnecessarily (longer than 1·5 seconds) then a plateau of alveolar pressure will be produced during which no further gas flow occurs

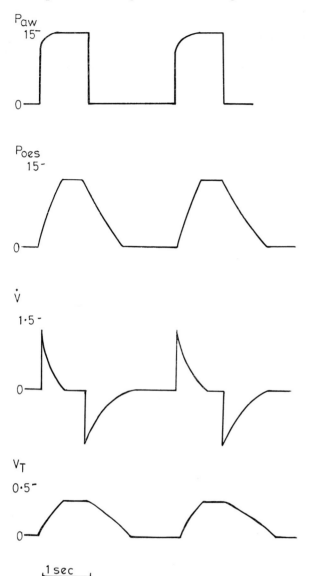

FIG. 2. Pressure flow and volume patterns produced by the East Radcliffe ventilator against the lungs of a patient with a low compliance. Note the rapid rise of oesophageal pressure to the plateau and the cessation of flow into the lungs when this plateau is reached. The resulting fall in tidal volume can be seen.

into the lungs. This is of no benefit to the patient and indeed may be harmful as it raises the mean intra-thoracic pressure and may reduce the cardiac output.

Let us now consider examples of commercially available versions of this type of device.

## THE EAST RADCLIFFE VENTILATOR

The mechanism of this instrument is shown in Fig. 4. During the inspiratory phase the bellows I are emptied into the patient by the descent of the weight W on the arm when it comes off the lift of the cam 5, the non-return valve 1 closes. At the same time the inspiratory poppet valve 2 is opened by the lift of the cam rotating on the shaft AB which is driven by an electric motor.

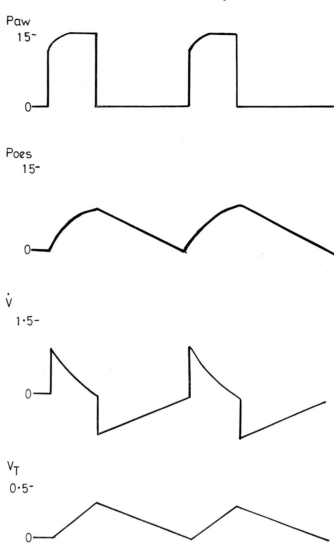

FIG. 3. Patterns produced by the East Radcliffe ventilator acting against a patient with a high airways resistance. Note the slow rise of oesophageal pressure and that its final end inspiratory value is lower than in Fig. 1 due to the pressure loss required to overcome airway resistance. Note also the very prolonged expiratory flow and pressure decay patterns.

The constant pressure applied to the airway during inspiration is therefore dependent on the mass of the weight W placed on the beam and the distance this weight is from the fulcrum, the constant pressure generated by this machine is therefore adjustable. The cycling from inspiration to expiration occurs when the rotation of the shaft AB lifts the cam and expiratory valve 3 and closes the inspiratory valve 2, the patient then expires passively to atmosphere through the non-return valve 4. The termination of the inspiratory phase is therefore time cycled because it depends upon the rotation of the shaft. During the inspiratory period the expiratory bellows E and spring S are compressed by the lift of the cam 6. During expiration these bellows are then free to expand and as the expiratory flow from the patient is directed into them, a sub-atmospheric pressure is generated, the magnitude of which depends upon the adjustable tension of the spring S. If the tension of this spring is set to a minimum,

constant pressure generators and time cycled in which the desired minute volume is set directly by the flow of gases per minute which are delivered to the ventilator. The minute volume delivered to the patient is therefore set, but the machine may determine how this minute volume is divided up and delivered. This group of machines are therefore known as *minute volume dividers*. The machine may set the length of the inspiratory phase, the pressure at which the inspired gases are delivered and their flow rate, but regardless of the manipulation of these controls the

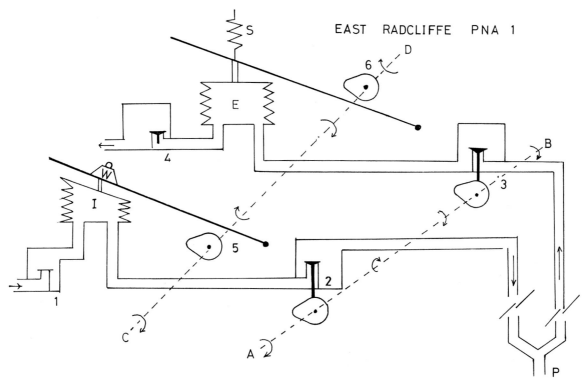

FIG. 4. Schematic diagram of the East Radcliffe ventilator.

| | | |
|---|---|---|
| *I* | inspiratory bellows | *W* weight |
| *E* | expiratory bellows | *S* spring |
| *AB* | inspiratory and expiratory valve cam shaft | |
| *CD* | bellows cam shaft | |

1. Inspiratory non return valve
2. Inspiratory poppet valve
3. Expiratory poppet valve
4. Expiratory non return valve
5. Inspiratory bellows cam
6. Expiratory bellows cam

the pressure generated is so small that after some 100 ml of gas has passed into the bellows the airway pressure returns to atmospheric and expiratory flow is unassisted. During expiration the inspiratory bellows are refilled with gas because the lift of the cam 5 expands the bellows and gas is entrained via the non-return valve 1.

Consideration of the mechanism of this instrument shows that the tidal volume delivered is very dependent upon the compliance of the patient, the adjustment of the weight applied to the inspiratory bellows, and the length of the inspiratory phase. The inspiratory to expiratory ratio is fixed at 1 to 1·7 by the position of the cams on the shafts *AB* and *CD*. The frequency of ventilation can be varied by step increments by means of a gear box.

There is an important group of ventilators that are

minute volume received by the machine will be delivered to the patient. If such a ventilator has a patient triggering device then it cannot be considered to be truly patient cycled because the patient has no control over the minute volume of gas which is delivered during inspiration. Thus, the minute volume delivered by such a machine may be inadequate to meet the demands of the patient's respiratory centre. For this reason, patient triggering devices are potentially dangerous in these machines.

## MANLEY

This is a minute volume divider and a constant pressure generator in which the power is supplied by the compressed gases, either from an anaesthetic machine or a pipe line

(Fig. 5). The duration of the inspiratory phase, the pressure at which the gases are delivered to the airway and their flow rate can be varied by adjusting the machine. However, as it is a minute volume divider the ventilator will deliver the metered minute volume from the anaesthetic machine to the patient regardless of any manipulation of the controls. Fresh gases enter continually at the port 1 but during the inspiratory phase are stored in the bellows $A$ under a pressure created by the spring

bellows, expiration then occurs through the expiratory valve 4, and out to the atmosphere through the non-return valve 5. A sub-atmospheric expiratory phase is obtained by the insertion of an expiratory bellows in the expiratory circuit. This bellows $E$ is linked to the inspiratory bellows $I$ so that as the inspiratory bellows rises by filling with fresh gas during the expiratory phase it expands the expiratory bellows and creates a sub-atmospheric pressure. This sub-atmospheric pressure

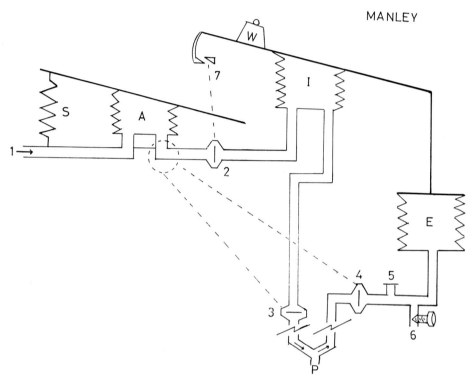

MANLEY

FIG. 5. Schematic diagram of the Manley ventilator.

| | |
|---|---|
| $A$ Storage bellows | 1. Fresh gas port |
| $I$ Inspiratory bellows | 2. Dumping valve from storage bellows to inspiratory bellows |
| $E$ Expiratory bellows | 3. Inspiratory valve |
| $W$ Weight | 4. Expiratory valve |
| $S$ Spring | 5. Non return expiratory valve |
| Dotted lines indicate valves operated from the toggle mechanism. | 6. Adjustable bleed valve for subatmospheric phase |
| | 7. Tidal volume stop |

$S$ of 110–150 cm. $H_2O$. A toggle switch positively operates valve 2 both by the arm of the storage bellows $A$ and the stop on the inspiratory bellows ($I$) beam. The inspiratory and expiratory valves 3 and 4 are closed by compressed gas which is re-directed against them by the same toggle switch along narrow bore tubes between bellows $A$ and $I$. During inspiration valve 3 is open and valve 4 is closed so that the inspiratory bellows $I$ empties into the patient under the influence of the weight $W$. The inspiratory phase ends when the storage bellows $A$ fills to a certain height with the fresh gas. When this height is reached it operates the toggle switch thereby closing the inspiratory valve 3, opening the expiratory valve 4 and the delivery valve 2 so that the storage bellows empties into the inspiratory

is adjustable by the variable bleed valve 6. The expiratory phase ends when the adjustable stop on the bellows beam 7 operates the toggle switch which opens the inspiratory valve 3, closes the delivery valve 2, and the expiratory valve 4.

We can now use the simplified mechanical description of the action of the Manley ventilator to analyse its functional behaviour. The machine acts as an almost constant pressure generator during inspiratory phase, and this phase must be time cycled at the rate by which the initial gas flow fills the storage bellows $A$, before it operates the toggle switch. The height to which the bellows can fill before operating the toggle is adjustable. The expiratory to inspiratory cycling is determined by the rate at which the gas flow from the storage bellows fills the main inspiratory bellows and also by the adjustable tidal volume stop 7.

We can see how the Manley acts as a minute volume divider and how its timing is altered by the various controls. The tidal volume is directly controlled by adjusting the excursion of the inspiratory bellows by the stop 7, and this tidal volume will be delivered to the patient providing the pressure applied by the weight is sufficient to overcome the compliance and airways resistance of the

overdistended. This can be overcome by adding additional weights to the beam but the distensibility of the bellows tends to defeat this manœuvre.

In spite of the interaction of the controls the instrument is simple to use and the bellows distension gives an obvious indication if the pressure setting is below that necessary to deliver the required tidal volume. It has, however, insufficient reserves of power for use in the Intensive Therapy Unit where marked and rapid changes in compliance and airways resistance are met. The effect of

BARNET 2

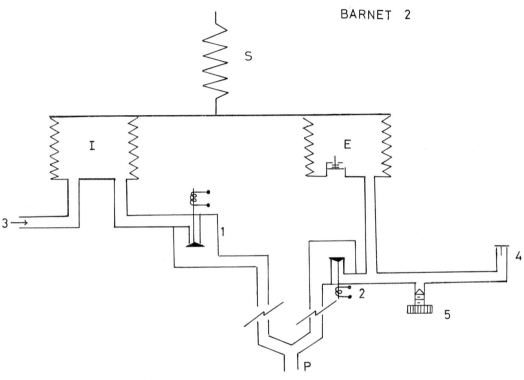

FIG. 6. Schematic diagram of the Barnet ventilator.

| I | Inspiratory bellows | 1. Solenoid operated inspiratory valve |
| E | Expiratory bellows | 2. Solenoid operated expiratory valve |
| S | Spring | 3. Gas or air inlet port |
| | | 4. Expiratory non return valve |
| | | 5. Subatmospheric pressure control bleed valve |

patient. The machine is a minute volume divider and therefore, if the tidal volume is increased by movement of the stop 7, then as the total ventilation per minute is unaltered this must decrease the respiratory frequency. The inspiratory time is dependent on the filling of the storage bellows A and will be unaltered by any changes in the setting of tidal volume, therefore any changes in the respiratory frequency must take place from the length of the expiratory phase. This instrument has considerable interaction of its controls and any changes in the settings of the tidal volume will alter the inspiratory/expiratory ratio. If the Manley ventilator is working against a greatly decreased compliance then the pressure applied by the weight to the inspiratory bellows I may be insufficient to empty the bellows and the storage bellows A will fill before the inspiratory bellows have delivered the tidal volume to the patient. The result is that the inspiratory bellows do not empty completely and gradually become

changes in compliance occurring during anaesthesia altering the tidal volume delivered by the Manley ventilator could be overcome by greatly increasing the weight on the beam. However, if the compliance is relatively normal this would lead to the tidal volume being emptied into the lungs rapidly with a high flow during the early part of the inspiratory phase and the maintenance of an alveolar pressure plateau as in Fig. 2. This would serve no useful purpose and might reduce the cardiac output.

The interaction of the controls seen in the Manley is not so evident in another type of constant pressure generator time cycled, minute volume divider, the Barnet.

## THE BARNET

A simplified diagram of the mechanism of the Barnet ventilator is shown in Fig. 6. The inspiratory phase commences when the solenoid operated valve 1 opens and the solenoid operated expiratory valve 2 closes. The gas in the inspiratory bellows which is under the action of the spring $S$ then drives its contents into the patient but at the same time fresh gas which is being fed to the machine is still entering at the port 3 and being driven to the patient. The inspiratory phase is terminated by the closure of the solenoid valve 1, and the opening of the expiratory valve 2. The timing of these solenoid valves is controlled by an electronic circuit. Expiration occurs passively to the atmosphere via the expiratory valve 2, and the non-return valve 4. During the expiratory period the incoming fresh gas is stored in the bellows $I$ which therefore expand, but as they are mechanically linked to the expiratory bellows these also expand, and if the patient's expiratory flow is directed to the expanding expiratory bellows then a sub-atmospheric phase occurs. The magnitude of the sub-atmospheric phase created is dependent upon the bleed to the bellows from the atmosphere. This is controlled by the adjustable valve 5.

If the pressure applied by the spring to the inspiratory bellows is high enough to overcome the patient's compliance for the tidal volume required and the patient's airway resistance for the particular flows delivered during the inspiratory period, then the tidal volume is set by the timing mechanism which divides up the minute volume of gas delivered to the instrument. The instrument is, therefore relatively easy to use and for this reason is popular both in the Intensive Therapy Unit and the operating theatre. The duration of the inspiratory/expiratory phases may be varied independently between 0·6 and 5 seconds by adjustment of the electronic timing circuit. It follows, therefore, that the respiratory frequency can be varied from 7 to 60 per minute and the inspiratory/expiratory ratio between 1 to 9 and 9 to 1. The Barnet Mark III ventilator is a development of the Barnet Mark II ventilator, and has three methods of cycling at the end of inspiration; can be time cycled, volume cycled or pressure cycled. This instrument is of considerable complexity, the original inspiratory bellows has now become a driving bellows for an open circuit bellows and an additional closed circuit bellows has been added. Any attempt to analyse the functional behaviour of the Barnet Mark III ventilator when working in its many modes is very confusing and does not assist in the use of the machine. Although there are functional differences between the various methods of operation it is the author's opinion that in this instance the manufacturer's technological achievement exceeds clinical requirements. The Barnet Mark II already had the attributes of being able to control the timing of the inspiratory/expiratory periods, and as it was a minute volume divider both the tidal volume and the minute volume could be readily ascertained.

Another form of constant pressure generator is that in which the constant pressure is obtained by taking the high pressure gas source through a reducing valve and then delivering the reduced pressure to the patient's airway. This is the method used with the Bennett ventilator. The cycling from inspiration to expiration in the Bennett

occurs when the pressure applied to the patient's airway is so near to the alveolar pressure that the flow into the patient becomes very low, the Bennett valve senses this low flow and terminates the inspiratory phase. Alternatively, the timing mechanism overrides this and cuts off flow through the Bennett valve which ends the inspiratory phase.

The pressure applied to the airway during the inspiratory phase need not be constant, it can either increase or decrease. The effects of either increasing or decreasing pressure applied to the airway will affect the flow pressure and volume patterns in a manner that can be predicted from Fig. 1. If the pressure decreases towards the end of the inspiratory period then the flow will also decrease towards the end of the inspiratory period and the rate of rise of the oesophageal pressure will also decrease. Conversely, if the pressure increases during the inspiratory period then the flow pattern will be reversed from that in Fig. 1, and will gradually increase during the inspiratory period and then fall off again as the alveolar pressure rises and flow decreases. Provided there has been sufficient time during the inspiratory period for distribution of the inspired gas then despite assertions to the contrary the author does not believe that any particular pattern of flow has an effect on the distribution of the inspired gas. The Engström ventilator can be regarded as an increasing pressure generator during inspiration. It uses a bag in a bottle and possesses tremendous reserves of power. The undoubted advantages of this instrument appear to come from the fact that it will deliver a pre-set tidal volume of gas at a respiratory frequency set by the user, irrespective of changing conditions in the patient. The volume pre-set behaviour of the Engström is not unique and is also shared by the Blease Pulmoflator, for these reasons both these ventilators will be discussed later.

If the energy obtained from the compressed anaesthetic gases is stored in an anaesthetic reservoir bag and then released to inflate the patient's lungs it is possible to make a simple cheap automatic lung ventilator. An example of this is the Mini-Vent (Fig. 7). The anaesthetic gases are fed into the reservoir bag 1 at a pressure varying between 40 and 60 pounds per square inch. During expiration the bobbin is held against the stops 3 by the airway pressure and by the action of the magnet 4, and thus the bobbin shuts off the inspiratory ports 5, the patient then breathes out passively via the expiratory port 6, and through the centre of the adjustable stops 9, to atmosphere via the large opening 7. The distance between the magnet and the stop 3 is controlled by the bobbin carrier 8. When this is screwed further into the housing via the movement of the knurled knob 11 the pressure required to move the bobbin 2 away from the magnet will be greater and therefore the pressure built up in the reservoir bag increases. During the period that the patient is breathing out to atmosphere, the reservoir bag is filling at a rate which is dependent upon the fresh anaesthetic gas flow and when the pressure in the bag is high enough to overcome the pull of the magnet the bobbin is forced away from it and closes the expiratory port 6. The anaesthetic reservoir bag then empties into the patient's lungs, the pressure at which it does this decreases as the bag empties. When the pressure in the anaesthetic reservoir bag falls to a low level the bobbin 2 is attracted back to the magnet, thus ending the inspiratory phase. The pressure to which that in the reservoir bag has to fall before the bobbin returns to 3 is adjustable by the stop 9 and the aluminium screw knob 10. If the stops are moved further out less pressure will be required in the reservoir bag before the bobbin

the inspiratory phase ends when a certain volume in a reservoir bag has been delivered to the patient and the ventilator might therefore be considered as being volume cycled between inspiration and expiration. Unfortunately this is not strictly true because the pressure on the bag side of the bobbin may not be the same as the bag pressure; it is usually quite close to it but the pressure may be very different if resistance to flow around the magnets has

MINIVENT

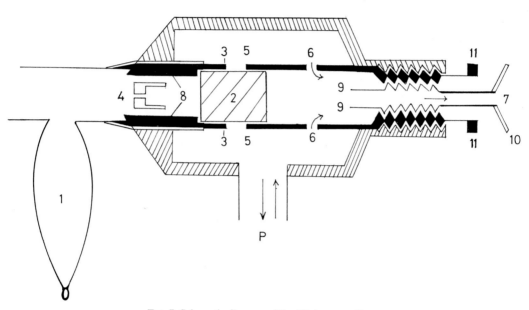

FIG. 7. Schematic diagram of the Minivent ventilator.

1. Anaesthetic reservoir bag
2. Bobbin
3. Expiratory bobbin stops
4. Magnet
5. Inspiratory ports

6. Expiratory ports
7. Expiratory channel
8. Bobbin carrier and adjusting knob
9. Inspiratory bobbin stops
10. Inspiratory stop adjusting knob

is pulled back to the position against the stops 3. Thus, the setting of the two controls 7 and 11 determines the pressure range within which the reservoir bag activates the instrument. Therefore, when the fresh gas flow has been set for any patient with a particular compliance and airways resistance, the duration of inspiration and expiration and the tidal volume will be determined by these controls. The minute volume of ventilation, of course, depends upon the inflating gas flow, so that this instrument is also a minute volume divider. The instrument acts as a decreasing pressure generator during the inspiratory phase which causes little change in the physiological effects from that of a constant pressure generator. The change over from expiration to inspiration occurs when the pressure in the bag rises sufficiently for the force which is being exerted on the bobbin to overcome the attraction of the magnet. It could, therefore, be said that

changed, which can easily occur if the parts become occluded by mucus.

The change from inspiration to expiration, therefore, is a hybrid of flow cycling and pressure cycling. The expiratory period is a pure constant atmospheric generator with the patient breathing out to atmosphere, and the change from expiration to inspiration occurs when the pressure in the reservoir bag rises to a level where the force it exerts on the bobbin is sufficient to overcome the attraction of the magnet. It might therefore be thought that the change over is pressure cycled but once again the pressure in the bag at this time is unrelated to any pressure in the patient and in fact the change over occurs when a tidal volume which enters the lungs during the previous inspiratory phase has been replaced by the fresh gas flow, therefore the change over is dependent both upon the compliance of the patient and upon the fresh gas flow. These small ventilators are relatively cheap and simple to use but it is obvious that their modes of cycling are affected by many different aspects of the ventilatory cycle. For this reason patients being ventilated by this type of machine require

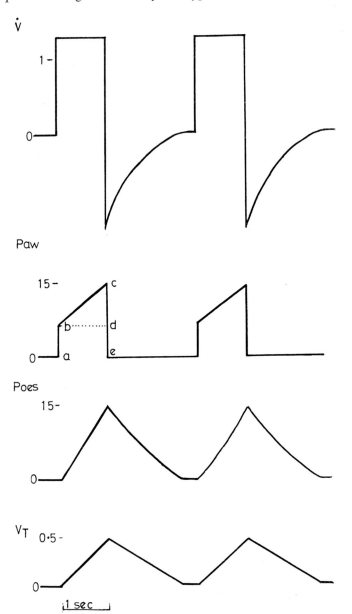

FIG. 8. Theoretical patterns produced against 'normal' lungs by a constant flow generator, which is time cycled both at inspiratory and expiratory cycling.

very close and constant surveillance. They illustrate the importance of having a clear understanding of how a particular machine acts so that any changes in its behaviour can readily be understood and corrected.

### Inspiratory Flow Generation

If the pressure supplied to a ventilator is extremely high, such as in the piped gas system of a hospital where it is approximately 4,000 cms of water pressure, then even if the patient's lungs were to be inflated to a pressure of 40 cms

of water by this gas supply the relatively small drop in pressure delivered to the machine would be insignificant and will have virtually no effect upon the gas flow. This means that instruments such as the Bird or the Harlow ventilator which take the pipe line pressure and deliver it to the patient, act as constant flow devices during the inspiratory period. It follows that the flow pattern into the patient's lungs is uninfluenced by any change in the lung characteristics of that patient. The airway and alveolar pressure patterns and the volume patterns will be a result of this constant flow acting against the patient's lung characteristics. The simplest forms of constant flow generators are those in which the patient is connected directly to a high pressure gas source and the gas flow is limited by the placing of an adjustable high resistance, such as a needle valve, which limits the flow to suitable levels. This is the system which is used in the Bird, the Sheffield and the Loosco Infant Ventilators. A compressor or positive displacement pump can also supply a constant flow as they all supply a small volume of gas with each stroke at a high frequency and so give an almost continuous flow. This type of constant flow device is used to drive the bellows in the bottle of the Blease Pulmoflator. The constant inspiratory flow generator has many theoretical functional advantages, particularly if it is time cycled from inspiration to expiration. It is apparent that if a suitable constant flow can be selected and the length of the inspiratory phase also adjusted then the machine in effect behaves as a volume pre-set device, because the integral of the constant inspiratory flow and the duration of the inspiratory phase must equal the tidal volume. This is the method employed in the Loosco and Sheffield Infant Ventilators and is one of the reasons for their popularity. Other constant flow devices are pressure cycled at the end of the inspiratory phase and this can be a source of difficulty.

Another advantage of the constant flow inspiratory generator is that the volume and pressure patterns produced are readily observed, and these parameters can be used to detect changes in the compliance of the patient being ventilated. When the constant flow is applied, as seen in Fig. 8, there is a sharp rise in the airway pressure from *a* to *b* due to the constant flow having to raise the airway pressure to a value *b*, when the airway resistance will be overcome and gas will flow into the lungs. When gas enters the lungs the alveolar pressure rises in a linear fashion which is superimposed upon the initial rise *ab*. The rate of rise of the oesophageal pressure from *b* to *c* is a measure of the compliance of the patient.

If the airways resistance is high, as in Fig. 9, the rise in airway pressure before flow occurs into the lungs *ab* and the oesophageal pressure rises will be unchanged. Conversely, if the airways resistance is normal but the compliance is low, as in Fig. 10, then the rate of rise of airway pressure before the oesophageal pressure rises (i.e. *ab*) is normal, but thereafter the rate of rise of airway pressure (*bc*) is greatly increased because of the low compliance. In the three examples, Figs. 8, 9 and 10, the instrument was time cycled and in each case the duration of the inspiratory period was 1 second. As has already been stated a constant flow generator which is time cycled at the end of the inspiratory phase will produce a set tidal volume, no matter what the compliance or airways resistance of the patient, provided the flow and

note that the final airway pressure of the patient with the low compliance (Fig. 9) is very much higher than that of the normal patient (Fig. 8). This means that if the instrument is cycled by a pressure reached in the patient's airway then any changes in airways resistance or compliance must

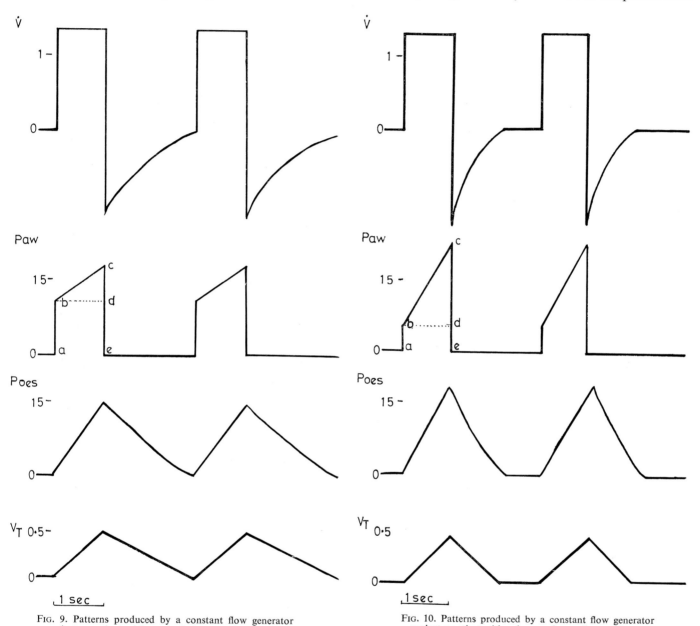

FIG. 9. Patterns produced by a constant flow generator against a patient with a raised airway resistance. Note the increase in the airway pressure *ab* necessary to overcome the resistance before flow occurs into the lungs. The increased work done against resistance is equivalent to area *abde*.

FIG. 10. Patterns produced by a constant flow generator against a patient with a decreased compliance. The steep rise *bc* is due to the decreased compliance and the work done against the decreased compliance is equivalent to area *bcd*.

the length of the inspiratory phase remain constant. This is evident in the three traces 8, 9 and 10, in which a 1 second inspiratory period was maintained with a constant flow of 1·25 litres per second; note that the tidal volume of one half litre remains the same no matter whether the airways resistance rises, as in Fig. 9, or the compliance falls, as in Fig. 10. Perhaps even more important is to

reduce the tidal volume because the final airway pressure remains the same unless it is altered by the operator when the changes in lung characteristics are noted. However, it should be remembered that changes in lung characteristics during prolonged artificial ventilation of patients are often rapid and not easy to detect. The pressure cycled machine needs constant surveillance and measurement of the tidal and minute volume. The reasons for this are evident if we examine Fig. 11, which is a trace of flow pressure and volume obtained from an asthmatic patient being ventilated with a Harlow ventilator, in which the inspiratory flow rate had been set too high (over 1·5 litres per second). The very rapid rise in airway pressure is very obvious, but even the high set cycling pressure is insufficient to overcome the airways resistance so that the oesophageal pressure rises to less

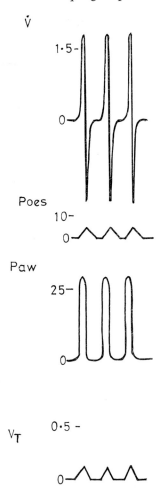

FIG. 11. Pressure, flow and volume patterns produced by a Harlow ventilator acting against a patient with a very high airways resistance. The flow is set too high and the rapid rise in airway pressure causes the machine to cycle at a high airway pressure before much flow of gas has entered the lungs.

than 5 cms of water. The tidal volume achieved is only 100 ml. It is very obvious from these traces that when a constant flow generator which is pressure cycled has the cycling process set too low to allow sufficient flow to enter the lungs, then the inspiratory phase will also be considerably shortened as it was in Fig. 1. These are some of the reasons why instruments such as the Bird ventilators are considered by many anaesthetists to be difficult to use.

If a constant flow, time cycled device is used to ventilate patients and an oscilloscope trace of airway pressure is obtained then changes in compliance and airways resistance can be recognized immediately from the oscilloscope

trace. Examination of Fig. 8, shows that an approximation of the work done against airways resistance is given by the oblong, *abde*, and that done against compliance by the triangle, *ebd*. The increase in work done against airways resistance is evident in Fig. 9, as the increase in the area of the oblong, *abde*, but because the compliance is unchanged the approximation of the work done against compliance, the area of triangle *bcd* remains unaltered from Fig. 8. Similarly, in Fig. 10, the work done against airways resistance is normal (area *abde*) but that done against compliance is very considerably increased as is evident by the increase in the area of triangle *bcd*.

The time cycled, constant flow generator such as the Loosco or Sheffield Ventilators are relatively simple devices. The valve which terminates the inspiratory flow from a constant flow generator is a solenoid operated valve the timing of which is controlled by an electronic circuit, there is no need therefore to describe these instruments in detail. Conversely, the pressure cycled constant flow generator is a difficult instrument to use correctly and therefore a description of one of these may not be out of place.

## THE BIRD VENTILATOR (Fig. 12)

During the inspiratory period the slide valve 1 and the bobbins 2 and 3 are held by the magnet 4 in the position shown in the diagram so that compressed gas entering at 5 passes through the ports in the slide valve to the venturi 6. If the venturi is open (depending upon the position of the control 7), then it may either entrain air or allow the flow to continue to raise the pressure in the chamber on the right hand side of the diaphragm 15. Pressure and flow are transmitted down the wide bore breathing hose to the patient via the inflating valve 8. A separate pressure lead 9 goes to the inflating valve 8 from the slide valve 1, and this maintains the balloon in the valve 8 inflated, and so closes the expiratory port. When the pressure in the chamber on the right of the diaphragm reaches that necessary to overcome the pull of the magnet 10, the slide valve is moved over to the left so that it then comes under the influence of the other magnet 4. When it is in this position the bobbin 2 on the slide valves cuts off the inflow of gas from the supply and the pressure in the chamber starts to fall to atmosphere because the inflating valve 8 is no longer held closed and the patient exhales to atmosphere. During this time the pressure in the small chamber 11 is held trapped and is released slowly by the adjustable bleed valve 12. When the pressure in this chamber falls to a sufficiently low level its piston, under the influence of the spring, moves across and pulls the lever 13 across to the right pushing the slide valve back until it is under the influence of the magnet 10, and is again held in the inspiratory position.

The analysis of the machine shows that it is a constant flow generator during inspiration because of the reserves of power contained in the compressed gas supply and that the rate of the flow can be adjusted by the resistance 14. Thus, the rate of inflation of the lungs can be controlled. The inspiratory to expiratory cycling occurs when a certain pressure is reached in the chamber, and this pressure is dependent upon the adjustable pull of the magnet 4. The length of the inspiratory phase, therefore, can be adjusted by the flow control and the tidal volume will be adjusted by the cycling pressure. If, however, during the inspiratory phase the air mix venturi is used then the machine will no longer behave as a constant flow generator because when a venturi works against a rising pressure the flow decreases as the pressure increases, therefore when the air mix is in use the latter part of

## THE CAPE VENTILATOR (Fig. 13)

The instrument is driven by an electric motor which compresses the inspiratory bellows $I$ by the Yorkshire linkage $Y$ and a rocking beam 1. The distance to which the beam compresses the bellows is adjustable by the movable fulcrum $F$. As the inspiratory bellows rise air is drawn in through the one-way valve 2 to fill the bellows and then during the compression stroke this valve closes and the inspiratory poppet valve 3 is opened by a camshaft driven

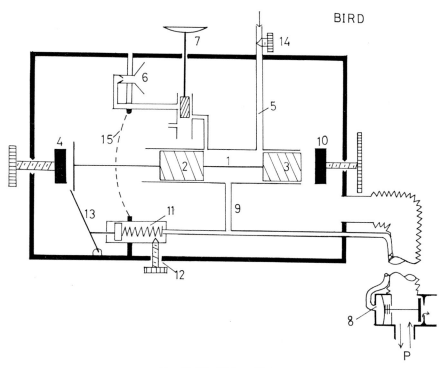

FIG. 12. The Bird ventilator.

1. Slide valve
2. } Bobbins
3. }
4. Magnet
5. High pressure "gas line"
6. Air entrainment venturi
7. "Air mix" control
8. Pressure controlled expiratory valve
9. Pressure lead to expiratory valve and timer
10. Magnet
11. Expiratory timer chamber
12. Bleed valve
13. Arm controlling expiratory movement of slide valve
14. Flow control
15. Diaphragm

inspiration will be prolonged because this decreasing flow will increase the time taken for the machine to reach its cycling pressure. The type of decrease in flow pattern described has no obvious clinical benefit.

There are a number of machines which are non-constant flow generators but because of their reserves of power, the pattern of flow is still dictated by the machine and is unaltered by the patient's characteristics. The commonest form of these non constant flow generators are derivations of the piston and cylinder machines which are driven by electric motors. One of the oldest examples of these which after considerable development is still in common use is that derived from the Smith Clarke ventilator, the Cape.

from the same motor. Inspiration then occurs when the bellows is driven downwards, the expiratory valve 4 being closed under the influence of another cam. The inspiratory phase is terminated when the position of the cams 3 and 4 are reversed and the speed at which this occurs is dependent upon the speed of the electric motor which is driving both the cam shaft and the bellows. The speed of these shafts is adjustable through a variable gear box. Expiration can occur passively through the non-return valve 5 out to atmosphere and is timed when the bellows $I$ has reached the end of its stroke, the inspiratory valve 3 closes and the expiratory valve 4 opens. A sub-atmospheric phase may be created by the beam 6 which drives an expiratory bellows so that when the patient's expired gases are directed into it, a sub-atmospheric phase is created. These expiratory bellows are always in operation, but the amount of gas that they take is dependent upon the variable resistance 7, which in its fully open position allows no sub-atmospheric phase to be created. The functional analysis of this machine therefore shows that it is time cycled both in the inspiratory/expiratory and expiratory/inspiratory change over and the ratio of inspiration to expiration is set by the position of

wave pattern of flow reaching a value of 1·2 litres per second can be predicted, as this flow pattern is set by the machine. The airway pressure follows a similar pattern to that of flow and it should be noted that the oesophageal pressure reaches some 12 cms of water, and the tidal volume is 0·5 litres. In trace 15, the machine is acting against a patient with a low compliance. Note that the pattern of flow remains exactly the same but now the airway pressure rises above 15 cm of water as does the oesophageal pressures. This must occur if the decreased

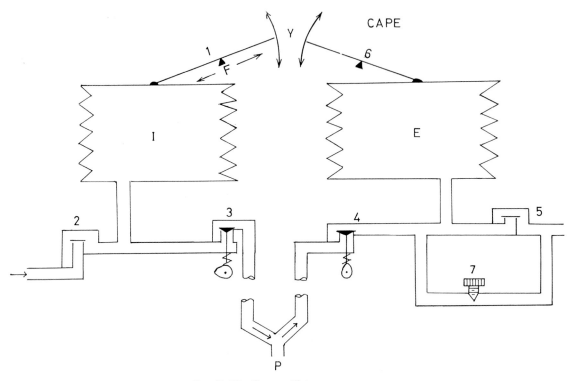

FIG. 13. The Cape ventilator.

| | |
|---|---|
| Y Yorkshire linkage | 1. Rocking beam |
| F Movable fulcrum | 2. Non return valve and fresh gas port |
| I Inspiratory bellows | 3. Inspiratory poppet valve |
| E Expiratory bellows | 4. Expiratory poppet valve |
| | 5. Expiratory non return valve |
| | 6. Rocking beam |

the cams on the cam shaft which controls the inspiratory and expiratory valves 3 and 4, this fixes the inspiratory/expiratory ratio to 1 to 2. The pattern of flow which is obtained from a piston moving down a cylinder from a crank shaft is that of a half sine wave and the Yorkshire linkage of the Cape produces an exactly similar pattern of flow. The machine is time cycled but it is volume pre-set, because this is adjusted by the position of the fulcrum and unless the pressure safety valve opens the set volume will be delivered by the machine.

Let us consider what volume pre-set really means by examining the flow, pressure and volume traces obtained with the Cape Ventilator in different situations. In Fig. 14 a Cape ventilator is being used to ventilate a patient with normal compliance and airway resistance. The half sine

compliance is to be overcome and the tidal volume maintained at 0·5 litres. In Fig. 16, the instrument is shown acting against a patient with a greatly increased airways resistance. The pattern of flow remains the same, but the airway pressure rises very significantly to 60 cms of water. It should be noted that this very high pressure applied to the airway does not reach the oesophagus, most of the pressure being lost in overcoming airways resistance. The tidal volume still remains the same

The Cape ventilator therefore compensates for changes in compliance and airways resistance because its reserves of power and mode of inspiratory to expiratory cycling are such that, the set tidal volume is always delivered to the patient. However, there are other machines which are not of the same functional behaviour but produce exactly similar results as far as the delivery of a set tidal volume is concerned. The two commonest examples are the Engström ventilator and the Blease Pulmoflator.

## THE ENGSTRÖM VENTILATOR

In this instrument, the piston 1 reciprocates in the cylinder, being driven by a variable speed gear box and

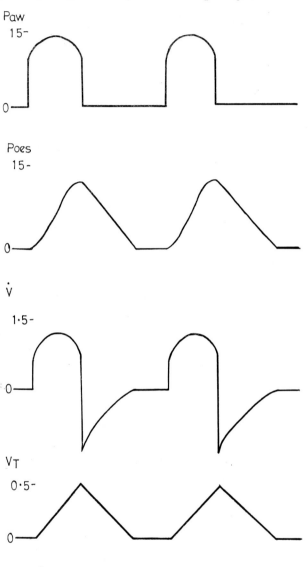

Fig. 14. Patterns produced by the Cape ventilator imposing its half sine wave flow against a patient with normal lungs.

electric motor. As the piston is driven to the right in the diagram (Fig. 17) the pressure rises on the right hand side of the piston and is transmitted to the reservoir bag 3 in the bottle so that the bag empties its contents via the non-return valve 4 into the patient. The rate at which this bag is emptied is determined by how much of the compressing gas from the cylinder is lost to atmosphere via the variable bleed valve 2. The volume of gas delivered by the piston is very greatly in excess of that required to compress

completely the bag in the bottle so that most of it is ejected to atmosphere through the valve 2. The pressure in the inspiratory circuit is measured by the water manometer 5, which can also act as a safety valve because the water level can be adjusted by the scissor legs 6. When the

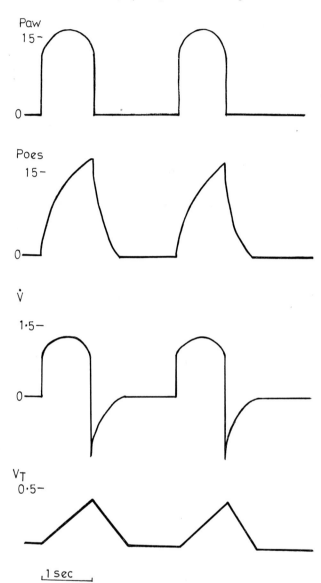

Fig. 15. Patterns produced by the Cape ventilator against a patient with a low compliance. Note that because the instrument is volume preset the tidal volume is unaltered but because of the decreased compliance the end inspiratory airway and oesophageal pressures are higher than Fig. 14, which also accounts for the short period required for expiratory flow. The machine will compensate for changes in compliance.

piston has travelled some 72 per cent of its way down the cylinder and before its velocity starts to decrease, a port in the connecting rod is opened to atmosphere, the pressure of the bag in the bottle returns to atmosphere and the inspiratory phase ends. The analysis of the inspiratory phase of the instrument therefore shows that because most of the flow from the cylinder is vented to atmosphere through the throttle, it acts as a pressure generator which increases during the inspiratory phase. The change from inspiratory to expiratory phase is time cycled being dependent upon the rate at which the piston moves down the cylinder until the port in the connecting rod

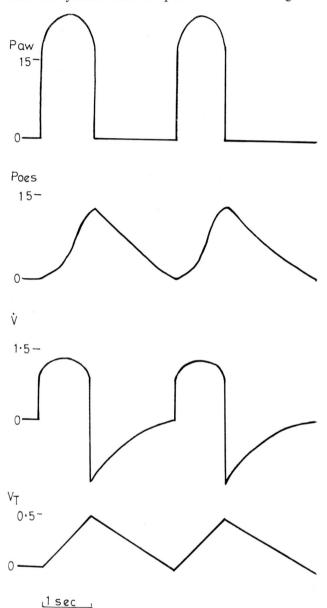

FIG. 16. Patterns produced by the Cape ventilator against a patient with a high airways resistance. Note the very high airway pressure which does not get through to the oesophagus because of the airways resistance. The slow expiratory flow and pressure decay patterns are obvious. Again the tidal volume does not alter because of the volume preset characteristics of the Cape.

opens, and this is controlled by the variable gear box and motor. Expiration will occur passively via the non-return valve 7, but a sub-atmospheric pressure can be produced if the compressed gas from the left hand side of the cylinder is directed to the venturi 8, which will then generate a sub-atmospheric phase in the expiratory circuit. The degree of sub-atmospheric pressure can be

regulated by the throttles 9 and 10. During the expiratory period the travel of the piston to the left will also create a sub-atmospheric phase from the right hand side of the cylinder and in the bag in the bottle which will therefore fill with air or anaesthetic gases via the port 11. The amount of gas which enters will be dependent upon the variable resistance 12, this is known as the dosing valve.

The machine has a fixed inspiratory/expiratory ratio of 1:2 which is set by the movement of the piston in the cylinder and by the ports in the connecting rod. The machine will only deliver that volume of gas which is allowed to be entrained by the dosing valve, but the reserves of pressure from the piston and cylinder are such that the volume that is in the bag will always be delivered to the patient, therefore the machine is a volume pre-set device.

## THE BLEASE PULMOFLATOR

In this machine (Fig. 18), a flow of air from a compressor enters the large chamber 1, via the port 2, and this constant flow from the compressor raises the pressure in the main chamber and pushes the diaphragm 3 over to the right. At the same time as the pressure is rising in the main chamber it is also compressing the bellows in the bottle 4, and driving the contents of that bellows on to the patient via the non-return valve 5. The pressure to which the bellows rise is dependent on the adjustment of the spring 13, but when the pressure has reached a level sufficient to move the diaphragm over to the right it moves the toggle mechanism 7, which opens the dumping valve 8, and allows the chamber pressure to return to atmospheric pressure. The rate at which the pressure in the chamber 1 rises is dependent upon how much of the gas from the compressor is allowed to bleed out to atmosphere through the adjustable throttle 12. Expiration occurs passively through the non return valve 9, into the chamber and out to atmosphere through valve 8. During the expiratory phase the flow of gas from the compressor can be directed to the left hand side of the venturi 10, in which case it will create a sub-atmospheric phase in the expiratory circuit. Conversely, it may be directed to the right hand side of the venturi assembly where it will cause a positive expiratory phase. During the expiratory phase the diaphragm starts to move back to the left and the rate at which it does this depends upon the leakage of atmospheric air inwards through the throttle 11, until the diaphragm has moved sufficiently over to the left to activate the toggle mechanism and close valve 8. The functional analysis of this machine shows that it is a constant flow generator during inspiration and the timing of the inspiratory phase can be controlled by the throttle 12. It is pressure cycled at the end of the inspiratory phase, and this is adjustable by the spring 13. It is possible, however, to limit the travel of the bellows 4, so that the volume delivered to the patient is limited. This means that the machine can behave in several different ways, for example, if the bellow's travel is not limited and the inflation pressure of the spring 13 is set to a low level, cycling will occur at a pressure which is closely related to that in the patient's airway but insufficient to empty the bellows. If, on the other hand, the bellows are set to limit the volume delivered and the inspiratory pressure is set to a maximum the volume will be expelled rapidly into the patient but the bellows pressure will continue to rise until the cycling pressure is reached. Most anaesthetists when they use this instrument ensure that the bleed valve from the main chambers is set to give a rapid rate of inflation which means that the machine is effectively volume cycled because once the volume has been delivered the pressure

because the constant atmospheric pressure then allows the higher alveolar pressure to fall by generating gas flow along the pressure gradient thus causing gas to leave the lungs. The flow, volume, airways and oesophageal pressure patterns which would result from this form of an expiratory phase can be seen in Figs. 1, 8 and 14. The only factors of importance are that if the compliance is reduced then the decay of alveolar pressure is faster because the oesophageal pressure reached at the end of inspiration is higher as in Figs. 2, 10 and 15. Conversely,

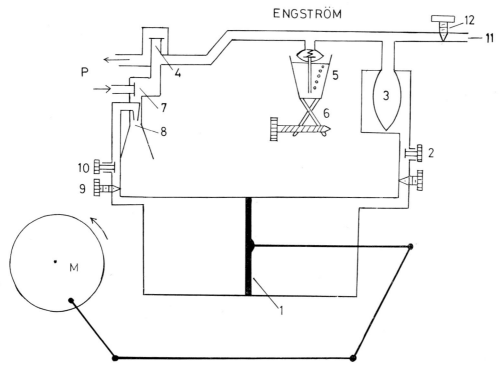

FIG. 17. The Engström ventilator.

M Shaft driven from electric motor and gear box
1. Piston
2. Adjustable bleed to atmosphere
3. Bag in bottle
4. Inspiratory non return valve
5. Water manometer
6. Height adjustment of manometer
7. Expiratory non return valve
8. Subatmospheric phase venturi
9. } Throttles controlling the magnitude of the sub-
10. } atmospheric phase
11. Fresh gas port
12. Dosing valve

will rise in the chamber 1 to reach the cycling pressure so rapidly that cycling occurs almost as soon as the volume has been delivered. This machine, therefore, can be regarded as a volume pre-set device.

### THE EXPIRATORY PHASE

We have seen that the tidal volume may enter the lungs under the influence of either pressure or flow generation and therefore it can only leave the lungs under the influence of one of these forces.

**Pressure Generation**

The most obvious method of pressure generation is to open a valve and allow the patient to vent to the atmosphere

if the airway resistance is increased then the decay of alveolar pressure is prolonged (Figs. 3, 9 and 16). Many anaesthetists are understandably reluctant to apply large airway pressures to patients because they consider that these pressures may greatly increase the mean intra-thoracic pressure and reduce the output of the heart. Consideration of Figs. 2, 10 and 15, however, shows that with a decreased compliance the duration of elevated alveolar pressure during the expiratory phase is greatly reduced so that some of the increased airway pressure is compensated for by the shortened expiratory period. Similarly, it will be noted that the very high airway pressures necessary to overcome high airways resistance do not lead to an increase in oesophageal pressure, but that there is a marked prolongation of the time taken for the oesophageal pressure to fall during expiration. (Figs. 3, 9 and 15). There is therefore a theoretical benefit in applying a sub-atmospheric phase to patients with a high airways resistance if it decreases the length of the expiratory phase by assisting expiratory flow.

We have seen that the gas from an inspiratory flow generator can be used during the expiratory phase to produce a sub-atmospheric pressure by directing it through a venturi (the Engström, the Loosco, the Bird and the Blease). Conversely, the inspiratory flow generator

such a constant flow device could produce a dangerous sub-atmospheric pressure in the airway. This is why such instruments have pressure limiting valves to prevent the airway and alveolar pressures ever becoming dangerously sub-atmospheric.

The various methods of obtaining sub-atmospheric expiratory phases either by constant pressure generation such as the venturi methods, or by flow generation such as the expanding bellows, all have varying effects on the expiratory flow and volume patterns, and they also alter

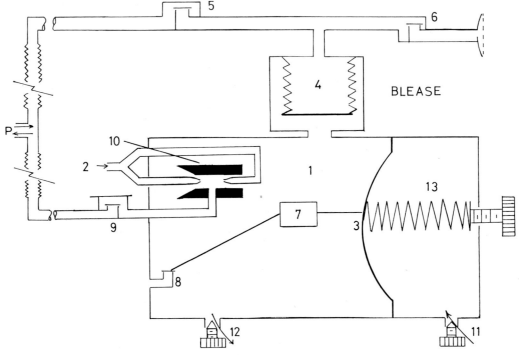

FIG. 18. The Blease Pulmoflator.

1. Large chamber
2. Pressure line from compressor
3. Diaphragm
4. Bellows in bottle
5. } Non return inspiratory valves
6. }
7. Toggle mechanism

8. Chamber pressure dumping valve
9. Expiratory non return valve
10. Expiratory phase venturi
11. Bleed valve timing expiratory phase
12. Bleed valve timing inspiratory phase
13. Spring controlling inspiratory pressure

can have its gas redirected against the expiratory flow to hold a small constant pressure above that of atmosphere during the expiratory phase, and this device is to be found on the Loosco Infant Ventilator, and the Blease Pulmoflator. This facility is of use during thoracic surgery to prevent collapse of the lower lung and may prevent the lungs reaching their 'closing volume' (*vide infra*) during artificial ventilation of the lungs.

We have also seen that in the Manley and the Barnet ventilators the constant flow of inspiratory gas can be harnessed to an expiratory bellows to produce a sub-atmospheric phase. However, when this method of flow generation is used to create a sub-atmospheric phase then it maintains a flow out of the lungs (because of the expansion of the bellows) irrespective of the pressure that results. Therefore if the compliance was decreased

the airway and alveolar pressure decay patterns in a complex manner. This complexity is increased by the addition of the necessary pressure limiting valves so that a general attempt to analyse the particular patterns is quite impossible, but if one has the knowledge of how the expiratory phase is controlled in the ventilator then it is relatively simple to describe the likely patterns which will occur. Finally, there is very little evidence to show that the different methods of obtaining a sub-atmospheric phase have any real clinical differences. What is of importance is the level of sub-atmospheric pressure which is applied and its duration, and in all instruments this can be controlled.

There are advantages in being able to retard expiration and maintain an end expiratory pressure above atmosphere to prevent mediastinal shift during thoracic surgery. The

Blease Pulmoflator and the Engström both have this facility. The use of the sub-atmospheric phase undoubtedly reduces the mean intrathoracic pressure, but it must be realized that most patients can compensate for increases in mean intrathoracic pressure, and that the sub-atmospheric phase should not be used routinely. Patients whose cardiac output falls during artificial ventilation have a cardio-vascular deficit. It is possible to overcome the effects of controlled ventilation on the circulation in these patients by the use of a sub-atmospheric phase but it should be stressed that this is a symptomatic form of treatment and should not be allowed to disguise the real physiological disturbance and a negative phase should not be used as a substitute for prompt and energetic treatment of the cardiovascular deficit.

The application of a sub-atmospheric expiratory phase in a patient with a very high airways resistance, such as those in status asthmaticus may, by increasing the pressure gradient between the alveoli and the airway during the expiratory phase, assist expiration so that the greatly increased functional residual capacity in these patients may be diminished.

However, it must not be forgotten that it is possible by the use of a sub-atmospheric expiratory phase to cause actual airway closure. It has been shown by Milic Emili *et al.*, 1970, that airway closure can occur in elderly patients at lung volumes which are near to their functional residual capacity and this will produce trapping of gas in the lungs which will adversely affect distribution of inspired gas. Obviously the use of sub-atmospheric phases in such patients will bring them much nearer to the 'closing volume' The traces seen in Fig. 19, were obtained when a chronic bronchitic patient was ventilated with the Cape Ventilator which was applying a 'negative phase'. The sub-atmospheric airway and oesophageal pressures can be clearly seen in the traces. When the negative phase was terminated, it can be seen that the expired tidal volume exceeded the inspired tidal volume and the tidal volume trace descends. This is due to the fact that the gas which had been trapped during the negative phase was released.

## CONCLUSIONS

A ventilator with sufficient reserves of power being operated by a person with a close understanding of its mechanical principles, will be capable of ventilating patients no matter what the condition of the lungs. It is necessary, of course, to adjust the machine so that any limiting factors in its performance can be overcome and the desired tidal volume delivered in the correct inspiratory period. It is because there are many limiting factors in the performance of these ventilators that some machines are easier to use than others. These difficulties are increased if any alterations in the characteristics of the patient markedly affect the function of the machine so that the minute volume of ventilation delivered may alter. However, there are certain basic principles common to all ventilators and once the user has gained an understanding of these principles and applied them to the

mechanism of the ventilator which he wishes to operate in clinical practice, then it is hoped many of the difficulties will be overcome. Volume preset machines which have large reserves of power such as the Engström, the Cape and the Blease are deservedly popular both in the operating theatre and the Intensive Therapy Unit because they are capable of ventilating patients no matter what the lung characteristics.

There are a large number of machines which are being marketed today which are capable of being used in almost

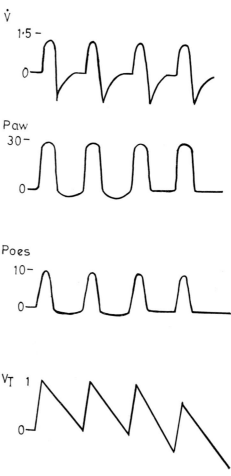

FIG. 19. Patterns produced by a chronic bronchitic patient when ventilated with and without a sub-atmospheric (negative) expiratory phase. When the sub-atmospheric phase was terminated the expired tidal volume exceeds the inspired due to release of gas 'trapped' in the lungs.

all the clinical situations in which they are required. However, there appears to be a tendency on the part of manufacturers to introduce technological innovations in the ventilators which allow the applied respiratory patterns to be varied within very wide limits. It seems to the author that these technological achievements have outstripped our clinical knowledge because there has as yet been no objective evidence showing the value of some of the respiratory patterns which have been described. It is hoped that this chapter may have given the user an understanding of some of the basic principles concerned in the operation of any ventilator so that it may be possible to allow him to use it to its best advantage.

### REFERENCES

Bergman, N. A. (1969), "Effect of Varying Respiratory Waveforms on Distribution of Inspired Gas during Artificial Ventilation," *Amer. Rev. of Resp. Dis.*, **100**, 518.

Milic-Emili, J., Leblanc, P. and Ruff, F. (1970), "Effects of Age and Body Position on Airway Closure in Man," *Brit. J. Anaesth.*, **42**, 86.

Mushin, W. W., Rendell-Baker, L., Thompson, P. W. and Mapleson, W. W. (1969), *Automatic Ventilation of the Lungs*, Oxford: Blackwell.

Otis, A. B., McKerrow, C. B., Bartlett, R. A., Mead, J., McIlroy, M. B., Selverstone, N. J. and Radford, E. P., Jr. (1956), "Mechanical Factors in Distribution of Pulmonary Ventilation," *J. appl. Physiol.*, **8**, 427.

Watson, W. E. (1962), "Observations on Physiological Dead Space during Intermittent Positive Pressure Respiration," *Brit. J. Anaesth.*, **34**, 502.

*CHAPTER* 2

# HUMIDIFICATION

## JOHN S. ROBINSON

The mucous membrane lining the respiratory tract from the anterior nares down to the alveoli is important in ensuring smooth pathways for the passage of respiratory gases, helping to prevent foreign particles entering the lungs and maintaining the humidity of the inspired gas. In the normal lung mucus lines the respiratory tract, with the exception of the alveoli and respiratory bronchioles, which are lined with a fluid containing surfactant. This respiratory mucus is derived from the uni-cellular goblet cells secreting mucin, and multi-cellular glands with both mucoid and serous secretions. The respiratory mucous membrane varies in different parts of the respiratory tract, in its thickness, its glands, blood supply and presence or absence of cilia. It seems likely that the differences are due to exposure to differing flow rates of respiratory gas and also to the water content of this gas. It is known that when major changes occur in the character or nature of gas flow for prolonged periods of time, alterations will occur in the mucous membrane of the area most involved. Thus a patient with a permanent tracheostomy is eventually able to humidify the inspired gas sufficiently to escape the problems of drying of secretions so evident in the immediate post-operative period.

Numerous studies of the humidification of inspired air, have shown that by the time the gas reaches the sub-glottic region of the trachea, it is not only warmed to 37°C, but also fully saturated with water vapour. This means that the water content is 44 mg per litre (44 grams per meter³ in SI units), which is the 'absolute' humidity at 37°C. Another way of expressing water content is to calculate the 'relative' humidity; that is, the water content of the gas expressed as a percentage of that of the gas fully saturated with water vapour at the same temperature. For example, air with a water content of 22 mg/l at 37°C has a relative humidity of 50 per cent at that temperature. Although both methods of expressing humidity are used,

when considering artificial methods of humidification of the inspired gas it is better to consider the water content of the inspired gas and its temperature because several types of humidifiers produce a water content above that of saturation at 37°C. Let us consider what happens when a person takes in a tidal volume of a litre of room air which has a temperature of 20°C, and a water content of 16 mg per litre. Heat and water must be transferred from the mucosa of the upper respiratory tract to the inspired air, the temperature must be raised from 20° to 37° and a further 28 mg of water vapour added to the gas. The mucosa becomes cooled during inspiration, both from the loss of heat required to raise the temperature of the inspired gas and by the provision of the latent heat of evaporation of the water entering the inspired gas. This cooling of the mucosa is counteracted by the return of the heat and water to the mucosa during expiration, because the alveolar air rewarms it and so undergoes a decrease in temperature and, therefore, a decrease in its water content before its exit to the atmosphere. If the relationship of the temperature of air to its possible water content is plotted, Fig. 1, it can be seen that the water content of the air rises exponentially with temperature, note that the steep portion of the exponential curve occurs at 37°C, these are the conditions in the trachea so that the mechanism of cooling of the upper respiratory tract will be maximally efficient at returning both heat and water to the mucosa. Under normal resting conditions, man looses some 250 ml of water and 350 calories per day from the respiratory tract. During severe exercise or ventilation of the lungs by dry gases, as in an extremely cold environment (where the water content of the air at 0°C or below is negligible), the subjects often complain of sore throats and severe thirst due to the drying of the mucosa and the excessive loss of water from the respiratory tract. The fact that there is little water in air at 0°C or below, means that a considerable quantity of heat is required from the upper respiratory tract, not only to warm the air, but to add extra water vapour to the inspired gas, however, when a person breathes out into a cold environment the mucosa of the upper respiratory tract does not fall to 0°C and therefore the condenser effect which conserves water and heat in the normal person is not as efficient and water conservation only reaches about 40 per cent efficiency. The upper respiratory tract does not suffer cold injury in an arctic environment because water has a high specific

that is a water content above 44 mg per litre of gas is desired, then the water must be carried as a micro-aerosol otherwise the gas temperature would have to be raised to a level at which injury to respiratory mucosa would occur. Further discussion, therefore, of the humidification of inspired gas evolves upon the physical principles and the methods of increasing the water content of gas delivered to the patient. The clinical significance of the results and efficiency of these methods will be discussed where appropriate.

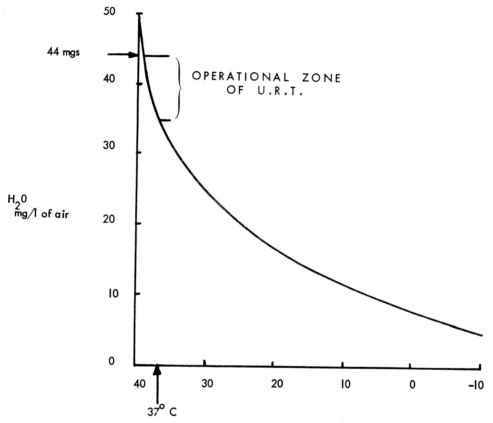

FIG. 1. The relationship of the temperature of air to its possible water content. The arrows indicate 100% relative humidity (saturation) at 37°C. The temperature and water content range found in the upper respiratory tract are also indicated.

heat) 1 calorie per gram) but air has a low specific heat of 0·34 calories per gram, so that the cold dry air requires but little energy to raise its temperature.

The efficiency of the upper respiratory tract as a means of humidification, is therefore very great, and it has long been recognized that when the naso-pharynx has been by-passed by endotracheal intubation or tracheostomy, there is a need for humidification of the inspired gases (Cushing and Miller, 1958; Burton, 1962; Sara, 1965). The precise value of water content that should be added to the inspired gases is still a matter of controversy. However, there is general agreement that the water content of the inspired gases should approach 44 mg per litre (100 per cent saturation) but whether this water should be entirely in the vapour phase by heating the inspired gas to 37°C, or whether it can be carried as micro-droplets in a colder gas is debatable. Certainly if super humidification is desired,

There are only three major methods of humidifying inspired gas.

1. A condenser can be introduced to the gas circuit close to the endotracheal tube or tracheostomy tube.

2. Micro droplets of water may be produced by an energy source, gas pressure, spinning disc or acoustic energy and these droplets added to the inspired gas as an aerosol.

3. Water may be added as vapour by passing the inspired gases over or through heated water.

**Condenser Humidifiers**

A condenser humidifier is simply an extension of the mechanism for conservation of water and heat of the upper respiratory tract. The humidifier consists of either a wire gauze or a tube consisting of a large number of small-bore tubes. During expiration the warm, wet gas from the patient passes over the gauze element which is at a lower temperature and therefore, the gas is cooled and water condenses out on to the element which itself warms up. During the following inspiration the gas entering the humidifier is warmed by the element and the water condensed on the element evaporates to humidify the gas.

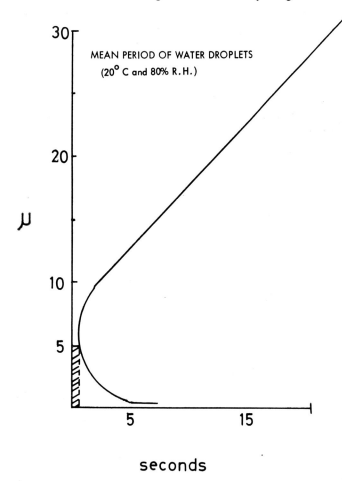

FIG. 2. The mean life period of water droplets in still air of 80% RH plotted against time. The range of droplet size produced by commercially available nebulizers lies in the hatched area. Note that the life period does not significantly increase until droplet sizes of 10 $\mu$ are reached. The increase in life period below 1 $\mu$ is due to the large increase in surface tension at such droplet size which increases its stability. Data from Green and Lane, 1957.

The dead space of these devices can be as low 17 ml and they may have a resistance to gas flow of one-tenth of that of the airways (0·1 cm $H_2O$/l/sec at 0·5 l/sec). The use of condenser humidifiers in small children is inappropriate because of the large dead space as well as the small, but significant increase in resistance. These humidifiers will be most efficient when the inspired gas is much colder than the expired gas, which is not the situation in which these humidifiers are usually used. Even so, if the patient is breathing room air at 20°C containing some 6 or 7 mg of water per litre (50 per cent RH), a good condenser

humidifier should be able to produce almost 42 or 43 mg per litre of water content in the inspired air (RH almost 100 per cent). However, if the patient is breathing dry gas from a cylinder or a piped gas supply, then the humidifier will not saturate the inspired gas with water, in fact only about 26 mg per litre of water (RH 60 per cent) are added to the inspired gas.

Condenser humidifiers have not found much favour in clinical practice, because they quickly become coated with secretions which raise their resistance to an unacceptable level, and as most patients requiring humidification are receiving dry gas from a high pressure supply their clinical efficiency is poor. Furthermore, Pennington et al. (1965) stated that to prevent colonization of the gauze with bacteria they should be changed three-hourly, which is impracticable.

### Aerosol of Water Droplets

Before considering the operational features of the humidifiers which produce micro-droplets of water in the inspired gas, it is worth studying the behaviour of such mists. When a micro-droplet of water is suspended in still air, the length of time that the droplet will remain before undergoing complete evaporation is dependent upon its diameter. In Fig. 2, the life period of a droplet in still air has been plotted against size and it can be seen that the mean life period of water droplets does not increase greatly until they are over 10 microns in diameter. Even so, it should be remembered that a droplet of 20 microns diameter will evaporate completely in still air at 20°C with an 80 per cent relative humidity within 2·4 seconds. (It can also be seen from Fig. 2, that when the droplet diameter is below 1 micron that the life period of the droplet increases.) The humidity of the gas medium is important, water drops of 10 $\mu$ diameter at 20° in still dry air would disappear in 60 milli seconds, but if the relative humidity of the air were raised to 80 per cent the life period would increase to 2·5 seconds. Microaerosols of water droplets therefore can only produce a level of water content in the inspired gas air of saturation or above, if the carrier gas is partially saturated with water vapour by passing it over heated water, or if there are a sufficient number of droplets present to produce saturation when the droplets evaporate.

Apart from the satisfaction of seeing dense clouds of mist issuing from a nebulizer, the stability of a micro aerosol of water in air has other advantages. If it is desired that droplets of water should precipitate out in the peripheral airways of the lung to loosen secretions by dissolving them in a water solvent, or by carrying drugs such as isoprenaline to portions of the lungs where they are more readily absorbed, then an understanding of the physical principles governing the life period of such droplets and their penetration into the lung fields is important. It is well known that although a visible fog or mist exists in the atmosphere, the relative humidity can be less than 78 per cent. This is because the vapour pressure above mists of small droplets is higher than elsewhere due to the high surface tension in the drops, which prevents their

*Established 1870*

## P. H. POPE & SON
**STOCK AND SHARE BROKERS**

Partners:
L. F. ROBERTS
W. H. LOWE, F.C.A.

Associate:
J. E. HARPER, F.C.A.

TEL. No. STOKE-ON-TRENT 25154 (4 LINES)

V.A.T. No. 278 9217 11

*6 Pall Mall,*

*Hanley,*

*Stoke-on-Trent*

ST1 1EU

BH

14th February, 1984.

Dear Dr. Matthew,

    We refer to your purchase of 1,000 Brunswick Oil NL Ordinary Shares of $1.00 on 24th January, we enclose herewith Bought Transfer Form relating to this stock and would be obliged if you would sign this where indicated and return it to this office as soon as possible.

Yours faithfully,

Dr. Matthew,
35, Hilton Road,
Harpfields,
Stoke-on-Trent,
Staffs.

J. H. POPE & SON
STOCK AND SHARE BROKERS

MEMBERS OF THE STOCK EXCHANGE

HH                                    14th February, 1984.

Dear Dr. Matthew,

We refer to your purchase of 1,000 Brunswick Oil N.L. ordinary shares of £1.00 on 24th January. We enclose herewith Bought Transfer form relating to this stock and would be obliged if you would sign this where indicated and return it to this office as soon as possible.

Yours faithfully,


Dr. Matthew,
35, Hilton Road,
Harpfields,
Stoke-on-Trent,
Staffs.

evaporation to raise the relative humidity to 100 per cent. When a cold water mist is generated by a nebulizer, the temperature of the mist may be a little below that of the room and although the mist appears dense there may not be enough mass of particulate water present to raise the humidity of the gas (that is water in the vapour phase) to the level of 44 mg per litre at 37°C, i.e. 100 per cent saturation. It is worth remembering when considering these droplet concentrations that a town fog which gives a visibility of only about 20 metres contains but $10^4$ particles/cm$^3$ so that a dense fog from a nebulizer is in itself inadequate indication that the water content of the inspired gas is high. The life period of a droplet may be increased by the use of a monolayer to increase its surface tension, such as the addition of propylene glycol to the water.

Another factor must be considered, other than that of the droplets evaporating to produce saturation of the inspired gas, that is the stability of the droplets themselves. They must not precipitate out in the upper airways before the inspired gas is warmed sufficiently for the particulate water to enter the vapour phase. Consideration of the life period of a droplet of water in the inspired gas is complicated by the fact that the air is moving and is turbulent. However, it is simpler to consider first the half life of the droplet in still air, and then to see how turbulence will affect it. The half life of the droplet in still air is given by the relationship of the Smoluchowski theory (Davis and Rideal, 1963), the relationship is:

$$t/_2 = \frac{(3\,\eta)}{4k\,Tno} \frac{(a\quad\quad)}{a + 0\cdot9\,f}$$

where $a$ is the radius of the droplet
$\quad\quad no \quad$ the number of droplets
$\quad\quad \eta \quad$ the viscosity of the gas medium
$\quad\quad k, \quad$ the Boltzman constant
$\quad\quad T, \quad$ the temperature °Kelvin
$\quad\quad f, \quad$ the mean free path

This is really a derivation of Stokes' Law, which is an expression of the velocity at which a sphere drops in a viscous medium. However, Stokes' Law needs to be corrected in several respects, particularly because of the inhomogeneity of the medium; by this, it is meant that the drops are so small that they fall in between the molecules of the carrier gas and therefore are not continually opposed by the viscous medium. It is important to note that the half life of a droplet cloud is very dependent upon the number of drops present because this appears twice in the equation, as the number of droplets, and also as the mean free path which is the distance between the droplets. It seems therefore, that we can expect that drops dispersed in a dense mist will disappear more rapidly due to collision and precipitation. In fact the Smoluchowski equation gives values of 3·7 sec for water when nebulized by ultrasonic means but the mist produced by a gas-driven nebulizer might in part be expected to last up to 5 or 6 seconds. It might be thought, therefore, that the gas-driven nebulizer, by producing a more stable mist has greater clinical usefulness but unfortunately the density of the mist in most of these devices (*vide infra*) is insufficient to raise the

saturation of the inspired gas to 100 per cent and therefore although the dense mist from ultrasonic nebulizers has a short life, its very density makes it useful for spontaneously-breathing patients. But well-designed heated gas-driven nebulizers producing an aerosol in a gas of high relative humidity can produce supersaturation far more cheaply and with a more stable mist.

We must now consider the important effects of the turbulent gas flow in the airways. It is known that the deposition of droplets is governed by the relationship found by Friedlander and Johnson (1957). This states that the inertial impaction of the deposition of droplets is directly proportional to the number of droplets, the fourth power of the velocity of the droplet, the fourth power of the diameter of the droplet and inversely proportional to the distance to be travelled across the gas stream. The relationship allows us to determine where droplets of particular diameters will be deposited in an idealized respiratory tract and this is given in Fig. 3. It can be seen that the alveolar sacs and ducts are reached by droplets of between 1 and 3 $\mu$, bronchioles by droplets of approximately 6 $\mu$ and the bronchi and upper airways by droplets of about 10 $\mu$. Thus, if deposition of water droplets is desired throughout the airways, it is necessary to have a spectrum of droplet sizes between 2 and 10 $\mu$ with a total water content over 44 mg/l. The advantages of deposition of particulate water in the bronchial tree may be questioned but there is good clinical evidence that the deposition of particulate water may act as a solvent to viscid sputum which is retained in the bronchi and bronchioles so that it may be moved to the major bronchi where it can be voided.

It must be remembered however, that the use of ultrasonic nebulizers which are capable of producing super saturation of the gas inspired into the airways is not without its dangers. Butler and Cheney, (1969), showed that the use of an ultrasonic nebulizer increased the airways resistance and also there are dangers of water intoxication when ultrasonic nebulizers are used on infants. Jones, Clarke and Oliver (1969) have shown the importance of the fluid lining layer in increasing the resistance to gas flow in tubes due to two-phase liquid flow. The increase in resistance to gas flow is not due to the fluid reducing the diameter of the tube but to energy losses from the gas due to the formation of standing waves in the liquid layer. This may be the cause of the reported increase in airway resistance when high-density mists are inhaled, which may increase the thickness of the fluid lining.

Using these facts and theories, it is possible to appraise critically the various types of nebulizers and humidifiers in clinical use.

### Ultrasonic Nebulizers

There are two types of ultrasonic nebulizers in use. In the first type, Fig. 4A, a layer of water of 2 cms or more in depth lies on top of the transducer, which vibrates at 1·5 MH₃ (1,500,000 cycles per second). The very high frequency and intensity of the energy produces a cavity in the layer of water and where this cavity reaches the surface the droplets escape. The count median diameter (C.M.D.)

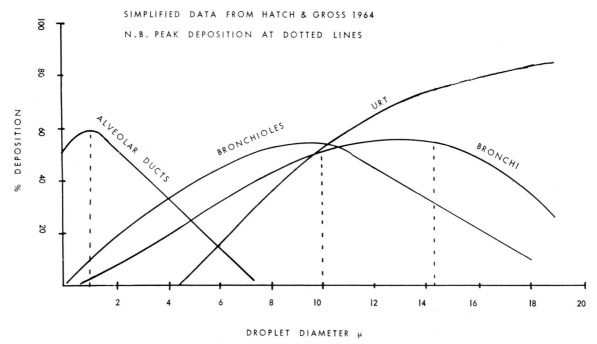

FIG. 3. The sites of maximum deposition of droplets expressed as percentage deposition against droplet size.

of the droplets produced by this form of nebulization is given by the relationship

$$C.M.D. = 0.34 \sqrt[3]{\frac{8k\pi\sigma}{\rho f^2}} \quad (\text{Lang 1962})$$

where $f$ is the frequency of the exciting sound in HZ, $\sigma$ is the surface tension of dynes per cm and $\rho$ density is in grams/cm³.

In the other type of nebulizer, Fig. B, the water is added

drop by drop on to the surface of the transducer and it immediately breaks up into capillary waves and microdroplets. The droplet size has been shown to be almost directly related to the frequency of the exciting sound (Lane and Green, 1969), and as these nebulizers (e.g. the LKB) run at 3·5 MHz the droplet size is more uniform and of approximately 1 micron in diameter. In the other type of nebulizer the viscosity and density of the liquid are important. Obviously, if the viscosity of the liquid is low

**A**

$$C.M.D. = 0.34 \sqrt[3]{\frac{8k\pi\delta}{\rho f_2}}$$

**B**

$$C.M.D. \propto f$$

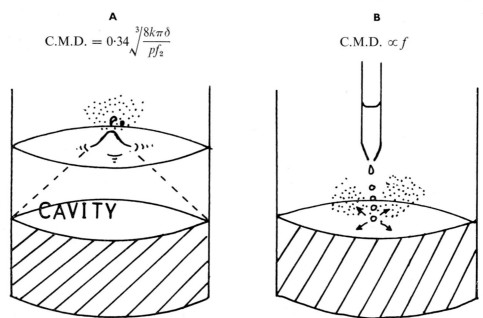

FIG. 4. The two methods of ultrasonic generation of a micro aerosol. Type A, acoustic energy produces cavitation in a layer of liquid and the aerosol escapes at the surface. The count median diameter of the droplets is given by the equation. In type B, the liquid is dropped upon the surface of the transducer, and is broken up into a micro aerosol and the count median diameter of the droplets is almost directly proportional to the frequency at which the transducer vibrates.

and the density high, then very small droplets may be formed (e.g. with alcohol). The density of the mist produced by ultrasonic nebulizers is dependent upon the flow of gas through the nebulizer, but most well-designed ultrasonic humidifiers can give a mist (water) density of between 100 and 200 mg/l.

### The Gas-driven Nebulizer

Gas-driven nebulizers produce droplets of a larger diameter than those produced by ultrasonic means. The principle of the action of these humidifiers is that a high-pressure gas source (20 to 60 psi) issues as a jet through a fine nozzle (Fig. 5). By the Bernoulli effect the pressure at the jet will be low because it is least where the velocity of gas flow is greatest, therefore, because this gas jet passes across the tip of another tube which extends down into the liquid reservoir, a suction effect draws up the water which is then broken up into a spray. This spray contains a very large spectrum of droplets from 5 to 20 $\mu$ but the number of small droplets is entirely dependent upon the

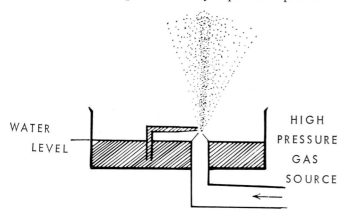

BERNOULLI EFFECT NEBULIZER

Fig. 5

pressure driving the jet. It is for this reason that efficient nebulizers require to be run at high pressure (60 psi). The large droplets produced from such a primary spray are quickly baffled out by the walls of the nebulizer. This is particularly so if as in Fig. 6, the gas stream is made to turn through 90°. There is a further method of reducing the spectrum of droplet sizes and producing an almost uniform mist of droplets of approximately 5 microns: i.e. to direct and impact the jet of gas and water onto an anvil. The inertial impaction of the droplets on the anvil removes the larger droplets proportionately to the square of their diameter, in other words, four times as many droplets are removed if their diameter is doubled. Furthermore, the removal of the droplets is directly proportional to their velocity so that once again a high-pressure gas source is necessary. The smaller droplets are swept to either side of the gas stream and, by using such a system a well-designed nebulizer can produce a mist density of up to 38 mg/l. However, few nebulizers reach this performance. (*Vide infra.*)

### Spinning-disc Humidifier

In this device, water is drawn up from the reservoir by means of an Archimedean screw so that it impinges on the surface of the rapidly rotating disc which flings water particles into the delivery system by the influence of centrifugal force. These methods produce a very wide range of droplet sizes and consequently very low mist density.

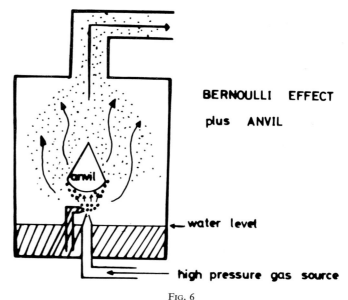

BERNOULLI EFFECT plus ANVIL

← water level

← high pressure gas source

Fig. 6

### Heated Water Humidifiers

In these devices, a water reservoir is heated by a thermostatically controlled electric heating element and the gas is driven over the surface of the water with or without baffling before delivery to the patient (Marshall and Spalding, 1953; Spalding, 1956). These humidifiers are surprisingly efficient and not particularly susceptible to changes in flow of gas being passed through them (e.g. within the clinical range). These humidifiers can produce a water content of between 35 and 40 mg./l. However, there are certain disadvantages.

Although they are able to produce a state of relative humidity of 90 per cent, this is usually at the point of emergence from the humidifier, and by the time the inspired air has passed down the delivery tube to the patient, the temperature may well have dropped considerably from the temperature of the humidifier resulting in loss of $H_2O$ by condensation. This difficulty has been overcome by lagging of the delivery tubes, but this makes them cumbersome. Alternatively, as in the Bennett cascade humidifier, the heater of the water bath is controlled by a thermostat: in the inspiratory limb of the delivery tube, so that the inspired air has a temperature of 37° and a humidity of 44 mg/l. Continued breathing of inspired air at 37°C has been reported to be the cause of hyperexia in several patients, but if the temperature of the inspired air is reduced to 32°C little harm should result, because this is the temperature that would be expected in the trachea of a spontaneously breathing patient without tracheostomy or endotracheal intubation and the reduction in humidity is only 10 mg/l of water at 32°C.

Heated water humidifiers, if they are to be efficient at high gas flows must either present a large surface area of heated water to the gas or the water must be heated to a level which causes the inspired air to have a temperature above 37°C. For this reason efficient heated water humidifiers have a large compressible volume of gas; above the water level which so raises the internal compliance of the ventilator that the set inspiratory flow and pressure patterns may be altered to unacceptable forms. Most of these defects are overcome in the humidifier designed by Spence and Melville (1972). The surface area of the heated water is greatly increased by passing the inspired gas over a large area, anodized, heated aluminium scroll lined with absorbent paper. The compressible volume ranges from 520–710 ml. The delivery hose is also heated and thermostatically controlled to deliver a gas mixture to the trachea of 37°C under standard conditions of gas flow. The instrument is capable of producing relative humidities in excess of 90 per cent under normal conditions of use.

### Performance of Various Humidifiers

The data that follow are taken from the work of Hayes and Robinson (1970), in which the delivery of water to a model lung system was measured by means of a mass spectrometer. A summary of the results appear in Table 1.

### Humidification by Aerosols

From the table, it can be seen that the small anvil-type gas-driven nebulizers which are intended to be run at 20 psi (Wright, 1958) have a performance which is so poor it must be regarded as inadequate because it is scarcely capable of humidifying dry gases beyond the saturation found in the ambient air. The nebulizers in the Bird apparatus can be seen to be very flow-dependent. This is particularly so because the flow control on the Bird ventilator not only controls the supply of gas to the patient but also that required to drive the nebulizer. This effect can be overcome by interposing the Bird 'low flow cartridge' between the gas supply and the ventilator which re-routes the supply to the nebulizer independently of that going through the ventilator. Nebulizers may be inserted into a circuit so that all the gas passes through the nebulizer (mainstream, Fig. 7) or sidestream in which the water aerosol is injected into the main gas stream. Sidestream humidification is quite inadequate and should only be used for administering drugs. It might also be noticed that when a Bird circuit includes a mainstream and sidestream micro nebulizer then the baffling of the droplets by this nebulizer causes precipitation and reduces the mist density. The common practice of leaving the micro nebulizer in the circuit should therefore be avoided. The ability of Ohio heated, gas-driven nebulizer to produce supersaturation (51 mg/l) reinforces the arguments about mist stability and relative humidity of the carrier gas. Amongst the other gas-driven humidifiers, it might be noted that the clouds of cold mist produced by the floating jet humidifiers, (e.g. The Win Liz, Fig. 8) have a very disappointing per-

TABLE 1

| Humidifier | Ventilator | Range of water content g/m³ | Range of water saturation % |
|---|---|---|---|
| Harlow gas-driven nebulizer | Harlow | 20–30 | 45–68 |
| Bird gas-driven nebulizer mainstream | Bird | 22–23 | 49–53 |
| Bird gas driven neublizer plus low flow cartridge | Bird | 23–32 | 53–72 |
| East Heated blow over | Barnet Mk III | 34–40 | 77–91 |
| Cape heated blow over | Cape | 26–28 | 60–64 |
| Bennett Cascade | Bennett PR2 | 70–76 | 31–33 |
| Loosco heated bubble through | Loosco Infant | 72 | 32 |
| De Vilbiss ultrasonic | Harlow | 23–92 | 53–209 |
| Mist-o-Gen Ultrasonic | Bourns Infant | 22–27 | 49–174 |
| Saline Drip | Harlow Spontaneous | 15 | 34 |
| Bird mainstream | Spontaneous | 20–24 | 45–55 |
| Air Shields gas-driven nebulizer | Spontaneous | 21 | 47 |
| Air Shields Spinning disc | Spontaneous | 20 | 45 |
| Puritan bubble through | Spontaneous | 6 | 14 |
| Wright gas-driven nebulizer | Spontaneous | 16 | 36 |
| Ohio heated gas-driven nebulizer | Spontaneous | 42–51 | 96–116 |
| Win Liz gas-driven nebulizer | Spontaneous | 17–20 | 36–43 |
| Marshall Spalding heated blow over | Spontaneous | 31 | 70 |
| DeVilbiss ultrasonic blow over | Spontaneous | 21–55 | 47–126 |

formance, which bears out the contention that cold mists are not always adequate to produce saturation of the inspired gas. These nebulizers produce a mist by siting a high-pressure gas jet within a thin film of water held in position by surface tension; providing the jet is sufficiently fine the film is broken up into tiny particles which are carried along by the gas stream, while the continuity of the film is maintained by more water drawn towards the jet by the Bernoulli effect. The position of the jet relative

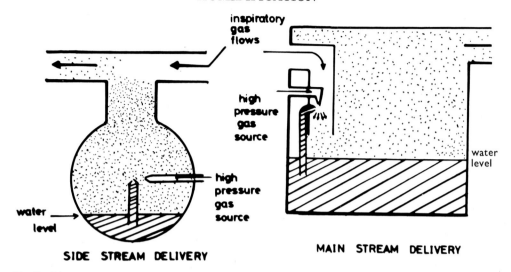

FIG. 7. Sidestream and Mainstream methods of interposing a gas driven nebulizer in the inspiratory limb of a ventilator circuit.

to the water level is critical and therefore the former floats within the reservoir.

The cascade type of humidifier (Fig. 9), which is incorporated in the Bennett circuit is of high efficiency when adjusted to deliver gases to the temperature of 37°C. This ingenious arrangement allows gas under pressure to push down the water level in the cascade tower until the foot of the tower is cleared. The pathway is then created for

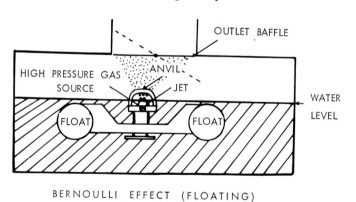

FIG. 8. The floating Bernoulli effect nebulizer.

the gas to pass to the underside of the floor of the cascade chamber and escape through the perforation; simultaneously, the general water level in the container rises slightly so that a small quantity spills into the tower by way of the port in the side of the tower. The water is intercepted therefore, by the gas stream which gives rise to a foam which is delivered as a mist to the inspiratory flow (Waynans and Rigley, 1966).

## Hot-water Humidifier

The hot-water humidifiers are surprisingly efficient even in the unsophisticated bubble through heated arrangements of the Loosco infant ventilator, because of the small flow of gas being bubbled through they are adequately humidified.

## Ultrasonic Nebulization

The ultrasonic nebulizers are capable of producing up to 100 g water/m³ and it is suggested that the setting of the output of these humidifiers is critical if over- or under-humidification is to be avoided. The correct setting for any given gas flow through such an ultrasonic nebulizer

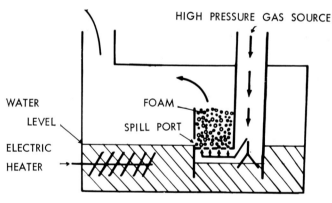

FIG. 9. The cascade humidifier.

may be determined by immersing the delivery hose in water at a temperature of 37°C in such a manner that only the outlet protrudes above the surface. The gain of the transducer amplifier is then decreased until the issuing mist is no longer visible, this method gives a mist density approximately that of the saturated vapour pressure of water at 37°C.

## Other Methods of Humidification

There are still some humidifiers available in which gas is meant to be humidified by bubbling the gas directly through the water without this being heated. These bubble humidifiers are dangerously inadequate and are best ignored as a means of humidification. Similarly, although in wide clinical use, the installation of saline or the water by a drip into the trachea should not be relied on to produce humidification of the inspired gas.

## Conclusions

Theory and practical measurement show that there are only three types of humidifiers of any practical clinical value. The most efficient, the ultrasonic humidifier is capable of producing any range of humidification. The precise value of the density of the mist delivered must be adjusted to the clinical needs of the patient. The gas-driven heated nebulizer-type of humidifier can be extremely efficient: as they may be one-sixth of the cost of ultrasonic humidifiers, and their droplet size is theoretically of greater advantage than the small uniform droplet size of the ultrasonic humidifier. Their value for the humidification of gases during mechanical ventilation of the lungs should be more closely examined, but they do require a high-pressure gas source. Moreover, because such humidifiers tend to be more flow-dependent than the ultrasonic humidifiers, they require greater care in the delivery of the vapour to the tracheostomy of a spontaneously breathing patient.

The ultrasonic humidifiers produce a greater mist density which allows inefficient delivery and greater dilution of the micro aerosol by the carrier gas. The hot-water humidifiers, although often decried as being old-fashioned, are surprisingly efficient and have a definite place, particularly when incorporated in a ventilator circuit. They must be provided with efficient safety devices because of the danger of overheating due to thermostat failure.

## REFERENCES

Burton, J. D. K. (1962), "Effect of Dry Anaesthetic Gases on the Respiratory Mucosa," *Lancet*, i, 235.
Cheney, F. W. and Butler, J. (1969), "The Effect of Ultrasonically Produced Aerosols on Airway Resistance in Man," *Anaesthesiology*, **29**, 1099.
Cushing, I. E. and Miller, W. F. (1958), "Considerations in Humidification by Nebulisation," *Dis. Chest.*, **34**, 388.
Davies, J. T. and Rideal, E. K. (1963), *Interfacial Phenomena*, p. 355. London: Academic Press.
Green, H. L. and Lane, W. R., (1957) *Particulate Clouds, Dust, Smoke and Mist*, 3rd ed. Princeton: D. Van Nostrand.
Harch, T. F. and Gross, P. (1964), *Pulmonary Deposition and Retention of Inhaled Aerosols*. New York: Academic Press.
Hayes, B. and Robinson, J. S. (1970), "An Assessment of Methods of Humidification of Inspired Gas," *Brit. J. Anaesth.*, **42**, 94.
Johnstone, H. F. and Friedlander, (1961), *Inhaled Particles and Vapour*, Ed. Davies, C. N. N. York: Permagon Press.
Jones, J. G., Clarke, S. W. and Oliver, R. W. (1969), "Two-phase Gas-liquid Flow in Airways," *Brit. J. Anaesth.*, **41**, 192.
Lang, R. J. (1962), "Ultrasonic Atomisation of Liquids," *J. acoust. Soc. Amer.*, **34**, 6.
Marshall, J. and Spalding, J. M. K. (1953), "Humidification in Positive Pressure Respiration for Bulbo Spinal Paralysis," *Lancet*, **2**, 1022.
Pennington, J. H., Lumley, J. and O'Grady, F. (1966), "The Growth of Ps.Pyocyanea in Garthur Condenser Humidifiers," *Anaesthesia*, **21**, 211.
Sara, C. (1965), "The Management of Patients with a Tracheostomy," *Med. J. Aus.* **1**, 99.
Spalding, J. M. K. (1956), "Humidifier for Patients Breathing Spontaneously," *Lancet*, **2**, 1140.
Spence, M. and Melville, A. W. (1972), "A New Humidifier," *Anesthesiology*, **36**, 89.
Wright, B. M. (1958), "A New Nebuliser," *Lancet*, **2**, 24.
Wynands, J. E. and Wrigley, F. R. H. (1966), "A Simple Method of Humidifying Gases," *Canad. Anaesth. Soc. J.*, **13**, 403.

*CHAPTER* 3

# THE DESIGN AND CALIBRATION OF VAPORIZERS FOR VOLATILE ANAESTHETIC AGENTS

## D. W. HILL

The saturated vapour pressure of most volatile anaesthetic agents at room temperature is generally much greater than the partial pressure required to produce clinical anaesthesia. The function of an anaesthetic vaporizer is to bring about dilution of the saturated vapour in a controlled fashion which is reasonably independent of both changes in the ambient temperature and the volume flow of gas perfusing the vaporizer.

### The Variation of the Saturated Vapour Pressure with Temperature

When a liquid is in contact with its vapour inside a closed container, a state of equilibrium is attained in which as many molecules leave the liquid by evaporation per second to escape into the vapour phase as rejoin the bulk liquid per second. Under these conditions, the vapour above the liquid is said to be fully saturated. This is the condition that is obtained in the vaporizing chamber of a calibrated vaporizer. The vapour molecules bombard the walls of the vessel and give rise to a definite pressure, known as the Saturated Vapour Pressure (s.v.p.). The s.v.p. depends only upon the nature of the liquid and its temperature. For practical purposes, within the range of ambient pressures encountered during surgery, its value is usually taken to be independent of the barometric pressure. This fact is important in discussing the performance of vaporizers under hypobaric and hyperbaric conditions.

For a given volatile anaesthetic agent, the graph of s.v.p. (P) against ambient temperature (t) is a smooth curve. An equation can be fitted to each curve, those for diethyl ether and halothane being:

Ether: $\log_{10} P = 6.78574 - (994.195)/(t + 220)$

Halothane: $\log_{10} P = 6.8468 - (1079.74)/(t + 222.06)$

In these equations, the s.v.p. ($P$) is given in torr and the temperature ($t$) in °C. The saturated vapour pressure of halothane is 243 torr at 20°C. From a knowledge of the s.v.p. (Table 1) of a particular agent over the required

Table 1

Vapour Pressure of Volatile Anaesthetics
at 20°C.

| | |
|---|---|
| diethyl ether | 442 mmHg |
| trichlorethylene | 58 mmHg |
| chloroform | 160 mmHg |
| halothane | 243 mmHg |

temperature range, it is now possible to arrange to systematically dilute the saturated vapour to levels commensurate with clinical requirements.

When a gas stream is passed through the vaporizing chamber, it will sweep away the most 'energetic molecules', where these will have overcome the inwardly-directed attractive forces present at the liquid-vapour interface. As a result the mean energy, and hence the temperature, of the liquid falls as evaporation proceeds.

**Plenum Vaporizers**

The glass bottle vaporizers found on anaesthetic machines are of the plenum type which are perfused with fresh gas from the machine. The term is derived from the plenum system of ventilation in which gas is forced into the system. The vaporizer (Fig. 1) consists basically of a vaporization chamber which is perfused with a fraction of the fresh gas flow and adds to this a proportion of anaesthetic vapour. At low flows through the vaporizer care must be taken to ensure that the gas picks up sufficient of the vapour, particularly in the case of a heavy vapour such as halothane. The larger fraction of the fresh gas flow is then added to the output from the vaporizing chamber in order to dilute the issuing vapour to the required clinical concentration.

**The Boyle Bottle Vaporizer**

The simplest type of plenum vaporizer is seen in the well-known Boyle bottle vaporizer. A cylindrical tap splits the gas into bypass and vaporizing chamber flows. Movement of a plunger allows the distance between the port delivering gas into the chamber and the surface of the liquid anaesthetic to be varied. The vaporizing chamber is a simple glass bottle which does not contain any wicks. The variation of the output from an ether Boyle bottle with the setting of the tap control lever and the position of the plunger has been discussed by Macintosh, Mushin and Epstein (1958). Stability of the output of a vaporizer with time really means stability with regard to a fall in temperature of the vaporizing liquid. Since glass is a poor

conductor of heat, there is insufficient inflow of heat to hold the temperature of the liquid constant. As the temperature falls, so the output concentration decreases significantly with time. Halothane is not as volatile as ether (its saturated vapour pressure at 20°C is approximately one-third of an atmosphere compared with one-half for ether). Thus cooling problems are not so serious when halothane is vaporized. Since lower concentrations are required for halothane than for ether, the halothane Boyle bottle uses only the control tap and has no moving plunger, the gas entering the bottle from fixed holes in the inlet pipe, above the surface of the halothane. A simple glass bottle holding the liquid agent does not always produce fully saturated vapour, so that the calibration

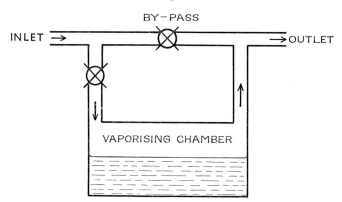

FIG. 1. Simple plenum vaporizer.

from this type of vaporizer is not reproducible. In addition, when the vaporizer has been standing for some time, a considerable concentration of vapour builds up above the liquid. This gives rise to a significant 'surge' of vapour when the vaporizer is first turned on (Jennings and Hersant, 1965). A surge of vapour may also be delivered if the vaporizer is shaken. Seed (1967) describes a baffle device fitted into the bottle of a Boyle halothane vaporizer to prevent agitation of the halothane when the anaesthetic machine is moved.

These deficiencies have led to the development of a number of more sophisticated, although more expensive, vaporizers usually having wicks and some method of compensation for the fall in temperature which occurs as the liquid vaporizes. For the low flow rates encountered in small animal anaesthesia the cooling effect is minimal. Parbrook (1966) describes an all-glass simple by-pass vaporizer for such applications.

**Improved Plenum Vaporizers**

Pearce (1962) describes a version of the Boyle halothane vaporizer in which the temperature of the halothane is measured by a small bimetallic strip type of thermometer. A chart is provided in the model sold by the Loosco Company of Amsterdam so that the correct tap setting can be chosen to give the required halothane concentration for a given gas flow and temperature. But, of course, the tap requires resetting if vaporization lowers the temperature of the liquid halothane.

Although a degree of manual temperature compensation is provided in this system, the design of the tap will not ensure a constant by-pass ratio over a wide range of flow rates. A refinement is achieved in the Drager 'Vapor' range of vaporizers by using two special conical taps, one to control the by-pass and the other to control the chamber flow (Fig. 2). The body of the vaporizer is made from a heavy block of copper having a high thermal capacity. This acts as a reservoir of heat and helps to hold the temperature of the halothane constant. The actual

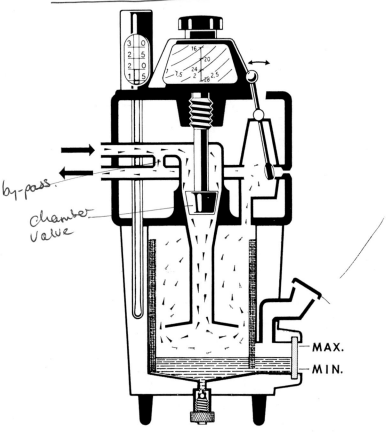

FIG. 2. Cross-section of a Drager 'Vapor' vaporizer.

temperature of the halothane is read from a built-in mercury-in-glass thermometer. The dial used for setting the concentration of halothane delivered by the vaporizer carries a number of scales each corresponding to a particular concentration. In use the dial is rotated until the required concentration scale intersects a fixed temperature scale at the temperature shown on the thermometer. The assembly opening of the by-pass valve is pre-set by the manufacturer, the chamber valve acting as the concentration control. Each consists of a male and a female cone, the ratio of the length of a cone to its gap being of the order of 100 : 1; filters are provided to prevent the ingress of particulate matter into the valves. The pressure drop across each valve is linearly related to both the forward and reverse flows. As a result, the flow-splitting ratio is little changed over the fresh gas flow range of 100 ml to 10 l./min. The vaporizing chamber of this machine contains wicks. The Vapor vaporizers are the most accurate yet

made, and they are extremely useful in the laboratory as sources of accurate concentrations of anaesthetic vapours (Hill, 1963). However, they are very heavy and tend to be expensive. A pressure relief valve is fitted to the vaporizing chamber in order to prevent any build-up of vapour pressure.

The need for a manual adjustment to compensate for temperature changes of the liquid can be eliminated by the use of a temperature-sensitive valve. The disadvantage of this type of apparatus is that the output concentration is sometimes dependent upon the perfusing gas flow rate at the lower flows.

Automatic temperature compensation is used in the well-known Fluotec Mark 2 vaporizer (Fig. 3) (Mackay, 1957; Brennan, 1957). The concentration control adjusts the splitting ratio between the chamber and by-pass flows. The gas going into the chamber passes over a series of wicks in order to ensure that it emerges fully saturated. The size of the outlet port from the chamber is controlled by a bimetallic strip valve. As evaporation proceeds and the temperature of the halothane falls so the strip bends back, opening the valve and allowing more vapour to emerge in order to hold the output concentration from the vaporizer reasonably constant. The output is independent of flow rate above 4 l./min (Fig. 4). At lower flow rates, the output rises to a peak at about 1 l./min due to non-linearity of the flow-splitting ratio, and falls to zero if the fresh gas flow is reduced to 500 ml/min. There is then insufficient pressure drop developed across the by-pass to force gas through the vaporizing chamber. A calibration card for use at flow rates below 4 l./min is provided with the instrument. A vaporizer employing similar principles is the MIE. 'Halothane 4'. This employs a mercury-expansion type of thermal compensation device and does not exhibit a peak in its flow calibration curve like the Fluotec. Massa and Zander (1964) found that the Halothane 4 vaporizer gave output concentrations lower than the indicated calibration.

The design of the new Mark 3 Fluotec is aimed at producing a vaporizer whose calibration is almost independent of temperature over the range 18–36°C and of flow from 250 ml/min to 10 l/min. Figure 5 is a cross-section of the Mark 3 vaporizer in the 'on' position. The fresh gas inflow is split into two streams in the rotary valve C. One stream passes through port H and enters the vaporizing chamber. It then passes over nickel-plated copper helix wicks. The gas saturated with halothane vapour leaves the chamber at J, passes into control channel F and rejoins the second gas stream in the sump cover D. The mixed gas and vapour leaves at G. The output concentration is set by the relative resistances to flow of the two gas streams, that is the relative restrictions of the temperature sensitive valve E and the control channel F. The resistance of F is changed by turning control knob K. F is a long, wide, but very shallow groove which gradually deepens from 0·002 in. to 0·011 in. to add more vapour to the by-pass at the higher percentage settings. The bimetallic strip valve E opens as the temperature falls. The control channel F is machined into the face of the rotary valve C, the opposite face is coated with polytetrafluorethylene (PTFE) to provide a

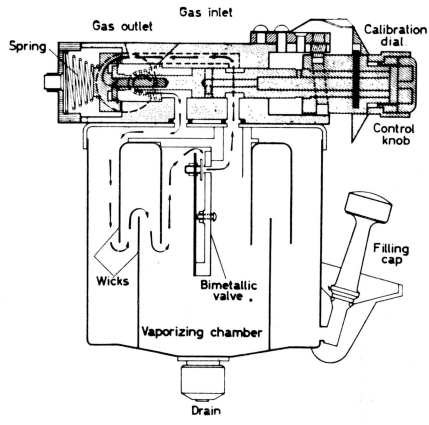

FIG. 3. Cross-section of a Mark 2 Fluotec vaporizer.

non-stick surface. Paterson *et al.* (1969) reported test figures obtained with the Fluotec Mark 3. They report that its flow resistance (approximately 50 cm. $H_2O$ at 10 l./min) is high and that it is heavy. The design of the control valve is such as to virtually eliminate the possibility of it sticking due to accumulation of thymol from the halothane.

The Pentec Mark 2 is made on similar principles and can provide a methoxyflurane concentration in the range 0·2–2·0 per cent v/v.

The problem of holding the calibration of a vaporizer reasonably constant with changing flow rates when an automatic temperature compensation system is employed has been tackled in an ingenious fashion in the New Foregger 'Fluomatic' halothane vaporizer. A sectional diagram of the Fluomatic in the 'on' position is given in Figure 6. The fresh gas flowing into the vaporizer at (1) is divided in the usual way, the by-pass stream passing through the fixed restriction (2) to the outlet (3). The vaporizing chamber stream flows through the wicks and chamber which has a small gas volume and emerges through the variable control valve (4) which is in series with a fixed restriction (5), to merge with the by-pass flow. The relief valve (6) limits the pressure of the inlet gas if high flows are applied to the vaporizer. The control needle valve (4) has a relatively large needle made from a plastic material which has a high coefficient of thermal expansion relative to the valve seating. As the temperature of the emerging gas and vapour stream from the chamber alters,

so the valve opens or closes to adjust the flow in such a way as to hold the output concentration constant. A similar

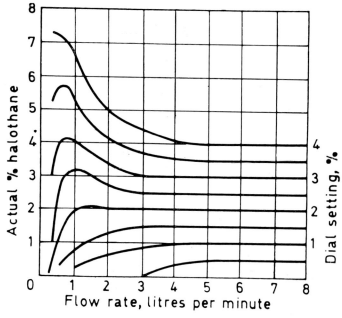

FIG. 4. Calibration curve for a Mark 2 Fluotec vaporizer.

arrangement operates with the fixed restriction (5) in series with the control valve. The advantage of this arrangement is that no additional moving parts are needed.

Figures 7 and 8 show the performance of the Fluomatic under conditions of varying temperature and flow rate.

The lower saturated vapour pressure of methoxyflurane means that a vaporizer for this substance must pass more of the fresh gas through the vaporizing chamber than would occur for vaporizers designed to work with other

low-resistance channel completely by-passes the vaporizing chamber, and the chamber is vented to atmosphere at (8). The pressure applied to the vaporizer is limited by the relief valve (6).

The mode of operation of plenum vaporizers can be clearly seen in the following calculation. Suppose that the

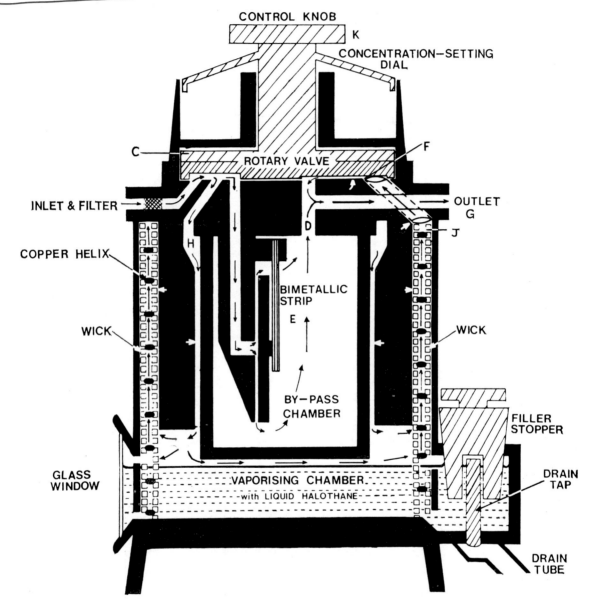

FIG. 5. Cross-section of a Mark 3 Fluotec vaporizer.

agents. Figure 9 shows a section of the Foregger 'Pento-matic' vaporizer. The upper section (2) of the control valve controls the by-pass flow, whilst the lower section (4) controls the outlet from the vaporizing chamber. The two sections move up or down as a unit when the concentration setting dial (5) is adjusted. The valves provide automatic temperature compensation as described for the Fluomatic vaporizer. The isolation valve (7) is moved through a linkage to the control knob (5) to close both the inlet and outlet of the vaporizing chamber (Fig. 9). A

vaporizer is required to produce a 1 per cent v/v concentration of halothane in a total minute volume (gas + vapour) of 6 l. If the ambient temperature is 22°C, the saturation concentration of halothane in the vaporizing chamber is 35·5 per cent v/v. To produce the required 1 per cent v/v concentration, 1 part of the saturated vapour must be added to 34·5 parts of fresh gas. Thus, of the total volume flow of 6000 ml, 170 ml must emerge from the vaporizing chamber, and 5830 ml of gas must pass through the by-pass per minute. Of the 170 ml, 35·5 per cent is halothane

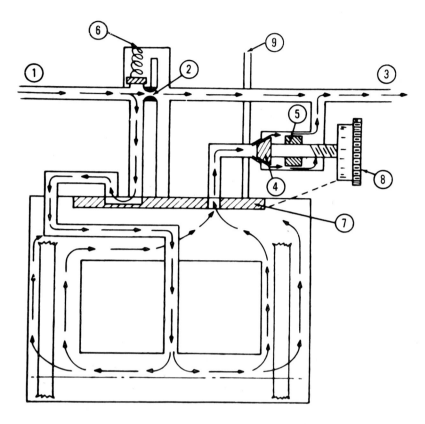

FIG. 6. Cross-section of a Fluomatic vaporizer in the 'on' position.

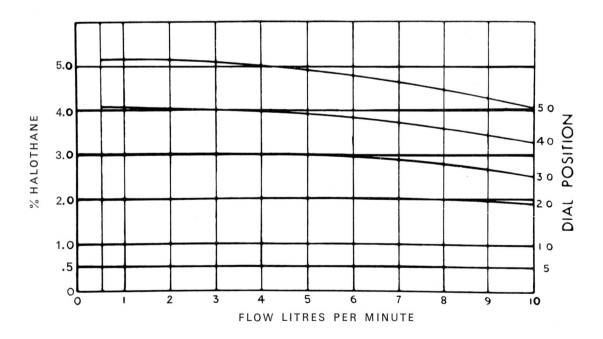

FIG. 7. The variation of the output from a Fluomatic vaporizer with gas flow at constant temperature of 20°C.

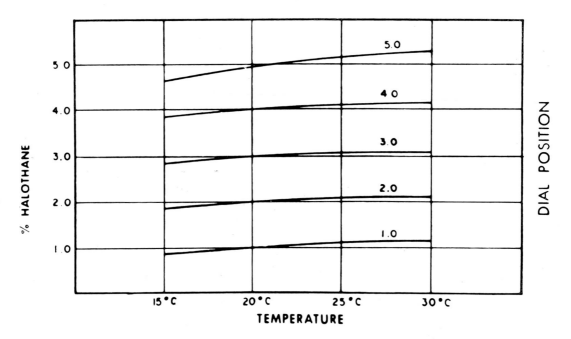

Fig. 8. The variation of the output with temperature with a Fluomatic vaporizer at a series of different flow rates.

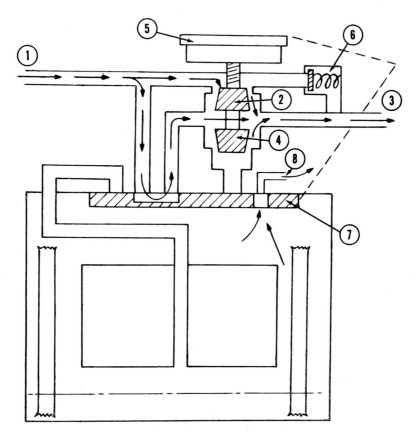

Fig. 9. Cross-section of a Pentomatic vaporizer in the 'on' position.

vapour, i.e. 60 ml. of halothane vapour. This corresponds to the vaporization of 0·26 ml. of liquid halothane per minute. The gas flow into the vaporizing chamber is (170 − 60) = 110 ml/min.

In the case of the temperature-compensated vaporizers so far described, it has not been required to measure the by-pass and vaporizing chamber flows separately. However, if these are both known, together with the temperature of the liquid, and the vaporizing chamber delivers saturated vapour, then both the output concentration and the mass of agent delivered per minute can be calculated. This principle is used in the well-known Foregger 'Copper Kettle' vaporizer (Morris, 1952), in which the vaporizing chamber is constructed of copper and is fixed to a copper plate on the anaesthetic machine. This provides a good reservoir of heat when ether is used. Figure 11 shows the Copper Kettle vaporizer in section. The flow of oxygen enters the vaporizer through tube (1) and surge chamber (2). It leaves the chamber via the concentric tube (3) which leads into the annular chamber (4) of the sintered bronze disc diffuser (5). The many fine bubbles formed give rise to fully saturated vapour. The bubbles rise through the liquid agent (6) and pass into the chamber (7) above the liquid, the saturated vapour emerging via the exit tube (8) to join the main by-pass gas flow stream from the anaesthetic machine gas flow meters. The kettle inlet (1) is fed from its own oxygen flow meter. A copper kettle of 400 ml capacity is normally used for the vaporization of ether and methoxyflurane, a 160 ml. capacity kettle being used with halothane (Feldman and Morris, 1958). The British Oxygen 'Halox' vaporizer works on similar principles (Young, 1966) but has an all-glass construction since it is only intended for use with halothane. An additional oxygen flow meter fitted to the Boyle anaesthetic machine measures the oxygen fed through a sintered glass disk to bubble through the halothane (Fig. 11). If it is required to produce an output of 2·5 l./min. containing 3·1 per cent v/v of halothane, there must be a flow of 172 ml./min. into the chamber and a by-pass flow of 2250 ml./min. if the saturation concentration of halothane is 31·2 per cent at 20°C. Calculators are available to help the anaesthetist set up the required flows (Collis, 1966; Jennings, Taylor and Young, 1967). Martin (1968) has evaluated the performance of the Halox vaporizer. He finds that at flows greater than 4 l./min. the fall in temperature of the Halox is troublesome. In his opinion, under these circumstances the Halox offers no advantages over the Boyle bottle type of halothane vaporizer.

**Draw-over Vaporizers or Inhalers**

The plenum vaporizers so far described are designed to work with the uni-directional gas flows obtained from anaesthetic machines or gas cylinders; their resistance is too high for use as draw-over vaporizers where the patient's respiratory efforts pull the gas through the vaporizer, and their calibration would not hold under intermittent flow conditions. The EMO vaporizer was developed as a calibrated, low-resistance, draw-over vaporizer for use in under-developed countries and in emergency conditions (Epstein and Macintosh, 1956;

Leatherdale, 1966). The water jacket surrounding the vaporizing chamber provides a reservoir of heat, and a metal bellows filled with ether vapour acts as a temperature-compensation valve at the chamber outlet. As the temperature falls the bellows contracts and opens the valve. The calibration of the EMO only holds for intermittent flows.

The Oxford Miniature Vaporizer (OMV) employs stainless steel wicks and a water-filled base, and can be used

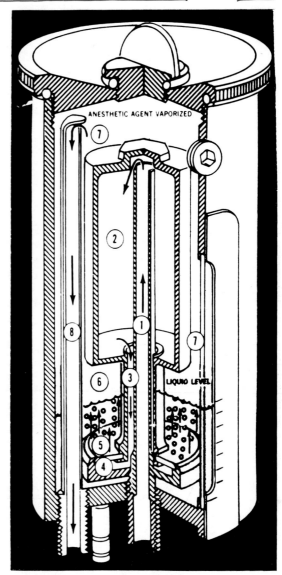

FIG. 10. Cross-section of a Copper Kettle vaporizer.

with halothane, chloroform or trichlorethylene under continuous or intermittent flow conditions. Its clinical performance for halothane is discussed by Parkhouse (1966) and Jensen (1967).

Compact draw-over vaporizers lend themselves to incorporation in portable anaesthetic apparatus. Stephens (1965) describes the performance of the Cyprane 'Halothane air' apparatus which incorporates a compact halothane inhaler, and Hedstrand (1966) describes the AGA 'Anestor Militar' emergency anaesthetic apparatus

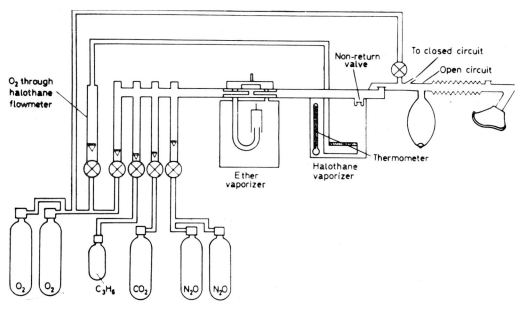

FIG. 11. The connection of a Halox vaporizer to the manifold of a Boyle anaesthetic machine.

which uses the SOCSIL draw-over vaporizer for ether, halothane or chloroform (Hallen and Norlander, 1966; Martinez, Norlander and Santos, 1966). The Blease Universal Vaporizer can be used as a plenum or draw-over vaporizer, and can be provided with a series of interchangeable control cams so that it can be used with almost any volatile anaesthetic agent (Fig. 12). The pressure drop across it is 10 cm. $H_2O$ at a gas flow rate of 30 l./min. It offers the advantage that it can be used with an anaesthetic machine in order to familiarize anaesthetists with its characteristics. It can then be used with confidence by these anaesthetists under draw-over conditions. A detailed study of the Blease Universal Vaporizer is that of Merri-

field, Hill and Smith (1967). Although it performed in a satisfactory manner for plenum and draw-over conditions, the concentration fell off rapidly with time when it was placed inside a circle. Schreiber and Weis (1965) report inaccuracies present in the calibration of a Blease Universal Vaporizer.

The Cyprane inhaler for methoxyflurane (Fig. 13) is designed as a small portable analgesia apparatus for minor surgery and obstetrical practice. During inspiration air is entrained through the mixture adjusting collar F. It is directed down into the vaporizing chamber through slots in G, or directed upwards to the face piece through slots in E, or through both depending upon the setting of F

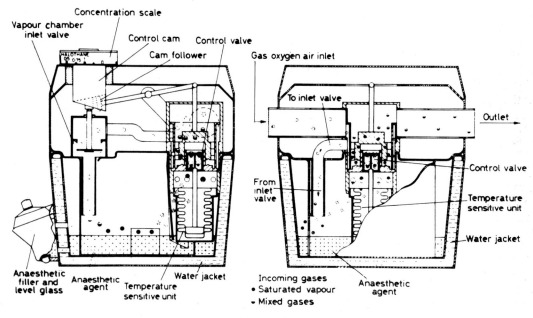

FIG. 12. Cross-section of the Blease Universal vaporizer.

which alters the relative areas of the ports in *G* and *E*. The position of the collar *F*, and hence the concentration, can be locked with a key. On expiration the gases pass to the atmosphere through valve *B* and the holes in the side of cover *A*, The non-return valve *D* prevents the expired gases passing through the vaporizing chamber. Filling is via cap *H*.

### The Use of Vaporizers with Circle Anaesthetic Systems

A vaporizer can either be placed outside a circle absorption circuit (VOC) or a semi-open circuit in the fresh gas supply line, or it can be placed inside the circle. In the first case it receives only the fresh gas flow rate in the form of dry gas. In the second it receives the patient's expired minute volume of gas which will be fully saturated with water and will contain exhaled anaesthetic vapour. The two conditions are quite different, the first requiring a high-efficiency vaporizer which can deliver a high output concentration at low flows, the second requiring a low-efficiency vaporizer which will only add small increments of vapour to the minute volume recirculating through it.

A detailed account of the functioning of vaporizers in circle systems is given by Mapleson (1960), and Mushin and Galloon (1960). One advantage of using a circle system lies in the economy of consumption of the anaesthetic agent which is possible at low fresh gas flow rates. When flows through the vaporizer of one l./min or less are used, attention must be paid to the so-called 'pumping effect' (Hill and Lowe, 1962; Gordh *et al.*, 1964). Unless the vaporizer is designed to eliminate this effect when intermittent positive pressure ventilation is employed, the inflation pressure is transmitted up the fresh gas pipe from the circle into the vaporizing chamber of the vaporizer. During the expiratory phase when the pressure is released, the contents of the chamber return to the by-pass not only via the normal exit port of the chamber but via the inlet port as well. This additional increment of vapour gives rise to an enhanced outlet concentration. For example, Hill and Lowe found that at 500 ml/min, the effect of IPPR at 10 breaths per minute with a 20 cm. $H_2O$ inflation pressure was to increase the output of a Mark 2 Fluotec vaporizer from the 3 per cent v/v set on the dial to 4·1 per cent. If requested to do so, the makers of the Fluotec can supply a model which has a miniature pressure regulator fitted to its outlet (Edmondson and Hill, 1962; Kapfhammer and Atabas, 1965). This prevents pressure fluctuations from the circle getting back into the vaporizer. Another possibility is to fit a uni-directional valve to the outlet of the vaporizer (Keenan, 1963). A different approach has been adopted in the case of the Mark 3 Fluotec. Firstly, the volume of the vaporizing chamber has been reduced from about 750 ml. in the Mark 2 Fluotec to 270 ml in the Mark 3. In addition the resistance of the chamber outlet is higher than the inlet. As a result, during compression the additional gas forced into the by-pass enters the vaporizing chamber through its inlet. The length and volume of the expansion chamber are such, together with the fact that the wicks are not near the inlet, as to prevent this gas from picking up halothane vapour. During decompression this gas returns to the by-pass and does not

add to the output concentration. The Drager 'Vapor' vaporizer is fitted with a long inlet tube to the vaporizing chamber. When the pressure in the vaporizing chamber due to IPPR is released, the vapor does not emerge into the by-pass from this long tube, and is forced back into the chamber during the next inflation (Fig. 14). A method tried by Hill and Lowe (1962) and Lowe *et al.* (1962) was to place a needle valve distal to the Fluotec and by this means raise the pressure in the vaporizer to 40 cm. $H_2O$ which is well above normal inflation pressures. Keet, Valentine and Riccio (1963) describe an arrangement designed to prevent pressure effects on the Vernitrol vaporizer.

Two design features are claimed to eliminate the

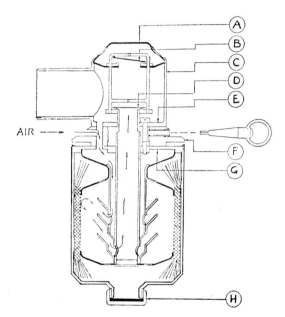

FIG. 13. Cross-section of the Cyprane inhaler for methoxyflurane.

'pumping effect' in the case of the Foregger 'Fluomatic' vaporizer. The gas volume of the vaporizing chamber has been deliberately kept to a minimum so that no serious volumes of halothane vapour can be discharged from the chamber into the by-pass during the deflationary phase. The Fluomatic also operates with a significant pressure drop of 8 cm. $H_2O$/l./min of gas flow into it. This discourages any flow of vapour out of the normal inlet of the vaporizing chamber when the pressure in the chamber is released.

The Rowbotham and Goldman dental vaporizers (Goldman, 1962) have found favour for use as halothane vaporizers *inside a circle* (VIC) (Burton, 1958; Gusterson, 1959; Hall *et al.*, 1966). The Goldman vaporizer is so constructed that even at high flow rates it cannot produce more than 3 per cent v/v of halothane and offers little resistance to gas flow. Bodman, Gerson and Smith (1967) measured the inspired concentration in a circle system using a Goldman vaporizer and a halothane meter. With this simple type of vaporizer, there is an appreciable surge of vapour when it is first used, and the cooling effect is

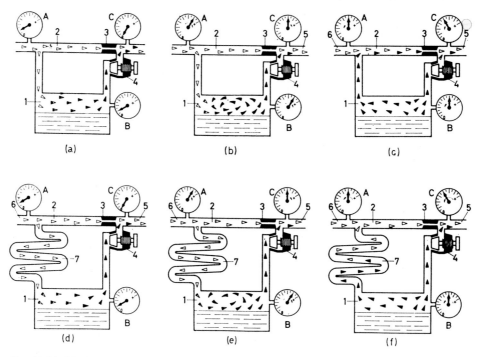

FIG. 14 (a), (b), (c). The release of positive pressure from the vaporizing chamber allows vapour to rejoin the by-pass from the normal inlet to the chamber; (d) this effect is eliminated by the use of a long inlet pipe to the vaporizing chamber.

not negligible. However, it works well and was never designed as a precision vaporizer (Goldman, 1966). It is usual to allow the patient to breathe spontaneously with the vaporizer inside the circle. Should he lighten, a compensatory action occurs, his increased ventilation vaporizing more anaesthetic. If IPPR is used, there is a risk of vaporizing an excessive amount of anaesthetic (Marret, 1959; Mushin and Galloon, 1960). This risk can be minimized by using some form of halothane analyser in the circuit to measure the inspired concentration.

### Dental Vaporizers

Young (1969) reports that the addition of a blotting paper wick to a Goldman or McKesson dental vaporizer increased the halothane output concentration by about 1 per cent and improved the clinical efficiency.

### Vaporizers under Hyperbaric and Hypobaric Conditions

The saturated vapour pressure of a volatile anaesthetic agent is a function only of the ambient temperature. It increases by only approximately 1 per cent per atmosphere. For halothane it is 243 torr at 20°C giving a saturation concentration of 32 per cent v/v. When the ambient pressure is increased by 1 atmosphere to 2 atmospheres absolute (2 a.t.a.) the saturation concentration is halved to 16 per cent. Although the concentration is halved, the mass delivered per minute remains sensibly constant, since the density of the vapour mixture is now doubled at the higher pressure and the *tension remains the same*. Thus little clinical difference would be expected in the settings

of anaesthetic vaporizers used in hyperbaric operating rooms. This is borne out by McDowall (1964) and Vermeulen-Cranch (1964). There will be some slight differences, since the flow-splitting ratios will be affected by the pressure. Similar, but reverse, considerations apply under hypobaric conditions encountered at high altitudes (Safar and Tenicella, 1964).

### The 'Pressure Pot' Vaporizer

The idea of pressurizing an anaesthetic vaporizer has been developed by Bracken, Brooks and Goldman (1968). They apply 4 atmospheres pressure, i.e. 4·2 kg./sq. cm. (60 lb./sq. in. on the gauge) from a pipeline containing oxygen, or premixed 50 per cent oxygen and 50 per cent nitrous oxide (Entonox) to a stout metal 'pot' of 0·5 litre capacity (Fig. 15). Assuming that the saturation concentration of halothane contained in the pot is approximately 33 per cent at room pressure, then by bringing the pot pressure up to 5 atmospheres absolute, i.e. 4 atmospheres on the gauge, the halothane concentration is reduced to 6·7 per cent. Assume that 500 ml./min. of gas at 4 atmospheres (gauge pressure) is fed into the pot, on expanding to atmospheric pressure this becomes 2·5 litres. If it is required to produce a 2 per cent concentration, the 6·7 per cent from the pot must be diluted by adding a by-pass gas flow of 5·9 l./min at atmospheric pressure, so that a total volume of gas plus vapour of 8·4 l./min. is available. Titel *et el*, (1968) describe an interesting pressurized vaporizer fitted with a compensator for temperature changes. The output is calibrated directly in ml. of halothane vapour per minute (Fig. 16).

## The Calibration of Anaesthetic Vaporizers

Nearly all manufacturers of calibrated vaporizers use an optical method of calibration based upon the measurement

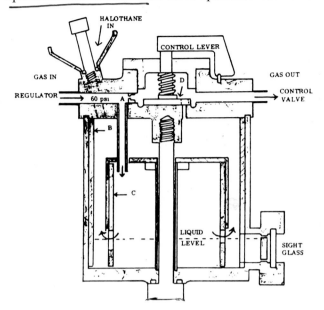

FIG. 15. Cross-section of a pressurized vaporizer.

of the refractive index of the emergent vapour mixture by means of a Rayleigh refractometer (Edmondson, 1957; Luder, 1964), air being used as the carrier gas. The method

has the advantage from the manufacturer's viewpoint that the calibration of the refractometer, once established, is very stable. The instrument can be calibrated from known vapour mixtures or from a knowledge of the refractive indices of the vapours concerned. It is, however, only suitable for use with binary gas and vapour mixtures. For accurate work, with other gases and water vapour present, it is convenient to use a non-dispersive infra-red gas analyser (Hill, 1958). Gas chromatography can also be used for the measurement of halothane and other volatile agents in anaesthetic circuits (Hill, 1960), and is particularly useful for the measurement of the concentrations of volatile agents in blood (Butler and Hill, 1962).

For an absolute *calibration of vaporizers*, it is best to use known vapour concentrations prepared in alloy cylinders under pressure as described by Hill (1961).

### Servicing of Vaporizers

With any anaesthetic vaporizer, it is necessary to carry out a regular routine servicing procedure. The vaporizing chamber should be drained off periodically; in the case of halothane vaporizers this will avoid a build-up of thymol in the container. The interior of the vaporizer should be inspected for any incipient corrosion, and the tap checked for sticking. Grease should not be used as oxygen will be present when the vaporizer is in use. In the case of calibrated vaporizers, the control knob should not bind, and the calibration should be checked by the manufacturers at yearly intervals. Adner and Hallen (1965) discuss reliability aspects of anaesthetic vaporizers.

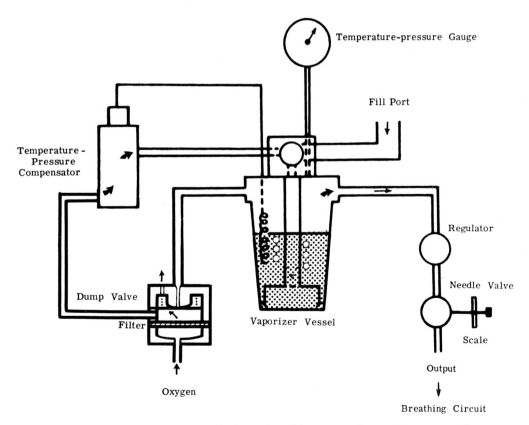

FIG. 16. Cross-section of a pressurized vaporizer with pressure and temperature compensation.

# REFERENCES

Adner, M. and Hallen, B. (1965), "Reliability of Halothane Vaporizers," *Acta anaesth. scand.*, **9**, 233.

Bodman, R. I., Gerson, G. and Smith, K. (1967), "A Simple Closed Circuit for Halothane Anaesthesia," *Anaesthesia*, **22**, 476.

Bracken, A. B., Brookes, R. C. and Goldman, V. (1968), "New Equipment for Dental Anaesthesia using Pre-mixed Gases and Halothane," *Brit. J. Anaesth.*, **40**, 903.

Brennan, H. J. (1957), "A Vaporizer for Fluothane," *Brit. J. Anaesth.*, **29**, 332.

Burton, P. J. C. (1958), "Halothane Concentrations from a Rowbotham's Bottle in a Circle Absorption System," *Brit. J. Anaesth.*, **30**, 312.

Butler, R. A. and Hill, D. W. (1962), "Estimation of Volatile Anaesthetics in Tissues by Gas Chromatography," *Nature (Lond.)*, **189**, 488.

Collis, J. M. (1966), "Concentration Graphs for the Halox Vaporizer," *Anaesthesia*, **21**, 558.

Edmondson, W. (1957), "Gas Analysis by Refractive Index Measurement," *Brit. J. Anaesth.*, **29**, 570.

Edmondson, W. and Hill, D. W. (1962), "A Pressurizing Valve for the Fluotec Vaporizer," *Brit. J. Anaesth.*, **34**, 741.

Epstein, H. G. and Macintosh, R. (1956), "An Anaesthetic Inhaler with Automatic Thermo-compensation," *Anaesthesia*, **11**, 83.

Feldman, S. A. and Morris, L. E. (1958), "Vaporization of Ether and Halothane in the Copper Kettle," *Anesthesiology*, **19**, 650.

Goldman, V. (1962), "The Goldman Halothane Vaporizer Mark 2," *Anaesthesia*, **17**, 537.

Goldman, V. (1966), "Correspondence," *Brit. J. Anaesth.*, **38**, 980.

Gordh, T., Hallen, B., Okmian, L., Wahlin, A. and Stern, B. (1964), "The Concentration of Halothane by the Combined Use of Fluotec Vaporizer and Engstrom Respirator," *Acta anaesth. scand.*, **8**, 97.

Gusterson, F. R. (1959), "Halothane in the Closed Circuit, with Special Reference to Prostatectomy," *Anaesthesia*, **14**, 35.

Hall, J. M., Hellewell, J., Fischer, E. L., Burns, T. H. S. and Fuzzy, G. J. J. (1966), "A Test of Two Types of Halothane Vaporizer," *Brit. J. Anaesth.*, **38**, 484.

Hallen, B. and Norlander, O. P. (1966), "Performance of the Aga-Socsil Vaporizer for Volatile Anaesthetics Studied by Gas Chromatography," *Acta anaesth. scand.*, Suppl. 26, 43.

Hedstrand, U. (1966), "Aga Anestor Militar in Clinical Use," *Acta anaesth. scand.*, Suppl. 26, 53.

Hill, D. W. (1958), "Halothane Concentrations Obtained with a Fluotec Vaporizer," *Brit. J. Anaesth.*, **30**, 563.

Hill, D. W. (1960), "The Application of Gas Chromatography to Anaesthetic Research," in *Gas Chromatography*, ed. Scott, R. P. W., p. 334. London: Butterworths.

Hill, D. W. (1961), "Production of Accurate Gas and Vapour Mixtures," *Brit. J. appl. Physics*, **12**, 410.

Hill, D. W. (1963), "Halothane Concentrations Obtained from a Drager Vapor Vaporizer," *Brit. J. Anaesth.*, **35**, 285.

Hill, D. W. and Lowe, H. J. (1962), "Comparison of Concentrations of Halothane in Closed and Semi-closed Circuits during Controlled Ventilation," *Anesthesiology*, **23**, 291.

Jennings, A. M. C. and Hersant, M. E. (1965), "Increase of Halothane Concentrations following Refilling of Certain Vaporizers," *Brit. J. Anaesth.*, **37**, 137.

Jennings, A. M. C., Taylor, T. H. and Young, J. V. I. (1967), "Nomograms for the Halox Vaporizer," *Brit. J. Anaesth.*, **39**, 598.

Jensen, J. K. (1967), "Halothankonzentrationen erreight durch den 'Oxford Miniature Inhaler'," *Anaesthesist*, **16**, 54.

Kapfhammer, V. and Atabas, A. (1965), "Der Fluotec Mark 2 mit angebrauten Druckausgleich Ventil," *Anaesthesist.*, **14**, 18a.

Keenan, R. L. (1963), "Prevention of Increased Pressures in Anaesthetic Vaporizers with a Uni-directional Valve," *Anesthesiology*, **24**, 732.

Keet, J. E., Valentine, G. W. and Riccio, J. S. (1963), "An Arrangement to Prevent Pressure Effect on the Vernitrol Vaporizer," *Anesthesiology*, **24**, 734.

Leatherdale, R. A. L. (1966), "The EMO Ether Inhaler (Clinical Experience in a Series of over 1000 Anaesthetics)," *Anaesthesia*, **21**, 504.

Lowe, H. J., Beckham, L. M., Han, Y. H. and Evers, J. L. (1962), "Vaporizer Performance: Closed Circuit Fluothane Anesthesia," *Curr. Res. Anesth.*, **41**, 742.

Luder, M. (1964), "Bestimmungen von Halothandampkonzentrationen mit dem Laboratoriumsinterferometer. 1: Mitseilung, Methodik," *Anaesthesist*, **13**, 360.

McDowall, R. G. (1964), "Anaesthesia in a Pressure Chamber," *Anaesthesia*, **19**, 331.

Macintosh, R., Mushin, W. W. and Epstein, H. G. (1958), *Physics for the Anaesthetist*, 2nd ed. Oxford: Blackwell.

Mackay, J. M. (1957), "Clinical Evaluation of Fluothane with Special Reference to a Controlled Percentage Vaporizer," *Canad. Anaesth. Soc. J.*, **4**, 235.

Mapleson, W. W. (1960), "The Concentration of Anaesthetics in Closed Circuits with Special Reference to Halothane. 1: Theoretical Study," *Brit. J. Anaesth.*, **32**, 298.

Marrett, H. R. (1959), "Halothane in Use in the Closed Circuit," *Anaesthesia*, **14**, 28.

Martin, L. V. H. (1968), "Observations on the Halox Vaporizer," *Anaesthesia*, **23**, 119.

Martinez, L. R., Norlander, O. P. and Santos, A. (1966), "Laboratory Evaluation of a Socsil Vaporizer," *Acta anaesth. scand.*, Suppl. 26, 75.

Massa, L. S. and Zander, (1964), "Calibration of a New Vaporizer," *Anesthesiology*, **25**, 708.

Merrifield, A. J., Hill, D. W. and Smith, K. (1967), "Performance of the Portablease and the Fluoxair Portable Anaesthetic Equipment, with Reference to Use under Adverse Conditions," *Brit. J. Anaesth.*, **39**, 50.

Molyneux, L. (1959), "Acoustic Gas Analyser," *J. Sci. Instrum.*, **36**, 118.

Morris, L. E. (1952), "A New Vaporizer for Liquid Anesthetic Agents," *Anesthesiology*, **13**, 587.

Mushin, W. W. and Galloon, S. (1960), "The Concentration of Anaesthetics in Closed Circuits with Special Reference to Halothane. 3: Clinical Aspects," *Brit. J. Anaesth.*, **32**, 324.

Parbrook, G. D. (1966), "A Halothane Vaporizer for Small Animal Anaesthesia," *Anaesthesia*, **21**, 403.

Parkhouse, J. (1966), "Clinical Performance of the O.M.V. Vaporizer," *Anaesthesia*, **21**, 504.

Paterson, C. M., Hulands, G. H. and Nunn, J. F. (1969), "Evaluation of a New Halothane Vaporizer: The Cyprane Fluotec Mark 3," *Brit. J. Anaesth.*, **41**, 109.

Pearce, C. (1962), "A Versatile Halothane Vaporizer," *Anaesthesia*, **17**, 540.

Safar, P. and Tenicella, R. (1964), "High Altitude Physiology in Relation to Anesthesia and Inhalational Therapy," *Anesthesiology*, **25**, 515.

Schreiber, P. and Weis, K. H. (1965), "Konzentrationsmessungen mit dem Gardner-Universal-Verdampfer," *Anaesthesist*, **14**, 289.

Seed, R. F. (1967), "Vaporization of Halothane during Movement," *Brit. J. Anaesth.*, **22**, 659.

Stephens, K. F. (1965), "Transportable Apparatus for Halothane Anaesthesia," *Brit. J. Anaesth.*, **37**, 67.

Titel, J. M., Lowe, H. J., Elam, J. O. and Glosholz, J. R. (1968), "Quantitative Closed-circuit Halothane Anaesthesia," *Anesth. & Analg.*, **47**, 560.

Vermeulen-Cranch, D. M. E. (1964), "Anaesthesia in a High Pressure Chamber," in *Clinical Application of Hyperbaric Oxygen*, ed. Boerema, I., Brummelkamp, W. H. and Meijne, N. J., p. 206. Amsterdam: Elsevier.

Young, J. I. V. (1966), "The Practical Use of the Halox Vaporizer," *Anaesthesia*, **21**, 551.

Young, T. M. (1969), "Vaporizers for Dental Anaesthesia Modified by the Addition of a Wick: an Evaluation of Performance," *Brit. J. Anaesth.*, **41**, 120.

# CHAPTER 4

# ANAESTHETIC CIRCUITS

### C. M. CONWAY

## Introduction

The modern anaesthetic machine is usually equipped with calibrated rotameters and accurate vaporizers in order to supply known volumes and concentrations of oxygen, anaesthetic gases and volatile agents. The concentration of gases and vapours actually delivered to the patient may be considerably modified by the anaesthetic circuit used to connect the patient to the anaesthetic machine. In order to predict the patient's inspired atmosphere accurately a knowledge of the functional behaviour of anaesthetic circuits is necessary.

Functional analysis of anaesthetic circuits is usually directed to a prediction or measurement of the degree of rebreathing present. This is a reflection of the functional apparatus dead space and the extent of this is presented in terms of carbon dioxide accumulation. Alteration in carbon dioxide levels in any anaesthetic circuit, due to rebreathing of alveolar gas, will always be accompanied by a reduction in inspired oxygen concentration, and is usually associated with a reduced inspired concentration of any volatile or gaseous agents used.

It is an unfortunate historical fact that many commonly used anaesthetic circuits have been designed or have evolved with a disregard for function. Valves and conducting tubing have often been arranged for convenience and ease of access rather than for functional reasons. It is also true that in the description of gas circuits there is considerable ambiguity of nomenclature, the terms semi-open, semi-closed, and closed often appearing to have synonymous meanings. For descriptive purposes in this chapter the following classification will be adhered to.

1. Open. A circuit with infinite boundaries and no restriction upon the entry of fresh gas.
2. Semi-open. A partially bounded circuit with some restriction of fresh gas entry.
3. Closed. A fully bounded circuit with no provision for gas overflow.
4. Semi-closed. A fully bounded circuit with provision for venting of excess gas:
   (a) semi-closed rebreathing circuits
   (b) semi-closed absorption circuits
   (c) non-rebreathing circuits.

This classification allows rigid definition of any circuit under any given conditions of use. However, the behaviour of many circuits can be drastically altered by small changes in circuit arrangement or fresh gas flow-rate. Thus a T-piece circuit usually behaves as a semi-closed rebreathing circuit, but with low gas flows and an unduly short expiratory limb atmospheric air may be entrained and the circuit

is then semi-open. Similarly, increasing fresh gas flow to any closed circuit will convert it to a semi-closed circuit, with a consequent alteration in functional analysis.

## Open Circuits

Unbounded open circuits offer minimal control over inspired concentration of gases and vapours and for this reason are nowadays rarely used. The simplest open circuit exists when an anaesthetic agent is administered from a mask or delivery tube held a discrete distance from the face, as when a child is induced by surrounding him with an atmosphere of nitrous oxide, or when volatile liquids are administered in an open-drop fashion on to a mask held some inches from the face.

No rebreathing occurs in an open circuit. The inspired gas consists of a mixture of the administered agents and atmospheric air. The inspired concentration of anaesthetics so delivered will be a function of the rate and mode of delivery of anaesthetic agent, the density of the gases used, the rate of atmospheric dilution and the pattern of ventilation, and is not amenable to simple mathematical analysis

## Semi-open Circuits

The simplest semi-open circuit is a gauze-covered Schimmelbusch mask applied to the face. The mask behaves as an extension of the patient's deadspace and the degree of rebreathing depends on the mask volume and the thickness of material on and around the frame. Rebreathing is increased when a towel is wrapped round the mask.

Diethyl ether is the agent used most commonly on such masks. As air is the vaporizing gas, and as high concentrations of diethyl ether may be achieved under the mask, reduction of the inspired oxygen concentration commonly occurs in this system. This reduction is due to displacement of air by ether vapour, and is accentuated by rebreathing of expired air of lower oxygen content. The danger of hypoxaemia may be reduced by administering a stream of oxygen beneath the mask. This will not only enrich the inspired atmosphere in respect of oxygen but will also tend to flush the mask and reduce rebreathing.

## Closed Circuits

Although closed methods of administering anaesthetics were in use from the middle of the nineteenth century, the safe and controlled use of closed-circuit apparatus was not possible until the introduction of practicable methods of carbon dioxide absorption, by Jackson in laboratory animals in 1915, and by Waters in man in 1923. Typical examples of closed-circuit apparatus preceding the use of carbon dioxide absorption were the ether inhalers of

Clover and Ormsby. In both of these the patient breathed to and fro from a reservoir bag, over an ether vaporizer. No adequate provisions were made to counteract the rising carbon dioxide content and falling oxygen content of the system, and these factors, together with the high concentrations of ether which could be obtained, accounted for the rapidity with which anaesthesia could be induced with these inhalers. Similar uncontrolled rebreathing occurs in the Goldman and Oxford vinesthene inhalers of more recent times.

Two basic patterns of closed-circuit absorption apparatus are possible, the to-and-fro, and the circle systems (Fig. 1). In the to-and-fro system of Waters there are no

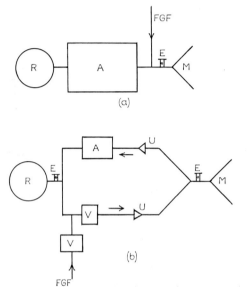

FIG. 1. Schematic diagrams of (a) to-and-fro circuit and (b) circle system.

A = Absorber
E = Expiratory valve
FGF = Fresh gas flow
M = Mask or endotracheal tube
R = Reservoir bag
U = Unidirectional valves
V = Vaporizer

unidirectional valves. The patient breathes to and fro from a rebreathing bag and through a carbon-dioxide absorber. Fresh gas is introduced into the circuit near the patient's mouth. The reservoir bag may be separated from the absorber by a suitable length of wide-bore tubing, but the absorber itself must be placed near to the mask or endotracheal tube.

The circle system was introduced by Sword in 1926. Here the direction of gas flow is controlled by two unidirectional valves, so that expired gas passes through an absorber, into a reservoir bag and thence back to the patient. Numerous variations of circle arrangement are possible, depending on the site of entry of fresh gas into the circuit and the relative positions of unidirectional valves, overspill valves, the reservoir bag and the absorber. These factors of circuit arrangement can assume considerable importance when the circle is used as a semi-closed system, but are of less significance in the fully closed circuit used with basal fresh gas flow. Of greater importance in

any closed circuit is the position and efficiency of any vaporizer used.

The principal reason for the introduction and early popularity of the closed circuit was the economy possible in the consumption of gases and anaesthetic vapours. Other advantages of these systems are the conservation of heat and water vapour, the limitation of fire hazard when inflammable or explosive agents are used, and the ability to perform efficient controlled ventilation with these circuits. The to-and-fro system, although much simpler and less cumbersome than the circle, has certain deficiencies. Its dead space extends as far as the proximal boundary of the carbon dioxide absorbent. As absorption occurs soda-lime nearest to the patient is exhausted first, and this leads to a progressive increase in apparatus dead space and fall in circuit efficiency. With this circuit, there is also a risk of inhalation of irritant soda-lime dust. In the circle system, initial soda-lime exhaustion has no effect on apparatus dead space, and the risk of dust inhalation is greatly reduced. The circle has an appreciably greater resistance than the to-and-fro system, and is less efficient in retaining both heat and water vapour. The resistance of a circle system can be reduced by removing the unidirectional valves and incorporating a circulating fan into the system.

The basic principle governing the use of closed systems of anaesthesia is that at equilibrium there is no net exchange of anaesthetic agent between the patient and his ambient atmosphere. Thus when equilibrium is attained, anaesthesia can theoretically be maintained indefinitely by providing a supply of oxygen to meet the patient's basal requirements and by efficiently absorbing carbon dioxide. Under these circumstances no additional anaesthetic agent need be added to the circuit.

This theoretical approach is complicated by several factors. In practice, even with the most insoluble anaesthetic agents, several hours are needed for full equilibrium. Even when equilibrium is approached, any small alteration in alveolar concentration of anaesthetic, produced by such factors as changes in the respiratory pattern or small changes in the proportion of gases added to the circuit, may have a marked effect upon anaesthetic uptake. Uptake or excretion of any one component of the gas mixture within the circuit will affect the concentrations of all other components of that mixture and may thereby alter their uptake and excretion.

Although closed-circuit anaesthesia with basal oxygen flows and no added anaesthetic can rarely if ever be attained, these circuits can be used with very low gas flows and minimal added volatile anaesthetic, and are therefore more economical than other methods of administering inhalation anaesthetics. However, an overriding danger of the closed circuit is that because of varying anaesthetic uptake, varying efficiency of carbon dioxide absorption and the difficulty of accurately calculating basal oxygen requirements, it is never possible to predict the concentrations of gases within the circuit. The greatest variations of gas concentration occur during induction, when anaesthetic uptake is high, and when nitrogen excreted by the patient dilutes the gases in the circuit. Dangerous variations of gas composition can occur if anaesthetic gases have to be added in unduly large volumes, as with the closed-circuit use of nitrous oxide, when small alterations in nitrous oxide uptake can markedly affect the concentration within the circuit and may lead to hypoxia. Complex variations occur when volatile agents are used in a closed circuit, with the vaporizer either in the circuit or in the fresh gas supply-line. For these reasons the circle and to-and-fro systems are more commonly used as semi-closed systems with a fresh gas flow greater than basal, for as fresh gas flow to such systems is increased gas composition within the system tends to approach that in the fresh gas line.

### Semi-closed Rebreathing Circuits

The widely accepted classification of these circuits by Mapleson (1954) is illustrated in Fig. 2. The Magill (Mapleson A) circuit has been extensively studied. During spontaneous ventilation, rebreathing may be prevented in this circuit by relatively low fresh gas flows. During the initial phase of exhalation the patient end of the tubing is filled first with dead space gas and then with alveolar gas. This gas stream from the patient meets fresh gas flowing into the circuit, increasing pressure under the expiratory valve. When this valve opens alveolar gas from both patient and tubing are discharged from the circuit. If fresh gas flow is sufficient, dead space gas will also be vented, followed finally by fresh gas. Mapleson (1954) predicted that rebreathing would be prevented by a fresh gas flow equal to the patient's alveolar ventilation. Under these circumstances, at the moment inspiration commences the circuit will contain only fresh gas and dead space gas, of identical composition. Mapleson based his predictions on a number of assumptions concerning, most importantly, the absence of linear mixing of gas streams and ideal characteristics of the expiratory valve. He recommended that in practice a fresh gas flow equal to minute volume should be used. In clinical practice Kain and Nunn (1968) have shown that in spontaneously breathing lightly anaesthetized patients fresh gas flow could be reduced to an average of 71 per cent of minute volume before rebreathing occurred.

The efficiency of system A depends on the flushing effect of fresh gas flow to expel expired gas. Mapleson (1958) and Nunn and Newman (1964) have shown that in this circuit when fresh gas flow falls below alveolar ventilation the degree of carbon dioxide retention will be an inverse function of fresh gas flow rate, and that under these circumstances hyperventilation by the patient will not affect alveolar gas composition.

During controlled ventilation the Mapleson A circuit behaves in a different manner. In order to ventilate the patient the expiratory-valve opening pressure must be increased. Venting of gas from the circuit now occurs during inspiration. During exhalation alveolar gas is retained in the tubing, and this alveolar gas is the first component delivered to the patient in inspiration. When pressure is raised high enough to open the valve, a mixture of exhaled and fresh gases are discharged from the circuit. The degree of rebreathing will be a complex function of fresh gas flow, tidal volume, respiratory rate, and the rate of pressure rise during inspiration, and can be reduced by using high fresh gas flows, increasing tidal volume, reducing respiratory rate, and applying a high pressure early in inspiration in order to vent a greater amount of alveolar gas from the circuit.

In circuits B, C, and D, fresh gas is introduced close to the patient. Although at first sight this would appear to be beneficial, during spontaneous ventilation these circuits all behave in a less efficient manner than system A. In

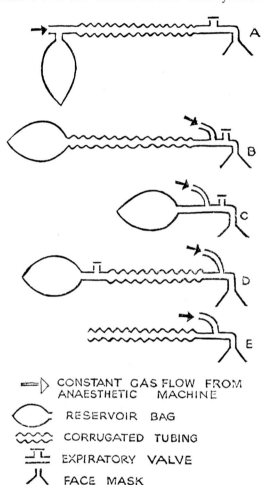

CONSTANT GAS FLOW FROM ANAESTHETIC MACHINE

RESERVOIR BAG

CORRUGATED TUBING

EXPIRATORY VALVE

FACE MASK

FIG. 2. The five semi-closed rebreathing circuits. (Reproduced from Mapleson, W. W., 1954, *British Journal of Anaesthesia*).

system B there is a closed limb unflushed by fresh gas. The tubing may be considered as an extension of the reservoir bag. During expiration fresh and expired gas flows into the reservoir and a mixture of fresh and alveolar gas will be discharged when the valve opens. During inspiration, the patient receives fresh gas from the machine and a mixture of fresh gas and alveolar gas from the reservoir. Prevention of rebreathing requires a fresh gas flow greater than twice the minute volume.

System C (Water's circuit without absorber) may be regarded as a limiting case of either systems A or B in which tube length has been reduced to zero. The conditions for eliminating rebreathing in this circuit are the same as in system B. The absence of tubing in system C effectively reduces the volume of the reservoir, and allows more effective mixing of fresh and expired gas. If rebreathing does occur, carbon dioxide will build up at a slower rate than in system B.

In system D both fresh and expired gas flow back along the tubing during expiration, initially into the bag and later out through the valve. During inspiration, the patient will therefore receive not only fresh gas from the machine but also mixed fresh and alveolar gas from the tubing. Rebreathing can be prevented by a fresh gas flow in excess of twice minute volume. When rebreathing does occur in system D, $CO_2$ will tend to build up at a slower rate than in systems B and C. When the volume of the tubing is

It will be seen that the order of merit of these four circuits during spontaneous ventilation is A, D, C, B. During controlled ventilation the order of merit becomes D, B, C, A. Gas deposition at end-expiration in these circuits is illustrated in Fig. 3.

System E of Mapleson's classification is the valveless T-piece circuit described by Ayre in 1937. During expiration in this circuit fresh gas and expired gas from the patient flow down the expiratory limb. Because peak expiratory flow occurs early in expiration, the proportion of fresh gas added to expired gas in this limb increases as expiration progresses. In the expiratory pause fresh gas

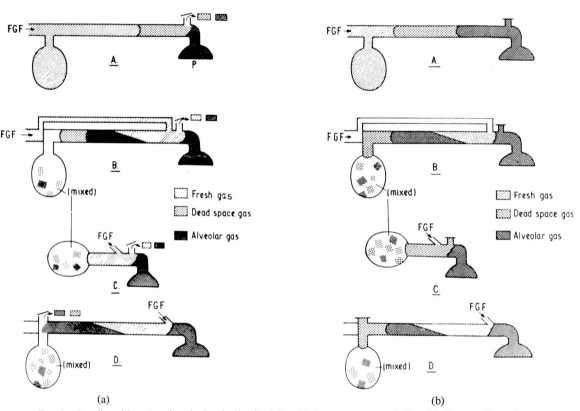

(a)                                         (b)

FIG. 3. Gas disposition at end-expiration in circuits A-D. (a) Spontaneous ventilation (b) Controlled ventilation. (Reproduced from Sykes, M.K. (1968) *British Journal of Anaesthesia*).

greater than the patient's tidal volume, system D will behave as a T-piece circuit, described below.

During controlled ventilation systems B and C behave in a manner similar to that described for spontaneous ventilation. Rebreathing is slightly reduced as fresh gas can accumulate at the patient end of the tubing during the expiratory pause. This gas will be delivered to the patient at the start of inspiration, whilst mixed expired gas will tend to be vented from the circuit. This improved behaviour is less marked in system C because of the absence of tubing to act as a fresh-gas reservoir. Fresh gas flows of at least twice minute volume are still necessary to minimize rebreathing with both circuits. During controlled ventilation with system D nearly all the fresh gas input is delivered to the patient during inspiration. This system therefore causes less rebreathing than systems B and C during controlled ventilation.

accumulates at the patient end of the limb (Fig. 4). During inspiration, gas can be drawn from both the expiratory

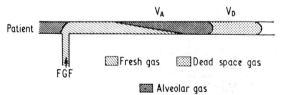

FIG. 4. T-piece (Mapleson E circuit). Gas disposition at end expiration. (Reproduced from Sykes, M. K. (1968) *British Journal of Anaesthesia*.)

limb and the fresh-gas supply. If fresh gas flow is greater than the peak inspiratory flow rate, all the inspirate will consist of fresh gas. This requires a fresh gas flow of about three times minute volume. When smaller fresh gas flows than this are provided, some gas from the expiratory limb will be reinhaled. The initial portion of this will be fresh gas which accumulated during the expiratory pause; but as inspiration continues, gas containing an increasing concentration of $CO_2$ will be inhaled. Two factors reduce the effects of rebreathing which occurs late in inspiration in this circuit. As inspiration continues inspiratory flow rate falls, so that late in inspiration the incoming fresh gas supply may satisfy inspiratory requirements. Moreover, although rebreathing of contaminated gas is potentially maximal at the end of inspiration, this gas will come to occupy the patient's dead space and will not take part in gas exchange.

The efficiency of the T-piece is improved when the expiratory pause is prolonged, when inspiratory flow-rate rises slowly and falls rapidly, and when late expiratory flow-rate is low. Under favourable conditions fresh gas flow may be reduced to $2-2\frac{1}{2}$ times minute volume without rebreathing occurring.

Controlled ventilation with system E is most simply performed by intermittent occlusion of the expiratory limb. The inspired gas will then consist entirely of fresh gas. During exhalation fresh gas and expirate are lost through the open expiratory limb. Under these circumstances the circuit has no reservoir and minute volume must be related to fresh-gas flow and inspiratory-expiratory ratio. To maintain a normal value for this last ratio will usually require a fresh gas flow of about three times minute volume. The principle of mechanical intermittent occlusion of the expiratory limb of a T-piece is used by several paediatric ventilators.

Many modifications of the T-piece circuit have been described, most of them concerned with the form of the expiratory limb. When this limb is shortened rebreathing can be reduced, but at a risk of dilution of fresh gas with atmospheric air and thus conversion of the system from semi-closed to semi-open. When the volume of the expiratory limb exceeds the patient's tidal volume, air dilution cannot occur. Further increase of expiratory-limb volume will not affect functional performance but may add expiratory resistance. The addition of an open-tailed bag to the expiratory limb, as in Jackson-Rees' modification of the circuit does not affect function provided that patient and bag are separated by a length of tubing of internal volume greater than the patient's tidal volume. Under these conditions the circuit resembles system D. If the interposed tubing is of insufficient volume rebreathing of mixed gases from the bag can occur, as in system C.

### Semi-closed Absorption Circuit

Increasing fresh-gas flow to a closed absorption circuit above basal levels converts it to a semi-closed system. It is possible in such a system to control the inspired atmosphere, at the expense of increased wastage of fresh gas and anaesthetic vapours.

For the inspired atmosphere to be the same as that in the fresh-gas inflow in such a system, it is necessary for alveolar gas to be preferentially vented from the circuit. Under these circumstances use of soda-lime will be minimal. To obtain such advantageous circumstances, careful

attention must be paid to the relative position of the various components of a circuit. The studies of Brown, Seniff and Elam (1964) and Eger and Ethans (1968) have clarified the effects of circuit arrangement upon gas concentrations within the semi-closed circle system. During spontaneous ventilation in the circle, maximum efficiency occurs if the overflow valve is close to the patient. Fresh gas should enter the system between absorber and inspiratory unidirectional valve and the reservoir bag should be connected between absorber and expiratory unidirectional

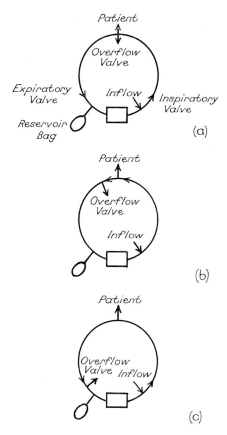

FIG. 5. Three common circle arrangements. (a) Overflow close to patient. Efficiency high during spontaneous ventilation but low in controlled ventilation. (b) Overflow and undirectional valves close to patient. Efficiency high during both spontaneous and controlled ventilation. (c) Overflow remote from patient. Efficiency during spontaneous ventilation less than system (a) but unchanged during controlled ventilation.

valve. An efficient arrangement is shown in Fig. 5a. The circuit illustrated in Fig. 5b differs only in having the unidirectional valves near the patient rather than near the absorber, and functions with equal efficiency. Figure 5c shows a system with overflow remote from the patient, and this circuit is less efficient than the other two.

During controlled ventilation, when gas venting will occur during inspiration, the efficiency of the first system (5a) drops to zero, as all alveolar gas passes through the absorber and only fresh gas is vented. System 5b retains its high efficiency, and the efficiency of system 5c is also unchanged during controlled ventilation. System 5b, though theoretically ideal, has a number of practical disadvantages. Arrangements of unidirectional valves and an overflow placed near the patient tend to be cumbersome, and such valves tend to have a higher resistance, and function less efficiently than large valves placed away from the patient. The efficiency of system 5a during controlled ventilation can be improved if overflow is vented through a dump valve which closes when sudden rises in pressure occur. Venting of excess then occurs during late expiration and the efficiency of the system does not differ during spontaneous and controlled ventilation. Valves of this design may however remain permanently closed if inflow and pressure within the system are high. In practice, it is usually possible to change the site of the overflow from the Y-piece of the circuit to a position nearer the absorber when controlled ventilation is initiated.

### Semi-closed Non-rebreathing Circuits

These circuits contain some form of non-rebreathing valve placed close to the patient. Many different designs of such valves are available (Sykes, 1959), and they are most conveniently used in modifications of Mapleson's A, B, or C rebreathing circuits, where they replace the expiratory valve. Under ideal circumstances a non-rebreathing circuit will allow full control over the inspired atmosphere when fresh gas flow is equal to minute ventilation, the valve merely increasing apparatus dead space by 10–15 ml. In practice, reflux of expired gas into the inspiratory limb often occurs, due to sluggish closure or inefficient seating of the valve. This reflux can amount to 70 per cent of tidal volume, though usually it is only the dead space portion of expired gas which is reinhaled. Sticking of the expiratory valve during spontaneous ventilation can lead to inhalation of air, whilst in controlled ventilation some slip of gas past the expiratory valve often occurs in the initial part of inspiration, reducing tidal volume delivered.

During spontaneous ventilation with a non-rebreathing circuit serious dysfunction of the circuit can occur if there is even a small discrepancy between fresh gas flow and the patient's minute volume. If fresh gas flow is inadequate the inspiratory reservoir will become depleted of gas, limiting and finally preventing inspiration. An excess of fresh gas will raise pressure in the inspiratory reservoir: this will eventually cause the valve to jam in an inspiratory position and prevent exhalation. It is usual in these circuits to supply a small excess of fresh gas supply over minute ventilatory requirements, and to incorporate some form of overflow valve in the inspiratory limb. This will vent excess gas from the circuit and also prevent pressure rising in the inspiratory limb.

### Vaporizer Position in Absorption Circuits

Interest in this problem was stimulated by the introduction of halothane into clinical practice and its early use in closed and semi-closed absorption circuits—techniques primarily designed for purposes of economy. It became apparent that halothane concentrations delivered to the patient could be greatly influenced by the position of the vaporizer within the circuit, and were also affected by fresh gas flow rates and by ventilation, as well as by vaporizer settings. Although initially directed towards halothane anaesthesia, the theory that has been developed to explain variations of inspired anaesthetic concentrations with different vaporizer positions can be applied to any gas or vapour (Mapleson, 1960). It is only in the circle system that vaporizer position assumes practical importance. Such systems can be classified as to whether the vaporizer is within the circle portion of the circuit (VIC), or outside the circle and in the fresh gas line (VOC).

### Vaporizer Setting

*VOC.* With the vaporizer in the fresh gas line, vaporization is effected by fresh gas flow alone. Anaesthetic concentrations within the circuit will depend upon anaesthetic uptake. When uptake is occurring fresh gas will be diluted by gas within the circle and inspired concentration of anaesthetic will be lower than the vaporizer setting. At a later stage of anaesthesia, when equilibrium is being approached, inspired concentration will rise, eventually to equal vaporizer setting.

*VIC.* In this system, vaporization is effected by mixed fresh and expired gases passing through the vaporizer. With basal or low fresh gas flows, high proportions of expired gas containing anaesthetic will recirculate through the vaporizer. Thus the concentration of anaesthetic delivered to the patient will always be higher than the vaporizer setting.

### Fresh Gas Flow Rate

*VOC.* The mass of anaesthetic added to the circuit will be a function of fresh gas flow rate. As fresh gas flow rises, so anaesthetic concentration within the circuit will rise eventually to equal vaporizer setting.

*VIC.* Fresh gas flow here acts as a diluent of anaesthetic concentration within the circuit. As fresh gas flow is increased, so inspired anaesthetic concentration falls, eventually to equal vaporizer setting.

### Ventilation

*VOC.* When ventilation increases, a greater mass of anaesthetic will be removed from the circuit due to enhanced uptake by the patient. Inspired anaesthetic concentrations will therefore fall. This, however, will not necessarily result in a lighter plane of anaesthesia. Increased ventilation will tend to raise alveolar anaesthetic concentration and thus increase depth of anaesthesia.

*VIC.* The mass of anaesthetic vaporized is now a function of ventilation, and at basal flows both inspired and alveolar anaesthetic concentrations will be directly proportional to ventilation. As fresh gas flow is increased this dependence will diminish until, when fresh gas flow is high enough to produce non-rebreathing conditions, concentrations within the circuit will be virtually independent of ventilation.

When anaesthetics such as halothane are used in VOC systems with low or basal fresh gas flows, achievement of adequate initial anaesthetic concentrations within the system may be time-consuming unless vaporizers capable of delivering high concentrations are used. In contrast, VIC systems require vaporizers of low efficiency and limited output. Vaporizers used within a circle must also offer low resistance to gas flow.

VIC arrangements are capable of producing high inspired concentrations of anaesthetic. During spontaneous ventilation with such circuits, excessive depth of anaesthesia, by depressing ventilation, will reduce gas flow through the vaporizer and allow concentrations within the circuit to fall. This built-in safety factor of VIC systems is obviously of limited utility. Respiratory depression occurring during anaesthesia with VOC systems will allow anaesthetic concentrations within the circuit to rise, as anaesthetic is being continuously added to the system. This rise will be opposed by a tendency for the alveolar anaesthetic concentration to fall due to decreased alveolar ventilation. When controlled ventilation is performed with a VIC system, any small measure of inherent safety within the circuit is abolished: very high concentrations of anaesthetic agent may now be produced within the circuit and excessive depth of anaesthesia can easily and rapidly be produced.

### Apparatus Deadspace

Any anaesthetic circuit imposes a deadspace upon the patient. Simple anaesthetic apparatus such as masks and catheter mounts acts as an extension of anatomical deadspace. Apparatus deadspace will be equal to the effective volume of such apparatus. This may be less than, but cannot exceed, apparatus volume as measured by water displacement.

With more complex circuits contamination of fresh gas with expired gas may occur. Effective apparatus deadspace will then be a function not only of apparatus volume, but also of fresh gas flowrate and the pattern of respiration, and will also depend on the phase of respiration in which contamination occurs. Changes in ventilation often occur in response to the imposition of anaesthetic apparatus on a patient, and these changes may modify effective apparatus deadspace. Measurement of apparatus deadspace is often only possible by use of model lungs to simulate respiration, by studies in trained conscious volunteers breathing at a constant rate and tidal volume, and by measuring the volume of expired gas that is inhaled.

### Resistance in Anaesthetic Circuits

### Apparatus resistance

All anaesthetic apparatus other than the open system will offer some degree of increased resistance to respiration. To overcome this apparatus resistance the spontaneously breathing patient will have to generate greater pressure gradients between his alveoli and the atmosphere. These alterations in alveolar pressure may have adverse effects on the cardiovascular system. Excessively high apparatus resistance will markedly increase the work cost of respiration and may lead to hypoventilation.

Flow in anaesthetic tubing may be laminar or turbulent. When flow is laminar resistance will be inversely proportional to the fourth power of tube radius and directly proportional to tube length, gas flow rate and gas viscosity. During turbulent flow resistance is proportional to the square of volume flow and to gas density. In smooth straight tubes turbulent flow only occurs at high gas velocity, but areas of turbulent flow may easily arise at local constrictions and sharp bends. Minimal apparatus resistance requires that all gas-conducting pathways should be of minimal practicable length and greatest practicable diameter, and should be designed to avoid sharp bends or sudden variations in diameter. As resistance is a function of flow, flow rates must always be stated when values of resistance are described. During normal spontaneous ventilation in adult man peak inspiratory flows of from 20 to 60 l/min may be met.

The resistance of any apparatus will be critically affected by that portion of it with the smallest internal diameter. Endotracheal tubes and their connectors, being limited in internal diameter, are usually responsible for the predominant portion of apparatus resistance. At steady flows of 50 l/min the resistance of a Magill (Mapleson A) semi-closed system is such as to cause a pressure drop across the system of 0·25 cm $H_2O$ (25 Newtons/square meter). Addition to the system of a 10 mm. i.d. endotracheal tube with a suitable curved (Magill) connector and catheter mount will increase this pressure drop to 2·5 cm $H_2O$ (250 $Nm^{-2}$), and replacement of the curved connector by a right angled (Cobb) connector further increases the pressure drop to over 5 cm $H_2O$ (500 $Nm^{-2}$).

Expiratory valves incorporated in anaesthetic systems will only open to vent gas when pressure within the circuit exceeds a certain minimum valve opening pressure. The ideal expiratory valve will open at a low opening pressure and will pass high gas flows at that opening pressure. If this opening pressure is too low any reservoir bag in the system may fail to fill before gas venting occurs. The pressure-volume characteristics of commonly used rubber reservoir bags are such that these reservoirs are comfortably filled at interval pressures of less than 0·5 cm $H_2O$ (50 $Nm^{-2}$). Minimum expiratory valve opening pressures in excess of this value are unneccessary and potentially dangerous.

### REFERENCES

Brown, E. S., Seniff, A. M. and Elam, J. O. (1964), "Carbon Dioxide Elimination in Semiclosed Systems," *Anesthesiology*, **25**, 31.

Eger, E. I. and Ethans, C. T. (1968), "The Effects of Inflow, Overflow and Valve Placement on Economy of the Circle System," *Anesthesiology*, **29**, 93.

Kain, M. L. and Nunn, J. F. (1968), "Fresh Gas Economics of the Magill Circuit," *Anesthesiology*, **29**, 964.

Mapleson, W. W. (1954), "The Elimination of Rebreathing in Various Semiclosed Anaesthetic Systems," *Brit. J. Anaesth.*, **26**, 323.

Mapleson, W. W. (1958), "Theoretical Considerations of the Effect of Rebreathing in Two Semiclosed Anaesthetic Systems," *Brit. med. Bull.*, **14**, 64.

Mapleson, W. W. (1960), "The Concentration of Anaesthetics in Closed Circuits, with Special Reference to Halothane: I. Theoretical study," *Brit. J. Anaesth.*, **32**, 298.

Nunn, J. F. and Newman, H. C. (1964), "Inspired Gas, Rebreathing and Apparatus Dead Space," *Brit. J. Anaesth.*, **36**, 5.

Sykes, M. K. (1959), "Non-rebreathing Valves," *Brit. J. Anaesth.*, **31**, 450.

Sykes, M. K. (1968), "Rebreathing Circuits: a Review," *Brit. J. Anaesth.*, **40**, 666.

# CHAPTER 5

# EXPLOSIONS

## J. P. BLACKBURN

Anaesthetic fires and explosions occur infrequently because of the widespread use of intravenous agents, halothane and other non-flammable inhalational agents, and improved safety precautions in modern anaesthetic practice. However, a potentially explosive mixture is present if ether, cyclopropane, ethyl chloride or ethylene are administered, and the use of hyperbaric oxygen during surgery, or for other forms of treatment, has created a new fire hazard.

Two conditions are required for the production of a fire or explosion:

(i) the presence of a flammable mixture,
(ii) a source of ignition of sufficient energy.

Table 1 shows the limits of flammability of some anaesthetic agents (Coward and Jones, 1952).

TABLE 1

| Drug | Air % | Oxygen % | Nitrous Oxide % | Density |
|------|-------|----------|-----------------|---------|
| Diethyl ether | 1·9 to 48 | 2·0 to 82 | 1·5 to 24 | 2·56 |
| Divinyl ether | 1·7 to 27 | 1·8 to 85 | 1·4 to 25 | 2·42 |
| Ethyl chloride | 4·0 to 15 | 4·0 to 67 | 2·0 to 33 | 2·23 |
| Cyclopropane | 2·4 to 10 | 2·5 to 60 | 1·6 to 30 | 1·45 |
| Ethylene | 3·0 to 28 | 3·0 to 80 | 2·0 to 40 | 0·97 |

Trichoroethylene and methoxyflurane are normally considered to be non-flammable, as flammable concentrations cannot be obtained from vaporizers under clinical conditions.

Combustion is initiated by supplying 'activation energy', in some form, to heat the mixture above its ignition temperature. This increases the energy of the molecular collisions occurring in the mixture, and initiates the chemical reaction. Vigorous oxidation, which can occur in flammable anaesthetic mixtures when the activation energy is supplied, leads to the production of heat and light. Flames produced by oxidation may be static, like a candle flame, or may travel through the mixture. If the rate of combustion is very fast the temperature rises rapidly and the flame travels with high velocity through the mixture, producing shock waves. The rapid rise in pressure causes additional heating and an explosion occurs. Such explosions may result in severe injury or death of the patient or theatre personnel.

If the mixture contains very little of the flammable agent, then a flame cannot travel away from the source of ignition, because relatively few molecules react per unit volume, and insufficient heat is produced to raise the temperature of adjacent areas of the mixture above their ignition temperature. Also, in mixtures with a high concentration of the flammable agent, heat production is low because there is insufficient oxygen to react with the agent and the mixture does not burn.

In general, the agents shown in Table 1 burn with a static or travelling flame when mixed with air in suitable proportions, but explode when mixed with oxygen, nitrous oxide, or nitrous oxide/oxygen mixtures.

Most flammable anaesthetic agents mixed with air ignite at about 400°C, although suitable mixtures of diethyl ether with air may ignite at only 200°C, when a cool flame can travel slowly through the mixture and may ignite an explosive mixture some distance away. When mixed with oxygen the minimum ignition temperature is about 350°C.

In general, an explosive mixture with oxygen requires about 1 micro-joule of energy to ignite it, this is 1/100th of the energy required to ignite a mixture with air.

The characteristics of the source of ignition are important. The faster the energy is supplied to the mixture from the ignition source and the smaller the volume to which it is supplied, the lower will be the minimum ignition energy.

Some concern has been expressed about the use of flammable agents which are then discontinued. Vickers (1965) has used ether or cyclopropane with oxygen for induction and intubation. The patient was subsequently ventilated with a non-explosive mixture using a semi-open circuit and the gas mixture at the expiratory valve was found to be non-explosive within three minutes of discontinuing the explosive agent in the case of ether and one minute in the case of cyclopropane.

Furthermore, Coste and Chaplin (1937) have demonstrated that the gas mixture obtained 2 ins. away from the mask of a patient anaesthetized with open ether was non-flammable. When a 4 ounce bottle of ether was emptied on the floor a sample of gas taken 1 in. above the pool of ether ignited (ether concentration 2·12 per cent), but a sample taken 8 ins. above the ether did not burn (ether concentration 0·19 per cent) and the ether could not be ignited by a gas flame $3\frac{1}{4}$ in. above the pool. This work has been extended by Vickers (1970) who analysed gas mixtures at various distances from the expiratory valve. Ether 15 per cent at 8 l./min. or cyclopropane 50 per cent at 1 l./min. was discharged into still air in a room. The lower explosive limit was defined as 1 and concentrations of 0·9 were detected in each case at the closest sampling point 10 cm. × lateral to the expiratory valve. The concentrations decreased very rapidly as distance from the outlet valve increased and were only a small fraction of the lower explosive limit.

It would therefore appear that the 'zone of risk' as originally defined was unnecessarily wide and that: 'an area extending for 25 cm. around any part of the anaesthetic circuit, or the gas paths of an anaesthetic apparatus should be regarded as a 'zone of risk' (Recommendations of the Association of Anaesthetists of Great Britain and Ireland, 1971). Full precautions should be taken against all sources of ignition within this zone.

### Source of Ignition

1. Static electricity. This is the most important cause of anaesthetic explosions, and sparks which occur on connecting or disconnecting the breathing circuit are particularly dangerous.

2. Electric arcs from diathermy, switches, motors, faulty apparatus and short circuits.

3. Hot filaments of endoscope bulbs and cautery. Open flames or fires.

A spark is an efficient ignition source as the gas is heated to a high temperature. Anaesthetic mixtures with air cannot be ignited by sparks arising from the discharge of static electricity as insufficient energy is supplied to initiate combustion, but explosive anaesthetic mixtures with oxygen can be ignited in this way. However, diathermy, electric motors, switches and other devices can arc repeatedly so that considerable energy can be supplied which may ignite any suitable gas mixture.

### Prevention

Explosions can be prevented (i) by avoiding flammable anaesthetic agents, particularly when mixed with oxygen, (ii) by rendering explosive mixtures non-flammable, (iii) by eliminating all sources of ignition.

1. If air is used instead of oxygen, flammable anaesthetic mixtures will burn but not explode.

2. Efficient air conditioning of the operating theatre will reduce the concentration of flammable mixture in the atmosphere, and 15–20 air changes per hour are recommended. As all the flammable anaesthetic agents except ethylene are heavier than air (see Table 1), air should be extracted near floor level, preferably near the anaesthetic machine. The use of closed circuit systems will also limit the escape of flammable agents (H.M.S.O., 1956).

3. Diluents such as nitrogen or helium (Stephens and Bourne 1960, Hingson 1958) and energy-absorbing substances may be added to anaesthetic mixtures. When nitrogen or helium are used the oxygen concentration of the inspired gas mixture may have to be reduced to unacceptably low levels. Free radical absorbers like carbon tetrafluoride and bromine containing fluoro-carbons may be used, but these substances are toxic, and careful control of the mixture is necessary.

4. Sources of ignition should be eliminated wherever possible.

(i) Static electricity is difficult to eliminate completely, but a number of precautions should be taken.

(a) Earthing. If every piece of equipment in an operating theatre were connected directly to earth

through a low resistance pathway, static charges would leak to earth and would not accumulate. However, in this situation, if more than one fault developed in an electrical apparatus, theatre personnel and patients may run the risk of electrocution. If a piece of equipment was not effectively grounded and its case became live, then anyone connected through a low resistance pathway to earth who touched the faulty apparatus would experience a severe electric shock, as a large current could flow through his body to earth. In practice, a compromise is reached whereby static charges are dissipated quickly by providing a resistance path to earth of 50 K$\Omega$–100 M$\Omega$. This reduces the risk of electrocution, by limiting the current which can flow to earth.

(b) Materials which readily acquire static charge, like non-conducting rubbers, wool, nylon and many other plastics are avoided. Conducting rubber is used for face masks, tubing footwear, trolley wheels and most other purposes (Hospital Technical Memorandum No. 1). Endotracheal tubes are not made of conducting rubber since, when in use, they are covered with a conducting film of water that prevents the accumulation of static charges. Also, drip sets and diathermy quivers are not made of conducting material. Antistatic rubber should have the following specification:

New Anaesthetic tubing 25 K$\Omega$–1 M$\Omega$ per 5 ft. length
New footwear              50 K$\Omega$–1 M$\Omega$
New castor tyres            0    –10 K$\Omega$
After use, the upper acceptable limit is increased to 100 M$\Omega$.

(c) Floors should be made of conducting materials with the following electrical properties (Hospital Technical Memorandum No. 2):

Dry test: The resistance between 2 electrodes of area 4 sq. ins. each weighing 2 lbs. placed on the floor 2 ft. apart should not exceed 2 M$\Omega$ on average and all areas tested should have resistances of less than 5 M$\Omega$.

Wet test: Water is applied to the floor under one electrode and the resistance measured between this electrode and a known earth. The resistance should be not less than 50 K$\Omega$ on average and all areas should have resistance of greater than 20 K$\Omega$.

(d) If possible, relative humidity should not be allowed to fall below 50 per cent. The generation of static electricity is more difficult under conditions of high humidity as the surface film of moisture will conduct away static charges to earth.

(e) Radioactive sources can be used to ionize the air in a localized area and so dissipate any static charges.

(ii) Electric arcs are capable of igniting anaesthetic agents mixed with air, oxygen or nitrous oxide.

The diathermy is used routinely during surgery and is, of course, a good ignition source. If the gut is opened using diathermy, explosions due to the ignition of hydrogen sulphide, methane or hydrogen may occur.

Switches on electrical equipment used close to anaesthetic apparatus should be of the sparkless locking variety, but wall mounted switches and socket outlets can be of normal construction regardless of fixing height (Department of Health and Social Security).

Electrically powered ventilators for use with flammable anaesthetic mixtures must have the electric circuits in gas tight enclosures with sealed electric motors and switches. Suckers should be similarly protected, although in practice it should only be necessary to vent the exhaust gases to the atmosphere well away from the motor. Intrinsically safe circuits have been developed, where it is possible to arrange that an arc which might occur has insufficient energy to ignite an explosive mixture. The current flowing in an intrinsically safe circuit is usually limited by a series resistor, so that ignition cannot occur under most fault conditions. These circuits are only suitable for small battery operated devices such as endoscopes.

(iii) Cautery or open flames should not be allowed in the presence of explosive anaesthetic mixtures and, for additional safety, endoscope bulbs should be battery-operated and under-run so that overheating or bursting of the bulb cannot occur.

### Conclusions

Prevention of anaesthetic explosions is of paramount importance and it is essential that appropriate safety measures are enforced. On the other hand, it is important that the subject is viewed in perspective and that unnecessary precautions, which may jeopardize the patient in other ways, are avoided.

During the last ten years in Great Britain no anaesthetic explosions attributable to static electricity have been reported to the Department of Health and Social Security. This is due partly to the widespread use of non-flammable agents and also to the use of conducting rubber and other antistatic precautions. The use of antistatic rubber in the anaesthetic breathing circuit is of particular importance, as otherwise sparks may occur when parts of the circuit are connected or disconnected.

Only two anaesthetic explosions from other causes have been reported during the last five years. These involved the use of cyclopropane/oxygen or ether/oxygen mixtures in close proximity to a diathermy electrode or cautery.

It appears that only sources of ignition in close proximity to the anaesthetic circuit, conducting airways and the lung are likely to cause explosions. In an adequately air conditioned theatre, flammable gas mixtures are rapidly diluted by room air and become non-explosive. Thus, electrical apparatus used at a normal distance from the patient or the anaesthetic machine can be regarded as safe, particularly if it is operated above floor level. This includes non-spark proof E.C.G. and X-ray machines.

The department of Health and Social Security has recently recommended that wall-mounted switches and socket outlets in anaesthetizing areas need no longer be of the spark-proof locking variety, which have plugs which are not interchangeable with those in general use. As the explosion risk is extremely remote, it is far more likely that the patient may be endangered because resuscitation equipment (especially suckers) with standard plugs cannot be connected to existing locking sockets in the operating theatre in an emergency.

The Recommendations of the Association of Anaesthetists of Great Britain and Ireland (1971) concerning explosion hazards have now been published, based on the work of Vickers (1965, 1970). These recommendations cover the 'Zone of Risk' and antistatic precautions not only in operating theatres but in recovery rooms, X-ray departments and other sites in which anaesthetics are not normally given.

## REFERENCES

Coste, J. H. and Chaplin, C. A. (1937), "An Investigation into the Risks of Fire or Explosion in Operating Theatres," *Brit. J. Anaesth.*, **14**, 115.

Coward, H. F. and Jones, G. W. (1952), "Limits of Flammability of Gases and Vapours," *U.S. Bur. Mines*, Bull. No. 503.

Department of Health and Social Security (1969), "Switches and Socket-outlets in Anaesthetising Areas." G/H39/6.

Hingson, R. A. (1958), "The Western Reserve Anesthetic Machine, Oxygen Inhalator and Resuscitator," *J. Amer. Med. Ass.*, **167**, 1077.

H.M.S.O. (1956), *Report of a Working Party on Anaesthetic, Explosions, including Safety Code for Equipment and Installations.* London: H.M.S.O.

Hospital Technical Memorandum No. 1 (1968). *Anti-static Precautions: Rubber, Plastics and Fabrics.* London: H.M.S.O.

Hospital Technical Memorandum No. 2 (1965), *Anti-static Precautions: Flooring in Anaesthetising Areas.*" London: H.M.S.O.

Recommendations of the Association of Anaesthetists of Great Britain and Ireland (1971), "Explosion Hazards," *Anaesthesia*, **26**, 155.

Stephens, K. F. and Bourne, J. G. (1960), "Anaesthesia for Mass Casualties," *Lancet*, **ii**, 481.

Vickers, M. D. (1965), "Duration of the Explosion Hazard following Induction with Ether or Cyclopropane," *Anaesthesia*, **20**, 315.

Vickers, M. D. (1970), "Explosion Hazards," *Anaesthesia*, **25**, 482.

*SECTION V*

# APPENDIX

CHAPTER 1

# MATHEMATICS AND SHAPES

## D. STRICKLAND

### Introduction

The object of this chapter is to find an underlying pattern of thought that may help those readers to whom mathematics is formidable. Einstein is reputed to have collected and played with puzzles of the bent nail and inter-locking shape variety in order to clarifiy his mind while wrestling with abstruse problems. Although some pure mathematicians may insist that their subject can be formally divorced from the real world, there can be little doubt that it is more rewarding to look for pattern in mathematics, and to relate mathematics where possible to human experience.

To a great extent, understanding a mathematically biased paper in a medical journal is an excercise in translation from one language to another. It is hoped that the use of symbols in some way increases the efficiency of transfer of information, and that the result is not analogous to the excessive use of Latin tags in English prose. At its worst, the use of mathematics obscures what would have been obvious in English. At its best, it illuminates an argument or a conclusion by rendering it concise and general. Whatever the reason for the mathematics, it is certain that the reader will be involved in the translation from a symbolic language into concepts with which he is more familiar.

The underlying theme of this chapter is suggested by the use of the word 'shapes' in its title. An anaesthetist may be confronted by a shape when recognizing a pattern in a recorded waveform, or he may summarize the relationship between two physiological parameters by recalling a linear or other graph relating them. To provide a framework for revising mathematics, continual reference to this theme of relating problems to shapes will be used. It is also helpful to observe the inevitability of basic mathematical concepts and operations and to relate them to the manner in which human beings have come to understand the physical universe, just as the developing child comes to understand his environment. Being aware of pattern and inevitability helps to free the non-mathematician from the somewhat numbing suspicion that mathematics is esoteric, tortuous and in some unpleasant way infinite.

### Linear Relationships, $y = kx$

Early observations, such as that to cry twice as loud causes double the disturbance, and that an increase in reach increases the number of objects acquired seems to predispose the developing individual to seek for linear relationships between cause and effect. The straight line graph (Fig. 1) may illustrate the fact that some physical quantity ($x$), such as the force acting freely on a body, causes another ($y$), the acceleration produced, to vary in proportion, (Newton). The graph may on the other hand represent an idealized situation—for example it may represent the best straight line for a series of experimental observations for which statistical analysis confirms a supposition that $y$ is proportional to $x$. Again, it may summarize a more complex situation. For example the application of a positive pressure to a face mask will certainly not produce a change of lung volume which is precisely proportional to the pressure applied, but it may be useful to think in terms of a linear relationship over a restricted range.

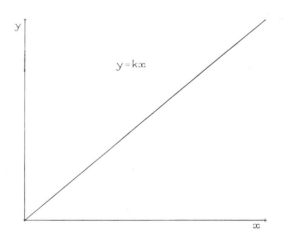

FIG. 1. This graph expresses the human tendencies to define and to look for effects which are proportional to causes.

The obvious appeal of the formula $y = kx$ is that it accords with the strong human impression that one thing often depends on another in a proportional way. However, it goes deeper than this, because we find in science a recurring drive to *define* new quantities on the basis of proportionality to previously defined quantities. In the development of Mechanics (the success of which has strongly influenced later subjects) new quantities such as *force* and *energy* were given precise formulation by definitions based on proportionality. For example it is a rudimentary observation that the harder an object is pushed the more it accelerates. The statement that force equals mass times acceleration does not summarize a fact about the physical universe that was waiting to be discovered by Newton. Rather it shows that primitive observations on pushing things about could only be put on a satisfactory quantitative basis when force was *defined* in this way. This approach has proved extremely fruitful and has suggested new quantities worth defining. It also explains why the experimental discovery that two previously defined quantities (such as pressure and flow) are approximately proportional to one another leads to the application of a Newton-type law, and to the definition of their ratio as a new parameter.

### New Shapes—Powers of $x$

The example of pressure applied to a face mask and the resulting change of lung volume is illustrative of the fact that physiological variables are often not related linearly

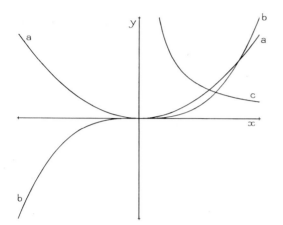

FIG. 2. (a) The parabola, $y = kx^2$. (b) The cubic curve, $y = kx^3$. (c) The reciprocal, or rectangular hyperbola curve, $y = k/x$ (shown for positive $x$).

except over small ranges. When the straight line ceases to describe the relationship between two quantities, we find that the mathematician has a formidable arsenal of 'functions'. For example there is $y = x^2$, $y = x^n$ (any n), $y = \sin x$, $y = \log x$, $y = \tanh x$ . . . the list seems endless. However, when most commonly encountered functions are examined in detail an interesting fact emerges. They can often be built-up from functions having simple shapes. Fig. 2 illustrates three such shapes, (a) the parabola (square law), (b) the cubic, and (c) the

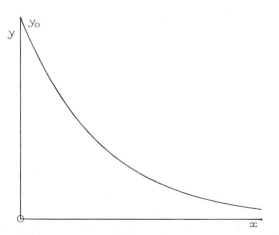

FIG. 3. Exponential decay curve, $y = e^{-\alpha x}$.

rectangular hyperbola. Shape c exemplifies the fact that some quantities decrease as others increase. A shape that is of considerable importance is the 'exponential decay' curve (Fig. 3) which is encountered in the wash-out in time of indicator dye in cardiac output measurements, reactions obeying the Law of Mass Action, in the decrease of light intensity with concentration in photometric measurements and in the recovery of systems embodying stiffness and viscosity. It can be stated that this curve is described by the mathematical formula

$$y = y_0 e^{-\alpha x}$$

where $y_0$ is the initial value and $e$ is a number to be considered in more detail later. However, it can also be expressed as follows:

$$y = y_0 - ax + bx^2 - cx^3 + dx^4 - \ldots \text{ etc.}$$

where $a, b, c, d \ldots$ are numerical coefficients that can be calculated if needed. For our present purpose we need

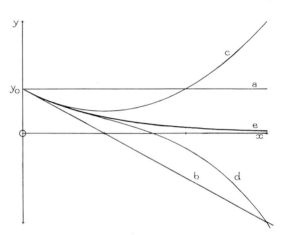

FIG. 4. Successive approximations as an interpretation of power series. (a) $y = y_0$ for all $x$. (b) $y = y_0 - ax$. (c) $y = y_0 - ax + bx^2$. (d) $y = y_0 - ax + bx^2 - cx^3$. (e) $y = y_0 - ax + bx^2 - cx^3 + \ldots = y_0 e^{-\alpha x}$.

only concern ourselves with the interpretation of this result. Clearly it is not true to say that $y = y_0$, since this says that $y$ is always $y_0$ (Fig. 4, curve a) no matter what value is taken on by $x$. If we take the next term ($-ax$), this attempts to correct, but soon gets out of hand (Fig. 4, curve b). To correct for the downward plunge, we try adding a square-law term (Fig. 4, curve c), but $x^2$ begins to increase rapidly with $x$, and the curve swings the other way. Subtracting the next term brings the rapidly increasing $x^3$ term to bear, and this overcomes the excesses of the $x^2$ term, but in turn it too gets out of control (Fig. 4, curve d). It transpires that if the coefficients $a$, $b$, $c$, etc., decrease rapidly enough, each succeeding term exercises its control over the previous ones, and in turn is kept under control by those that follow. Two things are illustrated by this example. The first is that 'power series' give the basic structure of many important shapes (and their mathematical relationships). The second is that it is often useful to get away from symbols and employ words to describe what is happening.

### 'Function' Notation

Equations such as $y = x^2$ may often be thought of in terms of cause ($x$) and effect ($y$). $x$ may be thought of as an 'independent' variable whose variations force the 'dependent' variable $y$ to take on corresponding values. When discussing functions in general it is common to write $y = f(x)$, which should be read as '$y$ is some function of $x$'. Any letter may be used in place of $f$, so $z = g(x)$ can be read as '$z$ is some other function of $x$'. If a constant (2, $k$, etc.) is put in parentheses, as in $y = f(2)$, this means that $y$ equals the value the function $f$ takes when the independent variable equals 2. For example if the function being discussed were $\log_{10} x$, then $f(2)$ would mean $\log_{10} 2$.

### Rates of Change—Differentiation

An infant who has discovered the reality of distance by experimental groping, and has experienced time by waiting for an adult to fetch something out of reach, is ripe to discover velocity as the rate of change of displacement

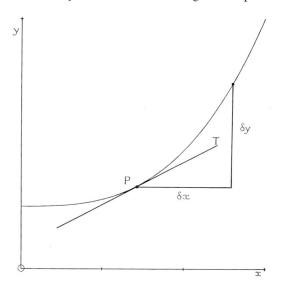

FIG. 5. Differentiation. The slope of the tangent at $P$ is estimated by $\delta y / \delta x$ with greater precision the smaller $\delta x$ is made.

with time. In the development of science, the process of defining new quantities (such as velocity) as the rates of change of previously defined ones (such as displacement), mirrors this personal experience. Time is only one reference for this concept of 'differentiation'. There can obviously be a temperature differential such as occurs with respect to distance between skin and deep tissue, and one is aware of the rate of change of committments with income.

Fig. 5 illustrates the ideas underlying the formal definition of differential coefficient. Taking a finite change of the variable $x$ (written as $\delta x$, an 'increment' of $x$), the corresponding change of $y$ is shown as $\delta y$. The ratio $\delta y / \delta x$ gives a measure of the extent to which $y$ changes as a consequence of altering $x$. If we wish to assess how rapidly $x$ is forcing $y$ to change over a smaller section of the range, the ratio of the relatively large $\delta y$ and $\delta x$ is obviously not a reliable estimator, and the solution is to

take a smaller increment $\delta x$. The underlying concept of the differential calculus is that by extending this process indefinitely we can assess more and more precisely the trend *at a particular point* on the curve. Clearly one cannot make a physical measurement from a graph in which the measured quantities are infinitely small, but for a known mathematical function it is possible to calculate what would result if we could do this. Differential coefficient can be regarded as the limit of the ratio

$$\frac{\text{change in } y, (\delta y)}{\text{the change in } x, (\delta x), \text{ which causes the change } \delta y}$$

if $\delta x$ is made vanishingly small. It is useful to think of such a mathematical statement as detailing the necessary analytical steps to be taken. The corresponding graphical operation consists of estimating the slope of the tangent PT at the point for which the rate of change is required.

Text-books go on from this point to establish standard results for a number of common functions. For example, if $y = x^n$, the rate of change of $y$ with respect to $x$ (the differential coefficient) is $nx^{n-1}$, and if $y = \sin x$ it is $\cos x$, and so on. The actual analytical procedure used in deriving these results is no more than deriving an expression for the estimator $\delta y / \delta x$ and correcting it by finding what is left when $\delta x$ is made vanishingly small. The usual symbol $dy/dx$ may be taken to imply that this analytical process has been accomplished.

The particular result, that if $y = x^n$, $dy/dx = nx^{n-1}$ is important. In words it states that if $y$ is a power of $x$, so is the rate of change of $y$ with respect to $x$ (with a numerical scaling factor $n$). An immediate consequence is that a large family of common shapes which can be constructed from a power series in $x$ have rates of change which can be similarly constructed. In fact the most commonly encountered functions form a closely knit family, as the examples in Table 1 show. In passing, notice that the seventh example has a special property not shared by the others. Also notice that the first is truly a member of the family since putting $n = 1$ in the result for $x^n$ gives $1 . x^{1-1}$, and since $x^{1-1}$ means $x/x$.

TABLE 1

| Function $y$ | $\dfrac{dy}{dx}$ |
|:---:|:---:|
| $x$ | $1$ |
| $x^2$ | $2x$ |
| $x^3$ | $3x^2$ |
| $x^n$ | $nx^{n-1}$ |
| $\sin x$ | $\cos x$ |
| $\cos x$ | $-\sin x$ |
| $e^x$ | $e^x$ |
| $\log_e x$ | $x^{-1}$ |

### Differentiating Techniques

In following some mathematics involving differentiation, one is likely to encounter the use of simplifying techniques for dealing with awkward functions. Suppose that one has learned to differentiate a dozen functions such as sin $x$, $x^2$ and so on. It would be absurd to have to learn a new batch such as sin $2x$, $(2x)^2$. Obviously if at some value of $x$, sin $x$ is changing at a certain rate, sin $2x$ will be changing twice as rapidly with $x$, because the 2 is helping $x$ along. Expressed more formally

$$\frac{d[f(kx)]}{dx} = k\frac{d[f(u)]}{du}$$

where $f(x)$ is any function of $x$, and $u = kx$.

Another situation is illustrated by $y = \sin(x^2)$, in which $y$ is a function of $x^2$, which is in turn another function of $x$. To deal with this we may call $x^2$ '$u$' and write

$$y = \sin(u)$$
and
$$u = x^2$$

Now we know how rapidly $y$ changes with $u$ ($dy/du = \cos u$) and we know how rapidly $u$ changes with $x$ ($du/dx = 2x$). Suppose that at some value of $x$, $u$ changes with $x$ at the rate 10 units. Then this boosts the rate at which $y$ changes with $u$ ten-fold, to give

$$\frac{dy}{dx} = \frac{dy}{du} \cdot \frac{du}{dx}$$

A formal proof of this can only reinforce the obvious. To illustrate the difference between the result for $f(kx)$ and this last result, if the rate of earning from the yield of one apple tree is £10 per year, the rate for three trees is £30 per year: but when selling rabbits one must allow for the rate of increase in the number of rabbits during the year.

Other techniques, such as differentiation of products and ratios of functions are given in text-books to reduce the number of functions to be regarded as standard. On inspection these general results can be seen to be as reasonable as those dealt with above.

## Introduction to Integration

Equipped with a pedometer and a watch a hiker can calculate his speed ($v$) from the formula relating the unknown $v$ to distance and time ($x$ and $t$), i.e.

$$v = \frac{dx}{dt}$$

This contains (symbolically) the instructions necessary for the operation. We will now imagine the inverse situation, in which an observer is travelling in a vehicle equipped with a speedometer and a clock, but no distance-measuring device. Obviously the distance travelled is a function of speed and time, or $x = f(x, t)$ in mathematical symbols, and the problem is to discover what this function is. In this example we will measure distance in metres (m) and time in seconds (s) for numerical convenience, and fit the speedometer with a scale calibrated in m/s. Very roughly, 50 miles per hour (80 km/hr) is 20 m/s. Suppose that measurement started when $v$ is 20 m/s and that this speed is maintained for 15s, and then over the next 10s the speed is steadily increased to 30 m/s and this speed held for 12s. Fig. 6 shows a graph of speed versus time, the

measurement beginning at $B$ and ending at $E$. Over the first time interval (15s, or $\delta t_1$ as shown on the graph) the distance travelled is 20 m/s multiplied by 15s, or 300 m. This is seen to be given by the area of the rectangle between the graph and the time axis, and if this area is expressed in terms of the scale calibrations we can say that the distance covered in the first interval is

$$\delta x_1 = v_1 \, \delta t_1$$

where $v_1$, represents the 20 m/s. The third interval similarly gives

$$\delta x_3 = v_3 \, \delta t_3$$

corresponding to a distance of 360 m, and the only problem is to determine the distance $\delta x_2$ travelled during the interval $\delta t_2$ when the speed was changing. In this

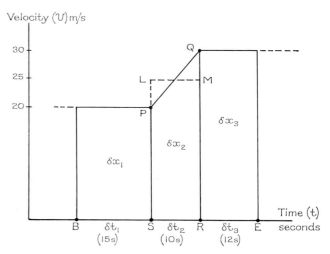

FIG. 6. Integration illustrated for graph made up of linear sections.

example the speed is assumed to have changed linearly so the average speed (say $v_2$) is 25 m/s. Distance $\delta x_2$ is given by

$$\delta x_2 = v_2 \, \delta t_2$$

which is given by the area of the rectangle LMRS superimposed on the graph. It will be seen that this is still the area between the graph and the time axis, since the trapezium PQRS has the same area as the rectangle LMRS. Consequently, the total distance $x$ is given by

$$x = \delta x_1 + \delta x_2 + \delta x_3$$
$$\text{or } x = v_1 \, \delta t_1 + v_2 \cdot \delta t_2 + v_3 \cdot \delta t_3$$

The symbol $\Sigma$ is used to denote summation of terms so we could write

$$x = \sum_{r=1}^{r=3} v_r \cdot \delta t_r$$

This formulation should be thought of in words. The suffix $r$ is known as a dummy suffix. The summation sign with its attendant '$r = 1$' and '$r = 3$' is to be interpreted as 'starting with $r$ equal to 1 in the following expression, find the result. Then repeat with $r$ equal to 2 and then 3, and add all the results together'.

It must be stressed that this formulation is purely for convenience, as would be clear if there were a hundred terms instead of three.

Now suppose that the velocity had altered in a way that was not simply linear and that the graph is as shown in Fig. 7. Concentrating on a representative interval $\delta t$, it is

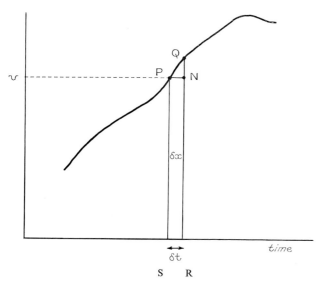

FIG. 7. Taking a thin slice of a graph to be integrated.

necessary to find the area $\delta x$. In the simpler case we imagined a rectangle having the same area as the trapezium, but now we are going to alter our approach slightly. The rectangle PNRS, whose area is $v \cdot \delta t$, differs in area from $\delta x$ by the small area PQN. Suppose that $\delta t$ is so small that we can regard PQN as approximately triangular, then

$$\delta x = v \cdot \delta t + \tfrac{1}{2} QN \cdot \delta t$$

As $\delta t$ is made smaller it will be seen that whereas only one term ($\delta t$) in $v \cdot \delta t$ is becoming small, *both* terms $QN$ and $\delta t$ are decreasing. As a result, the smaller we make $\delta t$ the more negligible the area of the approximately triangular part becomes *in proportion to* rectangular part. For example, if $v = 20$ m/s and $\delta t = 0.01$ s and if the velocity had been rising at the rate of 1 m/s in each second, $QN$ would be 0.01 m/s. The corresponding graph areas (expressed in terms of the distance travelled) are 0.2 m for the rectangle and 0.00005 m for the approximately triangular section. This is an error of 0.025 per cent, and if $\delta t$ is reduced ten-fold the area of the rectangle is reduced by a factor of 10 while the approximately triangular section is reduced by 100, giving an error of 0.0025 per cent.

We may express this as

$$\delta x = v \cdot \delta t + \text{ERROR}$$

where the error term becomes more and more negligible as $\delta t$ is reduced. The process of summing an increasingly large number of terms such as $v \cdot \delta t$, each of which is made progressively smaller, is called *integration*. In place of the $\Sigma$ symbol the integral sign $\int$ is used, and in conformity with the practice in differentiation $\delta t$ is changed to $dt$ to

remind us that the process is taken to limit. The answer to the question 'what function is distance of velocity and time?' is expressed by

$$x = \int v \cdot dt$$

which reads as '$x$ is the integral of $v$ *with respect to $t$*'.

### Three Approaches to Integration

Given graphs such as those shown in Fig. 6 and 7 (which are analogous to flow of gas versus time) the resulting required quantity (distance, or in the case of gas flow, volume) can be determined by measuring the area under the graph and expressing the result in terms of the problem-variables. For example, suppose that a graph of flow versus time has an area of 200 small squares on a piece of graph paper and that one graph division along the time-axis represents 5 seconds and one along the flow axis represents 0.1 litres per second.

Then    1 'small square' $\equiv$ (is equivalent to) 0.5 litres

Total volume = 100 litres

In passing it is worth noting that when interpreting the area under a graph, which may be of any size and may even have quite arbitrary scale marks (as in the case of many pen-recorder charts) confusion can be avoided by noting what the basic paper area corresponds to. For example, the flow graph may have had scale lines 2.3 mm apart in the flow direction and 0.2 inches in the time direction. Rather than expressing the area in square inches or square mm it is far simpler to say

Graph area = 200 small rectangles

1 small rectangle $\equiv$ 0.1 l/s times 5s

Result = 100 l.

Techniques have been developed for estimating areas of graphs and these will be discussed later.

A second approach involves the use of instruments (integrators) which keep a running tally of the products of one variable and increments of the other. These include many ingenious mechanical devices, the integrator circuits of electronic analogue computers and the combination of digital computer 'hardware' and the programmes ('software') that guide the computer through its calculations. All such devices do no more than carry out the calculations that are so tedious when performed by the human presented with a graph, and where possible do this in 'real time', rather than in retrospect.

The third approach to integration forms the subject matter of the integral calculus, and is concerned with establishing the results of integration without having to go through the process of area measurement. This is exactly analogous to the differential calculus, and is relevant when the shapes of the graphs can be expressed as known mathematical functions. For example, if a gas volume ($V$) were related to time ($t$) by

$$V = t^2$$

the differential calculus would enable us, without measuring slopes on a graph to write, for flow,

$$F = \frac{dV}{dt}$$
$$= 2t$$

In the same way if we knew that

$$F = 2t$$

the integral calculus would enable us, without measuring areas on a graph, to write

$$V = t^2$$

As a consequence there are two situations in which integration may be met:–

1. Where the quantity to be integrated (flow for example) is not a known mathematical function of the variable of integration (time in this example). Retrospective graphical assessment is then the solution if one is unfortunately unable to employ an integrating device 'on-line'.
2. When the mathematical function is known and the techniques of the integral calculus can take us directly to the formula for the result. The use of integrals, in a mathematical text is in essence similar to the use of algebra or trigonometry. It seeks to establish a result for a desired unknown quantity starting with premises that relate that quantity to others that are known.

### Integration by Graphical Techniques

All graphical methods of integration seek to assess the area under a graph by approximation. The simplest is the well-known *trapezium approximation* technique, in which the assumption is made that the shape can be broken down into trapezia such as *PQRS* in Fig. 6, even though the graph is not made up of straight line sections. More sophisticated methods exist that reduce the errors implied in this assumption by assuming that the sections are parabolic or involve higher order terms giving a better fit. While we are still discussing integrals in this pictorial manner it is useful to introduce some of the symbols encountered in the integral calculus.

Fig. 8 shows part of a graph of flow of a fluid versus time and we wish to know the volume that passes in the interval $t_1$ to $t_2$. The formula

$$V = \int F \cdot dt$$

states the general relationship, and is read as 'volume is the integral of flow with respect to time'. Now one cannot expect an answer to the question 'what volume has passed at some time (t)?' unless one specifies when the measurement commenced. The general relationship is said to be 'indefinite' and one may meet it in the form

$$V(t) = \int^t F \cdot dt$$

This formulation is intended to stress the indefinite

aspect and may be read as 'the volume that has passed up to some time $t$ may be found by integrating $F$ with respect to time up to time $t$'. As used by mathematicians this notation announces the derivation of a general rather than a particular result. It will be shown later how such general results can be used in numerical examples.

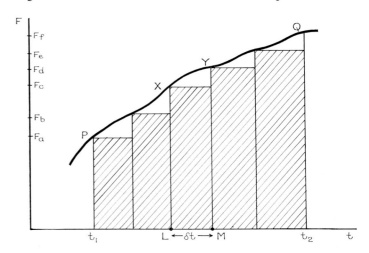

Fig. 8. Integration. The area under the curve between $P$ and $Q$ is estimated by that of the shaded rectangles with greater precision the smaller $\delta t$ is made.

Our problem is to find the volume passing between times $t_1$ and $t_2$, and this is expressed symbolically as

$$V = \int_{t_1}^{t_2} F \, dt$$

which is intended to remind us of the summation notation encountered in the discussion of Fig. 6. It reads 'volume passing is the integral of flow with respect to time, the integration being carried out between the limits $t = t_1$ and $t = t_2$'.

The trapezium technique makes the assumption that by taking samples of the ordinate ($F_a$, $F_b$, $F_c$ . . . $F_f$) at sufficiently frequent steps $\delta t$, the unshaded areas above the shaded rectangles can be assumed to be triangles.

The area of the trapezium $LXYM$, for example, is the width $\delta t$ multiplied by the average height $(F_c + F_d)/2$. Consequently the volume is

$$V = \int_{t_1}^{t_2} F \cdot dt$$

$$\simeq [(F_a + F_b)/2 + (F_b + F_c)/2 + \ldots + (F_e + F_f)/2] \cdot \delta t$$

Inspection shows that each of the terms $F_b/2 \ldots F_e/2$ occurs twice and that $F_a/2$ and $F_f/2$ occur only once each. The result can therefore be expressed as

[(MEAN OF FIRST AND LAST ORDINATES) + INTERMEDIATE ORDINATES] . WIDTH

It is the object of more elaborate graphical methods to obtain better assessment of the areas of the unshaded shapes in Fig. 8, and the object of the integral calculus is to obtain analytical results for as many shapes as possible.

## Integral Calculus

Given a table of results of differentiation, such as Table 1, it is possible to use them 'backwards' to obtain integrals. For example, suppose we need to find the area under the parabolic curve of Fig. 1 (a). We require

$$\int y \,.\, dx$$

where $y = x^2$. Now a known result is that the differential coefficient of $x^3$ with respect to $x$ is $3x^2$, or

$$\frac{d(x^3)}{dx} = 3x^2$$

Since integration is the inverse of differentiation we can say that, since $3x^2$ is the rate of change of $x^3$ with respect to $x$, $x^3$ is the integral of $3x^2$ with respect to $x$. Compare this with saying that, since flow is the rate of change of volume with respect to time, then volume is the integral of flow with respect to time. We therefore have

$$\int 3x^2 \,.\, dx = x^3$$

or

$$\int x^2 \,.\, dx = x^3/3$$

This is an example of an 'indefinite integral', a general result that can be tabulated with many others ready for use in a definite example. It can be stated that the object of the integral calculus is to extend the list of known integrals. For simple functions which are known to be the differential coefficients of other functions there is no problem. The art of using integral calculus is to extend the list, and there are techniques for manipulating functions in order to do this. For those without the aptitude or inclination for this decoding process, tables of integrals are published. When reading a mathematically biased treatment of a medical subject, one often encounters the steps between an initial formulation in terms of an integral and the desired result. This adds verisimilitude to the treatment, but the anaesthetist needs to decide for himself whether it contributes significantly to the understanding of the subject matter.

To illustrate how a definite integral is obtained we will take the area under a parabolic curve. Suppose that we need the area between the graph of $y = x^2$ and the $x$-axis, between $x = 3$ and $x = 5$. The indefinite result is known to be

$$\int x^2 \, dx = x^3/3$$

and the *meaning* of this is as $x$ increases, the area involved increases as $x^3/3$. Now suppose we ask what the area is *up to* some value of $x$ such as $x = 5$. Clearly the answer will depend on where one starts. This may be expressed as

$$\int x^2 \, dx = x^3/3 + K$$

where $K$ is known as a 'constant of integration'. The significance of this becomes clear in the case of measuring volume flow with a spirometer. At any value of time the volume is given by

VOLUME INDICATED
= VOLUME ACQUIRED + STARTING VOLUME

in which the starting volume of the spirometer (the base-line) is analogous to the constant of integration.

To find the change in volume between two instants one ignores the baseline. More formally,

VOLUME INDICATED AT $t_1$
= VOLUME ACQUIRED AT $t_1 + K$

VOLUME INDICATED AT $t_2$
= VOLUME ACQUIRED AT $t_2 + K$

Subtraction eliminates $K$ and yields the obvious result

DIFFERENCE BETWEEN INDICATED VOLUMES
= NETT VOLUME CHANGE

By analogy we have

$$\int^{x=3} x^2 \, dx = 3^3/3 + K$$

$$\int^{x=5} x^2 \, dx = 5^3/3 + K$$

So

$$\int_{x=3}^{x=5} x^2 \, dx = 5^3/3 - 3^3/3$$

$$= 41 \cdot 7 - 9 \cdot 0$$

$$= 32 \cdot 7$$

Often use is made of 'modulus' signs to indicate the steps in forming a definite integral. In this example

$$\int_{x=3}^{x=5} x^2 \, dx = \left| x^3/3 \right|_{x=3}^{x=5}$$

It is worth interpreting this in words. It states that as $x$ changes, the area under the graph of $x^2$ changes as $x^3/3$ (the result given in a table of integrals). In order to find the nett area between limits $x = 3$ and $x = 5$ it is necessary to evaluate $x^2/3$ at $x = 5$ and at $x = 3$ and subtract. This is merely a notation of course, and to appreciate what is happening it is simply necessary to relate it to the familiar spirometer baseline analogy.

## Logarithms

One way of multiplying 4 by 8 and obtaining 32 is to note that these numbers are $2^2$, $2^3$ and $2^5$ respectively, and to use the index law:–

$$2^2 \times 2^3 = 2^{2+3}$$

$$= 2^5$$

The index numbers 2, 3, 5 can be regarded as some sort of 'transform' or coded version of the original numbers 4, 8, 32. An encoding/decoding table which included more numbers would enable us to use addition as the transform operation corresponding to multiplication for numbers in between and beyond these simple ones. Such a table would be called the table of logarithms to the base 2 (and anti-logarithms for users who prefer not to use the encoder table backwards for decoding). The disadvantage of base 2 is that the simple steps of unity in the logarithms corresponds to increases in powers of 2. Fewer people can recall that $2^{15} = 32,768$ than that $10^5 = 100,000$ since people are conditioned to count in a scale of ten. The table of logarithms to base 10 is no more than a list of values of the indices of the powers to which 10 must be raised to equal (be a coded version of) the numbers being converted. Thus $\log_{10}3 = 0{\cdot}47712$ seems reasonable because $10^{\frac{1}{2}}$ is $\sqrt{10}$ which is slightly larger than 3. $\log_{10}30$ is $1{\cdot}47712$ because 30 is one (1) power of ten beyond 3, and so on. The use of the bar notation for logarithms of numbers below 1 has been known to confuse the essential simplicity of this logarithm/power-index relationship. It is convenient to write

$$\log_{10}0{\cdot}3 = -1 + 0{\cdot}47712 \text{ (or } \bar{1}{\cdot}47712)$$

rather than $\qquad \log_{10}0{\cdot}3 = -0{\cdot}52388$

because of the economy (both in time and paper) of having tables from 1–10 only. It might however obscure the fact that $10^{-0{\cdot}52388}$ is approximately $10^{-\frac{1}{2}}$ or $1/\sqrt{10}$, which is of the same order as $0{\cdot}3$.

All the well-known manipulative properties of logarithms are based on the definition, that the logarithm ($L$) of a number ($n$) to a given base ($b$) is the index of the power to which the base must be raised to equal that number. In symbols

$$L = \log_b n$$

is merely another way of writing that

$$b^L = n$$

Substituting 2, 5, 32 for $b$, $L$, $n$ takes us back to

$$2^5 = 32$$

or $\qquad 5 = \log_2 32$

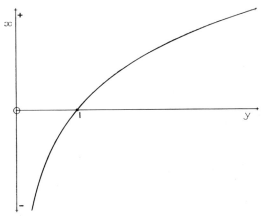

FIG. 9. Graph of $x = \log_b y$, showing the change of sign as $x$ passes through unity.

Since we have talked in terms of $x$ and $y$ when discussing simple shapes, let us use $x$ for 'logarithm' and $y$ for 'number' for comparison purposes. We may write

$$x = \log_b y \quad \text{(see Fig. 9)}$$

$$y = b^x \quad \text{(see Fig. 10)}$$

Now it happens that the shape described by $y = b^x$ occurs frequently in nature in processes where the rate of activity increases with the active population. Growth by cell-division and the proliferation of neutrons in atomic

explosions follow this sort of pattern, and since the logarithmic shape involved no more than a change of axis (that is shifting attention from one variable to the other, regarded as the independent one), we find that the logarithmic function occurs in situations far removed from the mundane exercise of multiplying and dividing using logarithm tables. If we regard $x$ as cause and $y$ as effect, we may expect to find the ('exponential') relationship $y = b^x$ wherever an effect depends on the cause as a power.

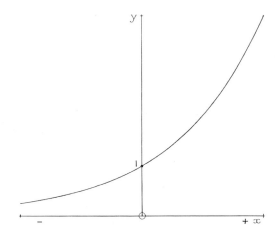

FIG. 10. Graph of $y = b^x$, showing that it is the same as the graph in Fig. 7 with the axes interchanged.

For example (Fig. 10) if $x$ is time and $y$ is number of bacteria at the point $y = 1$ and $x = 0$ on the graph, the rest of the graph to the right takes on some significance.

**The Exponential Decay Curve**

Concentrating our attention on the left-hand side of Fig. 10 this may be redrawn as in Fig. 11 in which it is scaled up in the $y$ sense and reversed in the $x$ sense, the latter manoeuvre enabling us still to think of $x$ as positive. It is therefore now the graph of $y = b^{-x}$ where $x$ is positive and the minus sign deals with keeping the index negative. This shape is of considerable importance. Examples include fall of concentration ($y$) with time ($x$) when an

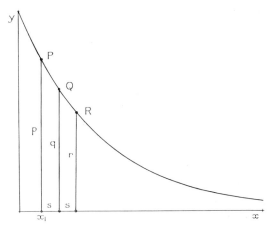

FIG. 11. Graph of exponential decay, $y = b^{-x}$, showing that the ordinates decrease by constant proportion for equal steps in the abscissae.

indicator such as dye in blood (or helium in air) is being washed out of a well-mixing chamber by a steady flow of untagged blood (or air). Other examples are the decrease of transmitted light intensity ($y$) with optical path length or with concentration of dye ($x$) in a photometric densitometer, and the decay of voltages and currents with time in some important electrical circuits. In mechanical devices the decay of velocity of bodies acted upon by friction, when kinetic energy is dissipated as heat, may follow the same law.

Before we show how this simple shape may be disguised by mathematics let us first show what is simple about it and list some of its important properties.

1. In words, it illustrates the law of decrease by constant proportion. For example if the ordinates marked $p\ q\ r$ are equally spaced in the $x$ direction, whatever proportion $q$ is of $p$, so $r$ will be the same proportion of $q$. Thus if $q$ is 80 per cent of $p$, $r$ is 80 per cent of $q$. This follows from

$$p = b^{-x_1}$$
$$q = b^{-(x_1 + s)}$$
$$r = b^{-(x_1 + 2s)}$$

which yield

$$q/p = b^{-s}$$

and $r/q = b^{-s}$ also.

2. Every section of the curve differs from any other section in scale only. For example, if the section $PQ$ were scaled down in the $y$ sense to 80 per cent in our example, it would exactly fit $QR$. The practical importance of this is that anything that may be said about any part of the curve applies (with the scaling proviso) to any other part. Having such accommodating geometry, this shape enables us to predict ahead or extrapolate back in a way that is rivalled only by the straight line.

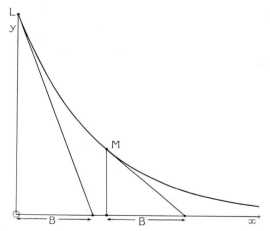

FIG. 12. $y = b^{-x}$, showing that the rate of change is proportional to the ordinate at any point.

3. The slope at any point is proportional to the ordinate at that point. For example (Fig. 12) if the ordinate at $M$ is one-third of that at $L$ the rate of decay at $M$ is also one-third of that at $L$.

4. As a consequence of this last fact, the bases $B$ of the triangles under the tangents are the same, no matter where the points $L$ and $M$ are. This becomes important in phenomena that decay with time, in which case $B$ is a time interval and is known as the 'time constant' of the process. It serves as a measure of the speediness or leisureliness of the process and may be thought of as the time the process would have taken to be completed had it been able to maintain its current rate of decrease. For example, suppose that the curve represents the wash-out section of a dye-curve in a cardiac output measurement and that the initial negative slope was such that $B$ is 20 seconds. Then as long as the curve remains an exponential decay, the rate of decay at every point is such that it would have reached the baseline in 20 seconds.

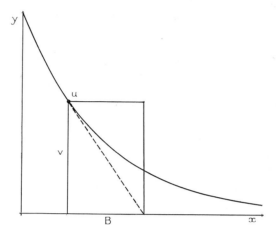

FIG. 13. Geometrical interpretation of the area from a point ($U$) to infinity.

5. The area under the curve from any point (such as $U$ in Fig. 13) to the infinitely remote point where the process may be thought of as having finished is proportional to the ordinate ($u$) and is in fact equal to the area of the rectangle $uB$. This means that operations involving integration (as in dye-curve cardiac output computers) are extremely simple, although the associated mathematics may not give that impression.

It might seem surprising that a shape with such obliging properties could generate large quantities of apparently erudite mathematics, and it is valuable to enquire why.

### Choice of Base ($b$) for Describing Exponential Decay

A practical example of exponential decay will have units and scales for $x$ and $y$ and be of the form

$$y = ab^{-cx} \text{($a$ is value at $x = 0$)}$$

For example, for a dye dilution curve, $x$ may be time in seconds and $y$ and $a$ may be in mg/100 ml. Since $-cx$ is an index, it is a pure number, so $c$ will be in seconds to the power $-1$. The number $b$ is a matter of choice, since any decision to alter it can always be allowed for by a compensating choice of $c$. This is no more than stating that any number can be expressed as the appropriate power of any other number, which is the same as saying that one can look up the logarithm of a number in any sort of logarithm tables and expect to find an entry. For example suppose that $b$ is 2 and that at some point on the graph $y$ is an eighth of $a$, then $cx$ must be 3 since $\frac{1}{8} = 2^{-3}$. Now the fraction $\frac{1}{8}$ can be expressed in an infinite number of ways, including $10^{-0.90309}, 8^{-1}, 64^{-0.5}, 100^{-0.45155}$ and so on. Each index is simply the logarithm of $\frac{1}{8}$ to the appropriate base. Now since every exponential decay curve in the universe is the same as every other except only in scale, it is convenient to choose a common base for describing them. A committee of binary digital computers might decide that 2 is the obvious choice, while a committee of human beings would probably choose 10. In contrast a committee of mathematicians would decide on $2.71818\ldots$, or '$e$', a number which cannot be exactly expressed in decimals and which is unrelated to the digital complement of mathematicians. The reason why $e$ is favoured is that all operations involving differentiation or integration are simpler for the mathematician to perform. If a graph of $2^x$ is plotted against $x$ and its slope measured and plotted on the same scale, the new graph will be the same shape but will be different in scale from the original. The same is true for $3^x$, $4^x$ and so on. The exponential $e$ is the only number for which $e^x$ and its rate of change with respect to $x$ are identical. This is very convenient, since the same applies if it is differentiated again with respect to $x$, and if it is integrated—the whole family of curves are identical. In contrast, every time $10^x$ is differentiated with respect to $x$ we must remember to scale up by a factor $(2.303)$ which is somewhat cumbersome.

Returning to the dye-curve example there will be some value of $c$ for which the result could be written

$$y = ae^{-cx}$$

and this is the form that is encountered in the literature. Although mathematical operations such as differentiation are simpler with this form, and numerical calculations are neither more nor less difficult with $e$ than with any other base number, the main effect of the appearance of $e$ on those less certain of their mathematics is to create the erroneous impression that this special number has something impressive to say. Relegating this idea to the realm of folk-lore we can go back to the basic geometrical facts about the shape whenever we need to understand it. One useful side effect of using $e$ is illustrated in time decay processes where it is convenient to think in terms of the *time constant* mentioned earlier. This comes in naturally when the equation is written with $1/T$ instead of $c$, as in

$$y = ae^{-t/T}$$

Here $T$ is the 'time constant' as described when the decay-rate geometry was discussed, and $T$ was interpreted as the time the process would have taken had its current rate of change been maintained. Another interpretation follows by setting $t = T$ in the above equation, since this gives

$$y = ae^{-1}$$

which means that after a time $T$ has elapsed, $y$ has fallen to $1/e$ (or $36.8$ per cent) of the initial value $a$. For some decay processes (such as decay of radio-active materials) the measure of lengthiness of the process is taken as the 'half-life', or the time taken to reach 50 per cent of the initial value. It might be felt that 50 per cent is easier to visualize (and remember) than $36.8$ per cent, but the advantages of the time constant measure show up when one is considering rates of change and integrals. For example the total area under the graph is immediately known to be $aT$, and the initial slope is $-a/T$. With a little thought much can be done with the exponential decay curve without resorting to any mathematics at all.

## Napierian Logarithms

Tables of logarithms to base $e$ are somewhat worse than those to base 2 for calculations by decimally conditioned beings, since they increase in steps of 1 for increases of powers of $e$. Their purpose is solely to give answers to results in the form $y = \log_e x$ without the need for scaling. In fact $\log_e x$ can be calculated from $\log_{10} x$ times $\log_e 10$ since one of the properties of logarithms is that

$$\log_b n = \log_u n \cdot \log_b u$$

for any bases $b$ and $u$.

The conversion factors of greatest interest are

$$\log_e n = 2.30259 \log_{10} n$$

and

$$\log_{10} n = 0.43429 \log_e n$$

## $e^{-x}$ and $e^x$ as Power Series

The coefficients in the power series of $e^{-x}$ are the rapidly decreasing ones referred to earlier.

$$e^{-x} = 1 - \frac{x}{1} + \frac{x^2}{2.1} - \frac{x^3}{3.2.1} + \frac{x^4}{4.3.2.1} - \cdots$$

Similarly $e^x$ has all positive terms, or

$$e^x = 1 + \frac{x}{1!} + \frac{x^2}{2!} + \frac{x^3}{3!} + \frac{x^4}{4!} + \cdots$$

where $n! = n(n-1)(n-2)\ldots 3.2.1$

The fact that $\frac{d(e^x)}{dx}$ is equal to $e^x$ is illustrated by taking any term, such as the $x^3$ term.

$$\frac{d}{dx}\frac{x^3}{3!} = \frac{3x^2}{3!}$$

$$= \frac{x^2}{2!}$$

so each term moves down one place and the first vanishes because 1 does not change with $x$.

A similar series can be written for $10^x$, but every term after the 1 is scaled up by a power of $\log_e 10$, which suggests that the mathematician may have some force behind his insistence that $e$ yields elegant results. The factorial type coefficients occur in many power series. For example

$$\sin x = x - \frac{x^3}{3!} + \frac{x^5}{5!} - \frac{x^7}{7!} + \cdots$$

$$\cos x = 1 - \frac{x^2}{2!} + \frac{x^4}{4!} - \frac{x^6}{6!} + \cdots$$

They have a somewhat forceful way with them as can be seen if one sets out to calculate 100! The idea of a series converging is brought home by realizing that $e^{1000}$ is a finite number, although a huge one. Since the expansion runs

$$1 + 1000 + \frac{(1000)^2}{2!} + \frac{(1000)^3}{3!} + \cdots$$

the persistence of the steadily growing denominators is impressive, because there will come a term $(1000)^n/n!$ where the steady increase in $n!$ overcomes the repeated multiplications by 1000, and succeeding terms are gradually rendered more and more trivial.

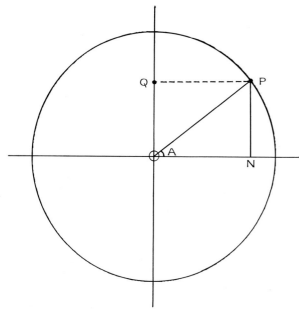

FIG. 14. Initial definition of sin $A$ as $PN/OP$.

### The Sinusoidal Function

At their most mundane, tables of sines and cosines seem primarily intended to enable surveyors to measure the widths of rivers without taking to boats. However, just as the logarithmic function is found to extend beyond the field of mere computation, so it is found that the sine function is vital to our description of the physical universe. Referring to Fig. 14, for an angle less than 90°, the sine of angle $A$ is taken as ratio of the length of the 'opposite' side $PN$ to the length of the hypotenuse $OP$ of a right-angled triangle $OPN$ containing the angle $A$. By associating signs with the axes as in Fig. 15 this definition is extended to angles beyond 90° by taking the projection $OQ$ of $OP$ on the vertical axis, and in general

$$\sin A = OQ/OP$$

$$\cos A = ON/OP$$

If a plot is made of sin $A$ versus $A$ the curve ($a$) of Fig. 16 is obtained. Similarly ($b$) is a plot of cos $A$. It is found that these shapes have an important property. If the slope (rate of change) of the sine curve ($a$) is plotted versus the angle $A$, it is found to follow the cosine curve ($b$), due

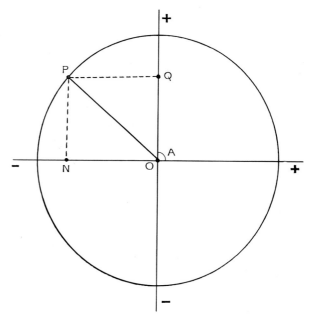

FIG. 15. Extended definition of sin $A$ as $OQ/OP$.

allowance being made for scale. If the slope of curve $b$ is plotted, curve $c$ results, and this is found to be curve $a$ inverted. These curves are all the same shape, differing only in phase (displacements along the angle axis). It is of considerable importance that of all conceivable repetitive shapes, only the sine function has this property. It is well-known that a large range of physical phenomena, such as currents in oscillatory circuits, displacements, velocities and pressures in mechanical oscillatory systems vary sinusoidally. That is, that graphs of such quantities plotted against time have the same shape as the curves in Fig. 16. The reason for this link between oscillatory phenomena and the trigonometrical tables is that many of the quantities which we define to describe the physical universe are

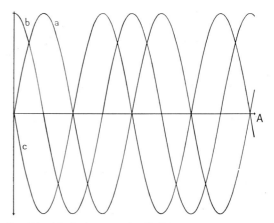

FIG. 16. ($a$) sin $A$ versus $A$. ($b$) The rate of change of sin $A$ = cos $A$. ($c$) The rate of change of cos $A$ = $-$sin $A$.

related to one another by being proportional to the rate of change of others. Furthermore oscillatory systems involve restraints which force the quantities we are measuring to vary so that the rate of change of one quantity must follow the same shaped variation as another. For example, when a pendulum swings, the force tending to bring it back increases with the displacement of the bob, and the deceleration is, by Newton's law, proportional to this force. Whatever movement takes place is constrained so that the rate of change of displacement (acceleration) follows the same pattern of variation as does the displacement itself. Since the sinusoid is the only oscillatory waveform that has this property, a freely swinging pendulum has no choice but to move with sinusoidally changing displacement.

If all oscillatory systems were as simple as that, we would be restricted in speech to emitting pure tones, and the E.C.G. would have little diagnostic significance. As a result of the work of Fourier we know that the complex

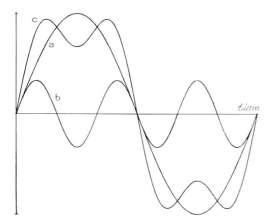

FIG. 17. (a) Fundamental waveform. (b) Third harmonic of a. (c) The result of adding a to b.

oscillations that are produced in speech, music, earthquake tremors, E.C.G. waveforms, and indeed anything in the universe that changes, can be broken down into component sinusoids. A very simple waveform will serve to introduce this idea. In Fig. 17 a new shape is built up by adding two sinusoids, the more rapidly alternating one being the third harmonic of the slower one, which means that it undergoes three cycles of variation while the 'fundamental' waveform undergoes one cycle. It will be noticed that the higher frequency has the result of steepening the sides of the waveform, and it is found that the more abrupt the change, the higher the order of harmonic is necessary to create this abruptness. If a waveform with sudden changes were handled by any medium (such as an electronic amplifier, or a badly designed stethoscope) that discriminated against the high frequency components, the sudden changes would not be adequately reproduced. This can be easily observed when one cannot clearly distinguish between sibilant consonants over a telephone link with inadequate high frequency

response, and exactly the same phenomenon accounts for the inability of some poorly designed E.C.G. recorders to reproduce a QRS complex adequately.

Fourier's analysis, as far as regularly repetitive waveforms are concerned, seems reasonable since we know that musical instruments emit harmonics which are sinusoids whose frequencies are multiples of the fundamental note. The fact that non-repetitive waveforms can similarly be regarded can be shown to be reasonable by firing a pistol near a piano. No matter how the strings are tuned they will all respond to their own particular frequency-components. The importance of this is that sinusoids are relatively simple to handle conceptually and mathematically, and from the work of Fourier is growing a vast science concerned with signal analysis, by which anything that changes and is measurable is becoming amenable to mathematical investigation. Whereas the far reaches of this science are somewhat complex, certain powerful simplifications are afforded by regarding regular or reasonably regular shapes, such as in the E.C.G. and respiratory flows and pressures, as built up from the simpler sinusoidal shapes.

It can quite generally be stated that if any waveform is altered in shape by any intervening medium or device then some combination of the following must have occurred:–

1. The original sinusoidal components have been altered in their relative magnitudes.
2. The relative timings (phases) have been altered.
3. New sinusoidal components have been introduced.

Appreciation of these facts makes it much easier to understand the defects and limitations of a wide range of devices and systems, such as recording systems, spirometers, stethoscopes and physiological transducers. It also helps in the understanding of physiological systems such as the circulation and the mechanics of respiration.

### The Mathematical Representation of Sinusoids

Since the sine function relates to angles we find that a sinusoidal quantity that varies in time describes the variation of the intercept $OQ$ in Fig. 14 as $OP$ rotates. In symbols:–

$$y = y_0 \sin (kt)$$

where $k$ is a conversion factor that produces an angle for the term in parentheses. Since the largest value that the sine of an angle can have is unity, the interpretation of $y_0$ is that it is the maximum (or 'peak') amplitude of $y$. To interpret $k$ we observe that the higher the frequency ($f$) the more rapidly the term $kt$ must vary, so $k$ is proportional to $f$. Finally the fact that the process is cyclic tells us that every time $ft$ changes by one unit (cycle) the angle must change by 360°, so

$$y = y_0 \sin (360 \, ft)°$$

It is more usual, however, to express angles in radians, for which $2\pi$ radians equals 360°. Just as in the use of $e$, so here the use of radians is a requirement of mathematical convenience unrelated to computation. The power-series expansion for $\sin x$ that was quoted earlier is true for

$x$ measured in radians. The introduction of a correction factor $2\pi/360$ to render this expansion valid for degree measure would make the result extremely unwieldy and disguise its simple pattern. Consequently the usual expression for a sinusoid is

$$y = y_0 \sin(2\pi ft)$$

or

$$y = y_0 \sin(\omega t)$$

where

$$\omega = 2\pi f$$

If the sinusoid does not happen to pass through zero at the time we chose as origin ($t = 0$) the value of the angle ($\phi$ at $t = 0$) can be added for complete generality to give

$$y = y_0 \sin(\omega t + \phi)$$

Fourier's expression for a repetitive waveform is simply the sum of terms like this, all having whole multiples of the fundamental value of $\omega$ and each with its appropriate amplitude and phase.

### Partial Differential Notation

In the chapter 'Physical Principles I' partial differential coefficients (rates of change) are met. In order to visualize these it is instructive to imagine a man climbing a hill towards a peak that is to the north-east. If he rests at a point of height $h$ where two paths meet, one running east and the other north he might well estimate the slopes of these two paths where he is resting. Denoting distance walked up the easterly path by $e$ and that along the northerly one by $n$, these slopes are written as:

$$\frac{\partial h}{\partial e} \quad \text{and} \quad \frac{\partial h}{\partial n}$$

Here the symbol $\partial$ (rather than $d$) is used to imply that he depends on two variables, not one. For example the first is read as 'the rate of change of $h$ with respect to $e$, $n$ being kept constant'.

More generally if a variable $V$ is a function of several variables

$$V = f(x, y, z, \text{etc.})$$

$\dfrac{\partial V}{\partial x}$ means the rate of change of $V$ with respect to $x$, for fixed values of the other variables.

Also in the hill-climbing example

$$\frac{\partial^2 h}{\partial e^2} \quad \text{means} \quad \frac{\partial}{\partial e}\left(\frac{\partial h}{\partial e}\right)$$

that is, the rate at which the easterly path becomes steeper as he goes further east. Conventionally

$$\frac{\partial^2 h}{\partial n \partial e} \quad \text{means} \quad \frac{\partial}{\partial n}\left(\frac{\partial h}{\partial e}\right)$$

This describes how rapidly easterly paths become steeper if he elects to go north.

### Conclusion

The anaesthetist has to decide on his objectives when revising or extending his knowledge in response to the steady increase of mathematics in medical literature. If he intends to generate mathematics himself, or if his requirement is to be able to follow the detailed steps of mathematical arguments, then there is no alternative but to acquire the manipulative skills presented in standard texts. If his intention is to be able to follow the general drift of a mathematical treatment while assuming the validity of the steps, he must acquire the comparable skill of selectivity. In either case, the realization that mathematics is primarily based on human experience and that its concepts, aims and operations can be expressed in words can be of great assistance. For example, when it is found that text-books on trigonometry devote many pages to evolving such formulae as

$$\sin(A + B) = \sin A \cos B + \cos A \sin B$$

it is as reasonable to ask a mathematician to explain the purpose behind evolving such conversion routines, as it is to ask an anaesthetist to state the object of administering a muscle relaxant. In this particular example the assurances that there are a limited number of such formulae, and that their purpose is to convert mathematical statements which are in an inconvenient or inelegant form into ones which are easier to comprehend, removes the spurious element of mystique and replaces it with purpose. It is valuable when asking advice of a mathematician on a particular point, to give some thought to the structure of your question. Instead of asking 'how do I convert logarithms in one base to logarithms in another?', it is better to state the immediate problem and ask for a resumé of similar manipulations. This will elicit the fact that there are a handful of similar useful conversion routines which all stem from the definition of logarithms, and that the logarithm itself is no more than an inverse way of regarding an index or power which has manipulative and conceptual usefulness.

A text-book which is written along these lines, and which combines helpfulness and entertaining readability, is *Mathematics in Medicine and the Life Sciences*, by G. R. Stibitz (Year Book Medical Publishers).

CHAPTER 2

# DATA HANDLING AND STATISTICS

## D. M. BURLEY

The purpose of this chapter is to give the reader some insight into the various methods which are used to extract meaning from the masses of recorded data which are now an integral part of modern scientific medicine. Gone are the days when an anaesthetic record consisted of a brief note such as 'gas, $O_2$, ether'. Measurements are now made of induction time, blood pressure and pulse rate, ECG's are monitored, anaesthetic levels in blood are determined; all being recorded as columns of figures or points on a graph. These remarks apply to all branches of medicine and nearly all walks of life. It hardly seems possible nowadays to enter an airport building or even walk down the street without a dedicated girl, holding a board with forms attached, stopping you to ask, 'where are you going?', 'when are you coming back?', 'have you been there before?'. All is noted down, but what happens to it one is tempted to ask? As an intelligent reader of this chapter your answer will be that the data will be classified, correlated and analysed appropriately; conclusions being drawn on the basis of that analysis for the formulation of an hypothesis or a plan for rational action.

The majority of doctors have some basic knowledge of mathematics, dimly remembered from school Vth or VIth Form studies. Therefore throughout this chapter the derivation of simple formulae will be explained, more complex ones being presented with examples for easy reference.

## Definitions

*Population and sample:* The *population* under study is the whole group of patients with a given characteristic or reaction which we wish to investigate. It may be all the patients udergoing a particular operation during the 5 years 1964–68, it may be all the patients admitted to a hospital for a given year, it may even be the whole population of the country. Whatever group is chosen it must be defined and written down. If we are lucky it may be possible to study every member of the population, but usually size precludes this and a *sample* has to be taken. This sample may be chosen by a number of methods such as taking every tenth patient who presents, or every patient admitted on a Monday. Whatever sampling method is chosen, however, it must be borne in mind that in the end we are going to reason from the results in the sample to the population as a whole and hence *bias* must be avoided. It is all to easy for bias to creep in by the back door if one is not alert to this possibility. My example of choosing patients admitted on a Monday could be a biased sample if we were studying the results of some anaesthetic procedure in E.N.T. operations generally, and it was found that tonsillectomies were never admitted on a Monday. A

method of overcoming bias when samples are being compared is by *randomization* and the techniques for random selection of patients or random allocation of treatments are dealt with in detail in other books such as Bradford Hill's classic work 'Principles of Medical Statistics' which has a table of random numbers in the appendix.

*Measurement Scales:* We are used to measuring things in pounds and ounces, feet and inches; where an inch is an inch from Land's End to John 'O Groats, and two inches is twice as long. This is an *interval* scale and the measurements are absolute, each being related to the other numerically. All this may seem obvious, but there is a tendency to assign numerical values to subjective observations; degrees of pain, tenderness of joints, etc., and forget that these are *ordinal.* In other words they give order or rank to the observations; such as 0 for 'no tenderness', 1 for 'slight tenderness', 2 for 'moderate tenderness' and 3 for 'severe tenderness', and we can say 3 is worse than 1. What we cannot say, however, is that 3 is three times as bad as 1. Finally there is the *nominal* scale where a number is used simply to distinguish one person from another, or one happening from another, without thought of ranking. This is just like a number in a telephone directory and, as Smart (1963) points out the telephone number 2222 is not twice as large as number 1111, it is just different.

*Parametric and non-parametric:* The numerical characteristics of a given population are known as *parameters* and as will be seen later the statistical methods for handling this type of data are different from those used for handling frequencies or scores which have no fixed numerical value. The great variety of non-parametric methods for the statistical examination of frequencies and scores have been dealt with and classified in Siegel (1956). A few of those techniques in more common use are also described later.

## The Recording of Data

It is not intended in this Chapter to go into details of the methods for presenting data in visual form. Whether to use graphs and histograms, whether to express as absolute figures or percentages, whether to use an arithmetic or a logarithmic scale. These problems are dealt with simply by Moroney (1951) and Bradford Hill (1967) and one cannot do better than quote the conclusions of the latter author. 'Tables and graphs must be entirely self-explanatory without reference to the text', and "Conclusions should be drawn from graphs only with extreme caution and only after careful consideration of the scales adopted'.

## The Normal and Binomial Distributions

Having cleared away a few definitions and mentioned methods of recording accumulated data, it is now essential to our understanding of statistical method to consider what we want the figures to provide information about. One of the basic questions requiring an answer is: could these findings have arisen by chance, or do they indicate changes brought about by some action on our part? To provide the answer one needs to understand something of the theory of probability and its connection with frequency distributions. A frequency distribution is simply a convenient way of expressing a mass of observations in a compact form. Two simple examples will suffice.

Some time ago I had occasion to toss 6 pennies in the air 100 times and record the frequency of heads or tails at each throw. The results were as follows:

| | |
|---|---|
| 6 heads | 1 |
| 5 heads, 1 tail | 9 |
| 4 heads, 2 tails | 32 |
| 3 heads, 3 tails | 29 |
| 2 heads, 4 tails | 22 |
| 1 head, 5 tails | 5 |
| 6 tails | 2 |

Note that the frequency of the central events is high with diminishing frequency in either direction.

On another occasion I measured the height of 100 randomly selected adult males to the nearest inch with the following results:

| Height (inches) | Number of Male Subjects |
|---|---|
| 62 | 2 |
| 63 | 3 |
| 64 | 5 |
| 65 | 8 |
| 66 | 10 |
| 67 | 13 |
| 68 | 18 |
| 69 | 15 |
| 70 | 9 |
| 71 | 6 |
| 72 | 5 |
| 73 | 3 |
| 74 | 2 |
| 75 | 1 |

In this second example note that the commonest height is 68″ and that on either side of this 'central' height there are decreasing numbers until at the extremes in either direction the occurrences are rare. In fact this information could be expressed in graphic form and an attractive curve smoothed in as in Figure 1. Note the characteristics of this curve, a convex top which part way down each side changes over into a concave tail. This curve is known as the *Normal* or *Gaussian Distribution*, and is characteristic of parameters which are subject to variation due to the interplay of many different factors. To obtain a completely smooth curve we would need to plot all the individual measurements to a fraction of an inch rather than grade them into discrete groups, but provided the number of measurements is large the latter method is much less laborious and the curve closely approximates to the true normal distribution curve.

Not all measurements of human parameters are suitable for expression as a normal distribution. In fact body weight, depending as it does on volume rather than a linear measurement, if plotted as a distribution curve, gives a peak value to the left of centre, a condition known as *positive skewness*. Those interested in these variations and other distributions such as the *Poisson Distribution* should study first Smart (1963), Moroney (1951) or Mather (1967).

To go back to the coin tossing example it will be clear that each coin when tossed can be in one of two conditions,

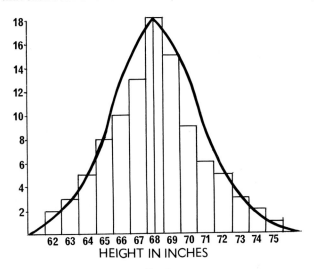

FIG. 1.

either 'heads' or 'tails', and that these events occur with equal frequency, provided the coin is not biased.

Call heads '$p$' and tails '$q$'. Then each coin is made of a head ($p$) or a tail side ($q$) and can be represented by $p + q$, with $p = \frac{1}{2}$ and $q = \frac{1}{2}$.

If two coins are tossed then the possible interactions are $(p + q) \times (p + q)$ or $(p + q)^2$.

| $(p + q)^2$ | $= p^2 +$ Both $p$'s (heads) | $2pq$ a '$p$' and a '$q$' (head and tail) | $+q^2$ Both $q$'s (tails) |
|---|---|---|---|
| frequency | $\frac{1}{2} \times \frac{1}{2} = \frac{1}{4}$ (25%) | $2 \times \frac{1}{2} \times \frac{1}{2} = \frac{1}{2}$ (50%) | $\frac{1}{2} \times \frac{1}{2} = \frac{1}{4}$ (25%) |

100%

Having set out the simplest example in detail the six coin situation can equally be worked out from:

$$(p + q)^6 =$$
$$p^6 + 6p^5q + 15p^5q + 20p^3q^3 + 15p^2q^4 + 6pq^5 + q^6$$

and expressed as a percentage

| | | |
|---|---|---|
| 6 heads ($p^6$) | = | 1·56% |
| 5 heads 1 tail ($p^5q$) | = | 9·38% |
| 4 heads 2 tails ($p^4q^2$) | = | 23·44% |
| 3 heads 3 tails ($p^3q^3$) | = | 31·25% |
| 2 heads 4 tails ($p^2q^4$) | = | 23·44% |
| 1 head 5 tails ($pq^5$) | = | 9·38% |
| 6 tails ($q^6$) | = | 1·56% |

If we look back at the results of my actual coin tossing we will see that some of the occurrences exceeded mathematical expectation and others were less. However, the longer one continued the experiment and the greater the amount of experimental data collected the nearer would the results have approximated to the mathematical expectation.

The mathematical expansion set out above is known as the *Binomial expansion* and the results can also be plotted as a frequency distribution curve as in Figure 2.

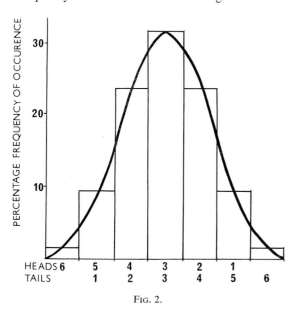

FIG. 2.

This is the *Binomial Distribution*. Note that it has a similar form to the normal distribution but of course the intervals are always discrete, (one cannot have $1\frac{1}{2}$ heads as one can have $1\frac{1}{2}$ inches). In fact as the number of observations increases so this distribution more and more closely approximates to the normal distribution.

If we do not wish to distinguish between heads and tails but merely need to know the frequency of 6 of a kind occurring together (in this case both 6 heads and 6 tails), the two probabilities are added, 1·56 per cent + 1·56 per cent = 3·12 per cent. Alternatively if we wish to know the frequency of any specific happening such as how likely is a Captain to win the toss 6 times in succession (irrespective of whether he calls heads or tails), this must be the same as the specific happening 6 tails *or* 6 heads, namely 1·56 per cent. Equally he could lose the toss 6 times in succession with a 1·56 per cent chance!

**Mean, Median and Mode**

The *mean value* of a set of observations is the sum of their values divided by the number of observations, usually expressed as:

$$\frac{\Sigma(x_1 \dots x_n)}{n} \quad \text{or simply} \quad \frac{\Sigma x}{n}$$

The Greek Sigma $\Sigma$ representing 'the sum of', $x_1 \dots x_n$ representing the values and $n$ representing the number of

values. This is obviously a useful piece of data to have, particularly if it is accompanied by a statement about the scatter or variability of the individual observations. There are occasions, however, when other types of average are required. For instance it is often useful to know the mid figure or *median*. That is the value which has an equal number of values on either side of it. It is the figure on the fiftieth percentile with 50 per cent of values on either side of it. Equally the fifth percentile divides the values into 95 per cent above the fifth percentile observation and 5 per cent below it. Growth in children for instance is often expressed in this way. Finally one may be more interested in the observation that is most frequent. To know that the average size of a family in a certain town is 2·4 children is a difficult concept to grasp and one might prefer to know that 2 children is the most popular size. The group with the largest number is known as the *mode* and may be to the left or right of the mean.

The calculation of the mean or median value could be tedious if there are a large number of observations. In this case division into discrete classes can simplify the arithmetic and an account of these methods can be obtained from Bradford Hill's 'Principles of Medical Statistics' (1967).

The relationship between mean, median and mode is approximately

$$\text{Mode} = \text{Mean} - 3 \, (\text{Mean} - \text{Median})$$

provided the distribution is not very skewed.

With a perfectly normal distribution the Median, Mean and Mode are all on the same line and hence the above formula can be used as a check on the normality of the distribution.

**Variance**

When defining the mean I said that a knowledge of this average was useful if accompanied by a statement about the scatter of the various values about it. This could be done partly by giving the total range, but this would still provide no information about the frequency of occurrence of values along this range. To take into account both factors it is necessary to calculate the average amount by which individual values depart from the mean value bearing in mind that the further they do depart from such a mean the more significant they are. To give correct weight to these points it can be calculated that it is necessary to take the *square* of the values by which each departs from the mean before finding the average.

This quantity is known as the *Variance* and is expressed as

$$\frac{\Sigma(x - \bar{x})^2}{n}$$

where $x$ represents each value

　　$\bar{x}$ represents the mean of the values

and　$n$ represents the total number of values.

The factor $\Sigma(x - \bar{x})^2$ known as the *sum of the squares* figures prominently in statistical calculations.

## Degrees of Freedom

If we have only one observation it is its own mean and there is nothing to compare it with. If there are two observations a mean can be calculated by averaging the two results and one comparison can be made: the first result against the second, with each being the same amount on either side of the mean value. With three observations there are two comparisons to be made and so on. Hence it isn't quite right to average the squared deviations by dividing by *n* as there is one less comparison than the total number of observations. This concept of numbers of comparisons is known as the number of *Degrees of Freedom* of the observations and is often denoted by the letter *N*.

$$N \text{ is therefore } n - 1$$

and the above formula for Variance should read

$$\frac{\Sigma(x - \bar{x})^2}{n - 1} \quad \text{or} \quad \frac{\Sigma(x - \bar{x})^2}{N}$$

## Standard Deviation and its Calculation

The Standard Deviation (S) is the square root of the variance.

$$S = \sqrt{\text{Var}}$$

but as

$$\text{Var} = \frac{\Sigma(x - \bar{x})^2}{N}$$

$$S = \sqrt{\frac{\Sigma(x - \bar{x})^2}{N}}$$

Worked Example:

Estimations of serum cholesterol were made in 10 apparently normal subjects with the following results:

270 240 200 255 305
250 215 275 220 170 mgs per cent

The calculation of the mean and standard deviation (S.D.) can be set out as in Table 1.

$$\text{Var} = \frac{\text{Sum of Squares}}{n - 1} = \frac{14200}{9} = 1578 \text{ (approx.)}$$

$$\text{S.D.} = \sqrt{\text{Var}} = \sqrt{1578} = \pm 39 \cdot 7$$

The value for the mean and standard deviation of serum cholesterol is therefore expressed as:

240 ± 39·7 mg per cent

or  240 ± 40 mg per cent to nearest whole number

Even from this fairly simple example it will be seen that the calculations can be time consuming and cumbersome and the use of a slide rule, calculating machine or computer becomes essential. To economize on the number of additions and subtractions which waste a lot of time when using a calculating machine the formula for the determination of variance needs to be modified.

TABLE 1

| Cholesterol Values $x$ | Value — Mean $(x - \bar{x})$ | Squares $(x - \bar{x})^2$ |
|---|---|---|
| 270 | +30 | 900 |
| 250 | +10 | 100 |
| 240 | 0 | 0 |
| 215 | −25 | 625 |
| 200 | −40 | 1600 |
| 275 | +35 | 1225 |
| 255 | +15 | 225 |
| 220 | −20 | 400 |
| 305 | +65 | 4225 |
| 170 | −70 | 4900 |
| Sum ($\Sigma x$) 2400 | Sum of Squares = 14200 $\Sigma(x - \bar{x})^2$ | |

Sum ($\Sigma x$) = 2400

Mean $\dfrac{(\Sigma x)}{n} = \dfrac{2400}{10} = 240$

Imagine that the mean of all sets of observations was zero. Then the sum of the squares would simply be the squares of all the values added up, $\Sigma x^2$ [the $\bar{x}$ in $\Sigma(x - \bar{x})^2$ being 0]. As this is rarely so we have to correct for the contribution made by the actual mean multiplied by the number of observations, i.e. $n\bar{x}^2$.

As the mean is $\dfrac{\Sigma x}{n}$

Then $\qquad n\bar{x}^2 = n \cdot \dfrac{\Sigma x}{n} \cdot \dfrac{\Sigma x}{n} = \dfrac{(\Sigma x)^2}{n}$

The term $\dfrac{(\Sigma x)^2}{n}$ is known as the *Correction Factor*.

$$\therefore \qquad \text{Sum of Squares} = \Sigma x^2 - \frac{(\Sigma x)^2}{n}$$

Let us check all this using the original observations (Table 2A).

TABLE 2

| | A | | B | |
|---|---|---|---|---|
| Cholesterol values $x$ | $x^2$ | $x - 250$ | $(x - 250)^2$ |
| 270 | 72900 | 20 | 400 |
| 250 | 62500 | 0 | 0 |
| 240 | 57600 | −10 | 100 |
| 215 | 46225 | −35 | 1225 |
| 200 | 40000 | −50 | 2500 |
| 275 | 75625 | 25 | 625 |
| 255 | 65025 | 5 | 25 |
| 220 | 48400 | −30 | 900 |
| 305 | 93025 | 55 | 3025 |
| 170 | 28900 | −80 | 6400 |
| Sum = 2400 | = 590200 | −100 | 15200 |

$$\Sigma x^2 - \frac{(\Sigma x)^2}{n} = 590200 - \frac{(2400)^2}{10}$$

$$= 590200 - 576000$$

$$= 14200$$

$$\left. \begin{array}{l} = 14200 \\ \text{Var} = \dfrac{14200}{9} \\ = 1578 \\ \text{S.D.} = \sqrt{1578} \\ = \pm 39{\cdot}7 \end{array} \right\} \text{as before}$$

Note also that if the arithmetic is further simplified by subtracting an *estimated* mean from each value of $x$, as in Table 2B, the result is the same. (I have deliberately chosen a slightly inaccurate mean as it is rarely possible to guess it correctly and it is preferable to choose a whole number.)

$$\Sigma x^2 = \frac{(\Sigma x)^2}{n} = 15200 - \frac{(100)^2}{10}$$

$$= 15200 - 1000$$

$$= 14200$$

$$\left. \begin{array}{l} \text{Var} = \dfrac{14200}{9} \\ = 1578 \\ \text{S.D.} = \sqrt{1578} \\ = \pm 39{\cdot}7 \end{array} \right\} \text{as before}$$

Therefore the addition or subtraction of a constant figure from all the values does not affect the calculation of S.D. and may well simplify it.

Finally if two observations have respectively Variance$_A$ and Variance$_B$ then the sum of the two observations will have Variance$_{A+B}$. Equally the difference between two observations having respectively Variance $_A$ and Variance$_B$ will also have a Variance $a + b$.

Some time has been spent on the calculation of standard deviation because it is fundamental to the understanding of calculations of probability. For instance if we are told that the serum cholesterol for 100 randomly selected apparently normal subjects was $240 \pm 40$, then how likely is it that the 101st subject with a serum cholesterol of 300 is normal. Or, if we are told that aspirin tablets normally disintegrate in gastric juice in $10 \pm 4$ minutes, how likely is it that a tablet disintegrating in 18 minutes has been badly made. To understand what the standard deviation can tell you about probability it is useful to study its relationship with the Normal Distribution pattern.

### The Connection between Standard Deviation and the Normal Distribution Pattern

Figure 3 is a repeat of Figure 1 without the columns. On it we see that two points have been marked with letters d. These are the points of inflection where the curve changes from convex to concave. With a symmetrical distribution these points are one standard deviation either side of the mean. If we now measure the proportion between the two d's, that is $\pm$ one standard deviation, it will be found to be just over 68 per cent of the total. Furthermore if another distance d is measured off this will embrace a further 27 per cent of values ($13\frac{1}{2}$ per cent on each side) making over 95 per cent of the total. Finally if 3d is measured off on each side the tiny remnant remaining is only a $\frac{1}{4}$ per cent of the total.

To go back to our two examples of cholesterol values and aspirin disintegration.

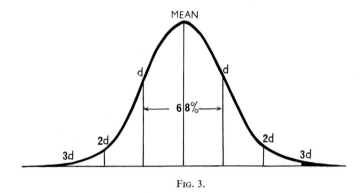

Fig. 3.

A value of 300 mg per cent, given the normal to be $240 \pm 40$, is $1\frac{1}{2}$ standard deviations away from the mean and $1\frac{1}{2}$ standard deviations or more from the mean will occur about once in every nine observations, so this is not so unusual. With our aspirin tablet the situation is a little more serious. 18 minutes is two standard deviations from $10 \pm 4$ minutes and hence would occur less than 5 per cent of the time (1 in 20), and so one would begin to think that there was something strange about the tablet. If the disintegration time had been 22 minutes or 3 standard deviations from the mean then this would occur about once in 400 occasions and make it a very rare event to have occurred by chance.

### Significance

How rare is a chance of one in twenty? This may seem a stupid question, but it is frequently overlooked that it means precisely what it says, namely that something unusual or different could have occurred by chance once in every 20 readings, observations, experiments, etc. What matters is the importance we attach to the occurrence of this unusual and different observation. In other words its *significance*. Statisticians have defined grades of statistical significance:

If a happening would have occurred by chance only once in 100 times or less it is termed 'Highly Significant' and is expressed in various ways ($P$ = probability).

$P \ll 0{\cdot}01$          (The probability is equal to or

$P \ll 1$ per cent          less than 1 in 100)

If a happening would have occurred by chance between

once in twenty times up to once in a hundred times it is termed Significant and expressed:

$$P < 0.05$$

or 
$$0.01 < P < 0.05$$

If a happening would have occurred by chance more frequently than once in twenty times it is said to be 'not significant' or in another context 'no significant difference'. In some ways it is unfortunate that these terms have become common parlance in medical writing because they are often used as judgements such as 'there is no significant difference between the treatments'.

What interpretation is put on the degrees of statistical significance will vary according to the circumstances. For instance if we were testing out an analgesic for the relief of post-operative pain and found it better than a placebo, but the results could have occurred by chance say with odds of 1 in 10 (10 per cent), then we might discard it and investigate another. On the other hand if we were treating leukaemia with a new antimetabolite and found it produced a longer period of remission than standard treatment, which could have occurred by chance once in ten times, it would be wrong to discard such a potentially valuable remedy and the proper procedure would be to treat another and perhaps larger group of cases.

Another way of looking at the matter is to consider what will happen if observations are made on 20 different parameters during the course of an investigation. By definition one of these may well give a result which seriously departs from the normal (1 in 20 = statistically significant). If 20 workers investigate an analgesic for the relief of post-operative pain, one of them may well find a statistically significant advantage for it. This incidentally is often the only one that is published!

I hope I have made it clear that words like 'not significant', 'significant' and 'highly significant' should only be used in the statistical sense in scientific papers when they indicate a degree of probability. In many instances it will be best to give the actual probability: $P = 0.02$ or whatever it is and say what conclusion is drawn.

### One Tailed or Two Tailed

If we look back at Figure 3 it will be seen that the distribution *tails off* either side of the mean. When one is assessing abnormal findings it is usual to assume they are equally important, whether abnormally low or abnormally high, hence the probability is a combined probability for both tails. If however one is concerned only with a high value, all other values being regarded as normal, then one can simply take the probability from one tail which will be a half the combined probability.

In most cases it is necessary to use two tailed values for probability but some tables give figures for one tail only, in which case these figures will need to be doubled.

### Application of the Standard Deviation

A knowledge of the mean and standard deviation of a wide variety of parameters for normal human subjects, enables one to form a good estimate of the degree of abnormality of any new individual result. To put it another way, it enables one to place an individual or an individual result in his or its correct place in the normal distribution curve.

For instance Wood *et al.* (1965) worked out the criteria for the Synacthen test of adrenal function by studying the plasma corticosteroid response to a given dose of tetracosactrin in 66 normal subjects. To allow up to a 1 in 20 chance for random error they quoted values for normality as a mean $\pm 2$ S.D. Any new patient for investigation whose values were outside this range was considered to have an abnormality of adrenal function. Because it approximates to the $P = 0.05$ level of significance $\pm 2$ S.D. is the most useful range to quote.

I say that 2 S.D. approximates to $P = 0.05$ because in fact the true values for the various levels of probability for the normal deviate are quoted in what is known as the table of 'c', part of which is as follows:

| Probability | 0.8 | 0.6 | 0.4 | 0.2 | 0.1 |
|---|---|---|---|---|---|
| 'c' | 0.25 | 0.52 | 0.84 | 1.28 | 1.64 |

| Probability | 0.05 | 0.02 | 0.01 | 0.001 |
|---|---|---|---|---|
| 'c' | 1.96 | 2.33 | 2.58 | 3.29 |

Note that $P = 0.05$ applies to $\pm 1.96$ S.D. for the normal deviate so $\pm 2$ S.D. is very close and convenient. Complete tables can be found in Fisher and Yates (1953) and Geigy Scientific Tables (1970).

### The Standard Error of the Mean

If we go back to our normal subjects with a cholesterol of $240 \pm 40$ we might reasonably ask how accurate is this mean.

In the same way as we can estimate how far individuals deviate from a mean and the probability of this, so we can determine how far sample means are likely to differ from a true population mean. Calculation of the *standard error of the mean* will give this answer. The Standard Error (S.E.) of the mean can be used to relate means to a true mean in the same way as the standard deviation can relate an individual to a group of individuals.

You will recall the method for working out the variance of a set of observations (p. 435). Now the variance of the mean itself or mean variance is $\dfrac{\text{Var}}{n}$, $n$ being the number of observations which made up that variance. Just as S.D. is $\pm\sqrt{\text{Var}}$,

so S.E. is 
$$\pm\sqrt{\frac{\text{Var}}{n}}$$

also 
$$\pm\sqrt{\frac{\text{Var}}{n}} = \frac{\sqrt{\text{Var}}}{\sqrt{n}} = \frac{S}{\sqrt{n}}$$

So we simply take the S.D. ($S$) and divide it by the square root of the number of observations.

With our cholesterol figures the mean and S.D. was

$$240 \pm 40 \text{ mg per cent, with } n = 10$$

so S.E. is     $\pm \dfrac{40}{\sqrt{10}} = \pm \dfrac{40}{3 \cdot 16} = \pm 12 \cdot 7$

If new means were taken using 10 values, 68 per cent would be within $\pm 12 \cdot 7$ mgs. of the true mean (1 S.E.) and over 95 per cent would be between $\pm 25 \cdot 4$ mg. per cent of the true mean (2 S.E.). A new mean which was outside this second figure could reasonably be considered to have come from an abnormal group (such as a group of diabetics).

Means of two or more sets of observations on the same parameter are very commonly the end result of various types of investigational work, but the total number of observations in each group may be different and the value of a true or population mean be unknown through lack of data. What is required is a method of comparing such means to see whether they differ significantly from each other. Provided the data are reasonably normally distributed this can be done by means of a '*t* test' which will be explained later.

**Comparison of Frequencies**

When we talked about the binomial distribution we showed that it was possible to calculate how frequently a certain event might occur from a knowledge of prior probabilities from the binomial expansion. At that time we dealt with occurrences of equal frequency (heads or tails), but probability can be calculated as well from happenings which are not equally probable. Tables of probability with the binomial distribution can be found in Mainland *et al.* (1956).

In medical investigations one is usually faced with the problem of comparing the frequency of happenings in patients receiving two or more kinds of treatment. For example:

> Using analgesic A toothache was relieved completely in 40 patients, partially in 22 and not at all in 6; with analgesic B toothache was relieved completely in 24 patients, partially in 36 and not at all in 9. Is there any statistically significant difference between the effects of these two analgesics?

In the example above it is impossible to relate toothache relief to any normal distribution so a test based on standard errors of the means is inappropriate. In this case recourse is made to the non-parametric frequency distribution known as $\chi^2$ (Chi-square).

**The '*t*' test and $\chi^2$ test**

These are grouped together because they are the commonest tests of significance applied to medical research. In the 1967 issues of the British Journal of Anaesthesia 30–50 per cent of all articles bore the results of some statistical operation of which 90 per cent involved the use of '*t*' or '$\chi^2$'. The '*t*' test was used whenever measurements were being recorded which could be averaged and compared. For example Usubiaga *et al.*

(1967) studied the effect of intravenous lignocaine on cardiac rates, Pauka and Sykes (1967) measured upper limb blood flow changes during thiopentone—halothane anaesthesia, Watts *et al.* (1967) measured recovery time after the use of muscle relaxants in both ventilated and hyperventilated patients, and there were many others.

Some authors worked out frequencies, often from some predetermined index, and applied the $\chi^2$ test. Davies and Doughty (1967) studied the effect of premedication in children in terms of demeanour, response to injection, etc., Hamilton *et al.* (1967) studied pentazocine given before anaesthesia using a scoring system for both the course of anaesthesia and emetic effects. Over the years numerous papers by Dundee (1960), Dundee and Moore (1960), Dundee and Riding (1960), Moore and Dundee (1961), Dundee and Rajagopalan (1962), etc., have investigated pain and its relief using measurements, such as time and local pressure, to invoke the '*t*' test, and scores and indices to invoke the $\chi^2$ test. The calculation of '*t*' and $\chi^2$ will, therefore, be explained in detail.

'*t*' TEST

The distribution of *t* was originally worked out by W. S. Gosset in 1908 who wrote at that time under the pseudonym of 'Student' and it came to be known as 'Student's *t* test'. Essentially it is an extension of our knowledge of the distribution of means and the normal deviate, to take into account that the variance of the quantity being measured is usually not precisely known because the sample being studied is small and can at best be only an estimate of the true population variance.

What we do is to compare means and see how much they depart from the Standard Error of these two means.

Hence     $t = \dfrac{\text{Difference between two means}}{\text{S.E. of that difference}}$

It has been mentioned already that the variance of both the sum and difference of two values is their combined variance $V_1 + V_2$.

$\therefore$ The variance of two means is $\dfrac{V_1}{n_1} + \dfrac{V_2}{n_2}$

where $n_1$ and $n_2$ are the number of values in each set. The S.E. is the square root of this quantity.

so     $t = \dfrac{\bar{x}_1 - \bar{x}_2}{\sqrt{\dfrac{V_1}{n_1} + \dfrac{V_2}{n_2}}}$

or     $t = \dfrac{\bar{x}_1 - \bar{x}_2}{\sqrt{\dfrac{S^2}{n_1} + \dfrac{S^2}{n_2}}}$ (since $V = S^2$)

Worked example:

When carrying out some research into the vital statistics of native women on two tropical islands I had occasion to measure the length of their necks and samples from each island were recorded in Table 3.

TABLE 3

| Island A | Island B |
|---|---|
| Length of necks in cms. | Length of necks in cms. |
| 11 | $14\frac{1}{2}$ |
| 12 | 10 |
| $11\frac{1}{2}$ | $12\frac{1}{2}$ |
| 13 | 15 |
| $9\frac{1}{2}$ | 9 |
| 8 | $13\frac{1}{2}$ |
| 9 | 17 |
| $10\frac{1}{2}$ | $13\frac{1}{2}$ |
| 10 | 19 |
| $10\frac{1}{2}$ | 16 |
| 105 | 140 |

The estimate of variance for each sample of 10 worked out as previously explained on page 435 is:

Island A 2·16 (S.D. ± 1·47)

Island B 9·18 (S.D. ± 3·03)

The variance of each mean is therefore 0·216 and 0·918 respectively. Combined variance = 1·134 with a standard error of $\sqrt{1\cdot134} = 1\cdot065$.

The difference between these two means is considerably greater, viz. $14 - 10\cdot5 = 3\cdot5$

and

$$t = \frac{3\cdot5}{1\cdot065} = 3\cdot3$$

If this figure of 3·3 represented the true factor for the number of deviations from the mean this would be highly significant statistically, but to allow for the smallness of the sample we have to look up the probability of $t$ in a table of $t$ values under the appropriate degree of freedom. As there were 9 comparisons in each group $(n - 1)$, there are 18 comparisons altogether. Hence we enter the tables under 18 degrees of freedom and note:

| Probability | 0·5 | 0·2 | 0·1 | 0·05 | 0·02 | 0·01 |
|---|---|---|---|---|---|---|
| '$t$' | 0·688 | 1·33 | 1·734 | 2·101 | 2·552 | 2·878 |

Hence the probability of a true difference between the two islands is very great $P < 0\cdot01$ and we have to look for a cause. In this instance we didn't have far to seek, because on Island B we found that women stretched their necks be wearing rings round them!

Out of interest compare the values of '$t$' with those of '$c$' on page 539

'$c$' at 0·05 is 1·96

'$t$' at 0·05 is 2·101 (18 degrees of freedom)

It is not by accident that as the number of comparisons, and therefore degrees of freedom, increases so $t$ gradually approaches 1·96 at the 0·05 level.

For examples of the $t$ test in action as applied specifically to anaesthetic work you are recommended to study some of the articles mentioned on the previous pages.

## CHI-SQUARE TEST ($\chi^2$)

This test can be used to compare frequencies. Going back to the toothache example of page 540 we set it out as in Table 4. This is known as a 'contingency table';

TABLE 4

| | Patients Relieved | Patients partly Relieved | Patients not Relieved | Total |
|---|---|---|---|---|
| Analgesic A | 40 | 22 | 6 | 68 |
| Analgesic B | 24 | 36 | 9 | 69 |
| Total | 64 | 58 | 15 | 137 |

in this case a 2 × 3 contingency table. What we wish to know is whether there is any difference between these two analgesics or whether such variation that is present is just due to chance.

To answer this we need to know the *expected* frequencies of patients falling into each group or 'cell' in the table.

Note first that 64 patients out of a total of 137 were relieved. So the expectation of being relieved as an individual is $\frac{64}{137} = 0\cdot47$. Also 68 individuals received analgesic A, therefore the number of individuals expected to be relieved would be $\frac{64 \times 68}{137} = 31\cdot8$. Working in this way through each of the other 5 cells we arrive at all the expected frequencies and a new table can be constructed (Table 5).

TABLE 5

| | Expected 'Relieved' | Expected 'partly Relieved' | Expected 'not Relieved' | Total |
|---|---|---|---|---|
| Analgesic A | 31·8 | 28·8 | 7·4 | 68 |
| Analgesic B | 32·2 | 29·2 | 7·6 | 69 |
| Total | 64 | 58 | 15 | 137 |

Note the totals are the same and if they are not, the sums have been done incorrectly.

We need now an expression which compares the observed frequency in each cell with the expected frequency and allows for its degree of departure from the expected value. Hence we take the *square* of the difference and divide by the expected value. This is Chi square and is expressed thus:

$$\chi^2 = \frac{(O - E)^2}{E}$$

The results are accumulated for each cell to give the total $\chi^2$ which is then sought in a table of distribution of $\chi^2$ under the appropriate degree of freedom. To obtain this degree of freedom one must realise that there are comparisons in two directions: A with B and 'relieved' with 'partly relieved' or 'not relieved'; one degree between the major classes and two between the subclasses. These are multiplied giving $1 \times 2 = 2$ degrees of freedom.

In general the number of degrees of freedom is $(m - 1)$ $(n - 1)$ where m is the number of rows and n the number of columns. For a $5 \times 4$ contingency table the number of degrees of freedom would be $(5 - 1)$ $(4 - 1) = 4 \times 3 = 12$.

In our example $\chi^2$ for the top left hand cell is :

$$\frac{(40 - 31 \cdot 8)^2}{31 \cdot 8} = \frac{8 \cdot 2 \times 8 \cdot 2}{31 \cdot 8} = 2 \cdot 1 \text{ (approx.)}$$

Proceeding in this way for each cell in turn the total $\chi^2 = 7 \cdot 9$ approx.

Entering the table of $\chi^2$ at 2 degrees of freedom we find

| P | 0·5 | 0·2 | 0·1 | 0·05 | 0·02 | 0·01 |
|---|-----|-----|-----|------|------|------|
| $\chi^2$ | 1·39 | 3·22 | 4·61 | 5·99 | 7·82 | 9·21 |

Hence $P = 0 \cdot 02$ very nearly, and such results would not be expected by chance more often than one in 50 times and one might reasonably conclude that there is a difference between analgesic A and analgesic B.

With $2 \times 2$ contingency tables a single formula can be used which gives the total $\chi^2$. Such a table would appear in general form as follows:

|  | Relieved | Not Relieved | Total |
|---|----------|--------------|-------|
| Analgesic A | a | b | a + b |
| Analgesic B | c | d | c + d |
|  | a + c | b + d | a + b + c + d |

and the formula

$$\chi^2 = \frac{(ad - bc)^2 (a + b + c + d)}{(a + c)(b + d)(a + b)(c + d)}$$

with *one* degree of freedom $[(2 - 1)(2 - 1) = 1]$.

Two errors may arise in the calculation of $\chi^2$ which have to be taken into account. First if the expected number in any cell is less than 5, variation will produce relatively large contributions to the total $\chi^2$ and give a falsely high and therefore significant result. With big tables it is usually possible to overcome this by amalgamating two or more subclasses.

A second source of error arises because $\chi^2$ is a continuous distribution and yet the observations are discontinuous (c.f. binomial and normal distributions). This should be corrected in the $2 \times 2$ contingency table where the total number of observations is less than 200 by adding 0·5 to any number less than expectation and subtracting 0·5 from any number greater than expectation. If there are more than 200 observations it makes little

difference to the final result. This correction is known as *Yates correction for continuity*.

The relationship between the normal deviate 'c', 't' and $\chi^2$ is dealt with in more detail by Mather (1967) and Croxton (1953).

### The Null Hypothesis, Type I and Type II Error

It is convenient when considering a statistical problem to put up a hypothesis which a particular statistical exercise will test. For instance in our neck measuring investigation the hypothesis might have been, 'that there is no difference between Islands A and B with respect to length of neck'. This type of hypothesis is known as *The Null Hypothesis*. The object of a particular statistical test (in this case the t test), is to test the hypothesis and to set a level of significance at which we would be prepared to reject the null hypothesis and say instead that the two islands were different. The level is usually set at $P = 0 \cdot 05$, but it can be at any level according to the importance we attach to not rejecting the null hypothesis wrongly. If $P = 0 \cdot 05$ then this hypothesis by definition will be rejected once in twenty times when it is true. If you cannot afford to be wrong that frequently a higher level will have to be set, say $P = 0 \cdot 02$ or $P = 0 \cdot 01$. The rejection error is often referred to as *Type I error* $(\alpha)$.

There is another type of error, however, and this is the risk of accepting the null hypothesis when it is false. Or put another way, no significant difference may be found between two treatments, when in fact one is superior to the other. This type of error is *Type II error* $(\beta)$. Clearly the lower the probability of Type I error for a given number of observations the higher will be the probability of Type II error. One could even have a situation with a small number of observations when it was virtually impossible to reach a desired level of significance and the null hypothesis would always be accepted. An important way therefore to increase the sensitivity of a statistical test and reduce the liability to error is to increase the number of observations. Also some statistical tests by their nature are less liable to give rise to Type II error. This factor is often referred to as the *Power* of the test, and it is $1 - \beta$.

### Sequential Analysis

This is a method of analysis whereby results are plotted as they come in rather than waiting for a fixed number to be obtained before analysis is performed. The significance of the results is decided by a plot crossing a number of pre-drawn boundaries. It is specially applicable for recording patient preferences; for example in a comparison of hypnotics.

A group of sleepless patients may be given two different hypnotics on alternate nights or for alternate pairs of nights and be asked to express preferences. Provided the two drugs are given in random sequence so that an equal number of patients receive hypnotic A first as receives hypnotic B, then the results as they come in can be recorded on a chart similar to the one shown in Figure 4. Every time there is a preference for hypnotic A a line is drawn diagonally across each square in a north-easterly direction and if the preference is for B the line is drawn in a south-easterly direction. Patients who are unable to express a preference are rejected. In time the line under construction will cross one of the boundaries and indicate whether a significant difference has been found in favour of one or other drug. The construction of these charts which can be of 'open' or 'closed' design, has been described by Bross (1952 and 1958) and Armitage (1960). The closed designs are more popular for medical work because the number of preferences recorded is limited by boundaries in all directions.

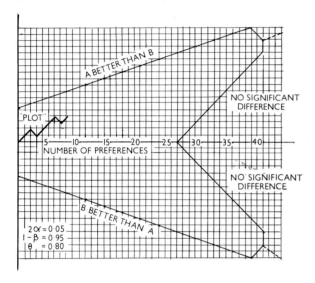

Fig. 4.

To prepare the chart or 'bat's wing' shown in Figure 4 a decision has to be made concerning 2 factors. First a Type I error $\alpha$ has to be set and it is usual to make this 0·025 for each of the upper and lower boundaries. Hence $2\alpha = 0·05$ (the customary level for the rejection of the null hypothesis). Secondly we have to know what degree of difference we are looking for in the two treatments. This can be set at any level but it must be borne in mind that it is going to be much harder to detect small differences than large ones. The factor is known as $\theta$ and if the two treatments are equal $\theta = \frac{1}{2}$ or 0·5. Usually we are looking for differences from $\theta = 0·75$ to $\theta = 0·85$ and the chart is constructed so as to give a 95% chance of obtaining a preference if $\theta$ is set between these limits. This factor is known as the Power of the test and is related to the avoidance of Type II error such that Power $= 1 - \beta = 0·95$. Values for $2\alpha$, $1 - \beta$ and $\theta$ for Figure 4 are shown in the bottom left hand corner.

### Other Useful Non-Parametric Statistical Tests

Instead of performing a sequential type of analysis preferences from a fixed sample can be examined by the use of the McNemar test.

40 sleepless patients took two hypnotics A and B in random order and were asked to express a preference for one or the other. 5 found neither hypnotic

effective and 12 found both equally effective. Of the remaining 23 patients, 16 preferred hypnotic A and 7 preferred hypnotic B.

It is clear that the 17 patients who for one reason or another couldn't express a preference provided no information of value and can be excluded. What we wish to know is whether 23 patients dividing themselves 16/7 in favour of hypnotic A is significant. As the expectation would have been $\frac{1}{2}$ if the hypnotics were equal in effectiveness, the proportion 16/7 can be looked up as a probability in an appropriate table of the binomial expansion. In this case 16 favourable results out of 23 has a probability of 0·047, but as this is only one tail and either hypnotic could have proved better, the actual probability of a difference of this magnitude is 0·094.

Another way of doing this calculation is to use the $\chi^2$ test with two cells only.

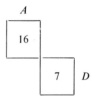

The simplified formula with Yates correction for continuity is:

$$\chi^2 = \frac{[(A - D) - 1]^2}{A + D}$$

$$= \frac{(16 - 7 - 1)^2}{23}$$

$$= \frac{8^2}{23}$$

$$= \frac{64}{23}$$

$$= 2·78$$

In the table of $\chi^2$ under 1 degree of freedom the 0·1 probability is 2·706 hence our probability is just below this. The $\chi^2$ distribution, however, is an approximation to the true distribution used in the first or exact method, although for all practical purposes the result is the same.

The sign test:
In crossover trials, that is trials where each patient receives both treatments, results may be expressed as plus or minus according to some method of rating.

Reaction times were tested before and after a dose of the well known anaesthetic agent ethyl alcohol. The method was to see if a threepenny piece placed in an appropriate machine could be arrested in its fall more quickly or more slowly when a red light appeared, before or after the consumption of a double whisky.

This was not a strictly controlled trial, but the results illustrate the method of analysis.

|  | Reaction time after $C_2H_5OH$ | (+ or −) (in time) |
|---|---|---|
| Subject 1 | Slower | + |
| 2 | Slower | + |
| 3 | Equal | 0 |
| 4 | Faster | − |
| 5 | Slower | + |
| 6 | Slower | + |
| 7 | Faster | − |
| 8 | Slower | + |
| 9 | Slower | + |
| 10 | Slower | + |

From the nine results giving useful information 7 were plus and 2 were minus. The one tail probability for 7 or more plusses in 9 subjects is 0·09 and therefore both tails 0·18, a result which could often occur by chance.

The Wilcoxon matched-pairs signed-ranks Test:

The sign test is rather insensitive as it only considers + and − values and takes no account of the degree of plus or minus. In the last example had we measured the fall of the threepenny piece in units of time the following results might have been obtained.

FALL IN UNITS OF TIME

|  | Before $C_2H_5OH$ | After $C_2H_5OH$ | Difference |
|---|---|---|---|
| Subject 1 | 10 | 15 | +5 |
| 2 | 12 | 15 | +3 |
| 3 | 8 | 8 | 0 |
| 4 | 12 | 11 | −1 |
| 5 | 17 | 25 | +8 |
| 6 | 8 | 9 | +1 |
| 7 | 11 | 9 | −2 |
| 8 | 10 | 13 | +3 |
| 9 | 13 | 14 | +1 |
| 10 | 14 | 20 | +6 |
|  | 115 | 139 | |
|  | Mean = 11·5 | Mean = 13·9 | |

The differences are now ranked irrespective of sign ignoring as before a difference of 0.

Values    −1 +1 +1 −2 +3 +3 +5 +6 +8
Rank      2  2  2  4  5·5 5·5 7  8  9
          average of    average of
          1 + 2 + 3    5 and 6

The ranks are now summed for each sign independently.

Values of + ranks = 2 + 2 + 5·5 + 5·5
                      + 7 + 8 + 9 = 39

Values of − ranks = 2 + 4 = 6

Having utilized information about the magnitude of the values as well as their direction it remains to consult an appropriate table. The smaller value is taken (here it is 6), and designated $T$. This is looked up under critical values of $T$ with $n = 9$. It is not quite significant at the 0·05 level, (two tailed), but this more sensitive test has utilized the additional information.

It will not have escaped the reader that the time values could have been analysed by means of a parametric $t$ test. It will, however be somewhat different from the $t$ test described above because the comparisons are paired in the same *subject*. Hence the mean of the *differences* is compared with its own standard error.

The mean of the differences = 2·4 units (13·9 − 11·5)

The variance           = 16·7 ($5^2 + 3^2 \ldots \div 9$)

The mean variance    = 1·67

The standard error    = $\sqrt{1·67}$ = 1·3 approx.

$$\therefore t = \frac{2·4}{1·3} = 1·85$$

With 9 degrees of freedom this is again not quite significant at the 0·05 level.

The performance of these calculations should now be quite familiar to readers. Although the operation of the Sign test and the Wilcoxon test were described using a crossover type of trial, they can also be used, as the full name of the latter test tells us for comparing pairs of patients who have been *matched* for all relevant characteristics before the trial starts, the only difference being in the nature of the treatment they are receiving.

**Analysis of Variance**

We considered earlier the calculation of variance and standard deviation for a set of observations such as serum cholesterol and we compared means and variances by means of a '$t$ test' in the 'long necks' example. Frequently in medical trials, however, we wish to examine variance in more detail and to partition that variance meaningfully between each of the factors which are making a contribution. For example we may give two different drugs at three different doses to an equal number of patients and in our analysis we will want to know whether there is any difference between the two drugs and whether there are any differences between the effect of the different doses used. The technique for partitioning the various effects is known as an *analysis of variance*.

In an experiment we gave an intravenous anaesthetic agent at a constant rate to males and females of different weights. We asked them to start counting at the beginning of the injection and noted how many seconds elapsed before they stopped and fell asleep. In six subjects the results were as follows:

| Subject | Sex | Weight | Time in seconds |
|---|---|---|---|
| 1 | Male | 140 lbs | 5 |
| 2 | Female | 140 lbs | 4 |
| 3 | Male | 180 lbs | 7 |
| 4 | Female | 180 lbs | 8 |
| 5 | Male | 220 lbs | 10 |
| 6 | Female | 220 lbs | 8 |
|  |  | Total | 42 |
|  |  | Average | 7 |

TABLE 9

| Subjects | Hb. | Alt. | Hb. | Alt. | Hb. | Alt. | Hb. | Alt. | Hb. | Alt. |
|---|---|---|---|---|---|---|---|---|---|---|
| 1–5 | 95 | 700 | 106 | 1600 | 107 | 2700 | 117 | 3600 | 112 | 4700 |
| 6–10 | 103 | 800 | 110 | 2000 | 110 | 2900 | 115 | 3700 | 122 | 4800 |
| 11–15 | 100 | 900 | 105 | 2000 | 103 | 3100 | 112 | 4200 | 116 | 5000 |
| 16–20 | 98 | 1200 | 99 | 2100 | 116 | 3100 | 115 | 4200 | 125 | 5200 |
| 21–25 | 104 | 1300 | 105 | 2300 | 114 | 3200 | 116 | 4300 | 125 | 5300 |

appear as in Table 9. If these values are plotted on a graph you will obtain a scatter diagram or 'plum pudding' as shown in Figure 7. It seems from this figure that there is some correlation between height above sea level and haemoglobin and possibly one could draw a straight line with approximately an equal number of points above and below it. What we would like to know is what is the best straight line, what is its formula and is there a significant correlation between height and haemoglobin?

We will deal with the last point first.

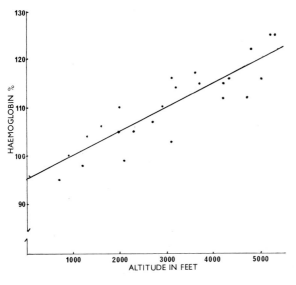

FIG. 7.

To decide whether there is a correlation between height and haemoglobin we have to calculate what is known as the *correlation coefficient* and this is represented by the letter $r$. It can be calculated from two types of formula. The first is:

$$r = \sqrt{1 - \frac{S^2}{\sigma^2}}$$

Where $S^2$ is the average of the squared deviations of the haemoglobin observations from the mean *at each unit of altitude*, and $\sigma$ is the average of the squared errors of each observation from the *total* mean.

This will be best understood by reference to Tables 7 and 8 and Figures 5 and 6. In Table 7/Figure 5 the errors from the mean (110) at altitudes 1,000 to 5,000 feet are respectively 0, +5, +10, −5 and −10 at each level and these numbers squared = 0, 25, 100, 25 and 100, totalling 250. As we are dealing with five levels of altitude the grand total is $5 \times 250 = 1,250$. This is $S^2$.

The mean of the whole table is also 110 and the errors are five lots of 0, five lots of +5, five lots of +10, five lots of −5 and five lots of −10. Once again if these values are squared and added up you get 1,250. This is $\sigma$.

So $\sigma^2$ and $S^2$ are the same and our formula $\sqrt{1 - \frac{S^2}{\sigma^2}}$

becomes
$$\sqrt{1 - \frac{1250}{1250}}$$
$$= \sqrt{1 - 1}$$
$$= \sqrt{0} = 0$$

hence $r = 0$

We have already agreed that there is no correlation in Table 7/Figure 5 so when there is no correlation $r = 0$.

Turning to Table 8/Figure 6 the errors at each unit of altitude are nil, so $S^2 = 0$. On the other hand the errors from the mean of all the observations (110) are as before, five lots of 0, five lots of +5, etc., and $\sigma$ squared = 1250.

So the formula $\sqrt{1 - \frac{S^2}{\sigma^2}}$

becomes
$$\sqrt{1 - \frac{0}{1250}}$$
$$= \sqrt{1 - 0}$$
$$= \sqrt{1}$$
$$= 1$$

Hence when there is perfect correlation $r = 1$. So $r$, the correlation coefficient runs from 0 to 1 with increasing direct correlation (if the correlation is negative it runs from 0 to −1). If we turn our attention to Table 9 the above formula can only be used if variations in haemoglobin are related to means of altitude at say each

1,000 ft. A second formula is however usually more useful when both $x$ and $y$ are varying.

$$r = \frac{\text{Covariance of } x \text{ and } y}{\sqrt{\text{Variance}_x \times \text{Variance}_y}}$$

$$= \frac{\Sigma(x - \bar{x})(y - \bar{y})}{\sqrt{\Sigma(x - \bar{x})^2 \cdot \Sigma(y - y)^2}}$$

From Table 9 this equation works out to be, in slightly simplified form

$$r = \frac{2567}{\sqrt{5177 \times 1534}}$$

$$= 0 \cdot 91$$

The correlation coefficient has a standard error just the same as a mean and its distribution from a sample population is like Student's '$t$' with $n - 2$ degrees of freedom, according to the following formula:

$$t = \frac{r \times \sqrt{n - 2}}{1 - r^2}$$

$$= \frac{0 \cdot 91 \times \sqrt{23}}{1 - 0 \cdot 91^2}$$

$$= \frac{0 \cdot 91 \times 4 \cdot 8}{1 - 0 \cdot 83} \text{ (approx.)}$$

$$= \frac{4 \cdot 37}{0 \cdot 17}$$

$$= 26 \text{ approx.}$$

In the table of '$t$' under 23 degrees of freedom 26 is far in excess of $P = \cdot 001$ and highly significant. Hence altitude and haemoglobin are positively correlated.

A note of warning needs to be sounded in that correlation is not synonymous with causation. There may for instance be a third common factor which is responsible for the correlation. With time correlations there may even be no actual link between correlated factors.

To return to the lines we drew in Figures 6 and 7, these are known as *regression lines* and can be calculated from the data. In fact there are always 2 lines; the regression of $x$ on $y$ and regression of $y$ on $x$.

The general formula for a straight line is $y = ax + b$.

Also the relationship between $y$ and $x$ in our correlation exercise is $(y - \bar{y}) = a(x - \bar{x})$

i.e.

$$y = ax + \begin{vmatrix} \bar{y} - a\bar{x} \\ \leftarrow b \rightarrow \end{vmatrix}$$

This is the *coefficient of regression*, and in the case of $y$ on $x$ can be calculated from

$$= \frac{\text{covariance of } x \text{ and } y}{\text{variance of } x}$$

$$= \frac{\Sigma(x - \bar{x})(y - \bar{y})}{(x - \bar{x})^2}$$

$$= \frac{2567}{517700}$$

$$= \frac{1}{200} \text{ approx.}$$

hence

$$y = \begin{vmatrix} \dfrac{1}{200x} + 110 - \dfrac{3000}{200} \\ ax \qquad \bar{y} - ax \\ (b) \end{vmatrix}$$

$$= \frac{1}{200x} + 95$$

$$= 0 \cdot 005x + 95 \text{ (as before)}$$

The regression equation for $x$ or $y$ can also be calculated, but unless the correlation between the two variables is perfect the line described will be a different one to that for $y$ on $x$, one line minimizing the values for the variance of $x$ and the other the variance of $y$.

For further studies of regression lines and regression equations the reader should go to Smart (1963), Mather (1967) or Moroney (1951) in the first instance. For more detailed treatment of all parametric tests, including analysis of covariance which is not treated in this chapter, Snedecor (1967) should be studied.

## Clinical Trials

The correct design of clinical trials is paramount if statistical tests are to give valid indications of probability. Details of such designs are beyond the scope of this chapter, although many of the references given include sections dealing with randomization procedures, how to match pairs, the validity of measurements, sample size and so on.

In the first instance the reader is directed to the classical work of Bradford Hill (1967), Mainland (1964) and an excellent primer by Maxwell (1969), who include chapters on the planning of studies, and with regard to sequential studies, Armitage (1960) and (1971).

## REFERENCES

Armitage, P. (1960), *Sequential Medical Trials.* Published by Blackwell's Scientific Publications.

Armitage, P. (1971), *Statistical Methods in Medical Research.* Published by Blackwell's Scientific Publications.

Bradford Hill, A. (1967), *Principles of Medical Statistics.* Published by The Lancet Limited.

Bross, I. (1952), "Sequential Medical Plans," *Biometrics,* **8,** 188.

Bross, I., (1958), "Sequential Clinical Trials," *J. chron. Dis.,* **8,** 349.

Croxton, F. E. (1959), *Elementary Statistics with Applications in Medicine and the Biological Sciences.* Published by Dover Publications Inc.

Davies, D. R. and Doughty, A. (1967), "Pre-medication of Children with Papaveretum—Hyoscine," *Brit. J. Anaesth.,* **39,** 638.

Documenta Geigy Scientific Tables (1970), Geigy Pharmaceutical Co. Ltd.

Dundee, J. W. (1960), "A Method for Assessing the Efficacy of Oral Analgesics: Its Application and Limitations," *Brit. J. Anaesth.,* **32,** 48.

Dundee, J. W. and Moore, J. (1960), "Alterations in Response to Somatic Pain Associated with Anaesthesia. I. An Evaluation of a Method of Analgesimetry," *Brit. J. Anaesth.,* **32,** 396.

Dundee, J. W. and Riding, J. E. (1960), "A Comparison of Inactin and Thiopentone as Intravenous Anaesthetics," *Brit. J. Anaesth.,* **32,** 206.

Dundee, J. W. and Rajagopalan, M. S. (1962), "Clinical Studies of Induction Agents. IV. A Comparison of G.29505 and Thiopentone as Main Anaesthetic Agents for a Standard Operation," *Brit. J. Anaesth.*, 34, 869.

Fisher, R. A. and Yates, F. (1953), *Statistical Tables for Biological, Agricultural and Medical Research*. Published by Oliver and Boyd.

Hamilton, R. C., Dundee, J. W., Clarke, R. S. J., Loan, W. B. and Morrison, J. D. (1967), "Studies of Drugs given before Anaesthesia. XIII. Pentazocine and other Opiate Antagonists," *Brit. J. Anaesth.*, 39, 647.

Mainland, D., Herrera, L., Sutcliffe, M. I. (1956), *Statistical Tables for use with Binomial Samples*. Published by the Department of Medical Statistics, New York University College of Medicine.

Mainland, D. (1964), *Elementary Medical Statistics*. Published by W. B. Saunders Company.

Mather, K. (1967), *The Elements of Biometry*. Published by Methuen and Company Ltd.

Maxwell, C. (1969), *Clinical Trial Protocol. A Primer for Clinical Trials*. Published by Stuart Phillips Publications.

Moore, J. and Dundee, J. W. (1961), "Alterations in Response to Somatic Pain Associated with Anaesthesia. VII. The Effects of Nine Phenothiazine Derivatives," *Brit. J. Anaesth.*, 33, 422.

Moroney, M. J. (1963), *Facts from Figures*. Published by Penguin Books.

Pauca, A., Sykes, M. K. (1967), "Upper Limb Blood Flow during Thiopentone-halothane Anaesthesia," *Brit. J. Anaesth.*, 39, 758.

Siegel, S. (1956), *Non-parametric Statistics for the Behavioural Sciences*. Published by McGraw-Hill Book Company Inc.

Smart, J. V. (1963), *Elements of Medical Statistics*. Published by Staples Press.

Usubiaga, J. E., Gustafson, W., Moya, F. and Goldstein, B. (1967), "The Effect of Intravenous Lignocaine on Cardiac Arrhythmias during Electro-convulsive Therapy," *Brit. J. Anaesth.*, 39, 867.

Watts, L. F., Lebowitz, M. and Dillon, J. B. (1967), "The Effects of Ventilation on the Action of Tubocurarine and Gallamine," *Brit. J. Anaesth.*, 39, 845.

Wood, J. B. *et al.* (1965), "A Rapid Test of Adrenocortical Function," *Lancet*, I, 244.

## CHAPTER 3

# COMPUTERS AND THE ANAESTHETIST

## J. P. BLACKBURN

Computers are increasingly used in all fields of activity for example, for routine clerical and accounting operations, for performing complex calculations which might take many years by other means and for controlling the course of an experiment, or analysing the results.

Sooner or later the impact of these machines will be felt in medicine, indeed in many research situations they have already made considerable contributions.

Computers fall naturally into two types, analogue and digital, although there are also hybrid computers which combine the advantages of both groups.

### ANALOGUE COMPUTERS

Analogue computers cannot work with alphanumeric data directly, but handle waveforms, which may be fixed or continually varying quantities. The input to the computer and the processed output are voltages proportional to the magnitude of the variables they represent.

The basic units of analogue computers are called operational amplifiers. These can be connected in different ways to perform a variety of tasks: addition, subtraction, multiplication, division, integration and so on. There are also a number of special purpose devices like function generators whereby a variety of non-linear operations may be handled.

The operational amplifiers have the following characteristics:

1. The gain (or amplification) is very large.
2. The output voltage is opposite in sign to the input voltage.
3. The input impedance is very large.

An operational amplifier is conventionally represented as a triangle with one side slightly rounded. A complete circuit is shown in Figure 1, where the amplifier is wired up to multiply $e_s$ by a constant. $e_0$ is also inverted.

The principle of operation is as follows. If point A is at zero volts, the output is also zero volts. Suppose $e_s$ now becomes positive, point A tries to follow, but there is immediately a large negative deviation of the output

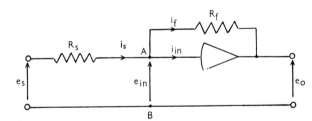

FIG. 1. Operational amplifier used to multiply by a constant.

voltage $e_0$, which is fed back to point A by the feedback resistor $R_f$ and tends to return point A to zero volts. Thus, the amplifier keeps its own input voltage very near zero volts.

We note that $i_{in}$ is negligibly small, as the input impedance of the amplifier is very large, and point A is at earth potential (it is often called a virtual earth). So the relationship of the output to the input is given by Ohm's Law

$$i_s = \frac{e_s}{R_s}$$

because $i_{in}$ is negligible

$$i_s = i_f$$

The output is inverted, and again by Ohm's Law

$$-e_0 = i_f R_f$$

$$\therefore \qquad e_0 = -\frac{R_f}{R_s} e_s$$

If several inputs are applied to the amplifier (Fig. 2) these are summed

$$e_0 = -\left( e_{s1}\frac{R_f}{R_{s1}} + e_{s2}\frac{R_f}{R_{s2}} + e_{s3}\frac{R_f}{R_{s3}} \right)$$

Similarly, the computer can integrate if we replace the resistor $R_f$ by a capacitor $C_f$ (Fig. 3).

When a charge $Q$ accumulates on a capacitor a proportional voltage $V$ is produced across the plates. The proportionality constant $C$ is the capacitance of the capacitor.

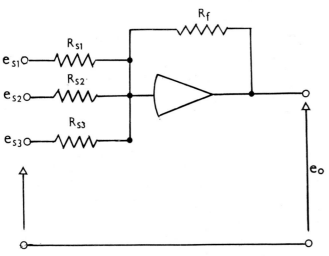

FIG. 2. Operational amplifier used for summation.

Thus $\qquad\qquad Q = CV$

But current $i$ is the rate of change of charge with time

So $\qquad\qquad i = \dfrac{dQ}{dt}$

$\therefore \qquad\qquad i = C\dfrac{dV}{dt}$

But the current flows as in the previous example

So $\qquad\qquad i_s = \dfrac{e_s}{R_s}$

$$-\frac{de_0}{dt} = \frac{i_f}{C_f}$$

$\therefore \qquad -\dfrac{de_0}{dt} = \dfrac{1}{C_f}\dfrac{e_s}{R_s}$

$\therefore \qquad e_0 = -\dfrac{1}{R_s C_f}\displaystyle\int e_s\, dt$

Non-linear functions may either be set up permanently in the machine by using logarithmic or square law function generators, or other devices may be adjusted by the user to simulate a variety of functions.

Multiplication of two signals, $x$ and $y$, can be achieved in various ways. One approach using square law networks together with addition, subtraction and division by a constant, is the so-called quarter square method,

where $\qquad \frac{1}{4}((x + y)^2 - (x - y)^2) = xy$

A typical analogue computer, shown in Figure 4, may have about 50 operational amplifiers which can be connected together quickly and easily and set up to perform any of the operations which have been described (Bellville and Hara, 1966).

### Applications

The applications of analogue computers are numerous and exist whenever the information that requires processing

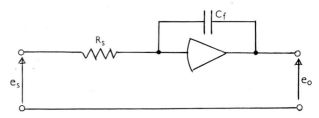

FIG. 3. Operational amplifier used for integration.

can be represented by voltages. Analogue devices will do several mathematical operations virtually instantaneously and at the same time, but it is relatively difficult and expensive to provide them with memory facilities and so are unsuitable for memorizing results. They cannot usually make many logical decisions.

Analogue outputs may be displayed on an oscilloscope, on an $x$–$y$ plotter or on a digital voltmeter.

In general, the analogue computer can be used in a variety of ways and investigation of medical problems may combine several methods of use.

### 1. Mathematical Computation

Analogue computers may be used to perform ordinary mathematical operations of addition, subtraction, multiplication, etc., but a particularly useful function is integration with respect to time. Thus, flow from a pneumotachograph can be integrated with respect to time with an operational amplifier to give volume, or acceleration may be integrated once to yield velocity and again to give displacement.

The analogue computer is useful in solving the differential equations which are often used to represent complex systems. Such equations commonly arise in the investigation of biological systems, in compartmental analysis and in calculations of the uptake, distribution and elimination of drugs from the body.

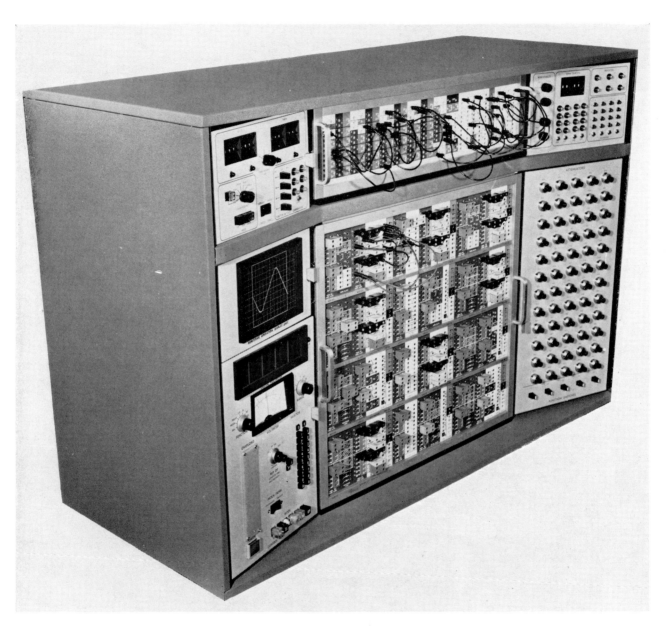

FIG. 4. Analogue computer (*courtesy of Electronic Associates Ltd.*).

## 2. Simulation of Biological Systems

Simulation of a system in the body using analogue computers is sometimes practised and can be used as a guide to the experimenter to suggest certain experiments and rule out the need for others. A model may allow the investigator to gain new insight through analogy with another physical system and the model may form the basis for extrapolation of results. Such models are usually dynamic and are modified in the light of results gained from new experiments. As analogue computers can be programmed quickly and easily, changes in the model can be made as new information becomes available.

Warner (1965), for example, has used analogue computer models of control systems to process flow and pressure information obtained from the aortic root of dogs exercising on a treadmill. The processed information is used to control reistance to outflow in the aorta by adjusting a semi-occlusive cuff placed round the distal aorta. In this investigation of the role of peripheral resistance in controlling cardiac output during exercise, a computer processed closed loop is established outside the animal which allows the investigator to have complete control of one or more variables in the experimental situation.

## 3. Data Processing

The analogue computer cannot be used to store data, but suitable signals can be processed in parallel and very fast, so that the answers are available while the experiment is in progress. When a computer is connected to the experimental preparation collecting and processing the data as it occurs, the machine is said to be used 'on-line'. Derived cardiovascular and respiratory information is usually computed in this way. Thus the time integral of aortic flow is stroke volume. Stroke volume multiplied by ventricular pressure gives power and the integral of power, for each stroke, is stroke work. Also, analogous to Ohm's law, arterial pressure divided by flow is equal to peripheral resistance (Osborn et al., 1963).

Similarly, analogue computers can be used for calculating respiratory volume, compliance, power, work and airway resistance from flow and pressure information (Osborn et al., 1963; Peters and Stacy, 1964; Fletcher and Bellville, 1966). In addition, the influence of air trapping in breathing mechanics has been investigated by deriving an equation which makes possible some measurement of airway elasticity (McWilliam and Adams, 1963).

Bellville et al. (1963) have used an analogue computer for calculating alveolar ventilation from tidal volume, physiological dead space and frequency of respiration, and plotting this against end-tidal $CO_2$ concentration. The alveolar-ventilation, end-tidal $P_{CO_2}$ response curve is considered by Bellville et al. to be a sensitive and reproducible method for assessing the effect of drugs upon respiration. The analogue computer not only gives a continuous plot of ventilation against $P_{CO_2}$ but also displays it while the experiment is in progress.

Another valuable use of analogue computers is in the calculation of cardiac output from indicator dilution curves. General purpose computers may be programmed to perform this calculation and there are several small special purpose computers developed for this application alone.

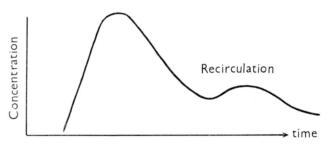

FIG. 5. Indicator dilution curve.

Cardiac output may be estimated by rapidly injecting an indicator, usually indocyanine green, into the circulation and sampling the arterial blood downstream from the injection site. The blood flow is calculated by dividing the dose of dye injected by the area under the indicator dilution curve, assuming there is no recirculation of dye. In practice, recirculation occurs (Fig. 5) but this is allowed for by assuming that the downslope of the curve, in the absence of recirculation, is exponential. Formerly, calculation of cardiac output was very time consuming because of the difficulty of measuring the area under the dye curve, but using an analogue computer this can now be done while the dye curve is being inscribed. Various techniques have been employed (Skinner and Gehrnlich, 1959; Moody et al., 1963; Wessel et al., 1964). One of the most elegant is as follows.

It is a property of an exponential that the area under the curve (A) Figure 6 from $t_2$ out to infinity, is the height of

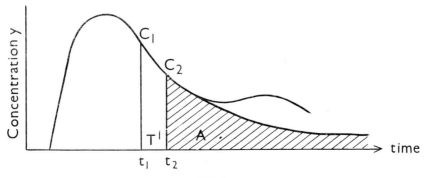

FIG. 6.

the curve ($C_2$) times the time constant which describes the steepness of the slope of the curve ($\tau$).

$$\text{Total area} = \int_0^\infty y \text{ corrected } dt = \int_0^{t_2} y \text{ uncorrected } dt$$
$$+ C_2\tau$$

Now $\qquad C_2 = C_1 e^{-T^1/\tau}$

$\therefore \qquad T^1/\tau = \ln(C_1/C_2)$

$\therefore \qquad C_2\tau = \dfrac{C_2/T^1}{\ln(C_1/C_2)}$

$$= \frac{C_2}{\ln(C_1/C_2)} \cdot \int_{t_1}^{t_2} dt$$

Suitable circuits can be built to use the computer as a low frequency oscillator, a filter or a wave shaper and various functions can be set up using the diode function generators.

## DIGITAL COMPUTERS

The digital computer works directly with numbers and all information is coded and stored in numerical form. Letters are also coded in a similar way, so that the machine can handle alphanumeric data. Almost all machines work serially through a set of instructions, which forms the programme, telling the machine what to do and calculations cannot be performed in parallel. Thus digital computers take a finite time to process data or perform a calculation.

However, modern machines work very fast, large

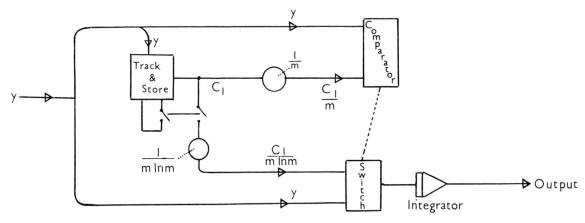

FIG. 7. Block diagram of indicator dilution curve analogue computer.

Let $\qquad C_1/C_2 = m, (m > 1)$

Then $\qquad C_2\tau = \dfrac{C_1/m}{\ln(C_1/C_2)} \displaystyle\int_{t_1}^{t_2} dt$

$$= \frac{1}{m \ln m} \int_{t_1}^{t_2} C_1 \, dt$$

$$\text{Total area} = \int_0^{t_1} y \, dt + \int_{t_1}^{t_2} \left[ y + \frac{C_1}{m \ln m} \right] dt$$

Hence the circuit adds in $\dfrac{C_1}{m \ln m}$ at time $t_1$ and the comparator cuts off the input at $t = t_2$ (Fig. 7). The dose of dye injected is now divided by the area to obtain the cardiac output.

### 4. General Purpose Laboratory Instrument

Finally, the analogue computer has some qualities which makes it able to replace a variety of laboratory instruments. Operational amplifiers make good low effective gain 'buffer amplifiers' which can be used to separate pieces of equipment and prevent undesirable interaction.

amounts of data can be stored or retrieved rapidly and also logical decisions can be taken when necessary.

Information is coded in a variety of forms and it might be thought reasonable to store information in the form of ten voltage levels, representing the numbers zero to nine, so that calculations can be performed in the decimal system. In practice, however, this has proved unreliable and only two states are recognized, normally designated '0' and '1'. These states can be represented as arbitrarily defined voltage levels, the presence or absence of an electrical pulse, the orientation of a magnet N–S or S–N, the open and closed positions of a switch, or the presence or absence of a hole in a punched card or punched paper tape. Because there are only two states this is called the binary system. Numbers are related in the binary and decimal systems as follows:

| Decimal | Binary |
|---------|--------|
| 0 | 0000 |
| 1 | 0001 |
| 2 | 0010 |
| 3 | 0011 |
| 4 | 0100 |
| 5 | 0101 |

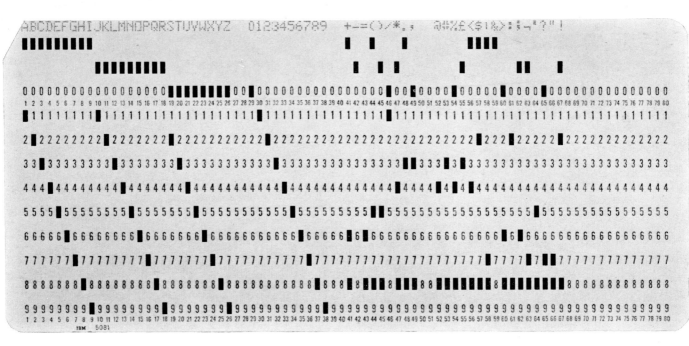

FIG. 8. Punched card (*courtesy of IBM (U.K.) Ltd.*).

and so on. In this example the binary 'word' 0000 is made up of 4 'bits' and the largest number which can be stored in a 4 bit word is 1111, equivalent to decimal 15. Each bit in a binary word represents a power of 2, so starting at the right hand bit, this is $2^0 = 1$, the next bit is $2^1$, the next $2^2$ and so on. Thus 1011 represents $2^0 + 2^1 + 2^3 = 11$.

The rules of binary arithmetic are very simple

$$0 + 0 = 0$$
$$1 + 0 = 1$$
$$1 + 1 = 0 \text{ and carry } 1$$

So

$$\begin{array}{ll} 0010 & 2 \\ + 0011 & +3 \\ \hline = 0101 & =5 \end{array}$$

Subtraction can be effected by forming the complement of the number to be subtracted and then performing addition.

The rules for multiplication are

$$0 \times 0 = 0$$
$$1 \times 0 = 0$$
$$1 \times 1 = 1$$

So

$$\begin{array}{l} 1001 \\ \times 101 \end{array} = \begin{array}{l} 9 \\ \times 5 \end{array}$$

$$\begin{array}{l} 1001 \\ 0000 \\ 1001 \end{array}$$

$$= 101101 = 45$$

Modern computers use words between 12 and 32 bits in length, word length may be fixed or variable and usually the left hand bit is used to designate the sign of a number. Using a 16 bit word with one sign bit integer numbers in the range $+32,767$ to $-32,768$ may be stored.

Fractional numbers, or 'real' numbers as they are called in one of the programming languages, are often stored in two parts using floating point notation. A binary number (the mantissa) with an implied binary point is used to represent the fractional part of the original number, while the exponent is represented by another binary number (the characteristic). Thus 34·73, equivalent to $0·3473 \times 10^2$, is stored in two words, one containing the binary equivalent of 0·3473 and the other the exponent 2 in binary form.

Digital computers can be divided into four main sections:

Input, Output, Control, Memory

## 1. Input Devices

These supply data or instructions to the machine. They may be keyboards or the information may be input from punched cards (Fig. 8) or punched paper tape. In addition, continuous signals like the ECG or a blood pressure waveform have to be broken down into a number of dis-

crete samples (analogue to digital conversion) so that the waveform is represented by a series of numbers (Fig. 9). The sampling rate is of crucial importance if the original signal is to be accurately reconstructed. Obviously if samples are taken infrequently the original signal cannot be recovered and there are theoretical reasons which govern the choice of sampling rate. In general, the sampling theorem states that if the continuous signal is sampled at a rate equal to twice the highest frequency present in

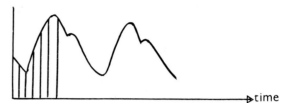

FIG. 9. Sampled version of analogue waveform.

the signal then no information is lost and the original data can be reconstructed. Figure 10 shows the effect of alterations in sampling rate. In practice, blood pressure traces are digitized at rates of about 100–200 samples/second, while ECG signals are sampled at 200–1,000 samples/ second.

Other forms of input are also available. For many people a typewriter keyboard is a barrier to communication with the machine, and although character readers and input devices linked to digital displays are available it will be a long time before typewritten or hand written data can be fed into the machine without passing through a slow intermediate stage where the input is translated into machine readable form.

## 2. Output Devices

These are units such as typewriters, high speed printers which may print up to 1,000 lines per minute, graph plotters and oscilloscopes for displaying alphanumeric data and analogue signals. The computer can also provide the processed information in the form of punched cards or write the output onto digital magnetic tape or other storage devices. Some machines can reconstitute continuous signals from stored sampled information using digital-to-analogue converters.

## 3. The Control Unit

This consists of devices which provide the arithmetic and decision-making capabilities of the computer and supervise the transfer of information between the memory and the input and output devices. The control unit also executes the instructions which form the programme. One of the important advances in digital computers was the development of stored programme machines, where the programme, as well as the data, was fed into the machine from the input devices, stored in memory and then executed.

## 4. Storage Devices

(i) **Rapid Access Store.** This is in direct communication with the control unit and is the working memory of

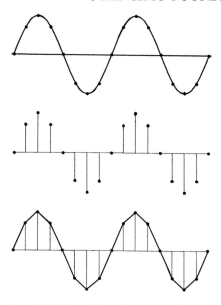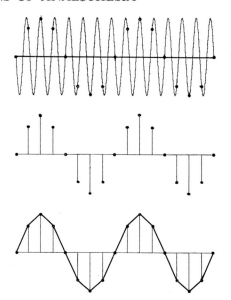

FIG. 10. Effect of alterations in sampling rate.

    (a) Correctly sampled signal.

        *Top:* Original signal, marked to show where samples will be taken.

        *Middle:* Sampled version, 8 samples per cycle.

        *Bottom:* Reconstructed signal. Linear interpolation between sample points.

    (b) Incorrectly sampled signal.

        *Top:* Original signal, 14 cycles of a sinusoid.

        *Middle:* Signal sampled at the same rate as (a). The samples are not obviously related to the signal from which they were obtained.

        *Bottom:* Reconstructed signal. This bears no resemblance to the original. This example has been chosen so that the middle and bottom traces in (a) and (b) are identical, to emphasize the misleading effect of inadequate sampling.

the system. This store consists of a number of small ferrite rings about 0·4 mm in diameter. A medium sized machine may have about half a million such rings, and each ring represents one bit of a word. Together these rings form the core storage. Magnetic core stores range in size from about 1,000 to over 100,000 words. Large machines will have more than 64,000 words and each word may have from 12 to 32 bits. One word of information can be stored or retrieved from such cores in less than one microsecond (one millionth of a second). The ferromagnetic rings have 3 wires wound round them, shown diagrammatically in Figure 11.

Let us assume that all the rings are magnetized N–S and this corresponds to state '0'. If a ring is magnetized S–N it is in state '1'.

Suppose it is desired to change the state of ring $x_3y_2$ from '0' to '1'. If currents of half the amount required to change the ring from a '0' to '1' state $(+\frac{1}{2})$ are applied to the input wires $x_3$ and $y_2$ simultaneously, then all the rings will remain in their original states except ring $x_3y_2$ which is remagnetized and changes from '0' to '1'.

Similarly when it is required to change a ring from a '1' to a '0' state currents of $-\frac{1}{2}$ are applied simultaneously through the appropriate $x$ and $y$ input lines.

During the read cycle currents of $+\frac{1}{2}$ are fed to the ring to be interrogated. If the ring is in a '1' state, no

change takes place and no voltage is induced in the sense winding. But if the ring is in a zero state, it is changed to a '1' and the changing magnetic field induces a voltage in the sense winding and a pulse is

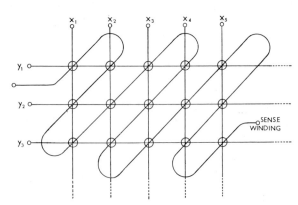

FIG. 11. Section of digital computer rapid access store.

output in the sense winding. This form of read-out is destructive, as all the rings read are in '1' states. If necessary the information can be written back into the rings immediately after interrogating them.

Although these operations sound cumbersome they are performed at great speed, and a modern digital computer can interrogate a number of rings in less than a millionth of a second.

(ii) **Backing Stores.** Bit patterns can be stored on a variety of magnetic materials. The most commonly employed are magnetic discs and magnetic tape. Magnetic discs are devices like gramophone records coated with magnetic oxide. About 500,000 words can be stored on a disc and retrieved within a few milliseconds. Single and multiple disc drives are available and discs may be interchangeable. Digital information can also be written on magnetic tape. Vast quantities of information can be stored cheaply, but access times vary from a few seconds to several minutes depending on the position of the data on the tape. About 400, 16 bit words, can be stored on one inch of tape.

## Digital Computer Programming

In early computers and in some special purpose computers the programme was 'wired in' and only data were stored in the memory. More recently stored programme machines became available where both instructions and data are stored. Also, with early machines the actual bit patterns corresponding to the various instructions had to be fed into the machine. Languages corresponding to machine instructions were then developed with statements such as 'load', 'store', 'add' and so on. This enabled programmers to write in nemonic code which was read by the machine and translated into machine instructions by a conversion programme called the 'assembler'.

High level languages are now available which are very easy to learn and instructions can be written in conventional mathematical symbols. One high level language instruction usually corresponds to many machine instructions, and a translation programme, called a 'compiler' converts the high level language instructions into the bit patterns required by the computer.

Computers will only do exactly what they are instructed and every eventuality has to be considered if correct results are to be obtained. However the time spent by the investigator in thinking analytically about his problem and specifying it in detail frequently gives him fresh insight and ideas.

## Uses of Digital Computers in Anaesthetics

Computers can be used to process different classes of data. We have already mentioned that information may be available as isolated numbers or as continuous signals which must be appropriately digitized. The data may be fed in from a typewriter or using punched cards or punched paper tape for retrospective analysis. Alternatively the computer may be used 'on-line' when the source of signals is connected directly to the machine and the data is processed as it arises.

## Anaesthetic Records

A number of workers have devised anaesthetic record cards (Hagelsten, 1968; Brueckner, 1968; Forrest *et al.*, 1963), where pre-operative assessment, anaesthetic course and post-operative comments can be recorded. Considerable discipline is necessary if the cards are to be filled in correctly, although the computer can be programmed to reject data which are obviously incorrect. These records must then be coded onto punched cards, or a similar medium, so that they are machine-readable. The stored data may be used for administrative purposes or research.

The object of such an exercise requires careful consideration from the outset and the forms must be designed so that the anaesthetist finds them convenient to fill in, and also so that the punch operator can code them efficiently.

## Statistical Calculations

Almost all computer centres have routine statistical programmes for analysing many kinds of data. Consultation with a statistician at an early stage is essential and if large amounts of data are to be processed careful design of the input documents is necessary. Forrest and Bellville (1967) have described computer assisted studies of analgesics and the relationship of halothane to massive hepatic necrosis. An essential part of these programmes is their ability to check errors arising in the original data or during transcription.

## Hospital Information Systems

A much more ambitious undertaking involves linking many of the hospital departments to a large central computer programmed to provide information of both an administrative and medical nature. Thus much of the patient record could be stored in the computer ready for immediate recall at a number of remote terminals. Operating theatre schedules, premedication administration, blood bank and pharmacy organization and the state of patients in the recovery room could all be appropriately processed and displayed. At the moment these installations have a large number of shortcomings. Suitable computers are very expensive, the system tends to be somewhat inflexible and input and output devices are inconvenient. Problems in data acquisition, particularly in updating the information and ensuring that it is accurate, have hampered some large scale systems.

## Literature Retrieval

A generally useful computer application is in the classification and storage of medical literature. The Medlars system classifies all the papers included in Index Medicus and lists of references on specific topics can be retrieved as required.

## Patient Data Analysis

When we consider results obtained from the patient, or signals (such as the ECG) arising directly from the patient, there are a number of different problems to be considered.

In one case there may be only a few results to be entered manually and processed. These may be pH blood gas values or electrolytes for instance. The volume of data is small and unreliable results can be eliminated by hand before the information is fed into the computer. Alternatively, if continuous waveforms are fed into the machine on-line, such as the ECG, blood pressure, or flow from a pneumotachograph, then not only must the computer be programmed to reject spurious data but also enormous numbers of samples from the analogue-to-digital converters have to be stored and processed within the machine. Computers are poor at pattern recognition because the data are processed serially. If the machine is to keep up with the incoming flow of data then signal processing has to be done rapidly, and because vast amounts of data are generated by the patient, problems of data reduction and presentation are important.

## 1. ECG Analysis

Computer processing of the ECG falls into two different categories. Typical of the first category are the detailed analysis programmes designed to examine one or two complexes of the conventional twelve lead or the orthogonal vector ECG (Caceres et al., 1964; Klingeman and Pipberger, 1967). An example of the second category is the completely different problem of analysing a single lead rapidly and continuously to detect arrhythmias in the intensive care situation.

The diagnostic ECG analysis programme, which examines only a limited amount of data in considerable detail, can separate normals from abnormals in over 90 per cent of cases and can classify the abnormals into a number of groups (Pordy et al., 1968). In general, most programmes do not analyse arrhythmias.

In the intensive care situation it is usually only possible to examine one lead and this has to be done rapidly and continuously. At the moment it is only possible to identify the QRS complex and recognize some changes in its shape and timing, so that ventricular ectopic beats can be located. Many workers have tried to identify P waves, but this is difficult as analysis is limited to the time before the next complex occurs.

The digital computer is useful, however, for deriving information which can be calculated from the timing of successive R waves. Alterations in rate and rhythm can be examined in detail and interleaved periodicities can be separated by various forms of signal analysis. These studies, based on instantaneous heart rate, may be of predictive value in patients likely to develop arrhythmias.

## 2. EEG Analysis

Computer assisted studies of the EEG have occupied the attention of many workers (Brazier, 1964; Adey and Walter, 1963; Walter, 1963) and at one time it was proposed to regulate the administration of anaesthetic automatically using changes in the EEG as the control signal (Bickford, 1950). The use of muscle relaxants has changed the emphasis on the signs of anaesthetic depth, and any control system making decisions based on the measurement and assessment of one variable is likely to be much inferior to an anaesthetist who uses multiple sources of information simultaneously to guide him in the anaesthetic management of a patient.

## 3. Blood Pressure Processing

The analysis of aortic, left ventricular, pulmonary artery and venous pressures has been attempted for a variety of purposes, some of which may be of interest to anaesthetists. Indices of myocardial contractility can be derived from pressure measurements and can be used to assess the effect of drugs upon the myocardium. In addition, some workers (Warner et al., 1966; Jones et al., 1966; Kouchoukos et al., 1970) claim that cardiac output can be computed on a beat by beat basis from central aortic pressure. The calculation involved is quite time consuming and computer processing is essential unless only a small number of beats require analysis.

## 4. Respiratory Physiology

On-line computation of pulmonary function has been used both for screening purposes (Shonfeld et al., 1964) and in the intensive care situation (Dammann, et al.,1964). Problems of using a pneumotachograph for long term studies in post-operative patients have limited the investigation of respiratory dynamics, but blood gas analysis and the analysis of expired air are performed routinely both for experimental and clinical purposes.

Temperature and other correction factors (Kelman, 1966; Kelman and Nunn, 1966) required for accurate blood gas analysis are often laborious to apply. If a digital computer is available it can easily be programmed to correct the measured blood gas values to the temperature of the patient and calculate the appropriate respiratory gas equations, with increased accuracy and considerable saving in time.

## 5. Computer Applications in Intensive Care

The prospect of using computers in intensive care wards offers new approaches to patient care in terms of predictive information, therapy and general management, but to be realistic the aims of any computer-assisted intensive care unit should be carefully defined from the outset.

Continuous signals such as the ECG, EEG, blood pressure and central venous pressure must be sampled rapidly by the analogue to digital converter and the values stored in the machine. The computer must be programmed to analyse the data and to reject artefacts arising from the transducers. The volume of data which can be collected in a short time is enormous and considerable thought must be given to suitable forms of data reduction and display.

Some information such as blood balance, urine output or body temperature will require less frequent recording and the results of blood gas analyses may be edited and entered by hand for subsequent processing. In addition, it is important to record general information about the patient, including therapy, and the method of data entry should be quick, efficient and suitable for ward use. The most convenient way to use the computer in this situation for entering data by hand is in the 'conversational mode'. The user communicates with the computer using a very simple keyboard to select options or enter doses or results and the computer displays on an oscilloscope screen either a list of options to be selected, or the data entered. The same system can be used to output the processed information in either alphanumeric or graphical form.

With such a display, plots of all the measured variables are rapidly available, but to use the computer in this way is to do nothing more than consider it as an efficient nurse charting pulse rate, blood pressure and so on. When a computer is available derived information is also rapidly obtainable, and plots of ejection time, the time between the Q or R wave and the onset of ventricular contraction, the rate of rise of arterial pressure, beat by beat cardiac output and so on may be of great value in the management of the patient and may provide predictive information which will lead to more precise treatment. All this information can be displayed on an oscilloscope at the bedside or may be printed or plotted for permanent storage.

It has been suggested that computers can be used directly to administer antiarrhythmic drugs or control fluid replacement post-operatively. It is important that the computer bases its decisions upon a large number of factors and it need hardly be stressed that such projects need to demonstrate complete reliability before they are adopted.

## Conclusion

Analogue computers are suitable for use in a variety of situations. They are relatively inexpensive, easy to programme and can perform calculations rapidly and in parallel. They are useful for modelling as well as for routine calculations and small general purpose computers are available for specific tasks, like the analysis of indicator dilution curves. They are limited by lack of memory facilities.

Digital computers can be used for a variety of purposes including all the applications for which analogue computers are normally employed.

The straightforward calculations and data analyses may be unexciting but can save enormous amounts of time and permit studies hitherto considered too laborious. Much more difficult is the analysis of signals derived directly from the patient and the greatest challenge lies in the operating theatre and intensive care unit. The use of computers in these situations will result in the ready availability of large amounts of derived information which may have far reaching effects on patient management. Finally, when the decision criteria involving the treatment of patients have been clarified, it is possible that computers may serve not only as data acquisition, processing and display devices, but may play a more active role in patient management (Forrest and Bellville, 1967).

The most flexible and powerful combination for scientific purposes is likely to be the hybrid computer, which combines both analogue and digital machines. Thus each device can do the tasks for which it is best suited. The analogue computer can perform rapid calculations under digital computer control and present the results to the digital machine for storage, or the analogue computer may pre-process the incoming signal so that the digital computer can work more efficiently.

## REFERENCES

Adey, W. R. and Walter, D. O. (1963), "Applications of Phase Detection and Averaging Techniques in Computer Analysis of EEG records in the Cat," *Expl. Neurol.*, 7, 186.

Bellville, J. W., Gilliland, M. C., Hara, H. H. and Mower, W. E. (1963), "Respiratory Carbon Dioxide Response Curve Computer," *Med. Electron. Biol. Engng.*, 1, 217.

Bellville, J. W. and Hara, H. H. (1966), "Use of Analog Computers in Anesthetic Research," *Anesthesiology*, 27, 70.

Bickford, R. (1950), "Electronic Control of Anaesthesia," *Electronics*, 23, 107.

Brazier, M. A. B. (1964), "Evoked Responses Recorded from the Depths of the Human Brain," *Ann. New York Acad. Sci.*, 112, 33.

Brueckner, J. B. (1968), "Routine Computer Application with a General Data Processing System in Anaesthesia." *Fourth World Congress of Anaesthesiologists, London.*

Caceres, C. A., Steinberg, C. A., Gorman, P. A., Calataynd, J. B., Dobrow, R. J. and Weihrer, A. L. (1964), "Computer Aids in Electrocardiography," *Ann. New York Acad. Sci.*, 118, 85.

Dammann, J. F., Grandine, J. D., Ryan, D. R., Updike, O. L. and Wright, D. J. (1964), "Data Acquisition and Interpretation System for Post-operative Patients," *Proc. San. Diego Symp. Bio-Med. Engng.*

Fletcher, G. and Bellville, J. W. (1966), "On-line Computation of Pulmonary Compliance and Work of Breathing," *J. Appl. Physiol.*, 21, 1321.

Forrest, W. H., Bellville, J. W., Seed, J. C., Houde, R., Wallenstein, S. L., Sunshine, A. and Laska, E. (1963), "A Uniform Method for Collecting and Processing Analgesia Data," *Psychopharm. Bull.*, 2, 1.

Forrest, W. H. and Bellville, J. W. (1967), "The Use of Computers in Clinical Trials," *Brit. J. Anaesth.*, 39, 311.

Hagelsten, J. O. (1968), "A Computer Based Anaesthetic Annual Report." *Fourth World Congress of Anaesthesiologists, London.*

Jones, W. B., Russell, R. O. and Dalton, D. H. (1966), "An Evaluation of Computed Stroke Volume in Man," *Amer. Heart J.* 72, 746.

Kelman, G. R. (1966), "Digital Computer Subroutine for the Conversion of Oxygen Tension into Saturation," *J. Appl. Physiol.*, 21, 1375.

Kelman, G. R. and Nunn, J. F. (1966), "Nomograms for Correction of Blood $P_{O_2}$, $P_{CO_2}$, pH and Base Excess for Time and Temperature," *J. Appl. Physiol.*, 21, 1484.

Klingeman, J. and Pipberger, H. V. (1967), "Computer Classification of Electrocardiograms," *Comput. Biomed. Res.*, 1, 1.

Kouchoukos, N. T., Sheppard, L. C. and McDonald, D. A. (1970), "Estimation of Stroke Volume in the Dog by a Pulse Contour Method," *Circ. Res.*, 26, 611.

McWilliam, R. and Adams, A. H. (1963), "Analogue Computer for Study of Breathing Mechanics," *Med. Electron. Biol. Engng.*, 1, 353.

Moody, N. F., Barber, H. D., Holmlund, B. A. and Merriman, J. E. (1963), "A Cardiac Output Computer for the Rapid Analysis of Indicator Dilution Curves," *I.E.E.E. Trans. Bio-Med. Elect. BME*, 10, 16.

Osborn, J. J., Badia W. and Gerbode, F. (1963), "Respiratory or Cardiac Work and other Analogue Computer Techniques," *J. Thoracic cardiovascular Surg.*, 45, 500.

Peters, R. M. and Stacy, R. W. (1964), "Automatized Clinical Measurement of Respiratory Parameters," *Surgery*, 56, 44.

Pordy, L., Jaffe, H., Chesky, K., Friedberg, C. K., Fallowes, L. and Bonner, R. E. (1968), "Computer Diagnosis of Electrocardiograms. IV. A Computer Program for Contour Analysis with Clinical Results of Rhythm and Contour Interpretation," *Comput. Biomed. Res.*, 1, 408.

Shonfeld, E. M., Kerekes, J., Rademacher, C. A., Weihrer, A. L., Abraham, S, Silver, H. and Caceres, C. A. (1964), "Methodology for Computer Measurement of Pulmonary Function Curves," *Dis. Chest*, 46, 427.

Skinner, R. L. and Gehrnlich D. K. (1959), "Analogue Computer Aids Heart Ailment Diagnosis," *Electronics*, 32, 56 (October).

Walter, D. O. (1963), "Spectral Analysis for Electroencephalograms," *Expl. Neurol.*, 8, 155.

Warner, H. R. (1965), "Control of the Circulation as Studied with Analog Computer Technics." In: *Handbook of Physiology*, Section 2, Circulation Vol. III, pp. 1825–1841. American Physiological Society.

Warner, H. R. (1966), "The Role of Computers in Medical Research," *JAMA*, **196**, 944.

Wessel, H. U., Hepner, C. F., James, G. W. and Kezdi, P. (1964), "Performance of a New On-line Computer for Indicator-dilution Curves," *J. Appl. Physiol.*, **19**, 1024.

*CHAPTER* 4

# MEASUREMENT AND RECORDING OF BIOLOGICAL ELECTRICAL SIGNALS

## J. P. BLACKBURN

In this chapter we will consider the sources of biological electrical potentials, the electrodes required to detect these, and the amplifiers and recorders used to display the signals. Finally problems of electrical interference and safety will be considered.

### Biological Electrical Signals

Electrical potentials can be detected in almost all parts of the body and it is well known that the inside of a cell is about 50 mV negative with respect to the outside, because of the differences in chemical composition between the inside and the outside of the cell. Changing potentials are associated with the depolarization of 'excitable tissues' and may be recorded from the central and peripheral nervous systems, the sense organs and skeletal, smooth or cardiac muscle. Electrical signals of interest to the anaesthetist are recorded from the heart, the central nervous system and the neuromuscular system.

### The Electrocardiogram

In spite of the complexities of different lead systems the electrocardiogram is essentially a measurement of the potential difference between two points. These may be two points on the body, as in the standard leads I, II and III, or with the chest leads, the potential difference is measured between the chest lead and a 'central terminal' obtained by combining signals from the right and left arms and the left leg in such a way as to derive their average.

The use of the conventional 12 lead electrocardiogram (ECG) is well established for diagnostic purposes, while for arrhythmia detection in the intensive therapy unit a single lead is commonly employed. In addition, the electrical changes in the heart may be recorded rather more efficiently and in more detail using an orthogonal vector system, the method described by Frank (1956) being most commonly employed. An array of eight electrodes is placed on the patient in such a way that the electrical signals originating from the heart are recorded in three planes at right angles. These three signals contain at least as much information as the 12 lead ECG if they are recorded simultaneously, so that phase information between the leads is not lost. The

problems of maintaining an array of electrodes on the patient limits the usefulness of the system for long term studies. Further details may be found in Chapter 5.

When recorded from the surface of the body, the ECG has a peak amplitude of about 1 mV and frequencies in the range 0·05–100 Hz are usually recorded. The sensitivity of the recorder is set so that 1 mV produces a pen deflection of 1 cm.

### The Electroencephalogram

This is a complex electrical signal conventionally recorded using a large array of electrodes. However during surgery or in the post-operative period a pair of electrodes is often adequate.

The electrical signal is about 50–200 $\mu$V in amplitude and for descriptive purposes the frequency range of the EEG is divided as follows:

| | |
|---|---|
| Delta waves | 0–4 Hz |
| Theta waves | 4–8 Hz |
| Alpha waves | 8–13 Hz |
| Beta waves | 13 Hz and above |

The EEG may be a useful guide to the adequacy of cerebral perfusion during open heart surgery and has been used in the assessment of cerebral death (Binnie *et al.*, 1970). The EEG has also been used to determine and control the depth of anaesthesia (Bickford, 1950), but the advent of muscle relaxants combined with light general anaesthesia has made such a system redundant. Changes associated with reduced cerebral perfusion, hypoxia or hypothermia are non-specific. Initially slow wave activity becomes more marked and increases in amplitude, then the electrical signals are reduced and finally no electrical activity is seen.

Artefact and interference free signals may be difficult to record under clinical conditions, and the signals may require expert analysis. However the cerebral activity monitor (Maynard *et al.*, 1969; Prior *et al.*, 1971) is considerably easier to use and the records can be readily interpreted. The EEG signal is recorded using two electrodes, band-pass filtered between 2–15 Hz to eliminate interference, and then amplitude limited, by logarithmic amplitude compression, and rectified. The output is displayed on a slow speed recorder as a smooth line drawn through the peaks of the compressed signal. A second channel is used to indicate the state of the electrodes and to record when the amplifier has been overloaded. Alterations in the amount or character of cerebral activity are easily visible (Fig. 1), but focal disturbances cannot be detected.

## The Electromyogram

As applied to anaesthesia, electromyography is still regarded primarily as a research tool for investigating various neurological conditions and determining the site and duration of action of muscle relaxants. For clinical purposes, assessment of the type and intensity of neuromuscular block is made by measuring the muscle contractions which occur when the appropriate motor nerve is stiulated. This is usually done by applying supramaximal twitch or tetanic stimuli to the ulnar nerve with surface electrodes and observing the contraction of the hypothenar muscles or adductor pollicis.

Electromyographic studies are used for a more detailed assessment of neuromuscular conduction. Again a supramaximal stimulus is applied to a motor nerve and the electrical activity of a group of muscle fibres is recorded using surface or needle electrodes. One nerve fibre typically supplies 100–300 muscle fibres which make up a 'motor unit', so when the nerve is stimulated a large number of muscle fibres are activated.

The response from a single muscle fibre is biphasic and lasts about 1 ms., while the response from a motor unit is more complex and has a duration of 5–10 ms. The amplitude of the response from a motor unit varies between 100 $\mu$V and 1·5 mV depending on the size of the unit and the position of the electrodes.

It should be noted that signals of this type are too rapidly changing to be displayed by a pen recorder. Cathode ray oscilloscopes can record such signals without distortion.

A more detailed account of electromyography and the changes which occur with neuromuscular blockade has been given by Wylie and Churchill-Davidson (1972).

## Electrodes

Electrical signals may be detected with intracellular electrodes, extracellular electrodes placed near the structure of interest, or most commonly using surface electrodes, such as those required for recording the ECG or the EEG. The main purpose of these electrodes is to detect biological electrical potentials from various sources, but in practice when a metal electrode is in contact with an electrolyte a number of electrochemical potentials are generated which may interfere with the signal of interest. These potentials often show slow fluctuations, but the effects can be greatly reduced by suitable filtering when a.c. coupled signals, such as the ECG, are recorded. Artefacts produced by the electrodes may be troublesome when small d.c. coupled signals are investigated.

## 1. Electrode Potential

The most obvious electrical effect occurring at the electrode is the electrode potential. This is the potential difference between the metal and the solution and in order to measure it some method of making electrical contact with the solution must be found, as the potential of a single electrode (half cell) cannot be measured in isolation. Electrode potentials are measured with respect to a standard electrode. The standard hydrogen electrode is used as a reference and is arbitrarily assumed to be at zero potential, although a calomel reference electrode is often more convenient to use. This has an electrode potential of about +0·3 V with respect to the hydrogen electrode, so allowance can be made for its contribution to the e.m.f. of the cell.

If a metal electrode is immersed in an electrolyte, which may be electrode jelly in the case of ECG or other surface

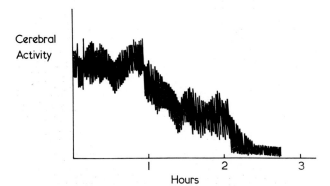

Fig. 1. Trace of cerebral activity, showing reduction in activity following hypotension and cardiac arrest. (Redrawn from Prior *et al.*, 1971.)

electrodes, or tissue fluid for electrodes placed in or near cells being investigated, there is a tendency of the metal to go into or come out of solution, depending on its position in the electrochemical series. Metals with negative electrode potentials (such as zinc, iron or tin) tend to ionize and pass into solution, leaving the electrode negatively charged with respect to the electrolyte, while the reverse reaction occurs with metals which develop positive electrode potentials.

Thus taking a silver electrode as an example:

$$Ag \rightleftharpoons Ag^+ + e^-$$

Metallic silver forms silver ions in solution, leaving electrons on the electrode. Also, silver ions in solution combine with these electrons, so that the electrode becomes positively charged. In practice the equilibrium is over to the left in the equation shown above and silver ions tend to come out of solution with the result that the electrode is about 0·8 V positive with respect to the electrolyte.

Ideally, when two identical electrodes are used in the same electrolyte, the potentials developed by the two half cells will be identical and should cancel when the electrodes are used together, although in practice small differences remain. Potential differences varying between a few microvolts and tens of millivolts have been described, depending on the type of electrode and the conditions under which the electrodes are prepared and used. In addition, the potential difference may not be stable, but may show marked fluctuations. If dissimilar metals are used for the two electrodes then there will be a potential difference between them which will depend on the positions of the metals in the electrochemical series.

The electrode potential will also be affected by the composition and concentration of the electrolyte.

## 2. Liquid-junction Potentials

When different electrolytes are in contact with each other without mixing, a liquid-junction potential is developed at the interface between the two solutions. This arises when the solutions have different concentrations and ionic mobilities. If the ions diffuse at different rates there will be a net separation of charges and a potential difference between the two solutions will result. If a solution of sodium chloride at 37°C is in contact with a similar solution which is ten times more concentrated, then a junction potential of 12·7 mV is produced, because of the differing mobilities of the sodium and chloride ions. If potassium chloride solutions are used instead of sodium chloride then the junction potential is only 1·1 mV because the mobilities of potassium and chloride ions are almost identical. Potassium chloride solution is used to connect the calomel electrode to the system under investigation, so the junction potential will be small. When electrolytes containing many different ions are in contact the liquid junction potential is very difficult to calculate, so where possible this situation is avoided by using a potassium chloride 'salt bridge' to connect different solutions.

## 3. Polarization Effects

When recording electrodes are connected to an amplifier, the current which flows depends on the potential difference between the electrodes and the input characteristics of the amplifier. This current causes a chemical reaction or a change in concentration at the interface between the electrode and the electrolyte. The change in composition may result in the deposition of metal or the formation of gas bubbles at the electrodes and the chemical reaction produces an e.m.f. which opposes the e.m.f. of the cell. Under these conditions the electrodes are said to be polarized and the potential difference which should exist between them as a result of the physiological process is reduced because of electrochemical events at the electrodes. Under some circumstances the current may be limited by the availability of ions at the electrode.

Non-polarizable (or reversible) electrodes are used whenever possible and can be made by keeping the metal electrode in contact with a solution of one of its own salts. Chemical changes still occur at the interface between the electrode and the electrolyte, but charge is carried freely by the common ions so electrochemical events at the electrodes should not limit the current which can be drawn from the system.

The commonest reversible system for physiological use is the silver/silver chloride electrode. Only small currents can be taken as silver chloride is virtually insoluble, but the electrode has the advantage that it is relatively non-toxic.

$$Ag \text{ (on electrode)} + Cl^- \rightleftharpoons AgCl \text{ (on electrode)} + e^-$$

Charge is carried freely by the chloride ions from the electrolyte to the electrodes. At one electrode chloride ions combine with metallic silver to form silver chloride and free electrons, while the opposite reaction occurs at the other electrode, where silver chloride dissociates into chloride ions and metallic silver. If heavier currents are to be passed, a soluble salt must be used. Salts of mercury or zinc can be employed, but are highly toxic to the tissues.

The subject of electrodes has been considered in some detail by Geddes (1972).

## Electrical Characteristics of the Source of Signals and the Amplifier

When recording electrical changes, the source of signals should have as low an impedance as possible, while the amplifier should have a high input impedance to minimize the current drawn from the preparation. The resistance of dry skin may be more than 1 M$\Omega$, but the skin impedance can be reduced to about 1,000 $\Omega$ by using electrode jelly. Alternatively the high impedance stratum corneum is breached using needle electrodes or multiple puncture electrodes (Lewes, 1966). In practice it is important that the impedances are approximately equal at the various electrodes when recording the ECG. Unequal skin impedances may cause distortion, particularly when the augmented limb leads or chest leads are recorded. For instance when a chest lead is recorded, the potential differences between the chest electrode and the 'central terminal' (made up of contributions from the left and right arms and left leg) is measured. The average of the limb potentials will depend on conditions at the individual electrodes and distortion of the signal may result if large differences are present.

More recently, capacitive electrodes, associated with suitable amplifiers, have been developed for long term use. When this arrangement is used, the electrode does not make contact with the skin directly but is insulated from it, so the body beneath the electrode forms one plate of a capacitor and the electrode forms the other plate. The advantage of the system is that no skin preparation is needed and electrode jelly is not used. Insulated gold electrodes are being developed, anodized aluminium electrodes have been described by Lopez and Richardson (1969), various types of electrodes have been reported by David and Portnoy (1972) and the subject has been reviewed by Bergey et al. (1971).

It is important to use an amplifier with an input impedance which is high in comparison with the signal source. If the input impedance of the amplifier is low, not only may an unacceptably large current be taken from the preparation leading to electrode artefacts, but also the voltage recorded by the amplifier will not be the true voltage which exists at the electrodes under open circuit conditions. Consider the case of a d.c. voltage generator (for simplicity), where the source resistance representing the tissue and total skin resistance is $S$ and the resistance presented by the amplifier is $R$ (Fig. 2). If the voltage developed by the generator is $E$ volts, this will also be the potential difference at two points $A$ and $B$ on the surface of the skin under open circuit conditions. When the amplifier is connected, however, a current $I$ will flow in the circuit.

$$I = \frac{E}{S + R}$$

$$V = IR$$

$$\therefore \qquad V = \frac{R}{S + R} \cdot E$$

Where $V$ is the voltage across the input terminals of the amplifier. (This is discussed fully in Chapter 2.) If the source resistance equals the amplifier input resistance the input voltage to the amplifier is half the source voltage.

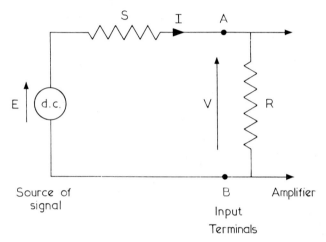

FIG. 2. Simple circuit showing the effect of source impedance $S$ and amplifier input impedance $R$. (For details *see* text.)

## Amplifiers

Suitable amplifiers must have adequate sensitivity, must remain stable and should have a suitable frequency response so that the input signal can be amplified without distortion. The importance of a high input impedance has already been stressed. ECG amplifiers, for instance, have input impedances ranging from 1 to 50 M$\Omega$. Amplifiers may be 'single-ended' in which case one of the connections is made to the 'active' input of the amplifier while the other input lead is connected to a reference, usually earth. This simple arrangement is adequate when signals of several volts are being considered and where one side of the input can be earthed, but electrical interference may be a problem when signals such as the ECG and EEG are being recorded. This problem will be discussed later.

More complex amplifiers may have two active inputs which are symmetrically arranged with respect to the earth reference. Differential amplifiers of this type are commonly used to record biological electrical potentials. Electrical signals applied as differences of voltage between the active inputs are amplified, but the amplifier does not respond appreciably to electrical changes affecting both inputs equally with respect to the earth reference. This feature is known as 'in-phase rejection', as in-phase signals affecting both inputs equally are ignored while out of phase signals appearing between the input terminals are amplified. The

in-phase rejection of a typical amplifier might be 10,000:1 meaning that a signal applied to both input terminals would need to be 10,000 times larger than a signal applied between them for the same change in the output. This technique is used to reduce a potent cause of electrical interference, because mains 'hum' affecting both inputs equally with respect to earth will not appear at the output.

Details of amplifiers will not be considered, but in general, amplifiers capable of amplifying d.c. or slowly changing signals operate in one of two ways. They may either be directly coupled, or they may convert their d.c. input into an a.c. signal which can then be amplified in a conventional a.c. coupled amplifier. This conversion is achieved either by 'chopping' the input signal using a relay or a solid state switch, or by modulating the input as in a so-called carrier amplifier. An amplified version of the original signal must be resynthesized at the output.

## Recording Devices

Once the signal has been amplified it must be displayed. One of the most useful general purpose displays is the cathode ray oscilloscope. In this instrument a beam of electrons is focussed onto a fluorescent screen and the beam is deflected by applying voltages to plates inside the oscilloscope tube (Fig. 3). The electrons can be deflected very

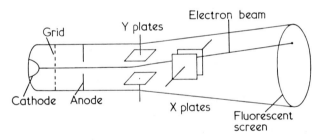

FIG. 3. Simplified diagram of cathode ray tube. The $X$ and $Y$ plates constitute the deflection system.

rapidly, so the instrument has a high frequency response and is virtually free from distortion, but permanent records are inconvenient to obtain as the trace has to be photographed. Storage oscilloscopes, where the trace may be stored on the tube and examined at leisure, are now available.

Other types of recorder include photographic instruments, where mirror galvanometers deflect white or ultra-violet light onto suitably sensitized paper (Fig. 4). Pen recorders are commonly employed (Fig. 5) and may use an ink system with pens or an ink jet (which has a higher frequency response), or thermal instruments write with a heated stylus on specially prepared paper (as in most ECG machines).

A pen attached to a galvanometer will normally sweep out an arc on the paper as it is deflected. The curved lines on the trace make timing of events difficult and the signals look distorted. With thermal recorders the paper is usually drawn over a knife edge on which the stylus rests, so that the trace is always at right angles to the paper (Fig. 6). The same effect may also be achieved by mechanically lengthening the pen as it is deflected so that it writes in rectilinear co-ordinates. These techniques produce amplitude distortion in the records, but this can either be corrected electrically in the amplifier or mechanically in the pen system.

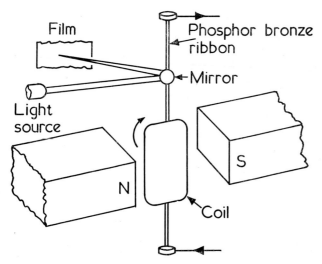

FIG. 4. Mirror galvanometer system.

The galvanometer and pen arm behaves as a complex mass-spring system which will resonate at a specific frequency and will overshoot if a step change is applied to it, in

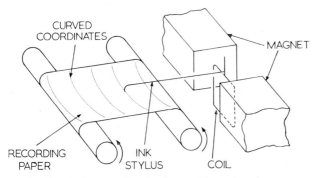

FIG. 5. Pen recorder, showing curvilinear distortion.

the same way as the catheter manometer system considered in chapter 3, page 42. Optimal damping should be applied to reduce overshoot and provide the best frequency response. This may be achieved electrically or by using oil as the damping medium.

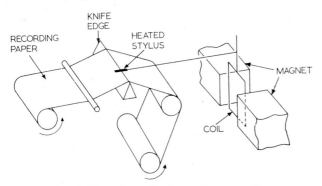

FIG. 6. Thermal recorder for rectilinear recording.

Although cathode ray oscilloscopes are capable of recording physiological signals without distortion (the frequency response is limited by the amplifiers and may be in the MHz range), pen recorders will only respond satisfactorily up to about 100 Hz and then only over a restricted range of amplitude. Ink jet recorders may be used up to about 500 Hz while mirror galvanometers may respond to frequencies of up to 3 kHz.

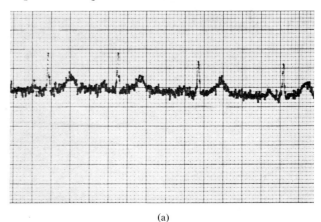

(a)

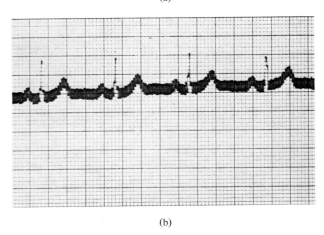

(b)

FIG. 7. Electrocardiogram showing:
(a) Skeletal muscle potential.
(b) 50 Hz mains interference.

## Electrical Interference

Biological electrical potentials may be contaminated by electrical interference produced by the patient or by the alternating current mains. Interference produced by the patient is caused by skeletal muscle action potentials which arise associated with movement or shivering. The trace has a characteristic appearance (Fig. 7a) and the ECG signal may be completely obscured by the interference. Slow base line wander on the ECG is usually associated with changes at the electrodes themselves.

Mains frequency interference, often called 'hum' may be troublesome during ECG or EEG recording, particularly in an environment where mains operated equipment is in use, such as an operating theatre or intensive therapy unit. Unlike small electronic components which can be 'screened' from some forms of mains interference, patients are physically large unscreened conductors, often in an environment in which electrical interference is present.

### Sources of Electrical Interference

#### (a) Capacitively Coupled Interference

Interference arises because of capacitative coupling between the source of interference and the patient from whom the signals are obtained, as shown in Fig. 8. The interference originates from a source of alternating emf, such as mains power cables. Often only one side of the mains supply is 'live' and the neutral line is at nearly the same potential as the local 'earth'.

The mains live conductor $L$ acts as one plate of the capacitor $C$, while the patient is the other plate. The other side of the mains is connected to earth through an impedance

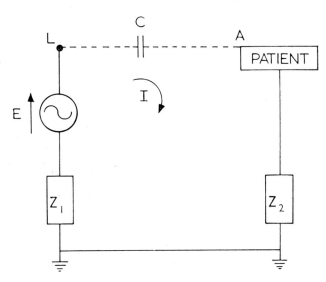

FIG. 8. Electrical interference produced by capacitative coupling.

$Z_1$ which usually has a low value. The patient is also connected to earth through the impedance $Z_2$. The size of $Z_2$ will depend very much on local conditions. It will be large if the patient is isolated from earth (for instance lying in bed) or may be very low if the patient is connected to earth (for instance by an earthed diathermy plate). When $L$ goes positive with respect to earth, negative charges will be attracted towards the surface $A$ and positive ones repelled. When $E$ reverses in polarity, negative charges will be repelled at $A$ and positive ones attracted. Thus a mains frequency current $I$ flows through the patient, even though there is no direct electrical connection between the patient and the mains. Interference of this type can also be picked up by signal leads and electrical components in the amplifier.

The factors affecting capacitance have been discussed in Chapter 2.

Capacitively coupled interference can be reduced by moving the patient away from the source of interference (in other words reducing $C$) and by 'screening' as much of the equipment as possible. The source of interference is

surrounded by a conductor connected by a low resistance pathway to earth as shown in Fig. 9. $C_1$ and $C_2$ represent the capacitance between $L$ and the screen and between screen and the patient, and $R$ represents the low resistance of the screen and the wire connecting it to earth. For greater generality the impedances $Z_1$ and $Z_2$ (which may be anything from direct connections to the high reactances of small stray capacitances) have been left in the circuit. A current $I_1$ flows from the source through the screen and there will thus

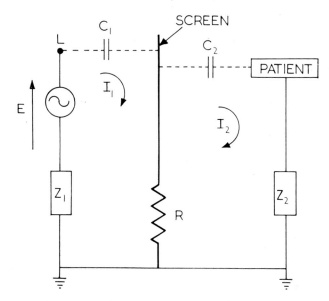

FIG. 9. Screening used to reduce capacitively coupled interference.

be a potential difference across resistance $R$. As far as the patient is concerned this small p.d. becomes the source instead of $E$, and consequently the lower $R$ is made the less p.d. appears across the patient. Notice that connecting the screen to earth does no more than virtually short circuit the output from $E$ via $C_1$, from the point of view of the patient. The screen can be a thin sheet of metal foil, a metal box or may be a wire mesh when flexibility is necessary, as with screened cables. Sources of interference should be screened as far as possible and signal leads and amplifiers should also be screened.

#### (b) Electromagnetically Induced Interference

As discussed in Chapter 2, when a magnet is moved in a coil an EMF is generated. Also when a current flows through a conductor, such as a mains lead, it generates a magnetic flux around the conductor and if 50 Hz mains alternating current is flowing the flux will change 100 times a second. If other conductors, such as the patient or the signal leads to the amplifier, lie in the changing magnetic flux, then voltages will be induced in the conductors. A simple circuit is shown in Fig. 10, where hum is induced in the signal lead to the amplifier.

Hum can also be induced in the earth wiring and this may cause trouble as shown in Fig. 11. The patient's right leg is connected to mains earth by an ECG recorder and the left leg is also connected to earth via a diathermy machine.

Lead II of the ECG is recorded using a differential input amplifier. Incidentally the ECG will be somewhat distorted because both right and left legs are connected to earth. An 'earth loop' ABCDE has been produced and as

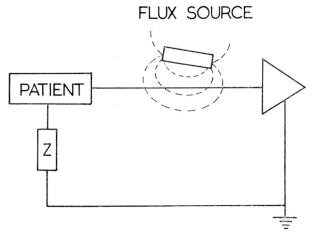

FLUX SOURCE

FIG. 10. Electromagnetically induced interference, showing a source of alternating magnetic flux which induces an alternating voltage in the signal lead between the patient and the amplifier.

part of the earth wiring lies alongside mains power cables it is inevitable that the earth conductors will be cut by changing electromagnetic flux and that a current will flow in the earth loop. This mains frequency current flows

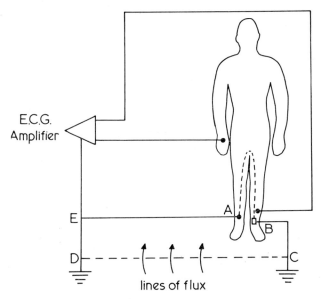

lines of flux

FIG. 11. Earth loop ABCDE involving the patient, producing electromagnetically induced interference.

through the patient, as shown by the dotted line and it is highly unlikely that it will affect the left leg and right arm electrodes equally. In other words, it will present an out of phase signal which will be amplified by the differential input amplifier.

The situation is improved considerably if the plate of the diathermy connected to earth is applied to the patient's

right leg, as shown in Fig. 12. There is now only one earth connection on the patient and, although current flows in the earth loop ABCDE, no mains induced current flows through the patient. Electromagnetically induced interference is generated in the same way as the effects produced in a transformer, where the source of interference represents the primary of the transformer and the patient, signal leads and earth connections take the place of the secondary winding.

We have already discussed one technique for reducing this type of interference, by avoiding multiple earths on the patient, so that earth loops involving the patient are not formed. Other methods involve deliberately making the transformer as inefficient as possible. Sources of interference should be kept as far away from the patient and associated equipment as is practicable. It is often impossible

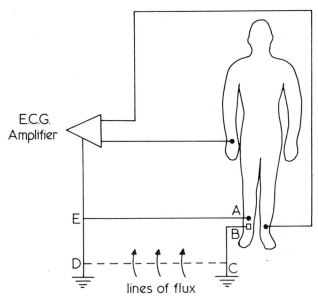

lines of flux

FIG. 12. Electromagnetically induced interference in the earth loop ABCDE no longer flows through the patient.

to screen the source as large amounts of soft iron would have to be used to confine the lines of flux. The area of the secondary winding should be reduced by keeping the leads close together and twisting the leads helps to cancel out induced voltages.

In spite of various precautions to reduce interference as much as possible, we are still left with a physically large and only partially screened conductor, comprising the patient, signal leads and amplifier, in a 50 Hz environment. In addition, this environment will not be constant as people and apparatus move about. As a result there will almost certainly be some interference present.

In Fig. 13, $I$ represents the current flowing through the patient as a result of this electrical interference. The current flows to earth through the impedance $Z$ and will produce a potential difference between electrodes $A$ and $B$ (a differential signal) which will be amplified along with the ECG and mains hum will be seen on the trace, unless the hum signal is small compared with the ECG signal.

In addition the whole patient will be varying in potential with respect to earth by $V = IZ$ volts. This in-phase signal (affecting both A and B equally) may be ten or a hundred times larger than the 1 mV ECG signal, but should not cause interference provided that the amplifier has good in-phase rejection.

In summary, the reduction of electrical interference depends on:

1. Careful electrode and signal lead technique.
2. Correct screening and earthing.
3. Well designed equipment, e.g. high in-phase rejection ratio.

### Electrical Safety of Patients

As more and more electrical equipment is used at the bedside or connected to the patient, it is important that doctors and nurses are aware of the electrical hazards which may arise (Starmer *et al.*, 1964; Bruner, 1967; Hopps, 1969; Loughman and Watson, 1971).

### (a) Electric Shock

When a voltage is applied between contacts placed on the surface of the body, a current will flow depending on the impedance of the pathway. The resistance between the surface of the skin and the underlying tissue varies between several megohms and tens of kilohms depending on the local conditions. As already mentioned, when electrode jelly is used to reduce the skin resistance it usually falls to about 1 kΩ, but may be as low as 300 Ω. The resistance of the underlying tissues is likely to be a few hundred ohms. It is important to note the variability of these figures, which makes dogmatic assertions suspect.

Mains frequency currents (50 Hz) are particularly effective in producing ventricular fibrillation and if the source is applied externally, for instance between the two arms, the following effects are found:

| | |
|---|---|
| Threshold of feeling | 0·5–2 mA |
| Muscular contraction | 25–100 mA |
| Ventricular fibrillation | 30–200 mA (typically 70 mA) |

The frequency of the stimulating current is important. If direct current is used, about five times the current is required, while when the diathermy is used, large high frequency currents pass through the body without ill effect.

Depolarization of excitable tissue depends on the current density (the current flowing per unit area) across the cell membrane. Current density is difficult to measure in practice and so the total current flowing between the electrodes is usually quoted. When surface electrodes are applied to the limbs, only about 1/1000th of the current flows through the heart because of the multiplicity of available pathways.

In order to appreciate the ways in which electrocution can arise, we must first consider the mains power supply (Dobbie, 1972a). The single phase 240 V a.c. mains supply normally provided at socket outlets and light fittings consists of:

1. A 'live' wire (*L*) which alternates at approximately 240 V with respect to local 'earth'.

2. A 'neutral' wire (*N*) carrying the return load current, and which is near 'earth' potential.

3. An 'earth' wire (*E*), not always present, which should be at local earth potential. This earth wire provides a return path for what are known as 'leakage currents' arising in the instrument. These are always present, because of capacitative and resistive coupling between live and earthed parts of the instrument. In addition, the earth wire is normally connected to the case of the instrument so that if, under fault conditions, some live part of the instrument comes in contact with the case, the earth wire can carry a large current and the case will remain near earth potential. Eventually if the fault current is large enough the fuse or circuit breaker will operate.

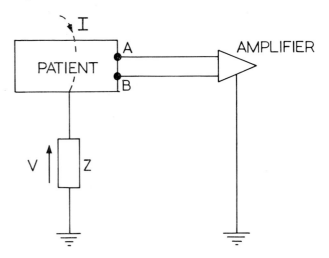

FIG. 13. Patient connected to differential input amplifier to illustrate in-phase and out of phase signals.

A current, limited by the resistance of the pathway and the rating of the fuses, will flow through the patient if he completes the circuit between the live and neutral or the live and earth wires.

It is possible for a current to reach the patient through the ECG or EEG electrodes if faults develop within the instrument, but equipment faults which endanger the patient in this way are very rare and usually two or more faults have to be present before the patient is at risk.

Manufacturers of electro-medical equipment in the U.K. are guided by publications and regulations of professional and official bodies, including the Department of Health and Social Security (1969). The provision of mains earth connection for reasons of safety relies on the mains plug being inserted into a three-pin mains socket. Even if patients are not involved, it is potentially dangerous for the user to ignore this requirement. In addition, the earthing serves as the first line of defence against capacitively coupled mains interference. The commonest electrical fault in mains operated equipment is disconnection of the earth wire. Usually the equipment will operate apparently normally in this condition so the operator is unaware that a potentially hazardous situation exists. However, if a second fault now develops, the case or other accessible parts of the instrument may become 'live' and constitute an electrical hazard both for the patient and the operator as shown in Fig. 14.

The current which can flow between the neutral and earth wires is likely to be much smaller but may endanger the

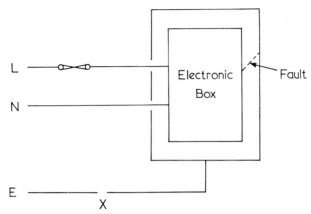

FIG. 14. Dangerous situation, showing broken earth lead X and live connection from electronics to outer metal case.

patient under some circumstances. The potential difference between the local earth and the mains supply neutral is likely to be a few volts because the latter, which completes the mains supply circuit, cannot be guaranteed to be at earth potential at all points along its length.

One way of improving the situation is to isolate the electrical supply to the equipment from earth by using an isolating transformer as shown in Fig. 15. Although 240 V

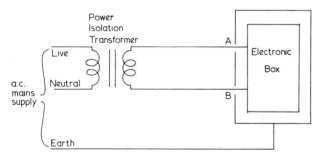

FIG. 15. Use of an isolating transformer.

is present between the supply wires A and B, the current which flows between A and Earth or B and Earth is very small and exists only because of the leakage within the transformer. In general however, isolating transformers are not used because they are expensive items of equipment which require leakage current monitors to establish that they are working effectively, and because they contribute only marginally to improved patient safety.

### (b) Microelectrocution

A more subtle cause of electrocution can arise when intracardiac electrodes are used or when a saline filled catheter forms a conducting pathway within the heart. When an intracardiac electrode is used all the current passes through the myocardium and the current density depends on the

size and position of the electrode. A small electrode in contact with ventricular muscle is most likely to produce ventricular fibrillation and a current of 180 μA has been reported to cause ventricular fibrillation in man (Whalen *et al.*, 1964). Usually much larger currents are required, however, and about 1 mA is needed to produce ventricular fibrillation with the electrode in the ventricle, while ventricular fibrillation cannot be produced with currents of up to 10 mA using an atrial electrode (Green *et al.*, 1972) in dogs. Small currents, which can endanger the patient, are found even when equipment is working normally and may be difficult to detect. The possibility of microelectrocution should always be considered when there is a catheter or other electrical connection in the ventricle, particularly if dysrhythmias occur in association with gross electrical interference on the ECG.

### Earth Points Having Different Potentials

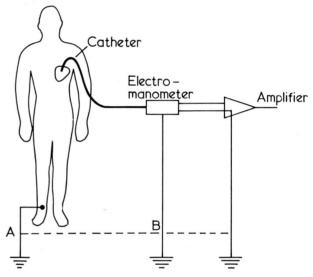

FIG. 16. Multiple earthing. If points A and B are at different potentials, then appreciable current may flow through the myocardium.

Ideally, two or more pieces of earthed equipment should be at the same potential. In practice, however, there may be significant differences in potential between earth terminals even in the same room. If earth leads from equipment earthed some distance away (for instance at a central monitoring station or computer) are applied to the patient together with locally earthed devices, then there may be several volts between the two earth points. Not only will there be large earth loops which may give rise to interference, but the patient may run the risk of electrocution. Combinations of equipment are frequently involved as shown in Fig. 16 and if the patient is earthed via the right leg lead of the ECG machine and via the saline filled electromanometer then the patient may be in danger if the earths are at different potentials, even though the equipment is operating normally. In addition, a current flowing down the mains earth conductor will alter the potentials of the earth sockets around the room. Small currents flow normally as 'leakage currents' from mains operated equipment, but larger 'fault currents' arising in faulty equipment may endanger the patient, even though there is no direct connection between the faulty equipment and the patient (Fig. 17).

Suppose the motor of a vacuum cleaner was faulty and allowed 1 A leakage current to flow to earth. The fuse would not blow and the user may not be aware of the fault.

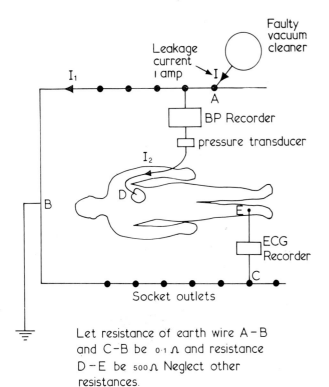

Let resistance of earth wire A–B and C–B be 0·1 Ω and resistance D–E be 500 Ω. Neglect other resistances.

$$V_{AB} \approx 1 \times 0.1$$
$$\approx 100 \text{ mv}$$

This is effectively across the patient.

$$So \ I_2 = \frac{0.1}{500}$$
$$= 200 \ \mu A$$

FIG. 17

However, if the cleaner is plugged in near the grounded electromanometer connected to a saline filled catheter and the patient is also earthed at another point by an ECG monitor plugged into a power socket some distance away, hundreds of microamps may flow across the myocardium. This is undoubtedly an extreme case, but it illustrates the way in which combinations of equipment, some of which are not faulty in any way and some of which are not directly connected to the patient, may produce a potentially dangerous situation.

### Safety Precautions

Measures which reduce interference will also increase patient safety. In general:

1. The patient should be isolated from earth wherever possible (Pocock, 1972a, b). Isolated pacemakers are used routinely and isolated ECG machines and electro-manometers are now available, Fig. 18. These may be battery driven, or special circuitry involving transformer or optical coupling may isolate the patient leads from mains earth. Specifications for these machines have not been finalized, but equipment is available where the leakage current to earth is less than 10 $\mu$A under the worst conditions. This specification is thought to be unrealistically stringent by some investigators (Dobbie, 1972b) and it is likely that 50–100 $\mu$A leakage current represents an acceptable and more realistic figure. Patient monitoring equipment must be capable of withstanding the voltages produced by surgical diathermy and defibrillation equipment and still maintain efficient patient isolation.

From the point of view of electrical safety, isolating the patient from earth means avoiding low impedance earth

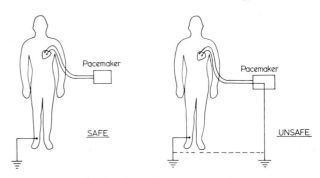

FIG. 18. Isolated equipment should be used if possible and direct earth connections avoided, particularly if a conducting pathway to the myocardium exists.

connections which may carry sufficiently large currents to endanger the patient. Connections involving the use of conducting rubber, which is of relatively high impedance, to avoid the build up of static electricity in the anaesthetic breathing circuit are of course desirable and will not increase the risk of electrocution.

2. When the patient must be earthed, then there should be only a single earth connection to the patient if possible. This will eliminate earth loops involving the patient and will reduce electrical interference as well as contributing to patient safety. All the equipment should be plugged into a single group of power sockets sharing a common earth. If necessary other metal objects within reach of the patient should also be connected to this common earth point. This ensures that all contacts made to the patient, either deliberate or accidental, are at the same potential and no current can flow through the patient.

3. Isolation of mains supply. The use of an isolating transformer has already been considered and the scheme is shown in Fig. 15. Contact between either of the floating supply wires and earth will not result in appreciable current flow. The leakage capacitance in the transformer and associated wiring will result in a current of a few milliamps flowing if one side of the isolated supply is short circuited to earth. If one wire of the isolated supply becomes accidentally grounded the system reverts to that

of the conventional mains supply. A line isolation monitor measures the impedance of both the isolated power lines to earth and triggers an alarm if the impedance drops below a pre-set level (such as 25 kΩ). Line isolation transformers are expensive and it is important to establish that such a system is justified in practice.

4. The commonest fault in mains operated equipment is disconnection of the earth wire in the mains lead. This can often pass unnoticed until a second fault develops which may cause electrocution. Careful maintenance of equipment is the only safeguard and at the moment the most efficient method of effecting this is under consideration (Editorial, 1972).

The subject of patient safety has received insufficient attention in the past. Now that the introduction of conducting devices within the heart has become relatively commonplace, it has become easy to produce ventricular fibrillation in patients with currents of only a few hundreds of microamps, which are likely to be completely undetected. There are numerous ways in which small currents can flow across the myocardium both when equipment appears to be operating normally and under fault conditions. It is important that manufacturers of monitoring equipment and those responsible for its installation and use are aware of these hazards and are able to avoid them in practice.

## REFERENCES

Bergey, G. E., Squires, R. D. and Sipple, W. C. (1971), "Electro-cardiogram Recording with Pasteless Electrodes," *IEEE Trans. Bio-Med. Engng.*, **18**, 206.

Bickford, R. G. (1950), "Automatic Electro-encephalographic Control of General Anaesthesia," *Electroenceph. clin. Neurophysiol.*, **2**, 93.

Binnie, C. D., Prior, P. F., Lloyd, D. S. L., Scott, D. F. and Margerison, J. H. (1970), "Electroencephalographic Prediction of Fatal Anoxic Brain Damage After Resuscitation from Cardiac Arrest," *Brit. med. J.*, **4**, 265.

Bruner, J. M. R. (1967), "Hazards of Electrical Apparatus," *Anesthesiology*, **28**, 396.

David, R. M. and Portnoy, W. M. (1972), "Insulated Electrocardiogram Electrodes," *Med. Biol. Eng.*, **10**, 742.

Department of Health and Social Security, Hospital Technical Memorandum No. 8, "Safety Code for Electro-medical Apparatus." London: H.M.S.O. Revised 1969.

Dobbie, A. K. (1972a), "Electricity in Hospitals," *Biomed. Engng.*, **7**, 12.

Dobbie, A. K. (1972b), "Is Money for Safety Unlimited?" *Med. Biol. Eng.*, **10**, 542.

Editorial (1972), "Equipment Maintenance," *Biomed. Engng.*, **7**, 219.

Frank, E. (1956), "An Accurate, Clinically Practical System for Spatial Vectorcardiography," *Circulation*, **13**, 737.

Geddes, L. A. (1972), *Electrodes and the Measurement of Bio-electric Events.* New York: Wiley-Interscience.

Green, H. L., Raftery, E. B. and Gregory, I. C. (1972), "Ventricular Fibrillation Threshold of Healthy Dogs to 50 Hz Current in Relation to Earth Leakage Currents of Electromedical Equipment," *Biomed. Engng.*, **7**, 408.

Hopps, J. A. (1969), "Shock Hazards in Operating Rooms and Patient-care Areas," *Anesthesiology*, **31**, 142.

Lewes, D. (1966), "Multipoint Electrocardiography Without Skin Preparation," *Wld. med. Electron. Instrum.*, **4**, 240.

Lopez, A. and Richardson, P. C. (1969), "Capacitive Electrocardiography and Bioelectric Electrodes," *IEEE Trans. Bio-Med. Engng.*, **16**, 99.

Loughman, J. and Watson, A. B. (1971), "Electrical Safety in Australian Hospitals and Proposed Standards," *Med. J. Aust.*, **2**, 349.

Maynard, D., Prior, P. F. and Scott, D. F. (1969), "Device for Continuous Monitoring of Cerebral Activity in Resuscitated Patients," *Brit. med. J.*, **4**, 545.

Pocock, S. N. (1972a), "Earth-free Patient Monitoring, Part I," *Biomed. Engng.*, **7**, 21.

Pocock, S. N. (1972b), "Earth-free Patient Monitoring, Part II," *Biomed. Engng.*, **7**, 67.

Prior, P. F., Maynard, D. E., Sheaff, P. C., Simpson, B. R., Strunin, L., Weaver, E. J. M. and Scott, D. F. (1971), "Monitoring Cerebral Function," *Brit. med. J.*, **2**, 736.

Starmer, C. F., Whalen, R. E. and McIntosh, H. D. (1964), "Hazards of Electric Shock in Cardiography," *Amer. J. Cardiol.*, **14**, 537.

Whalen, R. E., Starmer, C. F. and McIntosh, H. D. (1964), "Electrical Hazards Associated with Cardiac Pacemaking," *Ann. N.Y. Acad. Sci.*, **111**, 922.

Wylie, W. D. and Churchill-Davidson, H. C. (Eds.) (1972), "Normal Neuromuscular Transmission," p. 791, *et seq.*, in *A Practice of Anaesthesia*, 3rd edition. London: Lloyd-Luke Ltd.

*CHAPTER 5*

# PATIENT MONITORING

## J. P. BLACKBURN

The establishment of intensive therapy units has resulted from the need to concentrate the various highly specialized skills required in the treatment of critically ill patients within one functional unit. Monitoring devices have been developed for the collection of signals from patients by electronic or other means, although strictly speaking the term is derived from 'moneo' and thus some form of warning is implied. Monitoring devices are used to obtain

information which cannot be recorded in other ways, to reduce the demands on nurses when readings must be taken continuously or at frequent intervals and possibly to provide predictive information about the state of the patient.

Monitoring instruments have not proved to be acceptable in the general ward (Rawles and Crockett, 1969; Rawles, 1969), but patient monitoring is not confined to intensive therapy units, and the frequent use of hypotensive anaesthesia, hypothermia and more elaborate forms of cardiac and neurosurgery have made monitoring during the operative period essential.

In general, only a limited range of signals are recorded routinely. These include the ECG or some form of pulse monitor, the arterial blood pressure, central venous blood pressure, temperature and respiration. Blood gas analysis may also be important. Our present clinical knowledge allows interpretation of these signals and assessment of the state of the patient with a fair degree of confidence. However obtaining the signals reliably from a patient who may be hypotensive and restless may present unexpected difficulties and progress in this field is limited by difficulties at the patient/sensor interface (Crockett, 1970).

Invasive techniques for obtaining essential information from patients who are acutely ill are obviously justified, but there are many instances where reliable non-invasive methods would be advantageous. Some progress has been made in determining aortic blood flow (Light, 1969); while Weissler et al. (1969) and Reitan et al. (1972) and other workers have investigated systolic time intervals as indices of myocardial function. Automatic indirect methods for the determination of blood pressure are still somewhat unreliable, particularly in shocked and restless patients (Greatorex, 1971).

We will now consider some of the signals analysed routinely and then examine newer developments in the field.

## Electrocardiogram

This may be recorded as a conventional diagnostic 12 lead ECG or more usually as a single lead system for arrhythmia detection (see p. 188 et seq.). Vector systems have many advantages (von der Groeben et al., 1966) but the array of electrodes required is frequently difficult to maintain in practice. Early treatment of arrhythmias has significantly improved the mortality on many coronary units (Lown et al., 1967) and the ECG is frequently the only signal recorded. However, under these conditions a small percentage of patients may die because of pump failure, even though the ECG remains more or less unchanged.

Central monitoring stations may be used in coronary intensive care units. One nurse can watch the ECG traces from a number of patients, the nursing requirements for most of the patients are relatively modest and the patients benefit from being left undisturbed. In all other types of intensive therapy unit however, central monitoring stations are a disadvantage. Most patients require frequent nursing attention and information from the monitor should be displayed at the bedside where it can be seen easily by nurses and doctors and correlated immediately with changes in the condition of the patient.

Heart rate is frequently displayed on ECG monitors and may be charted by the nurse or recorded automatically. Arrhythmia monitors are now available which will detect abnormal beats either on the basis of prematurity or because of changes in the shape of the QRS complex. The QRS complex may be compared with a previously stored 'normal' beat for that patient and the shape of the typical stored complex may be modified automatically if appropriate. Artefacts such as excessive baseline wander or noise on the ECG are detected and inhibit the feature recognition process (Bushman, 1967; Horth, 1969; Neilson, 1971). Arrhythmia monitors are very complex internally but often have no controls requiring adjustment by the user. Well designed monitoring equipment is made self-adjusting as fas as possible so that it can be used easily in a clinical situation.

Intracardiac ECG recordings may be useful, particularly when automatic identification of the $P$ wave is attempted and His bundle electrograms have been used for investigating complex dysrhythmias and conduction defects (Smithen and Sowton, 1971).

Detailed analysis of interbeat intervals reveals a number of interesting features. In normal subjects, sinus arrhythmias can be easily identified and there are fluctuations related to the activity of the vasomotor centre and the thermoregulatory control system (Sayers, 1971). More detailed analysis of the effects of these nonlinear control systems may lead to earlier recognition of system malfunction in critically ill patients. In addition, a number of dysrhythmias show characteristic changes in the interbeat interval sequence (von der Groeben et al., 1966; Haisty et al., 1972).

The high frequency components of the ECG are also under investigation (Flowers et al., 1969; Sayers, 1967). ECG signals in the range 60–500 Hz, above the range of a normal ECG recorder, may provide a more detailed picture of the pattern of ventricular depolarization.

High frequency changes in the QRS complex are of very small amplitude, but may be extracted by a suitable averaging technique, Fig. 1. Changes in the pattern of ventricular depolarization may be caused by alterations in the excitability and size of an ischaemic area and this may be detected by the investigation of changes in the high frequency ECG. Excessive notching of the QRS complex in patients without other ECG evidence for infarction was shown to be an indication of intramural scarring in some cases (Flowers et al., 1969). At the moment changes in this complex electrical signal require further correlation with changes in the conditions of the patient. This signal may provide an earlier indication of ventricular malfunction than is at present available, but if this information is to be used effectively it is important that the cause of changes can be established, so that rational treatment can be instituted. A large number of cases will have to be investigated before useful conclusions can be drawn about the value of this new ECG signal in clinical practice.

Portable battery operated ECG monitors are now available which can be used easily under all conditions (Fig. 2). These are especially useful for patients who are being transferred from the operating theatre to the intensive therapy unit and are also valuable for mobile accident or myocardial infarction units. Portable d.c. defibrillators are also available, so patients with cardiac arrest may be diagnosed and treated under all conditions.

Problems of electrical interference and patient safety in ECG monitors and associated equipment, particularly when used with intracardiac electrodes or catheters, are discussed on p. 562 *et seq.*

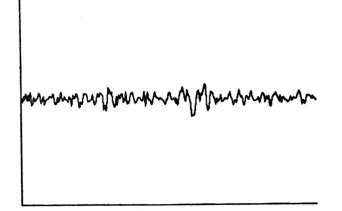

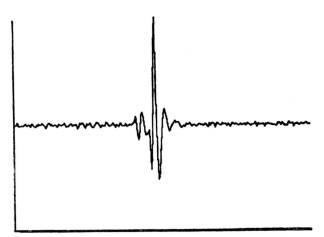

FIG. 1. High frequency ECG signal. Upper: ECG filtered 60–250 Hz. Lower: Average of 50 complexes. Abscissa 0·5 sec. The QRS complex would occur about the middle of the record.

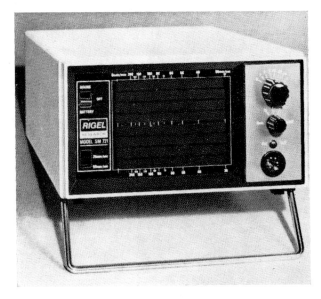

FIG. 2. Battery operated ECG monitor. (*Courtesy of Rigel Research Ltd.*)

## Pulse Monitors

A variety of devices are available for detecting the peripheral pulse. Most of them make use of the changes in light intensity reaching a photocell as a result of capillary pulsations. The devices are usually applied to the finger or the ear. An approximate indication of the systolic blood pressure can be obtained by inflating the sphygmomanometer cuff until the pulse is no longer detected. Finger plethysmographs or ultrasonic blood flow detectors can be used for the same purpose.

## Electroencephalogram

The electroencephalogram has been recorded during surgery and in the post-operative period. It is a useful guide to the adequacy of cerebral perfusion during cardiac bypass and has been used to assess and control the depth of anaesthesia (Bickford, 1950), but with the advent of muscle relaxants the classical signs of anaesthesia are no longer applicable. EEG records may also contribute to the assessment of cerebral death (Binnie *et al.*, 1970).

In general, artefact and interference free signals may be difficult to record under clinical conditions in intensive therapy units and the records may require interpretation by an experienced neurologist. The cerebral activity monitor described by Maynard *et al.* (1969) and Prior *et al.* (1971) overcomes many of these objections and presents the EEG signal in a form in which it can be readily interpreted. Further details may be found on p. 558.

## Blood Pressure

(a) **Indirect Methods.** There have been many attempts to automate the measurement of blood pressure using indirect methods (Geddes, 1970; Greatorex, 1971). Most of the methods work satisfactorily when applied to normal volunteers but are unreliable in hypotensive and restless patients. Systolic pressure can be detected more reliably than diastolic pressure. A large number of physical principles have been applied as mentioned on p. 43 *et seq.* A method recently developed which appears promising is to detect movements of the arterial wall using ultrasound (Ware and Laenger, 1967). The ultrasonic method appears to be easier to apply and less affected by artefacts than most of the other methods (Stegall *et al.*, 1968).

(b) **Direct Methods.** Transducers for measuring the arterial pressure are well established and there is no doubt that if arterial puncture is justified then such measurements are more reliable in the presence of hypotension than the indirect methods. In addition, arterial blood samples can be obtained for analysis. Miniature transducers less than 2·5 cm. long and 1·25 cm. in diameter (Fig. 3) can be attached to the patient at the arterial puncture site, thus eliminating long fluid filled catheters. Transducers are now available where the manometer chamber is electrically isolated from earth. Such instruments afford a greater measure of electrical safety for the patient.

Amplifiers with simple controls and easily read displays are available for use at the bedside. Systolic, diastolic and mean pressures may be presented on suitable meters or in digital form.

Catheterization of the right ventricle and pulmonary

artery can usually be accomplished quickly and easily if the Swan–Ganz catheter is used (Swan *et al.*, 1970). This balloon catheter can be floated through the right atrium and ventricle into the pulmonary artery. If the catheter is appropriately positioned in one of the branches of the pulmonary artery and the balloon is inflated, the pulmonary artery wedge pressure is obtained. Samples of mixed venous blood can be withdrawn from the pulmonary artery if required.

**Central Venous Pressure**

Traditionally, central venous pressure has been estimated using a catheter passed into the right atrium and connected to a saline manometer. Care must be taken that the reference zero of the system is maintained in the phlebostatic axis of the patient (Winsor and Burch, 1945; Debrunner and Bühler, 1969; Latimer, 1971). If an electrical output is required then the catheter is connected to a suitable electromanometer so that phasic or mean pressures may be displayed. A differential electromanometer for automatically correcting the reference level when the patient is tipped head up or down (Blackburn, 1968) has been used.

Changes in venous pressure are used to assist in the diagnosis of hypovolaemia, cardiac failure and tamponade. Further information can be obtained by observing the effect on the central venous pressure of the rapid infusion of 200 ml. dextrose (Sykes, 1963).

**Intracranial Pressure**

The measurement of intracranial pressure may be a valuable adjunct to the management of neurological cases in an intensive therapy unit. In cases of trauma or following neurosurgery it may be important to monitor intracranial pressure to indicate the onset of cerebral oedema or haemorrhage. This may be achieved by ventricular puncture using a water manometer, but this is difficult to maintain for long periods. Richardson *et al.* (1970) and Dorsch *et al.* (1971) have recently described implantable extradural pressure transducers which have remained *in situ* for several weeks. The transducers can be zeroed and calibrated while they are implanted, a feature which is particularly useful and which could possibly be incorporated in other implanted transducers.

**Temperature**

The measurement of temperature is generally straightforward and is described on p. 79 *et seq.*

Temperature measurements may be important during surgery when hypothermia is employed and are carried out routinely in the intensive therapy unit. Measurements can be made in a wide range of sites using rectal, oesophageal, nasopharyngeal and tympanic probes, needles for muscle temperature and skin loops.

The gradient between the core temperature and the peripheral skin temperature is of some interest and may be increased in shock (Joly and Weil, 1969).

**Respiration**

Monitoring respiration is often difficult unless the patient is receiving artificial ventilation, particularly if quantitative information is required. On some ventilators the tidal and minute volume can be read directly from the machine, although allowance may have to be made for gas compression and changes in volume of corrugated tubing connecting the patient to the ventilator.

An anemometer may be used intermittently to measure expired volume (Wright, 1955) and a pneumotachograph has also been used (Osborn *et al.*, 1968). Pneumotachographs are difficult instruments to use clinically, especially for long periods, because of condensation on the screen or in the pressure lines and the calibration of the instrument changes during inspiration and expiration (Grenvik *et al.*, 1966).

An ultrasonic spirometer has been developed similar in principle to the Doppler ultrasound blood flow detector.

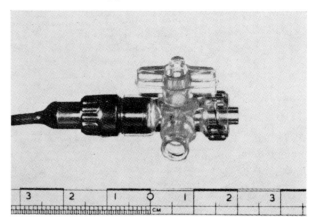

Fig. 3. Miniature blood pressure transducer. (*Courtesy of Statham Instruments Inc.*)

The transducer can easily be inserted in the airway, it has small dead space, low resistance and is unaffected by condensation or the accumulation of secretions. Alterations in gas composition and temperature will affect the calibration (Jackovitch and Eberhart, 1971).

Patients who are breathing spontaneously without an endotracheal or tracheostomy tube are more of a problem and usually only quantitative measures can be employed. Changes in the diameter of the chest or abdomen can be sensed in various ways. Impedance pneumography can be used to record changes in the electrical impedance of the chest during respiration (Baker and Hill, 1969). A temperature sensor placed in the airway will record changes in air temperature during respiration and thus indicate the onset of inspiration and expiration. Temperature probes may become displaced or covered with secretions and the impedance pneumogram may continue to record respiratory efforts made by the patient even though complete obstruction has occurred. This is due to changes in thoracic impedance caused by alterations in the shape of the chest and movement of gas within the lungs.

Respiratory rate has been derived from central venous pressure (Meagher *et al.*, 1966a) and a respiratory monitor has been developed for babies which is based on the movement of air within a segmented pneumatic mattress. Changes in the position of the infant with respiration cause alterations in the distribution of air within the mattress.

Air flow is detected by a heated thermistor and an alarm sounds if air movement within the mattress ceases (Fig. 4) (Lewin, 1969).

### Measurement of Cardiac Output

Measurement of cardiac output are often difficult to perform under clinical conditions. A number of methods have been described:

(a) **Fick Principle.** Under steady state conditions, the blood flow through an organ can be derived by measuring

*et al.,* 1965b) but this instrument is somewhat fragile. It has the advantage, however, that *in vivo* oxygen saturations may also be obtained (Monroe *et al.,* 1965a).

The technique of thermal dilution is being increasingly applied to the measurement of cardiac output. Dextrose or saline at room temperature is used as the indicator and is injected into the right atrium. The temperature is measured with a small thermistor bead mounted on a catheter and placed in the pulmonary artery. Thermal equilibrium between the indicator and the body occurs

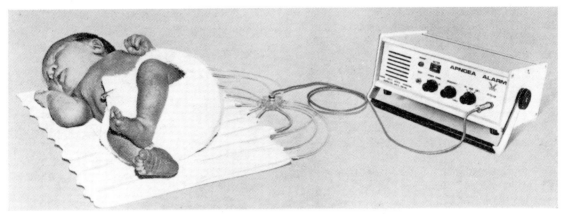

FIG. 4. Apnoea monitor using alterations in gas distribution within a segmented mattress to detect respiratory movement. (*Courtesy of Vickers Medical Ltd.*)

the amount of an indicator taken up by the organ per minute and dividing by the change in concentration of the substance at the input and output of the system. As applied to the measurement of cardiac output, the volume of blood flowing per minute through the heart (and thus through the lungs) is required. Oxygen uptake, or $CO_2$ output, is a convenient indicator and oxygen content must be measured both in mixed venous blood, preferably obtained from the pulmonary artery, and arterial blood. Then:

$$\text{Cardiac output} = \frac{\dot{V}_{O_2}}{Ca_{O_2} - C\bar{v}_{O_2}}$$

Where $\dot{V}_{O_2}$ is oxygen uptake in ml./min and $Ca_{O_2}$ and $C\bar{v}_{O_2}$ are the oxygen contents of arterial and mixed venous blood respectively.

Oxygen uptake is often difficult to measure and reliable estimates of blood oxygen content are somewhat difficult to obtain. Consequently the difference in oxygen saturation between arterial and venous blood has been employed alone as a guide to tissue perfusion. Oxygen extraction increases as tissue perfusion falls or the metabolic demands of the tissues increase.

(b) **Indicator Dilution Methods.** The principles involved in the use of non-diffusible indicators for estimating cardiac output have been discussed on p. 68. Indocyanine green is the most commonly used indicator, but in babies and children with small blood volume problems of sampling and reinjecting blood may limit the application of the method. Blood may be sampled and reinjected continuously using a roller pump (Cohn, 1969), alternatively blood sampling is avoided if a fibre-optic catheter is used (Monroe

relatively rapidly, so a recirculation peak is not seen on the indicator dilution curve. Thermal dilution methods are usually easy to apply in practice as no blood is withdrawn from the patient, and the estimation can be repeated quickly and conveniently as often as is required (Branthwaite and Bradley, 1968). Spontaneous temperature fluctuations, associated with respiration, may be found in the great veins, right heart and pulmonary artery because of alterations in the venous return from different parts of the body as a result of changes in intrathoracic pressure (Wessel *et al.,* 1966). These temperature fluctuations and loss of indicator as it equilibrates in the body may result in inaccurate estimations of cardiac output (Wessel *et al.,* 1971; Sanmarco *et al.,* 1971). A thermal dilution processor is shown in Fig. 5 and has been described by Cowell and Bray (1970).

(c) **Pressure Measurement Techniques.** The computation of aortic blood velocity based on differential pressure measurements has been described by Greenfield *et al.* (1962). In practice, the difficulties of setting up two accurately matched catheter manometer systems and uncertainty about the zero flow calibration limits the application of this technique in the clinical field (Greenfield and Fry, 1962).

A number of models have been developed from which stroke volume can be computed from a single aortic pressure measurement (Hamilton and Remington, 1947; Jones *et al.,* 1966; Kouchoukos *et al.,* 1969, 1970; Warner, 1966). Various assumptions are made in the application of these models and changes in heart rate and peripheral resistance are likely to alter the results (Greenfield *et al.,* 1971; Kouchoukos *et al.,* 1969, 1970).

A simple method for deriving stroke volume or cardiac output would be valuable clinically and the development of methods based on central aortic pressure pulse contour analysis are likely to be followed with interest by clinicians.

(d) **Ultrasonic Method.** An ultrasonic method for measuring aortic blood velocity has been described which is completely non-invasive (Light, 1969). A 2 M Hz ultrasonic beam is directed at the arch of the aorta from the suprasternal notch so that the beam is in the same axis as the blood flow. A Doppler shift in the reflected frequency occurs, as described on p. 56, and the signal received at the transducer is related to the velocity of the blood. There is a

to separate out a respiratory acidosis or alkalosis from a metabolic acid/base imbalance. It is defined as the concentration of bicarbonate in plasma, which may be separated from cells, with the haemoglobin completely oxygenated, at a $P_{CO_2}$ of 40 mm mercury and at a temperature of 37°C. If these conditions are standardized the influence of respiration on the acid-base content of the blood is eliminated.

Thus the $P_{CO_2}$ determines the respiratory component and the standard bicarbonate the metabolic component of acid-base imbalance.

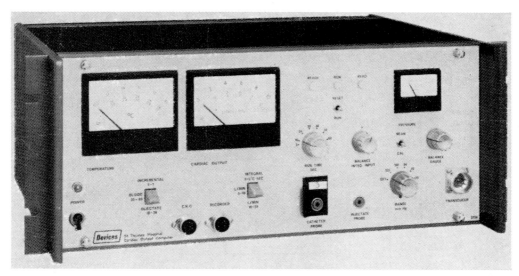

FIG. 5. Thermal dilution computer for deriving cardiac output. (*Courtesy of Devices Instruments Ltd.*)

change in blood velocity across the diameter of the aorta corresponding to the velocity profile, in addition to changes in velocity at different phases of the cardiac cycle. The complex reflected signal is passed through a frequency analyser to derive the quantity of blood flowing at each velocity during the cardiac cycle. If the arterial diameter is known and the mean velocity across the artery is averaged over one cardiac cycle, then the stroke volume can be derived.

### Blood Gas and Electrolyte Analysis

Rational management of acid base balance, oxygen therapy and parenteral nutrition depends on measurements made on arterial and venous blood samples.

Electrodes for the measurement of blood pH, $P_{O_2}$ and $P_{CO_2}$ are well established (Adams *et al.*, 1967) and are described on p. 107 *et seq.* and p. 98 *et seq.* A number of techniques are available for assessing the respiratory and metabolic state of the patient (Davenport, 1970; Siggaard-Andersen, 1963).

The usual procedure for blood gas analysis by the Astrup apparatus is to measure the pH of the specimen, and to equilibrate the blood with two $CO_2$ mixtures of known partial pressures after which the corresponding pH's are determined. From the three readings and by the use of a nomogram, the $P_{CO_2}$, the standard bicarbonate, the actual bicarbonate and the base excess or deficit are determined.

Astrup used the concept of standard bicarbonate in order

The Astrup nomogram is shown in Fig. 6 and is related to the Henderson-Hasselbalch equation

$$pH = pK + \log \frac{[HCO_3^-]}{0.03 \, P_{CO_2}}$$
$$= pK + \log [HCO_3^-] - \log 0.03 - \log P_{CO_2}$$
$$= \text{const.} - \log P_{CO_2} \text{ for a given bicarbonate}$$

i.e. $\log P_{CO_2} = \text{const.} - pH$ for a given bicarbonate

Thus if the equation is valid and $\log P_{CO_2}$ is plotted against pH a straight line results with a negative slope which can be made equal to unity if the scales of the axes are appropriately chosen. Moreover for different bicarbonate ion concentrations a series of parallel lines are obtained when pH is plotted against $\log P_{CO_2}$. These are known as bicarbonate isopleths.

In fact the Henderson equation does not take into account the buffering power of haemoglobin and the buffer line is affected by the haemoglobin concentration. The relationship is linear, however, over a restricted range of pH.

If a blood sample is equilibrated at two $CO_2$ tensions and the pH values measured, two points on the graph are determined and hence the buffer line for the sample may be drawn. If the pH of the original sample is measured its $P_{CO_2}$ can be read off.

The standard bicarbonate, corresponding to a $P_{CO_2}$ of 40 mm Hg can then be found from the nomogram, as the bicarbonate and pH scales are plotted together.

The fact that the slope of the buffer line varies with haemoglobin concentration implies that this information must be known when calculating acid-base values. However it has been shown experimentally that a base excess curve can be defined which will measure the non-respiratory component of the acid-base state independent of the haemoglobin concentration. The curve represents the points of intersection of the buffer lines of blood samples with different haemoglobin concentrations, but equal base deficit or excess as shown in Fig. 7.

The buffer base curve is determined similarly by drawing

can then be estimated to ±3 g/100 ml. This is obviously not a good method for determining haemoglobin concentration, but provides a useful check on the validity of the pH measurements used to define the buffer line.

Oxyhaemoglobin is more acidic than haemoglobin, so if the patient's blood is appreciably desaturated the buffer line will be displaced to the left (acid side) on the Astrup nomogram. This can be corrected using:

$$C = 0 \cdot 3 \times Hb \times \frac{(100 - O_2 \text{ saturation})}{100}$$

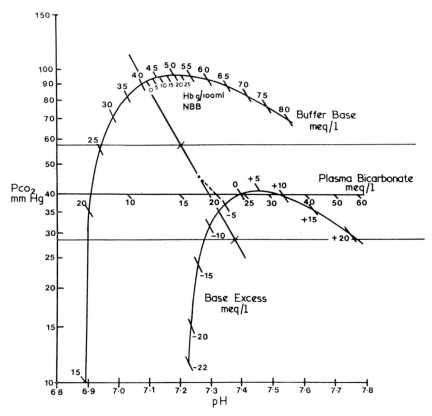

FIG. 6. Nomogram used with the Astrup interpolation technique. The buffer line obtained by equilibrating the blood sample with known gas mixtures is shown, together with the bicarbonate isopleth (dotted).

a line through the points of intersection of buffer lines representing samples with the same buffer base value but differing haemoglobin concentrations.

The buffer base depends on the haemoglobin concentration and the normal buffer base value for each haemoglobin concentration is shown on the haemoglobin scale situated on the buffer base curve. If the normal buffer base is subtracted from the buffer base of the sample, the value of the base excess if obtained.

The buffer line can be checked or the haemoglobin concentration can be found from the buffer line by artificially correcting the metabolic component of the acid base derangement and reading the haemoglobin concentration on the appropriate scale. This is done by moving along the buffer base line the appropriate number of mEq/l to correct the base excess to zero. The haemoglobin concentration

The corrected buffer line is then drawn C mEq/l to the right of the original line on the base excess and buffer base curves. $P_{CO_2}$, BE, BB and actual bicarbonate are read from the corrected line. Standard bicarbonate is defined when the blood is fully saturated and is therefore read from the original line.

The correction for desaturation only partially accounts for differences between the *in vivo* and *in vitro* buffer lines. The *in vivo* buffer line is also affected by the fact that some of the bicarbonate generated by the addition of $CO_2$ passes into the cells. The *in vivo* buffer line is therefore more horizontal than the *in vitro* line, as the body does not buffer a change in $P_{CO_2}$ as efficiently as occurs *in vitro*. If a blood sample is taken from a patient with a high $P_{CO_2}$ and then equilibrated *in vitro*, the *in vitro* buffer line will be displaced to the left and the patient will appear more acidotic than is actually the case. This error is about 4 mEq/l when the $P_{CO_2}$ is above 90.

Further details may be found in the chapters on 'Electrode systems for the measurement of blood gas tensions and contents', 'The determination of pH', 'Oxygen therapy at ambient pressure', 'Applied physiology of the body fluids' and 'The significance of acid base balance'.

### Computer Assisted Patient Monitoring

The operation of computers and some of their applications are considered on p. 549 et seq. The idea of using computers to assist the clinician in the management of the

These units are convenient to use under clinical conditions and can solve well defined problems.

When it comes to general purpose digital installations, however, only a small number of centres throughout the world are using computer based intensive care routinely. There are many difficulties in setting up such units for, unlike specific scientific projects, the problems to which the computer is harnessed may be poorly defined.

The computer can be employed in a number of ways:

1. Data collection. The ease with which data can be entered into the machine at the bedside is often of vital

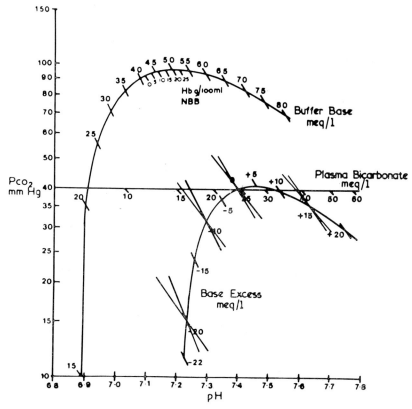

FIG. 7. Base excess line drawn through the points of intersection of buffer lines of blood samples with known base excess and variable haemoglobin concentration.

critically ill patient is attractive. The ability of analogue computers to process waveforms virtually instantaneously and to perform a number of operations in parallel is well known and digital machines are capable of storing vast amounts of data and retrieving it at high speed. Calculations can be performed and logical decisions made very rapidly and the data can be edited, correlated and displayed on a computer controlled oscilloscope terminal at the bedside. The information can also be presented in printed or graphical form for the patient's record.

Small special purpose processors, suitable for use at the bedside, are now available for performing specific tasks. Cardiac output computers for dye dilution (Moody et al., 1963) and thermal dilution estimations are well established and ectopic beat detectors have already been described.

importance to the medical and nursing staff. Information may be entered manually (William-Olsson et al., 1969) or automatically (Osborn et al., 1968; Sheppard et al., 1968; Warner et al., 1968). The keyboard should be linked with a computer controlled oscilloscope so that information can be presented quickly and conveniently.

2. Data processing. Large amounts of data can be processed at high speed. R-R intervals can be analysed from the ECG and characteristic patterns occur in various dysrhythmias and may be of predictive value (von der Groeben et al., 1966). Systolic time intervals may repay study and will be discussed below. There are many other examples.

3. Editing the data. The ability of the computer to

collect and process signals rapidly may be of doubtful benefit unless the information is presented to the clinician in readily assimilable form. An oscilloscope display capable of presenting both messages and graphs is essential. In one centre, base line readings are recorded on the patient and the nurses and doctors are only informed if significant alterations occur. The operator is then able to enter details about the patient (such as the administration of drugs) to explain the changes which have taken place (Warner et al., 1968).

4. Decision making. It is possible that the computer can assist directly in the treatment of the patient. If an adequate number of reliable signals can be fed into the machine and the decisions on which treatment is based can be rationalized, then the computer can control some forms of treatment, such as the rate of intravenous infusion (Sheppard et al., 1968). The administration of antidysrhythmic and cardiotonic drugs may also be controlled automatically. Even if the system were completely reliable, many clinicians would view such an installation with suspicion and maintain that clinical decisions are based on the assessment of many factors, some of which are unsuitable for computer collection and processing at the present time.

It is important when establishing a computer based intensive care system to display in the first instance the variables which the clinicians and nurses are used to seeing, such as pulse rate, blood pressure and central venous pressure. In this way they will be encouraged to use the display terminal and will then make use of derived information which was not previously available. In addition, the nurses must obtain information from the computer which is of direct use to them, so that they will consider it important to enter information into the system as required. An example is fluid balance. The fluid input and output are entered by hand or input automatically and the machine calculates the blood and crystalloid balance, draws attention to excessive loss, or suggests that drains may be blocked if the output is greater or less than prescribed limits.

A number of computer 'packages' are commercially available for patient monitoring systems. These are usually relatively small computers which may be programmed to tackle specific tasks such as intensive therapy, analysis of data obtained at cardiac catheterization, or the evaluation of respiratory function. When not in use as special purpose computers, the more flexible machines may be programmed by the user for other purposes.

In addition to providing routine information, computers can be used to perform simple analyses on long lengths of record, to extract signals from noise (such as the high frequency ECG), to perform calculations which would not normally be attempted by hand and to correlate and display the various types of derived data.

The aim of some of these forms of analysis is to provide predictive information about the state of the patient, but even when accurate prediction is possible, it must be combined with some guide to therapy, so that the patient can be treated effectively at an early stage.

## Telemetry

Single and multichannel systems have been used to telemeter signals from patients, although most systems have been confined to telemetry of the ECG using a single channel system. Battery operated telemetry equipment provides electrical isolation and so contributes to patient safety as described on p. 565 et seq. Telemetry is also useful for monitoring children, as such systems will avoid the need for leads connected directly to the patient. This is especially valuable when monitoring babies in incubators. Telemetry systems have also been used for patient monitoring under conditions of exercise (Mackay, 1970; Kuiper, 1971).

## Alarms

Many types of equipment for use in patient monitoring have become easier to use at the bedside. Controls are kept to a minimum, often as a result of considerable electronic complexity, and arrhythmia monitors and the cerebral activity monitor already described require virtually no setting up on the part of the user.

On the other hand, alarm systems are often unsatisfactory and the incidence of false alarms is unacceptably high. Raison et al. (1968) found that when 10 patients were observed for 44 hours there were 333 alarms produced from ECG and blood pressure signals. All these were false alarms resulting from mains interference, lead disconnection and excessive movement upsetting the ECG signal, and blood sampling or excessive damping of the arterial pressure waveform. A new system was therefore devised using combined signals and alarms were only registered when there was a fall in blood pressure associated with a rise or fall in pulse rate. An additional warning was actuated when the pulse pressure fell to less than 33 per cent of the mean pressure, indicating probable overdamping of the arterial line. As a result of these changes, only eight false alarms occurred in 92 hours and no clinically dangerous situations were missed.

## Recent Developments in Patient Monitoring

A number of developments have already been considered, particularly ectopic beat detection, cardiac interbeat-interval studies, the high frequency ECG, pulse contour methods for estimating stroke volume and computation of cardiac output from indicator dilution curves.

Systolic time intervals may be useful in assessing cardiac function (Weissler et al., 1969) and if the ECG, phonocardiogram and carotid pressure pulse are recorded externally, then these indices may be derived non-invasively, as described in the chapter on Cardiac Performance. Systolic time intervals have been used to assess left ventricular performance in myocardial infarction (Diamont and Killip, 1970; Samson, 1970), to investigate the effect of $\beta$-adrenergic blockade (Harris et al., 1967; Hunt et al., 1970), isoprenaline infusion (Leighton et al., 1970) and digitalis administration (Weissler et al., 1970). The pre-ejection period has also been shown to correlate well with ascending aortic blood flow acceleration (Reitan et al., 1972).

Various other methods are now available for investigating the performance of the heart. Left and right ventricular function curves have been plotted by Bradley et al. (1970)

using cardiac output estimated by thermal dilution and left and right atrial pressure measurements. Force-velocity relationships have been derived using cine-angiography (Hugenholtz et al., 1970), and a large number of indices of myocardial contractility have been developed (Mason et al., 1972). Left ventricular volume has been estimated ultrasonically in man by Gibson (1972) who derived pressure-volume relations on a beat-by-beat basis. This method is likely to be particularly useful as it is non-invasive and can be used for long periods without affecting ventricular function. Most of these indices require catheterization of the left ventricle and so can only be used for short periods of time.

As mentioned previously, respiratory function is difficult to evaluate. Osborn et al. (1968) have used a computer controlled pneumotachograph and rapid response oxygen and carbon dioxide analysers routinely following open heart surgery. In addition to deriving tidal volume and minute volume, physiological dead space, compliance and airway resistance could also be computed. This enabled the ventilator to be used more effectively and changes in the patient or ventilator performance could be detected at an early stage. In addition, oxygen uptake was monitored and increased oxygen uptake in hypothermic patients due to shivering was noted (Raison et al., 1970).

The interactions of the various biological control systems have been studied by Sayers (1971) and periodicities in heart rate and blood pressure due to cardiovascular, respiratory and thermal control systems have been described. These periodicities can be influenced by external stimuli and this may lead to new methods of testing the integrity and interactions of fundamental control systems in patients treated in intensive therapy units.

There is a growing interest in stress tests of various types. Rumball and Acheson (1963) described ECG changes produced by exercise in patients with latent heart disease and Elliott et al. (1970) have used a computer to study patients during exercise. Systolic time intervals have also been investigated during exercise by Aranow et al. (1971) and Pouget et al. (1971) in patients with angina. In normal controls on mild exercise there was a decrease in the pre-ejection period, largely due to a change in total electro-mechanical systole; while exercise in patients with angina caused a larger decrease in pre-ejection period, but this time the change was due to an increase in left ventricular ejection time.

Postural changes can be used to produce circulatory stress and systolic time intervals have been studied by Stafford et al. (1970). The Valsalva manoeuvre is well established in the diagnosis of heart failure and dysfunction of the autonomic nervous system, in addition Bushman (1971) has used the passive valsalva to investigate the circulatory response of patients under anaesthesia. Such methods could well be applied to the investigation of patients requiring intensive therapy. Another form of circulatory stress which can be applied conveniently is administration of a fluid load. Sykes (1963) has described the infusion of 200 ml. of fluid intravenously to differentiate normals and those with hypo or hypervolaemia and cardiac function curves have been obtained in patients with cardiogenic shock where right and left atrial pressures have been altered by trans-

fusion, venesection and the application of cuffs to the thighs (Bradley et al., 1970). Sheppard et al. (1968) infused fluid continuously under computer control following open heart surgery, provided the atrial and arterial pressures were below present limits.

The use of such stress tests is likely to be of growing importance in the investigation of patients who are critically ill. Variations in posture, fluid load or airway pressure can be effected easily at the bedside and alterations in responses to these tests are likely to occur at an earlier stage than is seen with conventionally recorded signals.

## Conclusions

Increasing use is being made of intensive therapy units for the treatment of critically ill patients and a large number of manufacturers offer equipment for patient monitoring. In general, this equipment can be used to record the ECG, blood pressure, central venous pressure and temperature, but problems arising at the patient/transducer interface may limit the reliability of the system at the present time.

Maloney (1968) has stressed many of the difficulties in patient monitoring and has emphasized the dangers which arise when the nurse is removed from the bedside to a central monitoring installation. The signals which can be recorded often contribute a great deal to the management of the patient, but nevertheless they provide only a small part of the overall clinical impression on which the doctors and nurses base their management of the case. At the moment clinical impressions (such as the patient's degree of alertness, colour, restlessness, abdominal distension, etc.) cannot be rationalized or transduced in such a way that they can be used as inputs to an automated patient monitoring system, although these signs provide valuable help to the clinicians.

In addition, when considering the installation of a patient monitoring system, the clinician may be confused by the conflicting claims of different manufacturers, he may be unable to work out the way in which different combinations of instruments may be used and he may be unable to assess the electrical safety of the installation.

In spite of these difficulties, intelligently used monitoring systems play an indispensable role in the management of critically ill patients. Sophisticated electronic systems which are easy to use under clinical conditions have been developed and new forms of derived data which may have predictive importance in the management of the patient are being investigated. Stress tests of various types can also be analysed rapidly and easily using automatic feature recognition systems. Perhaps the greatest challenge for the future lies in interpreting the complex interrelations between the physiological control systems, using the limited range of signals which can be conveniently recorded at the bedside.

## REFERENCES

Adams, A. P., Morgan-Hughes, J. O. and Sykes, M. K. (1967), "pH and Blood-gas Analysis," Anaesthesia, 22, 575.

Aranow, W. S., Bowyer, A. F. and Kaplan, M. A. (1971), "External Isovolumic Contraction Time and Left Ventricular Ejection Time/External Isovolumic Contraction Time Ratios at Rest and After Exercise in Coronary Artery Disease," Circulation, 43, 59.

Baker, L. E. and Hill, D. W. (1969), "The Use of Electrical Impedance

Techniques for the Monitoring of Respiratory Pattern, During Anaesthesia," *Brit. J. Anaesth.*, **41**, 2.

Bickford, R. G. (1950), "Automatic Electro-encephalographic Control of General Anaesthesia," *Electroenceph. clin. Neurophysiol.*, **2**, 93.

Binnie, C. D., Prior, P. F., Lloyd, D. S. L., Scott, D. F. and Margerison, J. H. (1970), "Electroencephalographic Prediction of Fatal Anoxic Brain Damage After Resuscitation from Cardiac Arrest," *Brit. med. J.*, **4**, 265.

Blackburn, J. P. (1968), "Self-levelling Venous Pressure Transducer," *Brit. med. J.*, **4**, 825.

Bradley, R. D., Jenkins, B. S. and Branthwaite, M. A. (1970), "The Influence of Atrial Pressure on Cardiac Performance Following Myocardial Infarction Complicated by Shock," *Circulation*, **42**, 827.

Branthwaite, M. A. and Bradley, R. D. (1968), "Measurement of Cardiac Output by Thermal Dilution in Man," *J. Appl. Physiol.*, **24**, 434.

Bushman, J. A. (1971), "Systems Response Testing in Cardiovascular Monitoring," in *Computer in der Schwerkranken überwachung.* Internationales Symposium, Düsseldorf.

Bushman, J. A. (1967), "Monitoring the ECG Waveform," *Biomed. Engng.*, **2**, 106.

Cohn, J. D. (1969), "A Pump System for Performing Indicator Dilution Curves Without Blood Loss," *J. Appl. Physiol.*, **26**, 841.

Cowell, T. K. and Bray, D. G. (1970), "Measuring the Heart's Output," *Electron. Power*, **16**, 150.

Crockett, G. S. (1970), "The Patient-sensor Interface," *Postgrad. Med. J.*, **46**, 378.

Davenport, H. W. (1970), *The ABC of Acid Base Chemistry*, 5th edition, University of Chicago Press.

Debrunner, F. and Bühler, F. (1969), "Normal Central Venous Pressure, Significance of Reference Point and Normal Range," *Brit. med. J.*, **3**, 148.

Diamont, B. and Killip, T. (1970), "Indirect Assessment of Left Ventricular Performance in Acute Myocardial Infarction," *Circulation*, **42**, 579.

Dorsch, N. W. C., Stephens, R. J. and Symon, L. (1971), "An Intracranial Pressure Transducer," *Biomed. Engng.*, **6**, 452.

Elliott, S. E., Miller, C. W., Armstrong, W. T. and Osborn, J. J. (1970), "The Use of the Digital Computer in the Study of Patients During Exercise-induced Stress," *Amer. Heart J.*, **79**, 215.

Flowers, N. C., Horan, L. G., Tolleson, W. J. and Thomas, J. R. (1969), "Localization of the Site of Myocardial Scarring in Man by High Frequency Components," *Circulation*, **40**, 927.

Geddes, L. A. (1970), "The Direct and Indirect Measurement of Blood Pressure." Chicago: Year Book Medical Publishers Inc.

Gibson, D. G. (1972), "Beat-by-beat Analysis of Left Ventricular Pressure Volume Relations in Atrial Fibrillation in Man," *Brit. Heart J.*, **34**, 204.

Greatorex, C. A. (1971), "Indirect Methods of Blood Pressure Measurement," in *IEE Medical Electronics Monograph 1–6* (B. W. Watson, Ed.). London: Peter Peregrinus Ltd.

Greenfield, J. C. and Fry, D. L. (1962), "Measurement Errors in Estimating Aortic Blood Velocity by Pressure Gradient," *J. Appl. Physiol.*, **17**, 1013.

Greenfield, J. C., Patel, D. J., Mallos, A. J. and Fry, D. L. (1962), "Evaluation of Kolin Type Electromagnetic Flowmeter and the Pressure Gradient Technique," *J. Appl. Physiol.*, **17**, 372.

Greenfield, J. C., Starmer, C. F. and Walston, A. (1971), "Measurement of Aortic Blood Flow in Man by the Computed Pressure Derivative Method," *J. Appl. Physiol.*, **31**, 792.

Grenvik, A., Hedstrand, U. and Sjogren, H. (1966), "Problems in Pneumotachography," *Acta Anaesth. Scandinav.*, **10**, 147.

Haisty, W. K., Batchlor, C., Cornfield, J. and Pipberger, H. V. (1972), "Discriminant Function Analysis of RR Intervals: An Algorithm for On-line Arrhythmia Diagnosis," *Comput. Biomed. Res.*, **5**, 247.

Hamilton, W. F. and Remington, J. W. (1947), "The Measurement of Stroke Volume from the Pressure Pulse," *Amer. J. Physiol.*, **148**, 14.

Harris, W. S., Schoenfeld, C. D. and Weissler, A. M. (1967), "Effects of Adrenergic Receptor Activation and Blockade on the Systolic Pre-ejection Period, Heart Rate and Arterial Pressure in Man," *J. clin. Invest.*, **46**, 1704.

Horth, T. C. (1969), "Arrhythmia Monitor," *Biomed. Engng.*, **4**, 308.

Hugenholtz, P. G., Ellison, R. C., Urschel, C. W., Mirsky, I. and Sonnenblick, E. H. (1970), "Myocardial Force Velocity Relationships in Clinical Heart Disease," *Circulation*, **41**, 191.

Hunt, D., Sloman, G., Clarke, R. M. and Hoffman, G. (1970), "Effects of Beta-adrenergic Blockade on the Systolic Time Intervals," *Amer. J. Med. Sci.*, **259**, 97.

Jackovitch, T. and Eberhart, R. C. (1971), "The Doppler Principle Applied to Respiratory Flow Measurement," *Proc. San Diego Biomed. Symp.*, **10**, 47.

Jones, W. B., Russell, R. O. and Dalton, D. H. (1966), "An Evaluation of Computed Stroke Volume in Man," *Amer. Heart J.*, **72**, 746.

Joly, H. R. and Weil, M. H. (1969), "Temperature of the Great Toe as an Indication of the Severity of Shock," *Circulation*, **39**, 131.

Kouchoukos, N. T., Sheppard, L. C. and McDonald, D. A. (1970), "Estimation of Stroke Volume in the Dog by a Pulse Contour Method, "*Circ. Res.*, **26**, 611.

Kouchoukos, N. T., Sheppard, L. C., McDonald, D. A. and Kirklin, J. W. (1969), "Estimation of Stroke Volume from the Central Arterial Pressure Contour in Postoperative Patients," *Surgical Forum*, **20**, 180.

Kuiper, J. (1971), "Medical Telemetry System," in *IEE Medical Electronics Monograph 1–6* (B. W. Watson, Ed.). London: Peter Peregrinus Ltd.

Latimer, R. D. (1971), "Central Venous Catheterisation," *Brit. J. Hosp. Med.*, **5**, 369.

Leighton, A. R., Tolumbo, A. A., Zaron, S. J. and Robinson, J. L. (1970), "The Use of Systolic Time Intervals in Predicting Hemodynamic Effects of Isoproterenol," *Clin. Res.*, **18**, 317.

Lewin, J. E. (1969), "An Apnoea-alarm Mattress," *Lancet*, **ii**, 667.

Light, L. H. (1969), "Transcutaneous Observations of Blood Velocity in the Ascending Aorta in Man," *J. Physiol.*, **204**, 1P.

Lown, B., Fakhro, A. M., Hood, W. B. and Thorn, G. W. (1967), "The Coronary Care Unit," *JAMA*, **199**, 188.

Mackay, R. S. (1970), *Bio-medical Telemetry*, 2nd edition. New York: John Wiley.

Maloney, J. V. (1968), "The Trouble with Patient Monitoring," *Ann. Surg.*, **168**, 605.

Mason, D. T., Zelis, R., Amsterdam, E. A. and Massumi, R. A. (1972), "Clinical Determination of Left Ventricular Contractility by Hemodynamics and Myocardial Mechanics," in *Progress in Cardiology* (P. N. Yu and J. F. Goodwin, Eds.). Philadelphia: Lea and Febiger.

Maynard, D., Prior, P. F. and Scott, D. F. (1969), "Device for Continuous Monitoring of Cerebral Activity in Resuscitated Patients," *Brit. med. J.*, **4**, 545.

Meagher, P. F., Jensen, R. E., Weil, M. H. and Shubin, H. (1966), "Measurement of Respiration Rate from Central Venous Pressure in the Critically Ill Patient," *IEEE Trans. Bio-Med. Engng.*, **13**, 54.

Monroe, R. G., Polanyi, M., Nadas, A. S., Gamble, W. J. and Hugenholtz, P. G. (1965a), "The Use of Fibreoptics in Clinical Cardiac Catheterisation. I. Intracardiac Oximetry," *Circulation*, **31**, 328.

Monroe, R. G., Polanyi, M., Gamble, W. J. and Hugenholtz, P. G. (1965b), "The Use of Fibreoptics in Clinical Cardiac Catheterisation. II. *In Vivo* Dye-dilution Curves," *Circulation*, **31**, 344.

Moody, N. F., Barber, H. D., Holmlund, B. A. and Merriman, J. E. (1963), "A Cardiac Output Computer for the Rapid Analysis of Indicator Dilution Curves," *IEEE Trans. Bio-Med. Engng.*, **10**, 16.

Neilson, J. M. (1971), "Hybrid Computer Monitoring of ECG Arrhythmias," *Computer in der Schwerkranken überwachung Internationales Symposium*, Düsseldorf.

Osborn, J. J., Beaumont, J. O., Raison, J. C. A., Russell, J. and Gerbode, F. (1968), "Measurement and Monitoring of Acutely Ill Patients by Digital Computer," *Surgery*, **64**, 1057.

Pouget, J. M., Harris, W. S., Mayron, B. A. and Naughton, J. P. (1971), "Abnormal Responses of the Systolic Time Intervals to Exercise in Patients with Angina Pectoris," *Circulation*, **43**, 289.

Prior, P. F., Maynard, D. E., Sheaff, P. C., Simpson, B. R., Strunin, L., Weaver, E. J. M. and Scott, D. F. (1971), "Monitoring Cerebral Function," *Brit. med. J.*, **2**, 736.

Raison, J. C. A., Beaumont, J. O., Russell, J. A. G., Osborn, J. J. and

Gerbode, F. (1968), "Alarms in an Intensive Care Unit: An Interim Compromise," *Comput. Biomed. Res.*, **1**, 556.

Raison, J. C. A., Osborn, J. J., Beaumont, J. O. and Gerbode, F. (1970), "Oxygen Consumption After Open Heart Surgery Measured by a Digital Computer System," *Ann. Surg.*, **171**, 471.

Rawles, J. M. (1969), "Patient Monitoring: A Clinician's Point of View," *Biomed. Engng.*, **4**, 264.

Rawles, J. M. and Crockett, G. S. (1969), "Automation on a General Medical Ward: Monitron System of Patient Monitoring," *Brit. med. J.*, **3**, 707.

Reitan, J. A., Smith, N. T., Borison, V. S. and Kadis, L. B. (1972), "The Cardiac Pre-ejection Period: A Correlate of Peak Ascending Aortic Blood Flow Acceleration," *Anesthesiology*, **36**, 76.

Richardson, A., Hide, T. A. H. and Eversden, I. D. (1970), "Long Term Continuous Intracranial Pressure Monitoring by Means of a Modified Subdural Pressure Transducer," *Lancet*, **ii**, 687.

Rumball, A. and Acheson, L. D. (1963), "Latent Coronary Heart Disease Detected by Electrocardiogram Before and After Exercise," *Brit. med. J.*, **1**, 423.

Samson, R. (1970), "Changes in Systolic Time Intervals in Acute Myocardial Infarction," *Brit. Heart J.*, **32**, 839.

Sanmarco, M. E., Philips, C. M., Marquez, L. A., Hall, C. and Davila, J. C. (1971), "Measurement of Cardiac Output by Thermal Dilution," *Amer. J. Cardiol.*, **28**, 54.

Sayers, B. McA. (1967), "Computers and Computing Methods: The Engineer's Viewpoint," *Proc. Roy. Soc. Med.*, **60**, 756.

Sayers, B. McA. (1971), "Systems Analysis in Intensive Care Problems," *Computer in der Schwerkranken überwachung*. Internationales Symposium, Düsseldorf.

Sheppard, L. C., Kouchoukos, N. T., Kurtts, M. A. and Kirklin, J. W. (1968), "Automated Treatment of Critically Ill Patients Following Operation," *Ann. Surg.*, **168**, 596.

Siggaard-Andersen, O. (1963), "The Acid-base Status of the Blood," *Scand. J. Clin. Lab. Invest.*, **15**, suppl. 70.

Smithen, C. S. and Sowton, E. (1971), "His Bundle Electrograms," *Brit. Heart J.*, **33**, 633.

Stafford, R. W., Harris, W. S. and Weissler, A. M. (1970), "Left Ventricular Systolic Time Intervals as Indices of Postural Circulatory Stress in Man," *Circulation*, **41**, 485.

Stegall, H. F., Kardon, M. B. and Kemmerer, W. T. (1968), "Indirect Measurement of Arterial Blood Pressure by Doppler Ultrasonic Sphygmomanometry," *J. Appl. Physiol.*, **25**, 793.

Swan, H. J. C., Ganz, W., Forrester, J., Marcus, H., Diamond, G. and Chonette, D. (1970), "Catheterization of the Heart in Man with Use of a Flow-directed Balloon-tipped Catheter," *New Engl. J. Med.*, **283**, 447.

Sykes, M. K. (1963), "Venous Pressure and Clinical Indication of Adequacy of Transfusion," *Ann. Roy. Coll. Surg.*, **33**, 185.

von der Groeben, J., Whitcher, C. E., Fitzgerald, J. W. and Omodt, L. (1966–68), "Computer Analysis and Monitoring of Cardiac Arrhythmias in Surgical Patients," Progress report to PHS grant HE 10202. Stanford University School of Medicine.

Ware, P. W. and Laenger, C. J. (1967), "Indirect Blood Pressure Measurement. Doppler Ultrasound Kinetoarteriography," *Proc. 20th Ann. Conf. on Engng. in Med. and Biol.* (Boston), Wellesley Press, Mass.

Warner, H. R. (1966), "The Role of Computers in Medical Research," *JAMA*, **196**, 944.

Warner, H. R., Gardner, R. M., Toronto, A. F. (1968), "Computer-based Monitoring of Cardiovascular Functions in Postoperative Patients," *Circulation*, **37**, suppl. II, 68.

Weissler, A. M., Harris, W. S. and Schoenfeld, C. D. (1969), "Bedside Technics for the Evaluation of Ventricular Function in Man," *Amer. J. Cardiol.*, **23**, 557.

Weissler, A. M. and Schoenfeld, C. D. (1970), "Effect of Digitalis on Systolic Time Intervals in Heart Failure," *Amer. J. Med. Sci.*, **259**, 4.

Wessel, H. U., James, G. W. and Paul, M. H. (1966), "Effects of Respiration and Circulation on Blood Temperature of the Anesthetized Dog," *Amer. J. Physiol.*, **211**, 1403.

Wessel, H. U., Paul, M. H., James, G. W. and Grahn, A. R. (1971), "Limitations of Thermal Dilution Curves for Cardiac Output Determinations," *J. Appl. Physiol.*, **30**, 643.

William-Olsson, G., Norlander, O., Norden, I. and Petterson, S. O. (1969), "A Patient Monitoring System with Display Terminals," *Opuscula Medica*, **14**, 39.

Winsor, T. and Burch, G. E. (1945), "The Phlebostatic Axis and Phlebostatic Level, Reference Levels for Venous Pressure Measurement in Man," *Proc. Soc. Exp. Biol. Med.*, **58**, 165.

Wright, B. M. (1955), "A Respiratory Anemometer," *J. Physiol.*, **127**, 25P.

# INDEX